Essentials of Exercise Physiology

Third Edition

Essentials of Exercise Physiology

Third Edition

William D. McArdle (Sound Beach, NY)
Professor Emeritus, Department of Family, Nutrition, and Exercise Science
Queens College of the City University of New York
Flushing, New York

Frank I. Katch (Santa Barbara, CA)
International Research Scholar, Faculty of Health and Sport
Agder University College
Kristiansand, Norway

Instructor and Board Member
Certificate Program in Fitness Instruction
UCLA Extension, Los Angeles, CA

Former Professor and Chair of Exercise Science
University of Massachusetts
Amherst, Massachusetts

Victor L. Katch (Ann Arbor, MI)
Professor, Department of Movement Science
Division of Kinesiology

Associate Professor, Pediatrics
School of Medicine
University of Michigan
Ann Arbor, Michigan

Acquisitions Editor: Emily Lupash
Managing Editor: Rebecca Keifer
Marketing Manager: Christen D. Murphy
Production Editor: Sirkka E. H. Bertling
Designer: Risa Clow
Illustrators: Sam Collins and Rob Duckwall
Compositor: Maryland Composition, Inc.
Printer: R. R. Donnelley & Sons--Willard

Library of Congress Cataloging-in-Publication Data

McArdle, William D.
    Essentials of exercise physiology / William D. McArdle, Frank I. Katch, Victor L. Katch. — 3rd ed.
        p. ; cm.
    Includes bibliographical references and index.
    ISBN 0-7817-4991-3
    1. Exercise—Physiological aspects. I. Katch, Frank I. II. Katch, Victor L. III. Title.
    [DNLM: 1. Exercise—physiology. 2. Physical Fitness—physiology. 3. Sports Medicine.   QT 260 M478eb 2005]
QP301.M1149 2005
612'.044

The publishers have made every effort to trace the copyright holders for borrowed material. If they have inadvertently overlooked any, they will be pleased to make the necessary arrangements at the first opportunity.

To those who provide great meaning to my life: my wife Kathleen; my children Theresa, Amy, Kevin, and Jennifer; their spouses Christian, Jeff, Nicole, and Andy; and my grandchildren Liam, Aidan, Quinn, Dylan, Owen, Henry, and Kelly Rose.
—Bill McArdle

To my beautiful wife Kerry, who has been there for me from the beginning, and our great children, David, Kevin, and Ellen.
—Frank I. Katch

To Heather, Erika, Leslie, and Jesse; you light up my life.
—Victor L. Katch

The third edition of *Essentials of Exercise Physiology* is a compact version of *Exercise Physiology: Energy, Nutrition, and Human Performance*. It is ideally suited for an undergraduate level one-semester introductory course in exercise physiology and related areas. This revision has the advantage of being less expensive and smaller, while maintaining many of the features that have made *Exercise Physiology: Energy, Nutrition, and Human Performance* a leading textbook in the field since 1981 and the First Prize winner in medicine of the British Medical Association's 2002 Medical Book Competition. This *Essentials* text maintains the same strong pedagogy, writing style, and graphics and flow charts of the prior edition, with considerable added material and exciting new features.

In preparing this edition, we incorporated feedback from students and faculty familiar with the first and second editions. We surveyed more than 30 exercise physiology instructors and chose material most often covered in their courses. We also added several topic areas that appeared on numerous instructors' "wish lists."

The results of the survey were revealing; the overall theme of the prior edition, *"understanding interrelationships among energy intake, energy transfer during exercise, and the physiologic systems that support that energy transfer,"* was embraced by all surveyed. We retained this theme in the third revision.

ORGANIZATION

We have rearranged material within and among chapters to make the information flow more logically. By combining topic headings that incorporate common materials and eliminating other material deemed too advanced or unnecessary for an essentials text, we have reduced the book from 21 chapters to 18. The restructuring now makes it possible to cover most of the chapters in a one-semester course. More in depth, advanced material appears in the larger and expanded sixth edition of *Exercise Physiology: Energy, Nutrition, and Human Performance*.

Section I. *Introduction to Exercise Physiology* introduces the historical roots of exercise physiology and delves into the basics of the scientific method, with emphasis on how theories, laws, and facts interrelate to create new knowledge. We also discuss professional aspects of exercise physiology and the interrelationship between exercise physiology and sports medicine in this section.

Section II. *Nutrition and Energy* is composed of three chapters and emphasizes the interrelationship between food energy and optimal nutrition for exercise. Also included in this section is a critical discussion of the alleged benefits of commonly promoted nutritional (and pharmacologic) aids to enhance performance.

Section III. *Energy Transfer* has four chapters that focus on energy metabolism and how energy transfers from stored nutrients to muscle cells to produce movement during rest and diverse forms of physical activity. Also included is a discussion of the measurement and evaluation of the different capacities for human energy transfer.

Section IV. *The Physiologic Support Systems* contains four chapters that deal with the major physiologic systems (pulmonary, cardiovascular, neuromuscular, and endocrine) that interact to support the body's response to acute and chronic physical activity and exercise.

Section V. *Exercise Training and Adaptations* includes three chapters that describe application of the scientific principles of exercise training, including the highly specific functional and structural adaptation responses to chronic exercise overload. The

body's response to resistance training and the effects of different environmental challenges on energy transfer and exercise performance are discussed. We also critique the purported performance-enhancing effects of various "physiologic" agents.

Section VI. *Optimizing Body Composition, Successful Aging, and Health-Related Exercise Benefits* contains three chapters featuring health-related aspects of regular physical activity. We include a discussion of body composition assessment; the important role physical activity plays in weight control, successful aging, and disease prevention; and clinical aspects of exercise physiology.

NEW WORKBOOK FORMAT

Our goal was to make the third edition more *student friendly* by incorporating up-to-date pedagogical activities to enhance learning. Based on our more than 90 years of combined in-class teaching experience, we know that students become more engaged and understand more thoroughly what they read when they write down major concepts, ideas, relationships, and facts to questions based on their reading. For greatest effectiveness, this pedagogical exercise must occur while reading the text, not sometime afterwards. To accomplish this objective, we added a Questions & Notes section on the right side of most odd-numbered pages. We encourage students to answer the different questions and take marginal notes as they read. This concurrent active reading/learning element enhances student understanding of text material to a greater extent than simply reading and underlining text material.

HIGHLIGHTS OF NEW AND EXPANDED CONTENT

The following points highlight new and expanded content of the third edition of *Essentials of Exercise Physiology*:

- The most current information on the new 2005 MyPyramid (*http://www.mypryamid.gov*) and guidelines concerning proper nutrition appear throughout the textbook.
- Each section has undergone a major revision, incorporating the most recent research and information about the topic.
- We have included new emerging topics within each chapter based on current research.
- We include important selected references at the end of every chapter.
- Where applicable, we include relevant Internet web sites related to exercise physiology.
- We include additional For Your Information (FYI) boxes and have added new and updated material to the Close Up boxes.
- The full-color art program continues to be a stellar feature of the textbook. We have updated and expanded art and tables within each section to enhance text information.

SPECIAL FEATURES

A variety of features throughout the book facilitate student learning:

- **Close Up Boxes.** This popular feature focuses on timely and important exercise, sport, and clinical topics in exercise physiology that relate to the chapter content. Many of the boxes present practical applications to related topics of interest. This material, often showcased in a step-by-step, illustrated format, provides relevance to the practice of exercise physiology. Some Close Up boxes contain self-assessment and/or laboratory-type activities.
- **FYI Boxes.** FYI boxes throughout the text highlight key information about different exercise physiology areas. We designed these boxes to help bring topics to life and make them relevant to student learning.
- **Thought Questions.** We include Thought Questions at the end of each chapter section summary to encourage integrative, critical thinking to help students

apply information from the chapter. The instructor can use these questions to stimulate class discussion about chapter content and possible application of material to practical situations.

- **Questions & Notes.** This new feature (see description on previous page) facilitates student learning by focusing on specific questions related to important material presented in the text.
- **Appendices.** Useful current information is at the student's fingertips:
  Appendix A: Reliable Information Resources and Exercise Physiology
  Appendix B: The Internet and Exercise Physiology
  Appendix C: The Metric System and Conversion Constants in Exercise Physiology
  Appendix D: Metabolic Computations in Open-Circuit Spirometry
  Appendix E: Frequently Cited Journals in Exercise Physiology
  Appendix F: Evaluation of Body Composition – Girth Method
  Appendix G: Evaluation of Body Composition – Skinfold Method

FOR THE EXERCISE PHYSIOLOGY STUDENT

To enhance the student learning experience outside the classroom, we have included a Student Resource CD-ROM. This CD-ROM includes a quiz tool with approximately 350 multiple choice and true/false quiz questions to help students test their knowledge and prepare for exams. The quiz tool is also available online at *http://connection. lww.com/go/MKKEssentials.*

LiveAdvise Exercise Physiology, online teaching advice and student tutoring, is also available with this textbook. Our tutors are handpicked exercise physiology educators trained to help you. They are very familiar with this book and its ancillary package. You can connect live with a tutor during certain hours of the week, or send e-mail style messages to which the tutor will respond quickly—often within 24 hours. *This service is free with the purchase of your textbook!*

See the brochure in the front of the book or visit *http://connection.lww.com/liveadvise* for more information.

FOR THE EXERCISE PHYSIOLOGY INSTRUCTOR

We understand the demand on an instructor's time, so to make your job easier, you have access to Instructor's Resources upon adoption of the third edition of *Essentials of Exercise Physiology.* An Instructor's Resource CD-ROM (ISBN: 0-7817-6220-0) includes the following:

- A Test Generator with approximately 540 multiple choice, true/false, and fill-in-the-blank questions.
- PowerPoint slides for every chapter.
- An Image Bank that contains all of the figures and tables from the textbook.
- Chapter Objectives from the book.

Materials are also availavble online at *http://connection.lww.com/go/MKKEssentials.*

Essentials of Exercise Physiology, Third Edition offers you the fundamental aspects of exercise physiology in a comprehensive package that integrates the basic concepts and relevant scientific information to provide a foundation for understanding nutrition, energy transfer, and exercise training. To help your comprehension of the material, the authors have included numerous features that reinforce concepts and enhance your learning experience. This guide introduces you to these features.

Chapter Objectives and Outlines

open each chapter and present learning objectives and chapter contents to help you focus on and retain the crucial topics presented within each chapter.

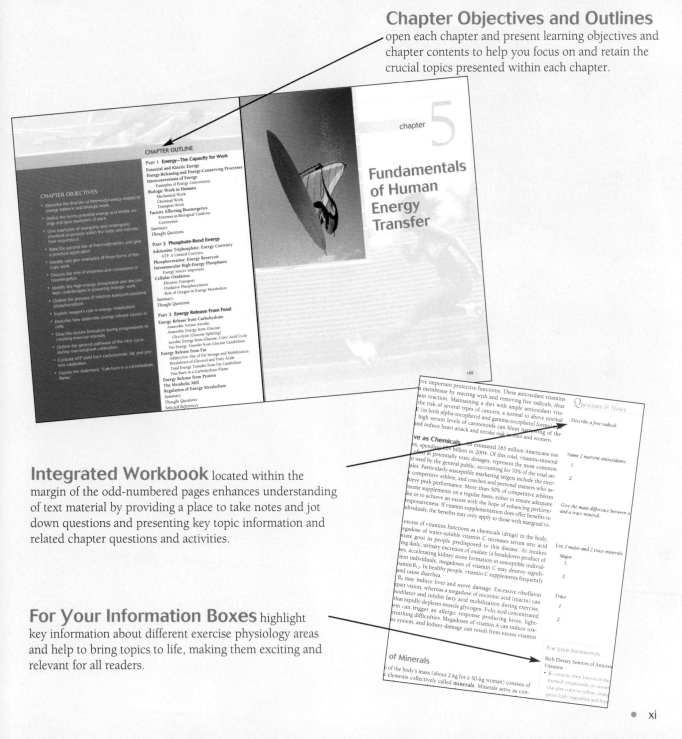

Integrated Workbook located within the

margin of the odd-numbered pages enhances understanding of text material by providing a place to take notes and jot down questions and presenting key topic information and related chapter questions and activities.

For Your Information Boxes highlight

key information about different exercise physiology areas and help to bring topics to life, making them exciting and relevant for all readers.

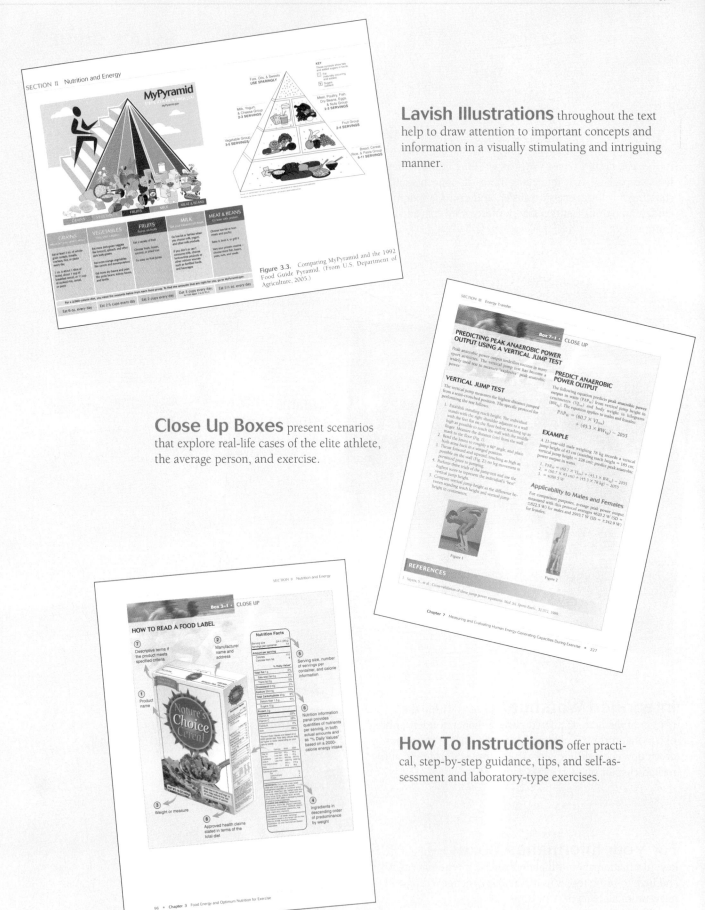

Lavish Illustrations throughout the text help to draw attention to important concepts and information in a visually stimulating and intriguing manner.

Figure 3.3. Comparing MyPyramid and the 1992 Food Guide Pyramid. (From U.S. Department of Agriculture, 2005.)

Close Up Boxes present scenarios that explore real-life cases of the elite athlete, the average person, and exercise.

How To Instructions offer practical, step-by-step guidance, tips, and self-assessment and laboratory-type exercises.

SECTION IV The Physiologic Support Systems

6. Pulmonary ventilation does not limit optimal alveolar gas exchange in healthy individuals who perform maximal exercise.

7. Airway resistance increases significantly after cigarette smoking. The added oxygen cost of breathing can

impair high-intensity, aerobic ⬚
Reversibility of these effects oc⬚
cigarette smoking abstinence.

THOUGHT QUESTIONS

1. How would the relationship change between $\dot{V}_E/\dot{V}O_2$ under the following conditions: (1) aging person who remains sedentary versus aging person who performs regular aerobic exercises; (2) transition from adolescence to young adulthood; and (3) person training for American football?

2. Present arguments to justify th⬚ does not limit aerobic exercise ⬚ healthy people.

3. In what ways are the terms lact⬚ of blood lactate accumulation ⬚ precise than the term anaerobi⬚

SELECTED REFERENCES

Abu-Hasan, M., et al.: Exercise-induced dyspnea in children and adolescents: if not asthma then what? Ann. Allergy Asthma Immunol., 94:366, 2005.

Agostoni, P., et al.: Exercise-induced pulmonary edema in heart failure. Circulation, 25;108:2666, 2003.

Ascensao, A.A., et al.: Cardiac mitochondrial respiratory function and oxidative stress: the role of exercise. Int. J. Sports Med., 26:258, 2005.

Baldari, C., et al.: Lactate removal during active recovery related to the individual anaerobic and ventilatory thresholds in soccer players. Eur. J. Appl. Physiol., 93:224, 2004.

Bassett D.R. Jr., Howley, E.T.: Limiting factors for maximum oxygen uptake and determinants of endurance performance.

Dempsey, J.A.: Crossing the apnoeic t⬚ consequences. Exp. Physiol., 90:13⬚

Gonzalez, J., et al.: A chest wall restric⬚ pulmonary function and exercise. 2⬚ restrictive breathing. Respiration, 6⬚

Hansen, J.E., et al.: Reproducibility of⬚ measurements in patients with pul⬚ hypertension. Chest, 126:816, 200⬚

Hashizume, K., et al.: Effects of abstin⬚ on the cardiorespiratory capacity. M⬚ 32:386, 2000.

Haverkamp, H.C., Dempsey, J.A.: On⬚ exchange efficiency during exercise⬚

Thought Questions located at the conclusion of each chapter part encourage critical thinking and problem-solving skills to help you utilize and apply information learned throughout the chapter in a practical and applicable manner.

Student Resource
CD-ROM to Accompany

Essentials of
Exercise Physiology

Version 1.0   Third Edition

LIPPINCOTT
WILLIAMS & WILKINS

William D. McArdle
Frank I. Katch
Victor L. Katch

Technical Support:
1-800-638-3030 or at techsupp@lww.com

Copyright © 2006 Lippincott Williams & Wilkins
A Wolters Kluwer Company
All rights reserved.

Live Advise

BONUS STUDENT CD-ROM

The CD-ROM packaged with the book includes a quiz tool with over 350 multiple choice and true/false questions that allows you to test your knowledge of text material and better prepare for exams. Quiz tool is also available at *http://connection.lww.com/go/MKKessentials.*

ONLINE TUTORING AND ASSISTANCE SERVICE

LiveAdvise Exercise Physiology

online tutoring and course assistance service is free with this textbook. Students and faculty members will have access to live assistance from experts in the field of exercise physiology. See the brochure in the front of this book or visit *http://connection.LWW.com/liveadvise* for more information.

Producing a book requires the coordinated efforts of many dedicated professionals. We are indebted to our publishing team at Lippincott Williams & Wilkins for their outstanding contributions during the text development and the production processes. We would like to acknowledge the expert talents of the following individuals: Sirkka Bertling, Production Editor; Risa Clow, Interior Design and Cover Design; Sam Collins, Artist; Rob Duckwall, Artist; Rebecca Keifer, Managing Editor; Emily Lupash, Acquisitions Editor; Mike Rosolio, Editorial Assistant; Marie Wayne, Permissions Department; and Pete Darcy, Executive Editor. A special thanks also goes to the many reviewers and users of the first two editions for their insightful comments and excellent suggestions for improvement.

WILLIAM D. MCARDLE
FRANK I. KATCH
VICTOR L. KATCH

Section I
INTRODUCTION TO EXERCISE PHYSIOLOGY 2

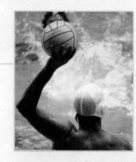

Section II
NUTRITION AND ENERGY 36

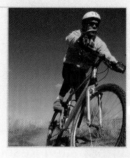

Section III
ENERGY TRANSFER 166

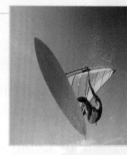

Section IV
THE PHYSIOLOGIC SUPPORT SYSTEMS 290

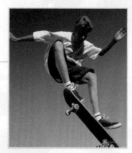

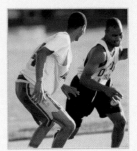

Section V
EXERCISE TRAINING AND ADAPTATIONS 432

Section VI
OPTIMIZING BODY COMPOSITION, SUCCESSFUL AGING, AND HEALTH-RELATED EXERCISE BENEFITS 556

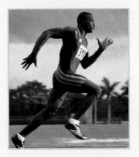

Essentials of Exercise Physiology

Third Edition

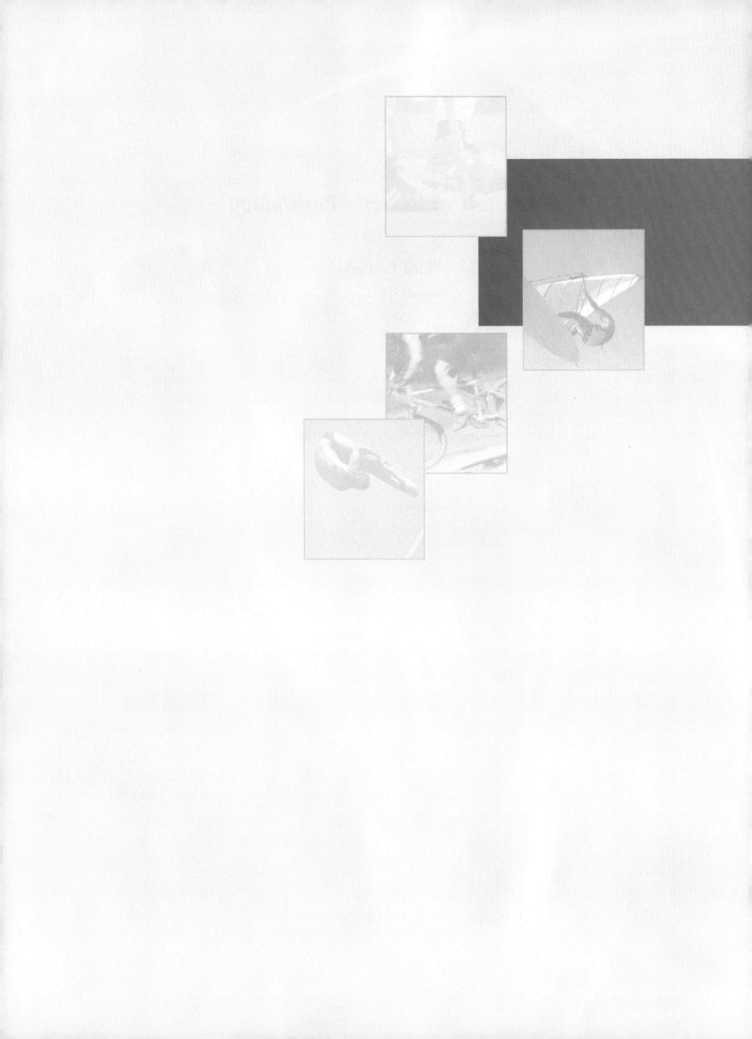

Section I

Introduction to Exercise Physiology

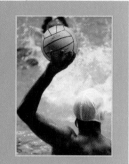

Exercise physiology enjoys a rich historical past, filled with engaging stories about important discoveries in anatomy, physiology, and medicine. Fascinating people and events have shaped our field. The ancient Greek physician Galen (131 to 201 A.D.) wrote detailed essays about improving health (proper nutrition), enhancing aerobic fitness (walking), and strengthening muscles (rope climbing and resistance training). From 776 B.C. to 393 A.D., the ancient Greek "sports nutritionists" planned the training regimens and diets for Olympic competitors. The diets were high in protein and meat, which were believed to improve overall fitness and competitive performance. New ideas about body functioning emerged during the Renaissance as anatomists and physicians exploded many notions inherited from antiquity. Gutenberg's printing press in the 15th century disseminated both classic and newly acquired knowledge. The average person could learn about local and world events, and education became more accessible as universities flourished throughout Europe.

The new anatomists went beyond simplistic notions of the early Greek scholar Empedocles' (c. 500–430 B.C.) four "bodily humors" and elucidated the complexities of the circulatory, respiratory, and digestive systems. Although the supernatural still influenced discussions of physical phenomena, many inquisitive people turned from dogma to experimentation as the source of knowledge. By the middle of the 19th century, fledgling U.S. medical schools began to graduate students, many of whom assumed positions of leadership in academia and the allied medical sciences. The pioneer physicians taught in medical school, conducted research, and wrote textbooks. Some became affiliated with departments of physical education and hygiene where they would oversee programs of physical training for students and sportsmen (athletes). These efforts helped to shape the origin of modern exercise physiology.

In **Part 1** of Chapter 1, we chronicle the achievements of several of the early American physician-scientists. The writing and research efforts (begun in 1860) by a college president and his physician son at Amherst College, MA, gave birth to exercise physiology as we know it today. Our history in America also includes the first exercise physiology laboratory at Harvard University begun in 1891 and the rigorous course of study for students in the Department of Anatomy, Physiology, and Physical Training. We also highlight scientific contributions of current American and Nordic researchers who have impacted the field of exercise physiology.

The study of exercise physiology pioneers and their two millennia of contributions in chemistry, nutrition, metabolism, physiology, and physical fitness helps us to more clearly understand our historical underpinnings. It also places in proper perspective the state and direction of our field today.

Part 2 of Chapter 1 explores the fundamentals of the scientific process, the basic notions about the scientific method and experimentation, and how science enables us to more fully comprehend the nature of the diverse phenomena related to exercise physiology. Understanding the systematic approach to problem solving provides both the practitioner and budding scholar a means to critically evaluate the scientific and popular literature related to the field.

Part 3 of Chapter 1 discusses the various roles of an exercise physiologist in the workplace and includes certification and education requirements necessary to achieve professional status.

"He who does not know what he is looking for will not lay hold of what he has found when he gets it."

—CLAUDE BERNARD

CHAPTER OBJECTIVES

- Briefly outline Galen's contributions to health and scientific hygiene.

- Discuss the beginnings of the development of exercise physiology in the United States. What were the roles of Austin Flint, Jr., and Edward Hitchcock, Jr.?

- Discuss the contributions of George Wells Fitz to the evolution of the academic field of exercise physiology.

- Outline the course of study for the first academic 4-year program in the United States from the Department of Anatomy, Physiology, and Physical Training at Harvard University.

- Describe the creation of the Harvard Fatigue Laboratory, its major scientists, and its contributions to the field of exercise physiology.

- List some major contributions of Nordic scientists to the field of exercise physiology.

- Describe the types of source materials in historical research and evaluative procedures in this type of research.

- Outline the general goals of science.

- Discuss the role of fact finding in the scientific process.

- Describe differences between causal and casual relationships.

- Identify important factors that determine the quality of experimental research in exercise physiology.

- Identify factors that affect relationships among variables.

- Describe differences and similarities among empirical, theoretical, basic, and applied research.

CHAPTER OUTLINE

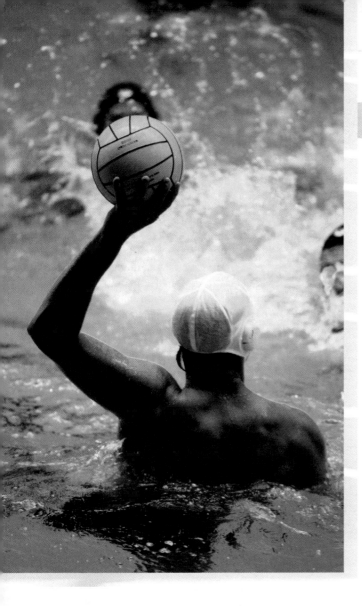

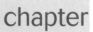

1

Exercise Physiology: From Past to Present

INTRODUCTION

The ability to impact the environment depends on our capacity for physical activity. Movement represents more than just a convenience; it is fundamental to our evolutionary development—no less important than the complexities of intellect and emotion.

In this century, we have amassed so much new knowledge about physical activity that exercise physiology is now a separate academic field of study within the biological and health-related sciences. Exercise physiology, as an **academic discipline**, consists of three distinct components (**Fig. 1.1**):

1. Body of knowledge built on facts and theories derived from research
2. Formal course of study in institutions of higher learning
3. Professional preparation of practitioners, future investigators, and leaders in the field

The current academic discipline of exercise physiology emerged from the influences of several traditional fields—primarily anatomy, physiology, and medicine. Each of these disciplines uniquely contributes to our understanding of human structure and function in health and disease. Human physiology integrates aspects of chemistry, biology, and physics to explain biological events and their sites of occurrence. Physiologists grapple with questions such as "What factors regulate body functions?" and "What sequence of events occurs between the stimulus and the response in the regulatory process?" The discipline of physiology compartmentalizes into subdisciplines, usually based on either a systems approach (renal, cardiovascular, neuromuscular, pulmonary) or a broad area of study (viral, cell, invertebrate, vertebrate, comparative, human).

Part 1 of this chapter briefly outlines the genesis of exercise physiology in the United States from antiquity to the present. We emphasize the growth of formal research laboratories and the publication of textbooks in the field. Although the roots of exercise physiology link to antiquity, the knowledge explosion of the late 1950s greatly increased the number of citations in the research literature. Consider the terms *exercise* and *exertion*. In 1946, only 12 citations appeared in 5 journals. By 1962, the number increased to 128 in 51 journals, and by 1981, 655 citations occurred in 224 journals. Since then, citations have increased progressively. In 1994, more than 3558 citations and topic headings appeared in 1288 journals. By October 1999, more than 6000 citation listings appeared in over 1400 different journals, and through July 2005, that number had swelled to 56,488! It is safe to say that exercise physiology currently represents a mature field of study.

The historical underpinnings of exercise physiology should be complemented by an introduction about the goals and process of science. This clarifies how scholars identify reliable information (facts) and generate hypotheses, laws, and theories related to a field and also explains how to critically evaluate the quality of information about a specific topic area. To this end, Part 2 of this chapter introduces basic concepts of the scientific process that guide discovery in the field of exercise physiology.

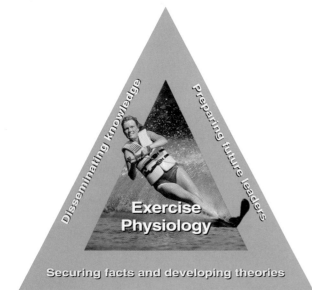

Figure 1.1 Science triangle. Three parts of the field of study of exercise physiology: (1) body of knowledge evidenced by experimental and field research engaged in the enterprise of securing facts and developing theories, (2) formal course of study in institutions of higher learning for the purpose of disseminating knowledge, and (3) preparation of future leaders in the field. (Adapted from Tipton, C.M.: Contemporary exercise physiology: Fifty years after the closure of the Harvard Fatigue Laboratory. *Exerc. Sport Sci. Rev.*, 26:315, 1998.)

PART 1 •
Origins of Exercise Physiology:
From Ancient Greece to the United States

The origins of exercise physiology begin with the influential Greek physicians of antiquity. We also highlight contributions from scholars in the United States and Nordic countries that fostered the scientific assessment of sport and exercise as a respectable field.

Earliest Development

The first real focus on the physiology of exercise likely began in early Greece and Asia Minor. Exercise, sports, games, and health concerned even earlier civilizations; the Minoan and Mycenaean cultures, the great biblical empires of David and Solomon, Assyria, Babylonia, Media, and Persia, and the empires of Alexander. The ancient civilizations of Syria, Egypt, Greece, Arabia, Mesopotamia, Persia, India, and China also recorded references to sports, games, and health practices (personal hygiene, exercise, training). The greatest influence on Western Civilization, however, came from the Greek physicians of antiquity—Herodicus (ca. 480 B. C.), Hippocrates (460 to 377 B. C.), and Claudius Galenus or **Galen** (131 to 201 A. D.). Herodicus, a physician and athlete, strongly advocated proper diet in physical training. His early writings and devoted followers influenced Hippocrates, the famous physician and "father of preventive medicine" who contributed 87 treatises on medicine, including several on health and hygiene.

Five centuries after Hippocrates, Galen emerged as the most well-known and influential physician that ever lived. Galen began studying medicine at about age 16. Over the next 50 years, he enhanced current thinking concerning health and scientific hygiene, an area some might consider "applied exercise physiology." Throughout his life, Galen taught and practiced "laws of health" (**Table 1.1**).

Galen wrote about 500 essays related to human anatomy and physiology, nutrition, growth and development, the benefits of exercise and deleterious consequences of sedentary living, and diverse diseases and their treatment. One of the first laboratory-oriented physiologists, Galen conducted original experiments in physiology, comparative anatomy, and medicine; he dissected animals (e.g., goats, pigs, cows, horses, and elephants). As physician to the gladiators (probably the first Sports Medicine physician), Galen treated gladiators' torn tendons and muscles using surgical procedures that he invented and recommended rehabilitation therapies and exercise regimens. Galen's writings about exercise and its effects might be considered the first formal "how to" manuals about such topics, which remained influential for the next 15 centuries.

Early United States Experience

By the early 1800s in the United States, European science-oriented physicians and experimental anatomists and physiologists strongly promoted ideas about health and hygiene. Before 1800, only 39 first-edition American-authored medical books had been published; several medical schools were founded (e.g., Harvard Medical School, 1782); seven medical societies existed (the first was the New Jersey State Medical Society in 1766); and only one medical journal existed (*Medical Repository*, initially published in 1797). Outside the United States, 176 medical journals were published, but by 1850, the number in the United States had increased to 117.

Medical journal publications in the United States increased tremendously during the first half of the 19th century. Steady growth in the number of scientific contributions from France and Germany influenced the thinking and practice of American medicine. An explosion of information reached the American public through books, magazines, newspapers, and traveling "health salesmen" who sold an endless variety of tonics and elixirs, promising to optimize health and cure disease. Many health reformers and physicians from 1800 to 1850 used "strange" procedures to treat disease and bodily discomforts. To a large extent, scientific knowledge about health and disease was in its infancy. Lack of knowledge and factual information spawned a new generation of "healers," who fostered quackery and primitive practices on a public who wanted almost anything that seemed to work. If a salesman could offer a "cure" to combat gluttony (digestive upset) and other physical ailments, the product or procedure would become the common remedy.

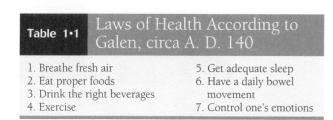

Table 1•1	Laws of Health According to Galen, circa A. D. 140
1. Breathe fresh air	5. Get adequate sleep
2. Eat proper foods	6. Have a daily bowel
3. Drink the right beverages	movement
4. Exercise	7. Control one's emotions

Questions & Notes

Name the most famous of the Greek physicians.

Name the "father" of preventive medicine.

Name the first U.S. physician to write that physical education should be based on a strong scientific foundation.

Name the first medical school in the United States.

FOR YOUR INFORMATION

Exercise Physiology
Much like biochemistry represents a field distinct from biology and chemistry, exercise physiology has become a separate field of study from physiology because of its focus on functional dynamics and consequences of movement. Exercise physiologists try to determine how the body (subcell, cell, tissue, organ, system) responds in function and structure to (1) acute exercise stress, and (2) chronic physical activity. The exercise physiologist also studies exercise and training responses related to environmental factors, such as heat, cold, altitude, microgravity, and underwater conditions.

The "hot topics" of the early 19th century (not much different than today) included nutrition and dieting (slimming), general information about exercise, how to best develop overall fitness, training (gymnastic) exercises for recreation and preparation for sport, and personal health and hygiene. Although many health faddists actually practiced "medicine" without a license, some enrolled in newly created medical schools (without entrance requirements), obtaining the M.D. degree in as little as 16 weeks. Despite this brief training, some pioneer physicians contributed to medical practice and subsequent development of exercise physiology as we know it today.

By the middle 19th century, fledgling medical schools began to graduate their students, and many assumed positions of leadership in academia and allied medical sciences. Interestingly, physicians either taught in medical school and conducted research (and wrote textbooks) or became affiliated with departments of physical education and hygiene and oversaw programs of physical training for students and athletes.

Austin Flint, Jr., M.D.: American Physician–Physiologist

Austin Flint, Jr., M.D. (1836–1915), a pioneer American physician–scientist, contributed significantly to the burgeoning literature in physiology (Fig. 1.2). A respected physician, physiologist, and successful textbook author, he fostered the belief among 19th century American physical education teachers that muscular exercise should be taught from a strong foundation of science and experimentation. Flint, a professor of physiology and physiological anatomy in the Bellevue Hospital Medical College of New York, chaired the Department of Physiology and Microbiology from 1861 to 1897. In 1866, he published a series of five classic textbooks; the first was entitled *The Physiology of Man; Designed to Represent the Existing State of Physiological Science as Applied to the Functions of the Human Body.*

Well trained in the scientific method, Dr. Flint received the American Medical Association's prize for basic research on the heart in 1858. His 1877 textbook (*The Principles and Practice of Medicine*) included many exercise-related details about the influence of posture and exercise on pulse rate, the influence of activity on respiration, and the effects of exercise on nitrogen elimination. Flint was well aware of scientific experimentation in France and England and cited the experimental works of leading European physiologists and physicians in his writings.

Through his textbooks, Austin Flint, Jr., influenced the first medically trained and science-oriented professor of physical education, Edward Hitchcock, Jr., M.D. (see next section). Hitchcock quoted Flint concerning the muscular system in his syllabus of *Health Lectures*, which became required reading for all students enrolled at Amherst College, MA, between 1861 and 1905.

Amherst College Connection

Two physicians, father and son, pioneered the American sports science movement. **Edward Hitchcock**, D.D., LL.D. (1793–1864), served as professor of chemistry and natural history at Amherst College and as president of the College from 1845 to 1854 (Fig. 1.3). He convinced the college president in 1861 to allow his son Edward (1828–1911), an Amherst graduate (1849) [Harvard Medical degree (1853)] to assume the duties of his anatomy course. Hitchcock Jr. replaced John D. Hooker (the first Professor of Physical Education in the United States who was forced to step down due to ill-health) on August 15, 1861, with full academic rank in the *Department of Physical Culture* at an annual salary of $1000—a position he held almost continuously to 1911.

The original idea of a Department of Physical Education with a professorship had been proposed in 1854 by William Augustus Stearns, D.D., the fourth President of Amherst College. Stearns considered physical education instruction essential for the health of students and useful to prepare them physically, spiritually, and intellectually. In 1860, the Barrett Gymnasium at Amherst College was completed and served as the training facility where all students were **required** to perform systematic exercises for 30 minutes daily, 4 days a week (Fig. 1.4). A unique feature of the gymnasium was Hitchcock's scientific laboratory, which included strength, anthropometric, and physiologic equipment. Dr. Hitchcock was first to statistically record basic data on a large group of subjects on a yearly

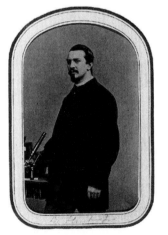

Figure 1.2 Austin Flint, Jr., M.D., American physician–physiologist.

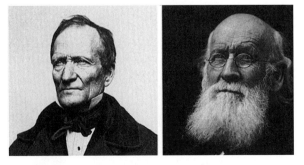

Figure 1.3 Drs. Edward Hitchcock (left), 1793–1864, and Edward Hitchcock, Jr., 1828–1911.

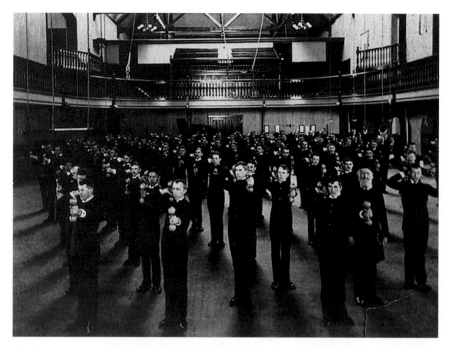

Figure 1.4   Dr. Edward Hitchcock, Jr. (second from right, with beard) and the entire class of students perform barbell exercises in the Pratt Gymnasium of Amherst College. (Photo courtesy of Amherst College Archives, and by permission of the Trustees of Amherst College, 1995.)

basis. These measurements provided solid information for his counseling duties (to students) concerning health, hygiene, and exercise training.

In 1860, the Hitchcocks coauthored an anatomy and physiology textbook geared to college physical education (Hitchcock, E., and Hitchcock, E., Jr.: *Elementary Anatomy and Physiology for Colleges, Academies, and Other Schools.* New York: Ivison, Phinney & Co., 1860); 29 years earlier, the elder Edward Hitchcock had published a science-oriented hygiene textbook. Interestingly, the anatomy and physiology book predated Flint's similar text by 6 years. This illustrated that an American-trained physician, with an allegiance to the implementation of health and hygiene in the curriculum, helped set the stage for the study of exercise physiology (and training) well before the medical establishment focused on this aspect of the discipline. **Figure 1.5** shows sample pages from the 1860 book on muscle structure and function.

George Wells Fitz, M.D.: A Major Influence   George Wells Fitz, M.D. (1860–1934), an early exercise physiology researcher (**Fig. 1.6**), helped establish the Department of Anatomy, Physiology, and Physical Training at Harvard University in 1891, shortly after he received his medical degree from Harvard Medical School (1891). One year later, Fitz developed the first formal exercise physiology laboratory in the United States where students investigated the effects of exercise on cardiorespiratory function, including muscular fatigue, metabolism, and nervous system functions. Fitz published his research in the prestigious *Boston Medical and Surgical Journal,* including studies on muscle cramping, efficacy of protective clothing, spinal curvature, respiratory function, carbon dioxide measurement, and speed and accuracy of simple and complex movements. He also wrote two textbooks (*Principles of Physiology and Hygiene* [New York: Holt, 1908]; and revised physiologist H. N. Martin's *The Human Body. Textbook of Anatomy, Physiology and Hygiene; with Practical Exercises* [New York: Holt, 1911]). Well-known researchers in the new program included distinguished Harvard Medical School physiologists Henry Pickering Bowditch, whose research produced the "all or none principle" of cardiac contraction and "treppe" (staircase phenomenon of muscle contraction).

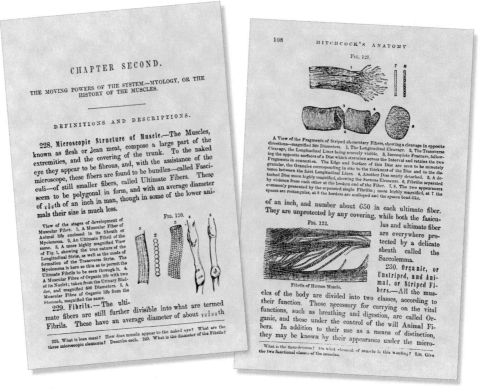

Figure 1.5 Examples from the Hitchcock text on structure and function of muscles. Note that study questions appear at the bottom of each page. (Reproduced from Hitchcock, E., and Hitchcock, E., Jr.: *Elementary Anatomy and Physiology for Colleges, Academies, and Other Schools.* New York: Ivison, Phinney & Co., 1860: pp., 132, 137. Materials courtesy of Amherst College Archives, and permission of the Trustees of Amherst College, 1995.)

The new 4-year course of study, well grounded in the basic sciences even by today's standards, provided students with a rigorous, challenging curriculum in what Fitz hoped would be a new science of physical education (sic, Exercise Physiology). The third year of study was taken at the medical school (see table in *Close Up* on page 11).

Prelude to Exercise Science: Harvard's Department of Anatomy, Physiology, and Physical Training (B.S. Degree, 1891–1898)

Harvard's new physical education major required students to take general anatomy and physiology courses in the medical school; after 4 years of study, graduates could enroll as second-year medical students and graduate in 3 years with an M.D. degree. Dr. Fitz taught the physiology of exercise course; thus, he deserves recognition as the first person to formally teach exercise physiology in an American university.

The new degree included experimental investigation and original work and a thesis, including 6 hours a week of laboratory study. The prerequisite for Fitz's physiology of exercise course included general physiology or its equivalent taken at the medical school. The physiology of exercise course introduced students to the fundamentals of physical education and provided training in experimental methods related to exercise physiology. In addition to the remedial exercise course, students took a required course in applied anatomy and animal mechanics. This thrice-weekly course, taught by Dr. Dudley Sargent, was the forerunner of modern biomechanics courses. Its prerequisite was general anatomy or its equivalent taken at the medical school.

Before its dismantling in 1900, nine men graduated with B.S. degrees from the Department of Anatomy, Physiology, and Physical Training. The first graduate, James Francis Jones (1893), became instructor in Physiology and Hygiene and Director of Gymnasium at Marietta College, Marietta, OH.

One year after Fitz's untimely resignation from Harvard in 1899, the department changed its curricular emphasis

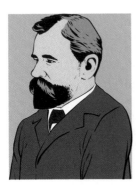

Figure 1.6 George Wells Fitz, M.D.

Box 1–1 • CLOSE UP

COURSE OF STUDY: DEPARTMENT OF ANATOMY, PHYSIOLOGY, AND PHYSICAL TRAINING, LAWRENCE SCIENTIFIC SCHOOL, HARVARD UNIVERSITY, 1893

Few of today's undergraduate Kinesiology major programs could match the strong science core required (for the Physical Education major) at Harvard in 1893. Below is the 4-year course of study as listed in the 1893 Harvard course catalog. Along with core courses, Professor Fitz established an exercise physiology laboratory. The following describes the laboratory's objectives:

"A well-equipped laboratory has been organized for the experimental study of the physiology of exercise. The object of this work is to exemplify the hygiene of the muscles, the conditions under which they act, the relation of their action to the body as a whole affecting blood supply and general hygienic conditions, and the effects of various exercises on muscular growth and general health."

First Year

Experimental Physics
Elementary Zoology
Morphology of Animals
Morphology of Plants
Elementary Physiology and Hygiene
General Descriptive Chemistry
Rhetoric and English Composition
Elementary German
Elementary French
Gymnastics and Athletics

Second Year

Comparative Anatomy of Vertebrates
Geology
Physical Geography and Meteorology
Experimental Physics
General Descriptive Physics
Qualitative Analysis
English Composition
Gymnastics and Athletics (Sargent & Lathrop)

Third Year (at Harvard Medical School)

General Anatomy and Dissection
General Physiology
Histology
Hygiene
Foods and Cooking [Nutrition] (at Boston Cooking School)
Medical Chemistry
Auscultation and Percussion
Gymnastics and Athletics

Fourth Year

Psychology
Anthropometry
Applied Anatomy and Animal Mechanics [Kinesiology]
Physiology of Exercise
Remedial Exercise
History of Physical Education
Forensics
Gymnastics and Athletics

to anatomy and physiology (dropping the term physical training from the department title). This terminated (at least temporarily) a unique experiment in higher education. For almost a decade before the turn of the century, the field of physical education was moving forward on a strong scientific foundation like other (more developed) disciplines at the university. Unfortunately, this occasion to nurture the next generation of students in exercise physiology (and physical education) was momentarily stymied. Twenty years would pass before the visionary efforts of Dr. Fitz to "study the physiological and psychological effects of exercise" and to establish exercise physiology as a bona fide field of study would revive, albeit outside of a formal physical education curriculum.

By 1927, 135 institutions in the United States offered bachelor's degree programs in Physical Education with coursework in the basic sciences; this included four master's degree programs and two doctoral programs (Teachers College, Columbia University, and New York University). Since then, programs of study with differing emphasis in exercise physiology have proliferated. Currently, more than 145 programs in the United States and 19 in Canada offer master's or doctoral degrees with specialization in a topic related to some aspect(s) of exercise physiology (*http://www.css.edu/users/tboone2/ asep/graduate.htm*).

Exercise Studies in Research Journals In 1898, three articles on physical activity appeared in the first volume of *The American Journal of Physiology*. Other articles and reviews subsequently appeared in prestigious journals, including the first published review in *Physiological Reviews* (2:310, 1922) on the mechanisms of muscular contraction by Nobel laureate A.V. Hill. The German applied physiology publication, *Internationale Zeitschrift für angewandte Physiologie einschliesslich Arbeitsphysiologie* (1929–1940; now *European Journal of Applied Physiology and Occupational Physiology*), became a significant journal for research in the area of exercise physiology. *The Journal of Applied Physiology*, first published in 1948, contained the classic paper by J.M. Tanner on ratio expressions of physiological data with reference to body size and function (a "must read" for every exercise physiologist). The official journal of the American College of Sports Medicine, *Medicine and Science in Sports*, first appeared in 1969. It aimed to integrate both medical and physiological aspects of the emerging fields of sports medicine and exercise science. The official name of this journal changed in 1980 to *Medicine and Science in Sports and Exercise*. Publications emphasizing applied and basic exercise physiology research have increased as the field has expanded into different areas. The World Wide Web offers unique growth potential in this regard. The first web-based exercise physiology journal (*Journal of Exercise Physiology–Online* http://www.asep.org/jeponline/JEPhome.htm*, Official Journal of the American Society of Exercise Physiologists) first appeared in April, 1998.

The scope of exercise physiology is expanding at such a rapid rate that it is now difficult to keep up with knowledge dissemination. Exercise physiology-related research commonly appears in journals representing almost every branch of medical/biological science. **Table 1.2** presents a partial list of research journals directly dealing with exercise physiology. Although the list is not inclusive, it does give an introductory list of relevant journals containing peer-reviewed research.

First Textbook in Exercise Physiology Debate exists over the question: "What was the first textbook in exercise physiology?" Several textbook authors give the distinction of being "first" to the English translation of Fernand Lagrange's *The Physiology of Bodily Exercise*, originally published in French in 1888. We disagree. To deserve such historical recognition, a textbook should meet at least the following three criteria in our opinion:

1. Provide sound scientific rationale for major concepts
2. Provide summary information (based on experimentation) about important prior research in a particular topic area (e.g., contain scientific references to research in the area)
3. Provide sufficient "factual" information about a topic area to give it academic legitimacy

The Lagrange book represents a popular book with a "scientific" title about health and exercise. Based on the aforementioned criteria, the book fails to exemplify a bona fide exercise physiology text; it contains less than 20 reference

Table 1·2	Partial Listing of Research Journals Publishing Exercise Physiology Research Articles
• Australian Journal of Physiotherapy • British Journal of Sports Medicine • British Medical Journal • Canadian Journal of Applied Physiology • Clinical Exercise Physiology • Coaching Science Abstracts • European Journal of Applied Physiology • Exercise Immunology Review • Health Sciences Library • Human Movement Science • Human Performance • International Journal of Epidemiology • International Journal of Psychophysiology • International Journal of Sport Nutrition • Internet Journal of Health Promotion	• Journal of the American Medical Association • Journal of Aging and Physical Activity • Journal of Applied Physiology • Journal of Exercise Physiology Online • Journal of Performance Enhancement • Journal of Science and Medicine in Sport • Journal of Sport Rehabilitation • Journal of Sport and Exercise Psychology • Journal of Athletic Training • Kinesiology Online • Medicine & Science in Sports & Exercise • New Zealand Journal of Physiotherapy • Pediatric Exercise Science

Box 1–2 • CLOSE UP

WHAT'S IN A NAME?

A lack of unanimity exists for the name of departments offering degrees (or even coursework) in exercise physiology. The table below lists 49 examples of names of departments in the United States that offer essentially the same area of study. Each provides some undergraduate or graduate emphasis in exercise physiology (e.g., one or several courses, internships, work-study programs, laboratory rotations, or in-service programs).

ALLIED HEALTH	LEISURE SCIENCE
Allied Health Sciences	Movement and Exercise Science
Exercise and Movement Science	Movement Studies
Exercise and Sport Science	Nutrition and Exercise Science
Exercise and Sport Studies	Nutritional and Health Sciences
Exercise Science	Performance and Sport Science
Exercise Science and Human Movement	Physical Culture
Exercise Science and Physical Therapy	Physical Education
Health and Human Performance	Physical Education and Exercise Science
Health and Physical Education	Physical Education and Human Movement
Health, Physical Education, Recreation & Dance	Physical Education and Sport Programs
Human Biodynamics	Physical Education and Sport Science
Human Kinetics	Physical Therapy
Human Kinetics and Health	Recreation
Human Movement	Recreation and Wellness Programs
Human Movement Sciences	Science of Human Movement
Human Movement Studies	Sport and Exercise Science
Human Movement Studies and Physical Education	Sport Management
Human Performance	Sport, Exercise, and Leisure Science
Human Performance and Health Promotion	Sports Science
Human Performance and Leisure Studies	Sport Science and Leisure Studies
Human Performance and Sport Science	Sport Science and Movement Education
Interdisciplinary Health Studies	Sport Studies
Integrative Biology	Wellness and Fitness
Kinesiology	Wellness Education
Kinesiology and Exercise Science	

citations. If not the Lagrange book, what text qualifies as the first exercise physiology text? Possible pre-1900 candidates for "first" include these four choices:

1. Combe's *The Principles of Physiology Applied to the Preservation of Health, and to the Improvement of Physical and Mental Education.* New York: Harper & Brothers, 1843
2. Hitchcock and Hitchcock's *Elementary Anatomy and Physiology for Colleges, Academies, and Other Schools.* New York: Ivison, Phinney & Co., 1860
3. Kolb's insightful book, *Physiology of Sport.* London: Krohne and Sesemann, 1893
4. Martin's text, *The Human Body. An Account of its Structure and Activities and the Conditions of its Healthy Working.* New York: Holt & Co., 1896

Contributions of the Harvard Fatigue Laboratory (1927–1946)

The real impact of laboratory research in exercise physiology (along with many other research specialties) occurred in 1927 at Harvard University, 27 years after Harvard closed the first exercise physiology laboratory in the United States. The

Questions & Notes

Name 3 exercise physiology journals.

1.

2.

3.

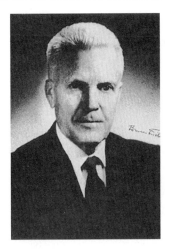

Figure 1.7 David Bruce Dill (1891–1986).

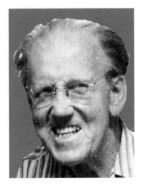

Figure 1.8 F.M. Henry (1904–1993), Director of the exercise physiology laboratory at U.C. Berkeley that produced some of the early work on oxygen kinetics during exercise and recovery.

800-square foot **Harvard Fatigue Laboratory** in the basement of Morgan Hall of Harvard University's Business School legitimized exercise physiology as an important area of research and study.

Many of the 20th century's great scientists with an interest in exercise affiliated with the Fatigue Laboratory. Renowned Harvard chemist and professor of biochemistry, **Lawrence J. Henderson, M.D.** (1878–1942), established the laboratory. **David Bruce Dill** (1891–1986), a Stanford Ph.D. in physical chemistry (**Fig. 1.7**), became the first and only scientific director of the Laboratory. While at Harvard, Dill refocused his efforts from biochemistry to experimental physiology and became the driving force behind the Laboratory's numerous scientific accomplishments. His early academic association with physician Arlie Bock (a student of famous high-altitude physiologist Sir Joseph F. Barcroft at Cambridge, England) and contact with 1922 Nobel laureate **Archibald Vivian Hill** provided Dill with the confidence to successfully coordinate the research efforts of dozens of scholars from 15 different countries.

Other Early Exercise Physiology Research Laboratories

Other notable research laboratories helped exercise physiology become an established field of study at colleges and universities. The Nutrition Laboratory at the Carnegie Institute in Washington, D.C. (established 1904) initiated experiments in nutrition and energy metabolism. The first research laboratories established in a department of physical education in the United States originated at George Williams College (1923), University of Illinois (1925), Springfield College (1927), and Laboratory of Physiological Hygiene at the University of California, Berkeley (1934) (**Fig. 1.8**).

Nordic Connection (Denmark, Sweden, Norway, and Finland)

Danish and Swedish scientists also pioneered the field of exercise physiology. In 1800, Denmark became the first

European country to require physical training (military-style gymnastics) in their school curriculum.

Danish Influence In 1909, the University of Copenhagen endowed the equivalent of a Chair in Anatomy, Physiology, and Theory of Gymnastics. The first Docent, **Johannes Lindhard, M.D.** (1870–1947), later teamed with **August Krogh, Ph.D.** (1874–1949), an eminent scientist who specialized in physiological chemistry and research instrument design and construction, to conduct many of the classic experiments in exercise physiology. For example, Lindhard and Krogh investigated gas exchange in the lungs, pioneered studies of the relative contribution of fat and carbohydrate oxidation during exercise, measured blood flow redistribution during different exercise intensities, and quantified cardiorespiratory dynamics in exercise.

By 1910, Krogh and his physician wife Marie (**Fig. 1.9**) had proven through a series of ingenious, decisive experiments that diffusion governed pulmonary gas exchange during exercise and altitude exposure, not oxygen secretion from lung tissue into the blood as postulated by British physiologists Sir John Scott Haldane and James Priestley. Krogh published a series of experiments (three appearing in the 1919 *Journal of Physiology*) concerning the mechanism of oxygen diffusion and transport in

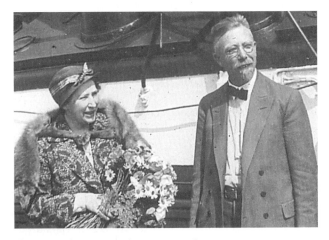

Figure 1.9 Marie and August Krogh.

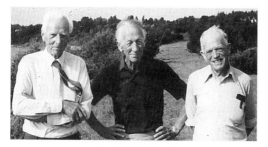

Figure 1.10 Erling Asmussen (left), Erik Hohwü-Christensen (center), and Marius Nielson (right), 1988.

Name the first and only director of the Harvard Fatigue Laboratory.

skeletal muscles. He won the Nobel Prize in physiology or medicine in 1920 for discovering the mechanism for capillary control of blood flow in resting and exercising muscle.

Three other Danish researchers—physiologists Erling Asmussen (1907–1991; ACSM Citation Award, 1976 and ACSM Honor Award, 1979), Erik Hohwü–Christensen (1904–1996; ACSM Honor Award, 1981), and Marius Nielsen (1903–2000)—conducted significant exercise physiology studies (**Fig. 1.10**). These "three musketeers," as Krogh called them, published voluminously during the 1930s to 1970s.

Christensen became Lindhard's student in Copenhagen in 1925. In his 1931 doctoral thesis, Christensen reported studies of cardiac output, body temperature, and blood sugar concentration during heavy exercise, compared arm versus leg exercise, and quantified the effects of training. Together with Krogh and Lindhard, Christensen published an important 1936 review article describing physiological dynamics during maximal exercise. Discovery of the concept of "carbohydrate loading" actually occurred in 1939. Experiments by physician Olé Bang in 1936, inspired by his mentor Ejar Lundsgaard, described the fate of blood lactate during exercise of different intensities and durations. Since 1973, Swedish-trained scientist **Bengt Saltin** (**Fig. 1.11**) (the only Nordic researcher besides Erling Asmussen to receive the ACSM Citation Award, 1980, and ACSM Honor Award, 1990; former student of Per-Olof Åstrand, discussed in the next section) has continued his significant scientific studies as professor and director at the Muscle Research Institute in Copenhagen.

Swedish Influence   Modern exercise physiology in Sweden can be traced to **Per Henrik Ling** (1776–1839), who in 1813 became the first director of Stockholm's Royal Central Institute of Gymnastics. Ling, a specialist in fencing, developed a system (incorporating his studies of anatomy and physiology) of "medical gymnastics," which became part of Sweden's school curriculum in 1820. Ling's son, Hjalmar, published a book on the kinesiology of body movements in 1866. As a result of the Lings' philosophy and influence, physical education graduates from the Stockholm Central Institute were well schooled in the basic biological sciences, in addition to proficiency in sports and games. Currently, the College of Physical Education (Gymnastik-Och Idrottshögskolan) and the Department of

Name 2 famous Danish exercise physiologists.

  1.

  2.

Name a famous Swedish exercise physiologist.

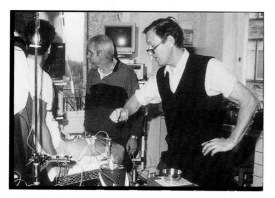

Figure 1.11 Bengt Saltin (hand on hip) during an experiment at the August Krogh Institute, Copenhagen. (Photo courtesy of Dr. David Costill.)

FOR YOUR INFORMATION

The Harvard Fatigue Laboratory
Over a 20-year span, Harvard Fatigue Laboratory scientists published at least 352 research papers, monographs, and a book dealing with basic and applied exercise physiology, including methodological refinements in blood chemistry analysis and simplified methods for analyzing fractional concentrations of expired air. Other research included acute responses and chronic adaptations to exercise under the environmental stress of altitude, heat, and cold exposure. Most of the physical activity experiments used humans exercising on either a treadmill or bicycle ergometer. These studies formed the cornerstone for future research efforts in exercise physiology; they included assessment of work capacity and physical fitness, cardiovascular and hemodynamic responses during maximal exercise, oxygen uptake and substrate utilization kinetics, exercise and recovery metabolism, and maximal oxygen uptake.

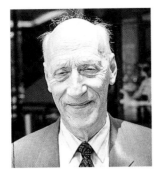

Figure 1.12 Per-Olof Åstrand, Department of Physiology, Karolinska Institute, Stockholm.

Physiology in the Karolinska Institute Medical School in Stockholm continue to sponsor studies in exercise physiology.

Per-Olof Åstrand, M.D., Ph.D. (b. 1922), is the most famous graduate of the College of Physical Education (1946); in 1952, he presented his doctoral thesis at the Karolinska Institute Medical School (**Fig. 1.12**). Åstrand taught in the Department of Physiology in the College of Physical Education from 1946–1977; it then became a department at the Karolinska Institute, where he served as professor and department head from 1977 to 1987. Christensen, Åstrand's mentor, supervised his thesis, which evaluated physical working capacity of men and women ages 4 to 33 years. This important study, among others, established a line of research that propelled Åstrand to the forefront of experimental exercise physiology for which he achieved worldwide fame. Åstrand has mentored an impressive group of exercise physiologists, including "superstar" Bengt Saltin.

Two Swedish scientists from the Karolinska Institute, **Dr. Jonas Bergström** and **Dr. Erik Hultman**, conducted important needle biopsy experiments. With this procedure, muscle was first studied under various conditions of exercise, training, and nutritional status. Collaborative work with other Scandinavian researchers and researchers in the United States provided new vistas from which to view the physiology of exercise.

Norwegian and Finnish Influence The new generation of exercise physiologists trained in the late 1940s analyzed respiratory gases with a highly accurate sampling apparatus that measured minute quantities of carbon dioxide and oxygen in expired air. Norwegian scientist Per Scholander (1905–1980) developed the method of analysis (and analyzer) in 1947.

Another prominent Norwegian researcher, **Lars A. Hermansen** (1933–1984; ACSM Citation Award, 1985) from the Institute of Work Physiology, made many contributions including a classic 1969 article entitled "Anaerobic energy release," which appeared in the initial volume of *Medicine and Science in Sports* (Volume 1, Number 1, pp. 32–38).

In Finland, Martti Karvonen, M.D., Ph.D. (ACSM Honor Award, 1991), from the Physiology Department of the Institute of Occupational Health, Helsinki, achieved notoriety for a method to predict optimal exercise training heart rate, now called the "Karvonen formula" (see Chapter 13). Paavo Komi, Department of Biology of Physical Activity, University of Jyväskylä, has been Finland's most prolific researcher, with numerous experiments published in the combined areas of exercise physiology and sport biomechanics.

Other Contributors to Exercise Physiology

In addition to the American and Nordic scientists who achieved distinction as exercise scientists, many other "giants" in the fields of physiology and experimental science made monumental discoveries that indirectly contributed to the knowledge base in exercise physiology. These include physiologists Antoine Laurent Lavoisier (1743–1794; fuel combustion), Sir Joseph Barcroft (1872–1947; altitude), Christian Bohr (1855–1911; oxygen–hemoglobin dissociation curve), John Scott Haldane (1860–1936; respiration), Otto Myerhoff (1884–1951; Nobel Prize, cellular metabolic pathways), Nathan Zuntz (1847–1920; portable metabolism apparatus), Carl von Voit (1831–1908) and his student, Max Rubner (1854–1932; direct and indirect calorimetry, and specific dynamic action of food), Max von Pettenkofer (1818–1901; nutrient metabolism), and Eduard F.W. Pflüger (1829–1910; tissue oxidation).

Closer to home, the field of exercise physiology owes a debt of gratitude to the pioneers of the physical fitness movement in the United States, notably **Thomas K. Cureton** (1901–1993; ACSM charter member, 1969 ACSM Honor Award) at the University of Illinois, Champaign (**Fig. 1.13**). Cureton, a prolific researcher, trained four generations of students beginning in 1941 who later established their research programs and influenced many of today's top exercise physiologists. These early graduates with an exercise physiology specialty soon assumed leadership positions as professors of physical education with teaching and research responsibilities in exercise physiology at numerous colleges and universities in the United States and throughout the world.

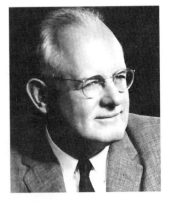

Figure 1.13 Thomas Kirk Cureton (1901–1993).

Contemporary Professional Exercise Physiology Organizations

Just as knowledge dissemination via publications in research and professional journals signals expansion of a field of study, development of professional organizations to certify and monitor professional activities becomes critical to continued growth. The American Association for the Advancement of Physical Education (AAAPE), formed in 1885, represented the first professional organization in the United States to include topics related to exercise physiology. This association predated the current **American Alliance for Health, Physical Education, Recreation, and Dance (AAHPERD)**.

Name a famous Norwegian and a famous Finnish exercise physiologist.

Norwegian:

Finnish:

Until the early 1950s, AAHPERD represented the preeminent professional organization for exercise physiologists. As the field began to expand and diversify its focus, a separate professional organization was needed to more fully respond to professional needs. In 1954, Joseph Wolffe, M.D., and 11 other physicians, physiologists, and physical educators founded the **American College of Sports Medicine (ACSM)**. Presently (August, 2005), with more than 30,000 members in more than 70 countries, the ACSM represents the largest professional organization in the world for exercise physiology (including allied medical and health areas). ACSM's mission *"promotes and integrates scientific research, education, and practical applications of sports medicine and exercise science to maintain and enhance physical performance, fitness, health, and quality of life."* ACSM publishes the research journal, *Medicine and Science in Sport and Exercise*, and other publications including the *ACSM's Health & Fitness Journal* and *Guidelines for Exercise Testing and Prescription*, a recognized reference standard for professionals in the field.

Name the pioneering physical fitness researcher from the University of Illinois.

Other important professional organizations related to exercise physiology include the International Council of Sport Science and Physical Education (ICSSPE), founded in 1958 in Paris, France, originally under the name International Council of Sport and Physical Education. ICSSPE serves as an international umbrella organization concerned with promoting and disseminating results and findings in the field of sport science. Its main professional publication, *Sport Science Review*, deals with thematic overviews of sport sciences research. The Federation Internationale de Medicine Sportive (FIMS), comprised of the national sports medicine associations of more than 100 countries, originated in 1928 during a meeting of Olympic medical doctors in Switzerland. FIMS promotes the study and development of sports medicine throughout the world and hosts major international conferences in sports medicine every 3 years; it also produces position statements on topics related to health, physical activity, and sports medicine. A 1995 joint position statement with the World Health Organization (WHO), entitled Physical Activity and Health, denotes one of their best-known documents. Other organizations representing exercise physiologists include the newly formed European College of Sport Science (ECSS) and British Association of Sport and Exercise Sciences (BASES). The most recent organization, the American Society of Exercise Physiology (ASEP), was formed in 1997 and held its first meeting in October, 1998.

What is the ACSM? Summarize its mission.

SUMMARY

1. Exercise physiology as an academic field of study consists of three distinct components: (1) a body of knowledge built on facts and theories derived from research, (2) a formal course of study at institutions of higher learning, and (3) professional preparation of practitioners and future leaders in the field.

2. Exercise physiology has emerged as a field separate from physiology because of its unique focus on the study of the functional dynamics and consequences of movement.

3. Galen (131–201 A. D.), one of the first "sports medicine" physicians, wrote prolifically, producing at

least 87 treatises on topics related to human anatomy and physiology, nutrition, growth and development, the benefits of exercise and deleterious consequences of sedentary living, and diseases and their treatment.

4. Austin Flint, Jr., M.D. (1836–1915), one of the first American pioneer physician–scientists, incorporated studies about physiological responses to exercise in his influential medical physiology textbooks.

5. Edward Hitchcock, Jr., (1828–1911), Amherst College Professor of Hygiene and Physical Education, devoted his academic career to the scientific study of physical exercise and training and body size and shape. His text on anatomy and physiology, coauthored with his father, significantly influenced the sports science movement in the United States after 1860. Hitchcock's insistence on the need for science applied to physical education undoubtedly influenced Harvard's commitment to create an academic Department of Anatomy, Physiology, and Physical Training in 1891.

6. George Wells Fitz, M.D. (1860–1934), created the first departmental major in Anatomy, Physiology, and Physical Training at Harvard University in 1891; the following year, he started the first formal exercise physiology laboratory in the United States. Fitz probably was first to teach a formal exercise physiology course at the university level.

7. The real impact of laboratory research in exercise physiology occurred in 1927 with the creation of the Harvard Fatigue Laboratory at Harvard University's business school. Two decades of outstanding work by this laboratory legitimized exercise physiology as a key area of research and study.

8. The Nordic countries played an important historical role in developing the field of exercise physiology. Danish physiologist August Krogh (1874–1949) won the 1920 Nobel Prize in physiology or medicine for discovering the mechanism that controlled capillary blood flow in resting or active muscle; Krogh's basic experiments led him to conduct other experiments with exercise scientists worldwide. His pioneering work in exercise physiology continues to inspire exercise physiology studies in many areas including oxygen uptake kinetics and metabolism, muscle physiology, and nutritional biochemistry.

9. Publications of applied and basic exercise physiology research have increased as the field expands into different areas. The World Wide Web offers unique growth potential for information dissemination in this area.

10. The American College of Sports Medicine, with over 30,000 members from North America and more than 70 other countries, represents the largest professional organization in the world for exercise physiology (including allied medical and health areas).

11. One theme unites the 2300-year history of exercise physiology: the value of mentoring by professors who spent an extraordinary amount of time "infecting" students with a love for science.

THOUGHT QUESTIONS

1. Discuss the benefits for fitness professionals to understand the historical roots of exercise physiology.

2. How has the historical link between exercise physiology and medicine benefited each field?

PART 2 •
Scientific Method and Exercise Physiology

Every exercise physiology student should become familiar with the methods of science to help separate fact from "hype"—most often encountered in advertising of health, fitness, and nutrition products. How does one know whether a product actually works? Does warming up really "warm" the muscles to prevent injury and enhance subsequent performance? Will breathing oxygen on the sidelines during a football game help the athlete recover? Does vitamin intake above recommended levels "supercharge" energy metabolism during exercise? Understanding the role of science in problem solving helps one to answer these and many other questions. The following section examines the goals of science, including different aspects of the scientific method of structured problem solving.

GENERAL GOALS OF SCIENCE

The two distinct goals of science often seem at odds. One goal serves mankind: to provide solutions to important problems and improve life's overall quality. This view of science, most prevalent among *nonscientists*, maintains that all scientific endeavors should exhibit practicality and immediate application. An opposing goal, predominant among *scientists*, maintains that science should describe and understand all occurrences without necessity for practical application; understanding phenomena becomes a worthy goal in itself. The desire for full knowledge implies being able to (1) account for (explain) behaviors or events, and (2) predict (and ultimately control) future occurrences and outcomes. Regardless of one's position concerning the major goal of science, its general objectives include being able to *understand*, *explain*, *predict*, and *control* phenomena. Scientists employ the scientific method to achieve these goals.

HIERARCHY IN SCIENCE

Full appreciation of science requires understanding its structure and its three levels of conceptualization (**Fig. 1.14**):

- Finding facts
- Developing laws
- Establishing theories

Fact Finding   The most fundamental level of scientific inquiry requires the systematic observation of measurable (**empirical**) phenomena. Often referred to as **fact finding**, this process requires standardized procedures and levels of agreement about what constitutes acceptable observation, measurement, and data recording procedures. In essence, fact finding involves recording information (data) about the behavior of objects. Facts provide the "building blocks" of science, although uncovering facts represents only the first level in the hierarchy of scientific inquiry.

Fact gathering occurs in many ways. We usually observe phenomena through visual, auditory, and tactile sensory input. Regardless of the observation method, to establish something as fact demands that different researchers reproduce observations under identical conditions on different occasions. For example, the healthy human heart's four chambers and the average sea level barometric pressure of 760 mm Hg represent indisputable, easily verifiable "facts." Facts usually take the form of objective statements about the observation, such as: "Jesse's body mass measured on a balance scale equals 70 kg (154 lb)," or "Jesse's heart rate on rising after 8 hours of sleep averages 63 beats per minute."

Interpreting Facts   Fact finding evaluates the observed object, occurrence, or phenomenon along a continuum, either imagined or real, that represents its

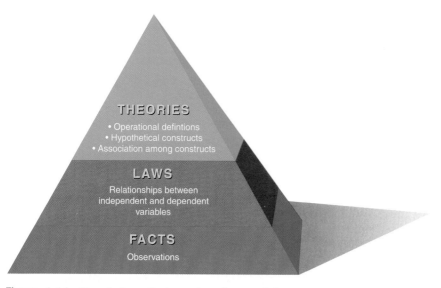

Figure 1.14   Foundations of science: facts, laws, and theories.

Questions & Notes

List the 3 building blocks of science.

1.

2.

3.

Give the major difference between a continuous and discrete variable.

Is body temperature measured on an ordinal or ratio scale?

FOR YOUR INFORMATION

A Fact is a Fact. . .
Facts exhibit no moral quality; once established, any question about facts arises only from interpretation. Although some may disagree with the meaning and implications of an established fact (e.g., the average woman possesses 50% less upper-body strength than the average man), no question exists about the "correctness" of the observation (that women have less upper-body strength than men). In essence, a fact is a fact. . . .

underlying measurable "dimension." The term **variable** identifies this measurable characteristic. Frequently, quantification of the variable occurs by assigning numbers to objects or events to describe their properties. For example, consider the variable percentage body fat with numerical values ranging from 3% to 60% of total body mass. Other examples include the weight of an object along a "heaviness" continuum, order of team finish in the NFL's American Conference, or heart rate from rest to maximal exercise.

Some variables like 50-m swim time or blood cholesterol level distribute in a continuous nature; they can take on any numerical value, depending on the precision of the measuring instrument. **Continuous variables** are further classified into ordinal, interval, and ratio numerical data. **Ordinal variables** have rank-ordered values (e.g., small, medium, large bone frame size; first through tenth place finish in a race; standings in league competition) according to some property about each person, group, object, or event compared with others studied. In ordered ranking, no inference exists of equal differences between specific ranks (e.g., race time difference between first and second place finish equals difference between ninth and tenth place). **Interval variables** exhibit similar properties as ordinal variables, except the distance between successive values on an unbroken scale from low to high represents the same amount of change. For example, in marathon running, the temporal 20-minute difference between a finish time of 2 h:10 min and 2 h:30 min equals that of 3 h:50 min and 4 h:10 min. The **ratio scale** possesses properties of interval and ordinal scoring but also contains an absolute zero point. Thus, a variable scored on a ratio basis with a value of 4 represents twice as much characteristic as a value of 2; this does not occur with interval-scored variables like temperature, in which 30°F is not twice as "hot" as 15°F.

In addition to continuous variables, some variables possess discrete properties. Scores for **discrete variables** fall only at certain points along a scale, like scores in most sporting events—"almost in" does not count in golf, soccer, basketball, or lacrosse. Discrete variables occur when the score's value simply reflects some characteristic of the object (e.g., male or female, hit or miss, win or lose, true or false, infected or not infected).

Casual and Causal Relationships

A fundamental scientific process involves observing and objectively measuring the quantity of a variable. However, it sometimes becomes important to consider how data from one variable relate to data from another variable. Understanding how variables change relative to each other represents a higher level of science than merely quantifying diverse isolated variables. For example, quantifying the degree of association between maximal oxygen uptake capacity (abbreviated $\dot{V}O_{2max}$) and chronological age reflects a higher level of understanding than describing the "facts" concerning each variable separately.

Figure 1.15, a scatter diagram between age and $\dot{V}O_{2max}$, shows that older people tend to have lower $\dot{V}O_{2max}$ values, whereas younger individuals possess higher scores. A science neophyte might interpret this inverse relationship as an indication that aging *causes* a decrease in $\dot{V}O_{2max}$, without considering an alternative possibility that decreases in $\dot{V}O_{2max}$ are caused by other variables like a sedentary lifestyle and/or a chronic disease that usually accompanies aging. A more extreme example to illustrate that association between variables does not necessarily **infer causality** considers the strong direct association in Western culture between the length of one's trousers and stature (i.e., taller individuals wear longer-length pants than shorter individuals). It seems highly unlikely that increasing trouser length causes increases in stature. In reality, this association is *casual* not *causal*, being driven more by cultural mores that "require" trousers to descend to ankle level—and leg length relates closely with overall body stature.

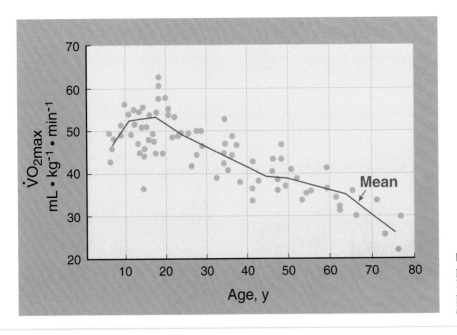

Figure 1.15 Generalized decline in peak $\dot{V}O_{2max}$ with age. (Modified from Robinson, S.: Experimental studies of physical fitness in relation to age. *Arbeitsphysiologie*, 10:18, 1938.)

The well-established positive relationship between increasing age and increasing systolic blood pressure among adults does not mean that hypertension remains inevitable with age. Rather, the relationship between aging and blood pressure exists because other factors, such as sedentary lifestyle, obesity, arteriosclerosis, increased stress, and poor diet, often increase with age. Each of these variables independently can elevate blood pressure. From a scientific perspective, a change in one variable (X) does not necessarily **cause** changes in the other variable (Y), simply because X and Y relate in a manner that seems to "makes sense."

Independent and Dependent Variables

Two categories of variables, independent and dependent, define the nature of relationships among occurrences. This categorization relates to the manner of the variable's use, not the nature of the variable itself. For causal relationships, manipulation of the value of the **independent variable** (X-variable) changes the value of the **dependent variable** (Y-variable). For example, increases in dietary saturated fatty acids (independent X-variable) increase levels of serum cholesterol (dependent Y-variable), whereas decreases in saturated fatty acid intake reduce serum cholesterol levels. In other words, the value of the dependent variable literally "depends on" the value of the independent variable.

For noncausal relationships, the distinction between dependent and independent variables becomes less clear. In such cases, the independent variable (e.g., the sum of five skinfolds or recovery heart rate on a step test) usually becomes the predictor variable, whereas the dependent variable (percentage body fat or $\dot{V}O_{2max}$) represents the quality predicted. In some cases, an independent variable becomes the dependent variable and vice versa. For example, body temperature represents the independent variable when used to predict change in regional blood flow or sweating response; body temperature assumes a dependent variable role when evaluating effectiveness of thermoregulation during heat stress.

Establishing Causality Between Variables

Scientists attempt to establish cause-and-effect relationships between independent and dependent variables by one of two methods:

1. Experimental studies
2. Field studies

Experimental Studies An **experiment** represents a set of operations to determine the underlying nature of the causal relationship between independent and dependent variables. *Systematically changing the value of the independent variable and measuring the effect on the dependent variable characterizes experimentation.* In some cases, the experiment evaluates the effect of combinations of independent variables (e.g., anabolic steroid administration plus resistance training; pre-exercise warm-up plus creatine supplementation) relative to one or more dependent variables. Regardless of the number of variables studied, an experiment's ultimate objective attempts to systematically isolate the effect of at least one independent variable related to at least one dependent variable. Only when this occurs can one decide which variable(s) really explains the phenomenon.

To illustrate the experimental method, consider two examples of seemingly straightforward studies of the effects of caffeine supplementation on endurance running performance.

1. In study one, the researcher randomly (chance selection of one subject does not affect selection of another subject) assigns 200 subjects to one of two independent groups of 100 subjects each. One group (experimental group) receives a known dose of caffeine in pill form 30 minutes before running to exhaustion at 75% of maximum heart rate; the other group (control group)

performs the identical endurance test without consuming caffeine. If time to exhaustion of the caffeine-supplemented experimental group exceeds the caffeine-free control group, caffeine may have enhanced performance. In this case, the results likely reflect a true effect of the independent variable and not chance occurrence.

2. In study two, the same experiment entails having only 100 subjects perform two run trials, one with and one without caffeine. For example, in the first trial, a subject consumes a known dose of caffeine in pill form 30 minutes before running. On another day, with sufficient time for recovery and for caffeine's effects to dissipate, the same subject runs without taking caffeine. Each of the 100 subjects would follow this procedure. To eliminate familiarization or training effects influencing test results, the order of testing alternates so that one-half of the subjects exercise first with caffeine, while the other 50 subjects perform first without caffeine.

The important feature of each experiment requires the researcher's ability to manipulate the independent variable (caffeine or no caffeine), while attempting to *control for* other important aspects such as test sequencing, environmental conditions, and perhaps even normal caffeine use before testing. *The control condition imposed by the experimenter represents the key feature of experimental research.* Control increases the likelihood that manipulation of the independent variable causes any observed change in the dependent variable.

Oftentimes, experimental results are not always as they appear. The two prior example experiments can be criticized on several grounds. Each of the research designs did not permit full control of potential intervening variables, thus a likelihood exists that variables other than the independent (treatment) variable could influence the observed change in performance. In both experiments, for example, subjects knew in which trial they received a treatment (regardless if they knew about caffeine). This creates the possibility of a **"placebo effect,"** in which a subject's performance improves largely from "expectation" or psychological factors. Many individuals perform at a higher level simply because of the suggestive power of believing the substance or procedure should produce an effect. To attribute a change in endurance to caffeine, unaffected by the subject's expectations, the researcher must use a placebo to provide appropriate control. In both preceding experiments, subjects in the no-caffeine trial should also receive an inert pill that looks, weighs, tastes, and smells the same as the caffeine-containing pill. An appropriate placebo condition controls the expectation effect and strengthens any conclusion that caffeine enhances endurance performance, should this occur.

Factors other than caffeine or a placebo effect also must be considered and controlled. For example, the experimenter needs to account for subjects' normal "background" level of caffeine consumption, particularly in the noncaffeine trials. Having subjects abstain from normal caffeine use for a predetermined duration before testing accomplishes this objective. To eliminate any possible effect of normal daily variation in performance, all testing should take place at the same time of day. To remove the potential for experimenter bias, subjects and researchers must remain unaware of the treatment condition (called a **double-blind** procedure). Some individuals might be "nonresponders" to caffeine's effects (habituation effect) because they regularly consume caffeine-containing foods and beverages. Thus, prior caffeine use becomes a potential confounding variable.

Controlling all potential factors that influence the effects of the independent variable(s) on the dependent variable(s) requires considerable effort, knowledge about the main factors, and creativity.

Field Studies   **Field studies** investigate events as they occur in normal living. Under such "natural" conditions, it becomes impossible to experimentally vary the independent variable or exert full control over potential interacting factors that might affect relationships. In medical areas, field studies (termed **epidemiologic research**) investigate group characteristics as they relate to the risks, prevalence, and severity of specific diseases. To a large extent, "risk profiles" for coronary artery disease, various cancers, and AIDS have emerged from associations generated from field studies. In exercise physiology, a field study might involve collecting data during a "real world" test of a new piece of exercise equipment (**Fig. 1.16**). The subject wears a wristband that receives signals from a chest-strap transmitter that sends the heart's electrical signals to the watch. The subject then pedals the "Surfbike" at different speeds to determine heart rate during different exercise intensities. Before the aquatic experiments, the subject's heart rate and oxygen uptake were determined in the laboratory while pedaling a bicycle ergometer at different speeds. A linear relationship between laboratory-determined heart rate and oxygen uptake allowed the researcher to "predict" the subject's oxygen uptake from heart rate measured during Surfbike exercise. An estimate of oxygen uptake permits calculation of caloric expenditure. In this particular experiment, Surfbike exercise at a heart rate of 178 beats per minute translated to 10.4 kCal expended per minute.

Although field studies provide objective insight about possible causes for observed phenomena, the lack of full control inherent in such research limits ability to infer causality. Because neither active manipulation of the independent variable by the experimenter nor control over potential intervening factors occurs, no certainty exists that any observed variation in the dependent variable necessarily resulted from variation in the independent variable.

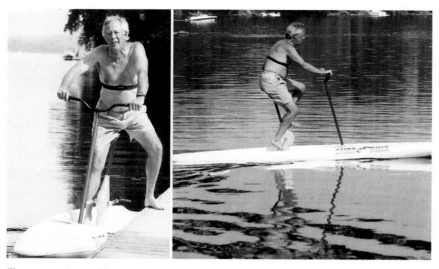

Figure 1.16   Field study in exercise physiology to estimate energy expenditure during Surfbike exercise from the heart rate-oxygen uptake relationship determined in the laboratory. Pedaling Surfbike during 400-m ride produced a heart rate of 178 beats per minute (equivalent to 10.4 kCal per minute energy expenditure). (Courtesy of F. Katch and P. Lagasse, Physical Activity Sciences, School of Medicine, Laval University, Québec City, Canada.)

Factors Affecting Relationships Among Variables

Many factors interact to causally affect relationships among variables. An understanding of the dynamics of relationships enables the educated science "consumer" to better evaluate research findings and possible limitations.

Experimental Testing Effects   Taking part in an experiment often changes subjects' behaviors, particularly if they know beforehand that someone is evaluating their performance. The potential for altered behavior raises the question of whether generalizability of results under structured laboratory conditions translates to behaviors in the "real world." Certainly, an appropriate control group that experiences the same laboratory environment and measurement procedures as the experimental group goes a long way in equalizing such effects across groups.

Measurement Errors   Measurement errors during data collection can be categorized into **technological error** and **recording error.** Technological errors include inherent instability of measuring devices (all mechanical and electronic instruments exhibit technological errors of different magnitudes) and the differential effects of external factors (temperature, humidity, electric current variations, air quality, proper calibration) on an instrument. Sometimes, technological errors remain constant relative to a standard—the machine always reads high or low—or they vary and the machine randomly reads high or low. Therefore, the researcher must identify the source of variable errors and minimize their effects; once identified, the constant error can be removed by calibrating the instrument or subtracting or adding the error component in subsequent computations. Proper and frequent instrument calibration minimizes most technological errors of measurement.

Recording errors include inaccuracies associated with improper observation and recording of phenomena. For example, measuring heart rate by pulse rate creates several potential sources of error: (1) location and timing of measurement, and (2) accuracy of measurement duration. Using a caliper to measure the thickness of subcutaneous fat (skinfolds) can introduce errors from nonstandardization of measurement sites, differences in technique for "pinching" the double

Questions & Notes

Briefly describe intravariability.

Briefly describe individual differences.

Give an example of a primary source in historical research.

Box 1-3 • CLOSE UP

HOW TO DISCERN RELIABLE HISTORICAL RESEARCH

The purpose of historical research has changed through the ages. The earliest writers of history focused on literary rather than scientific objectives; they preserved beloved folktales, created epics to entertain or inspire, defended and promoted numerous causes, zealously protected the privilege of a class, and glorified the state and exalted the church. In contrast, ancient Greek scholars envisioned history as a search for the truth—the application of exacting methods to select, verify, and classify facts according to specific standards that endure the test of critical examination and preserve an accurate record of past events. Historical research enlarges our world of experience; it provides deeper insights into what has been successfully and unsuccessfully tried.

Historical scholars collect and validate source materials to formulate and verify hypotheses. Unlike experimental research, their methods feature observations and insights that cannot be repeated under conventional laboratory conditions.

COLLECTING SOURCE MATERIAL

The historian's initial and most important problem-solving task seeks to obtain the best available data. The historian must distinguish between **primary source** and **secondary source** materials.

Primary Sources

Primary sources comprise the basic materials of historical research. This prized form of "data" derives from:

- Testimony from reliable eyewitnesses and earwitnesses to past events
- Direct examination of actual "objects" used in the past

A historian collects evidence from the closest witness to the past event or condition. Primary source materials include records preserved with the conscious intent of transmitting information. For example, a newspaper account of what transpired at a meeting has less intrinsic historical value than the meeting's official minutes. Records of past ideas, conditions, and events exist in written form (e.g., official records or executive documents, health records, licenses, annual reports, catalogs, and personal records—diaries, autobiographies, letters, wills, deeds, contracts, lecture notes, original drafts of speeches, articles, and books), visual or pictorial form (photographs, movies, microfilms, drawings, paintings, etchings, coins, and sculpture), mechanical form (tape recordings, phonograph records, and dictations), electronic form (digital "memory" on disc or tape), and sometimes oral form (myths, folktales, family stories, dances, games, ceremonies, and reminiscences by eyewitnesses to events).

---

layer of skin and underlying tissue, accurate caliper placement, and precisely when to read the caliper dial after the pinch. Experienced researchers attempt to eliminate all errors but realize this is nearly impossible.

Within-Subject (Intraindividual) Variability

Another source of measurement error relates to the inherent tendency for humans to exhibit a variable response from moment-to-moment and trial-to-trial. In a sense, **biological variation** should not be considered error, but rather a reality of life. All biological systems exhibit inherent variability, albeit small in some cases, depending on the variable. Resting blood flow, heart rate, and blood pressure fluctuate up to ±20% within the same person from day to day (and within the same day), even when measured under identical conditions. One explanation for normal variation in biological function lies in the body's ability to achieve an identical physiological result through diverse mechanisms. For example, blood flow from the heart (cardiac output) occurs from the interaction of heart rate and stroke volume (blood volume

pumped from the left ventricle with each beat). Consequently, increases or decreases in heart rate may have little impact on cardiac output if compensated by a proportionate alteration in the heart's stroke volume. All biological functions exhibit natural oscillations. These include easily measured variables, like heart rate, breathing rate, and body temperature, and more internal measures of electrical and chemical phenomena. These do not reflect error per se, but rather, they represent fluctuations of a normal state. Repeated measurements, or a single measurement for a prolonged duration, often dampen the variation effect and provide a more representative indication of normal functioning.

Individual Differences

Individuals differ from each other in subtle and complex ways. A sampling of exercise physiology variables showing considerable between-subject variation (**individual differences**) includes muscular strength, aerobic and anaerobic capacity, body composition, muscle fiber type, heart size, running economy, and training responsiveness. Individual differences in physio-

Box 1–3 • CLOSE UP *(Continued)*

Secondary Sources

Secondary sources include information provided by a person who did not directly observe the event, object, or condition. The original publication of a research report in a scientific journal represents a primary source (often used by modern researchers to provide context to their experiments), whereas summaries in encyclopedias, newspapers, periodicals, the Internet, and other references qualify as secondary materials. The more interpretations that separate a past event from the reader, the less trustworthy the evidence becomes; the transition often distorts and changes the facts. For this reason, secondary sources are less reliable. However, secondary sources acquaint a neophyte historian with major theoretical issues and suggest locations for uncovering primary source materials.

CRITICIZING SOURCE MATERIAL

Historians critically examine the trustworthiness of their source material. Through **external criticism**, the historian checks the authenticity and textual integrity of the "data" (time, place, and authorship) to determine its admissibility as reliable evidence. Enterprising and exacting investigation becomes part of external criticism—tracking down anonymous and undated documents, ferreting out forgeries, discovering plagiarism, uncovering incorrectly identified items, and restoring documents to their original forms.

After completing external criticism, the historian engages in **internal criticism** to establish the meaning and trustworthiness of a document's contents. Internal criticism determines the following:

- Conditions that produced the document
- Validity of the writer's intellectual premises
- Competency, credibility, and possible author bias
- Correctness of data interpretation

Careful historical research provides insight about how past facts influence current events. Whether an accurate record of the past predicts and influences future circumstances remains a hotly debated topic among historians.

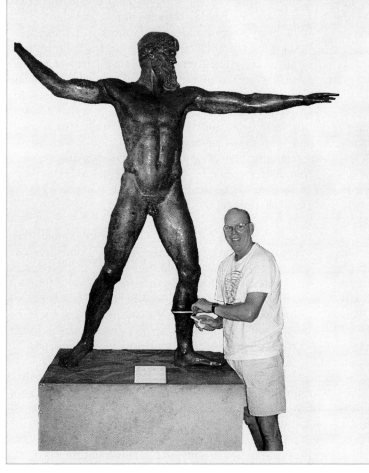

One of the authors taking anthropometric measurements on the original ancient Greek bronze statue Poseidon (460/450 B. C.; primary source–sculpted by either Kalamis or Onatas, and recovered intact in 1928 off Cape Artemision, Euobia, Greece) to determine anthropometric proportions compared with the modern reference man. For a stature of 207 cm, Poseidon's projected body mass using a prediction equation based on stature and six diameters equaled 133.7 kg. (Cooperative research project with Dr. Konstantine Pavlou, College of Sports Sciences and Hellenic Sport Science Institute, Athens, Greece and the National Archeological Museum of Athens.)

logical and performance responses reflect the existence of true biological differences among individuals.

Experimenter Expectation Effect   When the researcher anticipates (wishes) a particular outcome for an experiment, subtle "messages" and alterations in the testing environment may occur, which can influence subject behavior to achieve a desired outcome. Perception of researcher neutrality must be maintained during the research process.

Hawthorne Effect   The **Hawthorne effect** emerged from a series of experiments in the 1930s on worker productivity at the Western Electric Company in Hawthorne, New York. The research evaluated how work hours, pay, modification of lighting, and introduction of music related to job productivity. The data revealed that introducing a change produced noticeable productivity increases. Productivity increased even when reestablishing the original working conditions. In essence, care and attention shown to workers, not the nature of the specific change in working conditions, improved job performance. In this regard, researchers must remain vigilant to guard against a "Hawthorne effect." Personal attention to subjects, or the nature of the study and measurement variables, can cause subjects to modify behaviors and change the dependent variable regardless of the influence of the independent variable. One approach to minimize a Hawthorne effect allows experimental and control groups to interact equally among themselves and the research team.

Establishing Laws

Fact gathering does not generate much controversy; after all, facts are facts. Interpretation of facts, on the other hand, raises science to a level rife for debate. Interpreting facts leads to the second level of the scientific process—creating statements that describe, integrate, or summarize facts and observations. Such statements are termed **laws**. More precisely, a law represents a statement describing the relationships among independent and dependent variables. Laws generate from inductive reasoning (moving from specific facts to general principles). Many examples of laws exist in physiology. For example, blood flows through the vascular circuit in general accord with the physical laws of hydrodynamics applied to rigid, cylindrical vessels. Although true only in a qualitative sense when applied to the body, one law of hydrodynamics, termed Poiseuille's Law, describes the interacting relationships among a pressure gradient, vessel radius, vessel length, and fluid viscosity on the force impeding blood flow (see Chapter 9 for a description of Poiseuille's Law in action).

Laws are purposely not very specific; they remain powerful because they generalize to many different situations. A good (useful) law accounts for all of the facts among variables. Many laws have limits because they apply to only certain situations. A limited law proves less useful in predicting new facts. *A fundamental aspect of science tests*

predictions generated from a particular law. If the prediction holds up, the law expands to additional situations; if not, the law becomes restated in more restrictive terms. Developing new technologies often permits testing laws in situations heretofore thought impossible; this allows for development of a more comprehensive law.

Laws do not provide an explanation *why* variables behave the way they do; laws only provide a general summary of the relationship among variables. Theories explain the hows and whys about laws.

Developing Theories

Theories attempt to explain the fundamental nature of laws. **Theories** offer abstract explanations of laws and facts. They try to explain the "why" of laws. Theories involve a more complex understanding (and explanation) of variables than do laws. Examples of theories include Darwin's Theory of Natural Selection and Evolution, Einstein's Theory of Relativity, Canon's Theory of Emotions, Freud's Theory of Personality Formation and Development, and Helmholtz's Theories of Color Vision and Hearing.

Theories consist of the following three aspects: hypothetical construct, associations among constructs, and operational definitions.

Hypothetical Constructs   **Hypothetical constructs** represent nonobservable abstract entities, consciously invented and generalized for use in theories. For example, the construct of "intelligence" emerged from observations of presumably intelligent and nonintelligent behaviors. Several constructs comprise A.V. Hill's initial theory about "oxygen debt" in recovery from exercise (see Chapter 6). Hill proposed constructs, such as "oxygen deficit," "alactacid debt" and "lactacid debt," and "steady-state" and "non–steady-state" energy transfer, to explain his observations about oxygen uptake dynamics in recovery from different exercise intensities. "Physical fitness" represents another common construct in areas related to exercise physiology.

Associations Among Constructs   Scientific inquiry often requires defining relationships among constructs. For example, the construct "physical ability" becomes clarified by its association to the construct "physical fitness," which itself becomes operationally defined (see next section) by numerous specific "fitness" tests. In essence, the meaning of one construct becomes understood through its relationship to other more clearly defined variables.

Operational Definitions   The scientific process requires refinement of constructs into observable characteristics for objective quantification and recording. **Operational definitions** assign meaning to a construct by outlining the set of operations (like an instruction manual) to measure the quantity of that construct or to manipulate it. For example, the construct intelligence only becomes understood when operationally defined (i.e., score on a specific

IQ test). In exercise physiology, the construct anaerobic capacity becomes operationally defined as total work accomplished during 30 seconds of all-out exercise performed on an arm-crank or leg-cycle ergometer. Operational definitions permit constructs like muscular strength, aerobic capacity, flexibility, speed, anaerobic power, neuromuscular reaction speed, and physical fitness to emerge from the abstract to the concrete. Operational definitions permit testing of hypotheses and theories by providing a measurement link between an abstract construct and a concrete quantity or measurement. **Figure 1.17** shows the relations among theories, laws, and facts (observations).

The Burden of Disproof

Experimentation represents the scientific method for testing hypotheses; scientists either reject or fail to reject a hypothesis. Rejecting a hypothesis represents a powerful outcome because it may nullify a theory and specific predictions generated from the theory. Failure to reject a hypothesis indicates that the observable results appear to support the theory. The terms *reject* and *fail to reject* (in contrast to *prove* and *disprove*) deserve special attention. Failure to reject does not indicate confirmation or proof, only inability to reject a hypothesis. However, if other experiments (particularly from independent laboratories) also fail to reject a given hypothesis, a strong likelihood exists (high probability) for a correct hypothesis. The structure of science makes it impossible to totally confirm a theory's absolute "correctness" because scientists may still devise a future experiment to disprove a hypothesis based on a particular theory. The strength of the experimental method lies in rejecting hypotheses that have direct bearing on theories or predictions from theories. *The notion of disproof represents an important distinguishing feature of the scientific method.*

Publishing Results of Experiments: The Peer Review Process

Fact finding, law formulation, and theory development represent fundamental aspects of science. Allowing fellow scientists to critique one's research findings before general distribution completes the process of scientific inquiry. Most journals that disseminate research rely on the researcher's peers to review and pass judgment on the suitability and quality of methods, experimental design, appropriateness of conclusions, and contribution to new knowledge. Although this aspect of science is sometimes criticized for failing to achieve true objectivity and

Questions & Notes

Briefly describe the difference between a law and a theory.

FOR YOUR INFORMATION

Searching for Exercise Science Information: *The Web of Science*
Professionals in the field continually need to research information about a specific topic or must locate research articles by specific scientists. The **Web of Science** (*http://www.isinet.com/products/citation/wos/*) provides a unique web-based search tool, permitting extraordinary searching of many different databases. The Web of Science accesses multidisciplinary databases of bibliographic information gathered from thousands of scholarly journals. Each database is indexed so as to enable a search for a specific article by subject, author, journal, and/or author address. The information stored about each article includes the article's cited reference list (often called its bibliography), and searches can include the databases for articles that cite a known author or work. With the Web of Science you can: (1) search the databases for published works, (2) view full bibliographic records and add them to your Marked List for export to bibliographic management software, (3) save them to a file, (4) format them for printing, (5) e-mail them, (6) order the full text, (7) link directly to other articles on the same topic as the one you are viewing, even articles that have been published after the article you are viewing, and (8) save your search statements, which can be opened later and run again. Use the following URL for a tutorial on using the Web of Science: *http://www.isinet.com/tutorials/webofscience/*.

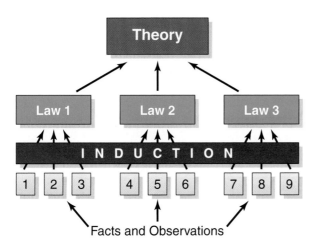

Figure 1.17   Relation among theories, laws, and facts.

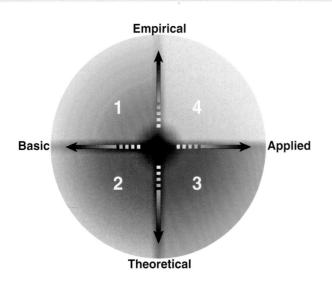

Figure 1.18   Research continuum in science.

freedom from professional bias, few would discount its importance. When executed properly, **peer review** maintains a level of "quality control" in disseminating new information.

Imagine the many instances in which an experimental outcome could be influenced by self-interest and/or professional bias. Athletic shoe and supplement manufacturers often sponsor laboratories to conduct detailed "research" on the efficacy of their products. To ensure credibility, research from such laboratories must be reviewed by experts having no affiliation (direct or indirect) with the company. Without a system of "checks and balances," such studies should be viewed with skepticism and lack trustworthiness as a legitimate source of new knowledge.

Empirical vs. Theoretical Research; Basic vs. Applied Research

Different approaches lead to successful experimentation and knowledge acquisition. **Figure 1.18** shows two different continuums for experimentation. The theoretical–empirical research continuum has at its foundation experimentation related to establishing laws and testing theories. Scientists conducting **theoretical research** maintain that fact finding alone represents an unfocused waste of energy if the process does not emanate from and contribute to theory building. Scientists at the opposite end of the continuum collect facts and make observations with little regard for building theory. The influential psychologist B.F. Skinner (1904–1990) exemplifies the proponent of the **empirical research** (experience-related) approach. His discoveries about reinforcement—a reward for suc-

cessful behavior increases the probability of success in subsequent trials—were uncovered by "accident." Skinnerian empiricists argue that theoretical scientists often fail to uncover meaningful relationships because they become too "locked into" theoretical formulations and abstract models.

Basic–applied research represents another continuum. **Applied research** incorporates scientific endeavors to solve specific problems, the solution of which directly applies to medicine, business, the military, sports performance, or society's general well-being. Applied research in exercise physiology might focus on methods for improving training responsiveness, facilitating fluid replenishment and optimizing temperature regulation in exercise, enhancing endurance performance, blunting the effects of fatigue byproducts, and countering the deterioration of physiological function during prolonged exposure to a weightless environment. **Basic research** lies at the other end of this continuum; no concern exists for immediate practical application of research findings. Instead, the researcher pursues a line of inquiry purely for the sake of discovering new knowledge. Oftentimes, uncovering facts that initially seem of little value fill a theoretical void, and like magic, a wonderful new practical solution (or product) emerges. Nowhere has this taken place with more regularity than with research related to the space program. Facts uncovered in a weightless environment about fundamental biological and chemical processes have contributed to practical outcomes that benefit humans. Experiments on how certain chemicals react in zero gravity, for example, have resulted in the discovery of at least 25 new medicines. Manned space missions have provided fresh insights into almost every facet of medicine and physiology, from the affects of weightlessness on bone dynamics, blood pressure, and cardiac, respiratory, hormonal, neural, and muscular function, to growth of genetically engineered plants and a new generation of polymers. Each new insight and observation spawns numerous new ideas and additional facts that help to create products with practical applications.

Research can be classified into one of four categories depicted by the quadrants in Figure 1.18. Basic–empirical research in Quadrant 1 has no immediate practical outcomes and little to do with theory. Research without immediate practical implications, but motivated by theory (establishing laws and conducting experiments that bear on theory), falls into Quadrant 2. Quadrant 3 contains theoretical–applied research primarily focused on problem solving within the framework of an existing theoretical model, and Quadrant 4 classifies empirical–applied research (not theory based), which is aimed at solving problems. Often, lines of demarcation are not as clear-cut as in the figure, and a particular research effort spans multiple quadrants.

SUMMARY

1. The ultimate aims of science include (1) explanation, (2) understanding, (3) prediction, and (4) control.

2. Fact finding, developing laws, and establishing theories represent three levels of scientific inquiry.

3. The term variable identifies measurable characteristics of an object, occurrence, or phenomenon. The values for discrete variables fall only at certain points along a scale (e.g., scores in most sporting events); continuous variables take on any numerical value, depending on the precision of the measuring instrument.

4. Variables are also categorized as either independent or dependent, depending on their use and not on their inherent nature. For causal relationships, manipulation of the independent X-variable changes the value of the dependent Y-variable. Understanding how variables change in relation to each other represents a higher level of science than simply describing and quantifying individual variables. Association between variables does not necessarily infer causality.

5. An experiment represents a set of operations to determine the underlying nature of the relationship between independent and dependent variables. Systematically changing the value of the independent variable and measuring the effect on the dependent variable characterizes experimentation (with control of other variables that might cause the relationship).

6. The key feature of experimental research involves the control of conditions imposed by the experimenter. Control increases the likelihood that manipulation of an independent variable causes any observed change in a dependent variable.

7. Subject selection, appropriate use of statistics, and ability to draw meaningful inferences and conclusions

from the data collected represent three important factors for evaluating the quality of research design.

8. Field or epidemiologic studies investigate events as they occur naturally. In exercise physiology, a field study might involve collecting data on the age, body mass, percentage body fat, and aerobic capacity of elite triathletes and their performance time during competition. Inability of the researcher to experimentally vary the independent variable or exert full control over potential interacting factors that might affect relationships limits research findings.

9. Many factors interact to affect relationships among variables. These include experimental testing effects, measurement errors, within-subject variability, individual differences, experimenter expectation effect, and the Hawthorne effect.

10. Interpreting facts leads to the second level of the scientific process—creating statements that describe (or summarize) relationships among facts. Laws only provide a general summary of the relationship among variables; they do not explain "why" variables behave the way they do.

11. Theories attempt to clarify the fundamental nature of laws—they attempt to explain the "why" of laws. Theories offer abstract explanations of laws and facts.

12. A theory's absolute "correctness" remains elusive. The strength of the experimental method lies in rejecting hypotheses that have direct bearing on theories or predictions from theories. The notion of disproof represents a key distinguishing feature of the scientific method.

13. Submitting research findings for critique by fellow scientists (peer review) before their dissemination completes the process of scientific inquiry.

THOUGHT QUESTIONS

1. How can an understanding of the scientific method enhance professional development in areas related to exercise physiology (e.g., physical fitness program development, athletic training, personal training)?

2. How would an experimental researcher attempt to show that a sedentary lifestyle causes coronary heart disease?

PART 3 •
The Exercise Physiologist

Many individuals view exercise physiology as representing an undergraduate or graduate academic major (or concentration) completed at an accredited college or university. In this regard, only those who complete this academic major have the "right" to be called "exercise physiologist." However, many individuals complete undergraduate and graduate degrees in related fields with considerable coursework and practical experience in exercise physiology (or related areas). Consequently, the title exercise physiologist could also apply so long as their academic preparation is adequate. Resolution of this dilemma becomes difficult because no national consensus exists as to what constitutes an acceptable (or minimal) academic program of course work in exercise physiology. In addition, there are no universal standards for hands-on laboratory experiences (anatomy, kinesiology, biomechanics, and exercise physiology), demonstrated level of competency, and internship hours that would stand the test of national certification or licensure. Moreover, because areas of concentration within the field are so broad, consensus certification testing becomes challenging. No national accreditation or licensure exists to certify exercise physiologists.

WHAT DO EXERCISE PHYSIOLOGISTS DO?

Exercise physiologists assume diverse careers. Some use their research skills primarily in colleges, universities, and private industry settings. Others are employed in health, fitness, and rehabilitation centers, whereas others serve as educators, personal trainers, managers, and entrepreneurs in the health and fitness industry.

Exercise physiologists also own health and fitness companies or are hands-on practitioners who teach and service the community including corporate, industrial, and governmental agencies. Some specialize in other types of professional work like massage therapy, while others go on to pursue professional degrees in physical therapy, occupational therapy, nursing, nutrition, medicine, and chiropractic.

Table 1.3 presents a partial list of different employment descriptions for a qualified exercise physiologist in one of six major areas.

THE EXERCISE PHYSIOLOGIST/ HEALTH-FITNESS PROFESSIONAL IN THE CLINICAL SETTING

The well-documented health benefits of regular physical activity have enhanced the exercise physiologist's role be-

yond traditional lines. A clinical exercise physiologist becomes part of the health/fitness professional team. This team approach to preventive and rehabilitative services requires different personnel depending on program mission, population served, location, number of participants, space availability, and funding level. A comprehensive clinical program can include the following personnel, in addition to the exercise physiologist:

- Physicians
- Certified personnel (exercise leaders, health-fitness instructors, directors, exercise test technologists, preventive and rehabilitative exercise specialists, preventive and rehabilitative exercise directors)
- Dietitians
- Nurses
- Physical therapists
- Occupational therapists
- Social workers
- Respiratory therapists
- Psychologists
- Health educators

Sports Medicine and Exercise Physiology: A Vital Link

The traditional view of **sports medicine** involves rehabilitating athletes from sports-related injuries. *A more contemporary view relates sports medicine to the scientific and medical (preventive and rehabilitative) aspects of physical activity, physical fitness, and exercise/sports performance.* Thus, a close link ties sports medicine to clinical exercise physiology. The sports medicine professional and exercise physiologist work hand-in-hand with similar populations. These include, at one extreme, the sedentary person who needs only a modest amount of regular exercise to reduce risk of degenerative diseases; at the other extreme are able-bodied and disabled athletes who strive to further enhance their performance.

Carefully prescribed physical activity significantly contributes to overall health and quality of life. In conjunction with sports medicine professionals, the clinical exercise physiologist tests, treats, and rehabilitates individuals with diverse diseases and physical disabilities. In addition, prescription of physical activity and athletic competition for the physically challenged plays an important role in sports medicine and exercise physiology, providing unique opportunities for research, clinical practice, and professional advancement.

TRAINING AND CERTIFICATION BY PROFESSIONAL ORGANIZATIONS

To properly accomplish responsibilities in the exercise setting, the health-fitness professional must integrate unique knowledge, skills, and abilities related to exercise, physical

Table 1·3	Partial List of Employment Opportunities for Qualified Exercise Physiologists					
SPORTS	COLLEGE UNIVERSITY	COMMUNITY	CLINICAL	GOVERNMENT MILITARY	BUSINESS	PRIVATE
Sports director Strength/ conditioning coach Director, manager of state/national teams Consultant	Professor Researcher Administrator Teacher Instructor	Manage/direct health/wellness programs Community education Occupational rehabilitation	Test/supervise cardiopulmonary patients Evaluate/supervise special populations (diabetes; obesity; arthritis; dyslipidemia; cystic fibrosis; cancer; hypertension; children; low functional capacity; pregnancy) Exercise technologist in cardiology practice Researcher	Fitness director/manager Health/fitness director in correctional institutions Sports nutrition programs	Sports management Health/fitness promotion Sport psychologist Health/ fitness club instructor	Personal health/ fitness consultant Own business

fitness, and health. Different professional organizations provide leadership in training and certifying health-fitness professionals at different levels. **Table 1.4** lists organizations offering training/certification programs with diverse emphases and specializations. The **ACSM** has emerged as the preeminent academic organization offering comprehensive programs in areas related to the health-fitness profession. ACSM certifications encompass cognitive and practical competencies that are evaluated by written and practical examinations. The candidate must successfully complete each of these components (scored separately) to receive the world-recognized ACSM certification. ACSM offers a wide variety of certification programs throughout the United States and in other countries (*http://www.acsm.org/ index.asp*).

ACSM QUALIFICATIONS AND CERTIFICATIONS

Health and fitness professionals should be knowledgeable and competent in different areas, including first-aid and CPR certification, depending on personal interest. **Table 1.5** presents content areas for different ACSM certifications. Each has general and specific learning objectives.

Health and Fitness Track

The **Health and Fitness Track** encompasses the Exercise Leader, Health/Fitness Instructor, and Health/Fitness Director categories.

Exercise Leader   An **Exercise Leader** must know about physical fitness (including basic motivation and counseling techniques) for healthy individuals and those with cardiovascular and pulmonary diseases. This category requires at least 250 hours of hands-on leadership experience or an academic background in an appropriate allied health field. Examples of general objectives for an Exercise Leader in exercise physiology include to:

- Define aerobic and anaerobic metabolism
- Describe the role of carbohydrates, fats, and proteins as fuel for aerobic and anaerobic exercise performance

Questions & Notes

List 3 possible job opportunities for exercise physiology graduates.

1.

2.

3.

List 3 different clinical personnel that exercise physiologists work with in the clinical setting.

1.

2.

3.

Give 2 differences between an exercise leader and a health/fitness director.

1.

2.

Table 1·4	Organizations Offering Training/Certification Programs Related to Physical Activity
ORGANIZATION	**AREAS OF SPECIALIZATION AND CERTIFICATION**
Aerobics and Fitness Association of America (AFAA) 15250 Ventura Blvd., Suite 200 Sherman Oaks, CA 91403	AFP Fitness Practitioner, Primary Aerobics Instructor, Personal Trainer & Fitness Counselor, Step Reebok Certification, Weight Room/Resistance Training Certification, Emergency Response Certification
American College Sports Medicine (ACSM) 401 West Michigan St. Indianapolis, IN 46202	Exercise Leader, Health/Fitness Instructor, Exercise Test Technologist, Health/Fitness Director, Exercise Specialist, Program Director
American Council on Exercise (ACE) 5820 Oberlin Dr., Suite 102 San Diego, CA 92121	Group Fitness Instructor, Personal Trainer, Lifestyle & Weight Management Consultant
Canadian Aerobics Instructors Network (CAIN) 2441 Lakeshore Rd. West, P.O. Box 70029 Oakville, ON L6L 6M9	CIAI Instructor, Certified Personal Trainer
Canadian Personal Trainers Network (CPTN) Ontario Fitness Council (OFC) 1185 Eglington Ave. East, Suite 407 North York, ON M3C 3C6	CPTN/OFC Certified Personal Trainer, CPTN Certified Specialty Personal Trainer, CPTN/OFC Assessor of Personal Trainers, CPTN/OFC Course Conductor for Personal Trainers
Canadian Society for Exercise Physiology 1600 James Naismith Dr., Suite 311 Gloucester, ON K1B 5N4	CFC-Certified Fitness Consultant, PFLC-Professional Fitness & Lifestyle Consultant, AFAC-Accredited Fitness Appraisal Center
The Cooper Institute for Aerobics Research 12330 Preston Rd. Dallas, TX 75230	PFS-Physical Fitness Specialists (Personal Trainer), GEL-Group Exercise Leadership (Aerobic Instructor), ADV.PFS-Advanced Physical Fitness Specialist, Biomechanics of Strength Training, Health Promotion Director
Disabled Sports USA 451 Hungerford Dr., Suite 100 Rockville, MD 20850	Adapted Fitness Instructor
International Weightlifting Association (IWA) P.O. Box 444 Hudson, OH 44236	CWT-Certified Weight Trainer
Jazzercise 2808 Roosevelt Blvd. Carlsbad, CA 92008	Certified Jazzercise Instructor
International Society of Sports Nutrition 600 Pembrook Dr. Woodland Park, CO 80863	Sports Nutrition Certification Body Composition Certification
National Strength & Conditioning Association (NSCA) P.O. Box 38909 Colorado Springs, CO 80937	Certified Strength & Conditioning Specialist, Certified Personal Trainer
YMCA of the USA 101 North Wacker Dr. Chicago, IL 60606	Certified Fitness Leader (Stage I-Theory, II-Applied Theory, III-Practical), Certified Specialty Leader, Trainer of Fitness Leaders, Trainer of Trainers

- Define the relationship of METs (multiples of resting metabolism) and kilocalories to levels of physical activity

Health/Fitness Instructor An undergraduate degree in exercise science, kinesiology, physical education, or appropriate allied health field represents the minimum education prerequisite for a **Health/Fitness Instructor**. These individuals must demonstrate competency in physical fitness testing, designing and executing an exercise program, leading exercise, and organizing and operating fitness facilities. The Health/Fitness Instructor has added responsibility for (1) training and/or supervising exercise leaders during an exercise program, and (2) serving as an exercise leader. Health/ Fitness Instructors also function as health counselors to offer multiple intervention strategies for lifestyle change.

Health/Fitness Director The minimum educational prerequisite for **Health/Fitness Director** certification requires a postgraduate degree in an appropriate allied health field. Health/Fitness Directors must acquire a Health/Fitness Instructor or Exercise Specialist certification. This level requires supervision by a certified program director and physician during an approved internship or at least 1 year of practical experience. Health/Fitness Directors require leadership qualities that ensure competency in training and supervising personnel and proficiency in oral presentations.

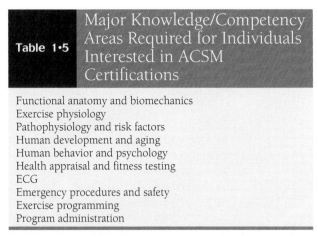

Table 1·5	Major Knowledge/Competency Areas Required for Individuals Interested in ACSM Certifications
	Functional anatomy and biomechanics
	Exercise physiology
	Pathophysiology and risk factors
	Human development and aging
	Human behavior and psychology
	Health appraisal and fitness testing
	ECG
	Emergency procedures and safety
	Exercise programming
	Program administration

From *ACSM's Guidelines for Exercise Testing and Prescription.* 7th Ed. Baltimore, MD: Lippincott Williams & Wilkins, 2005.

Clinical Track

The title **clinical track** indicates that certified personnel in these areas provide leadership in health and fitness and/or clinical programs. These professionals possess added clinical skills and knowledge that allow them to work with higher risk, symptomatic populations.

Exercise Test Technologist   **Exercise Test Technologists** administer exercise tests to individuals in good health and various states of illness. They need to demonstrate appropriate knowledge of functional anatomy, exercise physiology, pathophysiology, electrocardiography, and psychology. They must know how to recognize contraindications to testing during preliminary screening, administer tests, record data, implement emergency procedures, summarize test data, and communicate test results to other health professionals. Certification as an Exercise Test Technologist does *not* require prerequisite experience or special level of education.

Preventive/Rehabilitative Exercise Specialist   Unique competencies for the category **Preventive/Rehabilitative Exercise Specialist** include the ability to lead exercises for persons with medical limitations (particularly cardiorespiratory and related diseases) and healthy populations. The position requires a bachelor's or graduate degree in an appropriate allied health field and an internship of 6 months or more (800 hours), largely with cardiopulmonary disease patients in a rehabilitative setting. The Preventive/Rehabilitative Exercise Specialist conducts and administers exercise tests, evaluates and interprets clinical data and formulates an exercise prescription, conducts exercise sessions, and demonstrates leadership, enthusiasm, and creativity. This person can respond appropriately to complications during exercise testing and training and can modify exercise prescriptions for patients with specific needs.

Preventive/Rehabilitative Program Director   The **Preventive/Rehabilitative Program Director** holds an advanced degree in an appropriate allied health-related area. The certification requires an internship or practical experience of at least 2 years. This health professional works with cardiopulmonary disease patients in a rehabilitative setting, conducts and administers exercise tests, evaluates and interprets clinical data, formulates exercise prescriptions, conducts exercise sessions, responds appropriately to complications during exercise testing and training, modifies exercise prescriptions for patients with specific limitations, and makes administrative decisions regarding all aspects of a specific program.

Questions & Notes

List 2 competency areas for ACSM certification.

1.

2.

FOR YOUR INFORMATION

The American College of Sports Medicine
The ACSM has more than 30,000 International, National, and Regional Chapter members. ACSM's mission promotes and integrates scientific research, education, and practical applications of sports medicine and exercise science to maintain and enhance physical performance, fitness, health, and quality of life. The ACSM was founded in 1954. Since then, members have applied their knowledge, training, and dedication in sports medicine and exercise science to promote healthier lifestyles for people around the globe. In 1984, the National Center relocated to its current headquarters in Indianapolis, Indiana. The ACSM continues to grow and prosper both nationally and internationally. Working in a wide range of medical specialties, allied health professions, and scientific disciplines, ACSM is committed to the diagnosis, treatment, and prevention of sports-related injuries and the advancement of the science of exercise. The ACSM represents the largest, most respected sports medicine and exercise science organization in the world.

SUMMARY

1. A close link ties sports medicine to clinical exercise physiology. The sports medicine professional and exercise physiologist work side-by-side with similar populations. These include, at one extreme, the sedentary person who needs only a modest amount of regular exercise to reduce risk of degenerative diseases and patients recovering from surgery or requiring regular exercise to combat a decline in functional capacity brought on by serious illness. At the other extreme are able-bodied and disabled athletes who strive to enhance sports performance.

2. In their clinical role, exercise physiologists alongside sports medicine professionals test, treat, and rehabilitate individuals with diverse diseases and physical disabilities.

3. The American College of Sports Medicine (ACSM) has emerged as the preeminent academic organization offering comprehensive certification programs in several areas related to the health-fitness profession. ACSM certifications encompass cognitive and practical competencies that are evaluated by written and practical examinations.

THOUGHT QUESTIONS

1. Discuss advantages for personal trainers to become trained in exercise physiology and related areas and/ or obtain a special certification from a recognized organization. Why can't a person just have practical experience and learn to apply it to others?

2. How would you account for the differences that exist in quality of certification requirements of different organizations?

3. Discuss whether or not professionals in the field should be required by their certifying organization to take continuing education courses and subscribe to professional research journals.

SELECTED REFERENCES

ACSM's Guidelines for Exercise Testing and Prescription. 7th Ed. Baltimore: Lippincott Williams & Wilkins, 2005.

American Association for Health, Physical Education, and Recreation: *Research Methods Applied to Health, Physical Education, and Recreation.* Washington, D.C.: American Association for Health, Physical Education, and Recreation, 1949.

Asmussen, E.: Muscular exercise. In: *Handbook of Respiration.* Section 3. Respiration. Vol. II. Fenn, W.O. and Rahn, H. (eds.). Washington, D.C.: American Physiological Society, 1965.

Åstrand, P.O.: Influence of Scandinavian scientists in exercise physiology. *Scand. J. Med. Sci. Sports.,* 1:3, 1991.

Bagwell, C.E.: "Respectful image": revenge of the barber surgeon. *Ann. Surg.,* 241:872, 2005.

Bang, O., et al.: Contributions to the physiology of severe muscular work. *Skand. Arch. Physiol.,* 74(Suppl):1, 1936.

Barcroft, J.: *The Respiratory Function of the Blood. Part 1. Lesson From High Altitude.* Cambridge: Cambridge University Press, 1925.

Berryman, J.W.: *Out of Many, One. A History of the American College of Sports Medicine.* Champaign, IL: Human Kinetics, 1995.

Berryman, J.W.: The tradition of the "six things nonnatural": Exercise and medicine from Hippocrates through Ante-Bellum America. *Exerc. Sport Sci. Rev.,* 17:515, 1989.

Buskirk, E.R.: Early history of exercise physiology in the United States. Part 1. A contemporary historical perspective. In: *History of Exercise and Sport Science.* Messengale, J.D. and Swanson, R.A. (eds.). Champaign, IL: Human Kinetics, 1997.

Buskirk, E.R.: From Harvard to Minnesota: Keys to our history. *Exerc. Sport Sci. Rev.,* 20:1, 1992.

Christensen, E.H., et al.: Contributions to the physiology of heavy muscular work. *Skand. Arch. Physiol. Suppl.,* 10, 1936.

Consolazio, C.F.: *Physiological Measurements of Metabolic Functions in Man.* New York: McGraw-Hill Book Co., 1961.

Cureton, T.K., Jr.: *Physical Fitness of Champion Athletes.* Urbana, IL: University of Illinois Press, 1951.

Dill, D.B.: Arlie V. Bock, pioneer in sports medicine. December 30, 1888–August 11, 1984. *Med. Sci. Sports Exerc.,* 17:401, 1985.

Dill, D.B.: The Harvard Fatigue Laboratory: Its development, contributions, and demise. *Circ. Res.,* 20(Suppl I):161, 1967.

Dill, D.B.: *Life, Heat, and Altitude: Physiological Effects of Hot Climates and Great Heights.* Cambridge, MA: Harvard University Press, 1938.

Green, R.M.: *A Translation of Galen's Hygiene.* Springfield, IL: Charles C. Thomas, 1951.

Henry, F.M.: Aerobic oxygen consumption and alactic debt in muscular work. *J. Appl. Physiol.,* 3:427, 1951.

Henry, F.M.: Lactic and alactic oxygen consumption in moderate exercise of graded intensity. *J. Appl. Physiol.,* 8:608, 1956.

Henry, F.M.: Physical education: An academic discipline. *JOHPER,* 35:32, 1964.

Hermansen, L., and Andersen, K.L.: Aerobic work capacity in young Norwegian men and women. *J. Appl. Physiol.,* 20:425, 1965.

Hermansen, L.: Anaerobic energy release. *Med. Sci. Sports.,* 1:32, 1969.

Hoberman, J.M.: The early development of sports medicine in Germany. In: *Sport and Exercise Science.* Berryman, J.W., and Park, R.J. (eds.). Urbana, IL: University of Illinois Press, 1992.

Horvath, S.M., and Horvath, E.C.: *The Harvard Fatigue Laboratory: Its History and Contributions.* Englewood Cliffs, CA: Prentice-Hall, 1973.

Johnson, R.E., et al.: *Laboratory Manual of Field Methods for the Biochemical Assessment of Metabolic and Nutrition Conditions.* Boston, MA: Harvard Fatigue Laboratory, 1946.

Katch, V.L.: The burden of disproof. *Med. Sci. Sports Exerc.,* 18:593, 1986.

Khan, I.A., et al.: Evolution of the theory of circulation. *Int. J. Cardiol.* 98:519, 2005.

Krogh, A.: *The Composition of the Atmosphere; An Account of Preliminary Investigations and a Programme.* Kobenhavn, Denmark: A.F. Host, 1919.

Kroll, W.: *Perspectives in Physical Education.* New York: Academic Press, 1971.

Lusk, G.: *The Elements of the Science of Nutrition.* 2nd Ed. Philadelphia: W.B. Saunders, 1909.

Papavramidou, N.S. et al.: Galen on obesity: etiology, effects, and treatment. *World J. Surg.* 28:631, 2004.

Park, R.J.: Concern for health and exercise as expressed in the writings of 18th century physicians and informed laymen (England, France, Switzerland). *Res. Q.,* 47:756, 1976.

Park, R.J.: The emergence of the academic discipline of physical education in the United States. In: *Perspectives on the Academic Discipline of Physical Education.* Brooks, G.A. (ed.). Champaign, IL: Human Kinetics, 1981.

Park, R.J.: High-protein diets, "damaged hearts," and rowing men: antecedents of modern sports medicine and exercise science, 1867–1928. *Exerc. Sport Sci. Rev.* 25:137, 1997.

Park, R.J.: A long and productive career: Franklin M. Henry—Scientist, mentor, pioneer. *Res. Q. Exerc. Sports,* 65:295, 1994.

Park, R.J.: "Of the greatest possible worth": the Research Quarterly in historical contexts. *Res. Q. Exerc. Sport,* 76:55, 2005.

Park, R.J.: Physiologists, physicians, and physical educators: Nineteenth century biology and exercise, hygienic and educative. *J. Sport Hist.,* 14:28, 1987.

Park, R.J.: The rise and demise of Harvard's B.S. program in Anatomy, Physiology, and Physical Training. *Res. Q. Exerc. Sport,* 63:246, 1992.

Payne, J.F.: *Harvey and Galen. The Harveyan Oration. Oct. 19, 1896.* London: Frowde, 1897.

Ross, W.D.: Kinanthropometry: An emerging scientific technology. In: *Biomechanics of Sports and Kinanthropometry.* Book 6. Landry, F., and Orban, W.A. (eds.). Miami, FL: Symposia Specialists, Inc., 1978.

Schmidt-Nielsen, B.: *August and Marie Krogh: Lives in Science.* Washington, D.C.: American Physiological Society, 1995.

Schmidt-Nielsen, B.: August and Marie Krogh and respiratory physiology. *J. Appl. Physiol.,* 57:293, 1984.

Scholander, P.F.: Analyzer for accurate estimation of respiratory gases in one-half cubic centimeter samples. *J. Biol. Chem.,* 167:235, 1947.

Shaffel, N.: The evaluation of American medical literature. In: *History of American Medicine.* Marti-Ibanez, F. (ed.). New York: MD Publications, 1958.

Tipton, C.M.: Contemporary exercise physiology: Fifty years after the closure of the Harvard Fatigue Laboratory. *Exerc. Sport Sci. Rev.,* 26:315, 1998.

Tipton, C.M.: Exercise physiology, part II: A contemporary historical perspective. In: *The History of Exercise and Sports Science.* Messengale, J.D., and Swanson, R.A. (eds.). Champaign, IL: Human Kinetics, 1997.

Section II

Nutrition and Energy

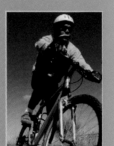

Proper nutrition forms the foundation for physical performance. The foods we consume provide fuel for biologic work and chemicals for extracting and using potential energy within this fuel. Food also provides essential elements for synthesizing new tissue and repairing existing cells. Often, individuals exercise for optimum performance, only to fall short due to inadequate, counterproductive, and sometimes harmful nutritional practices.

Chapter 2 reviews the six broad categories of nutrients: carbohydrates, lipids, proteins, vitamins, minerals, and water. Understanding each nutrient's role in energy metabolism and tissue synthesis clarifies one's knowledge of the interaction between food intake and storage and exercise performance. No nutritional "magic bullets" exist per se, yet the quantity and blend of nutrients in the daily diet profoundly affect exercise capacity, training responsiveness, and overall health. **Chapter 3** presents related information about food as an energy source and what constitutes an optimum diet for exercise and good health. **Chapter 4** concludes with a discussion of nutritional (and pharmacological) supplements and their possible role as ergogenic aids to physical performance.

What is a scientist after all? It is a curious man looking through a keyhole, the keyhole of nature, trying to know what's going on.

—JACQUES YVES COUSTEAU

CHAPTER OBJECTIVES

- Distinguish among monosaccharides, disaccharides, and polysaccharides.

- Discuss carbohydrate's role as an energy source, protein sparer, metabolic primer, and central nervous system fuel.

- Define and give an example of a triacylglycerol, saturated fatty acid, polyunsaturated fatty acid, monounsaturated fatty acid, and trans fatty acid.

- List major characteristics of high- and low-density lipoprotein cholesterol, and discuss the role of each in coronary heart disease.

- List four important functions of fat in the body.

- Define essential and non-essential amino acids, and give food sources for each.

- List one function for each fat- and water-soluble vitamin, and explain the potential risks of consuming these micronutrients in excess.

- Outline three broad roles of minerals in the body.

- Define osteoporosis, exercise-induced anemia, and sodium-induced hypertension.

- Describe how regular physical activity affects bone mass and the body's iron stores.

- Outline factors related to the female athlete triad.

- List the functions of water in the body.

- Define heat cramps, heat exhaustion, and heat stroke.

- Explain factors that affect gastric emptying and fluid replacement.

- List five predisposing factors to hyponatremia with prolonged exercise.

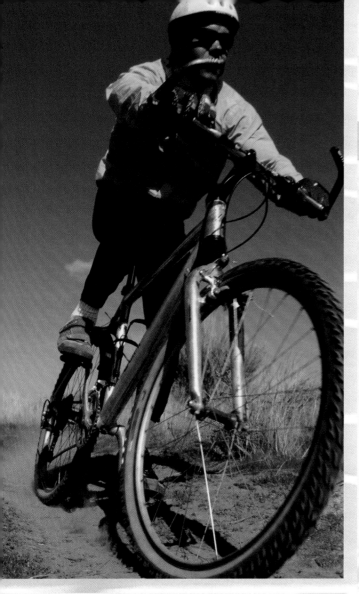

Macronutrients and Micronutrients

PART 1 •
Macronutrients: Energy Fuel and Building Blocks for Tissue Synthesis

The carbohydrate, lipid, and protein nutrients consumed daily supply the necessary energy to maintain bodily functions during rest and diverse physical activities. These nutrients, referred to as **macronutrients**, also maintain and enhance the organism's structural and functional integrity in response to exercise training. Part 1 discusses each macronutrient's general structure, function, and source in the diet and emphasizes their importance in sustaining physiologic function during physical activity.

CARBOHYDRATES

All living cells contain **carbohydrates**. With the exception of lactose and a small amount of glycogen obtained from animals, all dietary carbohydrate originates from plant sources. Atoms of carbon, hydrogen, and oxygen combine to form a carbohydrate (sugar) molecule, always in a ratio of 1 atom of carbon and 2 atoms of hydrogen for each oxygen atom. The general formula $(CH_2O)n$ represents a simple carbohydrate, where n equals from 3 to 7 carbon atoms.

Monosaccharides

The **monosaccharide** *molecule forms the basic unit of carbohydrates.* The molecule's number of carbon atoms determines its category. The Greek name for this number, ending with "ose," indicates sugars. For example, 3-carbon monosaccharides are **trioses**, 4-carbon sugars are **tetroses**, 5-carbon sugars are **pentoses**, 6-carbon sugars are **hexoses**, and 7-carbon sugars are **heptoses**. The hexose sugars, glucose, fructose, and galactose, represent the nutritionally important monosaccharides.

Glucose, also called dextrose or blood sugar, consists of 6 carbon, 12 hydrogen, and 6 oxygen atoms ($C_6H_{12}O_6$; **Figure 2.1**). It forms as a natural sugar in food or is produced in the body through the digestion (**hydrolysis**) of more complex carbohydrates. After absorption by the small intestine, glucose can be:

- Used directly by the cell for energy
- Stored as glycogen in the muscles and liver
- Converted to fats for energy storage
- Used to provide carbon skeletons for the synthesis of non-essential amino acids

Fruits and honey provide the main source of **fructose** (also called levulose or fruit sugar), the sweetest of the monosaccharides. Although the small intestine absorbs some fructose directly into the blood, the liver slowly converts it to glucose. **Galactose** does not exist freely in nature; rather, it forms milk sugar (**lactose**) in the mammary

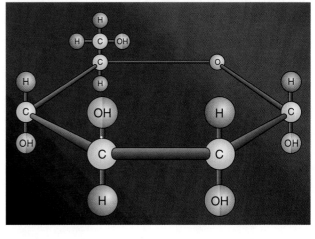

Figure 2.1 Three-dimensional ring structure of the simple sugar molecule glucose. The molecule resembles a hexagonal plate to which H and O atoms attach.

glands of lactating animals. In the body, galactose freely converts to glucose for energy metabolism.

Disaccharides

Combining two monosaccharide molecules forms a **disaccharide** or double sugar. The monosaccharides and disaccharides collectively make up the **simple sugars**.

Each of the disaccharides contains glucose as a principal component. The three disaccharides of nutritional significance include:

- **Sucrose:** glucose + fructose; the most common dietary disaccharide. It occurs naturally in most foods containing carbohydrate, particularly beet and cane sugar, brown sugar, sorghum, maple syrup, and honey
- **Lactose:** glucose + galactose; found in natural form only in milk and often called milk sugar
- **Maltose:** glucose + glucose; occurs in beer, cereals, and germinating seeds

Polysaccharides

Polysaccharides include plant and animal categories.

Plant Polysaccharides   Starch and fiber represent the two common forms of plant polysaccharides.

Starch   **Starch**, the storage form of plant polysaccharide, forms from hundreds of individual sugar molecules joined together. It appears as large granules in seed and corn cells and in grains that make bread, cereal, spaghetti, and pastries. Large amounts also exist in peas, beans, potatoes, and roots, in which starch stores energy for the plant's future needs. The term **complex carbohydrates** refers to dietary starch.

Fiber   **Fiber**, which is classified as a non-starch, structural polysaccharide, includes cellulose, the most abundant organic molecule on earth. Fibrous materials resist hydrolysis by human digestive enzymes. Plants *exclusively* contain fiber, which constitutes the structure of leaves, stems, roots, seeds, and fruit coverings. Fibers differ in physical and chemical characteristics and physiologic action; they occur primarily within the cell wall as cellulose, gums, hemicellulose, pectin, and noncarbohydrate lignins. Other fibers—mucilage and the gums—serve as integral components of the plant cell itself.

Animal Polysaccharides

During the process of **glucogenesis**, a few hundred to thousands of glucose molecules combine to form a **glycogen**, the large storage polysaccharide in mammalian muscle and liver. **Figure 2.2** illustrates that a well-nourished 80-kg person stores approximately 500 g of carbohydrate. Of this, approximately 400 g exist as muscle glycogen (largest reserve), 90 to 110 g exist as liver glycogen (highest concentration representing between 3% to 7% of the liver's weight), but only about 2 to 3 g exist as blood glucose. Because each gram of carbohydrate (glycogen or glucose) contains about 4 kCal of energy, the average person stores between 1500 and 2000 kCal as carbohydrate, which is enough total energy to power a 20-mile run.

Muscle glycogen serves as the major source of carbohydrate energy for active muscles during exercise. In contrast to muscle glycogen, liver glycogen reconverts to glucose for transport in the blood to the working muscles. **Glycogenolysis** describes this reconversion process (glycogen → glucose); it provides a rapid extramuscular glucose supply. Unlike liver, muscle cells do not contain the enzyme to reform glucose from stored glycogen. Thus, glucose (or glycogen) within a muscle cell cannot supply the carbohydrate needs of surrounding cells. Depleting liver and muscle glycogen through dietary restriction or heavy exercise stimulates glucose synthesis from structural components of the other macronutrients (principally protein's amino acids) through the process known as **gluconeogenesis** (glucose formation from non-glucose sources).

Hormones regulate liver and muscle glycogen stores by controlling the level of circulating blood sugar. Elevated blood sugar cause the pancreas' beta (β) cells to secrete additional **insulin**. Insulin facilitates the muscles' uptake of the glucose excess, yet it also inhibits further insulin secretion. This feedback regulation maintains blood glucose at an appropriate physiologic concentration. In contrast, if blood sugar falls below normal (**hypoglycemia**), the pancreas' alpha (α) cells

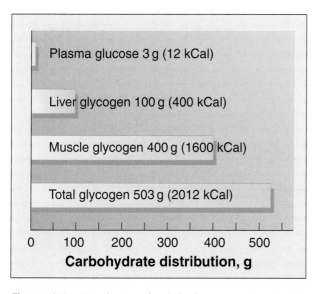

Figure 2.2   Distribution of carbohydrate energy in a typical 80-kg person.

Questions & Notes

List the 3 types of carbohydrates.

1.

2.

3.

List the 2 types of polysaccharides.

1.

2.

FOR YOUR INFORMATION
There are many terms that refer to monosaccharides and disaccharides or products containing these sugars. The following list includes names for sugars either naturally present in food products or added during their manufacture. Food labels (see Chapter 3) lump all these sugars under one category, listing them as "sugars."
- Sucrose
- Brown sugar
- Confectioner's sugar (powdered sugar)
- Turbinado sugar
- Invert sugar
- Glucose
- Sorbitol
- Levulose
- Polydextrose
- Lactose
- Mannitol
- Honey
- Corn syrup or sweeteners
- High-fructose corn syrup
- Molasses
- Date sugar
- Maple syrup
- Dextrin
- Dextrose
- Fructose
- Maltose
- Caramel
- Fruit sugar

Box 2–1 • CLOSE UP

HEALTH IMPLICATIONS OF DIETARY FIBER

Dietary fiber has received attention by researchers and the lay press because of studies that link high fiber intake with a lower occurrence of obesity, diabetes, hypertension, intestinal disorders, and heart disease. The diet in industrialized nations, which is high in fiber-free animal foods and low in natural plant fiber lost through processing (refining), contributes to intestinal disorders compared with a more primitive-type diet high in unrefined, complex carbohydrates. Americans typically consume about 12 to 15 g of fiber daily, far short of the recommendations of the Food and Nutrition Board of the National Academy of Sciences of 38 g for men and 25 g for women up to age 50 years and 30 g for men and 21 g for women over age 50 years.

Fibers hold considerable water and give "bulk" to the food residues in the intestines, often increasing stool weight and volume by 40% to 100%. This bulking-up action may aid gastrointestinal functioning and reduce the chances of contracting colon cancer and other gastrointestinal diseases later in life. Increased fiber intake, especially the **water-soluble fibers**, may modestly reduce serum cholesterol in humans. These include pectin and guar gum present in oats (rolled oats, oat bran, oat flour), legumes, barley, brown rice, peas, carrots, and diverse fruits.

For men with elevated blood lipids, adding 100 g of oat bran to their daily diets reduced serum cholesterol levels by 13% and lowered the low-density lipoprotein component of the cholesterol profile. In contrast, the **water-insoluble fibers**, cellulose, hemicellulose, and lignin, and cellulose-rich products, like wheat bran, did not reduce cholesterol levels. The precise mechanism by which dietary fibers favorably affect serum cholesterol remains unclear. The addition of fiber may simply replace cholesterol-laden items in the diet; fiber may actually hinder cholesterol absorption, or it may reduce cholesterol metabolism in the gut. These actions would depress cholesterol synthesis and simultaneously facilitate excretion of existing cholesterol bound to the fiber in the feces. Dietary fiber slows carbohydrate digestion, so it is absorbed more slowly into the bloodstream by the intestine. Fiber also decreases the total number of calories consumed in subsequent meals.

Current nutritional wisdom maintains that a dietary fiber intake of between about 20 to 40 g per day depending on your age and sex (ratio of 3:1 for water-insoluble to soluble fiber) plays an important part of a well-structured diet. Persons with marginal levels of nutrition should not consume excessive fiber because increased fiber intake decreases the absorption of calcium, iron, magnesium, phosphorus, and trace minerals. The accompanying table lists the fiber content of common foods listed by overall fiber content.

Fiber Content of Some Common Foods

FOOD	SERVING SIZE	TOTAL FIBER (G) PER SERVING
Avocado	1	22.9
Rice bran	1 oz	21.7
Pinto beans, dry, cooked	1 cup	19.5
100% Bran cereal	1 cup	16.4
Lima beans, fresh, cooked	1 cup	16.0
Wheat germ, toasted	1 cup	15.6
Longanberries, fresh	1 cup	9.3
Mixed veggies (corn, carrots, beans)	1 cup	7.2
Pumpkin pie	1 slice	5.4
Peas	1/2 cup	5.2
Cheerios cereal	1 cup	5.0
Spaghetti, whole wheat	1 cup	5.0
Barley, cooked, whole	1 cup	4.6
Pear, Bartlett	1	4.6
Kidney beans	1/2 cup	4.5
Oatmeal, cooked	1 cup	4.1
Bran muffin	1	4.0
Wild rice	1 cup	4.0
Apple	1 small	3.9
Blueberries	1 cup	3.9

Box 2–1 • CLOSE UP *(Continued)*

Fiber Content of Some Common Foods *(Continued)*

FOOD	SERVING SIZE	TOTAL FIBER (G) PER SERVING
Strawberries, fresh	1 cup	3.9
Potato	1 small	3.8
Almonds, dried	1 oz	3.5
Peanuts, dried, unsalted	1 oz	3.5
Corn on the cob	1	3.2
Broccoli, raw	1 cup	2.9
Green beans, raw, cooked	1 cup	2.5
Strawberries	3/4 cup	2.4
Carrot	1 medium	2.3
Whole wheat toast	1 slice	2.3
Macaroni, cooked, enriched	1 cup	2.2
Grapes, seedless	1 cup	1.9
Rye bread	1 slice	1.9
Onions, sliced, raw	1 cup	1.8
Pumpernickel bread	1 slice	1.7
Seven grain bread	1 slice	1.7
Walnuts, chopped, black	1 oz	1.6
Banana	1 small	1.3
Oatmeal bread	1 slice	1.0
Peanut butter	1 Tbsp	1.0
Spaghetti	1/2 cup	1.0
Danish pastry, plain	1	0.7
Fig bar cookie	1	0.6
Plum, small	1	0.6
White bread	1 slice	0.6
Lettuce	1/2 cup	0.5
Chocolate chip cookie	1	0.2

immediately secrete **glucagon** to normalize (increase) blood sugar level. Known as the *"insulin antagonist"* hormone, it stimulates liver glycogenolysis and gluconeogenesis to increase blood glucose.

Diet Affects Glycogen Stores The body stores comparatively little glycogen, so dietary intake can significantly affect its quantity. For example, a 24-hour fast or a low-carbohydrate, normal-calorie (isocaloric) diet dramatically reduces glycogen reserves. In contrast, maintaining a carbohydrate-rich isocaloric diet for several days doubles the body's carbohydrate stores compared with a normal, well-balanced diet. The body's upper limit for glycogen storage equals about 15 g per kilogram (kg) of body mass, equivalent to 1050 g for the average 70-kg man, or 840 g for a typical 56-kg woman. To determine your body's current glycogen content (in g), multiply your body weight in kilograms (lbs ÷ 2.205) by 15.

Carbohydrate's Role in the Body

Carbohydrates serve important functions related to energy metabolism and exercise performance.

Energy Source Energy from the breakdown of blood-borne glucose and muscle glycogen ultimately powers muscle action (particularly high-intensity exercise) and other more "silent" forms of biologic work. For physically active people, adequate daily carbohydrate intake maintains the body's limited glycogen stores. However, more is not necessarily better; if dietary carbohydrate intake exceeds the

Questions & Notes

Give the recommended fiber intake for men and women up to age 50 years.

Men:

Women:

For Your Information

Important Carbohydrate Conversions

Glucogenesis—glycogen synthesis from glucose (glucose → glycogen)

Gluconeogenesis—glucose synthesis largely from structural components of noncarbohydrate nutrients (protein → glucose)

Glycogenolysis—glucose formation from glycogen (glycogen → glucose)

cells' capacity to store glycogen, the carbohydrate excess readily converts to fat, triggering an increase in total body fat.

Protein Sparer   Adequate carbohydrate consumption preserves tissue proteins. Normally, protein contributes to tissue maintenance, repair, and growth and, to a lesser degree, serves as a nutrient energy source. With reduced glycogen reserves, gluconeogenesis synthesizes glucose from protein (amino acids) and the glycerol portion of the fat molecule (triacylglycerol). This metabolic process increases carbohydrate availability (and maintains plasma glucose levels) during dietary restriction, prolonged exercise, and repeated bouts of heavy training.

Metabolic Primer   Byproducts of carbohydrate breakdown serve as a "primer" to facilitate the body's use of fat for energy, particularly in the liver. Insufficient carbohydrate metabolism (either through limitations in glucose transport into the cell, as occurs in diabetes, or glycogen depletion through inadequate diet or prolonged exercise) increases dependence on fat utilization for energy. When this happens, the body cannot generate a sustained high level of aerobic energy transfer from fat-only metabolism. This consequence significantly reduces an individual's maximum exercise intensity.

Fuel for the Central Nervous System   The central nervous system requires carbohydrate for proper functioning. Under normal conditions, the brain uses blood glucose almost exclusively as its fuel without maintaining a backup supply of this nutrient. In poorly regulated diabetes, during starvation, or with a low carbohydrate intake, the brain adapts metabolically after about 8 days to use relatively large amounts of fat (in the form of ketones) as an alternative fuel source.

At rest and during exercise, the liver serves as the primary source to maintain normal blood glucose levels. In prolonged heavy exercise, blood glucose eventually falls below normal levels because of liver glycogen depletion and active muscles' continual use of available blood glucose. Symptoms of a modest hypoglycemia include feelings of weakness, hunger, and dizziness. This ultimately impacts exercise performance and may partially explain "central" or neurologic fatigue associated with prolonged exercise (or starvation).

Recommended Carbohydrate Intake

Figure 2.3 illustrates the carbohydrate content of selected foods. Rich carbohydrate sources include cereals, cookies, candies, breads, and cakes. Fruits and vegetables appear as less valuable sources of carbohydrates because the food's total weight (including water content) determines a food's carbohydrate percentage. The dried portions of fruits and vegetables exist as almost pure carbohydrate. For this reason, hikers and ultraendurance athletes rely on dried apricots, pears, apples, bananas, and tomatoes to provide a ready (but relatively lightweight) carbohydrate source.

Carbohydrates account for between 40% and 55% of the total calories in the typical American diet. For a sedentary 70-kg person, this translates to a daily carbohydrate intake of about 300 g. Average Americans consume about one-half of their carbohydrate as simple sugars, predominantly as sucrose and high-fructose corn syrup. Simple sugar intake represents the yearly intake equivalent to 60 pounds of table sugar (16 teaspoons of sucrose a day) and 46 pounds of corn syrup!

One hundred years ago, the average yearly intake of simple sugars equaled only 4 pounds per person. Consuming excessive fermentable carbohydrate (principally sucrose) contributes to tooth decay, but dietary sugar's contribution to diabetes, obesity, and coronary heart disease remains controversial.

For regular exercisers, carbohydrate should supply about 60% of total daily calories (400 to 600 g), predominantly as unrefined, fiber-rich, and nutrient-rich fruits, grains, and vegetables. During heavy training, carbohydrate intake may increase to 70% of the total daily energy intake.

Carbohydrate Confusion

Frequent and excessive consumption of more rapidly absorbed forms of carbohydrate (i.e., those with a high glycemic index; see next section) may alter the metabolic profile and possibly increase disease risk for obesity, type 2 diabetes, abnormal blood lipids, and coronary heart disease, particularly for individuals with excess body fat. For example, eating a high-carbohydrate, low-fat meal reduces fat breakdown and increases fat synthesis more in overweight men than lean men. Dietary patterns of women over 6 years showed that those who ate a starchy diet of potatoes and low-fiber, higher glycemic processed white rice, pasta, and white bread, along with non-diet soft drinks experienced 2.5 times the rate of type 2 diabetes than women who ate less of those foods and more fiber-containing unrefined whole-grain cereals, fruits, and vegetables. High blood glucose levels in type 2 diabetes can result from (1) decreased effects of insulin on peripheral tissue (insulin resistance), (2) inadequate insulin production by the pancreas to control blood sugar (relative insulin deficiency), or (3) the combined effect of both factors.

Metabolic Syndrome   Diet-induced insulin resistance/hyperinsulinemia often precedes manifestations of the **metabolic syndrome**, which is defined as having three or more of the criteria shown in **Table 2.1**. In essence, the syndrome reflects a concurrence of (1) disturbed glucose and insulin metabolism, (2) overweight and pattern of abdominal fat distribution, (3) mildly abnormal lipid profile (dyslipidemia), and (4) hypertension. These individuals exhibit a higher risk of cardiovascular disease, diabetes, and all-cause mortality. Estimates place the age-adjusted prevalence of the metabolic syndrome in the United States at 25% or about 47 million adult men and women. A particularly

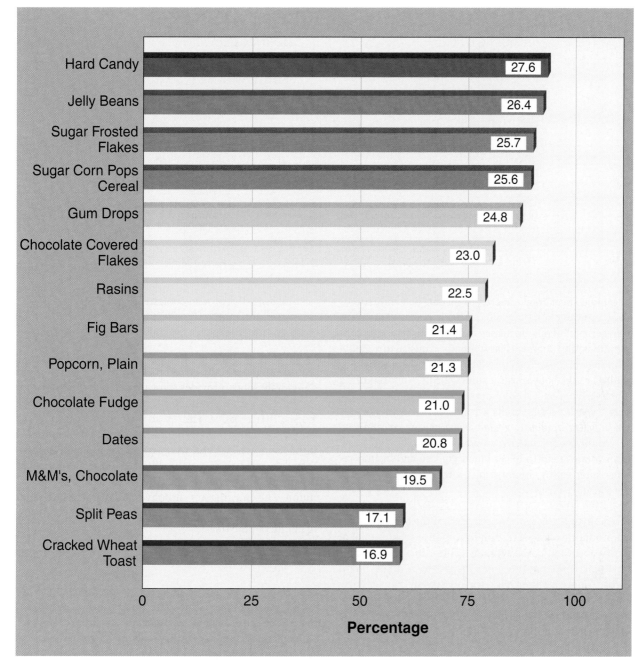

Figure 2.3   Percentage of carbohydrates in commonly served foods. The inset displays the number of grams of carbohydrate per ounce of food.

high prevalence occurs among Mexican-Americans and African-Americans. For children, estimates now indicate the incidence of metabolic syndrome at about 33%. In fact, one-third of all new diagnosed cases of type 2 diabetes occur in over-fat children under the age of 15 years.

All Carbohydrates Are Not Physiologically Equal   Digestion and absorption rates of different carbohydrate-containing foods might explain the carbohydrate intake–diabetes link. Low-fiber processed starches (and simple sugars in soft drinks) digest quickly and enter the blood at a relatively rapid rate (i.e., have a high glycemic index), whereas slow-release forms of high-fiber, unrefined complex carbohydrates (and carbohydrate foods rich in lipids) slow digestion, minimizing surges in blood glucose. The rapid rise in blood glucose that accompanies refined processed starch

Table 2·1 Identifying the Metabolic Syndrome	
RISK FACTOR	**DEFINING LEVEL**
Abdominal fatness (waist girth)[a]	
Men	>102 cm (>40 in)
Women	>88 cm (>35 in)
Triacylglycerols	≥150 mg/dL
High-density lipoprotein	
Men	<40 mg/dL
Women	<50 mg/dL
Blood pressure	≥130 / ≥85 mm Hg
Fasting glucose	≥110 mg/dL

[a]Overweight and overfatness are associated with insulin resistance and the metabolic syndrome. However, the presence of abdominal obesity is more highly correlated with the metabolic risk factors than an elevated body mass index (BMI). Therefore, the simple measure of weight girth is recommended to identify the body weight component of the metabolic syndrome.

and simple sugar intake increases insulin demand, stimulates overproduction of insulin by the pancreas to accentuate hyperinsulinemia, increases plasma triacylglycerol concentrations, and augments fat synthesis. Consistently eating such foods may eventually reduce the body's sensitivity to insulin (i.e., the body resists insulin's effects), thus requiring progressively greater insulin output to control blood sugar levels. *Type 2 diabetes results when the pancreas cannot produce sufficient insulin to regulate blood glucose causing it to rise.* On the other hand, diets with fiber-rich, low-glycemic carbohydrates tend to lower blood glucose and insulin response after eating, improve blood lipid profiles, and increase insulin sensitivity.

A Role in Obesity?   About 25% of the adult population produce excessive insulin in response to an intake of rapidly absorbed carbohydrates. These insulin-resistant individuals (i.e., require more insulin to regulate blood glucose) increase their risk for obesity by consistently consuming such a diet. Weight gain occurs because excessive insulin facilitates glucose oxidation at the expense of fatty acid oxidation; it also stimulates fat storage in adipose tissue.

The insulin surge in response to a sharp rise in blood glucose following ingestion of high-glycemic carbohydrates often abnormally decreases blood glucose. This "rebound hypoglycemia" sets off hunger signals that may cause overeating. A repetitive scenario of high blood sugar followed by low blood sugar exerts the most profound effect on sedentary obese individuals who show the greatest insulin resistance and, consequently, an exaggerated insulin response to a blood glucose challenge. For physically active people, on the other hand, regular low-to-moderate exercise produces the following (beneficial) effects:

1. Improves insulin sensitivity, thus reducing the insulin requirement for a given glucose uptake.
2. Stimulates plasma-derived fatty acid oxidation. This effect decreases fatty acid availability to the liver, thus depressing any increase in plasma very low-density lipoprotein cholesterol and triacylglycerol concentration.
3. Exerts a potent positive influence for weight control.

To reduce the risks for type 2 diabetes and obesity, consuming more slowly absorbed, unrefined complex carbohydrate foods provides a form of "slow-release" carbohydrate without producing rapid fluctuations in blood sugar. If rice, pasta, and bread remain the carbohydrate sources of choice, they should be consumed in unrefined form as brown rice and whole-grain pastas and multigrain breads. The same dietary modifications benefit individuals involved in heavy physical training and endurance competition. The daily dietary carbohydrate intake of these individuals often approaches 800 g (or approximately 8 to 10 g per kg of body mass).

Glycemic Index

The glycemic index serves as a relative (qualitative) indicator of carbohydrate's ability to raise blood glucose levels. Blood sugar increase, termed the glycemic response, is determined after ingesting a food containing 50 g of a carbohydrate (or carbohydrate-containing food) and comparing it over a 2-hour period to a "standard" for carbohydrate (usually white bread or glucose) with an assigned value of 100. The glycemic index expresses the percentage of total area under the blood glucose response curve for a specific food compared to glucose. Thus, a food with a glycemic index of 45 indicates that ingesting 50 g of the food raises blood glucose concentrations to levels that reach 45% compared to 50 g of glucose. The glycemic index provides a more useful physiologic concept than simply classifying a carbohydrate based on its chemical configuration as simple or complex, as sugars or starches, or as available or unavailable. A high glycemic index rating does not necessarily indicate poor nutritional quality, because carrots, brown rice, and corn, with their rich quantities of health-protective micronutrients, phytochemicals, and dietary fiber, have relatively high indices.

The revised glycemic index listing also includes the **glycemic load** associated with the consumption of specified serving sizes of different foods. Whereas the glycemic index compares equal quantities of a carbohydrate-containing food, the glycemic load quantifies the overall glycemic effect of a typical portion of food. This represents the amount of available carbohydrate in that serving and the glycemic index of the food. A high glycemic load reflects a greater expected elevation in blood glucose and a greater insulin response (release) to that food. Chronic consumption of a diet with a high glycemic load associates with an increased risk for type 2 diabetes and coronary heart disease.

Figure 2.4 lists the glycemic index for common items in various food groupings. For easy identification, foods are placed into high, medium, and low categories. Interestingly, a food's index rating does not depend simply on its classification as a "simple" (mono and disaccharides) or "complex" (starch and fiber) carbohydrate, because the plant starch in white rice and potatoes has a higher glycemic index than the simple sugars (particularly fructose) in apples and peaches. Because a food's fiber content slows digestion rate, many vegetables (e.g., peas, beans, and other legumes) have a low glycemic index. Ingesting lipids and proteins tends to slow the passage of food into the small intestine, reducing the glycemic load of the meal's carbohydrate content.

Carbohydrate Use During Exercise

The fuel mixture used during exercise depends on intensity and duration of effort, as well as the exerciser's fitness and nutritional status.

Questions & Notes

List 2 important functions of carbohydrates in the body.

1.

2.

Define hypoglycemia.

Name the type of carbohydrate that when consumed in excess may contribute to type 2 diabetes.

Give 2 variables, and their cut-off values, that are associated with the metabolic syndrome.

| *Variable* | *Cut-off* |
1.

2.

Box 2–2 • CLOSE UP

MORE FIBER MENU

The following table presents a sample daily 2200-kCal menu that includes 31 g of fiber (21 g insoluble fiber). In this particular meal plan, lipid calories account for 30% (saturated fat = 10%), protein calories account for 16%, and carbohydrate calories account for 54% of total calorie intake. Each 10-g increase in a subpar diet's fiber content reduces coronary risk by about 20%. Five daily servings of fruits and vegetables combined with six to 11 servings of grains (particularly whole grains) assures dietary fiber intake at recommended levels. Whole grains provide a nutritional advantage over refined grains in that they contain more fiber, vitamins, minerals, and diverse phytochemicals, all of which favorably impact health status.

2200-kCal Menu with 31 g of Fiber

Breakfast
  Whole grain cereal (0.75 cup)
  Whole wheat toast (2 slices)
  Margarine (2 tsp)
  Jelly, strawberry (1 Tbsp)
  Raisins (2 Tbsp)
  Orange juice (0.5 cup)
  Coffee or tea
Lunch
  Bran muffin (1)
  Milk, 2% (1 cup)
  Hamburger on bun, lean beef patty (3 oz) with 2
    slices tomato and lettuce, catsup (1 Tbsp) and
    mustard (1 Tbsp)

  Whole wheat crackers (4 small)
  Split-pea soup (1 cup)
  Coffee or tea
Dinner
  Green Salad (3.5 oz)
  Broccoli, steamed (0.5 cup)
  Roll, whole wheat (1)
  Margarine (2 tsp)
  Brown rice (0.5 cup)
  Chicken breast, skinless, broiled (3 oz)
  Salad dressing, vinegar and oil (1 Tbsp)
  Pear, medium (1)
  Yogurt, vanilla, lowfat (0.5 cup)

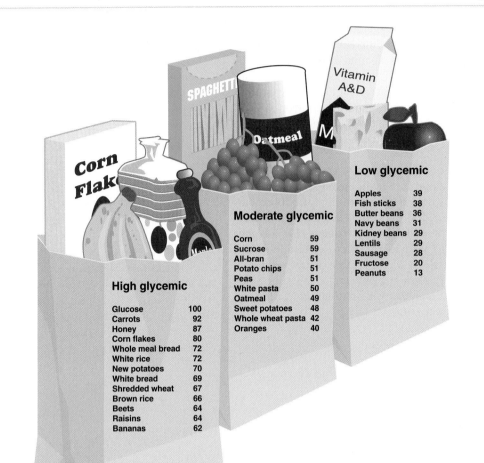

Figure 2.4 Categorization for glycemic index of common food sources of carbohydrates.

Low glycemic

Apples	39
Fish sticks	38
Butter beans	36
Navy beans	31
Kidney beans	29
Lentils	29
Sausage	28
Fructose	20
Peanuts	13

Moderate glycemic

Corn	59
Sucrose	59
All-bran	51
Potato chips	51
Peas	51
White pasta	50
Oatmeal	49
Sweet potatoes	48
Whole wheat pasta	42
Oranges	40

High glycemic

Glucose	100
Carrots	92
Honey	87
Corn flakes	80
Whole meal bread	72
White rice	72
New potatoes	70
White bread	69
Shredded wheat	67
Brown rice	66
Beets	64
Raisins	64
Bananas	62

Intense Exercise Stored muscle glycogen and blood-borne glucose primarily contribute to the total energy required during high-intensity exercise and in the early minutes of exercise when oxygen supply fails to meet the aerobic metabolism demands.

Figure 2.5 illustrates that, early in exercise, the muscles' uptake of circulating blood glucose increases sharply and continues to increase as exercise progresses. After 40 minutes, glucose uptake increases 7 to 20 times the uptake at rest, with the highest use occurring in more intense exercise. Carbohydrate's large energy contribution during all-out exercise occurs because it is the only macronutrient providing energy anaerobically (i.e., without oxygen). During high-intensity aerobic exercise, intramuscular glycogen becomes the preferential energy fuel. This provides an advantage because glycogen supplies energy for exercise twice as rapidly as fat and protein (see Chapter 8).

Moderate and Prolonged Exercise During the transition from rest to submaximal exercise, almost all energy comes from glycogen stored in active muscles. Over the next 20 minutes, liver and muscle glycogen provide about 40% to 50% of the energy requirement, with the remainder from fat breakdown plus some from blood glucose use. As exercise continues and glycogen stores deplete, fat catabolism increases its percentage contribution to the total energy for muscular activity. Additionally, blood-borne glucose becomes the major source of the limited carbohydrate energy. Eventually, liver glucose output does not keep pace with its use, and blood glucose concentration declines toward hypoglycemic levels.

Inability to maintain a desired level of performance (often referred to as **fatigue**) may occur if exercise progresses to the point where liver and muscle glycogen decrease severely, even with sufficient oxygen available to the muscles and almost unlimited potential energy from stored fat. Endurance athletes commonly refer to fatigue under these conditions as "**bonking**" or "**hitting the wall.**" Research does not explain why carbohydrate depletion coincides with the onset of fatigue in prolonged submaximal exercise. The answer may relate to (1) the key role of blood glucose in central nervous system function, (2) muscle glycogen's role as a "primer" in fat breakdown, and (3) the relatively slow rate of energy release from fat compared with carbohydrate breakdown.

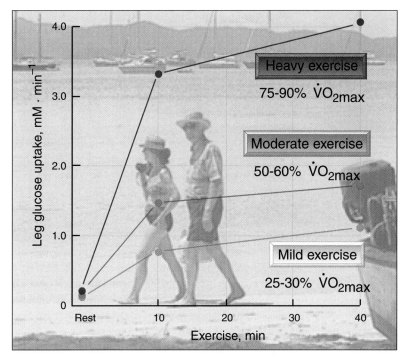

Figure 2.5   Blood glucose uptake by the leg muscles affected by exercise duration and intensity. Exercise intensity is expressed as a percentage of $\dot{V}O_{2max}$. (From Felig, P., Wahren, J.: Fuel homeostasis in exercise. *N. Engl. J. Med.*, 293:1078, 1975.)

Questions & Notes

Give the difference between the glycemic index and glycemic load.

Give one possible outcome of low muscle glycogen levels.

LIPIDS (OILS, FATS, AND WAXES)

A lipid (from the Greek *lipos*, meaning fat) molecule has the same structural elements as carbohydrate except that it differs in its linkage of atoms. Specifically, the lipid's ratio of hydrogen-to-oxygen considerably exceeds that of carbohydrate. For example, the formula $C_{57}H_{110}O_6$ describes the common lipid stearin, with an H-to-O ratio of 18.3:1; for carbohydrate, the ratio equals 2:1. Lipid, a general term, refers to a heterogeneous group of compounds that includes oils, fats, and waxes and related compounds. Oils remain liquid at room temperature, whereas fats remain solid. Approximately 98% of dietary lipid exists as triacylglycerols (see next section). Lipids can be placed into one of three main groups: **simple lipids**, **compound lipids**, and **derived lipids**.

Simple Lipids

The simple lipids or "neutral fats" consist primarily of **triacylglycerols**. They constitute the major storage form of fat; more than 90% of body fat exists as triacylglycerol predominantly in adipose (fat) cells. This molecule consists of two different clusters of atoms. A glycerol component has a 3-carbon molecule that itself does not qualify as a lipid because of its high solubility in water. The other component consists of three clusters of carbon-chained atoms, usually in an even number, termed fatty acids that attach to the glycerol molecule. Fatty acids contain straight hydrocarbon chains with as few as 4 carbon atoms or more than 20, although chain lengths of 16 and 18 carbons are most common.

Figure 2.6 illustrates the basic structure of saturated and unsaturated fatty acid molecules. All lipid-containing foods consist of a mixture of different proportions of saturated and unsaturated fatty acids.

Saturated Fatty Acids   **Saturated fatty acids** contain only single bonds between carbon atoms; all of the remaining bonds attach to hydrogen. The term saturated describes the fatty acid molecule because it holds as many hydrogen atoms

FOR YOUR INFORMATION

Carrots Versus Candy Bars: The Glycemic Index Does Not Tell All
Just because a food has a high glycemic index does not mean it should be avoided. For example, even though carrots have an index of 71 and candy bars rate lower at 65, it would take six or seven servings of carrots to match the blood glucose effect of one candy bar because measure for measure, candy bars contain far more carbohydrate. Looking at it another way, to achieve a caloric intake of 400 kCals requires eating 12 servings of carrots, four five-ounce potatoes, or three cups of corn but only one chocolate candy bar! The carrots also provide a considerably more nutritious food package (fiber, vitamins, minerals, and diverse phytochemicals) than the bar of candy.

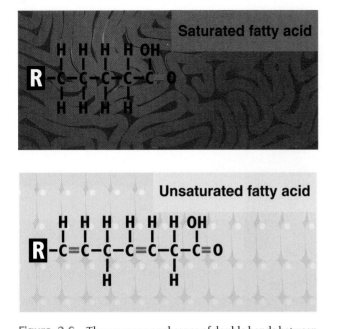

Figure 2.6 The presence or absence of double bonds between the carbon atoms constitutes the major structural difference between saturated and unsaturated fatty acids. *R* represents the glycerol portion of the triacylglycerol molecule.

as chemically possible (saturated with respect to hydrogen atoms).

Saturated fatty acids occur plentifully in animal products, such as beef, lamb, pork, chicken, and egg yolk, and in dairy fats of cream, milk, butter, and cheese. Saturated fatty acids from plants include coconut and palm oil, vegetable shortening, and hydrogenated margarine; commercially prepared cakes, pies, and cookies rely heavily on saturated fatty acids.

Unsaturated Fatty Acids   **Unsaturated fatty acids** contain one or more double bonds along the main carbon chain. Each double bond in the carbon chain reduces the number of potential hydrogen-binding sites; therefore, the molecule remains unsaturated relative to hydrogen. **Monounsaturated fatty acids** contain one double bond along the main carbon chain; examples include canola oil, olive oil, peanut oil, and oil in almonds, pecans, and avocados. **Polyunsaturated fatty acids** contain two or more double bonds along the main carbon chain; examples include safflower, sunflower, soybean, and corn oil.

Fatty acids from plant sources are typically unsaturated and liquefy at room temperature. Lipids with more carbons in the fatty acid chain and containing more saturated fatty acids remain firmer at room temperature.

Fatty Acids in the Diet   The average person in the United States consumes about 15% of their total calories as saturated fats (equivalent to more than 50 lb per year). This contrasts to the Tarahumara Indians of Mexico whose diet, which is high in complex, unrefined carbohy-

drate, contains only 2% of total calories as saturated fat. The strong relationship between saturated fatty acid intake and coronary heart disease risk has prompted health professionals to recommend replacing at least a portion of the saturated fatty acids in the diet with unsaturated fatty acids. Monounsaturated fatty acids lower coronary risk even below normal levels. Individuals should consume no more than 10% of total energy intake as saturated fatty acids. Ideally, fatty acid intake should include equal amounts of saturated, polyunsaturated, and monounsaturated fatty acids.

Compound Lipids

Compound lipids consist of neutral fat combined with other chemicals like phosphorus (**phospholipids**) and glucose (**glucolipids**). Another group of compound fats contains the **lipoproteins**, formed primarily in the liver from the union of triacylglycerols, phospholipids, or cholesterol with protein. *Lipoproteins serve important functions because they constitute the main form for lipid transport in the blood.* If blood lipids did not bind to protein, they literally would float to the top like cream in nonhomogenized milk.

High- and Low-Density Lipoprotein Cholesterol
Four types of lipo-proteins exist according to their gravitational densities: chylomicrons, and high-density, low-density, and very-low density lipoproteins. **Chylomicrons** form after emulsified lipid droplets leave the small intestine and enter the lymphatic vasculature. Normally, the liver takes up chylomicrons, metabolizes them, and delivers them to adipose tissue for storage.

The liver and small intestine produce **high-density lipoprotein (HDL)**. Of the lipoproteins, HDLs contain the greatest percentage of protein and the least total lipid and cholesterol. Degradation of a **very-low density lipoprotein (VLDL)** produces a **low-density lipoprotein (LDL)**. The VLDL contains the greatest percentage of lipid. VLDLs transport triacylglycerols (formed in the liver from fats, carbohydrates, alcohol, and cholesterol) to muscle and adipose tissue. The enzyme **lipoprotein lipase** acts on VLDL to transform it to a denser LDL molecule, with less lipid. LDL and VLDL contain the greatest lipid and least protein content.

"Bad" Cholesterol (LDL)   Among the lipoproteins, LDLs, which normally carry between 60% and 80% of the total serum cholesterol, have the greatest affinity for cells located in the arterial wall. LDL delivers cholesterol to arterial tissue; here, the LDL oxidizes to ultimately participate in the proliferation of smooth muscle cells and other unfavorable changes that damage and narrow the artery. Regular exercise, visceral fat accumulation, and the diet's composition influence serum LDL concentration.

"Good" Cholesterol (HDL)   Unlike LDL, HDL operates as so-called "good" cholesterol to protect against heart disease. HDL acts as a scavenger in the **reverse transport of**

cholesterol by removing it from the arterial wall for transport to the liver. There, it incorporates into bile where the intestinal tract excretes it.

The amounts of LDL and HDL cholesterol and their specific ratios (e.g., HDL/total cholesterol) and subfractions provide more meaningful indicators of coronary artery disease risk than just total cholesterol in blood. Regular aerobic exercise and abstinence from cigarette smoking increase HDLs and favorably affect the LDL/HDL ratio. We discuss the role of exercise on the blood lipid profile more fully in Chapter 17.

Derived Lipids

Derived lipids include substances formed from simple and compound lipids. **Cholesterol**, the most widely known derived lipid, exists only in animal tissue. Cholesterol does not contain fatty acids but shares some of the physical and chemical characteristics of lipids. Thus, from a dietary viewpoint, cholesterol is considered a lipid. Cholesterol, widespread in the plasma membrane of all animal cells, is obtained either through food intake (**exogenous cholesterol**) or from synthesis within the body (**endogenous cholesterol**). Even if an individual maintains a "cholesterol-free" diet, endogenous cholesterol synthesis usually varies between 0.5 to 2.0 g (50–200 mg·d^{-1}) daily. *The body forms more cholesterol with a diet high in saturated fatty acids because saturated fat facilitates the liver's cholesterol synthesis.* The rate of endogenous synthesis usually meets the body's needs; hence, severely reducing cholesterol intake, except in pregnant women and infants, causes little harm.

Cholesterol participates in many complex bodily functions, including the building of plasma membranes and as a precursor in synthesizing vitamin D, the adrenal gland hormones, and the sex hormones estrogen, androgen, and progesterone. Cholesterol serves as a component for bile (emulsifies lipids during digestion) and helps tissues, organs, and body structures form during fetal development.

Rich sources of cholesterol include egg yolk, red meats, and organ meats (liver, kidney, and brains). Shellfish, particularly shrimp, and dairy products (ice cream, cream cheese, butter, and whole milk) contain large amounts of cholesterol. *Foods of plant origin contain no cholesterol.*

Trans Fatty Acid: Perhaps the Most Dangerous Fat

During manufacturing, margarine and other vegetable shortenings, like corn, soybean, or sunflower oil, can become "partially hydrogenated" by bubbling hydrogen gas through the vegetable oil. This rearranges the chemical structure of the original polyunsaturated oil to a lipid not found in nature. The "partially hydrogenated" oils are termed a *trans* unsaturated fatty acid. This lipid forms when one of the hydrogen atoms along the restructured carbon chain moves from its naturally occurring *cis* position to the opposite side of the double bond that separates two carbon atoms (*trans* position). Although *trans* fatty acids are close in structure to most unsaturated fatty acids, the opposing hydrogens along its carbon chain make the physical properties similar to saturated fatty acids. Small amounts of naturally occurring *trans* fat can be found in some animal products such as butter, milk products, cheese, beef, and lamb; the richest *trans* fat sources comprise vegetable shortenings.

Margarine provides an example of a food containing a rich source of partially hydrogenated *trans* fat. A serving of French fries contains up to 3.6 g of *trans* fat, and doughnuts and poundcake can have 4.3 g. Liquid vegetable oils normally have no *trans* fatty acids, but they are sometimes added to extend the oil's shelf life. *Trans* fatty acids represent about 5% to 10% of the fat content of the typical American diet.

In July of 2003, the National Academy of Sciences' Institute of Medicine, which advises the government on health policy, made official what many researchers have

Questions & Notes

Give the major differences between a saturated and an unsaturated fatty acid.

List the 4 main functions of lipoproteins.

  1.

  2.

  3.

  4.

Describe the major differences between exogenous and endogenous cholesterol.

FOR YOUR INFORMATION

Triacylglycerol and Water
Three molecules of water form when glycerol joins with three fatty acids to synthesize a triacylglycerol. Conversely, during hydrolysis, when the fat molecule cleaves into its constituents by action of lipase enzymes, three molecules of water attach at the point where the fat molecule splits.

argued for years. *Trans* fatty acids *increase* low-density lipoprotein cholesterol concentration about the same as a diet high in saturated fatty acids. Unlike saturated fats, however, hydrogenated oils also *decrease* the concentration of beneficial high-density lipoprotein cholesterol. To worsen matters, *trans* fatty acids also elevate plasma triacylglycerols and may impair arterial wall flexibility. Estimates suggest that dietary *trans* fatty acids account for 30,000 deaths from heart disease annually. In addition, a prospective study of more than 84,204 healthy middle-aged women demonstrated that diets high in *trans* fatty acids promote insulin resistance, thus increasing risk for type 2 diabetes. Surprisingly, women with higher tissue levels of *trans* fatty acids experience a 40% greater likelihood of developing breast cancer than women with lower levels.

The Food and Drug Administration (FDA) has announced that by January 1, 2006 food producers must list a food's *trans* fat content (in grams) below the saturated fat line on all food labels. (Canada instituted such a requirement in early 2003 as part of its mandatory nutrition-labeling system.) The FDA estimates that this change in regulations "will save between $900 million and $1.8 billion a year in medical costs, lost productivity, and pain and suffering."

***Trans* Fat Recommendations**   Cutting back on saturated fat is important from a health standpoint. It is also important to significantly reduce the intake of *trans* fat. The following strategies can help with the difficult task of targeting *trans* fat in fast or processed foods:

1. Know the "suspect" types of foods high in *trans* fat. Small amounts of naturally occurring *trans* fat can be found in some animal products, such as butter, milk products, cheese, beef, and lamb. However, the richest sources comprise vegetable shortenings, some margarines, crackers, candies, cookies, snack foods, fried foods, baked goods, salad dressings, and other processed foods made with partially hydrogenated vegetable oils. While many brands of peanut butter contain small amounts of hydrogenated oil, they typically contain only traces of *trans* fatty acids.
2. Look for shortening or partially hydrogenated oil in the ingredients list. The higher they appear on the list and the more total fat on the label, the more *trans* fat the product contains.
3. In the minority of products that list the saturated, monosaturated, and polyunsaturated fats, you can roughly estimate *trans* fat content by totaling up those fats. If the numbers don't add up to the total fat and if partially hydrogenated oil is a main ingredient, then *trans* fat likely makes up the difference.
4. As a shortcut, look for products low in total fat; this means that *trans* fat also will be low.
5. Products can make claims such as "low saturated fat" and "extra lean" without considering *trans* fat.
6. Remember, deep-fried food, biscuits, and pie crusts are usually made with partially hydrogenated oils; avoid these products.

Fish Oils (and Fish) Are Healthful

Studies of the health profiles of Greenland Eskimos who consume large quantities of lipids from fish, seal, and whale, and yet have a low incidence of coronary heart disease, indicated the potential for two long-chain polyunsaturated fatty acids, eicosapentaenoic acid and docosahexaenoic acid, to confer diverse health benefits. These oils belong to an omega-3 fatty acid family found primarily in the oils of shellfish and cold-water herring, salmon, sardines, bluefish, and mackerel and sea mammals.

Regular intake of fish (2 weekly servings) and fish oil improve one's lipid profile (particularly plasma triacylglycerol) and decrease overall heart disease risk and mortality rate (chance of ventricular fibrillation and sudden death), inflammatory disease risk, and (for smokers) risk of contracting chronic obstructive pulmonary disease. Also, omega-3 fatty acids may also prove beneficial in the treatment of diverse psychological disorders.

Several mechanisms explain how eating fish protects against heart disease. Fish oil may act as an anti-thrombogenic agent to prevent blood clot formation on arterial walls. It also may inhibit the growth of atherosclerotic plaques, reduce pulse pressure and total vascular resistance (increase arterial compliance), and stimulate endothelial-derived nitric oxide to facilitate myocardial perfusion. The oil's lowering effect on triacylglycerol provides additional heart disease protection. On the negative side, concern exists that elevation in atherogenic low-density lipoprotein cholesterol may accompany the triacylglycerol-lowering effect of fish and fish oil supplements.

Lipids in Food

Figure 2.7 shows the approximate percentage contribution of common food groups to the total lipid content of the typical American diet. Plant sources contribute about 34% to the daily lipid intake, whereas the remaining 66% comes from lipids of animal origin.

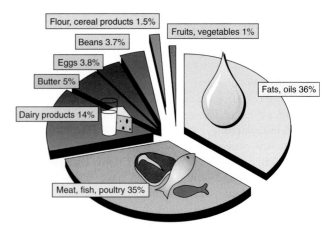

Figure 2.7 Contribution from the major food groups to the lipid content of the typical American diet.

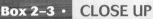

Box 2–3 · CLOSE UP

CHOLESTEROL IN FOODS: BE AWARE

Different foods contain different amounts of cholesterol. Meats and dairy products contain the most. Below is a listing of the cholesterol content of diverse foods. For comparison purposes, 100 grams equals 3.527 ounces or 0.22 pounds.

FOOD	SERVING SIZE	CHOLESTEROL PER SERVING (MG)
Pig brain	100 g	2530
Cow brain	100 g	2054
Duck egg	100 g	619
Pig kidney	100 g	480
Cow kidney	100 g	387
Liver	100 g	372
Pig liver	100 g	368
Lamb liver	100 g	323
Egg (whole or yolk only)	1 large	252
Prawns	6 medium	170
Mutton (fat)	100 g	138
Sardines	100 g	132
Hot Dog	2 (120 g)	112
Spare rib	100 g	105
Beef (lean)	100 g	99
Crab Meat	100 g	95
Mackerel	100 g	93
Pigeon	100 g	90
Chicken Dark (no skin)	100 g	86
Pork (lean)	100 g	77
Quail egg	1 large	74
Chicken White (no skin)	100 g	72
Tuna (canned)	100 g	61
Mussels	100 g	58
Cottage Cheese (4%)	1 cup	48
Oysters	12 (#)	42
Ice Cream	1 cup	42
Butter	1 Tbsp.	35
Milk (whole)	1 cup	34
Scallops	10 (#)	30
Cheese (hard)	30 g	28

Lipid's Role in the Body

Four important functions of lipids in the body include:

1. Energy reserve
2. Protection of vital organs and thermal insulation
3. Transport medium for fat-soluble vitamins
4. Hunger suppressor

Energy Reserve   Fat constitutes the ideal cellular fuel because each molecule (1) carries large quantities of energy per unit weight, (2) transports and stores easily, and (3) provides a ready energy source. At rest in well-nourished individuals, fat provides as much as 80% to 90% of the body's energy requirement. One gram of pure lipid contains about 9 kCal of energy, more than twice the energy available in a gram of carbohydrate or protein because of lipid's greater quantity of hydrogen.

Questions & Notes

Explain how to quickly estimate the Trans fat content of a food.

Box 2–4 • CLOSE UP

TRANS FAT IN COMMON FOODS

The following lists the *trans* fat and saturated fat in some top-selling foods:

PRODUCT	SERVING SIZE, GRAMS (PORTION)	SATURATED FAT, GRAMS	*TRANS* FAT, GRAMS
Dunkin' Donuts, glazed	53.5 (1 donut)	2.5	4
Entenann's Donut Shoppe Donuts, glazed	52 (4 pieces)	2.5	3
Burger King Dutch Apple Pie	113 (1 wedge)	2.5	2
I Can't Believe It's Not Butter Spread	14 (1 Tbsp)	1.5	2
Nabisco Chips Ahoy! Chocolate Chip Cookies	32 (3 cookies)	2	1.5
Nabisco Original Flavor Wheat Thins	31 (16 crackers)	1	2
Kellogg's Cracklin' Oat Bran Cereal	49 (3/4 cup)	2	1.5
Kellogg's Eggo Buttermilk Waffles, Frozen	70 (2 waffles)	1.5	1.5
Pillsbury Buttermilk Waffles, Frozen	68 (2 waffles)	1.5	1.5
Jell-O Pudding Snacks, Chocolate Flavor	113 (1 container)	1.5	1.5
Orville Redenbacher's Popping Corn, Movie Theater Butter	6.5 (1 cup popped)	0.5	1
General Mills Cinnamon Toast Crunch Cereal	30 (3/4 cup)	0	0.5
Jell-O Pudding Snacks	113 (1 container)	1.5	1.5

Approximately 15% of the body mass for men and 25% for women consists of fat. **Figure 2.8** illustrates the total mass (and energy content) of fat from various sources in an 80-kg young adult man. The amount of fat in adipose tissue triacylglycerol translates to about 108,000 kCal. Most of this energy remains available for exercise and would supply enough energy for a person to run from New York City to Madison, Wisconsin, assuming an energy expenditure of about 100 kCal per mile. Contrast this to the limited 2000 kCal reserve of stored glycogen that would provide energy for a 20-mile run. Viewed from a different perspective, the body's energy reserves from carbohydrate could power high-intensity running for only about 1.6 hours, but the fat reserves would last 75 times longer, or about 120 hours. As was the case for carbohydrates, fat as a fuel "spares" protein to carry out two of its three main functions of tissue synthesis and repair.

Protection and Insulation   Up to 4% of the body's fat protects against trauma to the vital organs such as the heart,

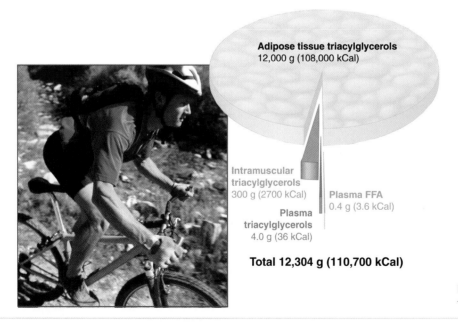

Adipose tissue triacylglycerols
12,000 g (108,000 kCal)

Intramuscular triacylglycerols
300 g (2700 kCal)

Plasma FFA
0.4 g (3.6 kCal)

Plasma triacylglycerols
4.0 g (36 kCal)

Total 12,304 g (110,700 kCal)

Figure 2.8 Distribution of fat energy within a typical 80-kg man.

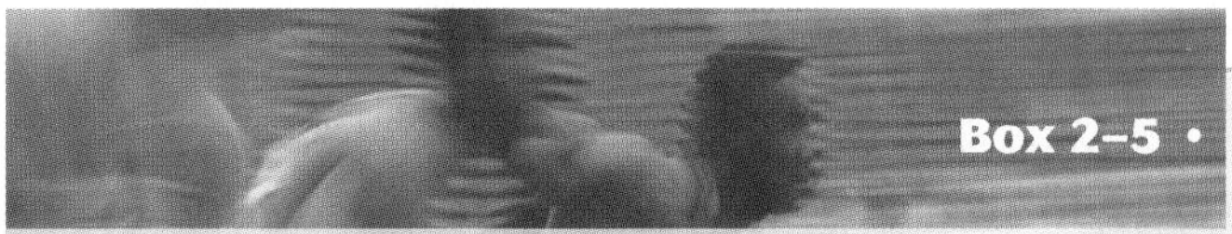

Box 2–5 • CLOSE UP

KNOW YOUR FISH (OIL)

The following list ranks the amount of omega-3 oils in cooked 4-oz servings of various fish.

Two Grams or More of Omega-3 Fatty Acids

• Pacific herring	2.4	• Atlantic salmon	2.1
• Atlantic herring	2.3	• Sablefish	2.0
• Pacific or jack mackerel	2.1		

One to Two Grams of Omega-3 Fatty Acids

• Canned pink salmon	1.9	• Coho salmon	1.2
• Whitefish	1.9	• Bluefish	1.1
• Pacific oysters	1.6	• Trout	1.1
• Pink salmon	1.5	• Eastern oysters	1.0
• Atlantic mackerel	1.4	• Rainbow smelt	1.0
• Sockeye or red salmon	1.4	• Whiting (hake)	1.0

Less than One Gram of Omega-3 Fatty Acids

• Freshwater bass	0.9	• Snapper	0.4
• Blue mussels	0.9	• Sturgeon	0.4
• Swordfish	0.9	• Atlantic perch	0.3
• Rainbow trout	0.8	• Clams, fresh or canned	0.3
• White canned tuna	0.8	• Haddock	0.3
• Canned sardines	0.7	• Light canned tuna	0.3
• Flounder or sole	0.6	• Yellowfin tuna	0.3
• Halibut	0.5	• Atlantic cod	0.3
• Rockfish	0.5	• Catfish	0.1
• Shrimp	0.4		

Low or No Oils with Omega-3 Fatty Acids

• Imitation crab, fish sticks, and fast food fish sandwiches

lungs, liver, kidneys, spleen, brain, and spinal cord. Fats stored just below the skin (subcutaneous fat) provide insulation, determining one's ability to tolerate extremes of cold exposure. This insulatory layer of fat probably affords little protection except to those in cold-related environments like deep-sea divers, ocean or channel swimmers, or Arctic inhabitants. In contrast, excess body fat hinders temperature regulation during heat stress, most notably during sustained exercise in air when the body's heat production can increase 20 times above resting. Under such conditions, the shield of insulation from subcutaneous fat retards the flow of heat from the body.

Vitamin Carrier and Hunger Suppressor   Dietary lipid serves as a carrier and transport medium for the fat-soluble vitamins A, D, E, and K, which require an intake of about 20 g of dietary fat daily. Thus, significantly reducing lipid intake depresses the body's level of these vitamins and may ultimately lead to vitamin deficiency. In addition to a vitamin carrier, dietary lipid delays the onset of "hunger pangs" and contributes to satiety after the meal. This occurs because

Questions & Notes

Give the 4 major functions of lipids in the body.

1.

2.

3.

4.

emptying of lipid from the stomach takes about 3.5 hours after its ingestion. This explains why reducing diets containing some lipid sometimes prove initially successful in blunting the urge to eat more than extreme "fat-free" diets.

Recommended Lipid Intake

In the United States, dietary lipid represents between 34% and 38% of total calorie intake. Most health professionals recommend that lipids should not exceed 30% of the diet's total energy content. Unsaturated fatty acids should supply at least 70% of total lipid intake.

For dietary cholesterol, the American Heart Association recommends that no more than 300 mg (0.01 oz) of cholesterol be consumed each day, which is an intake equivalent to about 100 mg per 1000 kCal of food ingested. Three hundred milligrams of cholesterol almost equals the amount in the yolk of one large egg and just about one-half of the daily cholesterol consumed by the average American male.

All Lipid Intake in Moderation In the quest for good health and optimal exercise performance, prudent practice entails cooking with and consuming lipids derived primarily from vegetable sources. This approach, however, may be too simplistic because total saturated and unsaturated fatty acid intake constitutes a risk for diabetes and heart disease. If so, then one should reduce the intake of lipids, particularly those high in saturated and *trans* fatty acids. Concerns also exist over the association of high-fat diets with ovarian, colon, endometrium, and other cancers. Another beneficial effect of reducing the diet's lipid content relates to weight control. The energy requirements of various metabolic pathways make the body particularly efficient in converting excess calories from dietary lipid to stored fat. Consequently, greater increases in body fat may occur with a high-fat diet compared to an equivalent caloric excess of carbohydrate.

Table 2.2 lists the saturated, monounsaturated, and polyunsaturated fatty acid content of various sources of dietary lipid. All fats contain a mix of each fatty acid type, yet different fatty acids predominate in certain foods. Several polyunsaturated fatty acids, most prominently linoleic acid (present in cooking and salad oils), must be consumed because they serve as precursors of other fatty acids that the body cannot synthesize (essential fatty acids). Humans require about 1% to 2% of total energy intake from linoleic acid (an omega-6 fatty acid). The best sources for alpha-linolenic acid or one of its related omega-3 fatty acids, eicosapentaenoic acid (EPA) and docosahexaenoic acid (KHA), are fatty fish (salmon, tuna, or sardines) or oils such as canola, soybean oil, safflower oil, sunflower oil, sesame oil, and flax oil.

Table 2•2	Examples of Foods High and Low in Saturated Fatty Acids, Foods High in Monounsaturated and Polyunsaturated Fatty Acids, and the Polyunsaturated to Saturated Fatty Acid (P/S) Ratio of Common Fats and Oils

High saturated	%	High monounsaturated	%	P/S Ratio, Fats & Oils	
Coconut oil	91	Olives, black	80	Coconut oil	0.2/1.0
Palm kernel oil	82	Olive oil	75	Palm oil	0.2/1.0
Butter	68	Almond oil	70	Butter	0.1/1.0
Cream cheese	57	Canola oil	61	Olive oil	0.6/1.0
Coconut	56	Almonds, dry	52	Lard	0.3/1.0
Hollandaise sauce	54	Avocados	51	Canola oil	5.3/1.0
Palm oil	51	Peanut oil	48	Peanut oil	1.9/1.0
Half & half	45	Cashews, dry roasted	42	Soybean oil	2.5/1.0
Cheese, Velveeta	43	Peanut butter	39	Sesame oil	3.0/1.0
Cheese, mozzarella	41	Bologna	39	Margarine, 100% corn oil	2.5/1.0
Ice cream, vanilla	38	Beef, cooked	33	Cottonseed oil	2.0/1.0
Cheesecake	32	Lamb, roasted	32	Mayonnaise	3.7/1.0
Chocolate almond bar	29	Veal, roasted	26	Safflower oil	13.3/1.0
Low saturated	**%**	**High polyunsaturated**	**%**		
Popcorn	0	Safflower oil	77		
Hard candy	0	Sunflower oil	72		
Yogurt, nonfat	2	Corn oil	58		
Crackerjacks	3	Walnuts, dry	51		
Milk, skim	4	Sunflower seeds	47		
Cookies, fig bars	4	Margarine, corn oil	45		
Graham crackers	5	Canola oil	32		
Chicken breast, roasted	6	Sesame seeds	31		
Pancakes	8	Pumpkin seeds	31		
Cottage cheese, 1%	8	Tofu	27		
Milk, chocolate, 1%	9	Lard	11		
Beef, dried	9	Butter	6		
Chocolate, mints	10	Coconut oil	2		

Data from the Science and Education Administration, Home and Garden Bulletin 72, Nutritive value of foods, Washington, DC: US Government Printing Office, 1985, 1986; Agricultural Research Service, United States Department of Agriculture. Nutritive value of American foods in common units. Agricultural Handbook no. 456. Washington, DC, US Government Printing Office, 1975.

Fat Use in Exercise

The contribution of fat to the energy requirements of exercise depends on fatty acid release from triacylglycerols in the fat storage sites and delivery in the circulation to muscle tissue as free fatty acids (FFA) bound to blood albumin. Triacylglycerols stored within the muscle cell also contribute to exercise energy metabolism. The data in **Figure 2.9** show that the FFA uptake of active muscles increases during 1 to 4 hours of moderate exercise. In the first 90 minutes, about 37% of the energy comes from fat catabolism. As exercise continues into the third hour (with accompanying glycogen depletion), FFA contributes up to 50% to 62% of the total exercise energy requirement.

PROTEINS

A normal size adult contains between 10 and 12 kg of protein, primarily located within skeletal muscle. Structurally, proteins resemble carbohydrates and lipids because they contain carbon, oxygen, and hydrogen. They differ because they also contain nitrogen (approximately 16% of the molecule) along with sulfur and occasionally phosphorus, cobalt, and iron.

Amino Acids

Just as glycogen forms from the linkage of many simple glucose subunits, protein molecules form from amino acid "building-block" linkages. Peptide bonds join amino acids in chains representing diverse forms and chemical combinations; combining two amino acids produces a dipeptide, and three amino acids linked together form a tripeptide. A linear configuration of up to as many as 1000 amino acids produces a polypeptide; combining more than 50 amino acids forms a polypeptide protein of which humans can synthesize about 80,000 different kinds. Single cells contain thousands of different protein molecules, whereas the body contains approximately 50,000 different protein-containing compounds. The biochemical functions and properties of each protein depend on the sequencing of its specific amino acids.

Of the 20 different amino acids required by the body, each contains a positively charged amine group at one end and a negatively charged organic acid group at

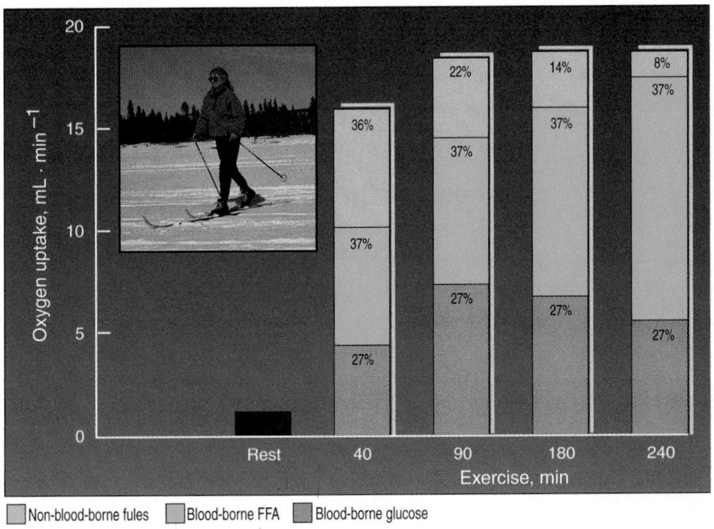

Figure 2.9 Uptake of oxygen and nutrients by the legs during prolonged exercise. Green and orange areas represent the proportion of the total oxygen uptake caused by oxidation of free fatty acids (FFA) and blood glucose. Blue areas indicate oxidation of non–blood-borne fuels (muscle glycogen and intramuscular fats and proteins). (From Ahlborg, G., et al.: Substrate turnover during prolonged exercise in man. *J. Clin. Invest.*, 53:1080, 1974.)

Questions & Notes

Give the recommended lipid intake as a percentage of the daily total kCal intake.

Give the recommended cholesterol intake as a percentage of the daily total kCal intake.

Give the amount of nitrogen contained in most protein molecules.

Give the general chemical structure of an amino acid.

State the major difference between an essential and a nonessential amino acid.

the other end. The amine group consists of 2 hydrogen atoms attached to nitrogen (NH_2), whereas the organic acid group (technically termed a carboxylic acid group) contains 1 carbon atom, 2 oxygen atoms, and 1 atom of hydrogen (COOH). The remainder of the amino acid molecule, its side chain, may take several different forms. *The specific structure of the side chain dictates the amino acid's particular characteristics.* **Figure 2.10** (top) shows the structure of the amino acid alanine.

Essential and Nonessential Amino Acids The body requires 20 different amino acids, although tens of thousands of the same amino acids may combine in a single protein compound. Of the different amino acids, eight (nine in infants) cannot be synthesized in the body at a sufficient rate to prevent impairment of normal cellular function. These make up the indispensable, or **essential, amino acids**, because they must be ingested preformed in foods. The body manufactures the remaining 12 **nonessential amino acids**. This does not mean they are unimportant; rather, they form from compounds already existing in the body at a rate that meets demands for normal growth and tissue repair.

Animals and plants manufacture proteins that contain essential amino acids. *No health or physiological advantage comes from an amino acid derived from an animal compared with the same amino acid derived from vegetable origin.* Plants synthesize protein (and thus amino acids) by incorporating nitrogen from the soil (along with carbon, oxygen, and hydrogen from air and water). In contrast, animals do not possess a broad capability for protein synthesis; they obtain much of their protein from ingested sources.

Constructing a body protein requires specific amino acid availability at the time of protein synthesis. **Complete proteins** or higher-quality proteins come from foods with all of the essential amino acids in their correct ratio. This maintains protein balance and allows tissue growth and repair. An **incomplete protein**, or lower-quality protein, lacks one or more of the essential amino acids. Diets that contain mostly incomplete protein eventually produce protein malnutrition (see following section on sources of protein), despite the food source's adequacy for energy value and protein quantity.

Sources of Proteins

Protein is derived from dietary sources or can be synthesized in the body.

Dietary Sources Complete proteins are in eggs, milk, meat, fish, and poultry. Eggs provide the optimal mixture of essential amino acids among food sources; hence, eggs receive the highest quality rating compared with other foods. Presently, almost two-thirds of dietary protein in the U.S. comes from animal sources, whereas 90 years ago, protein consumption occurred equally from plants and animals. Reliance on animal sources for dietary protein accounts for a relatively high current intake of cholesterol and saturated fatty acids.

The "**biologic value**" (protein rating) of food refers to its completeness for supplying essential amino acids. Animal sources contribute high-quality protein, whereas vegetables (lentils, dried beans and peas, nuts, and cereals) remain incomplete in one or more of the essential amino acids; thus, these rate lower in biologic value. Eating a variety of plant foods (grains, fruits, and vegetables), each providing a different quality and quantity of amino acids, contributes all of the required essential amino acids. **Table 2.3** lists examples of common food sources of protein and their relative protein rating.

Synthesis in the Body Enzymes in muscle facilitate nitrogen removal from certain amino acids and subsequently pass nitrogen to other compounds in the biochemical reactions of **transamination** (see Fig. 2.10, bottom). An amine group shifts from a donor amino acid to an acceptor acid, and the acceptor thus becomes a new amino acid. *This allows amino acid formation from non–nitrogen-carrying organic compounds formed in metabolism.*

Deamination represents the opposite process to transamination. It involves removal of an amine group from the amino acid molecule, with the remaining carbon skeleton converting to a carbohydrate or lipid or being used for energy. The cleaved amine group forms urea in the liver, which the kidneys excrete. Because urea must dissolve in water, excessive protein catabolism (involving increased deamination) promotes fluid loss.

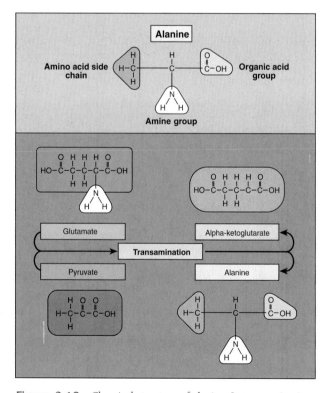

Figure 2.10 Chemical structure of alanine. In transamination, an amine group from a donor group transfers to an acceptor acid to form a new amino acid.

Table 2·3	Rating of Common Sources of Dietary Protein

FOOD	PROTEIN RATING
Eggs	100
Fish	70
Lean beef	69
Cow's milk	60
Brown rice	57
White rice	56
Soybeans	47
Brewer's hash	45
Whole-grain wheat	44
Peanuts	43
Dry beans	34
White potato	34

Questions & Notes

Give the RDA for protein for a college-age male and female.

Male:

Female:

For deamination and transamination, the resulting carbon skeleton of the non-nitrogenous amino acid residue further degrades during energy metabolism. In well-nourished individuals at rest, protein breakdown (**catabolism**) contributes between 2% to 5% of the body's total energy requirement. During its catabolism, protein first degrades into its amino acid components. The amino acid molecule then loses its nitrogen in the liver (via deamination) to form urea (H_2NCONH_2) for excretion.

Protein's Role in the Body

No body "reservoirs" of protein exist; all protein contributes to tissue structures or exists as constituents of metabolic, transport, and hormonal systems. Protein constitutes between 12% and 15% of the body mass, but its content in different cells varies considerably. A brain cell, for example, contains only about 10% protein, whereas protein represents up to 20% of the mass of red blood cells and muscle cells. The systematic application of resistance training increases the protein content of skeletal muscle, which represents about 65% of the body's total protein.

Amino acids provide the building blocks to synthesize diverse compounds such as RNA and DNA, the heme components of the oxygen-binding hemoglobin and myoglobin compounds, the catecholamine hormones epinephrine and norepinephrine, and the neurotransmitter serotonin. Amino acids activate vitamins that play a key role in metabolic and physiologic regulation.

Tissue synthesis (**anabolism**) accounts for more than one-third of the protein intake during rapid growth in infancy and childhood. As growth rate declines, so does the percentage of protein retained for anabolic processes. Continual turnover of tissue protein occurs when a person attains optimal body size and growth stabilizes. Adequate protein intake replaces the amino acids continually degraded in the turnover process.

Proteins serve as primary constituents for plasma membranes and internal cellular material. Proteins in cell nuclei (nucleoproteins) "supervise" cellular protein synthesis and transmit hereditary characteristics. Structural proteins comprise hair, skin, nails, bones, tendons, and ligaments, whereas globular proteins make up the nearly 2000 different enzymes that dramatically accelerate chemical reactions and regulate the catabolism of fats, carbohydrates, and proteins during energy release. Proteins also regulate the acid-base quality of the body fluids, which contributes to neutralizing (buffering) excess acid metabolites formed during vigorous exercise.

Vegetarian Approach to Sound Nutrition

True vegetarians (**vegans**) consume nutrients from only two sources—plants and dietary supplements. Vegans represent less than 1% of the U.S. population, al-

FOR YOUR INFORMATION

The Nine Essential Amino Acids
Histidine (infants)
Leucine
Lysine
Isoleucine
Methionine
Phenylalanine
Threonine
Tryptophan
Valine

FOR YOUR INFORMATION

Food Diversity: Crucial for Vegetarians
A vegan diet provides all of the essential amino acids if the RDA for protein includes 60% of protein from grain products, 35% from legumes, and the remaining 5% from green leafy vegetables. A 70-kg person who requires about 56 g of protein can obtain the essential amino acids by consuming approximately 1 1/4 cups of beans, 1/4 cup of seeds or nuts, about 4 slices of whole-grain bread, 2 cups of vegetables (half being green leafy), and 2 1/2 cups of diverse grain sources like brown rice, oatmeal, and cracked wheat.

though nearly 10% of Americans consider themselves "almost" vegetarians.

An increasing number of competitive and champion athletes consume diets consisting predominately of nutrients from varied plant sources, including some dairy and meat products. Considering the time required for training and competition, athletes often encounter difficulty planning, selecting, and preparing nutritious meals from predominantly plant sources without relying on supplementation. The fact remains that two-thirds of the world's population subsist on largely vegetarian diets with little reliance on animal protein. Well-balanced vegetarian and vegetarian-type diets can provide abundant carbohydrate, which is crucial when training intensely. *Vegetarian-type diets have the following characteristics: usually low or devoid of cholesterol, high in fiber, low in saturated and high in unsaturated fatty acids, and rich in fruit and vegetable sources of antioxidant vitamins and phytochemicals.*

Obtaining ample high-quality protein becomes the vegetarian's main nutritional concern. A **lactovegetarian** diet includes milk and related products like ice cream, cheese, and yogurt. The lactovegetarian approach minimizes the problem of acquiring sufficient high-quality protein and increases the intake of calcium, phosphorus, and vitamin B_{12} (produced by bacteria in the digestive tract of animals). Good meatless sources of iron include fortified ready-to-eat cereals, soybeans, and cooked farina, whereas cereals and wheat germ are relatively high in zinc. Adding an egg to the diet ensures an ample intake of high-quality protein (**ovolactovegetarian diet**).

Figure 2.11 displays the contribution of various food groups to the protein content of the American diet. By far, the greatest protein intake comes from animal sources, with only about 30% from plant sources.

Recommended Protein Intake

Eating excessive protein provides little benefit to sports performance despite the beliefs of many coaches, trainers, and athletes. Protein intake greater than 3 times the recommended level does not enhance work capacity during intensive training. *For athletes, muscle mass does not increase simply by eating high-protein foods.* If lean tissue synthesis resulted from all extra protein intake consumed

by the typical athlete, then muscle mass would increase tremendously. For example, eating an extra 100 g (400 kCal) of protein daily would translate to a daily 500 g (1.1 lb) increase in muscle mass. This obviously does not happen. Additional dietary protein, after deamination, provides for energy or recycles as components of other molecules including stored fat in subcutaneous depots. Dietary protein intake substantially above recommended values can prove harmful because excessive protein breakdown strains liver and kidney function through the production and elimination of urea and other solutes.

THE RECOMMENDED DIETARY ALLOWANCE: A LIBERAL STANDARD

The **Recommended Dietary Allowance (RDA)** for protein, vitamins, and minerals represents a standard for nutrient intake expressed as a daily average. These guidelines were initially developed in May 1942 by the Food and Nutrition Board of the National Research Council/National Academy of Science (*http://www.nas.edu/iom*) to evaluate and plan for the nutritional adequacy of groups rather than individuals. They have been revised 11 times. RDA levels represent a liberal yet safe excess to prevent nutritional deficiencies in practically all healthy people. In the 11th edition (1999), RDA recommendations included 19 nutrients, energy intake, and the **Estimated Safe and Adequate Daily Dietary Intakes (ESADDI)** for seven additional vitamins and minerals and three electrolytes. The ESADDI should be viewed as more tentative and evolutionary than the RDA. ESADDI recommendations for certain essential micronutrients (e.g., the vitamins biotin and pantothenic acid and trace elements copper, manganese, fluoride, selenium, chromium, and molybdenum) required sufficient scientific data to formulate an intake range considered adequate and safe, yet insufficient for a precise single RDA. Any intake within this range is considered acceptable for maintaining adequate physiologic function and sufficient enough to prevent under- or overexposure. No RDA or ESADDI exists for sodium, potassium, and chlorine; instead, recommendations refer to a minimum requirement for health.

The RDA reflects an ongoing evaluation based on available data of the nutritional needs of a population over a prolonged time period. Only laboratory measurements can determine the specific individual requirements. Malnutrition occurs from cumulative weeks, months, and even years of inadequate nutrient intake. Also, someone who regularly consumes a diet containing nutrients below the RDA standards may not become malnourished. Rather, the RDA represents a probability statement for adequate nutrition; as nutrient intake falls below the RDA, the statistical probability for malnourishment increases for that person. The chance progressively increases with lower nutrient intake. In Chapter 3, we discuss the Dietary Reference Intakes, which represent the current set of standards for recommended intakes of nutrients and other food components.

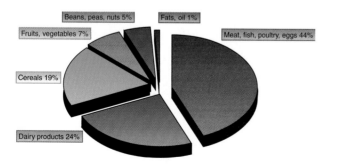

Figure 2.11 Contribution from the major food sources to the protein content of the typical American diet.

Table 2.4 lists the protein RDAs for adolescent and adult men and women. On average, 0.83 g protein per kg body mass represents the recommended daily intake. To determine the protein requirement for men and women ages 18 to 65 years, multiply body mass in kg by 0.83. Thus, for a 90-kg man, the total protein requirement equals 75 g (90 × 0.83). The protein RDA holds even for overweight people; it includes a reserve of about 25% to account for individual differences in protein requirement for about 98% of the population. Generally, the protein RDA (and the quantity of the required essential amino acids) decreases with age. In contrast, the protein RDA for infants and growing children equals 2.0 to 4.0 g per kg body mass to facilitate growth and development. Pregnant women should increase daily protein intake by 20 g/d, and nursing mothers should increase intake by 10 g/d. *A 10% increase in the calculated protein requirement, particularly for a vegetarian-type diet, accounts for dietary fiber's effect in reducing the digestibility of many plant-based protein sources.* Stress, disease, and injury usually increase the protein requirement.

Protein Requirements for Physically Active People

Any discussion of protein requirement must include the assumption of adequate energy intake to match the added needs of exercise. *If energy intake falls below the total energy expended during heavy training, even augmented protein intake may fail to maintain nitrogen balance.* This occurs because a disproportionate quantity of dietary protein catabolizes to balance an energy deficit rather than augment tissue maintenance and/or muscle development.

The common practice among weight lifters, body builders, and other power athletes who consume liquids, powders, or pills of predigested protein represents a waste of money and may actually be counterproductive for producing the desired outcome. For example, many of these preparations contain proteins predigested to simple amino acids through chemical action in the laboratory. Available evidence does not support the notion that simple amino acids absorb more easily or facilitate muscle growth. In fact, the small intestine absorbs amino acids rapidly when they are part of more complex di- and tripeptide molecules. The intestinal tract handles protein effectively in their more complex form. In contrast, a concentrated amino-acid solution draws water into the small intestine, which can cause irritation, cramping, and diarrhea in susceptible individuals.

Debate focuses on the necessity of a larger protein requirement for growing adolescent athletes, athletes involved in resistance training (to enhance muscle growth) and endurance training programs (to counter increased protein breakdown for energy), and wrestlers and football players subjected to recurring muscle trauma. Inadequate protein intake can reduce body protein, particularly from muscle, with concomitant impairment in performance. If athletes do require additional protein, then more than likely their increased food intake will compensate for training's increased energy expenditure. However, this may not occur in

FOR YOUR INFORMATION

Mix and Match

Obtain complete proteins with the following complementary combinations in a vegetarian diet:

- Beans and rice
- Peas and corn
- Bread and lentils
- Potatoes with milk or egg
- Cereals with milk or egg

FOR YOUR INFORMATION

Hunger and Undernutrition

Hunger is often described as an uneasiness and pain resulting from insufficient food consumption to meet the body's energy needs. Chronic hunger can lead to undernutrition, which retards growth in children and promotes weakness in adults. Also, risk of infection increases and nutrient-deficiency disease occurs as a result of undernutrition. The primary cause of undernutrition is poverty; the critical periods for undernutrition occur during pregnancy, infancy, childhood, and old age. Chronic undernutrition decreases exercise and sports performance, depresses overall motivation, and compromises immune function.

Table 2·4	Recommended Dietary Allowances of Protein for Adolescent and Adult Men and Women			
RECOMMENDED AMOUNT	**MEN**		**WOMEN**	
	ADOLESCENT	**ADULT**	**ADOLESCENT**	**ADULT**
Grams of protein per kg body weight	0.9	0.8	0.9	0.8
Grams of protein per day based on average weight[a]	59.0	56.0	50.0	44.0

[a]Average weight based on a "reference" man and woman. For adolescents (ages 14-18), average weight equals 65.8 kg (145 lb) for males and 55.7 kg (123 lb) for females. For adult men, average weight equals 70 kg (154 lb); for adult women, average weight equals 56.8 kg (125 lb).

athletes with poor nutritional habits or who voluntarily diet and reduce energy intake to hopefully gain a competitive advantage.

Do Athletes Require More Protein?

Much of the current understanding of protein dynamics and exercise comes from studies that expanded the classic method of determining protein breakdown through urea excretion. For example, the output of "labeled" CO_2 from amino acids (either injected or ingested) increases during exercise in proportion to metabolic rate. As exercise progresses, the concentration of plasma urea also increases, coupled with a dramatic rise in nitrogen excretion in sweat (often occurring without changing urinary nitrogen excretion). Figure 2.12 illustrates that the sweat mechanism helps to excrete nitrogen produced from protein breakdown during exercise. Furthermore, oxidation of plasma and intracellular amino acids increases significantly during moderate exercise, independent of changes in urea production.

Figure 2.12 also shows that protein use for energy reached its highest level when subjects exercised in the glycogen-depleted state. This emphasizes the important role of carbohydrate as a protein sparer, suggesting that carbohydrate availability affects the demand on protein "reserves" in exercise. Protein breakdown and accompanying gluconeogenesis (glucose synthesis from protein) undoubtedly become important factors in endurance exercise (or in frequent heavy training) when glycogen reserves diminish. Eating a high-carbohydrate diet (with adequate energy intake) preserves muscle protein in athletes who train hard and for protracted durations.

A continuing area of controversy concerns whether the initial increased protein demand when training commences creates a true long-term increase in protein requirement above the RDA. A definitive answer remains elusive, but protein breakdown above the resting level does occur during intense endurance training and resistance training to a greater degree than previously believed. Unfortunately, research has not pinpointed protein requirements for individuals who train 4 to 6 hours daily by resistance exercise. Their protein needs may average only slightly greater than for sedentary individuals. In addition, despite increased protein use for energy during intense training, adaptations may augment the body's efficiency in using dietary protein to enhance amino acid balance. *Until research clarifies this issue, we recommend that athletes who train intensely consume between 1.2 and 1.8 g of protein per kg of body mass daily.* This protein intake falls within the range typically consumed by physically active men and women, thus obviating the need to consume supplementary protein. With adequate protein intake, consuming animal sources of protein does not facilitate muscle strength or size gains with resistance training compared to protein intake from plant sources.

PROTEIN MALNUTRITION

Protein deficiency usually accompanies dietary energy deficiency from insufficient food intake. This often is observed in developing areas of the world where peoples' diets are low in energy and protein or in individuals who chronically starve themselves (anorexia nervosa). Individuals who consume too little protein and food energy can develop **protein-energy malnutrition (PEM)**. In its mild form, it is difficult to recognize if a person with PEM consumes too few calories or protein or both. If the nutrient deficiency, especially for energy, is severe, it triggers the deficiency disease **marasmus**. In contrast, the disease **kwashiorkor** develops when a poor nutrient intake, protein included, is added to other problems from concurrent diseases and infections. These two conditions can be present in the same individual. Kwashiorkor (a word from Ghana meaning "the disease that the first child gets when the new child comes") occurs primarily in young children who have an existing disease and who consume too few calories and insufficient protein, despite high protein needs.

Marasmus (meaning "to waste away") typically occurs in infancy where the infant slowly starves to death. It is caused by diets containing insufficient protein, energy, and other nutrients. This condition typically characterizes older children and adults who have reduced fat stores, minimal muscle mass, and poor strength and stamina.

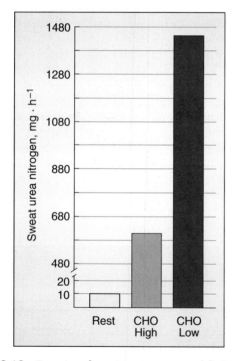

Figure 2.12 Excretion of urea in sweat at rest, and during exercise after carbohydrate loading (CHO High) and carbohydrate depletion (CHO Low). The largest utilization of protein (as reflected by sweat urea) occurs with low glycogen reserves. (From Lemon, P.W., Nagel, F.: Effects of exercise on protein and amino acid metabolism. *Med. Sci. Sports Exerc.*, 13:141, 1981.)

Box 2–6 • CLOSE UP

HOW TO LOWER HIGH BLOOD PRESSURE USING THE DASH DIET

About one-half of hypertensive individuals have their blood pressure treated, and only half of those individuals actually control it. One reason relates to the potential deleterious side effects of antihypertensive medication, including fatigue and impotence.

DIETARY APPROACH

Research with DASH (**Dietary Approaches to Stop Hypertension**) has shown that this diet lowers blood pressure similarly to drugs in some people and more than other lifestyle changes in most cases. After 2 months with DASH, individuals reduced systolic blood pressure by an average of 11.4 mm Hg and diastolic pressure by 5.5 mm Hg. Every decline of 2 mm Hg of systolic pressure typically lowers coronary disease risk by 5% and risk of stroke by 8%.

The DASH diet (**Table 1**) emphasizes fruits, vegetables, and dairy products and avoids fat.

SAMPLE DASH DIET

Table 2 shows a sample DASH diet consisting of approximately 2100 kCal. A 2100-kCal diet stabilizes weight in someone who is moderately active and weighs about 150 pounds. If the person is either more active or heavier than that and does not want to reduce weight, than that person should eat more servings than indicated by boosting either portion size or number of individual items. People who want to reduce weight or are lighter or less physically active should consume slightly fewer servings but no less than the minimum number for each range.

DASH-SODIUM

The successful DASH diet in combination with low daily sodium intake (<1500 mg·d^{-1}) reduced blood pressure even more than diet alone or a very low-salt diet. The DASH diet combined with low salt intake afforded the best approach to lowering blood pressure and helped reduce cancer risk, prevent osteoporosis, and protect against heart disease.

Table 1 — The DASH Approach to Lower Blood Pressure; Food Groups, Serving Sizes, and Number of Servings for Different Caloric Value Diets. The Number of Servings Per Day Corresponds to the Food Guide Pyramid Serving Sizes.

FOOD GROUP (ONE-SERVING EXAMPLE)	NUMBER OF SERVINGS PER DAY			
kCal Level	1600 kCal	2000 kCal	2600 kCal	3100 kCal
Grains (1 slice of bread; 1/2 cup of cold, dry cereal; 1 cup cooked rice or pasta)	6–7	7–8	10–11	12–13
Vegetables (1/2 cup of cooked or raw chopped vegetables; 1 cup of raw leafy vegetables; or 6 oz of juice)	3–4	4–5	5–6	6–7
Fruits (1 medium apple, pear, orange, or banana; 1/2 grapefruit; 1/3 cantaloupe; 1/2 cup of fresh frozen or canned fruit; 1/4 cup of dried fruit; or 6 oz of juice)	3–4	4–5	5–6	6–7
Low-fat dairy (1 cup of no-fat or low-fat milk or 1 1/2 oz of low-fat or part-skim cheese)	2–3	2–3	3–4	3–4
Meats, fish, poultry (a 3-oz chunk [roughly the size of a deck of cards])	1–2	1–2	2	2–3
Beans, nuts, and seeds (1/3 cup [1 1/2 oz] of nuts; 2 tablespoons of seeds; or 1/2 cup of cooked beans)	1/3	1/2	2/3	3/4
Limit fats and sweets				

Box 2–6 • **CLOSE UP** *(Continued)*

FOOD	AMOUNT
Table 2	**Sample DASH diet (2100 kCal)**
Breakfast	
Orange juice	6 oz
1% low-fat milk	8 oz (used with corn flakes)
Corn flakes (1 tsp sugar)	1 cup (dry) [equals 2 servings of grains]
Banana	1 medium
Whole-wheat bread	1 slice
Soft margarine	1 tsp
Lunch	
Low-fat chicken salad	3/4 cup
Pita bread	1/2 large
Raw vegetable medley	
carrot and celery sticks	3–4 sticks each
radishes	2
lettuce	2 leaves
Part-skim mozzarella	1 1/2 slices (1.5 oz)
1% low-fat milk	8 oz
Fruit cocktail	1/2 cup
Dinner	
Herbed baked cod	3 oz
Scallion rice	1 cup [equals 2 servings of grain]
Steamed broccoli	1/2 cup
Stewed tomatoes	1/2 cup
Spinach salad	
Raw spinach	1/2 cup
Cherry tomatoes	2
Cucumber	2 slices
Light Italian salad dressing	1 Tbsp [equals 1/2 fat serving]
Whole wheat dinner roll	1
Soft margarine	1 tsp
Melon balls	1/2 cup
Snack	
Dried apricots	1 oz (1/4 cup)
Mixed nuts, unsalted	1.5 oz (1/3 cup)
Mini-pretzels, unsalted	1 oz (3/4 cup)
Diet ginger ale	12 oz [does not count as a serving of any food]

REFERENCES

Appel, L.J., et al.: A clinical trial of the effects of dietary patterns on blood pressure. *N. Engl. J. Med.*, 336:1117, 1997.

Greenland, P.: Beating high blood pressure with low-sodium DASH. *N. Engl. J. Med.*, 344:53, 2001.

Sacks, F.M., et al.: Rationale and design of the dietary approaches to stop hypertension trial (DASH): A multicenter controlled feeding study of dietary patterns to lower blood pressure. *Ann. Epidemiol.*, 5:108, 1995.

Svetkey, L.P., et al.: Effects of dietary patterns on blood pressure: Subgroup analysis of the dietary approaches to stop hypertension (DASH) randomized clinical trial. *Arch. Intern. Med.*, 159:285, 1999.

SUMMARY

1. Carbon, hydrogen, oxygen, and nitrogen represent the primary structural units for most of the body's biologically active substances.

2. Specific combinations of carbon with oxygen and hydrogen form carbohydrates and lipids, whereas proteins consist of combinations of carbon, oxygen, and hydrogen, including nitrogen and minerals.

3. Simple sugars consist of chains of from 3 to 7 carbon atoms with hydrogen and oxygen in the ratio of 2 to 1. Glucose, the most common simple sugar, contains a 6-carbon chain: $C_6H_{12}O_6$.

4. Three classifications commonly define carbohydrates: monosaccharides (sugars such as glucose and fructose); disaccharides (combinations of two monosaccharides as in sucrose, lactose, and maltose); and polysaccharides, which contain three or more simple sugars to form plant starch and fiber and the large animal polysaccharide glycogen.

5. Glycogenolysis reconverts glycogen to glucose, whereas gluconeogenesis synthesizes glucose, most notably from the carbon skeletons of amino acids.

6. Fiber, a non-starch, structural plant polysaccharide, offers considerable resistance to human digestive enzymes. Although technically not a nutrient, water-soluble and water-insoluble dietary fibers confer health benefits for gastrointestinal functioning and cardiovascular disease.

7. Americans typically consume 40% to 50% of total calories as carbohydrates, with about one-half in the form of simple sugars, predominantly sucrose and high-fructose corn syrup.

8. Carbohydrates, stored in limited quantity in liver and muscle, serve four important functions: (1) major source of energy, (2) spares protein breakdown, (3) metabolic primer for fat metabolism, and (4) fuel for the central nervous system.

9. Muscle glycogen and blood glucose become the primary fuels for intense exercise. The body's glycogen stores also provide energy in sustained, intense aerobic exercise such as marathon running, triathlon-type events, long-distance cycling, and endurance swimming.

10. A carbohydrate-deficient diet rapidly depletes muscle and liver glycogen, profoundly affecting capacity for both high-intensity anaerobic exercise and long-duration aerobic exercise. Individuals who exercise regularly should consume at least 60% of daily calories as carbohydrates (400 to 600 g), predominantly in unrefined, fiber-rich complex form.

11. Like carbohydrates, lipids contain carbon, hydrogen, and oxygen atoms but with a higher ratio of hydrogen to oxygen. For example, the lipid stearin has the formula $C_{57}H_{110}O_6$. Lipid molecules consist of one glycerol molecule and three fatty acid molecules.

12. Plants and animals synthesize lipids into one of three groups: (1) simple lipids (glycerol plus three fatty acids), (2) compound lipids (phospholipids, glycolipids, and lipoproteins) composed of simple lipids in combination with other chemicals, and (3) derived lipids, like cholesterol, synthesized from simple and compound lipids.

13. Saturated fatty acids contain as many hydrogen atoms as chemically possible; thus, the molecule is considered saturated relative to hydrogen. Saturated fatty acids exist primarily in animal meat, egg yolk, dairy fats, and cheese. High saturated fatty acid intake elevates blood cholesterol and promotes coronary heart disease.

14. Unsaturated fatty acids contain fewer hydrogen atoms attached to the carbon chain. Fatty acids exist as either monounsaturated or polyunsaturated with respect to hydrogen. Increasing the diet's proportion of unsaturated fatty acids may offer protection against heart disease.

15. Lowering blood cholesterol, especially that carried by low-density lipoprotein cholesterol, provides significant coronary heart disease protection.

16. Dietary lipid represents between 34% and 38% of the typical person's total caloric intake. Prudent recommendations suggest a 30% level or lower, of which 70% to 80% should be unsaturated fatty acids.

17. Lipids provide the largest nutrient store of potential energy for biologic work. They also (1) protect vital organs, (2) provide insulation from cold, (3) transport fat-soluble vitamins, and (4) depress hunger.

18. During light and moderate exercise, fat contributes about 50% of the energy requirement. As exercise continues, fat becomes more important, supplying more than 70% of the body's energy needs.

19. Proteins differ chemically from lipids and carbohydrates because they contain nitrogen in addition to sulfur, phosphorus, and iron.

20. Subunits called amino acids form proteins. The body requires 20 different amino acids.

21. The body cannot synthesize eight of the 20 amino acids; they must be consumed in the diet and thus comprise the essential amino acids.

22. All animal and plant cells contain protein. Complete (higher-quality) proteins contain all the essential amino acids; the other protein type represents incomplete or lower-quality proteins. Examples of higher-quality, complete proteins include animal proteins found in eggs, milk, cheese, meat, fish, and poultry.

23. Consuming a variety of plant foods provides all the essential amino acids because each food source contains a different quality and quantity of amino acids.

24. The RDA represents the recommended quantity for nutrient intake. It serves as a liberal yet safe level of excess to meet the nutritional needs of practically all healthy people. For adults, the protein RDA equals 0.83 g per kg of body mass.

25. Protein breakdown above the resting level occurs during endurance and resistance training exercise to a degree greater than previously thought. Athletes in intense training (2 to 6 h·d^{-1}) should consume between 1.2 and 1.8 g of protein per kg of body mass daily.

26. Reduced carbohydrate reserves increase protein catabolism during exercise. Such findings support the wisdom of maintaining optimal levels of glycogen during strenuous training.

27. Undernutrition can lead to protein and energy malnutrition in the form of kwashiorkor or marasmus. Kwashiorkor results primarily from an inadequate energy and protein intake in comparison to body need. Marasmus results primarily from extreme starvation and low protein intake.

THOUGHT QUESTIONS

1. Outline a presentation to a high school class about how to eat well for a physically active, healthy lifestyle.

2. Many college students do not eat well-balanced meals. Give your recommendations concerning macronutrient intake to ensure proper energy reserves for moderate and intense physical activities. Are supplements of these macronutrients necessarily required for physically active individuals?

3. Explain the importance of regular carbohydrate intake when maintaining a high level of daily physical activity. Additionally, what are some "non-exercise" health benefits for a diet rich in food sources containing unrefined, complex carbohydrates?

4. Discuss a rationale for recommending adequate carbohydrate intake, rather than excess protein, for a person who wants to increase muscle mass through heavy resistance training.

PART 2 •
Micronutrients: Facilitators of Energy
Transfer and Tissue Synthesis

List the 2 classifications of vitamins.

1.

2.

Effective regulation of all metabolic processes requires a delicate blending of food nutrients in the cell's watery medium. Micronutrients have special significance in the metabolic mixture; they consist of the small quantities of vitamins and minerals that facilitate energy transfer and optimize normal growth and development. Consuming well-balanced meals ensures adequate nutrient intake, thus obviating the need to consume vitamin and mineral supplements. With proper food intake, such supplements offer little or no physiologic benefits and could be characterized as economically wasteful. Unfortunately, consuming micronutrients in excess can also pose significant dangers to health and well being.

Describe what generally happens to the excess intake of the B-complex vitamins.

VITAMINS
The Nature of Vitamins

The formal discovery of vitamins revealed that the body required these essential organic substances in minute amounts to perform highly specific metabolic functions. A person requires only about 350 g (12 oz) of vitamins from about 2000 lb of food consumed annually. Vitamins, often considered accessory nutrients, do not supply energy, are not basic building units for other compounds, and do not contribute substantially to the body's mass. Nevertheless, a prolonged inadequate intake of a particular vitamin can trigger symptoms of vitamin deficiency and lead to severe medical complications. For example, symptoms of thiamin deficiency occur after only 2 weeks on a thiamin-free diet, and symptoms of vitamin C deficiency appear after 3 or 4 weeks. At the other extreme, consuming some fat-soluble vitamins in excess can produce a toxic overdose manifested by hair loss, irregularities in bone formation, fetal malformation, hemorrhage, bone fractures, abnormal liver function, and ultimately death.

Give one major food source of antioxidant vitamins.

Classification of Vitamins

Thirteen different vitamins have been isolated, analyzed, classified, and synthesized, and had RDA levels established. Vitamins are classified as either **fat-soluble** (vitamins A, D, E, and K) or **water-soluble** (vitamin C and the B-complex vitamins: vitamin B_6 [pyridoxine], vitamin B_1 [thiamin], vitamin B_2 [riboflavin], niacin [nicotinic acid], pantothenic acid, biotin, folic acid, and vitamin B_{12} [cobalamin]).

Fat-Soluble Vitamins   Fat-soluble vitamins dissolve and store in the body's fatty tissues and do not require daily intake. In fact, symptoms of a fat-soluble vitamin insufficiency may not appear for years. Dietary lipid provides the source of fat-soluble vitamins. The liver stores vitamins A, D, and K; whereas vitamin E distributes throughout the body's fatty tissues. Prolonged intake of a "fat-free" diet accelerates a fat-soluble vitamin insufficiency. **Table 2.5** lists the major bodily functions, dietary sources, and symptoms of a deficiency or excess for the fat-soluble vitamins for males and females age 19 to 50 years. In chapter 3, we discuss the dietary reference intakes, including tolerable upper intake levels for all vitamins (and minerals) for different life-stage groups.

Water-Soluble Vitamins   Vitamin C (ascorbic acid) and the B-complex group constitute the nine water-soluble vitamins. They act largely as **coenzymes**—small molecules that combine with a larger protein compound (apoenzyme) to form an active enzyme that accelerates interconversion of chemical compounds. Coenzymes participate directly in chemical reactions; when the

| Table 2·5 | Food Sources, Major Bodily Functions, and Symptoms of Deficiency or Excess of the Fat-Soluble Vitamins for Healthy Adults (Ages 19 to 50 Years)[a] | | | |

VITAMIN	DIETARY SOURCES	MAJOR BODILY FUNCTIONS	DEFICIENCY	EXCESS
Vitamin A (retinol)	Provitamin A (beta–carotene) widely distributed in green vegetables; retinol present in milk, butter, cheese, fortified margarine	Constituent of rhodopsin (visual pigment); maintenance of epithelial tissues; role in mucopolysaccharide synthesis	Xeropthalmia (keratinization of ocular tissue), night blindness, permanent blindness	Headache, vomiting, peeling of skin, anorexia, swelling of long bones
Vitamin D	Cod-liver oil, eggs, dairy products, fortified milk, and margarine	Promotes growth and mineralization of bones; increases absorption of calcium	Rickets (bone deformities) in children; osteomalacia in adults	Vomiting, diarrhea, weight loss, kidney damage
Vitamin E (tocopherol)	Seeds, green leafy vegetables, margarines, shortenings	Functions as an antioxidant to prevent cell damage	Possibly anemia	Relatively nontoxic
Vitamin K (phylloquinone)	Green leafy vegetables, small amount in cereals, fruits, and meats	Important in blood clotting (helps form active prothrombin)	Conditioned deficiencies associated with severe bleeding, internal hemorrhages	Relatively nontoxic; synthetic forms at high doses may cause jaundice

[a]Food and Nutrition Board, National Academy of Sciences, 2002. (http://www.nal.usda.gov/fnic/etext/000105.html)

reaction runs its course, coenzymes remain intact and participate in further reactions. Water-soluble vitamins play an essential role as part of coenzymes in the cells' energy-generating reactions.

Because of their solubility in water, water-soluble vitamins disperse in the body fluids without appreciable storage, and the excess voids in urine. If the diet regularly contains less than 50% of the recommended values for water-soluble vitamins, marginal deficiencies may develop within 4 weeks. **Table 2.6** summarizes the RDA, food sources, major bodily functions, and symptoms resulting from both excess and deficiency of water-soluble vitamins.

The B-complex vitamins serve as coenzymes in energy-yielding reactions during carbohydrate, fat, and protein breakdown. They also contribute to hemoglobin synthesis and red blood cell formation. Vitamin C acts as a cofactor in enzymatic reactions and as a scavenger of free radicals in antioxidative processes and contributes to collagen synthesis and maintaining the intracellular matrix of bone and cartilage.

Vitamin Toxicity   Excess vitamins function as potentially harmful chemicals once enzyme systems catalyzed by specific vitamins saturate. A higher probability exists for overdosing with fat-soluble than water-soluble vitamins. Prolonged excessive intake of vitamins of either type can produce toxic effects and lead to death.

Fat-soluble vitamins should **not** *be consumed in excess without medical supervision.* Adverse reactions from excessive fat-soluble vitamin intake occur at a lower level than water-soluble vitamins. Women who consume excess vitamin A (as retinol but not in provitamin carotene form) early in pregnancy significantly increase risk of birth defects. Excessive vitamin A accumulation (called **hypervitaminosis A**) causes irritability, swelling of bones, weight loss, and dry itchy skin in young children. In adults, symptoms include nausea, headache, drowsiness, loss of hair, diarrhea, and bone brittleness from calcium loss. Discontinuing excessive vitamin A consumption reverses these symptoms. A regular excess of vitamin D can damage the kidneys. Although "overdoses" from vitamins E and K rarely occur, intakes above the recommended level provide no health or fitness benefits.

Vitamins' Role in the Body

Vitamins contain no useful energy for the body; instead, they link and regulate the sequence of metabolic reactions that release energy within food molecules. They also play an intimate role in tissue synthesis and other biologic processes. A vitamin participates repeatedly in metabolic reactions regardless of physical activity level; thus, the vitamin needs of athletes do not exceed those of sedentary counterparts. **Figure 2.13** summarizes the important functions of vitamins.

Individuals who expend considerable energy exercising do not need to consume special foods or supplements that increase the diet's vitamin content above the RDA. Also, at

| Table 2·6 | Food Sources, Major Bodily Functions, and Symptoms of Deficiency or Excess of the Water-Soluble Vitamins for Healthy Adults (Ages 19 to 50 Years)[a] | | | |

VITAMIN	DIETARY SOURCES	MAJOR BODILY FUNCTIONS	DEFICIENCY	EXCESS
Vitamin B$_1$ (thiamin)	Pork, organ meats, whole grains, legumes	Coenzyme (thiamin prophosphate) in reactions involving removal of carbon dioxide	Beriberi (peripheral nerve changes, edema, heart failure)	None reported
Vitamin B$_2$ (riboflavin)	Widely distributed in foods	Constituent of two flavin nucleotide coenzymes involved in energy metabolism (FAD and FMN)	Reddened lips, cracks at mouth corner (cheilosis), eye lesions	None reported
Niacin (nicotinic acid)	Liver, lean meats, grains, legumes (can be formed from tryptophan)	Constituent of two coenzymes in oxidation-reduction reactions (NAD$^+$ and NADP)	Pellagra (skin and gastrointestinal lesions, nervous mental disorders)	Flushing, burning and tingling around neck, face, and hands
Vitamin B$_6$ (pyridoxine)	Meats, vegetables, whole-grain cereals	Coenzyme (pyridoxal phosphate) involved in amino acid and glycogen metabolism	Irritability, convulsions, muscular twitching, dermatitis, kidney stones	None reported
Pantothenic acid	Widely distributed in foods	Constituent of coenzyme A, which plays a central role in energy metabolism	Fatigue, sleep disturbances, impaired coordination, nausea	None reported
Folate	Legumes, green vegetables, whole-wheat products	Coenzyme (reduced form) involved in transfer of single-carbon units in nucleic acid and amino acid metabolism	Anemia, gastrointestinal disturbances, diarrhea, red tongue	None reported
Vitamin B$_{12}$ (cobalamin)	Muscle meats, eggs, dairy products, (absent in plant foods)	Coenzyme involved in transfer of single-carbon units in nucleic acid metabolism	Pernicious anemia, neurologic disorders	None reported
Biotin	Legumes, vegetables, meats	Coenzymes required for fat synthesis, amino acid metabolism, and glycogen (animal starch) formation	Fatigue, depression, nausea, dermatitis, muscular pains	None reported
Vitamin C (ascorbic acid)	Citrus fruits, tomatoes, green peppers, salad greens	Maintains intercellular matrix of cartilage, bone, and dentine, important in collagen synthesis	Scurvy (degeneration of skin, teeth, blood vessels, epithelial hemorrhages)	Relatively nontoxic; possibility of kidney stones

[a]Food and Nutrition Board, National Academy of Sciences, 2002. (http://www.nal.usda.gov/fnic/etext/000105.html)

high levels of daily physical activity, food intake usually increases to sustain the added energy requirements of exercise. Additional food consumed through a variety of nutritious meals proportionately increases vitamin and mineral intake. This general rule has several possible exceptions. First, vitamin C and folic acid exist in foods that usually comprise only a small part of most Americans' total caloric intake; the availability of these foods also varies by season. Second, some athletic groups consume relatively low amounts of vitamins B$_1$ and B$_6$. If the daily diet con-

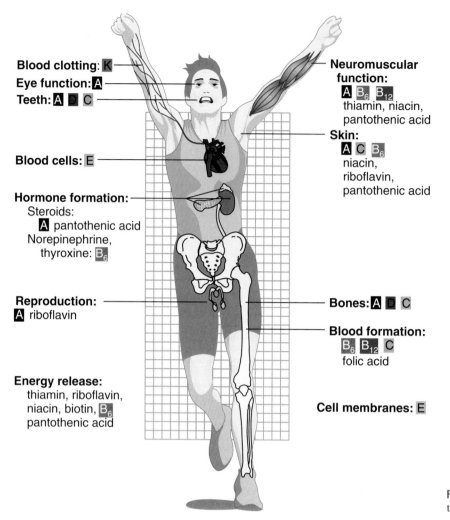

Blood clotting: K
Eye function: A
Teeth: A D C

Blood cells: E

Hormone formation:
Steroids:
A pantothenic acid
Norepinephrine,
thyroxine: B₆

Reproduction:
A riboflavin

Energy release:
thiamin, riboflavin,
niacin, biotin, B₆
pantothenic acid

Neuromuscular function:
A B₆ B₁₂
thiamin, niacin,
pantothenic acid

Skin:
A C B₆
niacin,
riboflavin,
pantothenic acid

Bones: A D C

Blood formation:
B₆ B₁₂ C
folic acid

Cell membranes: E

Figure 2.13 Biologic functions of vitamins.

tains fresh fruit, grains, and uncooked or steamed vegetables, an adequate intake of these two vitamins occurs. Individuals on meatless diets should consume a small amount of milk, milk products, or eggs (or a vitamin supplement) because vitamin B_{12} exists only in foods of animal origin.

Antioxidant Role of Specific Vitamins

Most of the oxygen consumed in the mitochondria during energy metabolism combines with hydrogen to produce water. Normally about 2% to 5% of oxygen forms oxygen-containing free radicals, like superoxide (O_2^-), hydrogen peroxide (H_2O_2), and hydroxyl (OH^-) radicals, due to electron "leakage" along the electron transport chain (see Chapter 5). A **free radical** represents a highly chemically reactive molecule or molecular fragment with at least one unpaired electron in its outer orbital or valence shell. These are the same free radicals produced by heat and ionizing radiation and carried in cigarette smoke, environmental pollutants, and even some medications.

A buildup of free radicals increases the potential for cellular damage (**oxidative stress**) to biologically important substances. Oxygen radicals exhibit strong affinity for the polyunsaturated fatty acids in the cell membrane's lipid bilayer. During oxidative stress, deterioration occurs in the plasma membrane's fatty acids. Membrane damage occurs through a chain-reaction series of events termed **lipid peroxidation**. These reactions, which incorporate oxygen into lipids, increase the vulnerability of the cell and its constituents. Free radicals also facilitate low-density lipoprotein cholesterol oxidation and thus accelerate the atherosclerotic process. Oxidative stress ultimately increases the likelihood of cellular deterioration associated with advanced aging, cancer, diabetes, coronary artery disease, and a general decline in central nervous system and immune function.

Nothing can stop oxygen reduction and free radical production, but an elaborate natural defense exists within the cell and extracellular space against its damaging effects. This defense includes diverse enzymatic and non-enzymatic mechanisms that work in concert to immediately counter potential oxidative damage. Three major antioxidant enzymes include **superoxide dismutase**, **catalase**, and **glutathione peroxidase**. The nutritive-reducing agents vitamins A, C, and E, and the vitamin A precursor β-carotene also serve important protective functions. These antioxidant vitamins protect the plasma membrane by reacting with and removing free radicals, thus squelching the chain reaction. Maintaining a diet with ample antioxidant vitamins may reduce the risk of several types of cancers; a normal to above normal intake of vitamin E (in both alpha-tocopherol and gamma-tocopherol forms) and β-carotene and/or high serum levels of carotenoids can blunt narrowing of the coronary arteries and reduce heart attack and stroke risk in men and women.

Vitamins Behave as Chemicals   An estimated 165 million Americans use dietary supplements, spending $24 billion in 2004. Of this total, vitamin–mineral pills and powders, often at potentially toxic dosages, represent the most common form of supplement used by the general public, accounting for 70% of the total annual supplement sales. Particularly susceptible marketing targets include the exercise enthusiast, the competitive athlete, and coaches and personal trainers who assist individuals achieve peak performance. More than 50% of competitive athletes in some sports consume supplements on a regular basis, either to ensure adequate micronutrient intake or to achieve an excess with the hope of enhancing performance and training responsiveness. If vitamin supplementation does offer benefits to physically active individuals, the benefits may only apply to those with marginal vitamin intakes.

Any significant excess of vitamins functions as chemicals (drugs) in the body. For example, a megadose of water-soluble vitamin C increases serum uric acid levels that precipitate gout in people predisposed to this disease. At intakes greater than 1000 mg daily, urinary excretion of oxalate (a breakdown product of vitamin C) increases, accelerating kidney stone formation in susceptible individuals. In iron-deficient individuals, megadoses of vitamin C may destroy significant amounts of vitamin B_{12}. In healthy people, vitamin C supplements frequently irritate the bowel and cause diarrhea.

Excess vitamin B_6 may induce liver and nerve damage. Excessive riboflavin (B_2) intake can impair vision, whereas a megadose of nicotinic acid (niacin) can act as a potent vasodilator and inhibit fatty acid mobilization during exercise, which is an effect that rapidly depletes muscle glycogen. Folic acid concentrated in supplement form can trigger an allergic response producing hives, lightheadedness, and breathing difficulties. Megadoses of vitamin A can induce toxicity to the nervous system, and kidney damage can result from excess vitamin D intake.

MINERALS

The Nature of Minerals

Approximately 4% of the body's mass (about 2 kg for a 50-kg woman) consists of 22 mostly metallic elements collectively called **minerals**. Minerals serve as constituents of enzymes, hormones, and vitamins; they combine with other chemicals (e.g., calcium phosphate in bone and iron in the heme of hemoglobin) or exist singularly (e.g., free calcium in body fluids). In the body, minerals are classified as **trace minerals** (those required in amounts ≤ 100 mg a day) and **major minerals** (those required in amounts ≥100 mg a day). Excess minerals serve no useful physiologic purpose and can produce toxic effects.

Kinds, Sources, and Functions of Minerals

Most major and trace minerals occur freely in nature, mainly in the waters of rivers, lakes, and oceans, in topsoil, and beneath the earth's surface. Minerals exist in the root systems of plants and in the body structure of animals who consume plants and water-containing minerals. **Table 2.7** lists the major bodily functions, dietary sources, and symptoms of a deficiency and excess for important major and trace minerals.

| | Table 2·7 | Important Major and Trace Minerals for Healthy Adults (Ages 19 to 50 Years): Their Food Sources, Functions, and Effects of Deficiencies and Excesses[a] | | |

MINERAL	DIETARY SOURCES	MAJOR BODILY FUNCTIONS	DEFICIENCY	EXCESS
Major				
Calcium	Milk, cheese, dark green vegetables, dried legumes	Bone and tooth formation; blood clotting; nerve transmission	Stunted growth; rickets, osteoporosis; convulsions	Not reported in humans
Phosphorus	Milk, cheese, yogurt, meat, poultry, grains, fish	Bone and tooth formation; acid-base balance	Weakness, demineralization of bone; loss of calcium	Erosion of jaw (phossy jaw)
Potassium	Leafy vegetables, cantaloupe, lima beans, potatoes, bananas, milk, meats, coffee, tea	Fluid balance; nerve transmission; acid-base balance	Muscle cramps; irregular cardiac rhythm; mental confusion; loss of appetite; can be life-threatening	None if kidneys function normally; poor kidney function causes potassium buildup and cardiac arrhythmias
Sulfur	Obtained as part of dietary protein, and present in food preservatives	Acid-based balance; liver function	Unlikely to occur with adequate dietary intake	Unknown
Sodium	Common salt	Acid-based balance; body water balance; nerve function	Muscle cramps; mental apathy; reduced appetite	High blood pressure
Chlorine (chloride)	Part of salt-containing food; some vegetables and fruits	Important part of extracellular fluids	Unlikely to occur with adequately dietary intake	With sodium, contributes to high blood pressure
Magnesium	Whole grains, green leafy vegetables	Activates enzymes in protein synthesis	Growth failure; behavioral disturbances; weakness, spasms	Diarrhea
Trace				
Iron	Eggs, lean meats, legumes, whole grains, green leafy vegetables	Constituent of hemoglobin and enzymes involved in energy metabolism	Iron deficiency anemia (weakness, reduced resistance to infection)	Siderosis; cirrhosis of liver
Fluorine	Drinking water, tea, seafood	May be important to maintain bone structure	Higher frequency of tooth decay	Mottling of teeth; increased bone density; neurologic disturbances
Zinc	Widely distributed in foods	Constituent of digestive enzymes	Growth failure; small sex glands	Fever, nausea, vomiting, diarrhea
Copper	Meats, drinking water	Constituent of enzymes associated with iron metabolism	Anemia, bone changes (rare in humans)	Rare metabolic condition (Wilson's disease)
Selenium	Seafood, meat, grains	Functions in close association with vitamin E	Anemia (rare)	Gastrointestinal disorders; lung irritation
Iodine (iodide)	Marine fish and shellfish, dairy products, vegetables, iodized salt	Constituent of thyroid hormones	Goiter (enlarged thyroid)	Very high intakes depress thyroid activity
Chromium	Legumes, cereals, organ meats, fats, vegetable oils, meats, whole grains	Constituent of some enzymes; involved in glucose and energy metabolism	Rarely reported in humans; impaired glucose metabolism	Inhibition of enzymes; occupational exposures; skin and kidney damage

[a]Food and Nutrition Board, National Academy of Sciences, 2002. (http://www.nal.usda.gov/fnic/etext/000105.html)

Box 2–7 • CLOSE UP

CHEMICAL CUISINE: USER BEWARE

Factory-made foods have made chemical additives a significant part of the diet. It is important to identify and know what these chemicals do, which ones are safe, and which are poorly tested or dangerous. Below, we list products that research suggests may be unsafe in the amounts consumed or that have been poorly tested. Products in the AVOID column are known to cause problems in humans. From: Center for Science in the Public Interest. Washington, D.C. (*http://www.cspinet.org/*)

CAUTION ADVISED

ARTIFICIAL COLORINGS [RED NO. 40 (most widely used food dye, mostly in junk foods); YELLOW NO. 5 (second most widely used dye; causes allergic reactions, primarily in aspirin-sensitive persons; the only dye that must be labeled by name on food label)]

ASPARTAME [Artificial sweetener (drink mixes, diet pop, gelatin desserts, other foods); made up of two amino acids; was thought to be perfect artificial sweetener, but recent links to cancer and hyperactivity in some individuals raise concerns]

CARRAGEENAN [Thickening and stabilizing agent (ice cream, jelly, chocolate milk, infant formula); obtained from seaweed; research with animals shows problems; tests with humans appear safe]

HEPTYL PARABEN [Preservative in beer and non-carbonated soft drinks]

INVERT SUGAR [Sweetener (candy, soft drinks); combined from dextrose and fructose; contributes to tooth decay; empty calories]

MONOSODIUM GLUTAMATE (MSG) [Flavor enhancer (soup, seafood, poultry, cheese, sauces, stews); amino acid, which in sensitive individuals can cause "Chinese Restaurant Syndrome," a burning sensation in the back of the neck, forearms, tightness of the chest, headache]

PHOSPHORIC ACID; PHOSPHATES [Acidulant, chelating agent, buffer, emulsifier, nutrient, discoloration inhibitor (baked goods, cheese, powdered foods, cured meat, soda pop, dehydrated potatoes); phosphates are non-toxic, but their widespread use has led to dietary imbalances that may contribute to osteoporosis]

AVOID

ARTIFICIAL COLORINGS [Most are synthetic chemicals that do not occur in nature. Some safer than others. Colorings are not listed by name on labels. Because colorings are used almost solely in foods of low nutritional value (candy, pop, gelatin desserts), avoid all artificially colored foods. Some colorings may cause hyperactivity in sensitive children. Avoid the following coloring agents: BLUE NO. 1 (beverages, candy, baked goods); BLUE NO. 2 (pet food, beverages, candy); CITRUS RED NO. 2 (skin of some Florida oranges only); GREEN NO. 3 (candy, beverages); RED NO. 3 (cherries in fruit cocktail, candy, baked goods); YELLOW NO. 6 (beverages, sausage, baked goods, candy, gelatin)]

BROMINATED VEGETABLE OIL (BVO) [Emulsifier, clouding agent in soft drinks; keeps flavor oils in suspension and gives a cloudy appearance to citrus-flavored soft drinks.]

BUTYLATED HYDROXYTOLUENE (BHT) [In cereals, chewing gum, potato chips, oils; retards rancidity in oils]

PROPYL GALLATE [In vegetable oil, meat products, potato sticks, chicken soup base, chewing gum; retards spoilage of fats and oils and often used with BHT; need more studies on safety]

QUININE [Flavoring agent (tonic water, quinine water, bitter lemon); poorly tested; may cause birth defects]

SACCHARIN [Artificial sweetener (drink mixes, diet pop, gelatin desserts, other foods); 350 times sweeter than sugar; may cause cancer]

SODIUM CAUSING CHEMICALS (NITROSAMINES) [particularly in bacon]; SODIUM NITRATE [Preservative, coloring, flavoring (bacon, ham, hot dogs, lunch meats, smoked fish, corned beef); leads to the formation of small amounts of potent cancer-causing agents]

SULFUR DIOXIDE, SODIUM BISULFITE [Preservative, bleach (sliced fruit, wine, processed potatoes); prevents discoloration; destroys vitamin B_1 and causes severe reactions, especially in asthmatics; implicated in numerous deaths]

Whereas vitamins activate chemical processes without becoming part of the byproducts of the reactions they catalyze, minerals often become part of the body's structures and existing chemicals. Minerals serve three broad roles:

1. They provide *structure* in forming bones and teeth.
2. In terms of *function*, they help maintain normal heart rhythm, muscle contractility, neural conductivity, and acid-base balance.
3. They help *regulate* cellular metabolism by becoming part of enzymes and hormones that modulate cellular activity.

Figure 2.14 lists minerals that participate in catabolic and anabolic cellular processes. Minerals activate numerous reactions releasing energy during carbohydrate, fat, and protein catabolism. Minerals help to synthesize biologic nutrients—glycogen from glucose, triacylglycerols from fatty acids and glycerol, and proteins from amino acids. Without the essential minerals, the fine balance would be disrupted between catabolism and anabolism. Minerals also form important constituents of hormones. For example, an inadequate thyroxine production from iodine deficiency significantly slows resting metabolism. In extreme cases, this predisposes a person to obesity. The synthesis of insulin, the hormone that facilitates glucose uptake by cells, requires zinc (as do approximately 100 enzymes), whereas the mineral chlorine forms hydrochloric acid.

Minerals and Physical Activity

Food sources in a well-balanced diet readily provide the minerals required by the body. In the next sections, we de-

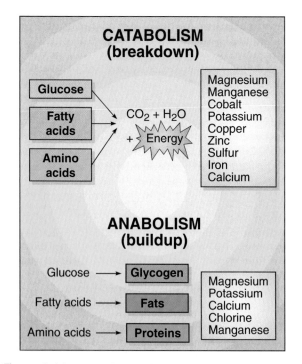

Figure 2.14   Minerals contribute to macronutrient catabolism (breakdown) and anabolism (build-up).

scribe specific functions for important minerals related to physical activity.

Calcium   Calcium, the most abundant mineral in the body, combines with phosphorus to form bones and teeth. These two minerals represent about 75% of the body's total mineral content of about 2.5% of body mass. In ionized form (about 1% of the body's 1200 mg of calcium), calcium plays an important role in muscle action, blood clotting, nerve impulse transmission, activation of several enzymes, synthesis of calciferol (active form of vitamin D), and fluid transport across cell membranes.

Osteoporosis: Calcium Intake and Exercise   The skeleton contains more than 99% of the body's total calcium. With calcium deficiency, the body draws on its calcium reserves in bone to replace the deficit. With prolonged negative imbalance, osteoporosis (literally meaning "porous bones") eventually develops as the bones lose calcium mass (mineral content) and calcium concentration (mineral density) and progressively become porous and brittle. Osteoporosis affects persons of all ages.

Osteoporosis currently afflicts 28 million Americans, of whom 80% to 90% are women, with another 18 million individuals with low bone mass (osteopenia). Fifty percent of all women eventually develop osteoporosis, owing to their relatively low calcium intake and the loss of the calcium-conserving hormone estrogen at menopause. Men are not immune, as 1.5 to 2.0 million men (1 in 8 men older than 50 years) suffer from this disease. Osteoporosis is a silent disease, sometimes going undetected for many years until a fracture occurs. It accounts for more than 1.55 million fractures yearly, including 700,000 spinal fractures, 250,000 wrist fractures, 300,000 hip fractures, and 300,000 fractures at other sites. Among women older than age 60, osteoporosis has reached near-epidemic proportions. On average, 24% of hip-fracture patients over 50 years of age die in the year following their fracture.

Dietary Calcium Crucial   As a general guideline, adolescent boys and girls (9 to 13 years) and young adult males and females (14 to 18 years) require 1300 mg of calcium daily or about as much calcium in six 8-oz glasses of milk. For adults between the ages of 19 and 50 years, the daily requirement decreases to 1000 mg. Although growing children require more calcium per unit body mass on a daily basis than adults, many adults remain deficient in calcium intake. For example, the typical adult's daily calcium intake ranges between 500 and 700 mg. More than 75% of adults consume less than the recommended amount, and about 25% of females in the United States consume less than 300 mg of calcium daily. Among athletes, female dancers, gymnasts, and endurance competitors are most prone to calcium dietary insufficiency.

Exercise Helps   *Regular exercise slows the rate of skeletal aging.* Regardless of age or gender, young children and adults who maintain physically active lifestyles have significantly greater bone mass compared with sedentary counterparts. For men and women who remain physically active, even at ages 70 and 80 years, bone mass exceeds that of inactive individuals of similar age. The decline in vigorous exercise as one ages closely parallels the age-related loss of bone mass.

Exercise of moderate intensity provides a safe and potent stimulus to maintain and even increase bone mass. **Weight-bearing exercise** represents a particularly desirable form of exercise; examples include walking, running, dancing, and rope skipping. Resistance training, which generates significant muscular force against the long bones of the body, also proves beneficial. The benefits of exercise depend on adequate calcium availability for the bone-forming process.

Female Athlete Triad: An Unexpected Problem for Women Who Train Intensely

A paradox exists between exercise and bone dynamics for athletic, premenopausal women. Women who train intensely and emphasize weight loss often engage in **disordered eating behaviors**, which are serious ailments that, in extreme cases, cause life-threatening complications (see *How to Recognize Warning Signs of Disordered Eating* in Chapter 16). Disordered eating decreases energy availability, reducing body mass and body fat to a point where the menstrual cycle becomes irregular (**oligomenorrhea**) or ceases, a condition termed **secondary amenorrhea**. The tightly integrated continuum that begins with disordered eating and that results in energy drain, amenorrhea, and eventual osteoporosis, reflects the clinical entity labeled the **female athlete triad** (**Fig. 2.15**).

Many girls and young women engaged in sports have at least one of the triad's disorders, particularly disordered eating behavior. Female athletes of the 1970s and 1980s believed the loss of normal menstruation reflected hard training and the inevitable consequence of athletic success. The prevalence of amenorrhea among female athletes in body weight-related sports (distance running, gymnastics, ballet, cheerleading, figure skating, and body building) probably ranges between 25% and 65%, whereas no more than 5% of the general population has this condition.

Sodium, Potassium, and Chlorine

The minerals sodium, potassium, and chlorine, collectively termed **electrolytes**, dissolve in the body as electrically charged particles called **ions**. Sodium and chlorine represent the chief minerals contained in blood plasma and extracellular fluid. Electrolytes modulate fluid movement within the body's various fluid compartments. This allows for a constant, well-regulated exchange of nutrients and waste products between the cell and its external fluid environment. Potassium represents the chief intracellular mineral.

Establishing proper electrical gradients across cell membranes represents the most important function for sodium and potassium ions. A difference in electrical balance between the cell's interior and exterior allows nerve impulse transmission, muscle stimulation and contraction, and proper gland functioning. Electrolytes maintain plasma membrane permeability and also regulate the acid and base qualities of body fluids, particularly blood.

Sodium: How Much Is Enough? The wide distribution of sodium in foods makes it easy to obtain the daily requirement without adding salt to foods. In the United States, sodium intake regularly exceeds the daily level recommended for adults of 2400 mg or the amount of one heaping teaspoon of table salt (sodium makes up about 40% of salt). The typical Western diet contains about 4500 mg of sodium (8 to 12 g of salt) each day. This represents 10 times the 500 mg of sodium the body actually needs. Heavy reliance on table salt in processing, curing, cooking, seasoning, and preserving common foods accounts for the large sodium intake. Aside from table salt, common sodium-rich dietary sources include monosodium glutamate (MSG), soy sauce, condiments, canned foods, baking soda, and baking powder.

Give the recommended calcium intake for a college-age male and female.

Male:

Female:

Name the components of the female athlete triad.

1.

2.

3.

Name 3 electrolyte minerals.

1.

2.

3.

FOR YOUR INFORMATION

Megavitamins

Although physically active individuals who eat a well-balanced diet do not need additional vitamins, most nutritionists believe that taking a multivitamin capsule that contains the recommended allowance of each vitamin does little harm. For some people, the psychological effects may even be beneficial. Some athletes "supercharge" with megavitamins, or doses of at least tenfold and up to 1000 times the RDA to improve exercise performance. This practice is potentially harmful, except in medically supervised treatment of a specific vitamin deficiency.

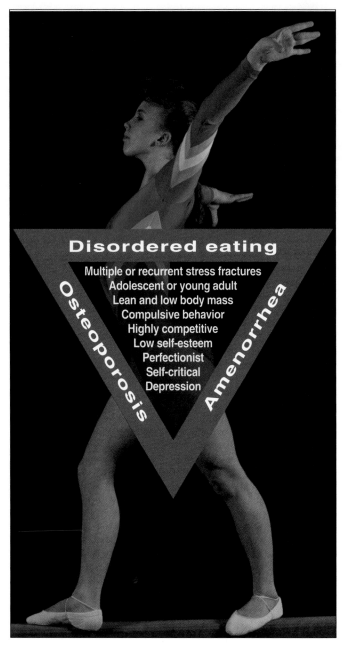

Disordered eating

Multiple or recurrent stress fractures
Adolescent or young adult
Lean and low body mass
Compulsive behavior
Highly competitive
Low self-esteem
Perfectionist
Self-critical
Depression

Osteoporosis   Amenorrhea

Figure 2.15 Female athlete triad: disordered eating, amenorrhea, and osteoporosis.

A normal sodium balance in the body usually occurs throughout a range of dietary intakes. For some individuals, excessive sodium intake becomes inadequately regulated. A chronic excess of dietary sodium can increase fluid volume and possibly increase peripheral vascular resistance; both factors could elevate blood pressure to levels that pose a health risk. **Sodium-induced hypertension** occurs in about one-third of hypertensive individuals in the United States.

For decades, the first-line of defense in treating high blood pressure attempted to eliminate excess sodium from the diet. Conventional wisdom maintains that by reducing sodium intake, perhaps the body's sodium and fluid levels would be reduced, thereby lowering blood pressure. Although sodium restriction does not lower blood pressure in people with normal blood pressure (and only mini-

mally affects those with high blood pressure), certain individuals remain "**salt sensitive**"—by reducing dietary sodium, their blood pressure decreases.

Iron   The body normally contains between 3 to 5 g (about one-sixth oz) of iron. Of this amount, approximately 80% exists in functionally active compounds, predominantly combined with hemoglobin in red blood cells. This iron-protein compound increases the oxygen-carrying capacity of blood approximately 65 times. Aside from its role in oxygen transport in blood, iron serves as a structural component of myoglobin (about 5% of total iron), a compound similar to hemoglobin that stores oxygen for release within muscle cells. Small amounts of iron also exist in cytochromes, the specialized substances that transfer cellular energy.

Iron Stores   About 20% of the body's iron does not combine in functionally active compounds. **Hemosiderin** and **ferritin** constitute the iron stores in the liver, spleen, and bone marrow. These stores replenish iron lost from the functional compounds; they also provide the iron reserve during periods of insufficient dietary iron intake. A plasma protein, **transferrin**, transports iron from ingested food and damaged red blood cells to tissues in need. Plasma levels of transferrin often reflect the adequacy of the current iron intake.

Athletes should include normal amounts of iron-rich foods in their daily diets. People with inadequate iron intake or with limited rates of iron absorption or high rates of iron loss often develop a reduced concentration of hemoglobin in red blood cells. This extreme condition of iron insufficiency, commonly called **iron deficiency anemia**, produces general sluggishness, loss of appetite, and reduced capacity to sustain even mild exercise. "Iron therapy" normalizes hemoglobin content of the blood and exercise capacity. **Table 2.8** lists recommendations for iron intake for children and adults.

Intestinal absorption of iron varies closely with iron need, yet considerable variation in absorption (bioavailability) occurs in relation to diet composition. For example, the small intestine usually absorbs between 2% and 10% of iron from plants (non-heme iron), whereas iron absorption from animal sources (heme iron) increases to between 10% and 35%.

Of Concern to Vegetarians   *The relatively low bioavailability of non-heme iron places women on vegetarian-type diets at risk for developing iron insufficiency.* Female vegetarian runners have a poorer iron status than counterparts who consume the same quantity of iron from predominantly animal sources. Including vitamin C-rich food in the diet enhances dietary iron bioavailability. This occurs because ascorbic acid increases the solubility of non-heme iron, making it available for absorption at the alkaline pH of the small intestine. The ascorbic acid in one glass of orange juice, for example, stimulates a threefold increase in non-heme iron absorption from a breakfast meal.

Females: A Population at Risk   Inadequate iron intake frequently occurs among young children, teenagers, and females of childbearing age, including physically active women.

Iron loss during a menstrual cycle ranges between 5 and 45 mg. This produces an additional 5-mg dietary iron requirement daily for premenopausal females, increasing the average monthly dietary iron intake need by about 150

Table 2·8	Recommended Dietary Allowances for Iron[a]	
	AGE (y)	**IRON (mg/d)**
Children	1–3	7
	4–8	10
Males	9–13	8
	14–18	11
	19–70	8
Females	9–13	8
	14–18	15
	19–50	18
	51–70	8
Pregnant	<19	27
	≥19	27
Lactating	<19	10
	≥19	9

[a]Dietary Reference Intakes: Recommended Intakes for Individuals. Food and Nutrition Board. Institute of Medicine. National Academies, 2002. (http://www.iom.edu/Object.File/Master/21/372/0.pdf)

Questions & Notes

Give the recommended iron intake for a college-age male and female.

Male:

Female:

FOR YOUR INFORMATION

Regular Exercise and Increased Muscle Strength Slow Skeletal Aging
Moderate- to high-intensity aerobic exercise (weight-bearing) performed 3 days per week for 50 to 60 minutes each builds bone and retards its rate of loss. Muscle-strengthening exercises also benefit bone mass. Individuals with greater back strength and those who train regularly with resistance exercise have a greater spinal bone mineral content than weaker and untrained individuals.

FOR YOUR INFORMATION

Six Principles to Promote Bone Health
1. *Specificity:* Exercise provides a local osteogenic effect
2. *Overload:* Progressively increasing exercise intensity promotes continued improvement
3. *Initial Values:* Individuals with the smallest total bone mass have the greatest potential for improvement
4. *Diminishing Returns:* As one approaches the biologic ceiling for bone density, further gains require greater effort
5. *More Not Necessarily Better:* Bone cells become desensitized in response to prolonged mechanical-loading sessions
6. *Reversibility:* Discontinuing exercise overload reverses the positive osteogenic effects of exercise

mg. The small intestine absorbs only about 15% of ingested iron, depending on one's iron status, form of iron ingested, and meal composition. Thus, an additional 20 to 25 mg of iron becomes available each month (from the additional 150-mg monthly dietary requirement) for synthesizing red blood cells lost during menstruation. Not surprisingly, 30% to 50% of American women experience significant dietary iron insufficiencies from menstrual blood loss combined with a limited dietary iron intake.

Athletes and Iron Supplements   *If an individual's diet contains the recommended iron intake, supplementing with iron does not increase hemoglobin, hematocrit, or other measures of iron status.* Any increase in iron loss with exercise training (coupled with poor dietary habits) in adolescent and premenopausal women could strain an already limited iron reserve. This does not mean that individuals involved in strenuous training should take supplementary iron or that indicators of sports anemia result from dietary iron deficiency or exercise-induced iron loss. Iron overconsumption or overabsorption could potentially cause harm. Supplements should not be used indiscriminately; excessive iron can accumulate to toxic levels and contribute to diabetes, liver disease, and heart and joint damage. Iron excess may even facilitate growth of latent cancers and infectious organisms. Athletes' iron status should be monitored by periodic evaluation of hematologic characteristics and iron reserves.

Minerals and Exercise Performance

Consuming mineral supplements above recommended levels on an acute or chronic basis does not benefit exercise performance or enhance training responsiveness. Loss of water and the mineral salts sodium chloride and potassium chloride in sweat poses an important challenge in prolonged, hot-weather exercise. Excessive water and electrolyte loss impairs heat tolerance and exercise performance and can trigger heat cramps, heat exhaustion, or heat stroke. The yearly number of heat-related deaths during spring and summer football practice provides a tragic illustration of the importance of replacing fluids and electrolytes. During practice or competition, an athlete may sweat up to 5 kg of water. This corresponds to about 8.0 g of salt depletion because each kg (1 L) of sweat contains about 1.5 g of salt (of which 40% represents sodium). Replacement of water lost through sweating becomes the crucial and immediate need.

Defense Against Mineral Loss in Exercise

Vigorous exercise triggers a rapid and coordinated release of the hormones **vasopressin** and **aldosterone** and the enzyme **renin** to minimize sodium and water loss through the kidneys and sweat. An increase in sodium conservation by the kidneys occurs even under extreme conditions like running a marathon in warm, humid weather where sweat output often reaches 2 L per hour. Adding a slight amount of salt to fluid ingested or food consumed usually replenishes electrolytes lost in sweat. In one study of runners during a 20-day road race in Hawaii, plasma minerals remained normal when the athletes consumed an unrestricted diet without mineral supplements. This finding (and the findings of others) indicates that ingesting "athletic drinks" provides no special benefit in replacing the minerals lost through sweating compared with ingesting the same minerals in a well-balanced diet. Taking extra salt may prove beneficial for prolonged exercise in the heat when fluid loss exceeds 4 or 5 kg. This can be achieved by drinking a 0.1% to 0.2% salt solution (adding 0.3 tsp of table salt per L of water). Intense exercise during heat stress can produce a mild potassium deficiency. A diet that contains the recommended amount of this mineral corrects any deficiencies. Drinking an 8-oz glass of orange or tomato juice replaces the calcium, potassium, and magnesium lost in 3 L (7 lb) of sweat, a sweat loss not likely to occur if an individual performs less than 60 minutes of vigorous exercise.

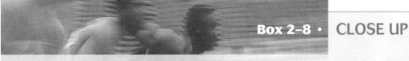

Box 2–8 • CLOSE UP

EXERCISE-INDUCED ANEMIA: FACT OR FICTION?

Research has focused on the influence of hard training on the body's iron status, primarily due to interest in endurance sports and increased participation of women in such activities. The term "**sports anemia**" frequently describes reduced hemoglobin levels approaching **clinical anemia** (12 g per 100 mL of blood for women and 14 g per 100 mL for men) attributable to intense training. Some researchers maintain that exercise training creates an added demand for iron that often exceeds its intake. This taxes iron reserves, which eventually slows hemoglobin synthesis and/or reduces iron-containing compounds within the cell's energy transfer system. Individuals susceptible to an "iron drain" could experience reduced exercise capacity because of iron's crucial role in oxygen transport and utilization.

Heavy training could theoretically create an augmented iron demand (facilitating development of clinical anemia). This loss of iron could come from iron loss in sweat and hemoglobin loss in urine due to red blood cell destruction with increased temperature, spleen activity, and circulation rates, and from mechanical trauma (**footstrike hemolysis**) from the feet repetitively pounding the running surface. Gastrointestinal bleeding also may occur with long-distance running. Such iron loss, regardless of cause, stresses the body's iron reserves for synthesizing 260 billion new red blood cells daily in the bone marrow of the skull, upper arm, sternum, ribs, spine, pelvis, and upper legs. Iron losses pose an additional burden to women because they have the greatest iron requirement yet lowest iron intake.

Suboptimal hemoglobin concentrations and hematocrits occur frequently among endurance athletes, thus supporting the possibility of an exercise-induced anemia. On closer scrutiny, however, transient reductions in hemoglobin concentration occur in the early phase of training and then return toward pretraining values.

A decrease in hemoglobin concentration with training parallels the disproportionately large expansion in plasma volume compared with total hemoglobin. Thus, total hemoglobin (an important factor in endurance performance) remains the same or increases somewhat with training, yet hemoglobin concentration (expressed mg per 100 mL blood) decreases in the expanding plasma volume.

Aerobic capacity and exercise performance normally improve with training despite the apparent dilution of hemoglobin. Although vigorous exercise may induce some mechanical destruction of red blood cells (including minimal iron loss in sweat), these factors do not appear to strain an athlete's iron reserves to precipitate clinical anemia, as long as iron intake remains within the normal range. Applying stringent criteria for what constitutes anemia and insufficiency of iron reserves makes "true" sports anemia much less prevalent among highly trained athletes than believed. For male collegiate runners and swimmers, large changes in training volume and intensity during various phases of the competitive season did not reveal the early stages of anemia. Data from female athletes also confirm that the prevalence of iron deficiency anemia did *not* differ in comparison with specific athletic groups or with nonathletic controls.

SUMMARY

1. Vitamins neither supply energy nor contribute to body mass. These organic substances serve crucial functions in almost all bodily processes and must be obtained from food or dietary supplementation.

2. Thirteen known vitamins are classified as either water soluble or fat soluble. Vitamins A, D, E, and K comprise the fat-soluble vitamins; vitamin C and the B-complex vitamins constitute the water-soluble vitamins.

3. Excess fat-soluble vitamins can accumulate in body tissues and increase to toxic concentrations. Except in relatively rare instances, excess water-soluble vitamins remain nontoxic and eventually pass in the urine.

4. Vitamins regulate metabolism, facilitate energy release, and serve important functions in bone formation and tissue synthesis.

5. Vitamins C and E and β-carotene serve key protective antioxidant functions. A diet with appropriate levels of these micronutrients reduces the potential for free radical damage (oxidative stress) and may protect against heart disease and cancer.

6. Vitamin supplementation above the RDA does not improve exercise performance or the potential for sustaining hard, physical training. Serious illness occurs from regularly consuming excess fat-soluble and, in some instances, water-soluble vitamins.

7. Approximately 4% of body mass consists of 22 elements called minerals. They distribute in all body tissues and fluids.

8. Minerals occur freely in nature, in the waters of rivers, lakes, oceans, and in soil. The root system of plants absorbs minerals; minerals eventually incorporate into the tissues of animals that consume plants.

9. Minerals function primarily in metabolism as important parts of enzymes. Minerals provide structure to bones and teeth and aid in synthesizing the biologic macronutrients—glycogen, fat, and protein.

10. A balanced diet provides adequate mineral intake, except in geographic locations with inadequate iodine in the soil.

11. Osteoporosis has reached epidemic proportions among older individuals, especially women. Adequate calcium intake and regular weight-bearing exercise and/or resistance training protect against bone loss at any age.

12. Women who train intensely often do not match energy intake to energy output. Reduced body weight and body fat can adversely affect menstruation, often causing advanced bone loss at an early age. Restoration of normal menses does not necessarily restore bone mass.

13. About 40% of American women of childbearing age have dietary iron insufficiency. This could lead to iron-deficiency anemia, which negatively affects aerobic exercise performance and ability to perform heavy training. For women on vegetarian-type diets, the relatively low bioavailability of non-heme iron increases risk for iron insufficiency. Vitamin C (in food or supplement form) increases intestinal non-heme iron absorption.

14. Regular physical activity probably does not create a significant drain on the body's iron reserves. If it does, then females (greatest iron requirement and lowest iron intake) could show increased risk for anemia. Assessment of the body's iron status should evaluate hematologic characteristics and iron reserves.

15. Excessive sweating during exercise produces significant losses of body water and related minerals; these should be replaced during and following exercise. Sweat loss during exercise usually does not increase mineral requirements above recommended values.

THOUGHT QUESTIONS

1. Discuss some specific conditions that justify vitamin and mineral supplementation.

2. Discuss factors that might contribute to sex-specific recommendations for vitamin and mineral intakes.

3. Outline the dynamics of bone loss and give suggestions to high school females regarding protection against osteoporosis.

4. If vitamin and minerals are intimately involved in the combustion of the macronutrients for energy, why isn't the recommended dietary intake of these chemicals related to daily activity level?

WATER IN THE BODY

Age, gender, and body composition influence an individual's body water content, which can range from 40% to 70% of total body mass. Water constitutes 72% of muscle weight and approximately 50% of the weight of body fat (adipose tissue). Thus, differences among individuals in relative percentage of total body water largely result from variations in body composition (i.e., differences in fat-free versus fat tissue).

The body contains two fluid "compartments." The first compartment, **intracellular**, refers to fluid inside cells; the second compartment, **extracellular**, includes (1) blood plasma (about 20% of total extracellular fluid) and (2) interstitial fluids, which primarily comprise fluid flowing in the microscopic spaces between cells. Interstitial fluid also includes lymph, saliva, fluids in the eyes, fluids secreted by glands and the digestive tract, fluids that bathe the nerves of the spinal cord, and fluids excreted from the skin and kidneys. *Much of the fluid lost through sweating comes from extracellular fluid, predominantly blood plasma.*

Describe the term "sports anemia" and those most susceptible.

Name the 2 fluid compartments of the body.

  1.

  2.

Functions of Body Water

Water serves six important functions:

1. Water provides the body's transport and reactive medium.
2. Diffusion of gases always takes place across surfaces moistened by water.
3. Transport of nutrients and gases occurs in aqueous solution, whereas waste products leave the body through the water in urine and feces.
4. Water, due to its significant heat-stabilizing qualities, absorbs considerable heat with only minimal changes in temperature.
5. Watery fluids lubricate joints, keeping bony surfaces from grinding against each other.
6. Being noncompressible, water provides structure and form to the body through the turgor it imparts to diverse tissues.

Water Balance: Intake Versus Output

The water content of the body remains relatively stable over time. Although considerable water loss occurs in physically active individuals, appropriate fluid intake rapidly restores any imbalance. **Figure 2.16** displays the sources of water intake and water loss (output). The bottom panel illustrates that fluid balance can change dramatically during exercise, especially in a hot, humid environment.

Water Intake In a normal environment, a fairly sedentary adult requires about 2.5 L of water each day. For an active person in a warm environment, the water requirement often increases to between 5 and 10 L daily. Three sources provide this water:

1. Liquids
2. Foods
3. Metabolic processes

The average individual normally consumes 1200 mL (41 oz) of water daily. Fluid intake can increase 5 or 6 times above normal during exercise and thermal stress. At the extreme, an individual lost 13.6 kg (30 lb) of water weight during a 2-day, 17-hour, 55-mile run across the desert in Death Valley, California. However, proper fluid ingestion with salt supplements kept body weight

For Your Information

Hydration Terminology
- *Euhydration:* Normal daily water variation
- *Hyperhydration:* New steady-state condition of increased water content
- *Hypohydration:* New steady-state condition of decreased water content
- *Rehydration:* Process of gaining water from hypohydrated state toward euhydration

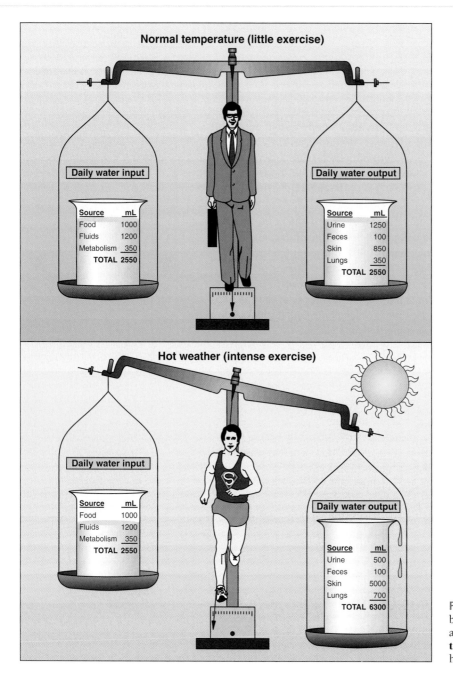

Figure 2.16 Water balance in the body. **Top:** Little or no exercise in normal ambient temperature and humidity. **Bottom:** Moderate to intense exercise in a hot, humid environment.

loss to only 1.4 kg. In this example, fluid loss and replenishment represented between 3.5 and 4 gallons of liquid!

Most foods, particularly fruits and vegetables, contain considerable water (e.g., lettuce, watermelon and cantaloupe, pickles, green beans, and broccoli); in contrast, butter, oils, dried meats, and chocolate, cookies, and cakes contain relatively little water.

Catabolizing food molecules for energy forms carbon dioxide and water. For a sedentary person, this **metabolic water** provides about 25% of the daily water requirement. This includes 55 g of water from the complete breakdown of 100 g of carbohydrate, 100 g of water from 100 g of protein breakdown, and 107 g of water from 100 g of fat catab-

olism. Additionally, each gram of glycogen joins with 2.7 g of water as the glucose units link together; glycogen subsequently releases this water during its catabolism for energy.

Water Output   The body loses water in four ways:

1. In urine
2. Through the skin
3. As water vapor in expired air
4. In feces

The kidneys normally reabsorb about 99% of the 140 to 160 L of filtrate formed each day, leaving from 1000 to 1500 mL or about 1.5 quarts of urine for excretion daily. Every 1 g of solute (e.g., the urea end-product of protein breakdown) eliminated by the kidneys requires about 15 mL of water. From a practical standpoint, using large quantities of protein for energy via a high-protein diet accelerates dehydration during exercise.

A small amount of water (perhaps 350 mL), termed **insensible perspiration**, continually seeps from the deeper tissues through the skin to the body's surface. Subcutaneous sweat glands also produce water loss through the skin. Evaporation of sweat's water component provides the refrigeration mechanism to cool the body. Daily sweat rate under most conditions amounts to between 500 and 700 mL. This by no means reflects sweating capacity; for example, a well-trained, acclimatized person produces up to 12 L of sweat (equivalent of 12 kg) at a rate of 1 L per hour during prolonged exercise in a hot environment.

Insensible water loss of 250 to 350 mL per day occurs through small water droplets in exhaled air. This loss results from the complete moistening of all inspired air passing down the pulmonary airways. Exercise affects this source of water loss. For physically active individuals, the respiratory passages release 2 to 5 mL of water each minute during strenuous exercise, depending on climatic conditions. Ventilatory water loss happens least in hot, humid weather and most in cold temperatures (inspired air contains little moisture) or at altitude because the less dense inspired air volumes (which require humidification) significantly increase compared with sea-level conditions.

Intestinal elimination produces between 100 and 200 mL of water loss because water constitutes approximately 70% of fecal matter. The remainder comprises nondigestible material, including bacteria from the digestive process, and the residues of digestive juices from the intestine, stomach, and pancreas. With diarrhea or vomiting, water loss can increase to between 1500 and 5000 mL.

Figure 2.17 shows that, in addition to the 2.0 L of water ingested daily by the typical sedentary adult, saliva, gastric secretions, bile, and pancreatic and intestinal secretions contribute an additional 7 L each day. This means that the intestinal tract takes up a total daily water quantity of about 9 L. Of concern to athletes is the fact that ingesting concentrated fluid solutions blunts the rate of water absorption and increases the potential for gastrointestinal distress. This can occur when ingesting salt tablets, concentrated mixtures of simple amino acids, or a

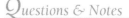

Questions & Notes

Give the amount of salt needed per liter of water to make a "homemade" fluid replacement drink.

List the 4 ways water is lost from the body.

1.

2.

3.

4.

Give the major physiologic defense against overheating.

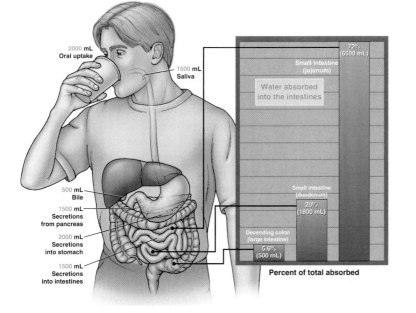

Figure 2.17   Estimated daily volumes of water that enter the small and large intestines of a sedentary adult and the volumes absorbed by each component of the intestinal tract. (Data from Gisolfi, C.V., and Lamb, D.R., (eds.). *Perspectives in Exercise and Sports Medicine: Fluid Homeostasis During Exercise*. Indianapolis: Benchmark Press, 1990.)

FOR YOUR INFORMATION

Don't Rely on Oral Temperature
Oral temperature does not usually provide an accurate measure of deep body temperature after strenuous exercise. Large and consistent differences occurred between oral and rectal temperatures; for example, the average rectal temperature of 103.5°F after a 14-mile race in a tropical climate differed from a "normal" 98°F when temperature was assessed orally. This 5.5°F discrepancy partly results from evaporative cooling of the mouth and airways during relatively high ventilatory volumes immediately after heavy exercise.

"sports drink" containing a large percentage of simple sugars and minerals (see page 115).

WATER REQUIREMENT IN EXERCISE

The loss of body water represents the most serious consequence of profuse sweating. Three factors determine water loss through sweating:

1. Severity of physical activity
2. Environmental temperature
3. Humidity

The major physiologic defense against overheating comes from evaporation of sweat from the skin's surface. The evaporative loss of 1 L of sweat releases about 600 kCal of heat energy from the body to the environment. **Relative humidity** (water content of the ambient air) impacts the efficiency of the sweating mechanism in temperature regulation. At 100% relative humidity, the ambient air becomes completely saturated with water vapor. This blocks evaporation of fluid from the skin surface to the air, thus minimizing this important avenue for body cooling. When this happens, sweat beads on the skin and eventually rolls off without generating a cooling effect. The air can hold considerable moisture, and fluid evaporates rapidly from the skin. This enables the sweat mechanism to function at optimal efficiency to regulate body temperature. Interestingly, sweat loss equal to 2% to 3% of body mass decreases plasma volume. This amount of fluid loss strains circulatory functions and ultimately impairs exercise capacity and thermoregulation. Chapter 15 presents a more comprehensive discussion of thermoregulatory dynamics during exercise in hot climates.

Exertional Heat Stroke

Heat stroke, the most serious and complex heat-stress malady, requires immediate medical attention. Heat stroke syndrome reflects a failure of heat-regulating mechanisms triggered by excessively high body temperatures. With thermoregulatory failure, sweating usually ceases, the skin becomes dry and hot, body temperature increases to 41°C or higher, and the circulatory system becomes strained. Unfortunately, subtle symptoms often confound the complexity of exertional hyperthermia. Instead of ceasing, sweating can occur during intense exercise (e.g., 10-km running race) in young, hydrated, and highly motivated individuals. Because of high metabolic heat production, the body's heat gain greatly exceeds avenues for heat loss. If left untreated, circulatory collapse and damage to the central nervous system and other organs can lead to death.

Heat stroke represents a medical emergency. While awaiting medical treatment, only aggressive treatment to rapidly lower elevated core temperature can avert death; the magnitude and duration of hyperthermia determine organ damage and mortality. Immediate treatment includes alcohol rubs and application of ice packs. Whole-body cold- or ice-water immersion remains the most effective treatment for a collapsed hyperthermic athlete.

Practical Recommendations for Fluid Replacement in Exercise

Depending on environmental conditions, total sweat loss during a marathon run at world record pace averages about 5.3 L (12 lb). The fluid loss corresponds to an overall reduction of 6% to 8% of body mass. *Fluids must be consumed regularly during physical activity to avoid dehydration and its life-threatening consequences.*

Fluid replacement maintains plasma volume so that circulation and sweating progress at optimal levels. Ingesting "extra" water before exercising in the heat provides some thermoregulatory protection. Pre-exercise hyperhydration delays dehydration, increases sweating during exercise, and blunts the rise in body temperature compared with exercising without prior fluids. As a practical step, a person should consume 400 to 600 mL (13 to 20 oz) of cold water 10 to 20 minutes before exercising. This prudent practice should be combined with continual fluid replacement during exercise.

Gastric Emptying   The small intestine absorbs fluids after they pass from the stomach. The following seven factors influence gastric emptying:

1. **Fluid temperature.** Cold fluids (5°C; 41°F) empty from the stomach at a faster rate than fluids at body temperature.
2. **Fluid volume.** Keeping fluid volume in the stomach at a relatively high level speeds gastric emptying and may compensate for any inhibitory effects of the beverage's carbohydrate or electrolyte content. Optimizing the effect of stomach volume on gastric emptying occurs by consuming 400 to 600 mL of fluid immediately before exercise. Then, regularly ingesting 150 to 250 mL of fluid (at 15-minute intervals) throughout exercise continually replenishes the fluid passed into the intestine and maintains a large gastric volume during exercise.
3. **Caloric content.** Increased energy content decreases gastric emptying rate.
4. **Fluid osmolarity.** Gastric emptying slows when the ingested fluid contains concentrated electrolytes or simple sugars, whether in the form of glucose, fructose, or sucrose. For example, a 40% sugar solution empties from the stomach at a rate 20% slower than plain water. *As a general rule, between a 5% and 8% carbohydrate-electrolyte beverage consumed during exercise in the heat contributes to temperature regulation and fluid balance as effectively as plain water.* As an added bonus, this drink helps maintain glucose metabolism and glycogen reserves in prolonged exercise.
5. **Exercise intensity.** Exercise does not negatively affect gastric emptying up to an intensity of about 75% of maximum, at which point the stomach's emptying rate becomes restricted.

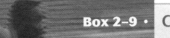

Box 2–9 • CLOSE UP

HOW TO DISTINGUISH BETWEEN HEAT CRAMPS, HEAT EXHAUSTION, AND HEAT STROKE

Human heat dissipation occurs by (1) redistribution of blood from deeper tissues to the periphery and (2) activation of the refrigeration mechanism provided by evaporation of sweat from the surface of the skin and respiratory passages. During heat stress, cardiac output increases, vasoconstriction and vasodilation move central blood volume towards the skin, and thousands of previously dormant capillaries threading through the upper skin layer open to accommodate blood flow. Conduction of heat away from warm blood at the skin's cooled surface provides about 75% of the body's heat-dissipating functions. Heat production during physical activity often strains heat-dissipating mechanisms, especially under high ambient temperature and humidity. This triggers a broad array of physical signs and symptoms collectively termed heat illness, ranging in severity from mild to life threatening.

CONDITION	CAUSES	SIGNS AND SYMPTOMS	PREVENTION
Heat Cramps	Intense, prolonged exercise in the heat; negative Na^+ balance	Tightening cramps, involuntary spasms of active muscles; low serum Na^+	Replenish salt loss; ensure acclimatization
Heat Syncope	Peripheral vasodilation and pooling of venous blood; hypotension; hypohydration	Giddiness; syncope, mostly in upright position during rest or exercise; pallor; high rectal temperature	Ensure acclimatization and fluid replenishment; reduce exertion on hot days; avoid standing
Heat Exhaustion	Cumulative negative water balance	Exhaustion; hypohydration, flushed skin; reduced sweating in extreme dehydration; syncope; high rectal temperature	Proper hydration before exercise and adequate replenishment during exercise; ensure acclimatization
Heat Stroke	Extreme hyperthermia leading to thermoregulatory failure; aggravated by dehydration	Acute medical emergency; includes hyperpyrexia (rectal temp > 41°C), lack of sweating, and neurologic deficit (disorientation, twitching, seizures, coma)	Ensure acclimatization; identify and exclude individuals at risk; adapt activities to climatic constraints

6. **pH**. Marked deviations from 7.0 decrease emptying rate.
7. **Hydration level**. Dehydration decreases gastric emptying and increases risk of gastrointestinal distress.

The trade-off between ingested fluid composition and gastric emptying rate must be evaluated based on environmental stress and energy demands. Exercise in a cold environment does not produce much fluid loss from sweating. In this case, reduced gastric emptying and subsequent water absorption are tolerated, and a more concentrated sugar solution (15 to 20 g per 100 mL of water) may prove beneficial. For survival, the primary concern during prolonged exercise in the heat becomes fluid replacement. Chapter 4 addresses the desirable composition of "sports drinks" and their effects on fluid replacement.

Adequacy of Rehydration Preventing dehydration and its consequences, especially a dangerously elevated body temperature (**hyperthermia**), requires adherence to an adequate water replacement schedule. This often becomes "easier said than done" because some individuals believe ingesting water hinders exercise performance. For wrestlers, chronic dehydration becomes a way of life during the competitive season. Competitors intentionally lose considerable fluid so they can wrestle in a lower weight class—often with fatal outcomes if dehydration becomes severe enough to precipitate cardiovascular abnormalities from electrolyte disturbances. Chronic dehydration also occurs in ballet, where dancers focus on body weight to appear thin. Many individuals on weight loss programs incorrectly believe that restricting fluid intake in some way accelerates body fat loss.

Monitoring change in body weight provides a convenient method to assess: (1) fluid loss during exercise and/or heat stress, and (2) adequacy of rehydration in recovery. In addition to having athletes "weigh in" before and after practice, coaches can minimize weight loss by providing scheduled water breaks during practice/training sessions and unrestricted access to water during competition. Each 0.45 kg (1 lb) of body weight loss corresponds to 450 mL (15 oz) of dehydration. After exercising, the thirst mechanism provides an imprecise guide to water needs. If rehydration depended entirely upon a person's thirst, it could take several days to reestablish fluid balance after severe dehydration.

Hyponatremia: Water Intoxication

Under normal conditions, a maximum of about 9.5 L (10 qt) of water can be consumed daily without unduly straining the kidneys or diluting chemical concentrations of body fluids. Consuming more than 9.5 L can produce **hyponatremia** (water intoxication), a condition related to significant dilution of the body's normal sodium concentration. In general, mild hyponatremia exists when serum sodium concentration falls below 135 $mEq \cdot L^{-1}$; serum sodium below 125 $mEq \cdot L^{-1}$ triggers severe symptoms.

A sustained low plasma sodium concentration creates an osmotic imbalance across the blood–brain barrier that causes rapid water influx into the brain. The resulting swelling of brain tissue produces a cascade of symptoms that range from mild (headache, confusion malaise, nausea, and cramping) to severe (seizures, coma, pulmonary edema, cardiac arrest, and death). The most important predisposing factors to hyponatremia include:

1. Prolonged high-intensity exercise in hot weather
2. Poorly conditioned individuals who experience excessive sweat loss with high sodium concentration
3. Physical activity performed in a sodium-depleted state due to "salt-free" or "low-sodium" diet
4. Use of diuretic medication for hypertension
5. Frequent intake of large quantities of sodium-free fluid during prolonged exercise

Extreme sodium loss (through prolonged sweating) coupled with dilution of existing extracellular sodium (and accompanying reduced osmolality) from consuming fluids with low or no sodium induces hyponatremia. Hyponatremia can occur in experienced athletes. The likely scenario includes high-intensity, ultramarathon-type, continuous exercise lasting 6 to 8 hours, although it can occur in only 4 hours. Nearly 30% of athletes who competed in an Ironman Triathlon experienced symptoms of hyponatremia; these occurred most frequently late in the race or in the recovery after competition. In a large study of more than 18,000 ultraendurance athletes (including triathletes), approximately 9% of collapsed athletes during or following competition presented with symptoms of hyponatremia. An experienced ultramarathoner required hospitalization after consuming nearly 20 L of fluid during a continuous 62-mile, 8.5 hour run.

SUMMARY

1. Water constitutes 40% to 70% of an individual's total body mass. Muscle contains 72% water by weight, whereas water represents only about 50% of the weight of body fat.

2. Approximately 62% of total body water occurs intracellularly (inside the cells), and 38% occurs extracellularly in the plasma, lymph, and other fluids outside the cell.

3. Aqueous solutions supply food and oxygen to the cells, and waste products always leave via a watery medium. Water gives structure and form to the body and regulates body temperature.

4. The normal average daily water intake of 2.5 L comes from (a) liquid intake (1.2 L), (b) food (1.0 L), and (c) metabolic water produced during energy-yielding reactions (0.3 L).

5. Daily water loss occurs through urine (1.0 to 1.5 L), through the skin as insensible perspiration (0.35 L) and sweat (500 to 700 mL), as water vapor in expired air (0.25 to 0.35 L), and in feces (0.10 L).

6. Exercise in hot weather greatly increases the body's water requirement because of fluid loss via sweating. In extreme conditions, fluid needs increase 5 or 6 times above normal.

7. Heat cramps, heat exhaustion, and heat stroke comprise the major forms of heat illness. Heat stroke represents the most serious and complex of these maladies.

8. Several factors greatly affect the rate of gastric emptying: (1) keeping fluid volume in the stomach at a relatively high level speeds gastric emptying, (2) concentrated sugar solutions impair gastric emptying and fluid

replacement, and (3) cold fluids empty from the stomach more rapidly than fluids at body temperature.

9. Maintaining plasma volume (so circulation and sweating progress optimally) represents the primary aim of fluid replacement. For the ideal replacement schedule during exercise, fluid intake should match fluid loss. Monitoring change in body weight during and following workouts indicates the effectiveness of fluid replacement.

10. Optimal gastric volume for fluid replacement occurs by consuming 400 to 600 mL of fluid immediately before exercise, followed by regular ingestion of 250 mL of fluid every 15 minutes during exercise.

11. Drinking concentrated sugar-containing beverages slows the rate of gastric emptying; this could disrupt fluid balance in exercise, especially during heat stress.

12. The ideal oral rehydration solution contains between 5% and 8% carbohydrates. This beverage concentration replenishes carbohydrate without adversely affecting fluid balance and thermoregulation.

13. Excessive sweating and ingesting large volumes of plain water during prolonged exercise sets the stage for hyponatremia or water intoxication. A decrease in extracellular sodium concentration causes this potentially dangerous malady.

THOUGHT QUESTIONS

1. What specific approaches might a coach establish for athletes to guard against dehydration and possible heat injury? Include those factors that optimize fluid replenishment.

2. Describe the ideal fluid (in terms of content and quantity) to consume prior, during, and following exhausting exercise.

SELECTED REFERENCES

Achten, J., Jeukendrup, A.E.: Optimizing fat oxidation through exercise and diet. *Nutrition*, 20:716, 2004.

Achten, J., Jeukendrup, A.E.: Relation between plasma lactate concentration and fat oxidation rates over a wide range of exercise intensities. *Int. J. Sports Med.*, 25:32, 2004.

Adams-Hillard, P.J., Deitch, H.R.: Menstrual disorders in the college age female. *Pediatr. Clin. North Am.*, 52:179, 2005.

Aguilo, A., et al.: Antioxidant diet supplementation influences blood iron status in endurance athletes. *Int. J. Sport Nutr. Exerc. Metab.*, 14:147, 2004.

Ahlborg, G., and Felig, P.: Influence of glucose ingestion on the fuel-hormone response during prolonged exercise. *J. Appl. Physiol.*, 41:683, 1976.

Albert, C.M., et al.: Blood levels of long-chain n-3 fatty acids and risk of sudden death. *N. Engl. J. Med.*, 346:1113, 2002.

Al-Delaimy, W.K., et al.: A prospective study of calcium intake from diet and supplements and risk of ischemic heart disease among men. *Am. J. Clin. Nutr.*, 72:814, 2003.

Alessio, H.M., et al.: Generation of reactive oxygen species after exhaustive aerobic and isometric exercise. *Med. Sci. Sports Exerc.*, 32:1576, 2000.

Almond, C.S., et al.: Hyponatremia among runners in the Boston Marathon. *N. Engl. J. Med.*, 352:1550, 2005.

American College of Sports Medicine, American Dietetic Association and Dietitians of Canada: Joint Position Statement. Nutrition and athletic performance. *Med. Sci. Sports Exerc.*, 32:2130, 2000.

American College of Sports Medicine: American College of Sports Medicine Position Stand. Osteoporosis and exercise. *Med. Sci. Sports Exerc.*, 27:i, 1995.

American College of Sports Medicine: Position stand on physical activity and bone health. *Med. Sci. Sports Exerc.*, 36:1985, 2004.

Andreoli, A., et al.: Effects of different sports on bone density and muscle mass in highly trained athletes. *Med. Sci. Sports Exerc.*, 33:507, 2001.

Androgué, H.J., and Madias, N.E.: Hyponatremia. *N. Engl. J. Med.*, 342:1581, 2000.

Ayus, J.C., et al.: Hyponatremia, cerebral edema, and noncardiogenic pulmonary edema in marathon runners. *Ann. Intern. Med.*, 132:711, 2000.

Barr, S.I., Rideout C.A.: Nutritional considerations for vegetarian athletes. *Nutrition*, 20:696, 2004.

Bazzano, L.A., et al.: Fruit and vegetable intake and risk of cardiovascular disease in US adults: The first National Health and Nutrition Examination Survey Epidemiologic Follow-up Study. *Am. J. Clin. Nutr.*, 76:93, 2002.

Beaton, L.J., et al.: Contraction-induced muscle damage is unaffected by vitamin E supplementation. *Med. Sci. Sports Exerc.*, 34:L798, 2002.

Beck, B.R., Snow, C.M.: Bone health across the lifespan—Exercising our options. *Exerc. Sport Sci. Rev.*, 31:117, 2003.

Bingham, S.A., et al.: Dietary fibre in food and protection against colorectal cancer in the European Prospective Investigation into Cancer and Nutrition (EPIC): an observational study. *Lancet*, 361:1496, 2003.

Brownlie, T. IV, et al.: Marginal iron deficiency without anemia impairs aerobic adaptation among previously untrained women. *Am. J. Clin. Nutr.*, 75:734, 2002.

Brownlie, T. IV, et al.: Tissue iron deficiency without anemia impairs adaptation in endurance capacity after aerobic training in previously untrained women. *Am. J. Clin. Nutr.*, 79:437, 2004.

Brutsaert, T.D., et al.: Iron supplementation improves progressive fatigue resistance during dynamic knee extensor exercise in iron-depleted, nonanemic women. *Am. J. Clin. Nutr.*, 77:441, 2003.

Burke, L.M., et al.: Effect of fat adaptation and carbohydrate restoration on metabolism and performance during prolonged cycling. *J. Appl. Physiol.*, 89:2413, 2000.

Carter, J.M., et al.: The effect of glucose infusion on glucose kinetics during a 1-h time trial. *Med. Sci. Sports Exerc.*, 36:1543, 2004.

Cases, N., et al.: Differential response of plasma and immune cell's vitamin E levels to physical activity and antioxidant vitamin supplementation. *Eur. J. Clin. Nutr.*, 59:781, 2005.

Cauley, J.A., et al.: Effects of estrogen plus progestin on risk of fracture and bone mineral density. *JAMA*, 290:1729, 2003.

Clarkson, P.M., and Thompson, H.S.: Antioxidants: What role do they play in physical activity and health? *Am. J. Clin. Nutr.*, 72:637, 2000.

Cobb, K.L., et al.: Disordered eating, menstrual irregularity, and bone mineral density in female runners. *Med. Sci. Sports Exerc.*, 35:711, 2003.

Coggan, A.R., and Coyle, E.F.: Metabolism and performance following carbohydrate ingestion late in exercise. *Med. Sci. Sports Exerc.*, 21:59, 1989.

Coyle, E.F.: Fluid and fuel intake during exercise. *J. Sports Sci.*, 22:39, 2004.

Coyle, E.F., and Coggan, A.C.: Effectiveness of carbohydrate feeding in delaying fatigue during prolonged exercise. *Sports Med.*, 1:446, 1984.

Coyle, E.F.: Improved muscular efficiency displayed as Tour de France champion matures. *J. Appl. Physiol.*, 98:2191, 2005.

Cullen, D.M., et al.: Bone-loading response varies with strain magnitude and cycle number. *J. Appl. Physiol.*, 91:1971, 2001.

Davies, J.H., et al.: Bone mass acquisition in healthy children. *Arch. Dis. Child.*, 90:373, 2005.

Dawson, B., et al.: Effect of vitamin C and vitamin E supplementation on biochemical and ultrastructural indices of muscle damage after a 21 km run. *Int. J. Sports Med.*, 23:10, 2002.

Deruisseau, K.C., et al.: Iron status of young males and females performing weight-training exercise. *Med. Sci. Sports Exerc.*, 36:242, 2004.

Duncan, C.S., et al.: Bone mineral density in adolescent female athletes: Relationship to exercise type and muscle strength. *Med. Sci. Sports Exerc.*, 34:286, 2002.

Earnest, C.P., et al.: Low vs. high glycemic index carbohydrate gel ingestion during simulated 64-km cycling time trial performance. *J. Strength Cond. Res.*, 18:466, 2004.

Eichner, E.R.: Fatigue of anemia. *Nutr. Revs.*, 59:S17, 2001.

Engel, S.G., et al.: Predictors of disordered eating in a sample of elite Division I college athletes. *Eat Behav.*, 4:333, 2003.

Erhardt, J.G., et al.: Lycopene, β–carotene, and colorectal adenomas. *Am. J. Clin. Nutr.*, 78:1219, 2003.

Erkkilá, A.T., et al.: N-3 Fatty acids and 5-y risks of death and cardiovascular disease events in patients with coronary artery disease. *Am. J. Clin. Nutr.*, 78:65, 2003.

Fallon, K.E.: Utility of hematological and iron-related screening in elite athletes. *Clin. J. Sport Med.*, 14:145, 2004.

Farajian, P., et al.: Dietary intake and nutritional practices of elite Greek aquatic athletes. *Int. J. Sport Nutr. Exerc. Metab.*, 14:574, 2004.

Fatouros, I.G., et al.: Oxidative stress responses in older men during endurance training and detraining. *Med. Sci. Sports Exerc.*, 36:2065, 2004.

Faulkner, R.A., et al.: Strength indices of the proximal femur and shaft in prepubertal female gymnasts. *Med. Sci. Sports Exerc.*, 35:513, 2003.

Feskanich, D., et al.: Walking and leisure-time activity and risk of hip fracture in postmenopausal women. *JAMA*, 288:2300, 2002.

Flemming, D.J., et al.: Dietary factors associated with the risk of high iron stores in the elderly Framingham Heart Study cohort. *Am. J. Clin. Nutr.*, 76:1375, 2002.

Fogelholm, M.: Dairy products, meat and sports performance. *Sports Med.*, 33:615, 2003.

Food and Nutrition Board, Institute of Medicine: *Dietary Reference Intakes for Energy, Carbohydrates, Fiber, Fat, Protein and Amino Acids.* Washington, D.C.: National Academy Press, 2002.

Friedmann, B., et al.: Effects of iron repletion on blood volume and performance capacity in young athletes. *Med. Sci. Sports Exerc.*, 33:741, 2001.

Fujimoto, T., et al.: Skeletal muscle glucose uptake response to exercise in trained and untrained men. *Med. Sci. Sports Exerc.*, 35:777, 2003.

Fung, T.T., et al.: Whole-grain intake and risk of type-2 diabetes: A prospective study in men. *Am. J. Clin. Nutr.*, 76:535, 2002.

Gardner, J.W.: Death by water intoxication. *Military Med.*, 5:432, 2002.

Gill, J.M.R., et al.: Effects of dietary monounsaturated fatty acids on lipoprotein concentrations, compositions, and subfraction distributions and on VLDL apolipoprotien B kinetics: dose-dependent effects on LDL. *Am. J. Clin. Nutr.*, 78:47, 2003.

Godek, S.F., et al.: Sweat rate and fluid turnover in American football players compared with runners in a hot and humid environment. *Br. J. Sports Med.*, 39:205, 2005.

Gross, T.S., et al.: Why rest stimulates bone formation: A hypothesis based on complex adaptive phenomenon. *Exerc. Sport Sci. Rev.*, 32:9, 2004.

Haub, M.D., et al.: Effect of protein source on resistive-training-induced changes in body composition and muscle size in older men. *Am. J. Clin. Nutr.*, 76:511, 2002.

Hawkins, S.A., et al.: Five-year maintenance of bone mineral density in women master runners. 35:137, 2003.

Hew, T.D., et al.: The incidence, risk factors, and clinical manifestations of hyponatremia in marathon runners. *Clin. J. Sports Med.*, 13:41, 2003.

Hill, R.J., and Davies, P.S.: Energy intake and energy expenditure in elite lightweight female rowers. *Med. Sci. Sports Exerc.*, 34:1823, 2002.

Hu, F.B.: Plant-based foods and prevention of cardiovascular disease: An overview. *Am. J. Clin. Nutr.*, 78(Suppl):544S, 2003.

Jacqmain, M., et al.: Calcium intake, body composition, and lipoprotein-lipid concentrations in adults. *Am. J. Clin. Nutr.*, 78:1448, 2003.

Janz, K.F., et al.: Everyday activity predicts bone geometry in children: The Iowa Bone Development Study. *Med. Sci. Sports Exerc.*, 36;1124, 2004.

Jeffery, R.W., et al.: Physical activity and weight loss: Does prescribing higher physical activity goals improve outcome? *Am. J. Clin. Nutr.*, 78:684, 2003.

Jentjens, R.L., et al.: Oxidation of combined ingestion of glucose and sucrose during exercise. *Metabolism*, 54:610, 2005.

Jentjens, R.L., Jeukendrup A.E.: High rates of exogenous carbohydrate oxidation from a mixture of glucose and fructose ingested during prolonged cycling exercise. *Br. J. Nutr.*, 93:485, 2005.

Jeukendrup, A.E.: Carbohydrate intake during exercise and performance. *Nutrition*, 20:669, 2004.

Jeukendrup, A.E., et al.: Nutritional considerations in triathlon. *Sports Med.*, 35:163, 2005.

Jeukendrup, A.E., Wallis, G.A.: Measurement of substrate oxidation during exercise by means of gas exchange measurements. *Int. J. Sports Med.*, 26 Suppl 1:S28, 2005.

Klungland Torstveit, M., Sundgot-Borgen, J.: The female athlete triad: are elite athletes at increased risk. *Med. Sci. Sports Exerc.*, 37:184, 2005.

Krauss, W.E., et al.: Effect of the amount and intensity of exercise on plasma lipoproteins. *N. Engl. J. Med.* 347:1483, 2002.

Kriska, A.: Can a physically active lifestyle prevent type 2 diabetes. *Exerc. Sport Sci. Rev.*, 1;132, 2003.

LaMothe, J.M., Zernicke, R.F.: Rest-insertion combined with high-frequency loading enhances osteogenesis. *J. Appl. Physiol.*, 96:1788, 2004.

Lanou, A.J., et al.: Calcium, dairy products, and bone health in children and young adults: a reevaluation of the evidence. *Pediatrics*, 115:736, 2005.

Lemaitre, R.N., et al.: n—3 Poly unsaturated fatty acids, fatal ischemic heart disease, and nonfatal myocardial infarction in obese adults. *Am. J. Clin. Nutr.*, 77:319, 2003.

Levine, B.D., Thompson P.D.: Marathon maladies. *N. Engl. J. Med.*, 352:1516, 2005.

Li, T.L., et al.: The effects of pre-exercise high carbohydrate meals with different glycemic indices on blood leukocyte redistribution, IL-6, and hormonal responses during a subsequent prolonged exercise. *Int. J. Sport Nutr. Exerc. Metab.*, 14:647, 2004.

Liese, A.D., et al.: Whole-grain intake and insulin sensitivity: the Insulin Resistance Atherosclerosis Study. *Am. J. Clin. Nutr.*, 78:965, 2003.

Lindsey, C., et al.: Association of physical performance measures with bone mineral density in postmenopausal women. *Arch. Phys. Med. Rehabil.*, 86:1102, 2005.

Liu, J.F., et al.: Blood lipid peroxides and muscle damage increased following intensive resistance training of female weightlifters. *Ann. N. Y. Acad. Sci.*, 1042:255, 2005.

Liu, S., et al.: Relation between changes in intakes of dietary fiber and grain products and changes in weight and development of obesity among middle-aged women. *Am. J. Clin. Nutr.*, 78:920, 2003.

Liu, S., et al.: Dietary glycemic load assessed by food-frequency questionnaire in relation to plasma high-density-lipoprotein cholesterol and fasting triacylglycerols in postmenopausal women. *Am. J. Clin. Nutr.*, 73:560, 2001.

Lonn, E., et al.: Effects of long-term vitamin E supplementation on cardiovascular events and cancer: a randomized controlled trial. *JAMA*, 293:1338, 2005.

Lukaski, H.C.: Vitamin and mineral status: effects on physical performance. *Nutrition*, 20:632–644, 2004.

Manetta, J., et al.: Fuel oxidation during exercise in middle-aged men: role of training and glucose disposal. *Med. Sci. Sports Exerc.*, 33:423, 2002.

Mauger, J-F, et al.: Effect of different forms of hydrogenated fats on LDL particle size. *Am. J. Clin. Nutr.*, 78:370, 2003.

Mensink, R.P., et al.: Effects of dietary fatty acids and carbohydrates on the ratio of serum total to HDL cholesterol and on serum lipids and apolipoproteins: a meta-analysis of 60 controlled trials. *Am. J. Clin. Nutr.*, 77:1146, 2003.

Michaëlsson, K., et al.: Serum retinol levels and the risk of fracture. *N. Engl. J. Med.* 348:287, 2003.

Modlesky, C.M., and Lewis, R.D.: Does exercise during growth have a long-term effect on bone health? *Exer. Sport Sci. Rev.*, 30:171, 2002.

Montain, S.J., et al.: Hyponatremia associated with exercise: Risk factors and pathogenesis. *Exerc. Sport Sci. Rev.*, 2:113, 2001.

Mozaffarian, D., et al.: Cereal, fruit, and vegetable fiber intake and risk of cardiovascular disease in elderly individuals. *JAMA*, 289:1659, 2003.

Nemet, D., et al.: Proteins and amino acid supplementation in sports: are they truly necessary? *Isr. Med. Assoc. J.*, 7:328, 2005.

Nogueira, J.A., Da Costa, T.H.: Nutrient intake and eating habits of triathletes on a Brazilian diet. *Int. J. Sport Nutr. Exerc. Metab.*, 14:684, 2004.

Onywera, V.O., et al.: Food and macronutrient intake of elite Kenyan distance runners. *Int. J. Sport Nutr. Exerc. Metab.*, 14:709, 2004.

Pattwell, D.M., Jackson M.J.: Contraction-induced oxidants as mediators of adaptation and damage in skeletal muscle. *Exer. Sport Sci. Rev.*, 32:14, 2004.

Pescatello, L.S., et al.: Daily physical movement and bone mineral density among a mixed racial cohort of women. *Med. Sci. Sports Exerc.*, 34:1966, 2002.

Pi-Sunyer, X.: Glycemic index and disease. *Am. J. Clin. Nutr.*, 76(Suppl):290S, 2002.

Pitkänen, H.T., et al.: Free amino acid pool and muscle protein balance after resistance exercise. *Med. Sci. Sports Exerc.*, 35:784, 2003.

Poppitt, S.D., et al.: Long-term effects of ad libitum low-fat, high-carbohydrate diets on body weight and serum lipids in overweight subjects with metabolic syndrome. *Am. J. Clin. Nutr.*, 75:11, 2002.

Quindry, J.C., et al.: The effects of acute exercise on neutrophils and plasma oxidative stress. *Med. Sci. Sports Exerc.*, 35:1139, 2003.

Ralston, S.H.: Genetic determinants of osteoporosis. *Curr. Opin. Rheumatol.*, 17:475, 2005.

Reinking, M.F., Alexander, L.E.: Prevalence of disordered-eating behaviors in undergraduate female collegiate athletes and nonathletes. *J. Athl. Train.*, 40:47, 2005.

Rowlands, A.V., et al.: Interactive effects of habitual physical activity and calcium intake on bone density in boys and girls. *J. Appl. Physiol.*, 97:1203, 2004.

Rozen, G.S., et al.: Calcium supplementation provides an extended window of opportunity for bone mass accretion after menarche. *Am. J. Clin. Nutr.,* 78:993, 2003.

Schenk, S., et al.: Different glycemic indexes of breakfast cereals are not due to glucose entry into blood but to glucose removal by tissues. *Am. J. Clin. Nutr.,* 78:742, 2003.

Schrauwen, P., et al.: Effect of 2 weeks of endurance training on uncoupling protein 3 content in untrained human subjects. *Acta. Physiol. Scand.,* 183:273, 2005.

Schumacher, Y.O., et al.: Hematological indices and iron status in athletes of various sports and performances. *Med. Sci. Sports Exerc.,* 34:869, 2002.

Sgouraki, E., et al.: Acute effects of short duration maximal endurance exercise on lipid, phospholipid and lipoprotein levels. *J. Sports Med. Phys. Fitness,* 44:444, 2004.

Shearer, J., Graham, T.E.: Novel aspects of skeletal muscle glycogen and its regulation during rest and exercise. *Exerc. Sport Sci. Rev.,* 32:120, 2004.

Siu, P.M., et al.: Effect of frequency of carbohydrate feedings on recovery and subsequent endurance run. *Med. Sci. Sports Exerc.* 36:315, 2004.

Stewart, K.J., et al.: Exercise effects on bone mineral density relationships to changes in fitness and fatness. *Am. J. Prev. Med.,* 28:453, 2005.

Sudi, K., et al.: Anorexia athletica. *Nutrition,* 20:657, 2004.

Torstveit, M.K., Sundgot-Borgen, J.: Low bone mineral density is two to three times more prevalent in non-athletic premenopausal women than in elite athletes: a comprehensive controlled study. *Br. J. Sports Med.,* 39:282, 2005.

Torstveit, M.K., Sundgot-Borgen, J.: The female athlete triad: are elite athletes at increased risk? *Med. Sci. Sports Exerc.,* 37:184, 2005.

Turner, C.H., and Robling, A.G.: Designing exercise regimens to increase bone strength. *Exerc. Sport Sci. Rev.* 31:45, 2003.

Uzunca, K.,et al.: High bone mineral density in loaded skeletal regions of former professional football (soccer) players: what is the effect of time after active career? *Br. J. Sports Med.,* 39:154, 2005.

Van Loon, L.J.C.: Use of intramuscular triacylglycerol as a substrate source during exercise in humans. *J. Appl. Physiol.,* 97 1170, 2004.

Van Remmen, H., et al.: Oxidative damage to DNA and aging. *Exerc. Sport Sci. Rev.,* 31:149, 2003.

Venables, M.C., et al.: Erosive effect of a new sports drink on dental enamel during exercise. *Med. Sci. Sports Exerc.,* 37:39, 2005.

Viitala, P., Newhouse, I.J.: Vitamin E supplementation, exercise and lipid peroxidation in human participants. *Eur. J. Appl. Physiol.,* 93:108, 2004.

Vincent, K.R., and Braith, R.W.: Resistance exercise and bone turnover in elderly men and women. *Med. Sci. Sports Exerc.,* 34:17, 2002.

Vivekananthan, D.P., et al.: Use of antioxidant vitamins for the prevention of cardiovascular disease: meta-analysis of randomised trials. *Lancet,* 362:920, 2003.

Vogt, M., et al.: Effects of dietary fat on muscle substrates, metabolism, and performance in athletes. *Med. Sci. Sports Exerc.,* 35:952, 2003.

Von Stengel, S., et al.: Power training is more effective than strength training for maintaining bone mineral density in postmenopausal women. *J. Appl. Physiol.,* 99:181, 2005.

Wallis, G.A., et al.: Oxidation of combined ingestion of maltodextrins and fructose during exercise. *Med. Sci. Sports Exerc.,* 37:426, 2005.

Wang, Q.J., et al.: Influence of physical activity and maturation status on bone mass and geometry in early pubertal girls. *Scand. J. Med. Sci. Sports,* 15:100, 2005.

Welsh, R.S., et al.: Carbohydrates and physical/mental performance during intermittent exercise to fatigue. *Med. Sci. Sports Exerc.,* 34;723, 2002.

Willett, A.M.: Vitamin D status and its relationship with parathyroid hormone and bone mineral status in older adolescents. *Proc. Nutr. Soc.,* 64:193, 2005.

Zanker, C.L., Cooke, C.B.: Energy balance, Bone turnover, and skeletal health in physically active individuals. *Med. Sci. Sports Exerc.,* 36:1372, 2004.

Zderic, T.W., et al.: Manipulation of dietary carbohydrate and muscle glycogen affects glucose uptake during exercise when fat oxidation is impaired by beta-adrenergic blockade. *Am. J. Physiol. Endocrinol. Metab.,* 287:E1195, 2004.

CHAPTER OBJECTIVES

- Define the following: (1) heat of combustion, (2) digestive efficiency, and (3) Atwater general factors.

- Compute the energy content of a meal from its macronutrient composition.

- Compare nutrient and energy intakes of physically active men and women with sedentary counterparts.

- Outline the MyPyramid recommendations.

- Describe the timing and composition of the preevent (precompetition) meal, including reasons for limiting lipid and protein intake.

- Summarize effects of low, normal, and high-carbohydrate intake on glycogen reserves and subsequent endurance performance.

- For endurance athletes, describe: (1) the potential negative effects of consuming a concentrated sugar drink 30 minutes before competition and (2) the ideal composition of a "sports drink."

- Discuss possible reasons why consuming high-glycemic carbohydrates during high-intensity aerobic exercise may enhance endurance performance.

- Define "glucose polymer," and give the rationale for adding these compounds to a sports drink.

- Make a general recommendation concerning carbohydrate intake for athletes in intense training.

- Describe the most effective way to replenish glycogen reserves after a hard bout of training or competition.

- Compare classic carbohydrate loading with the modified procedure.

CHAPTER OUTLINE

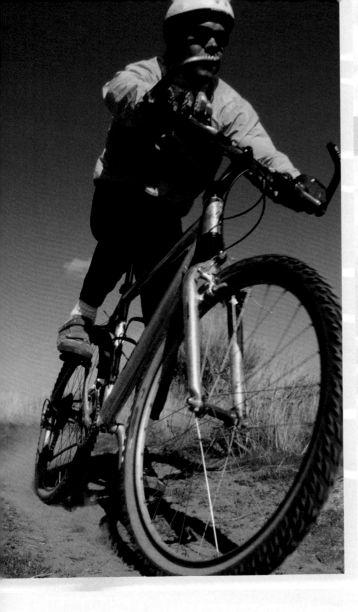

chapter 3

Food Energy and Optimum Nutrition for Exercise

PART 1 •
Food as Energy

CALORIE—A MEASUREMENT OF FOOD ENERGY

One kilogram–calorie (kilocalorie [kCal], or simply Calorie) expresses the quantity of heat necessary to raise the temperature of 1 kg (1 L) of water 1°C (specifically, from 14.5 to 15.5°C). For example, if a particular food contains 300 kCal, then releasing the potential energy trapped within this food's chemical structure increases the temperature of 300 L of water by 1°C. Different foods contain different amounts of potential energy kCals. One-half cup of peanut butter with a caloric value of 759 kCal contains the equivalent heat energy to increase the temperature of 759 L of water by 1°C.

Gross Energy Value of Foods

Laboratories use **bomb calorimeters**, similar to the one illustrated in **Figure 3.1**, to measure total (gross) energy value of various food macronutrients. Bomb calorimeters operate on the principle of **direct calorimetry**, measuring

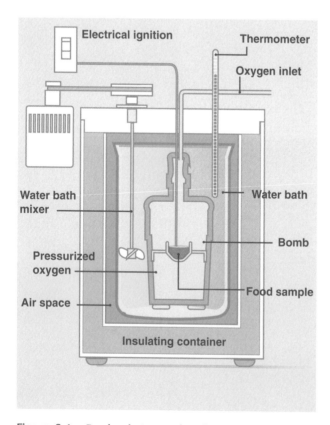

Electrical ignition

Thermometer

Oxygen inlet

Water bath mixer

Water bath

Bomb

Pressurized oxygen

Food sample

Air space

Insulating container

Figure 3.1. Bomb calorimetry directly measures the energy value of food.

the heat liberated as the food burns completely. The bomb calorimeter works as follows:

- A small, insulated chamber filled with oxygen under pressure contains a weighed portion of food.
- The food literally explodes and burns when an electric current ignites a fuse inside the chamber.
- A surrounding water bath absorbs the heat released as the food burns (termed the heat of combustion). Insulation prevents loss of heat to the outside.
- A sensitive thermometer measures the amount of heat absorbed by the water. For example, the complete combustion of one hot dog (beef, skinless, 2 oz), bun (1.4 oz), mustard, and small french fries (2.4 oz) liberates 512 kCal of heat energy. This would raise 5.12 kg (11.3 lb) of ice water to the boiling point.

Heat of Combustion   The heat liberated by burning (oxidizing) food in a bomb calorimeter represents its **heat of combustion** (total energy value of the food). *Burning 1 g of pure carbohydrate yields a heat of combustion of 4.20 kCal, 1 g of pure protein releases 5.65 kCal, and 1 g of pure lipid yields 9.45 kCal.* Because most foods in the diet consist of various proportions of these three macronutrients, the caloric value of a given food reflects the sum of the heats of combustion of each of the food macronutrients. The heats of combustion for the three macronutrients demonstrates that the complete oxidation of lipid (in the bomb calorimeter) liberates about 65% more energy per gram than protein oxidation and 120% more energy than carbohydrate oxidation.

Net Energy Value of Foods

Differences exist in the energy value of foods when comparing the heat of combustion (gross energy value) determined by direct calorimetry to the net energy actually available to the body. This pertains particularly to protein because its nitrogen component does not oxidize. In the body, nitrogen atoms combine with hydrogen to form urea, which excretes in urine. Elimination of hydrogen in this manner represents a loss of approximately 19% of protein's potential energy. The hydrogen loss reduces protein's heat of combustion in the body to about 4.6 kCal per gram instead of 5.65 kCal per gram in the bomb calorimeter. In contrast, identical physiologic fuel values exist for carbohydrates and lipids (which contain no nitrogen) compared with their heats of combustion in the bomb calorimeter.

Digestive Efficiency

The "availability" to the body of the ingested macronutrients determines their ultimate caloric yield. Availability refers to completeness of digestion and absorption. Normally, about 97% of carbohydrates, 95% of lipids, and 92% of proteins become digested, absorbed, and available for energy conversion. Large variation exists in the digestive efficiency for protein, ranging from a high of 97% for animal protein to a low of 78% for dried peas and beans. Furthermore, less energy becomes available from a meal with a high-fiber content.

Considering average digestive efficiencies, the **net kCal value** per gram available to the body equals 4.0 for carbohydrate, 9.0 for lipid, and 4.0 for protein. These corrected heats of combustion are known as the **Atwater general factors**, which were named after the scientist who first described energy release in the calorimeter (Wilbur Olin Atwater, 1844–1907).

Energy Value of a Meal

The caloric content of any food can be determined from Atwater values, as long as one knows its composition and weight. Suppose, for example, we wanted to determine the kCal value for 1/2 cup (3.5 oz or about 100 g) of creamed chicken. Based on laboratory analysis of a standard recipe, the macronutrient composition of 1 g of creamed chicken contains 0.2 g of protein, 0.12 g of lipid, and 0.06 g of carbohydrate.

Using the Atwater net kCal values, 0.2 g of protein contains 0.8 kCal (0.20 × 4.0), 0.12 g of lipid equals 1.08 kCal (0.12 × 9.0), and 0.06 g of carbohydrate yields 0.24 kCal (0.06 × 4.0). Therefore, the total caloric value of 1 g of creamed chicken equals 2.12 kCal (0.80 + 1.08 + 0.24). Consequently, a 100-g serving contains 100 times as much, or 212 kCal. **Table 3.1** presents another example of kCal calculations for 3/4 cup (100 g) of vanilla ice cream.

Fortunately, the need seldom exists to compute kCal values because the United States Department of Agriculture has already made these determinations for almost all foods.

Calories Equal Calories

Consider the following five common foods: raw celery, cooked cabbage, cooked asparagus spears, mayonnaise, and salad oil. To consume 100 kCal of each of these foods, one must eat 20 stalks of celery, 4 cups of cabbage, 30 asparagus spears, but only 1 tablespoon of mayonnaise or 4/5 tablespoon of salad oil. Thus, a small serving of some foods contains the equivalent energy value as a large quantity of other foods. Viewed from a different perspective, to meet daily energy needs, a sedentary young adult female would have to consume more than 420 stalks of celery, 84 cups of cabbage, or 630 asparagus spears, yet only 1.5 cups of mayonnaise or about 8 ounces of salad oil. The major difference among these foods is that high-fat foods contain more energy with little water. In contrast, foods low in fat or high in water tend to contain little energy.

Questions & Notes

Give the heat of combustion for 1 g each of carbohydrate, protein, and lipid.

Carbohydrate–

Protein–

Lipid–

Explain why 100 kCal from lipid is no more fattening than 100 kCal from protein.

Give the Atwater factors for:

Carbohydrate–

Protein–

Lipid–

Of the 3 major nutrients, which one has the highest digestive efficiency?

Give one major advantage of maintaining a low-fat diet.

For Your Information

More Lipid Equals More Calories
Lipid-rich foods contain a higher energy content than foods that are relatively fat free. One glass of whole milk, for example, contains 160 kCal, whereas the same quantity of skim milk contains only 90 kCal. If a person who normally consumes one quart of whole milk each day switches to skim milk, the total calories ingested each year would be reduced by the equivalent calories in 25 pounds of body fat. Thus, following this switch for just 3 years theoretically represents the equivalent energy in 75 pounds of body fat.

Table 3.1 Method of Calculating the Caloric Value of a Food from Its Composition of Macronutrients

Food: Ice cream (vanilla)
Weight: three-fourths cup = 100 grams

	PROTEIN	LIPID	CARBOHYDRATE
Percentage	4%	13%	21%
Total grams	4	13	21
In one gram	0.04 g	0.13 g	0.21 g
Calories per gram	0.16	1.17	0.84
	(0.04 × 4.0 kCal)	(0.13 × 9.0 kCal)	(0.21 × 4.0 kCal)

Total calories per gram: 0.16 + 1.17 + 0.84 = 2.17 kCal
Total calories per 100 grams: 2.17 × 100 = 217 kCal

Box 3-1 • CLOSE UP

HOW TO READ A FOOD LABEL

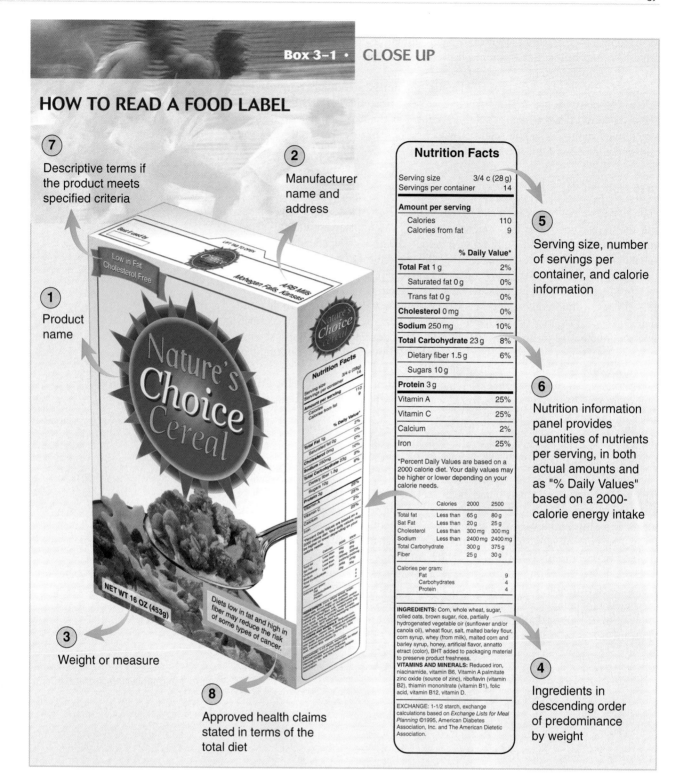

(7) Descriptive terms if the product meets specified criteria

(2) Manufacturer name and address

(1) Product name

(3) Weight or measure

(8) Approved health claims stated in terms of the total diet

(5) Serving size, number of servings per container, and calorie information

(6) Nutrition information panel provides quantities of nutrients per serving, in both actual amounts and as "% Daily Values" based on a 2000-calorie energy intake

(4) Ingredients in descending order of predominance by weight

Nutrition Facts

Serving size	3/4 c (28 g)
Servings per container	14

Amount per serving

Calories	110
Calories from fat	9

% Daily Value*

Total Fat 1 g	2%
Saturated fat 0 g	0%
Trans fat 0 g	0%
Cholesterol 0 mg	0%
Sodium 250 mg	10%
Total Carbohydrate 23 g	8%
Dietary fiber 1.5 g	6%
Sugars 10 g	
Protein 3 g	
Vitamin A	25%
Vitamin C	25%
Calcium	2%
Iron	25%

*Percent Daily Values are based on a 2000 calorie diet. Your daily values may be higher or lower depending on your calorie needs.

		Calories	2000	2500
Total fat	Less than		65 g	80 g
Sat Fat	Less than		20 g	25 g
Cholesterol	Less than		300 mg	300 mg
Sodium	Less than		2400 mg	2400 mg
Total Carbohydrate			300 g	375 g
Fiber			25 g	30 g

Calories per gram:

Fat	9
Carbohydrates	4
Protein	4

INGREDIENTS: Corn, whole wheat, sugar, rolled oats, brown sugar, rice, partially hydrogenated vegetable oir (sunflower and/or canola oil), wheat flour, salt, malted barley flour, corn syrup, whey (from milk), malted corn and barley syrup, honey, artificial flavor, annatto etract (color), BHT added to packaging material to preserve product freshness.
VITAMINS AND MINERALS: Reduced iron, niacinamide, vitamin B6, Vitamin A palmitate zinc oxide (source of zinc), riboflavin (vitamin B2), thiamin mononitrate (vitamin B1), folic acid, vitamin B12, vitamin D.

EXCHANGE: 1-1/2 starch, exchange calculations based on *Exchange Lists for Meal Planning* ©1995, American Diabetes Association, Inc. and The American Dietetic Association.

anced diet. *Physically fit Americans, including those involved in exceptional physical activities, consume diets that more closely approach dietary recommendations than peers of lower levels of fitness.*

Inconsistencies exist among studies that relate diet quality to physical activity level or physical fitness. Part of the discrepancy results from use of relatively crude and imprecise self-reported measures of physical activity, unreliable dietary assessments, and/or small sample size. **Table 3.2** contrasts the nutrient and energy intakes with national dietary recommendations of a large population-based cohort of nearly 7959 men and 2453 women who were classified as low, moderate, and high for cardiorespiratory fitness and who participated in the Aerobics Center Longitudinal Study. The most significant findings indicate:

- A progressively lower body mass index with increasing levels of physical fitness for both men and women.
- Remarkably small differences in energy intake in relation to physical fitness classification for women ($\leq$94 kCal per day) and men ($\leq$82 kCal per day); the moderate fitness group consumed the least calories for both sexes.
- A progressively higher dietary fiber intake and lower cholesterol intake across fitness categories.
- Men and women with higher fitness levels generally consumed diets that more closely approached dietary recommendations (with respect to dietary fiber, % energy from total fat, % energy from saturated fat, and dietary cholesterol) than peers of lower levels of fitness.

Attention to proper diet does not mean athletes must join the ranks of the more than 40% of Americans who take supplements (spending about $7 billion yearly) to micromanage their nutrient intake. *In essence, sound human nutrition represents sound nutrition for athletes.*

DIETARY REFERENCE INTAKES

Controversy surrounding use of the Recommended Dietary Allowances (RDAs) caused the Food and Nutrition Board and scientific nutrition community to reexamine the usefulness of these applications. This process, begun in 1997, led the National Academies' Institute of Medicine (in cooperation with Canadian scientists) to develop the **Dietary Reference Intakes (DRIs)**, a radically new and more comprehensive approach to nutritional recommendations for individuals. Think of the DRIs as the umbrella term encompassing an array of new standards—the **RDAs, Estimated Average Requirements (EARs), Adequate Intakes (AIs)**, and the **Tolerable Upper Intake Levels (UL)**—for nutrient recommendations for use in planning and assessing diets for healthy people.

Similarities of dietary patterns caused the inclusion of both Canada and the United States in the target population. Recommendations encompass not only daily intakes intended for health maintenance but also upper-intake levels that reduce the likelihood of harm from excess nutrient intake. The DRIs differ from their predecessor RDAs by focusing more on promoting health maintenance and risk reduction for nutrient-dependent diseases (e.g., heart disease, diabetes, hypertension, osteoporosis, various cancers, and age-related macular degeneration) rather than preventing deficiency diseases, such as scurvy (vitamin C deficiency) or beriberi (vitamin B_1 deficiency). In addition to including values for energy, protein, and the micronutrients, DRIs also provide values for macronutrients and food components of nutritional importance, such as phytochemicals. Whenever possible, nutrient intakes are recommended in four categories instead of one.

Unlike its RDA predecessor, the DRI value also includes recommendations that apply to gender and life stages of growth and development based on age and, when appropriate, pregnancy and lactation (*http://www.nap.edu/*; search for Dietary Reference Intakes).

Questions & Notes

In general, do athletes require different nutrients in different quantities than nonathletes?

Briefly explain how the DRIs differ from the RDAs.

Name the 4 different parts of the DRIs.

Table 3·2 Mean (±SD) Nutrient Intake Based on 3-Day Diet Records By Level of Cardiorespiratory Fitness in 7959 Men and 2453 Women

VARIABLE	Males Low Fitness (N = 786)	Females Low Fitness (N = 233)	Males Moderate Fitness (N = 2457)	Females Moderate Fitness (N = 730)	Males High Fitness (N = 4716)	Females High Fitness (N = 1490)
Demographic and health data						
Age (y)	47.3 ± 11.1^{a,b}	47.5 ± 11.2^b	47.3 ± 10.3^c	46.7 ± 11.6	48.1 ± 10.5	46.5 ± 11.0
Apparently healthy (%)	51.5^{a,b}	55.4^{a,b}	69.1^c	71.1^c	77.0	79.3
Current smokers (%)	23.4^{a,b}	12.0^{a,b}	15.8^c	9.0^c	7.8	4.2
BMI (kg·m^{-2})	30.7 ± 5.5^{a,b}	27.3 ± 6.7^{a,b}	27.4 ± 3.7^c	24.3 ± 4.9^c	25.1 ± 2.7	22.1 ± 3.0
Nutrient data						
Energy (kCal)	2378.6 ± 718.6^a	1887.4 ± 607.5^a	2296.9 ± 661.9^c	1793.0 ± 508.2^c	2348.1 ± 664.3	1859.7 ± 514.7
kCal·kg^{-1}	25.0 ± 8.1^a	27.1 ± 9.4^a	26.7 ± 8.4^c	28.1 ± 8.8^c	29.7 ± 9.2	31.7 ± 9.8
Carbohydrate (% kCal)	43.2 ± 9.4^b	47.7 ± 9.6^b	44.6 ± 9.1^c	48.2 ± 9.0^c	48.1 ± 9.7	51.1 ± 9.4
Protein (% kCal)	18.6 ± 3.8	17.6 ± 3.7^a	18.5 ± 3.8	18.1 ± 3.9	18.1 ± 3.8	17.7 ± 3.9
Total fat (% kCal)	36.7 ± 7.2^b	34.8 ± 7.6^b	35.4 ± 7.1^c	33.7 ± 6.8^c	32.6 ± 7.5	31.3 ± 7.5
SFA (% kCal)	11.8 ± 3.2^b	11.1 ± 3.3^b	11.3 ± 3.2^c	10.6 ± 3.2^c	10.0 ± 3.2	9.6 ± 3.1
MUFA (% kCal)	14.5 ± 3.2^{a,b}	13.4 ± 3.4^{a,b}	13.8 ± 3.1^c	12.8 ± 3.0^c	12.6 ± 3.3	11.9 ± 3.2
PUFA (% kCal)	7.4 ± 2.2^{a,b}	7.5 ± 2.2	7.5 ± 2.2	7.5 ± 2.2	7.4 ± 2.3	7.4 ± 2.4
Cholesterol (mg)	349.5 ± 173.2^b	244.7 ± 132.8^b	314.5 ± 147.5^c	224.6 ± 115.6^c	277.8 ± 138.5	204.1 ± 103.6
Fiber (g)	21.0 ± 9.5^b	18.9 ± 8.2^{a,b}	22.0 ± 9.7^c	20.0 ± 8.3^c	26.2 ± 11.9	23.2 ± 10.7
Calcium (mg)	849.1 ± 371.8^{a,b}	765.2 ± 361.8^{a,b}	860.2 ± 360.2^c	774.6 ± 342.8^c	924.4 ± 386.8	828.3 ± 372.1
Sodium (mg)	4317.4 ± 1365.7	3350.8 ± 980.8	4143.0 ± 1202.3	3256.7 ± 927.7	4133.2 ± 1189.4	3314.4 ± 952.7
Folate (mcg)	336.4 ± 165.2^b	301.8 ± 157.6^{a,b}	359.5 ± 197.0^c	319.7 ± 196.2	428.0 ± 272.0	356.2 ± 232.5
Vitamin B$_6$ (mg)	2.4 ± 0.9^b	2.0 ± 0.8^b	2.4 ± 0.9^c	2.0 ± 0.8^c	2.8 ± 1.1	2.2 ± 0.9
Vitamin B$_{12}$ (mcg)	6.6 ± 5.5^a	4.7 ± 4.2	6.8 ± 6.0	4.9 ± 4.2	6.6 ± 5.8	5.0 ± 4.2
Vitamin A (RE)	1372.7 ± 1007.3^{a,b}	1421.9 ± 1135.3^b	1530.5 ± 1170.4^c	1475.1 ± 1132.9^c	1766.3 ± 1476.0	1699.0 ± 1346.9
Vitamin C (mg)	117.3 ± 80.4^b	116.7 ± 7.5^b	129.2 ± 108.9^c	131.5 ± 140.0	166.0 ± 173.2	153.5 ± 161.1
Vitamin E (AE)	11.5 ± 9.1^b	10.8 ± 7.5	12.1 ± 8.6^c	10.3 ± 6.5^c	13.7 ± 11.4	11.5 ± 8.1

BMI, body mass index; SFA, saturated fatty acid; PUFA, polyunsaturated fatty acid; MUFA, monounsaturated fatty acid; RE, retinol equivalents; AE, alpha-tocopherol units.
^{a} Significant difference between low and moderate fit, $P < 0.05$.
^{b} Significant difference between low and high fit, $P < 0.05$.
^{c} Significant difference between moderate and high fit, $P < 0.05$.
From: Brodney, S. et al.: Nutrient intake of physically active fit and unfit men and women. *Med. Sci. Sports Exerc.* 33:459, 2001.

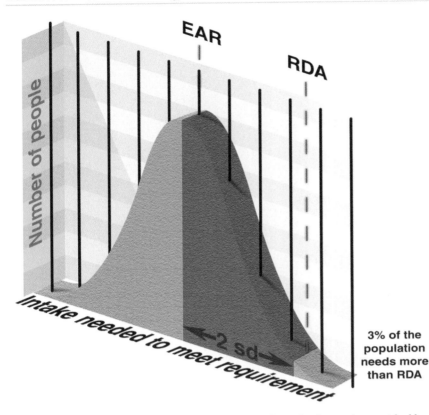

Figure 3.2. Theoretical distribution of the number of people adequately nourished by a given nutrient intake. For example, the number of people receiving adequate nutrition with 50 units of the nutrient is greater than those receiving only 15 units or who require 75 units. The RDA (Recommended Dietary Allowance) is set at an intake level that would meet the nutrient needs of 97% to 98% of the population (2 standard deviations [SD] above the mean). EAR is the Estimated Average Requirement, which represents a nutrient intake value estimated to meet the requirement of one-half (50%) of the healthy individuals in a gender and life-stage group.

The four different sets of values for the intake of nutrients and food components in the DRIs are as follows (**Fig. 3.2**):

- **Estimated Average Requirement (EAR):** Average level of daily nutrient intake to meet the requirement of one-half of the healthy individuals in a particular life stage and gender group. In addition to assessing nutritional adequacy of intakes of population groups, the EAR provides a useful value for determining the prevalence of inadequate nutrient intake by the proportion of the population with intakes below this value.
- **Recommended Dietary Allowance (RDA):** The average daily nutrient intake level sufficient to meet the requirement of nearly all (97% to 98%) healthy individuals in a particular life-stage and gender group. For most nutrients, this value represents the EAR plus two standard deviations of the requirement.
- **Adequate Intake (AI):** The AI provides a nutritional goal when no RDA exists. It represents a recommended average daily nutrient intake level based on observed or experimentally determined approximations or estimates of nutrient intake by a group (or groups) of apparently healthy people that are assumed to be adequate; the AI is used when an RDA cannot be determined. Low risk exists when intake is at or above the AI level.
- **Tolerable Upper Intake Level (UL):** The highest average daily nutrient intake level likely to pose no risk of adverse health effects to almost all individuals in the specified gender and life-stage group of the general population. As intake increases above the UL, the potential risk of adverse effects increases.

FOR YOUR INFORMATION

Recommended Meal Composition
Suggested composition of a 2500 kCal diet based on recommendations of an expert panel of the Institute of Medicine, National Academies.

	Carbo-hydrate	Lipid	Protein
Percentage	60	15	25
kCal	1500	375	625
Grams	375	94	69
Ounces	13.2	3.3	2.4

Table 3-3	Dietary Reference Intakes (DRIs): Recommended Intakes for Individuals: Vitamins												
LIFE STAGE GROUP	VITAMIN A (μg/d)[a]	VITAMIN C (mg/d)	VITAMIN D (μg/d)[b,c]	VITAMIN E (mg/d)[d]	VITAMIN K (μg/d)	THIAMIN (mg/d)	RIBOFLAVIN (mg/d)	NIACIN (mg/d)[a]	VITAMIN B6 (mg/d)	FOLATE (μg/d)[f]	VITAMIN B12 (mg/d)	PANTOTHENIC ACID (mg/d)	BIOTIN (μg/d)	CHOLINE (mg/d)[a]
Infants														
0–6 mo	400*	40*	5*	4*	2.0*	0.2*	0.3*	2*	0.1*	65*	0.4*	1.7*	5*	125*
7–12 mo	500*	50*	5*	5*	2.5*	0.3*	0.4*	4*	0.3*	80*	0.5*	1.8*	6*	150*
Children														
1–3 y	300	15	5*	6	30*	0.5	0.5	6	0.5	150	0.9	2*	8*	200*
4–8 y	400	25	5*	7	55*	0.6	0.6	8	0.6	200	1.2	3*	12*	250*
Males														
9–13 y	600	45	5*	11	60*	0.9	0.9	12	1.0	300	1.8	4*	20*	375*
14–18 y	900	75	5*	15	75*	1.2	1.3	16	1.3	400	2.4	5*	25*	550*
19–30 y	900	90	5*	15	120*	1.2	1.3	16	1.3	400	2.4	5*	30*	550*
31–50 y	900	90	5*	15	120*	1.2	1.3	16	1.3	400	2.4	5*	30*	550*
51–70 y	900	90	10*	15	120*	1.2	1.3	16	1.7	400	2.4[h]	5*	30*	550*
>70 y	900	90	15*	15	120*	1.2	1.3	16	1.7	400	2.4[h]	5*	30*	550*
Females														
9–13 y	600	45	5*	11	60*	0.9	0.9	12	1.0	300	1.8	4*	20*	375*
14–18 y	700	65	5*	15	75*	1.0	1.0	14	1.2	400[f]	2.4	5*	25*	400*
19–30 y	700	75	5*	15	90*	1.1	1.1	14	1.3	400[f]	2.4	5*	30*	425*
31–50 y	700	75	5*	15	90*	1.1	1.1	14	1.3	400[f]	2.4	5*	30*	425*
51–70 y	700	75	10*	15	90*	1.1	1.1	14	1.5	400	2.4[h]	5*	30*	425*
>70 y	700	75	15*	15	90*	1.1	1.1	14	1.5	400	2.4[h]	5*	30*	425*
Pregnancy														
≤18 y	750	80	5*	15	75*	1.4	1.4	18	1.9	600[f]	2.6	6*	30*	450*
19–30 y	770	85	5*	15	90*	1.4	1.4	18	1.9	600[f]	2.6	6*	30*	450*
31–50 y	770	85	5*	15	90*	1.4	1.4	18	1.9	600[f]	2.6	6*	30*	450*
Lactation														
≤18 y	1200	115	5*	19	75*	1.4	1.6	17	2.0	500	2.8	7*	35*	550*
19–30 y	1300	120	5*	19	90*	1.4	1.6	17	2.0	500	2.8	7*	35*	550*
31–50 y	1300	120	5*	19	90*	1.4	1.6	17	2.0	500	2.8	7*	35*	550*

Note: This table (taken from the DRI reports, see www.nap.edu) presents Recommended Dietary Allowances (RDAs) in **bold type** and Adequate Intakes (AIs) in ordinary type followed by an asterisk (*) RDAs and AIs may both be used as goals for individual intake. RDAs are set to meet the needs of almost all (97 to 98 percent) individuals in a group. For healthy breastfed infants, the AI is the mean intake. The AI for other life stage and gender groups is believed to cover needs of all individuals in the group, but lack of data or uncertainty in the data prevent being able to specify with confidence the percentage of individuals covered by this intake.

[a] As retinol activity equivalents (RAEs). 1 RAE = 1 mg retinol, 12 mg β-carotene, 24 mg α-carotene, or 24 mg β-cryptoxanthin. To calculate RAEs from REs of provitamin A carotenoids in foods, divide the REs by 2. For preformed vitamin A in foods or supplements and for provitamin A carotenoids in supplements, 1 RE = 1 RAE.

[b] Calciferol. 1 μg calciferol = 40 IU vitamin D.

[c] In the absence of adequate exposure to sunlight.

[d] As α-tocopherol, α-Tocopherol includes RRR-α-tocopherol, the only form of α-tocopherol that occurs naturally in foods, and the 2R-stereoisometric forms of α-tocopherol (RRR-, RSR-, RRS, and RSS-α-tocopherol) that occur in fortified foods and supplements. It does not include the 2S-stereoisomeric forms of α-tocopherol (SRR, SSR, SR-, and SSS-α-tocopherol), also found in fortified foods and supplements.

[e] As niacin equivalents (NE). 1 mg of niacin = 60 mg of tryptophan; 0–6 months = preformed niacin (not NE).

[f] As dietary folate equivalents (DFE). 1 DFE = 1 μg food folate = 0.6 μg of folic acid from fortified food or as a supplement consumed with food = 0.5 μg of a supplement taken on an empty stomach.

[g] Although AIs have been set for choline, there are few data to assess whether a dietary supply of choline is needed at all stages of the life cycle and it may be that the choline requirement can be met by endogenous synthesis at some of these stages.

[h] Because 10 to 30 percent of older people may malabsorb food-bound B12, it is advisable for those older than 50 years to meet their RDA mainly by consuming foods fortified with B12 or a supplement containing B12.

[i] In view of evidence linking folate intake with neural tube defects in the fetus, it is recommended that all women capable of becoming pregnant consume 400 μg from supplements or fortified foods in addition to intake of food folate from a varied diet.

[j] It is assumed that women will continue consuming 400 mg from supplements or fortified food until their pregnancy is confirmed and they enter prenatal care, which ordinarily occurs after the end of the periconceptional period—the critical time for formation of the neural tube.

Sources: Dietary Reference Intakes for Calcium, Phosphorous, Magnesium, Vitamin D, and Fluoride (1997); Dietary Reference Intakes for Thiamin, Riboflavin, Niacin, Vitamin B6, Folate, Vitamin B12, Pantothenic Acid, Biotin, and Choline (1998); Dietary Reference Intakes for Vitamin C, Vitamin E, Selenium, and Carotenoids (2000); and Dietary Reference Intakes for Vitamin A, Vitamin K, Arsenic, Boron, Chromium, Copper, Iodine, Iron, Manganese, Molybdenum, Nickel, Silicon, Vanadium, and Zinc (2001). These reports may be accessed via www.nap.edu. Copyright 2001 by the National Academy of Sciences. All rights reserved.

The DRI report indicates that fruits and vegetables yield about one-half as much vitamin A as previously believed. This means that individuals who do not eat vitamin A-rich, animal-derived foods should upgrade their intake of carotene-rich fruits and vegetables. The report also sets a daily maximum intake level for vitamin A, in addition to boron, copper, iodine, iron, manganese, molybdenum, nickel, vanadium, and zinc. Specific recommended intakes are provided for vitamins A and K, chromium, copper, iodine, manganese, molybdenum, and zinc. The report concludes that one can meet the daily requirement for the nutrients examined without supplementation. The exception is the mineral *iron* for which most pregnant women need supplements to obtain their increased daily requirement.

Table 3.3 presents the RDA, AI, and UL values for the different vitamins. Also shown are the functions of the different vitamins, sources of intake, and effects of excess intake. We present only data for the ages of 14 to 18 years and 19 to 70 years; for a more complete listing for other age groupings, see the original source (*http://nal.usda.gov/fnic/dga/index.html*). Well-balanced meals provide an adequate quantity of all vitamins, regardless of age and physical activity level. Similarly, mineral supplements generally confer little benefit because the required minerals occur readily in food and water. Indeed, individuals who expend considerable energy exercising generally do not need to consume special foods or supplements that increase micronutrient intake above recommended levels. Also, at high levels of daily physical activity, food intake generally increases to sustain the added energy requirements of exercise. Additional food through a variety of nutritious meals proportionately increases vitamin and mineral intakes. **Table 3.4** presents similar data for the different minerals.

MYPYRAMID REPLACES THE FOOD GUIDE PYRAMID

Key principles of good eating include *variety* and *moderation*. Lobbyists for the beef and dairy industries greatly influenced earlier approaches to formulating recommendations such as the Four-Food-Group Plan adopted in 1992. Research in nutrition, cancer, and heart disease over the past 40 years uncovered the shortcomings of this plan, with its overemphasis on meat and milk products. In the typical American diet, energy-dense but nutrient-poor foods frequently substitute for more nutritious foods. This pattern of food intake increases risks for obesity, marginal micronutrient intakes, depressed consumption of fiber and phytochemicals, a reduction in levels of HDL cholesterol, and elevated homocysteine levels.

To more clearly reflect the current state of nutritional knowledge, the U.S. Department of Agriculture (USDA) developed the "**Food Guide Pyramid**" as a model of *Dietary Guidelines for Americans* (see below) who are aged 2 years and older (**Figure 3.3**).

In April 2005, the federal government unveiled its latest attempt to personalize the approach of Americans to choose a healthier lifestyle that balances nutrition and exercise. It replaces the 1992 pyramid, which was criticized as broad and vague; it recommended, for example, that people eat 6 to 12 servings of grains, but gave no explanation as to who should eat 6 versus 12, and did not identify a serving size. The new color-coded food pyramid, termed **MyPyramid** (Figure 3.3), offers a fresh look and a complementary Web site (*http://www.mypyramid.gov*) to provide personalized and supplementary materials on food intake guidance (e.g., the recommended number of cups of vegetables) based on age, sex, and level of daily exercise. The pyramid is based on the 2005 Dietary Guidelines for Americans published by the Department of Health and Human Services and the Department of Agriculture (*http://www.healthierus.gov/dietaryguidelines/*). It provides a series of vertical color bands of varying widths with the combined bands for fruits (red band) and vegetables (green band) occupying the greatest width, followed by grains, with the narrowest bands occupied by fats, oils, meats, and sugars. A personalized pyramid is obtained by logging on to the Web site. For example, a 40-year-old man who exercises less than 30 minutes a day should consume about 2200 kcal daily, which includes 7 ounces of grains, 3 cups of vegetables, 2 cups of fruit, 3 cups of low-fat milk, and 6 ounces of lean meat. He can also consume 6 teaspoons of oil and another 290 kcal of fats and sweets. A new addition includes a figure walking up the left side of the pyramid to emphasize at least 30 minutes of moderate to vigorous daily physical activity. Critics maintain that the new approach shifts too much of the burden of responsibility to the individual, who must have access to a computer and the skills to navigate the relatively complicated government site. Also, much of what is contained in the guidelines is not readily conveyed in the pyramid. For example, the pyramid only hints about the necessity for eating fewer foods such as fats, sugars, and salt, and the concept of replacing unhealthy food (fast food, junk food, soda) with more desirable food is difficult to discern.

The *Dietary Guidelines for Americans 2005* provides recommendations on diet and lifestyle designed to promote health, support physically active lives, and reduce chronic disease risks. It also includes advice to exercise moderately for 30 minutes (e.g., walking, jogging, bicycling, and lawn, garden, and house work) "most, preferably all, days of the week." To help manage body weight and prevent gradual unhealthy body weight, 60 to 90 minutes per day of moderate physical activity is recommended. The *Dietary Guidelines* advise children to exercise moderately for 60 minutes daily. They acknowledge that good nutrition combined with regular exercise provides an important approach to ensure good health and combat the obesity epidemic in the United States. The *Dietary Guidelines* separate fruits and vegetables from grains and emphasize whole-grain consumption.

Table 3-4

Table 3-4 Dietary Reference Intakes (DRIs): Recommended Intakes for Individuals: Minerals

LIFE STAGE GROUP	CALCIUM (mg/d)	CHROMIUM (µg/d)	COPPER (µg/d)	FLUORIDE (mg/d)	IODINE (µg/d)	IRON (mg/d)	MAGNESIUM (mg/d)	MANGANESE (mg/d)	MOLYBDENUM (µg/d)	PHOSPHORUS (mg/d)	SELENIUM (µg/d)	ZINC (mg/d)
Infants												
0–6 mo	210*	0.2*	200*	0.01*	110*	0.27*	30*	0.003*	2*	100*	15*	2*
7–12 mo	270*	5.5*	220*	0.5*	130*	11*	75*	0.6*	3*	275*	20*	3
Children												
1–3 y	500*	11*	340	0.7*	90	7	80	1.2*	17	460	20	3
4–8 y	800*	15*	440	1*	90	10	130	1.5*	22	500	30	5
Males												
9–13 y	1,300*	25*	700	2*	120	8	240	1.9*	34	1,250	40	8
14–18 y	1,300*	35*	890	3*	150	11	410	2.2*	43	1,250	55	11
19–30 y	1,000*	35*	900	4*	150	8	420	2.3*	45	700	55	11
31–50 y	1,000*	35*	900	4*	150	8	420	2.3*	45	700	55	11
51–70 y	1,200*	30*	900	4*	150	8	420	2.3*	45	700	55	11
>70 y	1,200*	30*	900	4*	150	8	420	2.3*	45	700	55	11
Females												
9–13 y	1,300*	21*	700	2*	120	8	240	1.6*	34	1,250	40	8
14–18 y	1,300*	24*	890	3*	150	15	360	1.6*	43	1,250	55	9
19–30 y	1,000*	25*	900	3*	150	18	310	1.8*	45	700	55	8
31–50 y	1,000*	25*	900	3*	150	18	320	1.8*	45	700	55	8
50–70 y	1,200*	20*	900	3*	150	8	320	1.8*	45	700	55	8
>70 y	1,200*	20*	900	3*	150	8	320	1.8*	45	700	55	8
Pregnancy												
≤18 y	1,300*	29*	1,000	3*	220	27	400	2.0*	50	1,250	60	13
19–30 y	1,000*	30*	1,000	3*	220	27	350	2.0*	50	700	60	11
31–50 y	1,000*	30*	1,000	3*	220	27	360	2.0*	50	700	60	11
Lactation												
≤18 y	1,300*	44*	1,300	3*	290	10	360	2.6*	50	1,250	70	14
19–30 y	1,000*	45*	1,300	3*	290	9	310	2.6*	50	700	70	12
31–50 y	1,000*	45*	1,300	3*	290	9	320	2.6*	50	700	70	12

Note. This table presents Recommended Dietary Allowances (RDAs) in **bold type** and Adequate Intakes (AIs) in ordinary type followed by an asterisk (*). RDAs and AIs may both be used as goals for individual intake. RDAs are set to meet the needs of almost all (97 to 98 percent) individuals in a group. For healthy breastfed infants, the AI is the mean intake. The AI for other life stage and gender groups is believed to cover needs of all individuals in the group, but lack of data or uncertainty in the data prevent being able to specify with confidence the percentage of individuals covered by this intake.

Sources: Dietary Reference Intakes for Calcium, Phosphorous, Magnesium, Vitamin D and Fluoride (1997); Dietary Reference Intakes for Thiamin, Riboflavin, Niacin, Vitamin B₅ Folate, Vitamin B₁₂, Pantothenic Acid, Biotin, and Choline (1998); Dietary Reference Intakes for Vitamin C, Vitamin E, Selenium, and Carotenoids (2000); and Dietary Reference Intakes for Vitamin A, Vitamin K, Arsenic, Boron, Chromium, Copper, Iodine, Iron, Manganese, Molybdenum, Nickel, Silicon, Vanadium, and Zinc (2001). These reports may be accessed via www.nap.edu Copyright 2001 by the National Academy of Sciences. Reprinted with permission.

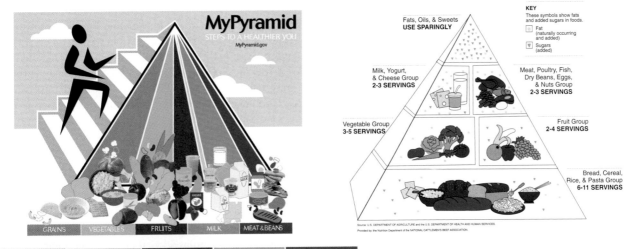

Figure 3.3. Comparing MyPyramid and the 1992 Food Guide Pyramid. (From U.S. Department of Agriculture, 2005.)

	MyPYRAMID	FOOD GUIDE PYRAMID
Calories	Individualized amounts from each food group based on age, gender, and PA	Broad range designed to fit the needs of the majorify of people
Physical Activity (PA)	Balance activity with food intake. PA for at least 30 min/d, and more for those trying to lose weight or prevent weight gain	No recommendations made
Grains	7-oz equivalents for a 2200 kCal diet; half the choices from whole grains	9 servings for a 2200 kCal diet (1 serving = 1 slice of bread or a 1/2 cup rice or pasta; choose whole grain bread, cereals and grains; limit high-fat and high-sugar baked foods
Vegetables	3 cups/d for a 2200 kCal diet; choose a variety of veggies each day. 3 cups/wk from dark green veggies; 2 cups/wk from orange veggies; 3 cups/wk from legumes; 6 cups/wk from starchy veggies, 7 cup/wk from other veggies	4 servings per day for 2200 kCal diet (1 serving = about 2 cups/d); eat a variety of vegetables, including dark green leafy vegetables, deep yellow vegetables, starchy vegetables, and other vegetables
Fruits	2 cups/d for a 2200 kCal diet; choose a variety of fruits; choose fresh, frozen, dried or canned; fruit juice should be less than 1/2 of total fruit intake	3 servings/d for a 2200 kCal diet (1 serving = about 1.5 cups); choose fresh fruit, frozen without sugar, dried, or fruit canned in water or juice; eat whole fruits more often than juices; regularly eat citrus fruits, melons, and berries
Milk, yogurt, cheese	3 cups/d for a 2200 kCal diet; choose fat-free or low-fat products	2–3 servings for a 2000 kCal diet (1 serving = 2–3 cups/d); use low-fat or nonfat milk and yogurt and part skim and low-fat cheeses
Meat, poultry, fish, dry beans, eggs, nuts	6 oz equivalents/d for a 2200 kCal diet; choose low-fat or lean; bake, broil, or grill; choose more fish, beans, peas, nuts, and seeds	6 oz for a 2200 kCal diet; eat lean meat, poultry without skin, and dry beans; trim fat and cook by broiling, roasting, grilling, or boiling; limit egg yolks (high cholesterol), and nuts and seeds (high kCal)
Oils	6 teaspoons/d on a 2200 kCal diet; choose from fish, nuts, and vegetable oils; limit solid fats (stick margarine, butter, shortening, and lard	Limit amount consumed; use unsaturated vegetable oils, and margarines that list liquid vegetable oils as first ingredients on label
Sugars and sweets	Choose foods and beverages with little added sugars	Limit amount consumed; limit high-sugar baked goods, sugar added as toppings and spreads, rinse fruits canned in heavy syrup

AN EXPANDING EMPHASIS ON HEALTHFUL EATING AND REGULAR PHYSICAL ACTIVITY

Scientists have responded to the rapidly rising number of overweight and obese adults and children and the increasing incidence of comorbidities associated with the overweight condition. In September 2002, the Institute of Medicine, the medical division of the National Academies, issued Guidelines as part of their Dietary Reference Intakes. Recommendations emphasized that Americans spend at least an *hour* (not 30 minutes as previously recommended—about 400 to 500 kCal) over the course of each day in moderately intense physical activity (brisk walking, swimming, or cycling) to maintain health and a normal body weight. This amount of regular physical activity, which was based on an assessment of the amount of exercise healthy people engage in each day, is twice as much as previously recommended in 1996 in a report from the United States Surgeon General! The advice, in agreement with the 2003 recommendations by the World Health Organization and the Food and Agriculture Organization of the United Nations (*http://www.who.int*), represents a bold increase in exercise duration considering the fact that 30 minutes of similar type exercise on most days has been shown to significantly decrease disease risk and more than 60% of the U.S. population fails to incorporate even a moderate level of exercise into their lives and 25% do no exercise at all. However, framing the Institute's 60-minute exercise recommendation is the belief that, to prevent weight gain, 30 minutes of daily exercise burns an insufficient number of calories.

The team of 21 experts also recommended for the first time a range for macronutrient intake plus how much dietary fiber to include in one's daily diet (previous reports over the past 60 years have dealt only with micronutrient recommendations). These recommendations are intended for use by professional nutritionists, as well as by the general public. To meet daily energy and nutrient needs while minimizing risk for chronic diseases, like heart disease and type 2 diabetes, adults should consume between 45% and 65% of their total calories from carbohydrates. This relatively wide range provides for flexibility, recognizing that both the high-carbohydrate, low-fat diet of Asian peoples and the higher fat diet of Mediterranean peoples, with its high monounsaturated fatty acid olive oil content, contribute to good health. The maximum intake of added sugars (i.e., the caloric sweeteners added to manufactured foods and beverages like soda, candy, fruit drinks, cakes, cookies, and ice cream) was placed at 25% of total calories. The panel suggested that this relatively high 25% level (considerably above the 2003 10% recommendation of the World Health Organization) represented the threshold above which there existed a significant decline in intake of certain important micronutrients such as vitamin A and calcium. The range of acceptable lipid intake was placed at 20% to 35% of caloric intake, which is a range lower at the lower end of most recommendations and higher at the upper end of the 30% limit set by the American Heart Association, American Cancer Society, and the National Institutes of Health. The panel noted that very low fat intake combined with high intake of carbohydrate tended to lower HDL cholesterol and raise triacylglycerol levels. Conversely, high intake of dietary fat (and accompanying increased caloric intake) contributes to obesity and the medical complications of obesity. Moreover, high-fat diets are usually associated with an increased saturated fatty acid intake, which raises plasma LDL cholesterol concentrations to further heighten coronary heart disease risk. "As low as possible" saturated fat intake was recommended; the panel also recognized that no safe level existed for *trans* fatty acid intake.

The panel recommended that adult men age 50 years and under consume 38 g of fiber daily and adult women consume 21 g a day, which are values that are significantly greater than the 12 to 15 g currently consumed. Particularly important is the consumption of water-soluble fibers (pectin from fruits and oat and rice bran), which reduce plasma cholesterol levels and slow digestion to increase satiety and decrease the risk of overeating.

Clearly, no one food or meal provides optimal nutrition and associated health-related benefits. Perhaps the following statement best summarizes the metabolic, epidemiologic, and clinical trial evidence over the past several decades regarding diet and lifestyle behaviors and coronary heart disease risk.

> *"Substantial evidence indicates that diets using nonhydrogenated unsaturated fats as the predominant form of dietary fat, whole grains as the main form of carbohydrates, an abundance of fruits and vegetables, and adequate omega-3 fatty acids can offer significant protection against coronary heart disease. Such diets, together with regular physical activity, avoidance of smoking, and maintenance of a healthy body weight, may prevent the majority of cardiovascular disease in Western populations."*

Mediterranean and Near-Vegetarian Diet Pyramids

Figure 3.4 presents the **Mediterranean Diet Pyramid**, a modification of the 1992 food-guide pyramid for application to individuals whose diet consists largely of (1) foods from the plant kingdom or (2) fruits, nuts, vegetables, and all manner of grains, and protein derived from fish, beans, and chicken, with dietary fat composed mostly of monounsaturated fatty acids and with mild alcohol consumption. Research findings indicate that a Mediterranean-type diet, possibly mediated via several plant foods in the diet, substantially reduces the rate of reoccurrence after a first myocardial infarction. Its high monounsaturated fatty acid content (generally in olive oil with its associated phytochemicals) also staves off age-related memory loss and the rate of overall mortality in healthy, elderly people. **Figure 3.5** presents the **Near-Vegetarian Diet Pyramid**, where no

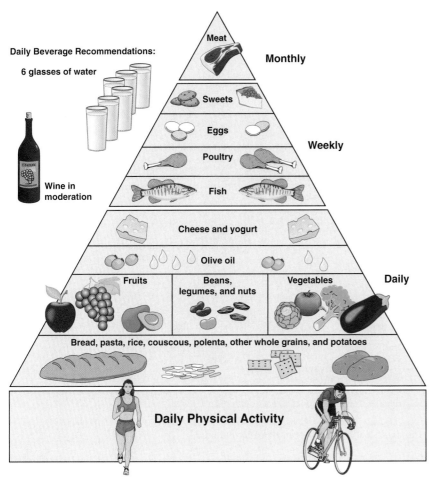

Daily Beverage Recommendations:

6 glasses of water

Wine in moderation

Meat — Monthly

Sweets

Eggs — Weekly

Poultry

Fish

Cheese and yogurt

Olive oil

Fruits | **Beans, legumes, and nuts** | **Vegetables** — Daily

Bread, pasta, rice, couscous, polenta, other whole grains, and potatoes

Daily Physical Activity

Figure 3.4. The Traditional Healthy Mediterranean Diet Pyramid.

List 2 major differences between the 1992 Food Guide Pyramid and the 2005 MyPyramid.

1.

2.

Give the recommended carbohydrate intake as a percentage of total kCal intake to minimize risk for chronic diseases.

Give the recommended maximum intake of added sugars as a percentage of total kCal.

Give the recommended acceptable range of lipid intake.

meat or dairy products are consumed. The focus of these two pyramids on fruits and vegetables, particularly cruciferous and green leafy vegetables and citrus fruit and juice, also reduces risk for ischemic stroke and may potentiate the beneficial effects of cholesterol-lowering drugs.

Diet Quality Index The **Diet Quality Index**, developed by the National Research Council Committee on Diet and Health, appraises the general "healthfulness" of one's diet. The index, presented in **Table 3.5**, offers a simple scoring scheme based on a risk gradient associated with diet and major diet-related chronic diseases. Respondents who meet a given dietary goal receive a score of 0; a score of 1 applies to an intake within 30% of a dietary goal; the score becomes 2 when intake fails to fall within 30% of the goal. The final score equals the total for all eight categories. The index ranges from 0 to 16, with a lower score representing a higher quality diet. A score of 4 or less reflects a more healthful diet; an index of 10 or higher indicates a less healthful diet that needs improvement.

EXERCISE AND FOOD INTAKE

Figure 3.6 illustrates the average energy intakes for males and females in the U.S. population grouped by age category. Mean energy intakes peaked between ages 16 to 29 years and declined thereafter. A similar pattern occurred for males and

Give the recommended fiber intake for adult men and women age 50 y and older.

Men:

Women:

FOR YOUR INFORMATION

Keep Them Unrefined, Complex, and Low Glycemic
Little health risk exists in subsisting chiefly on a variety of fiber-rich complex carbohydrates, as long as intake also supplies essential amino acids, fatty acids, minerals, and vitamins. The most desirable complex carbohydrates exhibit slow digestion and absorption rates. Such moderate- to low-glycemic types include whole-grain breads, cereals, pastas, legumes, most fruits, and milk and milk products.

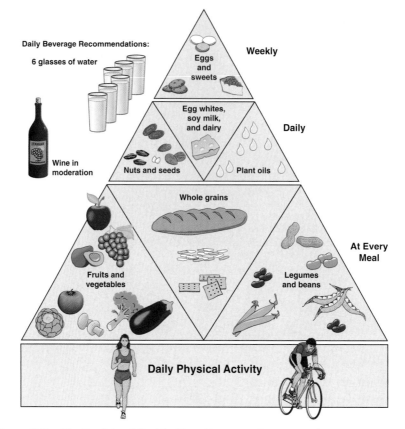

Figure 3.5. The Traditional Healthy Near-Vegetarian Diet Pyramid.

Table 3·5	The Diet Quality Index		
RECOMMENDATION		**SCORE**	**INTAKE**
Reduce total lipid intake to 30% or less of total energy		☐ 0 ☐ 1 ☐ 2	<30% >30–40% >40%
Reduce saturated fatty acid intake to less than 10% of total energy		☐ 0 ☐ 1 ☐ 2	<10% 10–13% >13%
Reduce cholesterol intake to less than 300 mg daily		☐ 0 ☐ 1 ☐ 2	<300 mg 300–400 mg >400 mg
Eat 5 or more servings daily of vegetables and fruits		☐ 0 ☐ 1 ☐ 2	≥5 servings 3–4 servings 0–2 servings
Increase intake of starches and other complex carbohydrates by eating 6 or more servings daily of breads, cereals, and legumes		☐ 0 ☐ 1 ☐ 2	≥6 servings 4–5 servings 0–3 servings
Maintain protein intake at moderate levels		☐ 0 ☐ 1 ☐ 2	100% RDA 100–150% RDA >150% RDA
Limit total daily sodium intake to 2400 mg or less		☐ 0 ☐ 1 ☐ 2	≤2400 mg 2400–3400 mg >3400 mg
Maintain adequate calcium intake (approximately the RDA)		☐ 0 ☐ 1 ☐ 2	≥100% RDA 67–99% RDA <67% RDA

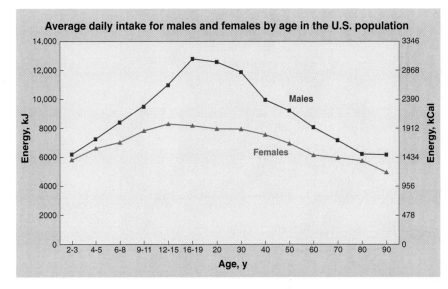

Figure 3.6. Average daily energy intake for males and females by age in the U.S. population during the years 1988 to 1991. (From Briefel, R.R., et al.: Total energy intake of the U.S. population: The Third National Health and Nutrition Examination Survey, 1988–1991. *Am. J. Clin. Nutr.,* 62(Suppl):10725, 1995; and Troiano, R.P.: Energy and fat intake of children and adolescents in the United States: Data from the National Health and Nutrition Survey. *Am. J. Clin. Nutr.,* 72:13435–13535, 2000.)

females, although males reported higher daily energy intakes than females at all ages. Between ages 20 to 29 years, women consumed 35% fewer kCal than men on a daily basis (3025 kCal vs. 1957 kCal). With aging, the gender difference in energy intake decreased; at age 70 years, women consumed 25% fewer kCal than men.

Physical Activity Makes a Difference

For individuals who regularly engage in moderate to intense physical activities, food intake balances easily with daily energy expenditure. Lumber workers, for example, who typically expend nearly 4500 kCal daily, unconsciously adjust energy intake to balance energy output. For them, body weight remains stable despite an extremely large food intake. The balancing of food intake to meet a new level of energy output takes 1 to 2 days to attain new energy equilibrium. The fine balance between energy expenditure and food intake does not occur in sedentary people, in whom caloric intake chronically exceeds their relatively low daily energy expenditure. Lack of precision in regulating food intake at the low end of the physical activity spectrum contributes to "creeping obesity" in highly mechanized and technologically advanced societies.

Figure 3.7 presents data on energy intake from a large sample of elite male and female endurance, strength, and team sport athletes in the Netherlands. For males, daily energy intake ranged between 2900 and 5900 kCal, whereas female competitors consumed 1600 to 3200 kCal. Except for the high-energy intake of athletes at extremes of performance and training, daily energy intake did not exceed 4000 kCal for men and 3000 kCal for women.

Extreme Energy Intake and Expenditure: The Tour de France

During competition or periods of high-intensity training, some sport activities require extreme energy output (sometimes in excess of 1000 kCal·h^{-1} in elite marathoners and professional cyclists) and a correspondingly high-energy intake. For example, the daily energy requirements of elite cross-country skiers during 1

Questions & Notes

Give the average energy intake for males and females between ages 16–29 years.

Males–

Females–

Briefly describe what happens to energy intake with aging.

Give the estimated energy expenditure for participants in the Tour de France.

List the 3 main food groups for the Traditional Mediterranean Diet Pyramid.

1.

2.

3.

List the 2 main food groups for the Near-Vegetarian Diet Pyramid.

1.

2.

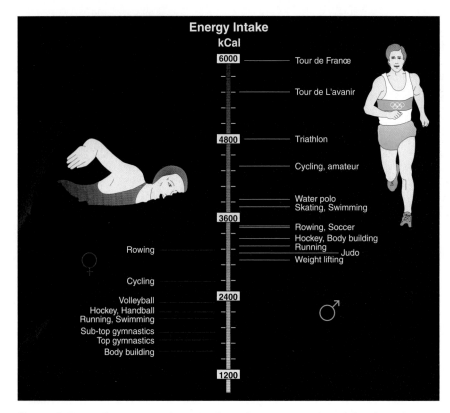

Figure 3.7. Daily energy intake in kCal per day in elite male and female endurance, strength, and team sport athletes. (From van Erp-Baart, A.M.J., et al.: Nationwide survey on nutritional habits in elite athletes. *Int. J. Sports Med.*, 10:53, 1989.)

week of training averaged 3740 to 4860 kCal for women and 6120 to 8570 kCal for men. **Figure 3.8** shows the variation in daily energy expenditure for a male competitor during the Tour de France professional cycling race. Energy expenditure averaged 6500 kCal daily for nearly 3 weeks during this event. Large daily variation occurred depending on the activity level for a particular day; the daily energy expenditure decreased to 3000 kCal on a "rest" day and increased to approximately 9000 kCal when cycling over a mountain pass. By combining liquid nutrition with normal meals, this cyclist nearly matched daily energy expenditure with energy intake.

The Precompetition Meal

Athletes often compete in the morning following an overnight fast. Significant depletion occurs in the body's carbohydrate reserves over 8 to 12 hours without eating (see Chapter 2), so precompetition nutrition takes on considerable importance even if the person follows appropriate dietary recommendations. *The precompetition meal provides the athlete with adequate carbohydrate energy and ensures optimal hydration.* Fasting before competition or intense training makes no sense physiologically because it rapidly depletes liver and muscle glycogen and ultimately

impairs exercise performance. Consider the following factors when individualizing an athlete's meal plans:

- Food preference
- Psychologic set
- Food digestibility

As a general rule, foods high in lipid and protein should not be consumed on competition days. These foods digest slowly and remain in the digestive tract longer than carbohydrate foods containing similar calories. Timing of the pre-competition meal also deserves consideration. Increased emotional stress and tension depress intestinal absorption because of a significant decrease in blood flow to the digestive tract. *Generally, 3 hours provides sufficient time to digest and absorb a carbohydrate-rich, precompetition meal.*

High Protein: Not the Best Choice Many athletes become accustomed to and even depend on the classic "steak and eggs" precompetition meal. Although this meal may satisfy the athlete, coach, and restaurateur, its benefits to exercise performance have yet to be demonstrated. In fact, this type of low-carbohydrate meal can actually hinder optimal performance.

The high-protein precompetition meal should be mod-

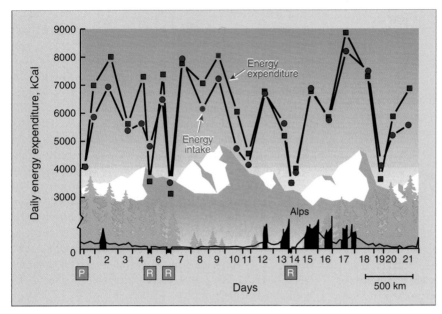

Figure 3.8.   Daily energy expenditure (purple squares) and energy intake (yellow circles) for a cyclist during the Tour de France competition. Note the extremely high energy expenditure values and the ability to achieve energy balance with liquid nutrition plus normal meals. P, stage; R, rest day. (Modified from Saris, W.H.M., et al.: Adequacy of vitamin supply under maximal sustained workloads: The Tour de France. In: *Elevated Dosages of Vitamins*. Walter, P., et al. (eds.). Toronto: Huber Publishers, 1989.)

Questions & Notes

List 2 food types that should be consumed during days of athletic competition.

   1.

   2.

Give 3 reasons the precompetition meal should be higher in carbohydrate than in protein.

   1.

   2.

   3.

Give the major purpose of the precompetition meal.

Give 2 benefits of a precompetition liquid meal.

   1.

   2.

ified or even abolished in favor of one high in carbohydrates for the following reasons:

- Dietary carbohydrates (not protein) replenish liver and muscle glycogen previously depleted from an overnight fast.
- Carbohydrates digest and become absorbed more rapidly than proteins or lipids; thus, carbohydrates provide energy faster and reduce the feeling of fullness.
- High-protein meals elevate resting metabolism more than high-carbohydrate meals due to greater energy requirements for protein's digestion, absorption, and assimilation. Additional metabolic heat places demands on the body's heat-dissipating mechanisms, which impairs exercise performance in hot weather.
- Protein catabolism for energy facilitates dehydration during exercise because the byproducts of amino acid breakdown require water for urinary excretion. Approximately 50 mL of water "accompanies" the excretion of each gram of urea in urine.
- Carbohydrate provides the main energy nutrient for short-duration anaerobic exercise and prolonged, high-intensity endurance activities.

Ideal Precompetition Meal

Ideal Precompetition Meal   *The ideal precompetition meal maximizes muscle and liver glycogen storage and provides glucose for intestinal absorption during exercise.* The meal should: (1) contain 150 to 300 g of carbohydrate (3 to 5 g per kg of body mass) in either solid or liquid form and (2) be consumed within 3 to 4 hours before exercising.

The benefit of a precompetition meal depends on the athlete maintaining a nutritionally sound diet throughout training. Pre-exercise food cannot correct existing nutritional deficiencies or inadequate nutrient intake during the weeks before competition.

Liquid Meals Commercially prepared **liquid meals** offer an alternative to the precompetition meal. Benefits include the following:

- Enhance energy and nutrient intake in training, particularly if daily energy output exceeds energy intake due to the athlete's lack of interest in food or nutrition mismanagement
- Provide a high glycemic carbohydrate for glycogen replenishment
- Contain some lipid and protein to contribute to satiety
- Supply fluid because these meals exist in liquid form
- Digest rapidly, leaving essentially no residue in the intestinal tract

Liquid meals prove particularly effective during day-long swimming and track meets or tennis, ice hockey, soccer, field hockey, martial arts, wrestling, volleyball, and basketball tournaments. During tournament competition, the athlete usually has little time for or interest in food. Athletes can also use liquid meals if they experience difficulty maintaining a relatively large body mass and as a ready source of calories to gain weight.

Carbohydrate Intake Before, During, and After Intense Exercise

High-intensity aerobic exercise continued for 1 hour decreases liver glycogen by about 55%, whereas a 2-hour strenuous workout almost depletes the glycogen in the liver and specifically exercised muscle fibers. Even maximal, repetitive, 1- to 5-minute bouts of exercise interspersed with brief rest intervals dramatically lowers liver and muscle glycogen levels (e.g., soccer, ice hockey, field hockey, European handball, and tennis). Carbohydrate supplementation improves both prolonged exercise capacity and intermittent, high-intensity exercise performance. The "vulnerability" of the body's glycogen stores during intense exercise has focused research on the potential "high performance" benefits of carbohydrate intake just before and during exercise. Current research also continues to delineate ways to optimize carbohydrate replenishment during the postexercise recovery period.

Before Exercise

The potential endurance benefits of ingesting simple sugars before exercise remain equivocal. One line of research contends that consuming rapidly absorbed, high-glycemic carbohydrates within 1 hour before exercising accelerates glycogen depletion and negatively affects endurance performance by (1) causing an overshoot in insulin release, thus creating low blood sugar, termed **rebound hypoglycemia**, that impairs central nervous system function during exercise and (2) facilitating glucose influx into muscle (through a large insulin release) to increase carbohydrate use as fuel during exercise. At the same time, high insulin levels inhibit lipolysis, which reduces free fatty acid mobilization from adipose tissue. Both augmented carbohydrate breakdown and blunted fat mobilization contribute to premature glycogen depletion and early fatigue.

Research in the late 1970s indicated that drinking a highly concentrated sugar solution 30 minutes before exercise precipitated early fatigue in endurance activities. These findings have not been replicated, however. More recent research indicates that consuming glucose before exercise increases muscle glucose uptake but reduces liver glucose output during exercise to a degree that actually *conserves* liver glycogen reserves. The discrepancy among research findings has no clear explanation. From a practical standpoint, one way to eliminate the potential for negative effects from pre-exercise simple sugars necessitates ingesting them at least 60 minutes before exercise. This allows sufficient time to re-establish hormonal balance prior to exercise.

Pre-Exercise Fructose Intake The small intestine absorbs fructose more slowly than glucose and causes only a minimal insulin response with essentially no decline in blood glucose. These observations have stimulated debate about whether fructose might provide a beneficial pre-exercise, exogenous carbohydrate fuel source for prolonged exercise. Although the theoretical rationale for fructose use appears plausible, its exercise benefits remain inconclusive. From a practical standpoint, consuming a high-fructose beverage often produces significant gastrointestinal distress (cramping, vomiting, and diarrhea), which negatively impacts exercise performance. *Also, once absorbed by the small intestine, fructose must be delivered to the liver for conversion to glucose. This time delay further limits fructose availability for energy.*

Glycemic Index and Pre-Exercise Food Intake

The glycemic index helps formulate the composition of the immediate pre-exercise meal to provide glucose to maintain blood sugar and muscle metabolism with minimal increase in insulin release. Maintaining normal plasma insulin levels should theoretically stabilize blood glucose and optimize fat mobilization and catabolism, thus sparing glycogen reserves. Consuming low-glycemic index foods immediately (<30 min) before exercise allows for a relatively slow rate of glucose absorption into the blood. This eliminates an insulin surge and yet provides a steady supply of "slow-release" glucose from the digestive tract during exercise, which is an effect that theoretically should benefit long-term, high-intensity exercise.

During Exercise

Consuming about 60 g of liquid or solid carbohydrates each hour during exercise benefits high-intensity, long-duration exercise and repetitive, short bouts of near-maximal effort. Sustained exercise below 50% of maximum intensity relies primarily on fat oxidation, with only a relatively small demand on carbohydrate breakdown. As such, consuming carbohydrate offers little benefit during such activity. In contrast, carbohydrate intake provides supplementary glucose during high-intensity, aerobic exercise when glycogen utilization increases greatly. Exogenous carbohydrate either (1) spares muscle glycogen because the ingested glucose powers the exercise or (2) helps to stabilize blood glucose, which prevents headache, lightheadedness, nausea, and other symptoms of central nervous system distress. Maintaining an optimal level of blood glucose also supplies muscles with glucose when their glycogen reserves deplete in the later stages of prolonged exercise.

Consuming carbohydrates while exercising at 60% to 80% $\dot{V}O_{2max}$ postpones fatigue by 15 to 30 minutes. This effect offers great potential for marathon runners who experience muscle fatigue within several hours after initiating exercise. **Figure 3.9** shows that a single, concentrated carbohydrate intake about 2 hours

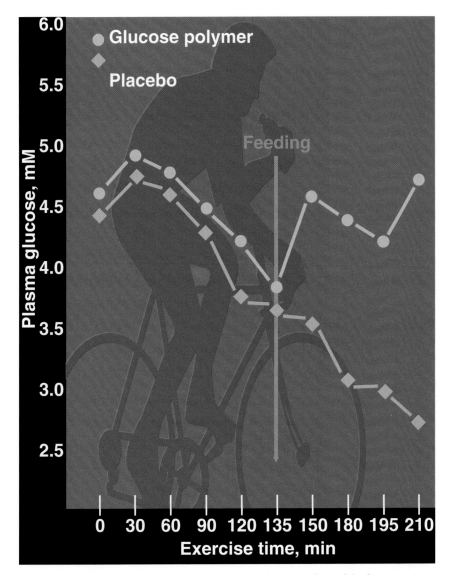

Figure 3.9. Average plasma glucose concentration during prolonged, high-intensity aerobic exercise when subjects consumed a placebo (green) or glucose polymer (gold; 3 g per kg body mass in a 50% solution). (Modified from Coggan, A.R., and Coyle, E.F.: Metabolism and performance following carbohydrate ingestion late in exercise. *Med. Sci. Sports Exerc.*, 21:59, 1989.)

into exercise (when blood glucose and glycogen reserves near depletion) restores blood glucose levels; this increases carbohydrate availability and delays fatigue because higher blood glucose levels help sustain the muscles' energy needs.

Post-Exercise Carbohydrate Intake

To speed glycogen replenishment after a hard bout of training or competition, one should immediately consume carbohydrate-rich (high-glycemic) foods. Specifically, consume 50 to 75 g (2 to 3 oz) of moderate- to high-glycemic carbohydrates every 2 hours, for a total of 500 g (7 to 10 g per kg body mass), or until a large, high-carbohydrate meal is consumed. If consuming carbohydrate immediately after exercise is impractical, meals containing 2.5 g of high-glycemic carbohydrates per kg of body mass consumed at 2, 4, 6, 8, and 22 hours after exercise rapidly restores muscle glycogen.

Avoid legumes, fructose, and milk products when trying to rapidly replenish glycogen reserves because of their slow rates of intestinal absorption. More rapid glycogen resynthesis results if the person remains inactive during recovery. *Under optimal carbohydrate intake conditions, glycogen replenishes at a rate of about 5% per hour. Thus, even under the best of circumstances, it requires at least 20 hours to re-establish glycogen stores after glycogen depletion.*

GLUCOSE INTAKE, ELECTROLYTES, AND WATER UPTAKE

Adding carbohydrate to the oral rehydration beverage provides additional glucose energy for exercise when the body's glycogen reserves deplete. Determining the optimal fluid/carbohydrate mixture and volume to consume during exercise takes on importance when the objectives are to reduce fatigue and prevent dehydration. Consuming a large, dilute fluid volume may lessen carbohydrate uptake, and concentrated sugar solutions diminish fluid replacement.

The rate of stomach emptying greatly affects the absorption of fluid and nutrients by the small intestine. Exercise up to an intensity of about 75% $\dot{V}O_{2max}$ has little negative effect on gastric emptying; but an exercise intensity of greater than 75% $\dot{V}O_{2max}$ slows the emptying rate considerably. Gastric volume, however, greatly influences gastric emptying; its rate decreases as stomach volume decreases. Consequently, maintaining a relatively large fluid volume in the stomach speeds gastric emptying.

Consider Fluid Concentration

Concern exists about the possible negative effects of sugar drinks on water absorption from the digestive tract. Gastric emptying slows when ingested fluids contain an excessive concentration of particles in solution (increased osmolality) or possess high caloric content. Any factor that impairs fluid uptake can negatively impact prolonged exercise in hot weather, when adequate water intake and absorption play prime roles in the participant's health and safety. Ingesting up to an 8% glucose-sodium oral rehydration beverage causes little negative effect on gastric emptying. In fact, it facilitates fluid uptake by the intestinal lumen, because rapid, active coupled or cotransport of glucose-sodium across the intestinal mucosa stimulates water's passive uptake by osmotic action. Water not only replenishes effectively, but the additional glucose uptake contributes to blood glucose maintenance. This glucose can then spare muscle and liver glycogen and/or provide for blood glucose reserves during the later stage of exercise.

Rehydration solutions combining two different, transportable carbohydrate substrates (glucose, fructose, sucrose, or maltodextrins) induce greater water uptake than solutions containing only one of the substrates. Adding the second substrate into the solution stimulates more intestinal transport mechanisms, thus facilitating net water absorption by osmosis. To optimize water and carbohydrate absorption, use a 6% carbohydrate-electrolyte solution containing a combination of fructose and sucrose, each of which is absorbed by separate, noncompetitive pathways.

Sodium's Potential Benefit

Adding a moderate amount of sodium to ingested fluid maintains plasma sodium concentration. This benefits the ultraendurance athlete at risk for hyponatremia (see Chapter 2), which results from significant sweat-induced sodium loss coupled with an unusually large intake of plain water. Adding sodium to the rehydration beverage maintains plasma osmolality, reduces urine output, and sustains the drive to drink. These factors promote continued fluid intake and fluid retention during recovery from exercise.

CARBOHYDRATE NEEDS IN INTENSE TRAINING

Repeated days of strenuous endurance workouts for distance running, swimming, cross-country skiing, and cycling can induce general fatigue that makes training progressively more difficult. Often referred to as "**staleness**," this physiologic state probably results from gradual depletion of glycogen reserves. In one experiment, in which athletes ran 16.1 km (10 miles) a day for 3 successive days, glycogen in the thigh muscles became nearly depleted, even though the athletes' diets contained about 50% carbohydrate. By the third day, glycogen usage during the run was less than on the first day, and fat breakdown supplied the predominant fuel to power exercise. No further glycogen depletion occurred when daily dietary carbohydrate increased to 600 g (70% of caloric intake). This demonstrates the importance of maintaining adequate carbohydrate intake during training.

Box 3–2 • CLOSE UP

RECOMMENDED ORAL REHYDRATION BEVERAGE

The ideal **oral rehydration beverage** has these five qualities:

1. Tastes good
2. Absorbs rapidly
3. Causes little or no gastrointestinal distress
4. Helps maintain extracellular fluid volume and osmolality
5. Offers potential to enhance exercise performance

Consuming a 5% to 8% carbohydrate-electrolyte beverage during exercise in the heat contributes to temperature regulation and fluid balance as effectively as plain water. The drink also maintains glucose metabolism and glycogen reserves in prolonged exercise.

To determine a drink's carbohydrate percentage, divide its carbohydrate content (in g) by the fluid volume (in mL) and multiply by 100. For example, 80 g of carbohydrate in 1000 mL (1 L) of water represents an 8%

solution. Of course, various environmental and exercise conditions interact to influence the optimal composition of the rehydration solution. With relatively short-duration (30 to 60 minutes), intense aerobic effort and high thermal stress, fluid replenishment takes on importance for health and safety; ingesting a more dilute carbohydrate-electrolyte solution (<5% carbohydrate) is advisable under such conditions. In cool weather, with less likelihood of significant dehydration, a more concentrated beverage of 15% carbohydrate suffices. Essentially, no differences exist among liquids containing glucose, sucrose, or starch as the preferred exogenous carbohydrate fuel source during exercise.

The optimal carbohydrate replacement rate ranges between 30 to 60 g (1 to 2 oz) per hour. The accompanying table compares the carbohydrate and mineral contents and solute concentrations (osmolality) of popular beverages used by athletes to replenish fluid during exercise.

BEVERAGES	CHO SOURCE	CHO %	NA (MG)	K (MG)	OTHER MINERALS/ VITAMINS[a]
Gatorade[b] [Quaker Oats Co]	Sucrose; glucose (powder)	6	110	25	Cl, Ph
Exceed[b] [Ross Laboratories]	Glucose polymers; fructose	7.2	50	45	—
Quickick[b] [Cramer Products, Inc.]	Fructose; sucrose	4.7	116	23	Cl, Ca, Mg, Ph
Sqwincher [Universal Products, Inc.]	Glucose; fructose	6.8	60	36	Cl, Ph, Ca, Mg, Vit C
10-K [Beverage Products, Inc.]	Sucrose; glucose; fructose	6.3	52	26	Vit C, Cl, Ph
USA Wet [Texas Wet, Inc.]	Sucrose	6.8	62	44	Cl, Ph
Coca-Cola [Coca-Cola, USA]	High-fructose corn syrup; sucrose	10.7–11.3	9.2	Trace	—
Sprite [Coca-Cola, USA]	High-fructose corn syrup; sucrose	10.2	28	Trace	Ph
Cranberry juice cocktail	High-fructose corn syrup	15	10	61	—
Orange juice	Fructose; sucrose; glucose	11.8	2.7	510	Ph, Vit C
Water	—	—	low[c]	low[c]	—
PowerAde	High-fructose corn syrup; maltodextrin	8	73	33	Ph, Ca, iron, Vit C and A, niacin, riboflavin, thiamin
All-Sport	High-fructose corn syrup	8–9	55	55	—
10 K	Sucrose; glucose; fructose	6.3	54	25	—
Cytomax	High-fructose corn syrup; sucrose	7–11	10	150	—
Breakthrough	Maltodextrin; fructose	8.5	60	45	—
Everlast	Sucrose; fructose	6	100	20	—
Hydra Charge	Maltodextrin; fructose	8	—	Trace	—
SportaLYTE	Maltodextrin; fructose; glucose	7.5	100	60	—

[a] When reported; [b] Serving size = 8 fluid oz; [c] Depends on water source; CHO, carbohydrate; Cl, chloride; Ph, phosphorus; Ca, calcium; Mg, magnesium; K, potassium; Na, sodium; Chart modified from Coleman, E.: Sports drink update. *Gatorade Sports Science Institute*, Vol. 1, No. 5, 1988.

Diet, Glycogen Stores, and Endurance Capacity

In the late 1960s, scientists observed that endurance performance significantly improved simply by consuming a carbohydrate-rich diet for 3 days prior to exercising. Conversely, endurance deteriorated if the diet consisted principally of lipids. In one series of experiments, subjects consumed one of three diets. The first diet maintained normal energy intake but supplied the majority of calories from lipids, with only 5% from carbohydrate. The second diet provided the normal allotment for calories with the typical percentages of the three macronutrients. The third diet provided 80% of calories as carbohydrate.

The results from this classic study illustrated in **Figure 3.10** show that the glycogen content of leg muscles, expressed as grams of glycogen per 100 g of muscle, averaged 0.6 for subjects who consumed the low-carbohydrate diet, 1.75 for subjects who consumed the typical diet, and 3.75 for subjects who consumed the high-carbohydrate diet. Furthermore, the subjects' endurance capacity varied greatly depending on the pre-exercise diet. When subjects consumed the high-carbohydrate diet, endurance more than tripled compared with the low-carbohydrate diet!

These findings highlight the important role nutrition plays in establishing appropriate energy reserves for exercise. A diet deficient in carbohydrate rapidly depletes muscle and liver glycogen. Glycogen depletion subsequently affects performance in maximal, short-term anaerobic exercise and prolonged, high-intensity aerobic effort. These observations pertain not only to athletes, but also to moderately active people who eat less than the recommended quantity of carbohydrate.

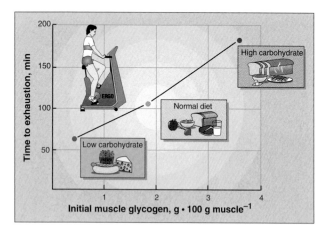

Figure 3.10. Classic experiment on the effects of a low-carbohydrate diet, mixed diet, and high-carbohydrate diet on glycogen content of the quadriceps femoris muscle and the duration of endurance exercise on a bicycle ergometer. With a high-carbohydrate diet, endurance time tripled compared with a diet low in carbohydrate. (Adapted from Bergstrom, J., et al.: Diet, muscle glycogen and physical performance. *Acta. Physiol. Scand.*, 71:140, 1967.)

Enhanced Glycogen Storage: Carbohydrate Loading

A particular combination of diet plus exercise produces a significant "packing" of muscle glycogen, a procedure termed "**carbohydrate loading**" or "**glycogen supercompensation**." The procedure increases muscle glycogen levels more than levels achieved by simply maintaining a high-carbohydrate diet. Glycogen loading packs up to 5 g of glycogen into each 100 g of muscle (in contrast to the normal value of 1.7 g). For athletes who follow the classic glycogen-loading procedure (see *How to Carbohydrate Load* on page 119), enhanced muscle glycogen levels are maintained (in a resting, nonexercising individual) for at least 3 days if the diet contains about 60% of total calories as carbohydrate during the maintenance phase.

Exercise facilitates both the rate and magnitude of glycogen replenishment. For sports competition and exercise training, a diet containing between 60% and 70% of calories as carbohydrates generally provides for adequate muscle and liver glycogen reserves. This diet ensures about twice the level of muscle glycogen compared with sedentary counterparts who consume a lower carbohydrate diet (50% to 60% carbohydrates). For well-nourished physically active individuals, the supercompensation effect remains relatively small. During intense training, however, individuals who do not upgrade daily caloric and carbohydrate intakes to meet increased energy demands may experience chronic muscle fatigue and staleness.

Individuals should learn all they can about carbohydrate loading before trying to manipulate their diet and exercise habits to achieve a supercompensation effect. If a person decides to supercompensate after weighing the pros and cons (see page 119), the new food regimen should be tried in stages during training and not for the first time before competition. For example, a runner should start with a long run followed by a high-carbohydrate diet. Keep a detailed log of how the dietary manipulation affects performance. Subjective feelings should be noted during exercise depletion and replenishment phases. With positive results, the person then tries the entire series of depletion, low-carbohydrate diet, and high-carbohydrate diet but maintains the low-carbohydrate diet for only 1 day. If no adverse effects appear, the low-carbohydrate diet should be gradually extended to a maximum of 4 days.

Modified Loading Procedure

The less-stringent, modified dietary protocol removes many of the negative aspects of the classic glycogen-loading sequence. This 6-day protocol does not require prior exercise to deplete glycogen. The athlete trains at about 75% of $\dot{V}O_{2max}$ (85% HR_{max}) for 1.5 hours and then gradually reduces (tapers) exercise duration on successive days. Carbohydrates represent about 50% of total caloric intake during the first 3 days. Three days before competition, the diet's carbohydrate content then increases to 70%

Box 3-3 •   CLOSE UP

HOW TO CARBOHYDRATE LOAD

The importance of muscle glycogen levels to enhance exercise performance remains unequivocal; time to exhaustion during intense aerobic exercise directly relates to the initial glycogen content of the liver and active musculature. In one series of experiments, muscle glycogen content increased six-fold and endurance capacity tripled for subjects fed a high-carbohydrate diet compared with feeding the same subjects a low-carbohydrate (high-fat) diet of similar energy content. Given muscle glycogen's importance in prolonged endurance performance, carbohydrate loading provides a strategy to increase initial muscle and liver glycogen levels.

CLASSIC CARBOHYDRATE LOADING PROCEDURE

Classic carbohydrate loading involves a two-stage procedure.

Stage 1—Depletion

Day 1: Perform exhaustive exercise to deplete muscle glycogen in specific muscles
Days 2, 3, 4: Maintain low-carbohydrate food intake (high percentage of protein and lipid in the daily diet)

Stage 2—Carbohydrate Loading

Days 5, 6, 7: Maintain high-carbohydrate food intake (normal percentage of protein in the daily diet)
Competition Day
Follow high-carbohydrate precompetition meal recommendation

SPECIFICS OF PRECOMPETITION DIET-EXERCISE PLAN TO ENHANCE GLYCOGEN STORAGE

- Employ high-intensity, aerobic exercise for 90 minutes about 6 days before competition to reduce muscle and liver glycogen stores. Because glycogen loading occurs only in the specific muscles depleted by exercise, athletes must engage the major muscles involved in their sport.
- Maintain a low-carbohydrate diet (60 to 100 g per day) for 3 days while training at moderate intensity to further deplete glycogen stores.
- Switch to a high-carbohydrate diet (400 to 700 g per day) at least 3 days before competition, and maintain this intake up to and as part of the precompetition meal.

Sample Meal Plans for Carbohydrate Depletion (Stage 1) and Carbohydrate Loading (Stage 2) Preceding an Endurance Event

Meal	Stage 1	Stage 2
Breakfast	1/2 cup fruit juice 2 eggs 1 slice whole-wheat toast 1 glass whole milk	1 cup fruit juice 1 bowl hot or cold cereal 1 to 2 muffins 1 Tbsp butter coffee (cream and sugar)
Lunch	6 oz hamburger 2 slices bread 1 serving salad 1 Tbsp mayonnaise and salad dressing 1 glass whole milk	2–3 oz hamburger with bun 1 cup juice 1 orange 1 Tbsp mayonnaise 1 serving pie or cake
Snack	1 cup yogurt	1 cup yogurt, fruit, or cookies
Dinner	2 to 3 pieces chicken, fried 1 baked potato with sour cream 1/2 cup vegetables 2 Tbsp butter iced tea (no sugar)	1–1 1/2 pieces chicken, baked 1 baked potato with sour cream 1 cup vegetables 1/2 cup sweetened pineapple iced tea (sugar) 1 Tbsp butter
Snack	1 glass whole milk	1 glass chocolate milk with 4 cookies

Carbohydrate intake averages approximately 100 g or 400 kCal during Stage 1; Stage 2 carbohydrate intake increases to 400 to 700 g or about 1600 to 2800 kCal.

Box 3–4 • CLOSE UP

NUTRIENT TIMING TO OPTIMIZE MUSCLE RESPONSE TO RESISTANCE TRAINING

An evidence-based nutritional approach has been proposed to enhance the quality of resistance training and facilitate muscle growth and strength development. This easy-to-follow new dimension to sports nutrition emphasizes not only the specific type and mixture of nutrients but also the timing of nutrient intake. Its goal is to blunt the catabolic state (release of the hormones glucagon, epinephrine, norepinephrine, and cortisol) and activate the natural muscle-building hormones (testosterone, growth hormone, IGF-1, and insulin) to facilitate recovery from exercise and maximize muscle growth. Three phases for optimizing specific nutrient intake are proposed:

1. The **energy phase** enhances nutrient intake to spare muscle glycogen and protein, optimizes muscular endurance, limits immune system suppression, reduces muscle damage, and facilitates recovery in the post-exercise period. Consuming a carbohydrate/protein supplement in the immediate pre-exercise period and during exercise extends muscular endurance; the ingested protein promotes protein metabolism, thus reducing demand for amino acid release from muscle. The carbohydrates consumed during exercise suppress the release of cortisol. This blunts the suppressive effects of exercise on immune system function and lessens the use of branched-chain amino acids generated by protein breakdown for energy.

The recommended *energy phase* supplement profile contains the following nutrients: 20 to 26 g of high-glycemic carbohydrates (glucose, sucrose, maltodextrin), 5 to 6 g of whey protein (rapidly digested, high-quality protein separated from milk in the cheese-making process), 1 g of leucine, 30 to 120 mg of vitamin C, 20 to 60 IU of vi-

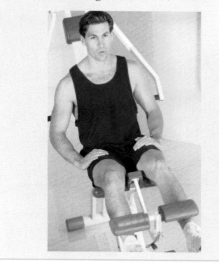

tamin E, 100 to 250 mg of sodium, 60 to 100 mg of potassium, and 60 to 220 mg of magnesium.

2. The *anabolic phase* consists of the 45-minute post-exercise metabolic window, which is a period of enhanced insulin sensitivity for muscle glycogen replenishment and the repair and synthesis of muscle tissue. This shift from catabolic to anabolic state occurs largely by depressing the action of the catabolic hormone cortisol and increasing the anabolic, muscle-building effects of the hormone insulin by consuming a standard high-glycemic carbohydrate/protein supplement in liquid form (e.g., whey protein and high-glycemic carbohydrates). In essence, the high-glycemic carbohydrate consumed after exercise serves as a nutrient activator to stimulate the release of insulin, which, in the presence of amino acids, increases muscle tissue synthesis and decreases protein degradation.

The recommended *anabolic phase* supplement profile contains the following nutrients: 40 to 50 g of high-glycemic carbohydrates (glucose, sucrose, maltodextrin), 13 to 15 g of whey protein, 1 to 2 g of leucine, 1 to 2 g of glutamine, 60 to 120 mg of vitamin C, and 80 to 400 IU of vitamin E.

3. The *growth phase* extends from the end of the anabolic phase to the beginning of the next workout. It represents the time period to maximize insulin sensitivity and maintain an anabolic state to accentuate gains in muscle mass and muscle strength. The first several hours (*rapid segment*) of this phase is geared to maintaining increased insulin sensitivity and glucose uptake to maximize glycogen replenishment. It also aims to speed the elimination of metabolic wastes via an increase in blood flow and stimulate tissue repair and muscle growth. The next 16 to 18 hours (*sustained segment*) maintains a positive nitrogen balance. This occurs with a relatively high daily protein intake (between 0.91 and 1.2 g of protein per pound of body weight) that fosters sustained but slower muscle tissue synthesis. An adequate carbohydrate intake emphasizes glycogen replenishment.

The recommended *growth phase* supplement profile contains the following nutrients: 14 g of whey protein, 2 g of casein, 3 g of leucine, 1 g of glutamine, and 2 to 4 g of high-glycemic carbohydrates.

REFERENCE

Ivy J,. Portman R. Nutrient timing: the future of sports nutrition. North Bergen, NJ: Basic Health Publ., Inc., 2004.

of energy intake, replenishing glycogen reserves to about the same point achieved with the classic loading protocol.

Rapid Loading Procedure: A One-Day Requirement

The 2 to 6 days required to achieve supranormal muscle glycogen levels represents a limitation of typical carbohydrate loading procedures. Research has evaluated whether a shortened time period that combines a relatively brief bout of high-intensity exercise with only 1 day of high-carbohydrate intake achieves the desired loading effect. Endurance-trained athletes cycled for 150 seconds at 130% of $\dot{V}O_{2max}$, followed by 30 sec of all-out cycling. In the recovery period, the men consumed 10.3 g·kg body mass^{-1} of high-glycemic carbohydrate foods. Biopsy data presented in **Figure 3.11** indicated that carbohydrate levels increased in all fiber types of the vastus lateralis muscle (82% increase) after only 24 hours. This increased glycogen storage equaled or exceeded values reported by others using a 2- to 6-day regimen. The short-duration loading procedure benefits individuals who do not wish to disrupt normal training with the time required and potential negative aspects of other loading protocols.

Limited Applicability and Negative Aspects

The potential benefits from carbohydrate loading apply only to intense and prolonged aerobic activities. *Unless the athlete begins competing in a state of depletion, exercise for less than 60 minutes requires only normal carbohydrate intake and glycogen reserves.* Carbohydrate loading and associated high levels of muscle and liver glycogen did not benefit athletes in a 20.9-km (13-mile) run compared with a run following a low-carbohydrate diet. Also, a single, maximal anaerobic exercise for 75 seconds also did not improve by increasing muscle glycogen availability above normal through dietary manipulation before exercise.

In most sport competition and exercise training, a daily diet of 60% to 70% of total calories as carbohydrates provides for adequate muscle and liver glycogen reserves. This diet ensures about twice the level of muscle glycogen compared with the 45% to 50% carbohydrate amount of the typical American diet. For well-nourished athletes, any supercompensation effect from carbohydrate loading remains relatively small. During

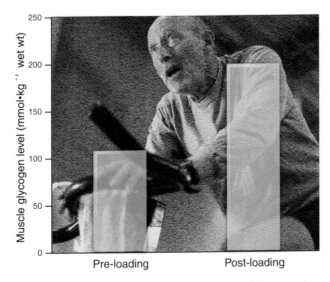

Figure 3.11. Muscle glycogen concentration of the vastus lateralis before (pre-loading) and after 180 seconds of near-maximal intensity cycling exercise followed by 1 day of high-carbohydrate intake (post-loading). (From Fairchild, T.J., et al.: Rapid carbohydrate loading after short bout of near maximal-intensity exercise. *Med. Sci. Sports Exerc.,* 34:980, 2002.)

intense training, however, athletes who do not upgrade daily caloric and carbohydrate intakes to meet energy demands may experience muscle fatigue and staleness.

The addition of 2.7 g of water stored with each gram of glycogen makes this a heavy fuel compared with equivalent energy as stored fat. A higher body mass due to water retention often makes the athlete feel heavy, "bloated," and uncomfortable; any extra load also directly adds to the energy cost of weight-bearing activities, such as running, racewalking, or cross-country skiing. The added energy cost may actually negate the potential benefits from increased glycogen storage. On the positive side, the water liberated during glycogen breakdown aids in temperature regulation to benefit exercise in the heat.

The classic model for supercompensation is ill advised for individuals with specific health problems. A dietary carbohydrate overload, interspersed with periods of high lipid or protein intake, may increase blood cholesterol and urea nitrogen levels. This could pose problems for individuals predisposed to type 2 diabetes and heart disease or with muscle enzyme deficiencies or renal disease. Failure to eat a balanced diet can produce deficiencies of some minerals and vitamins, particularly water-soluble vitamins; these deficiencies may require dietary supplementation. The glycogen-depleted state during the first phase of the glycogen-loading procedure certainly reduces one's capability to engage in intense training, possibly resulting in a detraining effect during the loading period. Dramatically reducing dietary carbohydrate for 3 or 4 days could also set the stage for lean tissue loss. This occurs because muscle protein serves as gluconeogenic substrate to maintain blood-glucose levels with low glycogen reserves.

SUMMARY

1. Within rather broad limits, a balanced diet from regular food intake provides the nutrient requirements of athletes and others engaged in exercise training and sports competition.

2. MyPyramid represents a model for good nutrition for all Americans, and includes regular physical activity. The guidelines emphasize diverse grains, vegetables, and fruits as major calorie sources, downplaying foods high in animal proteins, lipids, and dairy products.

3. For physically active individuals, 60% to 70% of daily caloric intake should come from carbohydrates (400 to 600 g), particularly unrefined, low-glycemic polysaccharides.

4. Volume of daily physical activity largely determines energy intake requirements. Under most circumstances, daily energy requirements for physically active individuals probably do not exceed 4000 kCal for men and 3000 kCal for women. Under extremes of training and competition, these values approach 5000 kCal for women and 9000 kCal for men.

5. The relatively high caloric intakes of physically active men and women usually increase protein, vitamin, and mineral intake above recommended values.

6. The ideal precompetition meal maximizes muscle and liver glycogen storage and enhances glucose for intestinal absorption during exercise. High-carbohydrate and relatively low-lipid and low-protein meals generally fill this requirement. A carbohydrate-rich pre-event meal requires about 3 hours for digestion and absorption.

7. Commercially prepared liquid meals offer a practical approach to precompetition nutrition and energy supplementation. These "meals" give balance in nutritive value, contribute to fluid needs, and absorb rapidly, leaving practically no residue in the digestive tract.

8. Consuming low-glycemic index foods immediately before exercise allows for a relatively slow rate of glucose absorption into the blood. This should eliminate an insulin surge, while providing a steady supply of "slow-release" glucose from the digestive tract during exercise.

9. Fluid volume within the stomach exerts the greatest effect on the rate of gastric emptying. To maintain a relatively large fluid volume in the stomach and speed gastric emptying, consume 400 to 600 mL of fluid immediately before exercise with subsequent regular ingestion of 250 mL at 15-minute intervals throughout exercise.

10. Consuming a 5% to 8% carbohydrate-electrolyte beverage during exercise in the heat contributes to temperature regulation and fluid balance as effectively as plain water. The drink also maintains blood glucose and glycogen reserves in prolonged exercise.

11. To speed glycogen replenishment after a bout of intense training or competition, consume 50 to 75 g of moderate- to high-glycemic carbohydrates every 2 hours for a total of 500 g. Even under optimal conditions, it takes at least 20 hours (5% per hour) to re-establish glycogen stores.

12. Successive days of intense training gradually deplete glycogen reserves, even with the typical carbohydrate

intake. This could lead to chronically reduced glycogen reserves and training "staleness."

13. A diet deficient in carbohydrate rapidly depletes muscle and liver glycogen. Glycogen depletion profoundly impairs performance in maximal, short-term anaerobic exercise and prolonged, high-intensity aerobic effort.

14. Carbohydrate loading can augment endurance performance. Athletes should become well informed about this procedure because of potential negative effects. Modifying the classic loading procedure augments glycogen storage without dramatically altering diet and exercise regimens.

THOUGHT QUESTIONS

1. Under what circumstances might an athlete require nutritional supplementation?

2. An athletic team has three matches scheduled on consecutive days. What should athletes consume after each day's competition, and why?

3. What advice would you give to a sprint athlete who plans to carbohydrate load for competition?

4. Among physically active men and women, how can individuals who consume the greatest number of calories weigh less than those who consume fewer calories?

SELECTED REFERENCES

Achten, J., et al.: Higher dietary carbohydrate content during interspersed running training results in a better maintenance of performance and mood state. *J. Appl. Physiol.*, 96:1331, 2004.

Akabas, S.R., Dolins, K.R.: Micronutrient requirements of physically active women: what can we learn from iron? *Am. J. Clin. Nutr.*, 81:1246S, 2005.

Barnett, C., et al.: Muscle metabolism during sprint exercise in man: influence of sprint training. *J. Sci. Med. Sport*, 7:314, 2004.

Bazzano, L.A., et al.: Fruit and vegetable intake and risk of cardiovascular disease in US adults: the first National Health and Nutrition Examination Survey Epidemiologic Follow-up Study. *Am. J. Clin. Nutr.*, 76:93, 2002.

Bosch, A.N., Noakes, T.D.: Carbohydrate ingestion during exercise and endurance performance. *Indian J. Med. Res.*, 121:634, 2005.

Burgomaster, K.A., et al.: Six sessions of sprint interval training increases muscle oxidative potential and cycle endurance capacity in humans. *J. Appl. Physiol.*, 98:1985, 2005.

Burke, L.M., et al.: Effect of fat adaptation and carbohydrate restoration on metabolism and performance during prolonged cycling. *J. Appl. Physiol.*, 89:2413, 2000.

Burns, S.F., et al.: A single session of resistance exercise does not reduce postprandial lipaemia. *J. Sports Sci.*, 23:251, 2005.

Cases, N., et al.: Differential response of plasma and immune cell's vitamin E levels to physical activity and antioxidant vitamin supplementation. *Eur. J. Clin. Nutr.*, 59:781, 2005.

Coggan, A.R., and Coyle, E.F.: Carbohydrate ingestion during prolonged exercise: Effects on metabolism and performance.

In: *Exercise and Sport Science Reviews*. Vol. 19. Holloszy, J.O. (ed.). Baltimore: Williams & Wilkins, 1991.

Cordain, L., et al.: Origins and evolutions of the Western diet: health implications for the 21st century. *Am. J. Clin. Nutr.*, 81:341, 2005.

Coyle, E.F.: Fluid and fuel intake during exercise. *J. Sports Sci.*, 22:39, 2004.

Cunha, T.S., et al.: Influence of high-intensity exercise training and anabolic androgenic steroid treatment on rat tissue glycogen content. *Life Sci.*, 77:1030, 2005.

Erlenbusch, M., et al.: Effect of high-fat or high-carbohydrate diets on endurance exercise: a meta-analysis. *Int. J. Sport Nutr. Exerc. Metab.*, 15:1, 2005.

Fiala, K.A., et al.: Rehydration with a caffeinated beverage during the nonexercise periods of 3 consecutive days of 2-a-day practices. *Int. J. Sport Nutr. Exerc. Metab.*, 14:419, 2004.

Food and Nutrition Board, Institute of Medicine: Dietary reference intakes for energy, carbohydrates, fiber, fat, protein and amino acids. Washington, D.C.: National Academy Press, 2002.

Fox, A.K., et al.: Adding fat calories to meals after exercise does not alter glucose tolerance. *J. Appl. Physiol.*, 97:11, 2004.

Grandjean, A.C.: Macronutrient intakes of US athletes compared with the general population and recommendations made for athletes. *Am. J. Clin. Nutr.*, 49:1070, 1989.

Helge, J.W., et al.: Interaction of training and diet on metabolism and endurance during exercise in man. *J. Physiol.*, 492:293, 1996.

Helge, J.W., et al.: Impact of a fat-rich diet on endurance in man: role of the dietary period. *Med. Sci. Sports Exerc.*, 30:456, 1998.

Hoffman, J.R., et al.: Effect of low-dose, short-duration creatine supplementation on anaerobic exercise performance. *J. Strength Cond. Res.*, 19:260, 2005.

Hoffman, J.R., et al.: Effects of beta-hydroxy beta-methylbutyrate on power performance and indices of muscle damage and stress during high-intensity training. *J. Strength Cond. Res.*, 18:747, 2004.

Horowitz, J.F., et al.: Energy deficit without reducing dietary carbohydrate alters resting carbohydrate oxidation and fatty acid availability. *J. Appl. Physiol.*, 98:1612, 2005.

Horowitz, J.F.: Fatty acid mobilization from adipose tissue during exercise. *Trends Endocrinol. Metab.*, 14:386, 2003.

Horowitz, J.F., et al.: Substrate metabolism when subjects are fed carbohydrates during exercise. *Am. J. Physiol.*, 276(5 Pt):E828, 1999.

Houmard, J.A.: Effect of volume and intensity of exercise training on insulin sensitivity. *J. Appl. Physiol.*, 96:101, 2004.

Ivy, J.L., et al.: Effect of a carbohydrate-protein supplement on endurance performance during exercise of varying intensity. *Int. J. Sport Nutr. Exerc. Metab.*, 13:388, 2003.

Jeffery, R.W., et al.: Physical activity and weight loss: does prescribing higher physical activity goals improve outcome? *Am. J. Clin. Nutr.*, 78:684, 2003.

Jenkins, D.J., et al.: Glycemic index: an overview of implications in health and disease. *Am. J. Clin. Nutr.*, 76(suppl):266S, 2002.

Jentjens, R.L., et al.: Oxidation of combined ingestion of glucose and fructose during exercise. *J. Appl. Physiol.*, 96:1277, 2004.

Jentjens, R.L., Jeukendrup, A.E.: High rates of exogenous carbohydrate oxidation from a mixture of glucose and fructose ingested during prolonged cycling exercise. *Br. J. Nutr.*, 93:485, 2005.

Jeukendrup, A.E., Wallis, G.A.: Measurement of substrate oxidation during exercise by means of gas exchange measurements. *Int. J. Sports Med.*, 26 Suppl 1:S28, 2005.

Khanna, G.L., Manna, I.: Supplementary effect of carbohydrate-electrolyte drink on sports performance, lactate removal & cardiovascular response of athletes. *Indian J. Med. Res.*, 121:665, 2005.

Kirwin, J.P., et al.: A moderate gycemic meal before endurance exercise can enhance performance. *J. Appl. Physiol.*, 84:53, 1998.

Lambert, C.P., et al.: Macronutrient considerations for the sport of bodybuilding. *Sports Med.*, 34:317, 2004.

Lasheras, C., et al.: Mediterranean diet and age with respect to overall survival in institutionalized, nonsmoking elderly people. *Am. J. Clin. Nutr.*, 71:987, 2000.

Leiper, J.B., et al.: The effect of intermittent high-intensity running on gastric emptying of fluids in man. *Med. Sci. Sports Exerc.*, 37:240, 2005.

Liu, S., et al.: A prospective study of dietary glycemic load, carbohydrate intake, and risk of coronary heart disease in US women. *Am. J. Clin. Nutr.*, 71:1455, 2000.

McArdle, W.D., et al.: *Sports and Exercise Nutrition.* 2nd Ed. Baltimore: Lippincott Williams & Wilkins, 2005.

Mori, Y., et al.: Weight loss-associated changes in acute effects of nateglinide on insulin secretion after glucose loading: results of glucose loading on 2 consecutive days. *Diabetes Obes. Metab.*, 7:182, 2005.

Morifuji, M., et al.: Dietary whey protein increases liver and skeletal muscle glycogen levels in exercise-trained rats. *Br. J. Nutr.*, 93:439, 2005.

Nybo, L.: CNS fatigue abnd prolonged exercise: effect of glucose supplementation. *Med. Sci. Sports Exerc.*, 35:589, 2003.

Pearce, P.Z.: Sports supplements: a modern case of caveat emptor. *Curr. Sports Med. Rep.*, 4:171, 2005.

Pi-Sunyer, X.: Glycemic index and disease. *Am. J. Clin. Nutr.*, 76(Suppl): 290S, 2002.

Riddell, M.C., et al.: Substrate utilization during exercise with glucose and glucose plus fructose ingestion in boys ages 10–14 yr. *J. Appl. Physiol.*, 90:903, 2001.

Roy, L.B., et al.: Oxidation of exogenous glucose, sucrose, and maltose during prolonged cycling exercise. *J. Appl. Physiol.*, 96:1285, 2004.

Sarris, W.W.M., et al.: How much physical activity is enough to prevent unhealthy weight gain? Outcome of the IASO 1st Stock Conference and consensus statement. *Obesity Reviews*, 4:1201, 2003.

Saunders, M.J., et al.: Effects of a carbohydrate-protein beverage on cycling endurance and muscle damage. *Med. Sci. Sports Exerc.*, 36:1233, 2004.

Sawka, M.N., et al.: Hydration effects on temperature regulation. *Int. J. Sports Med.*, 19(suppl 2):S108, 1998.

Shannon, K.A., et al.: Resistance exercise and postprandial lipemia: The dose effect of differing volumes of acute resistance exercise bouts. *Metabolism*, 54:756, 2005.

Shirreffs, S.M., et al.: Fluid and electrolyte needs for preparation and recovery from training and competition. *J. Sports Sci.*, 22:57, 2004.

Snyder, A.C.: Overtraining and glycogen depletion hypothesis. *Med. Sci. Sports Exerc.*, 30:1146, 1998.

Sparks, M.J., et al.: Pre-exercise carbohydrate ingestion: Effect of the glycemic index on endurance exercise performance. *Med. Sci. Sports Exerc.*, 30:844, 1998.

Stark, A.H., Madar, Z.: Olive oil as a functional food: epidemiology and nutritional approaches. *Nutr. Revs.*, 2002;60:170, 2002.

Stepto, N.K., et al.: Effect of short-term fat adaptation on high-intensity training. *Med. Sci. Sports Exerc.*, 34:449, 2002.

Tharion, W.J., et al.: Energy requirements of military personnel. *Appetite*, 44:47, 2005.

Theodorou, A.S., et al.: Effects of acute creatine loading with or without carbohydrate on repeated bouts of maximal swimming in high-performance swimmers. *J. Strength Cond. Res.*, 19:265, 2005.

Trichopoulou, A., et al.: Adherence to a Mediterranean diet and survival in a Greek population. *N. Engl. J. Med.*, 348:2599, 2003.

Utter, A.C., et al.: Effect of carbohydrate ingestion on ratings of perceived exertion during a marathon. *Med. Sci. Sports Exerc.*, 24:1779, 2002.

Vogt, M., et al.: Effects if dietary fat on muscle substrates, metabolism, and performance in athletes. *Med. Sci. Sports Exerc.*, 35:952, 2003.

Von Duvillard, S.P., et al.: Fluids and hydration in prolonged endurance performance. *Nutrition*, 20:651, 2004.

Wakshlag, J.J., et al.: Biochemical and metabolic changes due to exercise in sprint-racing sled dogs: implications for postexercise carbohydrate supplements and hydration management. *Vet. Ther.*, 5:52, 2004.

Welsh, R.S., et al.: Carbohydrates and physical/mental performance during intermittent exercise to fatigue. *Med. Sci. Sports Exerc.*, 34;723, 2002.

Williams, M.H.: *Nutrition for Health, Fitness, and Sport.* 7th Ed. New York: McGraw-Hill, 2005.

Zaryski, C., Smith, D.J.: Training principles and issues for ultra-endurance athletes. *Curr. Sports Med. Rep.*, 4:165, 2005.

CHAPTER OBJECTIVES

- List four examples of substances alleged to provide ergogenic benefits.

- Summarize research concerning caffeine's potential as an ergogenic aid.

- Discuss the physiologic and psychologic effects of alcohol and how alcohol affects exercise performance.

- Explain how glutamine and phosphatidylserine affect exercise performance and the training response.

- Describe any positive and negative ergogenic effects of creatine supplementation.

- Explain how carbohydrate–protein supplementation post exercise augments the response to resistance training.

- Give the rationale for medium-chain triacylglycerol supplementation as an ergogenic aid.

- Discuss the possible ergogenic benefits and risks of clenbuterol, amphetamines, chromium picolinate, beta-hydroxy-beta-methylbutyrate, and buffering solutions.

- Discuss the positive and negative effects of anabolic steroid use as an ergogenic aid.

- Discuss the positive and negative effects of androstenedione use as an ergogenic aid.

- Describe the medical use of human growth hormone, including its potential dangers when used by healthy athletes.

- Describe the rationale for DHEA use as an ergogenic aid.

CHAPTER OUTLINE

Used Since Antiquity
Functional Foods and Transgenic Nutraceuticals

PART 1 Nutritional Ergogenic Aids

Pangamic Acid — B_{15}
Buffering Solutions
    Effects Relate to Dosage and Degree
      of Exercise Anaerobiosis
Phosphate Loading
Anti-Cortisol–Producing Compounds
    Glutamine
    Phosphatidylserine
Chromium
    Chromium's Alleged Benefits
Creatine
    Important Component of High-Energy Phosphates
    Documented Benefits Under
      Certain Exercise Conditions
Ribose: The Next Creatine
on the Supplement Scene?
Ginseng and Ephedrine
    Ginseng
    Ephedrine
Amino Acid Supplements and Other Dietary
Modifications for an Anabolic Effect
    Prudent Means to Possibly Augment
      an Anabolic Effect
    Carbohydrate–Protein Supplementation Immediately
      in Recovery Augments Hormonal
      Response to Resistance Exercise
Bee Pollen
Boron
Coenzyme Q-10 (Ubiquinone)
Lipid Supplementation With Medium-Chain
Triacylglycerols
    Exercise Benefits Inconclusive
(—)-Hydroxycitrate: A Potential Fat Burner?
Vanadium
Pyruvate
    Effects on Endurance Performance
Glycerol
Summary
Thought Questions

PART 2 Pharmacologic Aids to Performance

Caffeine
    Caffeine's Ergogenic Effects
    Proposed Mechanism for Ergogenic Action

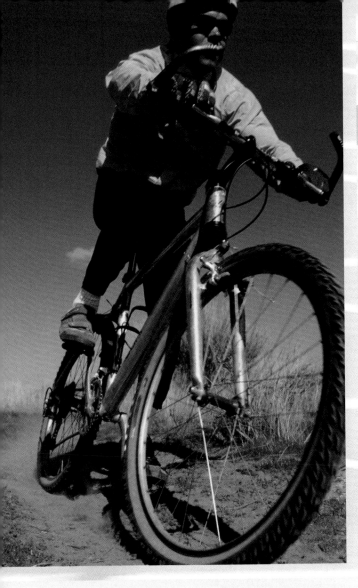

chapter 4

Nutritional (and Pharma- cologic) Aids to Performance

Ergogenic aids include substances and procedures believed to improve physical work capacity, physiologic function, or athletic performance. This chapter discusses the possible ergogenic role of some nutritional and pharmacological agents.

Considerable literature exists concerning the effects of different nutritional and pharmacological aids on exercise performance and training responsiveness. Product promotional materials often include testimonials and endorsements for untested products from sports professionals and organizations, media publicity, television infomercials, and Internet home pages. Frequently touted research studies quote potential performance benefits from steroids (and steroid substitutes), alcohol, amphetamines, hormones, carbohydrates, amino acids (either consumed singularly or in combination), fatty acids, caffeine, buffering compounds, wheat-germ oil, vitamins, minerals, catecholamine agonists, and even marijuana and cocaine. Athletes routinely use many of these substances, believing their use enhances performance or augments the effects of training.

Five mechanisms can explain how ergogenic agents exert their effects.

1. By acting as a central or peripheral stimulant to the nervous system (e.g., caffeine, choline, amphetamines, alcohol)
2. By increasing the storage and/or availability of a limiting substrate (e.g., carbohydrate, creatine, carnitine, chromium)
3. By acting as a supplemental fuel source (e.g., glucose, medium-chain triacylglycerols)
4. By reducing or neutralizing performance-inhibiting metabolic byproducts (e.g., sodium bicarbonate, citrate, pangamic acid, phosphate)
5. By facilitating recovery from strenuous exercise (e.g., high-glycemic carbohydrates, water)

USED SINCE ANTIQUITY

Ancient athletes of Greece reportedly used hallucinogenic mushrooms for ergogenic purposes, whereas Roman gladiators ingested the equivalent of "speed" to enhance performance in the Circus Maximus. Athletes of the Victorian era routinely used chemicals, such as caffeine, alcohol, nitroglycerine, heroin, cocaine, and even strychnine (rat poison), for a competitive edge. For today's exercise enthusiast, dietary supplements consist of nonprescription plant extracts, vitamins, minerals, enzymes, and hormonal products. To positively influence overall health and exercise performance, these supplements must provide a nutrient that is under-supplied in the diet or exert a drug-like influence on cellular function.

FUNCTIONAL FOODS AND TRANSGENIC NUTRACEUTICALS

An increasing belief in the potential for selected foods to promote health has led to the coining of the term **functional food.** Beyond meeting basic nutrition needs for survival, hunger satisfaction, and preventing adverse effects, functional foods comprise those foods and their bioactive components (e.g., olive oil, soy products, omega-3 fatty acids) that promote well-being, health, and optimal bodily function or reduce disease risk (**Fig. 4.1**). Primary physiologic targets for this expanding branch of food science include gastrointestinal functions, antioxidant systems, and macronutrient metabolism. Enormous pressure exists to understand nutrition's role in optimizing an individual's genetic potential, susceptibility to disease, and overall performance. Unfortunately, the science base generated by research in this field of human nutrition often falls prey to nutritional hucksters and scam artists.

Biotechnology also has created the emerging field of **transgenic nutraceuticals,** where genes introduced into a host plant or animal modify a biochemical pathway. This produces a new class of "natural" bioactive components of food in a non-food matrix with physiologic and therapeutic functions that often promote disease prevention and treatment. Nutraceuticals differ from functional foods that deliver their active ingredients within the food matrix. By definition, nutraceutical compounds fall along the continuum of food to supplements to drugs. Examples of such nutrient genetic engineering include remodeling of mammary gland milk of cows (adding or deleting specific milk proteins or adding oligosaccharides) to provide medical benefits and novel food oils that do not require chemical hydrogenation (and thus no harmful *trans* fatty acids). Undoubtedly, some of these biotechnology products will make their way into the exercise enthusiast's nutritional armamentarium to form the next wave of alleged performance enhancers.

PART 1 • Nutritional Ergogenic Aids

PANGAMIC ACID — B_{15}

Athletes often tout pangamic acid, commonly known as "vitamin B_{15}", for its alleged ergogenic benefits in aerobic exercise. Confusion exists as to the exact chemical structure of B_{15}. The products sold as **pangamic acid** contain a variety of different chemicals, although the original compound consisted of a mixture of calcium gluconate and N,N-dimethylglycine in a 60:40 ratio. Beginning in 1976 and reiterated in 1995, the Food and Drug Administration (FDA) stated that there was no identity established for a substance characterized by the name pangamic acid and that the chemical structure and nature of such a substance has not been definitely determined. The FDA also stated that they were unaware of any accepted scientific evidence that establishes the nutritional properties of pangamic acid or that has identified a deficiency of this substance in man or animals.

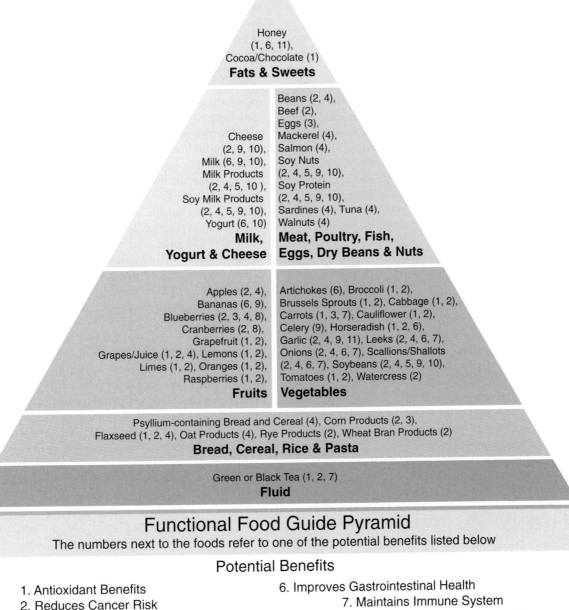

Honey
(1, 6, 11),
Cocoa/Chocolate (1)
Fats & Sweets

Cheese
(2, 9, 10),
Milk (6, 9, 10),
Milk Products
(2, 4, 5, 10),
Soy Milk Products
(2, 4, 5, 9, 10),
Yogurt (6, 10)
**Milk,
Yogurt & Cheese**

Beans (2, 4),
Beef (2),
Eggs (3),
Mackerel (4),
Salmon (4),
Soy Nuts
(2, 4, 5, 9, 10),
Soy Protein
(2, 4, 5, 9, 10),
Sardines (4), Tuna (4),
Walnuts (4)
**Meat, Poultry, Fish,
Eggs, Dry Beans & Nuts**

Apples (2, 4),
Bananas (6, 9),
Blueberries (2, 3, 4, 8),
Cranberries (2, 8),
Grapefruit (1, 2),
Grapes/Juice (1, 2, 4), Lemons (1, 2),
Limes (1, 2), Oranges (1, 2),
Raspberries (1, 2),
Fruits

Artichokes (6), Broccoli (1, 2),
Brussels Sprouts (1, 2), Cabbage (1, 2),
Carrots (1, 3, 7), Cauliflower (1, 2),
Celery (9), Horseradish (1, 2, 6),
Garlic (2, 4, 9, 11), Leeks (2, 4, 6, 7),
Onions (2, 4, 6, 7), Scallions/Shallots
(2, 4, 6, 7), Soybeans (2, 4, 5, 9, 10),
Tomatoes (1, 2), Watercress (2)
Vegetables

Psyllium-containing Bread and Cereal (4), Corn Products (2, 3),
Flaxseed (1, 2, 4), Oat Products (4), Rye Products (2), Wheat Bran Products (2)
Bread, Cereal, Rice & Pasta

Green or Black Tea (1, 2, 7)
Fluid

Functional Food Guide Pyramid
The numbers next to the foods refer to one of the potential benefits listed below

Potential Benefits

1. Antioxidant Benefits
2. Reduces Cancer Risk
3. Maintenance of Vision
4. Improves Heart Health
5. May Decrease Menopause Symptoms

6. Improves Gastrointestinal Health
7. Maintains Immune System
8. Maintains Urinary Tract Health
9. Reduces Blood Pressure
10. Improves Bone Health
11. Antibacterial Benefits

Figure 4.1.   Functional food guide pyramid. Different foods provide different benefits. (From Functional Foods for Health, University of Illinois at Chicago and the University of Illinois at Urbana-Champaign.)

Despite such admonitions, proponents of pangamic acid argue that studies conducted in Russia showed this compound increased cellular efficiency to use oxygen, reduced blood lactate buildup, and thus enhanced endurance. As with many proposed ergogenic aids, testimonials from athletes abound as to its effectiveness as a training aid and performance enhancer. On careful scrutiny of the early studies of pangamic acid, one cannot interpret the validity of the findings in light of the significant limitations in research design. Research in the United States has not shown any benefit of pangamic acid on $\dot{V}O_{2max}$, endurance performance, or circulating blood glucose and blood lactate levels. *From a nutritional perspective, pangamic acid has no vitamin or provitamin properties; it apparently serves no particular purpose in the body.* Concern has been expressed that synthetic mixtures sold as B_{15} may be harmful. The FDA guidelines prohibit the sale of this compound as a dietary supplement or drug.

BUFFERING SOLUTIONS

Dramatic alterations take place in the chemical balance of intracellular and extracellular fluids during all-out exercise of durations of between 30 and 120 seconds. This occurs because muscle fibers rely predominantly on anaerobic energy transfer, which significantly increases lactate formation and decreases intracellular pH. Increases in acidity inhibit the energy-transfer and contractile qualities of active muscle fibers. In the blood, increased concentrations of H^+ and lactate result in acidosis.

The bicarbonate aspect of the body's buffering system defends against an increase in intracellular H^+ concentration. Maintaining high levels of extracellular bicarbonate causes rapid H^+ efflux from cells and reduces intracellular acidosis. This fact has fueled speculation that increasing the body's bicarbonate (alkaline) reserve (pre-exercise

alkalosis) might enhance subsequent anaerobic exercise performance by delaying the decrease in intracellular pH. Research in this area, however, has produced conflicting results due to (1) variations in pre-exercise doses of sodium bicarbonate and (2) type of exercise to evaluate the ergogenic effects.

Attempting to correct previous limitations, one study evaluated the effects of acute induced metabolic alkalosis on short-term fatiguing exercise that generated significant lactate accumulation. Six trained middle-distance runners consumed a **sodium bicarbonate** solution (300 mg per kg body mass) or a similar quantity of calcium carbonate placebo before running an 800-m race or under control conditions (no exogenous substance). **Table 4.1** shows that ingesting the alkaline drink increased pH and standard bicarbonate levels before exercise. Study subjects ran an average of 2.9 seconds faster under alkalosis and achieved higher post-exercise blood lactate, pH, and extracellular H^+ concentration compared with the placebo or control subjects. Similar ergogenic effects of induced alkalosis also occur in short-term anaerobic performance using exogenous **sodium citrate** as the alkalinizing agent.

The ergogenic effect of pre-exercise alkalosis, either with sodium bicarbonate or sodium citrate, before high-intensity, short-term exercise probably results from increased anaerobic energy transfer during exercise. Increases in extracellular buffering provided by exogenous buffers may facilitate coupled transport of lactate and H^+ across muscle cell membranes into extracellular fluid during fatiguing exercise. This delays decreases in intracellular pH and its subsequent negative effects on muscle function. A 2.9-second faster 800-m race time represents a dramatic improvement; it transposes to a distance of about 19 m at race pace, bringing a last place finisher to first place in most 800-m races.

Table 4·1	Performance Time and Acid-Base Profiles for Subjects Under Control, Placebo, and Induced Pre-exercise Alkalosis Conditions Prior to and Following an 800-m Race			
VARIABLE	**CONDITION**	**PRE-TREATMENT**	**PRE-EXERCISE**	**POST-EXERCISE**
pH	Control	7.40	7.39	7.07
	Placebo	7.39	7.40	7.09
	Alkalosis	7.40	7.49[b]	7.18[a]
Lactate	Control	1.21	1.15	12.62
($mmol \cdot L^{-1}$)	Placebo	1.38	1.23	13.62
	Alkalosis	1.29	1.31	14.29[a]
Standard HCO_3^{-1}	Control	25.8	24.5	9.90
($mEq \cdot L^{-1}$)	Placebo	25.6	26.2	11.0
	Alkalosis	25.2	33.5[b]	14.30[a]
Performance time (min:s)	Control	2:05.8	Placebo	Alkalosis
			2:05.1	2.02.9[c]

[a] Alkalosis values were significantly higher than placebo and control values post exercise.
[b] Pre-exercise values were significantly higher than pre-treatment values.
[c] Alkalosis time was significantly faster than control and placebo times.
From Wilkes, D., et al.: Effects of induced metabolic alkalosis on 800-m racing time. *Med. Sci. Sports Exerc.*, 15:277, 1983.

Effects Relate to Dosage and Degree of Exercise Anaerobiosis

The interaction between bicarbonate dosage and the cumulative, anaerobic nature of exercise influences potential ergogenic effects of pre-exercise bicarbonate loading. *For men and women, dosages of at least 0.3 g per kg body mass (ingested 1 to 2 hours before competition) facilitate H^+ efflux from cells.* This significantly enhances a single maximal effort of 1 to 2 minutes or longer term arm or leg exercise that leads to exhaustion within 6 to 8 minutes. No ergogenic effect occurs for typical resistance training exercises (e.g., squat, bench press). All-out effort lasting less than 1 minute may improve only for repetitive exercise bouts. This form of intermittent anaerobic exercise produces high intracellular H^+ concentrations; consequently, buffering ability and power output capacity benefit from a higher pre-exercise bicarbonate level in extracellular fluids.

PHOSPHATE LOADING

The rationale concerning pre-exercise phosphate supplementation (**phosphate loading**) focuses on increasing extracellular and intracellular phosphate levels. This can produce three effects:

1. Increase ATP phosphorylation
2. Increase aerobic exercise performance and myocardial functional capacity
3. Augment peripheral oxygen extraction in muscle tissue by stimulating red blood cell glycolysis and subsequent elevation of erythrocyte 2,3-diphosphoglycerate (2,3-DPG)

The compound 2,3-DPG, which is produced within the red blood cell during anaerobic glycolytic reactions, binds loosely with subunits of hemoglobin, reducing its affinity for oxygen. This releases additional oxygen to the tissues for a given decrease in cellular oxygen pressure.

Despite the proposed theoretical rationale for ergogenic effects with phosphate loading, benefits are not consistently observed. Some studies show improvement in $\dot{V}O_{2max}$ and arteriovenous oxygen difference following phosphate loading, whereas other studies report no effects on aerobic capacity and cardiovascular performance.

One reason for inconsistencies in findings concerns variations in exercise mode and intensity, dosage and duration of supplementation, standardization of pretesting diets, and subjects' fitness level. *Presently, little reliable scientific evidence exists to recommend exogenous phosphate as an ergogenic aid.* On the negative side, excess plasma phosphate stimulates secretion of parathormone, the parathyroid hormone. Excessive parathormone production accelerates the kidneys' excretion of phosphate and facilitates resorption of calcium salts from bones to cause loss of bone mass. Research has not yet determined whether short-term phosphate supplementation jeopardizes normal bone dynamics.

ANTI-CORTISOL–PRODUCING COMPOUNDS

The anterior pituitary gland secretes adrenocorticotropic hormone (ACTH), which induces adrenal cortex release of the glucocorticoid hormone **cortisol** (hydrocortisone) (see Chapter 12). Cortisol decreases the transport of amino acid into cells. This effect depresses anabolism and stimulates protein breakdown to its building-block amino acids in all cells except the liver. The liberated amino acids circulate to the liver for synthesis to glucose (gluconeogenesis) for energy. Cortisol also serves as an insulin antagonist by inhibiting cellular glucose uptake and oxidation.

Prolonged, elevated serum concentrations of cortisol (usually resulting from exogenous intake) ultimately lead to excessive protein breakdown, tissue wasting, and negative nitrogen balance. The potential catabolic effect of exogenous

FOR YOUR INFORMATION

Supplement Use and Abuse Among Elite Athletes
Based on the latest survey of college student athletes by the National Collegiate Athletic Association (NCAA) in 2001, 29% of the respondents used nutritional supplements during the previous year. The most popular supplement was creatine (26%), followed by amino acids (10%), with androstenedione, chromium, and ephedra each used by about 4% of the athletes. The IOC initiated drug testing for stimulants in Olympic competition in the 1968 Mexico City games following the death of a famed Tour de France British cyclist from amphetamine overdose a year earlier. Testing has consistently expanded, with the initiation of random unannounced drug testing in track and field in 1989 to the administration of 3500 tests before the opening ceremonies of the 2002 Winter Games in Salt Lake City. The following categories comprise substances currently banned by the IOC:
- Stimulants
- Narcotic analgesics
- Androgenic anabolic steroids
- Beta-blockers
- Diuretics
- Peptide hormones and analogues
- Substances that alter the integrity of urine samples

cortisol has convinced bodybuilders and other strength and power athletes to use supplements believed to inhibit the body's normal cortisol release. Some believe that depressing cortisol's normal increase after exercise augments muscular development with resistance training because muscle tissue synthesis progresses unimpeded in recovery.

Athletes use the supplements glutamine and phosphatidylserine to produce an anti-cortisol effect.

Glutamine

Glutamine, a non-essential amino acid, exhibits many regulatory functions in the body, one of which provides an anticatabolic effect to augment protein synthesis. The rationale for glutamine's use as an ergogenic aid comes from findings that glutamine supplementation effectively counteracted protein breakdown and muscle wasting from repeated use of exogenous glucocorticoids. In one study with female rats, infusing a glutamine supplement for 7 days countered the normal depressed protein synthesis and atrophy in skeletal muscle with chronic glucocorticoid administration. However, no research exists concerning the efficacy of excess glutamine in altering the normal hormonal milieu and training responsiveness in healthy men and women. Thus, any objective decision about glutamine supplements for ergogenic purposes must await such studies.

Phosphatidylserine

Phosphatidylserine (PS) represents a glycerophospholipid typical of a class of natural lipids that comprise the structural components of biological membranes, particularly the internal layer of the plasma membrane that surrounds all cells. Speculation exists that PS, through its potential for modulating functional events in cell membranes (e.g., number and affinity of membrane receptor sites), modifies the body's neuroendocrine response to stress.

In one study, nine healthy men received 800 mg of PS derived from bovine cerebral cortex in oral form daily for 10 days. Three 6-minute intervals of cycle ergometer exercise of increasing intensity induced physical stress. Compared with the placebo condition, the PS treatment significantly diminished ACTH and cortisol release without affecting growth hormone release. These results confirmed earlier findings by the same researchers showing that a single intravenous PS injection counteracted hypothalamic-pituitary-adrenal axis activation with exercise. Soybean lecithin provides the majority of PS used for supplementation by athletes, yet the research showing physiologic effects used bovine-derived PS. Subtle differences in the chemical structure of these two forms of PS may create differences in physiologic action, including the potential ergogenic effects of this compound.

CHROMIUM

The trace mineral **chromium** serves as a cofactor for potentiating insulin function, although its precise mechanism of action remains unclear. Chronic chromium deficiency may trigger a rise in blood cholesterol and decrease the body's sensitivity to insulin, thus increasing the risk of type 2 diabetes. In all likelihood, some adult Americans consume less than the 50 to 200 μg of chromium, which is considered the estimated safe and adequate daily dietary intake. This occurs largely because chromium-rich foods (brewer's yeast, broccoli, wheat germ, nuts, liver, prunes, egg yolks, apples with skins, asparagus, mushrooms, wine, and cheese) do not usually constitute part of the regular daily diet. Food processing also removes significant chromium from foods in natural form. In addition, strenuous exercise and associated high carbohydrate intake promote urinary chromium losses, thus increasing the potential for chromium deficiency. For athletes with chromium-deficient diets, dietary modifications to increase chromium intake or prudent use of chromium supplements seem appropriate.

Chromium's Alleged Benefits

Chromium, touted as a "fat burner" and "muscle builder," represents one of the largest selling mineral supplements in the United States (second only to calcium). Supplement intake of chromium, usually as **chromium picolinate**, often reaches 600 μg daily. This picolinic acid combination supposedly improves chromium absorption compared with the inorganic salt chromium chloride. Millions of Americans believe the claims of health food faddists, television infomercials, and exercise zealots that additional chromium promotes muscle growth, curbs appetite, fosters body fat loss, and even lengthens life. Unfortunately, advertising mainly through magazine ads targets supplemental chromium to body builders and other resistance-trained athletes as a safe alternative to anabolic steroids.

Generally, studies suggesting beneficial effects of chromium supplements on body fat and muscle mass inferred body composition changes from changes in body weight (or anthropometric measurements), instead of a more appropriate assessment. One study observed that supplementing daily with 200 μg (3.85 mmol) of chromium picolinate for 40 days produced a small increase in fat-free mass and a decrease in body fat in young men who resistance trained for 6 weeks. No data were presented, however, to show increases in muscular strength.

Another study reported increases in body mass without a change in strength or body composition in previously untrained female college students (no change in males) receiving daily chromium supplements of 200 μg during a 12-week resistance training program compared with unsupplemented controls. When collegiate football players received daily supplements of 200 μg of chromium picolinate for 9 weeks, no changes occurred in body composition and muscular strength from intense weight-lifting training compared with a control group receiving a placebo. Among obese personnel enrolled in the U.S. Navy's mandatory remedial physical conditioning program, consuming 400 μg of additional chromium picolinate daily caused no greater loss in body weight or percentage of body fat and no increase in fat free mass (FFM) compared with a group receiving a placebo.

A comprehensive double-blind research design studied the effects of a daily chromium supplement (3.3 to 3.5 mmol either as chromium chloride or chromium picolinate) or a placebo for 8 weeks during resistance training in 36 young men. For each group, dietary intakes of protein, magnesium, zinc, copper, and iron equaled or exceeded recommended levels during training; subjects also had adequate baseline dietary chromium intakes. Chromium supplementation increased serum chromium concentration and urinary chromium excretion equally, regardless of its ingested form. **Table 4.2** shows that, compared with a placebo treatment, chromium supplementation did *not* affect training-related changes in muscular strength, physique, FFM, or muscle mass.

CREATINE

Meat, poultry, and fish provide rich sources of **creatine**; they contain approximately 4 to 5 g per kg of food weight. The body synthesizes only about 1 to 2 g of this nitrogen-containing organic compound daily, primarily in the kidneys, liver, and pancreas, from the amino acids arginine, glycine, and methionine. Thus, adequate dietary creatine becomes important for obtaining required amounts. Because the animal kingdom contains the richest creatine-containing foods, vegetarians experience a distinct disadvantage in obtaining ready sources of exogenous creatine. Skeletal muscle contains approximately 95% of the body's total 120 to 150 g of creatine.

FOR YOUR INFORMATION

Stop Caffeine When Using Creatine

Caffeine blunts the ergogenic effect of creatine supplementation. To evaluate the effect of pre-exercise caffeine ingestion on intramuscular creatine stores and high-intensity exercise performance, subjects consumed a placebo, a daily creatine supplement (0.5 g per kg body mass), or the same daily creatine supplement plus caffeine (5 mg per kg body mass) for 6 days. Under each condition, they performed maximal intermittent knee extension exercise to fatigue on an iso-kinetic dynamometer. Creatine supplementation, with or without caffeine, increased intramuscular PCr by between 4% and 6%. Dynamic torque production also increased 10% to 23% with creatine only compared with the placebo. Taking caffeine, however, totally negated creatine's ergogenic effect. Thus, athletes who load creatine should refrain from caffeine-containing foods and beverages for several days prior to competition.

| Table 4·2 | Effects of Two Different Forms of Chromium Supplementation on Average Values for Anthropometric, Bone, and Soft Tissue Composition Measurements Before and After Weight Training |

	PLACEBO		CHROMIUM CHLORIDE		CHROMIUM PICOLINATE	
	PRE	POST	PRE	POST	PRE	POST
Age (y)	21.1	21.5	23.3	23.5	22.3	22.5
Stature (cm)	179.3	179.2	177.3	177.3	178.0	178.2
Weight (kg)	79.9	80.5[a]	79.3	81.1[a]	79.2	80.5
Σ 4 skinfold thickness (mm)[b]	42.0	41.5	42.6	42.2	43.3	43.1
Upper arm (cm)	30.9	31.6[a]	31.3	32.0[a]	31.1	31.4[a]
Lower leg (cm)	38.2	37.9	37.4	37.5	37.1	37.0
Endomorphy	3.68	3.73	3.58	3.54	3.71	3.72
Mesomorphy	4.09	4.36[a]	4.25	4.42[a]	4.21	4.33[a]
Ectomorphy	2.09	1.94[a]	1.79	1.63[a]	2.00	1.88[a]
FFMFM (kg)[c]	62.9	64.3[a]	61.1	63.1[a]	61.3	62.7[a]
Bone mineral (g)	2952	2968	2860	2878	2918	2940
Fat-free body mass (kg)	65.9	67.3[a]	64.0	65.9[a]	64.2	66.1[a]
Fat (kg)	13.4	13.1	14.7	15.1	14.7	14.5
Body fat (%)	16.4	15.7	18.4	18.2	18.4	17.9

From Lukaski, H.C., et al.: Chromium supplementation and resistance training: Effects on body composition, strength, and trace element status of men. *Am. J. Clin. Nutr.,* 63:954, 1996.
[a] Significantly different from pretraining value.
[b] Measured at biceps, triceps, subscapular, and suptrailiac sites.
[c] Fat-free, mineral-free mass.

Creatine supplements sold as creatine monohydrate (CrH_2O) come as a powder, tablet, capsule, and stabilized liquid. A person can purchase creatine over the counter or via mail order as a nutritional supplement (without guarantee of purity). Ingesting a liquid suspension of creatine monohydrate at the relatively high daily dose of 20 to 30 g for up to 2 weeks increases intramuscular concentrations of free creatine and phosphorcreatine (PCr) by 30%. These levels remain high for weeks after only a few days of supplementation. The International Olympic Committee (IOC) and other sports governing bodies do not consider creatine an illegal substance.

Important Component of High-Energy Phosphates

The precise physiologic mechanisms underlying the potential ergogenic effectiveness of supplemental creatine remain poorly understood. Creatine passes through the digestive tract unaltered for absorption in the bloodstream from the intestinal mucosa. Just about all ingested creatine becomes incorporated within skeletal muscle (average concentration of 125 μM [range, 90 to 160 μM] per kg dry muscle) via insulin-mediated active transport. About 40% of the total exists as free creatine; the remainder combines readily with phosphate to form PCr. Type II, fast-twitch muscle fibers store about 4 to 6 times more PCr than ATP. PCr serves as the cells' "energy reservoir" to provide rapid phosphate-bond energy to resynthesize ATP. This becomes important in all-out effort lasting up to 10 seconds. Due to limited amounts of intramuscular PCr, it seems reasonable that any increase in PCr availability should accomplish the following:

1. Improve repetitive performance in muscular strength and short-term power activities
2. Augment short bursts of muscular endurance
3. Provide for greater muscular overload to enhance resistance training effectiveness

Documented Benefits Under Certain Exercise Conditions

Creatine received notoriety as an ergogenic aid when used by British sprinters and hurdlers in the 1992 Barcelona Olympic Games. Creatine supplementation at the recommended level exerts ergogenic effects in short-duration, high-intensity exercise (5% to 10% improvement) without producing harmful side effects (**Table 4.3**). However, anecdotes indicate a possible association between creatine supplementation and cramping in multiple muscle areas during competition or lengthy practice in football players. This effect may result from (1) altered intracellular dynamics from increased free creatine and PCr levels or (2) an osmotically induced enlarged muscle cell volume (greater cellular hydration) caused by the increased creatine content. Gastrointestinal tract disturbances, such as nausea, indigestion, and difficulty ab-

sorbing food, have also been linked to exogenous creatine ingestion.

Figure 4.2 illustrates the significant ergogenic effects of creatine loading on total work accomplished during repetitive sprint cycling performance. Active but untrained males performed sets of maximal 6-second bicycle sprints interspersed with various recovery periods (24, 54, or 84 s) between sprints to simulate sport conditions. Performance evaluations took place under creatine-loaded (20 g per day for 5 days) or placebo conditions. Supplementation significantly increased muscle creatine (48.9%) and PCr (12.5%) levels compared with the placebo levels. Increased intramuscular creatine produced a 6% increase in total work accomplished (251.7 kJ before supplement vs. 266.9 kJ after creatine loaded) compared with the group that consumed the placebo (254.0 kJ before test vs. 252.3 kJ after placebo). Creatine supplements have benefited an on-court "ghosting" routine of simulated positional play of competitive squash players. It also augments repeated sprint cycle performance after 30 minutes of constant load, submaximal exercise in the heat, without adversely affecting thermoregulatory dynamics. Creatine's benefits to muscular performance also occur in normally active older men.

Figure 4.3 outlines mechanisms of how elevating intramuscular free creatine and PCr with creatine supplementation might enhance exercise performance and the training response. Besides benefiting weight lifting and body building, improved immediate anaerobic power output capacity benefits sprint running, swimming, kayaking, cycling, jumping, football, and volleyball. Increased intramuscular PCr concentrations should also enable individuals to increase training intensity.

Oral supplements of creatine monohydrate (20 to 25 g per day) significantly increase muscle creatine and performance in high-intensity exercise, particularly repeated intense muscular effort. The ergogenic effect does not vary between vegetarians and meat eaters. Even daily doses as low as 6 g for 5 days improve repeated power performance.

For Division I football players, creatine supplementation during resistance training increased body mass, lean body mass, cellular hydration, and muscular strength and performance. Similarly, supplementation augmented muscular strength and size increases during 12 weeks of resistance training. For resistance-trained men who were classified as "responders" to creatine supplementation (i.e., an increase of $\geq$32 mmol·kg dry weight muscle^{-1}), 5 days of supplementation increased body weight and FFM and peak force and total force during repeated maximal isometric bench-presses. For men who were classified as "nonresponders" to supplementation (i.e., increase of $\leq$21 mmol·kg dry weight muscle^{-1}), no ergogenic effect occurred.

Taking a high dose of creatine helps replenish muscle creatine levels following heavy exercise. Such metabolic "reloading" should facilitate recovery of muscle contractile capacity, thus enabling athletes to sustain repeated ef-

Table 4·3	Selected Studies Showing an Increase in Exercise Performance Following Creatine Monohydrate Supplementation		
REFERENCE	**EXERCISE**	**PROTOCOL**	**EXERCISE PERFORMANCE**
d	Isokinetic, unilat. knee extensions ($180° \cdot s^{-1}$)	5 bouts of 30 ext. w/ 1-min rest periods	Reduction in decline of peak torque production during bouts 2, 3, and 4
e	Running	4 - 300 min w/ 4-min rest periods 4 - 300 m w/ 3-min rest periods	Improved time for final 300- and 100-m runs Improved total time for 4 - 1000-m runs; reduction in best time for 300- and 1000-m runs
a	Cycle ergometry (140 rev $\cdot$ min^{-1})	Ten 6-s bouts with 1-min rest periods	Better able to maintain pedal frequency during second 4-6 of each bout
f	Cycle ergometry (140 rev $\cdot$ min^{-1})	Five 6-s bouts w/ 30-s recovery followed by one 10-s bout	Better able to maintain pedal frequency near end of 10-s bout
b	Cycle ergometry (80 rev $\cdot$ min^{-1})	Three 30-s bouts w/ 4-min rest periods	Increase in peak power during bout 1 and increase in mean power and total work during bouts 1 and 2
c	Bench press	1-RM bench press and total reps at 70% 1-RM	Increase in 1-RM; increase in reps at 70% of 1-RM
g	Bench press	5 sets bench press w/ 2-min rest periods	Increase in reps completed during all 5 sets
g	Jump squat	5 sets jump squat w/ 2-min rest periods	Increase in peak power during all 5 sets
h	Bench press, squats, power clean	1-RM strength	Increase in 1-RM

From Volek, J.S., and Kraemer, W.J.: Creatine supplementation: Its effect on human muscular performance and body composition. *J Strength Cond. Res.,* 10:200, 1996.

[a]Balsom, P.D., et al.: Creatine supplementation and dynamic high-intensity intermittent exercise. *Scand. J. Med. Sci. Sports, 3:143, 1993.*

[b]Birch, R., et al.: The influence of dietary creatine supplementation on performance during repeated bouts of maximal isokinetic cycling in man. *Eur. J. Appl. Physiol., 69:268, 1994.*

[c]Earnest, C.P., et al.: The effect of creatine monohydrate ingestion on anaerobic power indices, muscular strength and body composition. *Acta Physiol. Scand., 153:207, 1995.*

[d]Greenhaff, P.L., et al.: Influence of oral creatine supplementation on muscle torque during repeated bouts on maximal voluntary exercise in man. *Clin. Sci., 84:565, 1993.*

[e]Harris, R.C., et al.: The effect of oral creatine supplementation on running performance during maximal short-term exercise in man. *J. Physiol., 467:74P,* 1993.

[f]Soderlund, K., et al.: Creatine supplementation and high-intensity exercise: Influence on performance and muscle metabolism. *Clin. Sci.,* 87 (suppl):120, 1994.

[g]Volek, J.S., et al.: Creatine supplementation enhances muscular performance during high-intensity resistance exercise. *J. Am. Diet. Assoc.,* 97:765, 1997.

[h]Pearson, D.R., et al.: Long-term effects of creatine monohydrate on strength and power. *J. Strength Cond. Res.,* 13:187, 1999.

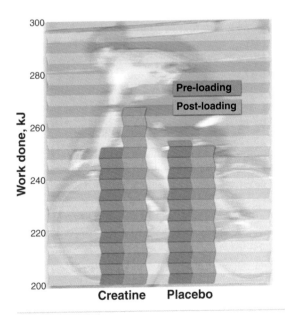

Figure 4.2. Effects of creatine loading versus placebo on total work accomplished during long-term (80-min) repetitive sprint-cycling performance. (From Preen, C.D., et al.: Effect of creatine loading on long-term sprint exercise performance and metabolism. *Med. Sci. Sports Exerc.,* 33:814, 2001.)

Effects on Body Mass and Body Composition

Body mass increases of between 0.5 and 2.4 kg often accompany creatine supplementation, independent of short-term changes in testosterone or cortisol concentrations. In fact, short-term creatine supplementation exerts no effect on the hormonal response to resistance training. It remains unclear how much of the weight gain occurs from (1) the anabolic effect of creatine on muscle tissue synthesis, (2) osmotic retention of intracellular water from increased creatine stores, or (3) other factors.

Creatine Loading   Many creatine users pursue a "loading" phase by ingesting 20 to 30 g of creatine daily (usually in tablet from or as powder added to liquid) for 5 to 7 days. A maintenance phase follows the loading phase, where the person supplements with as little as 2 to 5 g of creatine daily. Individuals who consume vegetarian-type diets show the greatest increase in muscle creatine because of the low creatine content of their diets. Large increases also characterize "responders," that is, individuals with normally low basal levels of intramuscular creatine.

Practical questions for the person desiring to elevate intramuscular creatine with supplementation concern (1) the magnitude and time course of intramuscular creatine increase, (2) the dosage necessary to maintain a creatine increase, and (3) the rate of creatine loss or "washout" following cessation of supplementation. To provide insight into these questions, researchers studied two groups of men. In one experiment, the men ingested 20 g of creatine monohydrate (approximately 0.3 g per kg of body mass) for 6 consecutive days, at which time supplementation ceased. Muscle biopsies were taken before supplement ingestion and at days 7, 21, and 35. Similarly, another group of men took 20 g of creatine monohydrate daily for 6 consecutive days. Instead of discontinuing supplementation, they reduced dosage to 2 g daily (approximately 0.03 g per kg body mass) for an additional 28 days. **Figure 4.4** illustrates that muscle creatine concentration increased by approximately 20% after 6 days. Without continued supplementation, muscle creatine content gradually declined to baseline in 35 days. The group that continued to supplement with reduced creatine intake for an additional 28 days maintained muscle creatine at the increased level (Fig. 4.4B).

For both groups, the increase in total muscle creatine content during the initial 6-day supplement period averaged about 23 mmol per kg of dry muscle, which represented about 20 g (17%) of the total creatine ingested. Interestingly, a similar 20% increase in total muscle creatine concentration occurred with only a 3-g daily supplement. However, this increase took place more gradually and required 28 days in contrast to only 6 days with the 6-g supplement.

A rapid way to "creatine load" skeletal muscle requires ingesting 20 g of creatine monohydrate daily for 6 days; then switching to a reduced dosage of 2 g per day keeps levels elevated for up to 28 days. If rapidity of "loading" is not a consideration, supplementing 3 g daily for 28 days achieves approximately the same high levels.

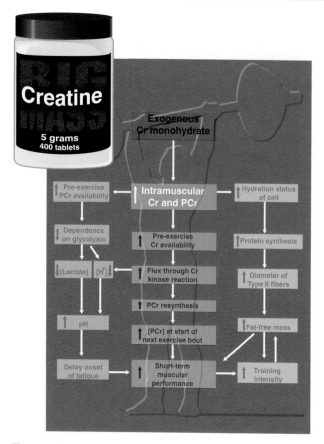

Figure 4.3. Possible mechanisms for how elevating intracellular creatine (Cr) and phosphocreatine (PCr) might enhance intense, short-term exercise performance and the exercise-training response. (Modified from Volek, J.S., and Kraemer, W.J.: Creatine supplementation: Its effect on human muscular performance and body composition. *J. Strength Cond. Res.*, 10:200, 1996.)

forts of high-intensity exercise. Whether this potential to maintain "quality" workouts enhances the strength and power training response awaits further research. Also, only limited information exists about long-term high doses of creatine supplementation in healthy individuals, particularly concerning the effects on cardiac muscle and kidney function (creatine degrades to creatinine before excretion in urine). Available data indicate that short-term use (e.g., 20 g per day for 5 consecutive days) in healthy men shows no detrimental effect on blood pressure, plasma creatine, plasma creatine kinase (CK) activity, or the renal response as measured by glomerular filtration rate and total protein and albumin excretion rates. For healthy subjects, no differences emerged in plasma contents and urine excretion rates for creatinine, urea, and albumin between control subjects and those who consumed creatine for between 10 months and 5 years.

Creatine supplementation does *not* improve exercise performance that requires high levels of aerobic energy transfer or cardiovascular and metabolic responses. It also exerts little effect on isometric muscular strength or dynamic muscle force measured during a single movement.

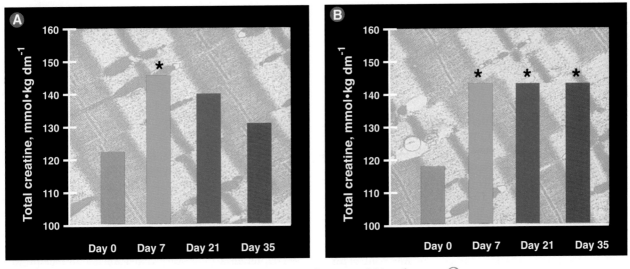

Figure 4.4.   A. Muscle total creatine concentration in six men who ingested 20 g of creatine for 6 consecutive days. **B.** Muscle total creatine concentration in nine men who ingested 20 g of creatine for 6 consecutive days and thereafter ingested 2 g of creatine per day for the next 28 days. In both **A** and **B**, muscle biopsy samples were taken before ingestion (day 0) and on days 7, 21, and 35. Values refer to averages per kg dry muscle mass (dm). *Significantly different from day 0. (From Hultman, E., et al.: Muscle creatine loading in men. *J. Appl. Physiol.*, 81:232, 1996.)

Questions & Notes

Give one condition in which creatine supplementation exerts ergogenic effects.

RIBOSE: THE NEXT CREATINE ON THE SUPPLEMENT SCENE?

Ribose has emerged as a competitor to creatine as a supplement to increase power and replenish high-energy compounds after intense exercise. The body readily synthesizes ribose, and the diet provides small amounts in ripe fruits and vegetables. Metabolically, the 5-carbon ribose sugar serves as an energy substrate for ATP resynthesis. Exogenous ribose ingestion has been touted as a means to quickly restore depleted ATP. To maintain optimal ATP levels and thus provide its ergogenic effect, recommended ribose doses range from 10 to 20 g per day. A compound that either increases ATP levels or facilitates its resynthesis could certainly benefit short-term, high-power physical activities. Unfortunately, only limited data exists to assess this potential. A double-blind randomized study evaluated the effects of oral ribose supplementation (4 doses per day at 4 g per dose) on repeated bouts of maximal exercise and ATP replenishment following intermittent maximal muscle contractions. No difference in any exercise performance measure (e.g., intermittent isokinetic knee extension force, blood lactate, and plasma ammonia concentration) emerged between ribose and placebo trials. Although the exercise significantly decreased intramuscular ATP and total adenine nucleotide content immediately after exercise and 24 hours later, oral ribose administration proved ineffective in facilitating recovery of these compounds. Further research is needed in this area.

Yes or No: Does creatine supplementation improve exercise performance requiring high levels of aerobic energy transfer?

GINSENG AND EPHEDRINE

The popularity of herbal and botanical remedies to improve health, control body weight, and improve exercise performance has soared. In 2003 alone, Americans spent $4.6 billion on such products. **Ginseng** and **ephedrine** are commonly marketed as nutritional supplements to "reduce stress," "revitalize," and "optimize mental and physical performance," particularly during times of fatigue and stress. Herbs such as ginseng also play a role as an alternative therapy in treating diabetes, stimulating immune function, and treating male impotence. Clinically, 1 to 3 g of ginseng administered 40 minutes before an oral glucose challenge reduces

FOR YOUR INFORMATION

Carbohydrate Ingestion Augments Creatine Loading
Research supports the common belief among athletes that consuming creatine with a sugar-containing drink increases creatine uptake and storage in skeletal muscle. For 5 days, subjects received either 5 g of creatine four times daily, or a 5-g supplement followed 30 minutes later by 93 g of a high glycemic index simple sugar four times daily. For the creatine-only supplement group, significant increases occurred for muscle PCr (7.2%), free creatine (13.5%), and total creatine (20.7%). However, much larger increases took place for the creatine plus sugar-supplemented group (14.7% increase in muscle PCr, 18.1% increase in free creatine, and 33.0% increase in total creatine).

postprandial glycemia in subjects without diabetes. As with caffeine, ephedrine and ginseng occur naturally and, for years, have been used in folk medicine to enhance "energy."

Ginseng

Used in Asian medicine to prolong life, strengthen and restore sexual functions, and invigorate the body, the ginseng root, often sold as Panax or Chinese or Korean ginseng, currently serves no recognized medical use in the United States except as a soothing agent in skin ointments. Commercial ginseng root preparations generally take the form of powder, liquid, tablets, or capsules; widely marketed foods and beverages also contain various types and amounts of ginsenosides. Because dietary supplements do not need to meet the same quality control for purity and potency as pharmaceuticals, considerable variation exists in the concentrations of marker compounds for ginseng, as well as levels of potentially harmful impurities and toxins like pesticide and heavy metal contamination. Neither the FDA nor other state or federal agencies routinely test ginseng-containing products or other supplements for quality.

Claims for ginseng in the Western world center around its ability to boost energy and diminish overall stress. Reports of an ergogenic effect often appear in the lay literature, but a review of the research provides little evidence to support the effectiveness of ginseng as an ergogenic aid. For example, volunteers consumed either 200 or 400 mg of the standardized ginseng concentrate each day for 8 weeks in a double-blind research protocol. Neither treatment significantly affected submaximal or maximal exercise performance, ratings of perceived exertion, or the physiologic parameters of heart rate, oxygen consumption, or blood lactate concentrations. Similarly, no ergogenic effects emerged on diverse physiologic and performance variables following a 1-week treatment with a ginseng saponin extract administered in two doses of either 8 or 16 mg per kg of body mass. When effectiveness has been demonstrated, the research has failed to use adequate controls, placebos, or double-blind testing protocols. *At present, no compelling scientific evidence exists that ginseng supplementation offers any ergogenic benefit for physiologic function or exercise performance.*

Ephedrine

Unlike ginseng, Western medicine had recognized the potent amphetamine-like compound ephedrine (with sympathomimetic physiologic effects) found in several species of the plant ephedra (dried plant stem called ma huang [ma wong; ephedra sinica]). The ephedra plant contains two major active components first isolated in 1928, ephedrine and pseudoephedrine, which exerts weaker effects than ephedrine. The medicinal role of this herb has included treating asthma, symptoms of the common cold, hypoten-

sion, and urinary incontinence and as a central stimulant to treat depression. Physicians in the United States discontinued ephedrine's use as a decongestant and asthma treatment in the 1930s in favor of safer medications.

Ephedrine exerts both central and peripheral effects, with the latter reflected in increased heart rate, cardiac output, and blood pressure. Due to its β-adrenergic effect, ephedrine causes bronchodilation in the lungs. High ephedrine dosages can produce hypertension, insomnia, hyperthermia, and cardiac arrhythmias. Other possible side effects include dizziness, restlessness, anxiety, irritability, personality changes, gastrointestinal symptoms, and difficulty concentrating.

FDA Bans Ephedrine In early 2004, the federal government announced a ban on the sale of ephedra, the latest chapter in a long story that gained national prominence after the deaths of two football players (professional all-Pro left tackle and University player) were linked to ephedra use in 2001. A little more than a month after the death of one of its players, the NFL added ephedra to its list of banned substances, becoming the first major sports body to do so.

The 2004 FDA ban was the culmination of a process that had started in June 1997 when the FDA first proposed to require a statement on dietary supplements with ephedra warning that they were hazardous and should not be used for more than 7 days. In February 2003, the FDA announced a series of measures that included strong enforcement actions against firms making unsubstantiated claims for their ephedra-containing products. In early 2004, the ban on ephedrine took effect (see *http://www.fda.gov/ola/2003/dietarysupplements1028.html* and *http://www.cfsan.fda.gov/~dms/ds-ephed.html*).

The FDA gathered and thoroughly reviewed a prodigious amount of evidence about ephedra's pharmacology, clinical studies of ephedra's safety and effectiveness, newly available adverse events reports, the published literature, and a seminal report by the RAND Corporation, an independent scientific institute. Published reports indicate nearly 1400 adverse effects from ephedra use reported to the FDA from January 1993 to February 2000. Incidents included 81 deaths, 32 heart attacks, 62 cases of cardiac arrhythmia, 91 cases of increased blood pressure, 69 strokes, and 70 seizures. During 2001, 1178 adverse reactions were reported to American poison control centers. In general, the cardiovascular toxic effects of ephedra (increased heart rate and blood vessel constriction) were not limited to massive doses but rather to the amount recommended by the manufacturer.

The totality of the available data showed little evidence of ephedra's effectiveness, except perhaps for short-term weight loss, while confirming that the substance raises blood pressure and otherwise stresses the circulatory system. These reactions were conclusively linked to significant adverse health outcomes, including heart ailments and strokes.

AMINO ACID SUPPLEMENTS AND OTHER DIETARY MODIFICATIONS FOR AN ANABOLIC EFFECT

Weight lifters, body builders, and fitness enthusiasts use **amino acid supplements** believing they boost the body's natural production of the anabolic hormones testosterone, growth hormone (GH), insulin, and insulin-like growth factor I (IGF-I) to improve muscle size and strength and decrease body fat. The rationale for trying nutritional ergogenic stimulants comes from the clinical use of amino acid infusion or ingestion in deficient patients to regulate anabolic hormones.

Research on healthy subjects does not provide convincing evidence for an ergogenic effect of oral amino acid supplements on hormone secretion, training responsiveness, or exercise performance. In studies with appropriate design and statistical analysis, supplements of arginine, lysine, ornithine, tyrosine, and other amino acids, either singularly or in combination, produced no effect on GH levels or insulin secretion or on diverse measures of anaerobic power and all-out running performance at $\dot{V}O_{2max}$. Furthermore, elite junior weight lifers that supplemented with all 20 amino acids did not improve physical performance or resting or exercise-induced responses of testosterone, cortisol, or GH. The indiscriminate use of amino acid supplements at dosage considered pharmacologic rather than nutritional increases risk of direct toxic effects or the creation of an amino acid imbalance.

Prudent Means to Possibly Augment an Anabolic Effect

With resistance training, muscle hypertrophy results from a shift in the body's normal dynamic state of protein synthesis and degradation to greater tissue synthesis. The normal hormonal milieu (e.g., insulin and GH levels) in the period following resistance exercise stimulates the muscle fiber's anabolic processes while inhibiting muscle protein degradation. Dietary modifications that increase amino acid transport into muscle, raise energy availability, or increase anabolic hormone levels would theoretically augment the training effect by increasing the rate of anabolism and/or depressing catabolism. Either effect should create a positive body protein balance for improved muscular growth and strength (see Close Up Box 3-4 on page 120).

Carbohydrate–Protein Supplementation Immediately in Recovery Augments Hormonal Response to Resistance Exercise

Studies of hormonal dynamics and protein anabolism indicate a transient but potential ergogenic effect (up to 4-fold increase in protein synthesis) of carbohydrate and/or protein supplements consumed *immediately following* resistance exercise workouts. This effect of supplementation in the immediate postexercise period of resistance exercise may also prove effective for tissue repair and synthesis of muscle proteins following aerobic exercise.

Drug-free male weightlifters with at least 2 years of resistance training experience consumed carbohydrate and protein supplements immediately after a standard resistance-training workout. Treatment included one of the following: (1) a placebo of pure water; or a supplement of (2) carbohydrate (1.5 g per kg body mass), (3) protein (1.38 g per kg body mass), or (4) carbohydrate/protein (1.06 g carbohydrate plus 0.41 g protein per kg body mass) consumed immediately following and then 2 hours after the training session. Compared with the placebo, each nutritive supplement produced a hormonal environment (elevated plasma concentrations of insulin and GH) in recovery conducive to protein synthesis and

(text continues on page 140)

Describe one situation where ginseng may provide an ergogenic effect.

Name one product known to augment the effects of creatine loading.

Discuss whether amino acid supplements, either alone or in combination, provide ergogenic effects.

Name 3 herbs and their purported beneficial effects.

Herb	Effect
1.	
2.	
3.	

FOR YOUR INFORMATION

Skip the Carnitine

Vital to normal metabolism, carnitine facilitates influx of long-chain fatty acids into the mitochondrial matrix where they enter beta-oxidation during energy metabolism. Patients with progressive muscle weakness benefit from carnitine administration, but healthy adults do not require carnitine supplements above that contained in a balanced diet. No research supports ergogenic benefits, positive metabolic alterations (aerobic or anaerobic), or body fat-reducing effects from carnitine supplementation.

Box 4–1 • CLOSE UP

HOW TO IDENTIFY HERBS AND THEIR USES

In seeking a competitive edge, athletes are particularly susceptible to fad diets and supplements whose ergogenic effects may not have been adequately validated. Many athletes fail to eat an optimal diet, especially when trying to control their body weight while training strenuously. These particular athletes often experience micronutrient deficiencies that, even if marginal, could negatively impact exercise performance, health, or both. The use of

HERB	OTHER NAME	PURPORTED USE
Astragalus	Huang qi	Supports immune system, benefits cardiovascular system, increases energy level, promotes tissue repair
Bilberry	Vaccinium myrtillus	Diabetes; macular degeneration; retinopathy
Bee Pollen	Buckwheat pollen; puhuang	Allergies; asthma; cholesterol and triacylglycerol lowering
Chamomile	Camomile, roman camomile	Stress reduction; supports immune function; assists sleep; promotes tissue repair
Echinacea	Echinacea purpurea; echinacea angustifolia	Common cold/sore throat; immune function; infection; influenza
Garlic	Allium sativum	High blood pressure; high triacylglycerols; intermittent claudication
Ginkgo Biloba	Maidenhair tree	Age-related cognitive decline; Alzheimer's disease; intermittent claudication; depression; atherosclerosis; impotence (of vascular origin)
Guarana	Paullinia cupana	Fatigue; weight loss
Kava Kava	Piper methysticum	Anxiety; restlessness; stress, muscle relaxing; improves sleep
Milk Thistle	Silybum marianum	Alcohol-related liver disease; hepatitis; liver support
Glucosamine Sulfate[a]		Osteoarthritis; joint inflammation; joint stiffness
Saw Palmetto	Serenoa repens, sabal serrulata	Benign prostatic hyperplasia; urination problems in males
St. John's Wort	Hypericum perforatum	Depression; anxiety or nervous unrest; mood disturbance of menopause
Witch Hazel	Hamamelis virginiana	Eczema; hemorrhoids; varicose veins
Yohimbe	Pausinystalia yohimbe	Impotence; depression
Valerian	Heliotrope; setwall; vandal root	Stress reduction; improves sleep; benefits cardiovascular system

[a]Not truly listed as an herb; usually listed as a supplement.

Box 4–1 • CLOSE UP *(Continued)*

herbs as nutritional supplements has expanded significantly during the last decade. Thus, knowledge of herbs, their purported beneficial effects, and their possible negative side effects takes on added importance.

The table below presents some popular herbs and their uses, active ingredients, common dosages, and precautionary information. The criteria for listing a purported use include those with reliable and relatively consistent scientific studies (3 or more) that show a beneficial outcome.

ACTIVE INGREDIENTS	COMMON DOSE	SIDE EFFECTS/INTERACTIONS
Flavonoids, polysaccharides, triterpene glycosides, amino acids and trace minerals	9–15 g per day	None
Anthocyanosides (bioflavonoid)	240–600 mg per day as herbal extract or 20–60 g of fruit daily	None
Protein, carbohydrates, minerals, and essential fatty acids	500–100 mg per day	Allergic reaction can occur; avoid with hypoglycemic agents
Alpha-bisabolol; bioflavonoids	Taken as tea drunk 3 to 4 times per day	Avoid if you have allergies to plants
Alkylamides, polyacetylenes	At onset of cold or flu: 3–4 mL every 2 h; or 300 mg powder per day	Increases production of interferon; do not use if allergic to sunflower plant family
Sulfur compound allicin	600–900 mg per day	Do not use with stomach problems such as heartburn, gastritis, or ulcers
Ginkgo flavone glycosides (bioflavonoid), terpene lactones	120–240 per day	Mild headaches lasting 1 or 2 days; mild upset stomach
Guaranine (identical to caffeine)	200–800 mg per day	Avoid if pregnant; glaucoma; heart disease; high blood pressure; history of stroke
Kava-lactones	200–250 mg per day	Avoid if pregnant or lactating; can cause drowsiness
Bioflavonoid complex- silymarin	200–400 mg per day 1500 mg per day	None Avoid if diabetic
Liposterolic extract of saw palmetto provides fatty acids, sterols, and esters	200–300 mg per day	None
Hypericin, flavonoids	900 mg per day	Can heighten sun sensitivity; can interfere with iron absorption
Tannins and volatile oils	As ointment or cream 3–4 times per day	Not for internal use–causes stomach irritation
Yohimbine (alkaloid)	15–30 mg per day	Use only under supervision of doctor
Essential oils	300–500 mg before sleep	None

REFERENCES

Therapeutic Research Faculty: Natural Medicines Comprehensive Database. 2nd Ed. Stockton, CA: Pharmacists Letter, 2004.

Schuyler, W., et al.: *The Natural Pharmacy.* 2nd Ed. Rocklin, CA: HealthNotes, Inc., 1999.

muscle tissue growth. Such data provide indirect evidence for a possible training benefit of increasing carbohydrate and/or protein intake immediately after a resistance-training workout.

BEE POLLEN

Bees gather pollen, the material from the fine, powder-like reproductive substance produced by flowering plants. Bee pollen's allure as a nutrient supplement for physically active individuals lies in its relatively rich mixture of vitamins, minerals, and amino acids required for energy-producing reactions. It also has the appeal of a compound directly synthesized in nature, making it an advertiser's dream as a cancer preventing, life-prolonging "perfect natural food." However, no reliable data attest to its effectiveness as an ergogenic aid. In one study, highly trained runners who received **bee pollen** supplements showed no improvement in recovery rate from repeated maximal treadmill runs to exhaustion. Furthermore, no effects of bee pollen supplementation occurred for maximal oxygen uptake, endurance performance, or other physiologic responses to exercise. In addition to a lack of scientific evidence to justify its use as an ergogenic aid, supplementing with bee pollen does not lack risk. Individuals allergic to specific pollens may experience extreme reactions when taking this supplement.

BORON

The actual biochemical function of the trace mineral **boron** remains unclear, although it appears in high concentrations in bone and in tissues of the spleen and thyroid gland. Boron deprivation significantly depresses bone tissue synthesis. Studies of postmenopausal women previously deprived of dietary boron showed that boron supplements augmented calcium and magnesium metabolism and increased testosterone levels. The promise of increased testosterone output tempts weight lifters and body builders to consume excess boron to promote an anabolic effect. Mail-order advertisements extol boron-containing supplements as a safe replacement for anabolic steroids without harmful side effects.

Limited information indicates that boron supplements do not affect testosterone levels in individuals adequately nourished for this mineral. For individuals undergoing resistance training, 6-mg supplements of boron (plus 800 μg of chromium picolinate) did not enhance lean tissue accretion or promote fat loss compared with a maltodextrin placebo. Until more research becomes available, we recommend that an individual's total intake of boron not exceed 10 mg daily.

COENZYME Q-10 (UBIQUINONE)

Coenzyme Q-10 (CoQ$_{10}$; ubiquinone in oxidized form and ubiquinol when reduced), which is found primarily in meats, peanuts, and soybean oil, functions as an integral component of the mitochondrion's electron transport system of oxidative phosphorylation. This lipid-soluble natural component of all cells exists in high concentrations within myocardial tissue. CoQ$_{10}$ has been used therapeutically to treat cardiovascular disease because of (1) its role in oxidative metabolism and (2) its antioxidant properties that promote scavenging of free radicals that damage cellular components. Due to its positive effect on oxygen uptake and exercise performance in cardiac patients, some consider CoQ$_{10}$ a potential ergogenic nutrient for endurance performance. Based on the belief that supplementation could increase the flux of electrons through the respiratory chain and thus augment aerobic resynthesis of ATP, the popular literature touts CoQ$_{10}$ supplements as a means to improve "stamina" and enhance cardiovascular function. However, no research data support such claims.

CoQ$_{10}$ supplementation increases serum CoQ$_{10}$ levels, but it does not improve a healthy person's aerobic capacity, endurance performance, plasma glucose or lactate levels at submaximal workloads, or cardiovascular dynamics when compared with a placebo. One study evaluated oral supplements of CoQ$_{10}$ on the exercise tolerance and peripheral muscle function of healthy, middle-aged men. Measurements included $\dot{V}O_{2max}$, lactate threshold, heart rate response, and upper-extremity exercise blood flow and metabolism. For 2 months, subjects received either CoQ$_{10}$ (150 mg per day) or a placebo. Blood levels of CoQ$_{10}$ increased significantly during the treatment period and remained unchanged in the controls. No differences occurred between groups for any of the physiologic or metabolic variables. Similarly, for trained young and older men, CoQ$_{10}$ supplementation of 120 mg per day for 6 weeks did not benefit aerobic capacity or lipid peroxidation, a marker of oxidative stress. Recent data indicate that CoQ$_{10}$ supplements (60 mg daily combined with vitamins E and C) did not affect lipid peroxidation during exercise in endurance athletes.

LIPID SUPPLEMENTATION WITH MEDIUM-CHAIN TRIACYLGLYCEROLS

Do high-fat foods or supplements elevate plasma lipid levels to make more energy available during prolonged aerobic exercise? One must consider several factors to achieve such an effect. For one thing, consuming triacylglycerols composed of predominantly long-chain fatty acids (12 to 18 carbons) significantly *delays* gastric emptying. This negatively affects the rapidity of exogenous fat availability; it also slows fluid and carbohydrate replenishment, both of which are crucial factors in high-intensity endurance exercise. In addition, after digestion and intestinal absorption (normally a 3- to 4-h process), long-chain triacylglycerols reassemble with phospholipids, fatty acids, and a cholesterol shell to form fatty droplets called chylomicrons. Chylomicrons then travel slowly to the systemic circulation via the lymphatic system. Once in the bloodstream, the tissues remove the triacylglycerols bound to chylomicrons. Consequently, the relatively slow rate of digestion, absorption, and oxidation of long-chain fatty acids make this energy source undesirable as a supplement to augment energy metabolism in active muscle during exercise.

Medium-chain triacylglycerols (MCT) provide a more rapid source of fatty acid fuel. MCTs are processed oils, frequently produced for patients with intestinal malabsorption and tissue-wasting diseases. Marketing for the sports enthusiast hypes MCTs as a "fat burner," "energy source," "glycogen sparer," and "muscle builder." Unlike longer chain triacylglycerols, MCTs contain saturated fatty acids with 8- to 10-carbon atoms along the fatty acid chain. During digestion, they hydrolyze by lipase action in the mouth, stomach, and intestinal duodenum to glycerol and medium-chain fatty acids (MCFA). The water solubility of MCFAs enables them to move rapidly across the intestinal mucosa directly into the bloodstream (portal vein) without necessity of slow transport in chylomicrons by the lymphatic system as required for long-chain triacylglycerols. Once in the tissues, MCFAs move through the plasma membrane and diffuse across the inner mitochondrial membrane for oxidation. They pass into the mitochondria largely independent of the carnitine-acyl-CoA transferase system; this contrasts with the slower transfer and mitochondrial oxidation rate of long-chain fatty acids. MCTs do not usually store as body fat because of their relative ease of oxidation. Because ingesting MCTs elevates plasma free fatty acids rapidly, some speculate that supplementing with these lipids might spare liver and muscle glycogen during high-intensity aerobic exercise.

Exercise Benefits Inconclusive

Consuming MCT does not inhibit gastric emptying, but conflicting research exists about their use in exercise. Ingesting 30 g of MCT before exercising (an estimated maximal amount tolerated in the gastrointestinal tract) contributed only between 3% and 7% of the total exercise energy cost.

Consuming a large quantity (86 g) of MCT (surprisingly well tolerated by subjects) provides interesting results. Endurance-trained cyclists rode for 2 hours at 60% $\dot{V}O_{2peak}$; they then immediately performed a simulated 40-km cycling time trial. During each of three rides, they drank 2 liters containing 10% glucose, a 4.3% MCT emulsion, or 10% glucose plus a 4.3% MCT emulsion. **Figure 4.5**

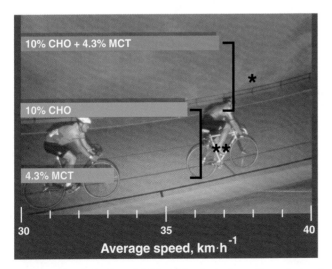

Figure 4.5. Effects of carbohydrate (CHO; 10% solution), medium-chain triacylglycerol (MCT; 4.3% emulsion), and carbohydrate + MCT ingestion during exercise on simulated 40-km time-trial cycling speeds after 2 hours of exercise at 60% of peak oxygen uptake. *Significantly faster than 10% CHO trials; **significantly faster than 4.3% MCT trials. (From Van Zyl, C.G., et al.: Effects of medium-chain triacylglycerol ingestion on fuel metabolism and cycling performance. *J. Appl. Physiol.*, 80:2217, 1996.)

Questions & Notes

Give the formal names for the following abbreviations:

   CoQ_{10} –

   MCT –

   HCA –

What is the function of coenzyme Q-10?

Give one negative effect of consuming medium-chain triacylglycerols.

Briefly describe how medium-chain triacylglycerols may act as an ergogenic supplement.

shows the effects of the beverages on average speed in the 40-km trials. Replacing the carbohydrate beverage with only the MCT emulsion impaired exercise performance by approximately 8%. The combined carbohydrate plus MCT solution consumed repeatedly during exercise significantly improved cycling speed by 2.5%. This small ergogenic effect occurred with (1) reduced total carbohydrate oxidation at a given level of oxygen uptake, (2) higher final circulating free fatty acid and ketone levels, and (3) lower final glucose and lactate concentrations.

The small endurance performance enhancement with MCT supplementation probably occurred because this exogenous fatty acid source contributed to the total exercise energy expenditure as well as total fat oxidation in exercise. Consuming MCTs does not stimulate the release of bile, the fat-emulsifying agent from the gall bladder. Thus, cramping and diarrhea often accompany an excess intake of this lipid form. Additional research must validate the ergogenic claims for MCT, including the tolerance level for these lipids during exercise. In general, the relatively small alterations in substrate availability and substrate oxidation by increasing the free fatty acid availability during moderately intense aerobic exercise had little effect on exercise capacity.

(—)-HYDROXYCITRATE: A POTENTIAL FAT BURNER?

(—)-Hydroxycitrate (HCA), a principal constituent of the rind of the fruit of Garcinia cambogia used in Asian cuisine, is the latest compound promoted as a "natural fat burner" to facilitate weight loss and enhance endurance performance. Metabolically, HCA operates as a competitive inhibitor of an enzyme that catalyzes the breakdown of citrate to oxaloacetate and acetyl-CoA in the cytosol. Inhibition of this enzyme limits the pool of 2-carbon acetyl compounds and, thus, reduces cellular ability to synthesize fat. Because inhibition of citrate catabolism also slows carbohydrate breakdown, HCA supplementation should provide a means to conserve glycogen and increase lipolysis during endurance exercise.

Research has evaluated acute effects of HCA ingestion on (1) HCA availability in the plasma and (2) fat oxidation rates at rest and during moderate-intensity exercise. Endurance-trained cyclists received either an HCA solution of 3.1 mL per kg of body mass ($19 \, g \cdot L^{-1}$; 6 to 30 times the dosage in weight-loss studies) or a placebo at 45 and 15 minutes before starting exercise (resting measure) and 30 and 60 minutes after a 2-hour exercise bout at 50% maximal working capacity. Supplementation increased plasma concentrations of HCA at rest and during exercise, but no change occurred in energy expenditure or in fat and carbohydrate oxidation between trials. These findings indicate that increasing plasma HCA availability with supplementation exerts no effect on skeletal muscle fat oxidation during rest or exercise, at least in endurance-trained humans. This casts serious doubt on the usefulness of large quantities of HCA as an anti-obesity agent or ergogenic aid.

VANADIUM

Vanadium, a trace element widely distributed in nature, comes from the bluish salt of vanadium acid. It was named in 1831 for the Norse goddess of beauty (Vanadis) because of its ability to form multi-colored compounds. This important element (no RDA established) exhibits insulin-like properties by facilitating glucose transport and utilization in skeletal muscle, stimulating glycogen synthesis, and activating glycolytic reactions. In animals, vanadium supplements attenuated the effects of diabetes, perhaps by augmenting the action of available insulin. In humans, administering 50 mg of vanadium twice daily for 3 weeks improved hepatic and skeletal muscle insulin sensitivity in type 2 diabetics, partly by enhancing insulin's inhibitory effect on fat breakdown. However, no altered insulin sensitivity occurred in non-diabetic subjects. Optimal iodine metabolism and thyroid function may also require an adequate vanadium intake. The best "natural" sources of vanadium include cereal and grain products and dietary oils; meat, fish, and poultry contain moderate amounts of this element.

Body builders ingest vanadium supplements, usually in its oxidized form as vanadyl sulfate, often combined with additional minerals or coatings or as bis-maltolato-oxo-vanadium (BMOV). Enthusiasts believe that vanadium provides the "pumped look" and gives the appearance of muscular hypertrophy (hardness, density, and size) because of enhanced muscle glycogen storage and amino acid uptake. No research supports an ergogenic role for vanadium supplements. Individuals should exercise extreme care when supplementing with this element because an excess of vanadium becomes toxic (particularly to the liver) in mammals.

PYRUVATE

Ergogenic effects have been extolled for **pyruvate**, the 3-carbon end product of the cytoplasmic breakdown of glucose in glycolysis. Exogenous pyruvate, as a partial replacement for dietary carbohydrate, allegedly augments endurance exercise performance and promotes fat loss. Pyruvic acid, a relatively unstable chemical, causes intestinal distress. Consequently, various forms of the salt of this acid (sodium, potassium, calcium, or magnesium pyruvate) are produced in capsule, tablet, or powder form. Supplement manufacturers recommend taking 2 to 4 capsules daily. One capsule usually contains 600 mg of pyruvate. The calcium form of pyruvate contains approximately 80 mg of calcium with 600 mg of pyruvate. Some advertisements recommend a dosage of one capsule per 20 pounds of body weight. Manufacturers also combine creatine monohydrate and pyruvate; one gram of creatine pyruvate provides about 80 mg of creatine and 400 mg of pyruvate. Recommended pyruvate doses range from 5 to 20 g per day. Pyruvate content in the normal diet ranges between 100 to 2000 mg daily. The largest dietary amounts occur in fruits and vegetables, particularly red apples (500 mg each), with smaller quantities in dark beer (80 mg per 12 oz) and red wine (75 mg per 6 oz).

Effects on Endurance Performance

Several reports indicate beneficial effects of exogenous pyruvate on endurance performance. Two double-blind, cross-over studies by the same laboratory showed that 7 days of daily supplementation of a 100-g mixture of pyruvate (25 g) plus dihydroxyacetone (DHA; 75 g, another 3-carbon compound of glycolysis) increased upper- and lower-body aerobic endurance by 20% compared with exercise with a 100-g supplement of an isocaloric glucose polymer. The pyruvate-DHA mixture increased cycle ergometer time to exhaustion of the legs by 13 minutes (66 min vs. 79 min), whereas upper-body arm-cranking exercise time increased by 27 minutes (133 min vs. 160 min). A reduction also occurred for local muscle and overall body ratings of perceived exertion when subjects exercised with the pyruvate-DHA mixture compared with the placebo. Dosage recommendations range between a total of 2 and 5 g of pyruvate spread throughout the day and taken with meals.

Proponents of pyruvate supplementation maintain that elevations in extracellular pyruvate augment glucose transport into active muscle. Enhanced "glucose extraction" from blood provides the important carbohydrate energy source to sustain high-intensity aerobic exercise while also conserving intramuscular glycogen stores. When the individual's diet contains a normal 55% of total kCals, pyruvate supplementation also increases pre-exercise muscle glycogen levels. Both of these effects (higher pre-exercise glycogen levels and facilitated glucose uptake and oxidation by active muscle) benefit high-intensity endurance exercise similar to how pre-exercise carbohydrate loading and glucose feedings during exercise exert ergogenic effects.

Effects of Body Fat Loss   Some research indicates that exogenous pyruvate intake can augment body fat loss when accompanied by a low-energy diet. Unfortunately, adverse side effects of a 30- to 100-g daily pyruvate intake include diarrhea as well as some gastrointestinal gurgling and discomfort. *Until additional studies from independent laboratories reproduce existing findings for exercise performance and body fat loss, one should view with caution conclusions about the effectiveness of pyruvate supplementation.*

GLYCEROL

Glycerol is a component of the triacylglycerol molecule, a gluconeogenic substrate, an important constituent of the cells' phospholipid plasma membrane, and an osmotically active natural metabolite. The 2-carbon glycerol molecule achieved clinical notoriety (along with mannitol, sorbitol, and urea) for its role in producing an osmotic diuresis. This capacity for influencing water movement within the body makes glycerol effective in reducing excess accumulation of fluid (edema) in the brain and eye. Glycerol's effect on water movement occurs because extracellular glycerol enters the tissues of the brain, cerebrospinal fluid, and eye's aqueous humor at a relatively slow rate; this creates an osmotic effect that draws fluid from these tissues.

Ingesting a concentrated mixture of glycerol plus water increases the body's fluid volume and glycerol concentrations in plasma and interstitial fluid compartments. This sets the stage for fluid excretion from an increase in renal filtrate and urine flow. However, because proximal and distal tubules reabsorb much of this glycerol, a large fluid portion of renal filtrate also becomes reabsorbed; this averts a marked diuresis. (Renal reabsorption does not occur with tissue dehydrators like mannitol and sorbitol, which produce a true osmotic diuresis.)

When consumed with 1 to 2 L of water, glycerol facilitates water absorption from the intestine and causes extracellular fluid retention, mainly in the plasma

Questions & Notes

Give one reason that long-chain fatty acids are undesirable as a supplement to augment energy metabolism.

Briefly describe how (–) - hydroxycitrate supposedly acts as an ergogenic supplement.

Briefly describe how pyruvate supposedly acts as an ergogenic supplement.

Briefly describe how glycerol supposedly acts as an ergogenic supplement.

fluid compartment. The hyperhydration effect of glycerol supplementation reduces overall heat stress during exercise as reflected by increased sweating rate; this lowers heart rate and body temperature during exercise and enhances endurance performance under heat stress. Reducing heat stress with hyperhydration using glycerol plus water supplementation prior to exercise increases safety for the exercise participant. The typically recommended pre-exercise glycerol dosage of 1.0 g of glycerol per kg of body mass in 1 to 2 L of water lasts up to 6 hours.

Not all research demonstrates meaningful thermoregulatory or exercise performance benefits of glycerol hyperhydration over pre-exercise hyperhydration with plain water. For example, exogenous glycerol diluted in 500 mL of water consumed 4 hours before exercise failed to promote fluid retention or ergogenic effects. Also, no cardiovascular or thermoregulatory advantages occurred when consuming glycerol with small volumes of water during exercise. Side effects of exogenous glycerol ingestion include nausea, dizziness, bloating, and light-headedness.

SUMMARY

1. Functional foods comprise those foods and their bioactive components (e.g., olive oil, soy products, omega-3 fatty acids) that promote well-being, health, and optimal bodily function or reduce disease health risk.

2. For transgenic nutraceuticals, genes introduced into a host plant or animal modify a biochemical pathway. This produces a new class of "natural" bioactive components of food in a non-food matrix with physiologic and therapeutic functions that often promote disease prevention and treatment.

3. By definition, nutraceutical compounds fall along the continuum from food to food supplements to drugs. Nutraceuticals differ from functional foods that deliver their active ingredients within the food matrix.

4. Ergogenic aids consist of substances or procedures that improve physical work capacity, physiologic function, or athletic performance.

5. Little scientific evidence exists to recommend exogenous phosphates or pangamic acid as ergogenic aids. From a nutritional perspective, pangamic acid has no vitamin or provitamin properties; it apparently serves no particular purpose in the body.

6. Increasing the body's alkaline reserve before anaerobic exercise by ingesting buffering solutions of sodium bicarbonate or sodium citrate improves performance. Buffer dosage and the cumulative anaerobic nature of the exercise interact to influence the ergogenic effect of bicarbonate (or citrate) loading.

7. Cortisol decreases amino acid transport into cells, depressing anabolism and stimulating protein catabolism. Some believe that blunting cortisol's normal increase after exercise in healthy, highly fit individuals augments muscular development with resistance training because muscle tissue synthesis progresses unimpeded in recovery.

8. An objective decision about the potential benefits and risks of glutamine, phosphatidylserine, and beta-hydroxyl-beta-methyl butyrate to provide a "natural" anabolic boost with resistance training for healthy individuals awaits further research.

9. Many tout chromium supplements (usually as chromium picolinate) for their fat-burning and muscle-building properties. Research fails to show any beneficial effect of chromium supplements on training-related changes in muscular strength, physique, fat-free body mass, or muscle mass.

10. In supplement form, creatine significantly increases intramuscular creatine and phosphocreatine, and enhances short-term anaerobic power output capacity and facilitates recovery from repeated bouts of intense effort. Creatine loading occurs by ingesting 20 g of creatine monohydrate for 6 consecutive days. Thereafter, reducing intake to 2 g daily maintains elevated intramuscular levels.

11. Because of its role in energy metabolism, exogenous ribose ingestion has been touted as a means to quickly restore depleted ATP. No significant difference in any exercise performance and physiologic measure emerged between ribose and placebo exercise trials.

12. No compelling scientific evidence exists to conclude that ginseng supplementation offers positive benefit for physiologic function or performance during exercise.

13. Accumulating evidence indicates that significant health risks accompany ephedrine use. Based on an analysis of existing data, on December 31, 2003, the FDA announced a ban on ephedra, which is the first time this federal agency has moved to ban a dietary supplement.

14. Many resistance-trained athletes supplement with amino acids, either singularly or in combination, to create a hormonal milieu to facilitate protein synthesis in skeletal muscle. Research generally shows no benefits of such supplementation on levels of anabolic

hormones or measures of body composition, muscle size, or exercise performance.

15. Carbohydrate-protein supplementation immediately in recovery from resistance training produces a hormonal environment conducive to protein synthesis and muscle tissue growth (elevated plasma concentrations of insulin and growth hormone). Such data provide indirect evidence for a possible training benefit of increasing carbohydrate and/or protein intake immediately after a resistance-training workout.

16. Bee pollen does not provide ergogenic effects compared to a well-balanced diet.

17. Boron supplements have no effect on anabolic hormone levels in individuals with adequate boron intake.

18. CoQ_{10} supplements in healthy individuals provide no ergogenic effect on aerobic capacity, endurance, submaximal exercise lactate levels, or cardiovascular dynamics.

19. Due to their relatively rapid digestion, assimilation, and catabolism for energy, some believe that consuming medium-chain triacylglycerols (MCT) enhances fat metabolism and conserves glycogen during endurance exercise. Ingesting about 86 g of MCT enhances performance by an additional 2.5%.

20. Increasing plasma (—)-hydroxycitrate (HCA) availability via supplementation exerts no effect on skeletal muscle fat oxidation at rest or during exercise.

21. The trace mineral vanadium exerts insulin-like properties in humans. However, no research documents an ergogenic effect, and extreme intake produces toxic effects.

22. Pyruvate supplementation purportedly augments endurance performance and promotes fat loss. Body fat loss is attributed to its small effect on increasing metabolic rate. A definitive conclusion concerning pyruvate's effectiveness requires verification by other investigators.

23. Pre-exercise glycerol ingestion promotes hyperhydration, which supposedly protects the individual from heat stress and heat injury during high-intensity exercise. Currently, the International Olympic Committee has banned the use of glycerol.

THOUGHT QUESTIONS

1. Respond to the question: "If the government allows the chemicals in food supplements to be sold over the counter, how could they possibly be harmful to you?"

2. Discuss the importance of the psychological or "placebo" effect in evaluating claims for the effectiveness of particular nutrients, chemicals, or procedures as ergogenic aids.

PART 2 •
Pharmacologic Aids to Performance

Many athletes at all levels of competition use pharmacologic and chemical agents believing a specific drug positively influences skill, strength, power, or endurance. When winning becomes all-important, cheating to win becomes pervasive. Often, despite scanty "hard" scientific evidence indicating a performance-enhancing effect of many of these chemicals, little can be done to prevent the use and abuse of drugs by athletes. We discuss here the most prominent of the pharmacologic agents and procedures used by athletes to enhance performance.

CAFFEINE

In January 2004, the IOC removed **caffeine** from its list of restricted substances. Caffeine belongs to a group of compounds called methylxanthines, which are found naturally in coffee beans, tea leaves, chocolate, cocoa beans, and cola nuts, and is added to carbonated beverages and nonprescription medicines (**Table 4.4**). Sixty-three plant species contain caffeine in their leaves, seeds, or fruit. In the United States, 75% (14 million kg) of caffeine intake comes from coffee, and 15% comes from tea. Depending on preparation, one cup of brewed coffee contains between 60 to 150 mg of caffeine, instant coffee contains about 100 mg, brewed tea contains between 20 and 50 mg, and caffeinated soft drinks contain about 50 mg. As a frame of reference, 2.5 cups of percolated coffee contain 250 to 400 mg, or generally between 3 and 6 mg per kg of body mass. Caffeine absorption by the small intestine occurs rapidly, reaching peak plasma concentrations between 30 and 120 minutes after ingestion to exert an influence on the nervous, cardiovascular, and muscular systems. Caffeine's metabolic half-life of 3 hours means that it clears from the body fairly rapidly, certainly after a night's sleep.

Caffeine's Ergogenic Effects

A strong base of evidence supports the use of caffeine to improve exercise performance. Ingesting the amount of caffeine (330 mg) in 2.5 cups of regularly percolated coffee 1 hour before exercising significantly extends endurance in intense aerobic exercise. Subjects who consumed caffeine exercised for an average of 90.2 minutes compared with 75.5 minutes in subjects who exercised without caffeine. Even though heart rate and oxygen uptake were similar during the two trials, the caffeine made the work seem easier.

Caffeine also provides an ergogenic benefit during maximal swimming performances completed in less than 25 minutes. In a double-blind, cross-over study, seven male and four female distance swimmers (<25 min for 1500 m) consumed caffeine (6 mg·kg body mass^{-1}) 2.5 hours before swimming 1500 m. **Figure 4.6** illustrates that the split times improved significantly with caffeine for each 500 m of the swim. Total swim time averaged 1.9% faster with caffeine than without it (20 min, 58.6 s vs. 21 min, 21.8 s). Lower plasma potassium concentration prior to exercise and higher blood glucose levels at the end of the trial accompanied enhanced performance with caffeine. This suggested that electrolyte balance and glucose availability might be key factors in caffeine's ergogenic effect.

Proposed Mechanism for Ergogenic Action

A precise explanation for the exercise-enhancing boost from caffeine remains elusive. In all likelihood, the ergogenic effect of caffeine (or other related methylxanthine compounds) in high-intensity, endurance exercise results from the facilitated use of fat as a fuel for exercise, thus sparing the body's limited glycogen reserves. In the quantities typically administered to humans, caffeine probably acts in one of the two following ways: (1) directly by stimulating adipose tissues to release fatty acids and (2) indirectly by stimulating epinephrine release from the adrenal medulla; epinephrine then facilitates fatty acid release from adipocytes into plasma. Increased plasma free fatty acid levels, in turn, increase fat oxidation, thus conserving liver and muscle glycogen. Caffeine also produces analgesic effects on the central nervous system and enhances motoneuronal excitability, facilitating motor unit recruitment.

Endurance Effects Often Inconsistent Prior nutrition may partly account for variation in response to exercise after individuals consume caffeine. Although group improvements in endurance occur with taking caffeine, individuals who maintain a high-carbohydrate intake show a diminished effect on free fatty acid mobilization. Individual differences in caffeine sensitivity, tolerance, and hormonal response from short- and long-term patterns of caffeine consumption also affect this drug's ergogenic qualities. *Beneficial effects do not consistently occur among habitual caffeine users; thus, a caffeine-using athlete should omit caffeine-containing foods and beverages 4 to 6 days before competition to optimize the potential for ergogenic benefits.*

Effects on Muscle Caffeine may act directly on muscle to enhance its capacity for exercise. A double-blind research design evaluated voluntary and electrically stimulated muscle actions under "caffeine-free" conditions and after oral administration of 500 mg caffeine. Electrically stimulating the motor nerve enabled researchers to remove central nervous system control and quantify caffeine's direct effects on skeletal muscle. Caffeine produced no effect on maximal muscle force during voluntary or electrically stimulated muscle actions. For submaximal effort, however, caffeine increased force output for low frequency electrical stimulation before and after muscle fatigue. This suggests that caffeine

Table 4•4	Caffeine Content of Some Common Foods, Beverages, and Over-the-Counter and Prescription Medications		

BEVERAGES AND FOOD		OVER-THE-COUNTER PRODUCTS	
SUBSTANCE	**CAFFEINE CONTENT, mg**	**SUBSTANCE**	**CAFFEINE CONTENT, mg**
Coffee[a]		**Cold Remedies**	
Coffee, Starbucks, grande, 16 oz	550	Dristan, Coryban-D, Triaminicin, Sinarest	30–31
Coffee, Starbucks, tall, 12 oz	375	Excedrin	65
Coffee, Starbucks, short, 8 oz	250	Actifed, Contac, Comtrex, Sudafed	0
Coffee, Starbucks, Americano, tall, 12 oz	70		
Coffee, Starbucks, Latte or Cappucinno, grande, 16 oz	70	**Diuretics**	
		Aqua-ban	200
Brewed, drip method	110–150	Pre-Mens Forte	100
Brewed, percolator	64–124		
Instant	40–108	**Pain Remedies**	
Expresso	100	Vanquish	33
Decaffeinated, brewed or instant; Sanka	2–5	Anacin, Midol	32
		Aspirin, any brand; Bufferin, Tylenol, Excedrin P.M.	0
Tea, 5 oz cup[a]			
Brewed, 1 min	9–33	**Stimulants**	
Brewed, 3 min	20–46	Vivarin tablet, NoDoz maximum strength caplet, Caffedrin	200
Brewed, 5 min	20–50	NoDoz tablet	100
Iced tea, 12 oz; instant tea	12–36	Energets lozenges	75
Chocolate			
Baker's semi-sweet, 1 oz; Baker's chocolate chips, and 5 1/4 cup	13	**Weight Control Aids**	
		Dexatrim, Dietac	200
Cocoa, 5 oz cup, made from mix	6–10	Prolamine	140
Milk chocolate canddy, 1 oz	6		
Sweet/dark chocolate, 1 oz	20	**Pain Drugs[b]**	
Baking chocolate, 1 oz	35	Cafergot	100
Chocolate bar, 3.5 oz	12–15	Migrol	50
Jello chocolate fudge mousse	12	Fiornal	40
Ovaltine	0	Darvon compound	32
Soft Drinks			
Jolt	100		
Sugar Free Mr. Pibb	59		
Mellow Yellow, Mountain Dew	53–54		
Tab	47		
Coca Cola, Diet Coke, 7-Up Gold	46		
Shasta-Cola, Cherry Cola, Diet Cola	44		
Dr. Pepper, Mr. Pibb	40–41		
Dr. Pepper, sugar free	40		
Pepsi Cola	38		
Diet Pepsi, Pepsi Light, Diet RC, RC Cola, Diet Rite	36		

[a] Brewing tea or coffee for longer periods slightly increases the caffeine content.
[b] Prescription required.
Data from product labels and manufacturers, and National Soft Drink Association, 1997. Caffeinism refers to caffeine intoxication characterized by restlessness, tremulousness, nervousness, excitement, insomnia, flushed face, diuresis, gastrointestinal complaints, rambling flow of thought and speech, tachycardia or cardiac arrhythmia, periods of inexhaustibility, and/or psychomotor agitation.

exerts a direct and specific ergogenic effect on skeletal muscle during repetitive low-frequency stimulation. Perhaps caffeine increases the sarcoplasmic reticulum's permeability to Ca^{++}, thus making this mineral readily available for contraction. Caffeine could also influence the myofibril's sensitivity to Ca^{++}.

ALCOHOL

Alcohol, more specifically ethyl alcohol or ethanol (a form of carbohydrate), is a depressant drug. Alcohol provides about 7 kCal of energy per gram (mL) of pure

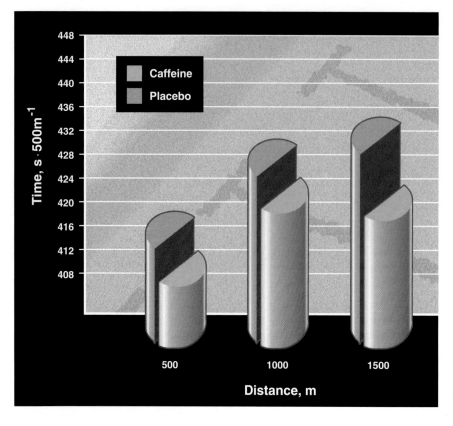

Figure 4.6. Split times for each 500 m of a 1500-m time trial for caffeine (*light purple*) and placebo (*dark purple*) trials. Caffeine produced significantly faster split times. (From MacIntosh, B.R., and Wright, B.M.: Caffeine ingestion and performance of a 1,500-metre swim. *Can. J. Appl. Physiol.*, 20:168, 1995.)

substance (100% or 200 proof). Adolescents and adults, both athletes and non-athletes, abuse alcohol more than any other drug in the United States. A standard drink refers to one 12-ounce bottle of beer or wine cooler, one 5-ounce glass of wine, or 1.5 ounces of 80-proof distilled spirits. Between 25% and 30% of males and 5% and 10% of females abuse alcohol. About 16% of alcohol abusers report a family history of alcoholism in first-, second-, or third-degree relatives. Among college students in the U.S., binge drinking contributes to 1400 unintended student deaths yearly (including motor vehicle accidents), and approximately 600,000 students are assaulted by a drinking student. Of particular concern are the more than 70,000 students between the ages of 18 and 24 years who become victims of alcohol-related sexual assault or date rape.

Use Among Athletes

Statistics remain equivocal about alcohol use among athletes compared with the general population. In a study of athletes in Italy, 330 male high school non-athletes consumed more beer, wine, and hard liquor and had greater episodes of heavy drinking than 336 young athletes. Interestingly, the strongest predictor of a participant's alcohol consumption related to the drinking habits of his or her best friend and boyfriend or girlfriend. In other research, physically active men drank less alcohol than sedentary counterparts. A self-reported questionnaire assessed alcohol intake of randomly selected students in a representative national sample of 4-year colleges in the

United States. Compared to non-athletic students, athletes were at high risk for binge drinking (≥ 5 alcoholic drinks on at least one occasion in the past 2 weeks for men and ≥ 4 for women), heavier alcohol use, and a greater number of drinking-related harms. Athletes were also more likely than non-athletes to surround themselves with (1) others who binge drink and (2) a social environment conducive to excessive alcohol consumption. These findings support the position that future alcohol prevention programs targeted to athletes should address the unique social and environmental influences that affect the current athletes' heavier alcohol use.

Table 4.5 compares serious male and female recreational runners and matched controls on responses to the Michigan Alcoholism Screening Test (MAST). Male runners drank more than nonexercising controls (14.2 vs. 5.4 drinks per week) and felt guiltier about their drinking (26.6%) than controls (13.8%). Male and female runners drank more frequently than controls (2.8 vs. 2.3 times per week), while runners with MAST scores suggesting a history of problem drinking drank significantly less than nonathletic controls with a similar score. Men also consumed more alcohol and drank more frequently (including binge drinking) than women. Control subjects reported that drinking alcohol did not interfere with sports participation and performance, but runners reported they were unsure of alcohol's effect on training and race performance. This study illustrates that problems associated with alcohol consumption do not exclude adult runners.

Table 4·5	Responses From Male and Female Recreational Runners and Matched Controls to the Shortened[a] and Brief[b] Versions of the Michigan Alcoholism Screening Test (MAST)			
	MEN (N = 536)		**WOMEN (N = 262)**	
MAST ITEM	**RUNNERS % (N)**	**CONTROLS % (N)**	**RUNNERS % (N)**	**CONTROLS % (N)**
1. I am not a normal drinker.[a,b]	19.1 (75)	22.8 (31)	12.1 (17)	13.9 (16)
2. My friends and relatives think I'm not a normal drinker.[a,b]	14.5 (56)	22.8 (31)	10.1 (14)	13.0 (15)
3. Attended Alcoholics Anonymous for drinking.[a,b]	4.5 (18)	8.9 (12)	2.1 (3)	4.3 (5)
4. Lost friends because of drinking.[a]	6.1 (24)	7.9 (11)	1.4 (2)	4.3 (5)
5. Trouble at work because of drinking.[a,b]	3.8 (15)	5.0 (7)	0.7 (1)	3.4 (4)
6. Feel guilty about drinking.[b]	26.6 (105)	13.8 (19)	16.7 (24)	15.5 (18)
7. Neglected obligations, family, work for 2 or more days in a row due to drinking.[a,b]	4.8 (19)	5.0 (7)	1.4 (2)	0.9 (1)
8. Experienced delirium tremens.[a]	4.3 (17)	2.9 (4)	0.7 (1)	3.4 (4)
9. Unable to stop drinking when desired.[b]	5.4 (21)	7.2 (10)	4.3 (6)	3.4 (4)
10. Sought help for drinking.[a,b]	5.3 (21)	7.2 (10)	2.1 (3)	6.0 (7)
11. Hospitalized for drinking.[a,b]	1.5 (6)	4.3 (6)	0.7 (1)	3.4 (4)
12. Drinking caused problems with spouse, parent, or other relative.[b]	20.6 (81)	21.0 (29)	2.8 (4)	8.5 (10)
13. Arrested for drunk driving.[a,b]	9.4 (37)	11.5 (16)	2.8 (4)	2.6 (3)
14. Arrested for drunken behavior.[b]	5.5 (22)	5.8 (8)	0.7 (1)	1.7 (2)

Adapted from Gutgesell, M., et al.: Reported alcohol use and behavior in long-distance runners. *Med. Sci. Sports. Exerc.,* 28:1063, 1996.

[a] Shortened MAST: From Binokur, A., and VanRooijen, I.: A self-administered short Michigan Alcoholism Screening Test (SMAST). *J. Studies Alcohol,* 36:117, 1975.

[b] Brief MAST: From Pokorny, A.D., et al.: The Brief MAST: A shortened version of the Michigan Alcoholism Screening Test. *Am. J. Psychiatry,* 129: 342, 1972.

Alcohol's Psychologic and Physiologic Effects

Some athletes use alcohol to enhance performance due to its supposed "positive" psychological and physiological effects. In the psychological realm, some have argued that alcohol before competition reduces tension and anxiety (**anxiolytic effect**), enhances self-confidence, and promotes aggressiveness. It also facilitates neurologic "disinhibition" through its initial, although transitory, stimulatory effect. Thus, the athlete may believe that alcohol facilitates physical performance at or close to physiologic capacity, particularly for maximal strength and power activities. *Research does not substantiate any ergogenic effect of alcohol on muscular strength, short-term maximal anaerobic power, or longer-term aerobic exercise performance.*

Although initially acting as a stimulant, alcohol ultimately depresses neurologic function (impaired memory, visual perception, speech, and motor coordination) in direct relationship to blood alcohol concentration. Damping of psychomotor function causes the anti-tremor effect of alcohol ingestion. Consequently, alcohol use has been particularly prevalent in sports that require extreme steadiness and accuracy such as rifle and pistol shooting and archery. Achieving an anti-tremor effect has also been the primary rationale among such athletes for using beta-blockers, such as propranolol, which blunt the arousal effect of sympathetic stimulation. Despite this specific potential for performance enhancement, the majority of research indicates that alcohol at best provides no ergogenic benefit; at worst, it can precipitate dangerous side effects that significantly impair performance (**ergolytic effect**). For example, alcohol's depression of nervous system function profoundly impairs almost all sports performances that require balance, hand-eye coordination, reaction time, and overall need to process information rapidly.

From a physiological perspective, alcohol impairs cardiac function. In one study, ingesting 1 g of alcohol per kg of body mass during 1 hour raised the blood alcohol level to just over $0.10 \text{ g} \cdot \text{dL}^{-1}$ (1 dL = 100 mL). This level, often observed among social drinkers, acutely depressed myocardial contractility. In terms of metabolism, alcohol inhibits the liver's capacity to synthesize glucose from non-carbohydrate sources via gluconeogenesis. These effects could significantly impair performance in high-intensity aerobic activities that rely heavily on cardiovascular capacity and energy from carbohydrate catabolism. Alcohol provides no benefit as an energy substrate and does not favorably alter the metabolic mixture in endurance exercise.

Alcohol Drinks for Fluid Replacement: Not a Good Idea

Alcohol exaggerates the dehydrating effect of exercise in a warm environment. It acts as a potent diuretic by (1) depressing anti-diuretic hormone release from the posterior pituitary and (2) diminishing the arginine-vasopressin response. These effects impair thermoregulation during heat stress, placing the athlete at greater risk for heat injury. Many athletes consume alcohol-containing beverages after exercising and/or sports competition; thus, one question concerns whether alcohol impairs rehydration in recovery.

Alcohol's effect on rehydration has been studied after exercise-induced dehydration equal to approximately 2% of body mass. The subjects consumed a rehydration fluid volume equivalent to 150% of fluid lost and containing 0%, 1%, 2%, 3%, or 4% alcohol. Urine volume produced during the 6-hour study period was directly related to the beverage's alcohol concentration; greater alcohol consumed produced more urine. The increase in plasma volume in recovery compared with the dehydrated state averaged 8.1% when the rehydration fluid contained no alcohol but only 5.3% for the beverage with 4% alcohol content. *The bottom line is that alcohol-containing beverages impede rehydration.*

Because of alcohol's action as a peripheral vasodilator, it should not be consumed during extreme cold exposure or to facilitate recovery from hypothermia. A good "stiff drink" does not warm you up. Current debate exists as to whether moderate alcohol intake exacerbates body cooling during mild cold exposure.

ANABOLIC STEROIDS

Anabolic steroids for therapeutic use became prominent in the early 1950s to treat patients deficient in natural androgens or with muscle-wasting diseases. Other legitimate steroid uses include treatment for osteoporosis and severe breast cancer in women and to counter the excessive decline in lean body mass and increase in body fat often observed among elderly men, HIV patients, and individuals undergoing kidney dialysis.

Anabolic steroids became an integral part of the high-technology scene of competitive American sports, beginning with the 1955 U.S. weightlifting team's use of Dianabol (modified, synthetic testosterone molecule, methandrostenolone). A new era of "drugging" competitive athletes was ushered in with the formulation of other anabolic steroids. An estimated 1 to 3 million athletes (e.g., 90% of male and 80% of female professional body builders) currently use androgens, often combined with stimulants, diuretics, and other drugs.

Steroid Structure and Action

Anabolic steroids function similarly to testosterone. By binding with special receptor sites on muscle and other tissues, testosterone contributes to male secondary sex characteristics, including gender differences in muscle mass and strength that develop at the onset of puberty. The hormone's androgenic (masculinizing) effects become minimized by synthetically manipulating the anabolic steroid's chemical structure to increase muscle growth from anabolic tissue building and nitrogen retention. Nevertheless, the masculinizing effect of synthetically derived steroids still occurs despite chemical alteration, particularly in females.

Athletes who take these drugs do so typically during the active years of their athletic careers. They combine multiple steroid preparations in oral and injectable form combined because they believe various androgens differ in their physiologic action. This practice, called "**stacking**," progressively increases the drug dosage (**pyramiding**) during 6- to 12-week cycles. The drug quantity far exceeds the recommended medical dose. The athlete then alters drug dosage and/or combines it with other drugs before competition to minimize chances of detection.

The difference between dosages used in research studies and the excess typically abused by athletes has contributed to a credibility gap between scientific findings (often, no effect of steroids) and what most in the athletic community believe to be true. **Table 4.6** lists examples of oral and injectable anabolic steroids, including typical retail cost and estimated range of black market prices. The latter vary considerably in different domestic regions and internationally. A conservative estimate would be at least twice the retail cost and up to 100 times more!

Table 4·6	Examples of Anabolic Steroids (Generic and Commercial Name), Including Typical Retail Costs and Black Market Prices[a]			
GENERIC NAME	**COMMERCIAL NAME**	**FORM**	**RETAIL PRICE**	**BLACK MARKET PRICE**
Oxymetholone	Anadrol	Oral	$90/100 tabs	$300/100 tabs
Testosterone cypionate	Testosterone	Injectable	$35/10 mL	$200/10 mL
Stanazolol	Winstrol V	Injectable	$250/30 mL	$400/30 mL
Boldenone	Equipoise	Injectable	$150/30 mL	$450/30 mL
Oxandrolone	Anavar	Injectable	$75/100 tabs	4150/100 tabs
Methandrostenolone	Dianabol	Oral	$100/100 tabs	$200/100 tabs

[a] 2005 estimated prices. Prices vary depending on location. Black market price reflects typical prices from various sources.

Steroid Use Estimates

Male and female athletes usually combine anabolic steroid use with resistance training and augmented protein intake because they believe this combination improves sports performance that requires strength, speed, and power. The steroid abuser often has the image of a massively developed body builder; however, abuse also occurs frequently in competitive athletes participating in road cycling, tennis, track and field, and swimming.

Federal authorities conservatively estimate that the emerging business of illegal trafficking in steroids exceeds $160 million yearly—a figure predicted to increase yearly. Because many competitive and recreational athletes obtain steroids on the black market, misinformed individuals take massive and prolonged dosages without medical monitoring. Particularly worrisome is steroid abuse among young boys and girls and its accompanying risks, including extreme masculinization and premature cessation of bone growth. In a 1999 study, as many as 175,000 high school girls, or 1.4% of girls in 9th to 12th grades nationwide, reported using steroids at least once in their lives, a rate that was up from 0.4% in 1991. Both male and female teenagers cite improved athletic performance as the most common reason for taking steroids, although 25% acknowledged enhanced appearance (more muscle in boys and less fat in girls) as the main reason.

Effectiveness of Anabolic Steroids

Much of the confusion about the ergogenic effectiveness of anabolic steroids results from variations in experimental design, poor controls, differences in specific drugs and dosages (50 to >200 mg per day vs. the usual medical dosage of 5 to 20 mg), treatment duration, training intensity, measurement techniques, previous experience as subjects, individual variation in response, and nutritional supplementation. Also, the relatively small residual androgenic effect of the steroid can make the athlete more aggressive (so-called "roid rage"), competitive, and fatigue resistant. Such disinhibitory central nervous system effects allow the athlete to train harder for a longer time or believe that augmented training effects actually occurred. Abnormal alterations in mood, including psychiatric dysfunction, have been attributed to androgen use.

Research with animals suggests that anabolic steroid treatment, when combined with exercise and adequate protein intake, stimulates protein synthesis and increases muscle protein content. In contrast, other research shows no benefit from steroid treatment on the leg muscle weight of rats subjected to functional overload by surgically removing the synergistic muscle. The researchers concluded that anabolic steroid treatment did not complement functional overload to augment muscle development. Effects of steroids on humans remain difficult to interpret. Some studies show augmented body mass gains and reduced body fat with steroid use in men who train, whereas other studies show no effects on strength and power or body composition, even with sufficient energy and protein

FOR YOUR INFORMATION

Caffeine Warning

Individuals who normally avoid caffeine may experience undesirable side effects when they consume it. Caffeine stimulates the central nervous system and can produce restlessness, headaches, insomnia and nervous irritability, muscle twitching, tremulousness, and psychomotor agitation and trigger premature left ventricular contractions. From the standpoint of temperature regulation, caffeine acts as a potent diuretic. Excessive consumption could cause an unnecessary pre-exercise fluid loss, negatively affecting thermal balance and exercise performance in a hot environment.

FOR YOUR INFORMATION

Alcohol Abuse

In 2002, the drinking rate for the total population aged 12 years and older was 51%. The current drinking rates by age group were as follows: 18% of those aged 12 to 17 years; 61% of those aged 18 to 25 years; and 54% of those aged 26 years and older.

Perhaps the depressing statistics about alcohol abuse partly reflect the tremendous amount of money spent to advertise alcoholic beverages on television and other media. For the first 12 months of 2002, The National Clearinghouse for Alcohol and Drug Information (*http://www.health.org/survey.htm*) reported that total dollars spent to advertise alcoholic beverages equaled $690 million.

Box 4–2 • CLOSE UP

HOW TO RECOGNIZE WARNING SIGNS OF ALCOHOL ABUSE

Alcohol consumption has been a socially acceptable behavior for centuries. It is consumed at parties, religious ceremonies, dinners, and sport contests and has also been used as a mild sedative or as a pain killer for surgery. Some athletes possess a negative attitude about drinking, but they, as a group, are not immune to alcohol abuse.

Addiction to alcohol develops slowly. Most people believe they can control their drinking habits and do not realize they have a problem until they become alcoholic; they develop a physical and emotional dependence on the drug, characterized by excessive use and constant preoccupation with drinking. Alcohol abuse, in turn, leads to mental, emotional, physical, and social problems.

ALCOHOL ABUSE: ARE YOU DRINKING TOO MUCH?

The following table can help identify problem behaviors with alcohol. Two or more "Yes" answers on this questionnaire indicate a potential for jeopardizing health through excessive alcohol consumption.

Identifying Alcohol Abuse[a]

Yes	No	Question
☐	☐	When you are holding an empty glass at a party, do you always actively look for a refill instead of waiting to be offered one?
☐	☐	If given the chance, do you frequently pour out a more generous drink for yourself than seems to be the "going" amount for others?
Yes	**No**	**Question**
☐	☐	Do you often have a drink or two when you are alone, either at home or in a bar?
☐	☐	Is your drinking ever the direct cause of a family quarrel, or do quarrels often seem to occur, if only by coincidence, after you have had a drink or two?
☐	☐	Do you feel that you must have a drink at a specific time every day (e.g., right after work, for your nerves)?
☐	☐	When worried or under unusual stress, do you almost automatically take a stiff drink to "settle your nerves?"
☐	☐	Are you untruthful about how much you have had to drink when questioned on the subject?
☐	☐	Does drinking ever cause you to take time off work or to miss scheduled meetings or appointments?
☐	☐	Do you feel physically deprived if you cannot have at least one drink every day?
☐	☐	Do you sometimes crave a drink in the morning?
☐	☐	Do you sometimes have "mornings after" when you cannot remember what happened the night before?

[a] Answer "Yes" or "No" to each question. **Evaluation:** One "Yes" answer should be viewed as a warning sign. Two "Yes" answers suggest an alcohol dependency. Three or more "Yes" answers indicate serious problems that require immediate professional help.

From: American Medical Association: *Family Medical Guide by the American Medical Association.* New York: Random House, 1982.

---

intake to support an anabolic effect. When steroid use produced body weight gains, the compositional nature of these gains (water, muscle, fat) remained unclear. The fact that steroid use remains widespread among top-level athletes (including body builders and weight lifters) suggests that it is a potent substance with considerable credibility.

Dosage Is an Important Factor

Variations in drug dosage contribute to the confusion (and credibility gap between scientist and steroid user) about the true effectiveness of anabolic steroids. Research studied 43 healthy men with some resistance training experience. Diet (energy and protein intake) and exercise (standard weight lifting, three times weekly) were controlled, with steroid dosage exceeding previous human studies (600 mg testosterone enanthate injected weekly or placebo).

Figure 4.7 illustrates changes from baseline average values for fat-free body mass (hydrostatic weighing), triceps and quadriceps cross-sectional muscle areas (magnetic resonance imaging), and muscle strength repetition maximum (1-RM) after 10 weeks of testosterone treatment. The men who received the hormone and continued to train gained about 0.5 kg (1 lb) of lean tissue weekly, with no increase in body fat over the relatively brief treatment period. Even the group that received the drug but did not train significantly increased muscle mass and strength compared with the group receiving the placebo, although their increases were less than the group that trained while taking testosterone.

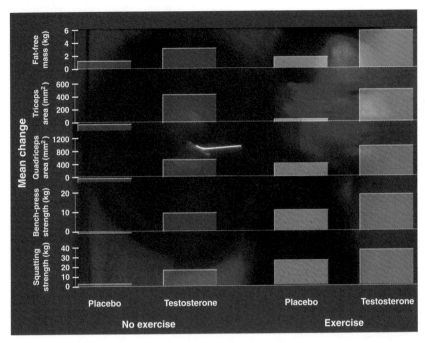

Figure 4.7. Changes from baseline in mean fat-free body mass, triceps and quadriceps cross-sectional areas, and muscle strength in the bench-press and squatting exercises over 10 weeks of testosterone treatment. (Data from Bhasin, S., et al.: The effects of supraphysiological doses of testosterone on muscle size and strength in normal men. *N. Engl. J. Med.*, 335:1, 1996.)

Risks of Steroid Use

Table 4.7 lists some of the known harmful side effects from abuse of anabolic steroids. Prolonged high dosages of steroids (often at levels 10 to 200 times the therapeutic recommendation) can impair normal testosterone-endocrine function. A study of five male power athletes showed that 26 weeks of steroid administration reduced serum testosterone to less than one-half the level measured when the study began, with the effect lasting throughout a 12- to 16-week follow-up period. Infertility, reduced sperm concentrations (azoospermia), and decreased testicular volume pose additional problems for the male steroid user.

Other accompanying hormonal alterations during steroid use in males include a sevenfold increase in the concentration of estradiol, the major female hormone. The higher estradiol level represents an average value for normal females and possibly explains the **gynecomastia** (excessive development of the male mammary glands, sometimes secreting milk) often reported among males who take anabolic steroids. Furthermore, steroids have been shown to cause:

1. Chronic stimulation of the prostate gland (increased size)
2. Injury and functional alterations in cardiovascular function and myocardial cell cultures
3. Possible pathologic ventricular growth and dysfunction when combined with resistance training
4. Increased blood platelet aggregation, which can compromise cardiovascular health and function and possibly increase risk of stroke and acute myocardial infarction (from blood clots)

Steroid Use and Life-Threatening Disease Concern regarding risk of chronic steroid use centers on evidence about possible links between androgen abuse and abnormal liver function. Because the liver almost exclusively metabolizes androgens, it becomes susceptible to damage from long-term steroid use and toxic excess. One of the serious effects of androgens on the liver occurs when it

Questions & Notes

Briefly describe how caffeine may act as an ergogenic supplement.

Name 2 substances with high caffeine content.

   1.

   2.

Briefly explain caffeine's effect on muscle function.

FOR YOUR INFORMATION

Alcohol in the Body

One alcoholic drink contains 1.0 ounce (28.4 g or 28.4 mL) of 100 proof (50%) alcohol. This translates into 12 ounces of regular beer (about 4% alcohol by volume) or 5 ounces of wine (11% to 14% alcohol by volume). The stomach absorbs between 15% and 25% of the alcohol ingested; the small intestine rapidly takes up the remainder for distribution throughout the body's water compartments (particularly the water-rich tissues of the central nervous system). The absence of food in the digestive tract facilitates alcohol absorption. The liver, the major organ for alcohol metabolism, removes alcohol at a rate of about 10 g per hour, equivalent to the alcohol content of one drink. Consuming two drinks in 1 hour produces a blood alcohol concentration of between 0.04 and 0.05 g·dL^{-1}. Age, body mass, body fat content, and gender influence blood alcohol level. The legal state limit for alcohol intoxication ranges between a blood alcohol concentration of 0.11 and 0.16 g·dL^{-1}. A blood alcohol concentration of greater than 0.40 g·dL^{-1} (19 drinks or more in 2 hours) can lead to coma, respiratory depression, and eventual death.

Table 4•7	Steroid Use and Associated Detrimental Side Effects	
SYSTEM	**ADVERSE EFFECT**	**REVERSIBILITY**
Cardiovascular	Increased LDL cholesterol	Yes
	Decreased HDL cholesterol	Yes
	Hypertension	Yes
	Elevated triglycerides	Yes
	Arteriosclerotic heart disease	No
	High blood pressure	Possible
Reproductive–Male	Testicular atrophy	Possible
	Gynecomastia (breast enlargement)	Possible
	Impaired spermatogenesis	Yes
	Altered libido (impotence)	Yes
	Male pattern baldness	No
	Enlarged prostate gland	Possible
	Pain in urinating	Yes
Reproductive–Female	Menstrual dysfunction	Yes
	Altered libido	Yes
	Clitoral enlargement	No
	Deepening voice	No
	Male pattern baldness	No
	Breast reduction	No
Hepatic	Elevated liver enzymes	Yes
	Jaundice	Yes
	Hepatic tumors	No
	Peliosis	No
Endocrine	Altered glucose tolerance	Yes
	Decreased FSH, LH	Yes
	Acne	Yes
Musculoskeletal	Premature epiphyseal closure (stunted growth)	No
	Tendon degeneration, ruptures	No
	Swelling of feet or ankles	Yes
Central Nervous	Mood swings	Yes
	Violent behavior	Yes
	Depression	Yes
	Psychoses/delusions	Yes
Other	Hepatoma	Yes
	Bad breath	Yes
	Nausea and vomiting	Yes
	Sleep problems	Yes
	Impaired judgment	Yes
	Paranoid jealous	Yes
	Increased risk of blood poisoning and infections	No

(and sometimes splenic tissue) develops localized blood-filled lesions (cysts), a condition called **peliosis hepatis**. In extreme cases, the liver eventually fails or intra-abdominal hemorrhage develops and the patient dies. These outcomes emphasize the potentially serious side effects even when a physician prescribes the drug in the recommended dosage. Although patients often take steroids for a longer duration than athletes, some athletes take steroids on and off for years, with dosages exceeding typical therapeutic levels.

Steroid Use and Plasma Lipoproteins Anabolic steroid use (particularly the orally active 17-alkylated androgens) in healthy men and women rapidly lowers high-density lipoprotein cholesterol (HDL-C), elevates both low-density lipoprotein cholesterol (LDL-C) and total cholesterol, and lowers the HDL-C:LDL-C ratio. Weight lifters who took anabolic steroids averaged an HDL-C of 26 mg·dL^{-1} compared with 50 mg·dL^{-1} for weight lifters not taking these drugs. Reduction of HDL-C to this level significantly increases risk of coronary artery disease.

ANDROSTENEDIONE: A LEGAL STEROID ALTERNATIVE IN SOME SPORTS

Many physically active individuals take an over-the-counter nutritional supplement, **androstenedione**, because they believe it produces endogenous testosterone, enabling them to train harder, build muscle mass, and repair injury more rapidly. Found naturally in meat and extracts of some plants, androstenedione is touted on the web as "a metabolite that is only one step away from the biosynthesis of testosterone." The National Football League, the National Collegiate Athletic Association, the Men's Tennis Association, and the IOC ban its use because they believe it provides an unfair competitive advantage and may endanger health, similar to anabolic steroids. The IOC banned for life the 1996 Olympic shot-put gold medalist because he used androstenedione, and it remains a banned substance by the IOC and U.S. Olympic Committee.

Originally developed by East Germany in the 1970s to enhance performance of their elite athletes, androstenedione was first commercially manufactured and sold in the U.S. in 1996. By calling the substance a supplement and avoiding any claims that it offers medical benefits, the 1994 FDA rules permit the marketing of androstenedione as a *food*. Because many countries consider androstenedione a controlled substance, athletes travel to the U.S. to purchase the compound, which contributes to the supplement industry's $12 billion yearly sales. Current androstenedione-containing products include chewing gum and a steroid lozenge that dissolves under the tongue.

Action and Effectiveness

Androstenedione, an intermediate or precursor hormone between DHEA and testosterone, aids the liver to synthesize other biologically active steroid hormones. Normally produced by the adrenal glands and gonads, it converts to testosterone through enzymatic action in diverse tissues of the body. Some androstenedione also converts into estrogens.

Little scientific evidence supports claims about this supplement's effectiveness or anabolic qualities. One study systematically evaluated whether short- and long-term oral androstenedione supplementation elevated blood testosterone concentrations and enhanced gains in muscle size and strength during resistance training. In one phase of the investigation, 10 young adult men received a single 100-mg dose of androstenedione or a placebo containing 250 mg of rice flour. With supplementation, serum androstenedione rose 175% during the first 60 minutes following ingestion and then rose further by about 350% above baseline values between minutes 90 and 270 minutes. However, no effect emerged for androstenedione supplementation on serum concentrations of either free or total testosterone.

In the experiment's second phase, 20 young, untrained men received either 300 mg of androstenedione daily or 250 mg of rice flour placebo daily during weeks 1, 2, 4, 5, 7, and 8 of an 8-week total body resistance-training program. Serum androstenedione increased 100% in the androstenedione-supplemented group and remained elevated throughout training. Although serum testosterone levels were significantly higher in the androstenedione-supplemented group than the placebo group before and after supplementation, serum free and total testosterone remained unaltered for both groups during the supplementation-training period. However, serum estradiol and estrone concentrations increased significantly during the training period only for the group receiving the supplement, suggesting an increased aromatization of the ingested androstenedione to estrogens. Furthermore, resistance training significantly increased muscle strength and lean body mass and reduced body fat for both groups, but *no synergistic effect* emerged for the group supplemented with androstenedione. The supplement did cause a 12% significant *reduction* in HDL-C after only 2 weeks, which remained lower for the 8 weeks of training and supplementation. Serum concentrations of liver function enzymes remained within normal limits for both groups throughout the experimental period.

Taken together, these findings indicate *no effect* of androstenedione supplementation on (1) basal serum concentrations of testosterone or (2) training responsiveness in terms of muscle size and strength and body composition. A worrisome outcome relates to the potential negative effects of the reduction of HDL-C

Questions & Notes

Give 2 legitimate (medical) uses of anabolic steroids.

1.

2.

Give the magnitude of the differences between a typical medical and a typical recreational dosage of steroids.

Give 3 associated detrimental side effects of steroid abuse.

1.

2.

3.

List 2 adverse side effects of steroid abuse that are not reversible.

1.

2.

FOR YOUR INFORMATION

It's Against the Law

A federal law makes it illegal to prescribe, distribute, or possess anabolic steroids for any purpose other than treatment of disease or other medical conditions. First offenders face up to 5 years in prison and a fine up to $250,000.

FOR YOUR INFORMATION

Summary of Research Findings Concerning Androstenedione

- Elevates plasma testosterone concentrations
- No favorable effect on muscle mass
- No favorable effect on muscular performance
- No favorable alteration in body composition
- Elevates a variety of estrogen subfractions
- No favorable effects on muscle protein synthesis or tissue anabolism
- Impairs the blood lipid profile in apparently healthy men
- Increases likelihood of testing positive for steroid use

Box 4–3 • CLOSE UP

AMERICAN COLLEGE OF SPORTS MEDICINE (ACSM) POSITION STATEMENT ON ANABOLIC STEROIDS

Based on the world literature and a careful analysis of claims about anabolic-androgenic steroids, ACSM issued the following statement:

1. Anabolic-androgenic steroids in the presence of an adequate diet and training can contribute to increases in body weight, often in the lean mass compartment.
2. The gains in muscular strength achieved through high-intensity exercise and proper diet can occur by the increased use of anabolic-androgenic steroids in some individuals.
3. Anabolic-androgenic steroids do not increase aerobic power or capacity for muscular exercise.

4. Anabolic-androgenic steroids have been associated with adverse effects on the liver, cardiovascular, reproductive system, and psychological status in therapeutic trials and in limited research on athletes. Until further research is completed, the potential hazards of the use of anabolic-androgenic steroids in athletes must include those found in therapeutic trials.
5. The use of anabolic-androgenic steroids by athletes is contrary to the rules and ethical principles of athletic competition as set forth by many of the sports governing bodies. The American College of Sports Medicine supports these ethical principles and deplores the use of anabolic-androgenic steroids by athletes.

on overall heart disease risk and elevated serum estrogen levels on risk of gynecomastia and possibly pancreatic and other cancers. One must view these findings within the context of this specific study because test subjects took dosages of androstenedione *far smaller* than those routinely taken by body builders and other athletes.

THG: THE (NEW) HIDDEN STEROID

Tetrahydrogestrinone (THG), a new drug listed by the FDA, is an anabolic steroid specifically designed to escape detection by normal drug testing. The drug was made public in 2003 when the United States Anti-Doping Agency (USADA; http://www.usantidoping.org), which oversees drug testing for all sports federations under the U.S. Olympic umbrella, was contacted by an anonymous track and field coach claiming several top athletes used the drug. The same coach subsequently provided the USADA with a syringe containing THG that the USADA then used to develop a new test for the substance. They then re-analyzed 350 urine samples from participants at the U.S. track and field championships held in June 2003, and 100 samples from random out-of-competition tests. Half a dozen athletes tested positive. In August 2003, Dwain Chambers, British sprinter and European 100-m champion, tested positive for THG. Its suspected use by Olympic athletes caused the IOC to begin re-testing urine samples from competitors at the 2002 Winter Games in Salt Lake City (no athletes tested positive). If found guilty of doping, any sportsman or woman who has won medals at either the 2003 World Athletics Championships or the 2002 Winter Olympics could have their medals rescinded and their performances scratched from the record books.

The source of the THG was traced to the Bay Area Laboratory Cooperative, BALCO, a U.S. company that analyses blood and urine from athletes and then prescribes a series of supplements to compensate for vitamin and mineral deficiencies. Among its clients are high-profile athletes in many professional and amateur sports. The ability to develop an undetectable steroid points to the disturbing ready market for such drugs among athletes who are prepared to do anything to achieve success.

CLENBUTEROL: ANABOLIC STEROID SUBSTITUTE

Extensive random testing of competitive athletes for anabolic steroid use has resulted in a number of steroid substitutes appearing on the illicit health food, mail order, and "black market" drug network. One such drug, the sympathomimetic amine **clenbuterol** (trade names Clenasma, Monores, Novegan, Prontovent, and Spiropent), has become popular among athletes because of its purported tissue-building, fat-reducing benefits. Typically, when body builders discontinue steroid use before competition to avoid detection and possible disqualification, they substitute clenbuterol in an attempt to maintain a steroid effect.

Clenbuterol, one of a group of chemical compounds classified as a beta-adrenergic agonist (albuterol, clenbuterol, salbutamol, salmeterol, and terbutaline), is not approved for human use in the United States but is commonly prescribed abroad as an inhaled bronchodilator for treating obstructive pulmonary disorders. Clenbuterol facilitates responsiveness of adrenergic receptors to circulating epinephrine, norepinephrine, and other adrenergic amines. A review of available animal studies (no human studies exist) indicates that when sedentary, growing livestock receive clenbuterol in dosages in excess of those prescribed in Europe for human use for bronchial asthma, clenbuterol increases skeletal and cardiac muscle protein deposition and slows fat gain by enhancing lipolysis. Clenbuterol has also been used experimentally in animals with some success to counter the wasting effects on muscle of aging, immobilization, malnutrition, and zero-gravity exposure. The enlarged muscle size from clenbuterol treatment resulted from a decrease in protein breakdown and an increase in protein synthesis. Reported short-term side effects in humans accidentally "overdosing" from eating animals that were treated with clenbuterol include muscle tremor, agitation, palpitations, muscle cramps, rapid heart rate, and headache. Despite such negative side effects, supervised use of clenbuterol may prove beneficial for humans with muscle wasting from disease, forced immobilization, and aging. Unfortunately, no data exist for its potential toxicity level in humans or its efficacy and safety in long-term use. Clearly, clenbuterol use cannot be justified or recommended as an ergogenic aid.

GROWTH HORMONE: THE NEXT MAGIC PILL?

Human growth hormone (hGH), also known as somatotropic hormone, now competes with anabolic steroids in the illicit market of alleged tissue-building, performance-enhancing drugs. This hormone, produced by the adenohypophysis of the pituitary gland, facilitates tissue-building processes and normal human growth. Specifically, hGH stimulates bone and cartilage growth, enhances fatty acid oxidation, and slows glucose and amino acid breakdown. Reduced hGH secretion (about 50% less at age 60 than age 30) accounts for some of the decrease in FFM and increase in fat mass that accompany aging; reversal occurs with exogenous hGH supplements produced by genetically engineered bacteria.

Children who suffer from kidney failure or hGH-deficient children take this hormone to help stimulate long bone growth. hGH use appeals to the strength and power athlete because, at physiologic levels, it stimulates amino acid uptake and protein synthesis by muscle, while enhancing fat breakdown and conserving glycogen reserves.

Research has produced equivocal results concerning the true benefits of hGH supplementation to counter the effects of aging, including loss of muscle mass, thinning bones, increase in body fat, particularly abdominal fat, and a depressed energy level. For example, 16 previously sedentary young men who participated in a 12-week resistance-training program received daily recombinant hGH (40 g·kg^{-1}) or a placebo. FFM, total body water, and whole body protein synthesis increased more in the hGH recipients, with no significant differences between groups in fractional rate of protein synthesis in skeletal muscle, torso and limb circumferences, or muscle function in dynamic and static strength measures. The researchers attributed the greater increase in whole body protein synthesis in the hGH group to a possible increase in nitrogen retention in lean tissue other than skeletal muscle (e.g., connective tissue, fluid, and non-contractile protein). One of the largest studies to date determined the effects of hGH on changes in the body composition and functional capacity of healthy men and women ranging in age from the mid-60s to late 80s. Men who took hGH gained 7 pounds of lean body mass and lost a similar amount of fat mass. Women gained about 3 pounds of lean body mass and lost 5 pounds of body fat compared to counterparts who received a placebo. The subjects remained sedentary and did not change their diet over the 6-month study period. Unfortunately, serious side effects afflicted between 24% and 46% of the subjects. These included swollen feet and ankles, joint pain, carpal tunnel syndrome (swelling of tendon sheath over a nerve in the wrist), and the development of a diabetic or prediabetic condition. As in previous research, no effects were noted for hGH treatment on measures of muscular strength or endurance capacity despite increases in lean body mass.

Briefly explain why steroid abuse relates to plasma lipoprotein levels.

Name the hormone for which androstenedione is a precursor.

Briefly explain how clenbuterol supposedly acts as an ergogenic aid.

Briefly explain how growth hormone supposedly acts as an ergogenic aid.

Name the gland that produces hGH.

Briefly explain how DHEA supposedly acts as an ergogenic aid.

Previously, healthy people could only obtain hGH on the black market, often in adulterated form. The use of human cadaver-derived hGH (discontinued by U.S. physicians, May, 1985) to treat children of short stature greatly increases the risk for contracting Creutzfeldt-Jakob disease, an infectious, incurable fatal brain-deteriorating disorder. A synthetic form of hGH (Protoropin and Humantrope), produced by genetic engineering, currently treats hGH-deficient children (cost about $10,000 per year). Undoubtedly, child athletes who take hGH believing they gain a competitive edge will suffer increased incidence of gigantism, while adults can develop acromegalic syndrome. Less visual side effects include insulin resistance leading to type 2 diabetes, water retention, and carpal tunnel compression. Additionally, once a drug reaches market, doctors can prescribe it at their discretion. For example, over a 4-year period from 1997 to 2001, prescriptions for hGH have more than tripled from 6,000 to 21,000. Men's fitness magazines currently advertise hGH, providing telephone numbers to call for a list of doctors who prescribe it.

DHEA: NEW DRUG ON THE CIRCUIT

Synthetic **dehydroepiandrosterone** (DHEA) use among athletes and the general population raises concerns among sports medicine personnel and the medical community because of issues related to safety and effectiveness. DHEA and its sulfated ester, DHEAS, are relatively weak steroid hormones synthesized primarily by primates in the adrenal cortex from cholesterol. The quantity of DHEA (commonly referred to as "mother hormone") produced by the body surpasses all other known steroids; its chemical structure closely resembles the sex hormones testosterone and estrogen, with a small amount of DHEA serving as a precursor for these hormones for men and women.

Because DHEA occurs naturally, the FDA has no control over its distribution or claims for its action and effectiveness. The lay press, mail order catalogs, and health food industry describe DHEA as a "superhormone" (even available as a chewing gum, each piece containing 25 mg) to increase testosterone production, preserve youth, protect against heart disease, cancer, diabetes, and osteoporosis, invigorate sex drive, facilitate lean tissue gain and body fat loss, enhance mood and memory, extend life, and boost immunity to a variety of infectious diseases, including AIDS. The IOC and U.S. Olympic Committee have placed DHEA on their banned substance lists at zero tolerance levels.

Figure 4.8 illustrates the generalized trend for plasma DHEA levels during a lifetime plus six common claims made by manufacturers for DHEA supplements. For boys and girls, DHEA levels are substantial at birth and then decline sharply. A steady increase in DHEA production occurs from age 6 to 10 years (an occurrence that some researchers feel contributes to the beginning of puberty and sexuality), followed by a rapid rise with peak production (higher in males than females) reached between ages 18 to 25 years.

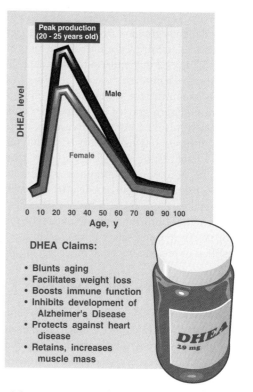

Figure 4.8. Generalized trend for plasma levels of DHEA for men and women during a lifetime.

In contrast to the glucocorticoid and mineralocorticoid adrenal steroids whose plasma levels remain relatively high with aging, a long, steady decline in DHEA occurs after age 30 years. By age 75, plasma levels decrease to only about 20% of the value in young adulthood. This fact has fueled speculation that DHEA plasma levels might serve as a biochemical marker of biologic aging and disease susceptibility. Popular reasoning concludes that supplementing with DHEA diminishes the negative effects of aging by raising plasma levels to more youthful concentrations. In fact, many people supplement with this hormone "just in case" it turns out to be beneficial without concern for safety.

DHEA Safety

In 1994, the Food and Drug Administration reclassified DHEA from the category of unapproved new drug (prescription required for use) to a dietary supplement for sale over the counter without a prescription. Despite its quantitative significance as a hormone, researchers know little about DHEA's relation to health and aging, cellular or molecular mechanisms of action, and possible receptor sites and the potential for negative side effects from exogenous dosage, particularly among young adults with normal DHEA levels. The appropriate DHEA dosage for humans has not been determined. Concern exists about possible harmful effects on blood lipids, glucose tolerance, and prostate gland health, particularly because medical problems associated with hormone supplementation often do not appear until years after their first use.

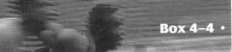

Box 4–4 • CLOSE UP

NCAA BANNED SUBSTANCES: COLLEGIATE ATHLETES BEWARE

NCAA BANNED DRUG CLASSES, 2003–2004 (http://www1.ncaa .org/ membership/ed_outreach/health-safety/ drug_testing/index.html)

The following table contains drug classes banned by the National Collegiate Athletic Association (NCAA). Many nutritional/dietary supplements contain NCAA banned substances. In addition, the U.S. Food and Drug Administration does not strictly regulate the supplement industry; therefore, purity and safety of nutritional/dietary supplements cannot be guaranteed. Impure or adulterated supplements may lead to a positive NCAA drug test. Supplement use is always at the student athlete's own risk.

STIMULANTS	ANABOLIC AGENTS	DIURETICS	STREET DRUGS	PEPTIDE HORMONES AND ANALOGUES
• Amiphenzzole • Amphetamine • Bemigride • Benzphetamine • Bromantan • Caffeine, Guarana (if urine conc. >15 $\mu \cdot mL^{-1}$) • Chlorphentemine • Cocaine • Cropropamide • Crothetamide • Diethylpropion • Dimethylamphetamine • Coxapram • Ephedrine (ma huang) • Ethamivian • Ethylamphetamine • Fencamfamine • Meclofenoxate • Methamphetamine • Methylenedioxy-methamphetamine (MDMA, ecstasy) • Methylphenidate • Nikethamide • Pemoline • Phendimetrazine • Phenetermine • Phenylephrine • Picrotoxine • Phenylpropanolamine (ppa) • Pipradol • Strychnine • Prolintane • Synephrine (citrus aurantium, zhi- shi, bitter orange)	• Anabolic steroids • Androstenediol • Androstenedione • Boldenone • Boldenone • Clenbuterol • Clostebol • Dehydrochlormethyl-testosterone • Dehydroepiandrosterone (DHEA) • Dihydrotestosterone (DHT) • Dromostanolone • Fluoxymesterone • Methandienone • Methenolone • Methyltestosterone • Nandrolone • Norandrostenedione • Norethandrolone • Oxandrolone • Oxymesterone • Oxymetholone • Stanozolol • Testosterone and related compounds	• Acetazolamine • Bendroflumethiazide • Benzthiazide • Bumetanide • Chlorothiazide • Chlorthalidone • Ethacrynic acid • Flumethiazide • Furosemide • Hydrochlorothiazide • Hydroflumethiazide • Methyclothiazide • Polythiazide • Quinethazone • Spironolactone • Tramterene • Trichlormethiazide	• Heroin • Marijuana (if conc. in urine exceeds 15 nanograms·mL^{-1}) • Tetrahydrocannabinol • THC	• Chorionic gonadrotrophin (GCG-human chorionic gonadotrophine) • Corticotrophin (ACTH) • Erythropoietin (EPO) • Growth hormone (hgGH, somatotrophin)—all the respective releasing factors of these substances are also banned • Sermorelin

AMPHETAMINES

Amphetamines, or pep pills, consist of pharmacologic compounds that exert a powerful stimulating effect on central nervous system function. Athletes most frequently use amphetamine (Benzedrine) and dextroamphetamine sulfate (Dexedrine). These compounds, referred to as **sympathomimetic**, mimic the actions of the sympathetic hormones epinephrine and norepinephrine, which trigger increases in blood pressure, heart rate, cardiac output, breathing rate, metabolism, and blood glucose. Taking 5 to 20 mg of amphetamine usually produces an effect for 30 to 90 minutes, although the drug's influence can persist much longer. Aside from causing an aroused level of sympathetic function, amphetamines supposedly increase alertness, wakefulness, and augment work capacity by depressing sensations of muscle fatigue. The deaths of two famed cyclists in the 1960s during competitive road racing were attributed to amphetamine use for just such purposes. In one of these deaths in 1967, British Tour de France rider Tom Simpson overheated and suffered a fatal heart attack during the ascent of Mont Ventoux. Soldiers in World War II commonly used amphetamines to increase alertness and reduce fatigue; athletes frequently use amphetamines for the same purpose.

Dangers of Amphetamines

Dangers of amphetamine use include the following:

- Continual use can lead to physiological or emotional drug dependency. This often causes cyclical dependency on "uppers" (amphetamines) or "downers" (barbiturates) (barbiturates blunt or tranquilize the "hyper" state brought on by amphetamines).
- General side effects include headache, tremulousness, agitation, insomnia, nausea, dizziness, and confusion, all of which negatively impact sports performance.
- Prolonged use eventually requires more of the drug to achieve the same effect because drug tolerance increases; this may aggravate and even precipitate cardiovascular and psychological disorders. Medical risks include hypertension, stroke, sudden death, and glucose intolerance.
- Amphetamines inhibit or suppress the body's normal mechanisms for perceiving and responding to pain, fatigue, or heat stress, severely jeopardizing health and safety.
- Prolonged intake of high doses of amphetamines can produce weight loss, paranoia, psychosis, repetitive compulsive behavior, and nerve damage.

Amphetamines and Athletic Performance

Athletes take amphetamines to get "up" psychologically for competition. On the day or evening before a contest, competitors often feel nervous, irritable, and have difficulty relaxing. Under these circumstances, a barbiturate induces sleep. The athlete then regains the "hyper" condition by taking an "upper." This undesirable cycle of depressant-to-stimulant becomes dangerous because the stimulant acts abnormally after barbiturate intake. Knowledgeable and prudent sports professionals urge banning amphetamines from athletic competition. Most athletic governing groups have rules regarding athletes who use amphetamines. Ironically, the majority of research indicates that amphetamines do not enhance physical performance. Perhaps their greatest influence pertains to the psychological realm, where naive athletes believe that taking any supplement contributes to superior performance. A placebo containing an inert substance often produces identical results as amphetamines.

SUMMARY

1. Caffeine exerts an ergogenic effect in extending aerobic exercise duration by increasing fat utilization for energy, thus conserving glycogen reserves. These effects become less apparent in individuals who (1) maintain a high-carbohydrate diet or (2) habitually use caffeine.

2. Consuming ethyl alcohol produces an acute anxiolytic effect because it temporarily reduces tension and anxiety, enhances self-confidence, and promotes aggression. Other than the antitremor effect, alcohol conveys no ergogenic benefits and likely impairs overall athletic performance (ergolytic effect).

3. Anabolic steroids compose a group of pharmacologic agents frequently used for ergogenic purposes. These drugs function like the hormone testosterone. Anabolic steroids may help to increase muscle size, strength, and power with resistance training in some individuals.

4. Significant side effects can accompany anabolic steroid use. These include infertility, reduced sperm concentrations, decreased testicular volume, gynecomastia, connective tissue damage that decreases the tensile strength and elastic compliance of tendons, chronic stimulation of the prostate gland, injury and functional alterations in cardiovascular function and myocardial cell cultures, possible pathological ventricular growth and dysfunction, and increased blood platelet aggregation that can compromise

cardiovascular system health and function and increase risk of stroke and acute myocardial infarction.

5. Research findings indicate no effect of androstenedione supplementation on basal serum concentrations of testosterone or training response in terms of muscle size and strength and body composition. Worrisome are the potentially negative effects of a lowered HDL-C on overall heart disease risk and the elevated serum estrogen level on risk of gynecomastia and possibly pancreatic and other cancers.

6. Tetrahydrogestrinone (THG) is designed to escape detection using normal drug testing. Its suspected use by competitive athletes caused the initiation of re-testing urine samples from competitors in diverse sports.

7. The beta$_2$-adrenergic agonist clenbuterol increases skeletal muscle mass and slows fat gain in animals to counter the effects of aging, immobilization, malnutrition, and tissue-wasting pathology. A negative finding showed hastened fatigue during short-term,

intense muscle actions. No data exist for its potential toxicity level in humans or its efficacy and safety in long-term use.

8. Debate exists about whether administration of growth hormone to healthy people augments muscular hypertrophy when combined with resistance training. Health risks exist for those who abuse this chemical.

9. Dehydroepiandrosterone (DHEA) is a relatively weak steroid hormone synthesized from cholesterol by the adrenal cortex. DHEA levels steadily decrease throughout adulthood, prompting many individuals to supplement, hoping to counteract the effects of aging. Despite its popularity among exercise enthusiasts, available research does not indicate an ergogenic effect of DHEA.

10. Little credible evidence exists that amphetamines ("pep pills") aid exercise performance or psychomotor skills any better than an inert placebo. Side effects of amphetamines include drug dependency, headache, dizziness, confusion, and upset stomach.

THOUGHT QUESTIONS

1. Respond to the question: "If hormones, such as testosterone, growth hormone, and DHEA, occur naturally in the body, what harm could exist in supplementing with these 'natural' compounds."

2. Outline the points you would make in a talk to a high school football team concerning whether or not they should consider using performance-enhancing chemicals and hormones.

3. A student swears that a chemical compound added to her diet profoundly improved weight-lifting performance. Your review of the research literature indicates no ergogenic benefits for this compound. How would you reconcile this discrepancy?

4. What advice would you give to a collegiate football player who "sees no harm" in replacing fluid lost during the first half with a few beers at half time?

SELECTED REFERENCES

Aagaard, P.: Making muscles "stronger": exercise, nutrition, drugs. *J. Musculoskelet. Neuronal. Interact.*, 4:165, 2004.

Abel, T., et al.: Influence of chronic supplementation of arginine aspartate in endurance athletes on performance and substrate metabolism - a randomized, double-blind, placebo-controlled study. *Int. J. Sports Med.*, 26:344, 2005.

Althuis, M.D., et al.: Glucose and insulin responses to dietary chromium supplements: A meta-analysis. *Am. J. Clin. Nutr.*, 76:148, 2002

Bahrke, M., Morgan, W.P.: Evaluation of the ergogenic properties of ginseng. *Sports Med.*, 29:113, 2000.

Bahrke, M.S., Yesalis, C.E.: Abuse of anabolic androgenic steroids and related substances in sport and exercise. *Curr. Opin. Pharmacol.*, 4:614, 2004.

Battra, D.S., et al.: Caffeine ingestion does not impede the resynthesis of proglycogen and macroglycogen after prolonged exercise and carbohydrate supplementation in humans. *J. Appl. Physiol.*, 96:943, 2004.

Bell, D.G., et al.: Effect of caffeine and ephedrine ingestion on anaerobic performance. *Med. Sci. Sports Exerc.*, 33:1399, 2001.

Bell, D.G., et al.: Effect of ingesting caffeine and ephedrine on 10-kn run performance. *Med. Sci. Sports Exerc.*, 34:344, 2002.

Bell, D.G., McLellan, T.M.: Effect of repeated caffeine ingestion on repeated exhaustive exercise endurance. *Med. Sci. Sports Exerc.*, 35:1348, 2003.

Bemben, M.G., Lamont, H.S.: Creatine supplementation and exercise performance: recent findings. *Sports Med.*, 35:107, 2005.

Bent, S., et al.: The relative safety of ephedra compared with other herbal products. *Ann. Intern. Med.*, 138:468, 2003.

Berardi, J.M., Ziegenfuss, T.N.: Effects of ribose supplementation on repeated sprint performance in men. *J. Strength Cond. Res.*, 17:47, 2003.

Berggren, A., et al.: Short-term administration of supraphysiological recombinant human growth hormone (GH) does not increase maximum endurance exercise capacity in healthy, active young men and women with normal GH-insulin-like growth factor I axes. *J. Clin. Endocrinol. Metab.*, 90:3268, 2005.

Bergstrom, J., et al.: Diet, muscle glycogen and physical performance. *Acta. Physiol. Scand.*, 71:140, 1967.

Bersheim, E., et al.: Effect of carbohydrate intake on net muscle protein synthesis during recovery from resistance exercise. *J. Appl. Physiol.*, 96:674, 2004.

Bhasin, S., et al.: Older men are as responsive as young men to the anabolic effects of graded doses of testosterone on the skeletal muscle. *J. Clin. Endocrinol. Metab.*, 90:678, 2005.

Biolo, G., et al.: An abundant supply of amino acids enhances the metabolic effect of exercise on muscle protein. *Am. J. Physiol.*, 273:E122, 1997.

Bird, S.P., Tarpenning, K.M.: Influence of circadian time structure on acute hormonal responses to a single bout of heavy-resistance exercise in weight-trained men. *Chronobiol. Int.*, 21:131, 2004.

Blackman, M.R., et al.: Growth hormone and sex steroid administration in healthy aged women and men: a randomized controlled trial. *JAMA*, 288:2282, 2002.

Blanchard, M.A., et al.: The influence of diet and exercise on muscle and plasma glutamine concentrations. *Med. Sci. Sports Exerc.*, 33:69, 2001.

Bohn, A.M., et al.: Ephedrine and other stimulants as ergogenic aids. *Curr. Sports Med. Rep.*, 2:220, 2003.

Branch, J.D.: Effect of creatine supplementation on body composition and performance: a meta-analysis. *Int. J. Sport Nutr. Exerc. Metab.*, 13:198, 2003.

Brown, G.A., et al.: Changes in serum testosterone and estradiol concentrations following acute androstenedione ingestion in young women. *Horm. Metab. Res.*, 36:62, 2004.

Brudnak, M.A.: Creatine: are the benefits worth the risk? *Toxicol. Lett.*, 150:123, 2004.

Bucci, L.R.: Selected herbals and human exercise performance. *Am. J. Clin. Nutr.*, 72(suppl):624S, 2000.

Burke, D.G., et al.: Effect of creatine and weight training on muscle creatine and performance in vegetarians. *Med. Sci. Sports Exerc.*, 35:1946, 2003.

Burke, L.M., et al.: Oral creatine supplementation does not improve sprint performance in elite swimmers. *Med. Sci. Sports Exerc.*, 27:S146, 1995.

Cabral de Oliveira, A.C., et al.: Protection of Panax ginseng in injured muscles after eccentric exercise. *J. Ethnopharmacol.*, 28;97:211, 2005.

Candow, D.G., et al.: Effect of glutamine supplementation combined with resistance training in young adults. *Eur. J. Appl. Physiol.*, 86:142, 2001.

Catlin, D.H., et al.: Trace contamination of over-the-counter androstenedione and positive urine test results for nandrolone metabolite. *JAMA*, 284:2618, 2000.

Catlin, D.H., et al.: Tetrahydrogestrinone: discovery, synthesis, and detection in urine. *Rapid Commun. Mass. Spectrom.*, 18:1245, 2004.

Chen, C.Y., et al.: Isoflavones improve plasma homocysteine status and antioxidant defense system in healthy young men at rest but do not ameliorate oxidative stress induced by 80% VO_{2peak} exercise. *Ann. Nutr. Metab.*, 49:33, 2005.

Chester, N., et al.: Physiological, subjective and performance effects of pseudoephedrine and phenylpropanolamine during endurance running exercise. *Int. J. Sports Med.*, 24:3, 2003.

Cheuvront, S.N., et al.: Branched-chain amino acid supplementation and human performance when hypohydrated in the heat. *J. Appl. Physiol.*, 97:1275, 2004.

Chilibeck, P.D., et al.: Effect of creatine ingestion after exercise on muscle thickness in males and females. *Med. Sci. Sports Exerc.*, 36:1781, 2004.

Chrusch, M.J., et al.: Creatine supplementation combined with resistance training in older men. *Med. Sci. Sports Exerc.*, 33:2111, 2001.

Chwalbinska-Moneta, J., et al.: Early effects of short-term endurance training on hormonal responses to graded exercise. *J. Physiol. Pharmacol.*, 56:87, 2005.

Clark, A.S., Henderson, L.P.: Behavioral and physiological responses to anabolic-androgenic steroids. *Neurosci. Biobehav. Rev.*, 27:413, 2003.

Clark, B.M., Schofield, R.S.: Dilated cardiomyopathy and acute liver injury associated with combined use of ephedra, gamma-hydroxybutyrate, and anabolic steroids. *Pharmacotherapy*, 25:756, 2005.

Colson, S.N., et al.: Cordyceps sinensis- and Rhodiola rosea-based supplementation in male cyclists and its effect on muscle tissue oxygen saturation. *J. Strength Cond. Res.*, 19:358, 2005.

Connes, P., et al.: Injections of recombinant human erythropoietin increases lactate influx into erythrocytes. *J. Appl. Physiol.*, 97:165, 2004.

Cunha, T.S., et al.: Influence of high-intensity exercise training and anabolic androgenic steroid treatment on rat tissue glycogen content. *Life Sci.*, 77:1030, 2005.

de Geus, B., et al.: Norandrosterone and noretiocholanolone concentration before and after submaximal standardized exercise. *Int. J. Sports Med.*, 25:528, 2004.

Doherty, M., et al.: Caffeine is ergogenic after supplementation of oral creatine monohydrate. *Med. Sci. Sports Exerc.*, 34:1785, 2002.

Doherty, M., et al.: Caffeine lowers perceptual response and increases power output during high-intensity cycling. *J. Sports Sci.*, 22:637, 2004.

Doherty, M., Smith, P.M.: Effects of caffeine ingestion on rating of perceived exertion during and after exercise: a meta-analysis. *Scand. J. Med. Sci. Sports*, 15:69, 2005.

Drakeley, A., et al.: Duration of azoospermia following anabolic steroids. *Fertil. Steril.*, 81:226, 2004.

Duarte, J.A., et al.: Strenuous exercise aggravates MDMA-induced skeletal muscle damage in mice. *Toxicology*, 206:349, 2005.

Earnest, C.P., et al.: Effects of a commercial herbal-based formula on exercise performance in cyclists. *Med. Sci. Sports Exerc.*, 36:504, 2004.

Eckerson, J.M., et al.: Effect of two and five days of creatine loading on anaerobic working capacity in women. *J. Strength Cond. Res.*, 18:168, 2004.

El-Sayed, M.S., et al.: Interaction between alcohol and exercise: physiological and haematological implications. *Sports Med.*, 35:257, 2005.

Engels, H.J., et al.: Effects of ginseng on secretory IgA, performance, and recovery from interval exercise. *Med. Sci. Sports Exerc.*, 35:690, 2003.

Esmarck, B., et al.: Timing of postexercise protein intake is important for muscle hypertrophy with resistance training in elderly humans. *J. Physiol.*, 535:301, 2001.

Evans, R.K., et al. Effects of warm-up before eccentric exercise on indirect markers on muscle damage. *Med. Sci. Sports Exerc.*, 34:1892, 2002.

Fairchild, T.J., et al.: Rapid carbohydrate loading after a short bout of near maximal-intensity exercise. *Med. Sci. Sports Exerc.*, 34:980, 2002.

Ferreira, S.E., et al.: Does an energy drink modify the effects of alcohol in a maximal effort test? *Alcohol Clin. Exp. Res.*, 28:1408, 2004.

Finn, J.P., et al.: Effect of creatine supplementation on metabolism and performance in humans during intermittent sprint cycling. *Eur. J. Appl. Physiol.*, 84:238, 2001.

Fleck, S.J., et al.: Anaerobic power effects of an amino acid supplement containing no branched amino acids in elite competitive athletes. *J. Strength Cond. Res.*, 9:132, 1995.

Fomous, C.M., et al.: Symposium: conference on the science and policy of performance-enhancing products. *Med. Sci. Sports Exerc.*, 34:1685, 2002.

Gallagher, P.M., et al.: b-hydroxy-b-methylbutyrate ingestion, Part I: effects on strength and fat free mass. *Med. Sci. Sports Exerc.*, 32:2116, 2000.

Gallagher, P.M., et al.: b-hydroxy-b-methylbutyrate ingestion, Part II: effects on hematology, hepatic and renal function. *Med. Sci. Sports Exerc.*, 32:2116, 2000.

Gaullier, J.M., et al.: Supplementation with conjugated linoleic acid for 24 months is well tolerated by and reduces body fat mass in healthy, overweight humans. *J. Nutr.*, 135:778, 2005.

Gleeson, M.: Interrelationship between physical activity and branched-chain amino acids. *J. Nutr.*, 135:1591S, 2005.

Godard, M.P., et al.: Oral amino-acid provision does not affect muscle strength or size gains in older men. *Med. Sci. Sports Exerc.*, 34:1126, 2002.

Gotshalk, L.A., et al.: Creatine supplementation improves muscular performance in older men. *Med. Sci. Sports Exerc.*, 34:537, 2002.

Goto, K., et al.: The impact of metabolic stress on hormonal responses and muscular adaptations. *Med. Sci. Sports Exerc.*, 37:955, 2005.

Goulet, E.D., Dionne, I.J.: Assessment of the effects of eleutherococcus senticosus on endurance performance. *Int. J. Sport Nutr. Exerc. Metab.*, 15:75, 2005.

Green, G.A., et al.: Analysis of over-the-counter dietary supplements. *Clin. J. Sports Med.*, 11:254, 2001.

Halson, S.L., et al.: Effects of carbohydrate supplementation on performance and carbohydrate oxidation after intensified cycling training. *J. Appl. Physiol.*, 97:1245, 2004.

Harkey, M.R., et al.: Variability in commercial ginseng products: an analysis of 25 preparations. *Am. J. Clin. Nutr.*, 73:1101, 2001.

Hartgens, F., et al.: Misuse of androgenic-anabolic steroids and human deltoid muscle fibers: differences between polydrug regimes and single drug administration. *Eur. J. Appl. Physiol.*, 86:233, 2002.

Hartgens, F., et al.: Prospective echocardiographic assessment of androgenic-anabolic steroids effects on cardiac structure and function in strength athletes. *Int. J. Sports Med.*, 24:344, 2003.

Hartgens, F., Kuipers, H.: Effects of androgenic-anabolic steroids in athletes. *Sports Med.*, 34:513, 2004.

Hellsten, Y., et al.: Effect of ribose supplementation on resynthesis of adenine nucleotides after intense intermittent training in humans. *Am. J. Physiol. Regul. Integr. Comp. Physiol.*, 286:R182, 2004.

Hingson, R.W., et al.: Magnitude of alcohol-related mortality and morbidity among U.S. college students ages 18–24. *J. Stud. Alcohol*, 63:136, 2002.

Hingson, R.W., and Howland, J.: Comprehensive community interventions to promote health: Implications for college-age drinking problems. *J. Stud. Alcohol Suppl.*, 14:226, 2002.

Hitchins, S., et al.: Glycerol hyperhydration improves cycle time trial performance in hot humid conditions. *Eur. J. Appl. Physiol.*, 80:494, 1999.

Hodges, A.N., et al.: Effects of pseudoephedrine on maximal cycling power and submaximal cycling efficiency. *Med. Sci. Sports Exerc.*, 35:1316, 2003.

Hoffman, J.R., et al.: Effect of low-dose, short-duration creatine supplementation on anaerobic exercise performance. *J. Strength Cond. Res.*, 19:260, 2005.

Hollidge-Horvat, M.G., et al.: Effect of induced metabolic alkalosis on human skeletal muscle metabolism during exercise. *Am. J. Physiol.*, 278:E316, 2000.

Hultman, E., et al.: Muscle creatine loading in men. *J. Appl. Physiol.*, 81:232, 1996.

Indig, D., et al.: Illicit drug-related harm during the Sydney 2000 Olympic Games: implications for public health surveillance and action. *Addiction*, 98:97, 2003.

Ivy, J.L., et al.: Contribution of medium and long chain triglyceride intake to energy metabolism during prolonged exercise. *Int. J. Sports Med.*, 1:15, 1980.

Ivy, J.L., et al.: Early post-exercise muscle glycogen recovery is enhanced with a carbohydrate-protein supplement. *J. Appl. Physiol.*, 93:1337, 2002.

Ivy, J.L.: Effect of pyruvate and dehydroxyacetone on metabolism and aerobic endurance capacity. *Med. Sci. Sports Exerc.*, 6:837, 1998.

Izquierdo, M., et al.: Effects of creatine supplementation on muscle power, endurance, and sprint performance. *Med. Sci. Sports Exerc.*, 34:332, 2002.

Izquierdo, M., et al.: Maximal strength and power, muscle mass, endurance and serum hormones in weightlifters and road cyclists. *J. Sports Sci.*, 22:465, 2004.

Jacobs, I., et al.: Effects of ephedrine, caffeine, and their combination on muscular endurance. *Med. Sci. Sports Exerc.*, 35:987, 2003.

Jowko, E., et al.: Creatine and beta-hydroxy-beta-methylbutyrate

(HMB) additively increase lean body mass and muscle strength during a weight training program. *Nutrition*, 17:558, 2001.

Juhn, M.: Popular sports supplements and ergogenic aids. *Sports Med.*, 33:921, 2003.

Kam, P.C., Yarrow, M.: Anabolic steroid abuse: physiological and anaesthetic considerations. *Anaesthesia*, 60:685, 2005.

Kamber, M., et al.: Nutritional supplements as a source for positive doping cases? *Int. J. Sport Nutr. Exerc. Metab.*, 11:258, 2001.

Kearns, C.F., et al.: Chronic administration of therapeutic levels of clenbuterol acts as a repartitioning agent. *J. Appl. Physiol.*, 91:2064, 2001.

Kearns, C.F., McKeever, J.: Clenbuterol diminishes aerobic performance in horses. *Med. Sci. Sports Exerc.*, 34:1976, 2002.

Kicman, A.T., and Gower, D.B.: Anabolic steroids in sport: Biochemical, clinical and analytical perspectives. *Ann. Clin. Biochem.*, 40(Pt 4):321, 2003.

Kilduff, L.P., et al.: The effects of creatine supplementation on cardiovascular, metabolic, and thermoregulatory responses during exercise in the heat in endurance-trained humans. *Int. J. Sport Nutr. Exerc. Metab.*, 14:443, 2004.

Kimball, S.R., et al.: Role of insulin in translational control of protein synthesis in skeletal muscle by amino acids or exercise. *J. Appl. Physiol.*, 2002;93:1168, 2002.

Kitaura, T., et al.: Inhibited longitudinal growth of bones in young male rats by clenbuterol. *Med. Sci. Sports Exerc.*, 34:267, 2002.

Koenigsberg, P.S., et al.: Sustained hyperhydration with glycerol ingestion. *Life Sci.*, 57:645, 1995.

Koh-Banerjee PK, et al. Effects of calcium pyruvate supplementation during training on body composition, exercise capacity, and metabolic responses to exercise. *Nutrition.*, 21:312, 2005.

Kreider, R.B., et al.: Long-term creatine supplementation does not significantly affect clinical markers of health in athletes. *Mol. Cell. Biochem.*, 244:95, 2003.

Labrie, F., et al.: Tetrahydrogestrinone induces a genomic signature typical of a potent anabolic steroid. *J. Endocrinol.*, 184:427, 2005.

Laure, P., et al.: Drugs, recreational drug use and attitudes towards doping of high school athletes. *Int. J. Sports Med.*, 25:133, 2004.

Levenhagen, D.K., et al.: Postexercise protein intake enhances whole-body and leg protein accretion in humans. *Med. Sci. Sports Exerc.*, 34:828, 2002.

Liang, M.T., et al.: Panax notoginseng supplementation enhances physical performance during endurance exercise. *J. Strength Cond. Res.*, 19:108, 2005.

Lieberman, H.R., et al.: Carbohydrate administration during a day of sustained aerobic activity improves vigilance, as assessed by normal ambulatory monitoring device, and mood. *Am. J. Clin. Nutr.*, 76:120, 2002.

Lieberman, H.R.: The effects of ginseng, ephedrine, and caffeine on cognitive performance, mood and energy. *Nutr. Revs.*, 50:91, 2001.

Lim, K., et al.: (-)-Hydroxycitrate ingestion and endurance exercise performance. *J. Nutr. Sci. Vitaminol.* (Tokyo), 51:1, 2005.

Liu, J.F., et al.: Blood lipid peroxides and muscle damage increased following intensive resistance training of female weightlifters. *Ann. N. Y. Acad. Sci.*, 1042:255, 2005.

Magkos, F., Kavouras, S.A.: Caffeine and ephedrine: physiological, metabolic and performance-enhancing effects. *Sports Med.*, 34:871, 2004.

Malinowski, K., et al.: Effect of chronic clenbuterol administration and exercise training on immune function in horses. *J. Anim. Sci.*, 82:3500, 2004.

McMurray, R.G., Hackney, A.C.: Interactions of metabolic hormones, adipose tissue and exercise. *Sports Med.*, 35:393, 2005.

Mendel, R.W., et al.: Effects of creatine on thermoregulatory responses while exercising in the heat. *Nutrition*, 21:301, 2005.

Mendes, R.R., et al.: Effects of creatine supplementation on the performance and body composition of competitive swimmers. *J. Nutr. Biochem.*, 15:473, 2004.

Miller, S.L., et al.: Independent and combined effects of amino acids and glucose after resistance exercise. *Med. Sci. Sports Exerc.*, 35:449, 2003.

Newman, J.E., et al.: Effect of creatine ingestion on glucose tolerance and insulin sensitivity in men. *Med. Sci. Sports Exerc.*, 35:69, 2003.

Nishijima, Y., et al.: Influence of caffeine ingestion on autonomic nervous system activity during endurance exercise in humans. *Eur. J. Appl. Physiol.*, 87:475, 2002.

Noakes, T.D.: Tainted glory--doping and athletic performance. *N. Engl. J. Med.*, 351:847, 2004.

Op'T Eijnde, B., et al.: No effects of oral ribose supplementation on repeated maximal exercise and de novo ATP resynthesis. *J. Appl. Physiol.*, 91:2275, 2001.

Ostojic, S.M.: Creatine supplementation in young soccer players. *Int. J. Sport Nutr. Exerc. Metab.*, 14:95, 2004.

Paddon-Jones, D., et al.: Potential ergogenic effects of arginine and creatine supplementation. *J. Nutr.*, 134:2888S, 2004.

Parise, G., et al.: Effects of acute creatine monohydrate supplementation on leucine kinetics and mixed-muscle protein synthesis. *J. Appl. Physiol.*, 91:1041, 2001.

Paul, G., et al.: Efficacy and safety of ephedra and ephedrine for weight loss and athletic performance: a meta-analysis. *JAMA*, 289:1537, 2003.

Percheron, G., et al.: Effect of 1-year oral administration of dehydroepiandrosterone to 60- to 80-year-old individuals on muscle function and cross-sectional area: a double-blind placebo-controlled trial. *Arch. Intern. Med.*, 163:720, 2003.

Plaskett, C.J., Cafarelli, E.: Caffeine increases endurance and attenuates force sensation during submaximal isometric contractions. *J. Appl. Physiol.*, 91:1535, 2001.

Porter, D.A., et al.: The effect of oral coenzyme Q10 on the exercise tolerance of middle-aged, untrained men. *Int. J. Sports Med.*, 16:421, 1995.

Price, M., et al.: Effects of sodium bicarbonate ingestion on prolonged intermittent exercise. *Med. Sci. Sports Exerc.*, 35:1303, 2003.

Ransone, J., et al.: The effect of beta-hydroxy beta-methylbutyrate on muscular strength and body composition in collegiate football players. *J. Strength Cond. Res.*, 17:34, 2003.

Rasmussen, B.B., Phillips, S.M.: Contractile and nutritional regulation of human muscle growth. *Exerc. Sport Sci. Rev.*, 31;127, 2003.

Raymer, G.H., et al.: Metabolic effects of induced alkalosis during progressive forearm exercise to fatigue. *J. Appl. Physiol.*, 96:2050, 2004.

Rennie, M.J., Tipton, K.D.: Protein and amino acid metabolism during and after resistance exercise and the effects of nutrition. *Ann. Rev. Nutr.*, 20:457, 2000.

Rogers, N.L., Dinges, D.F.: Caffeine: implications for alertness in athletes. *Clin. Sports Med.*, 24:1, 2005.

Rosell, M., et al.: The relation between alcohol intake and physical activity and the fatty acids 14:0, 15:0 and 17:0 in serum phospholipids and adipose tissue used as markers for dairy fat intake. *Br. J. Nutr.*, 93:115, 2005.

Roy, B.D., et al.: An acute oral dose of caffeine does not alter glucose kinetics during prolonged dynamic exercise in trained endurance athletes. *Eur. J. Appl. Physiol.* 85:280, 2005.

Roy, B.D., et al.: Macronutrient intakes and whole body protein metabolism following resistance exercise. *Med. Sci. Sports Exerc.*, 32:1412, 2000.

Sekera, M.H., et al.: Another designer steroid: discovery, synthesis, and detection of 'madol' in urine. *Rapid Commun. Mass Spectrom.*, 19:781, 2005.

Selsby, J.T., et al.: Mg2+-creatine chelate and a low-dose creatine supplementation regimen improve exercise performance. *J. Strength Cond. Res.*, 18:311, 2004.

Shekelle, P.G., et al.: Efficacy and safety of ephedra and ephedrine for weight loss and athletic performance: A meta-analysis. *JAMA*, 289:1537, 2003.

Shomrat, A., et al.: Effects of creatine feeding on maximal exercise performance in vegetarians. *Eur. J. Appl. Physiol.*, 82:321, 2000.

Slater, B., et al.: Beta-hydroxy-beta-methylbutyrate (HMB) supplementation does not affect changes in strength or body composition during resistance training in trained men. *Int. J. Sport Nutr. Exerc. Metab.*, 11:384, 2001.

Sleeper, M.M., et al.: Chronic clenbuterol, administration negatively alters cardiac function. *Med. Sci. Sports Exerc.*, 34:643, 2002.

Snow, R.J., Murphy, R.M.: Factors influencing creatine loading into human skeletal muscle. *Exerc. Sport Sci. Rev.*, 31:154, 2003.

Stacy, J.J., et al.: Ergogenic aids: human growth hormone. *Curr. Sports Med. Rep.*, 3:229, 2004.

Stephens, T.J., et al.: Effect of sodium bicarbonate on muscle metabolism during intense endurance cycling. *Med. Sci. Sports Exerc.*, 34:614, 2002.

Tagarakis, C.V., et al.: Anabolic steroids impair the exercise-induced growth of the cardiac capillary bed. *Int. J. Sports Med.*, 21:412, 2000.

Tarnopolsky, M.A., et al.: Gender differences in carbohydrate loading are related to energy intake. *J. Appl. Physiol.*, 91:225, 2001.

Tipton, K.D., et al.: Acute response of net muscle protein balance reflects 24-h balance after exercise and amino acid ingestion. *Am. J. Physiol.*, 284:E76, 2003.

Tipton, K.D., et al.: Ingestion of casein and whey proteins result in muscle anabolism after resistance exercise. *Med. Sci. Sports Exerc.*, 36:2073, 2004.

Tokish, J.M., et al.: Ergogenic aids: a review of basic science, performance, side effects, and status in sports. *Am. J. Sports Med.*, 32:1543, 2004.

Utter, A.C., et al.: Carbohydrate supplementation and perceived exertion during prolonged running. *Med. Sci. Sports Exerc.*, 36:1036, 2004.

van Loon, L.J., et al.: Effects of creatine loading and prolonged creatine supplementation on body composition, fuel selection, sprint and endurance performance in humans. *Clin. Sci. (Lond)*, 104:153, 2003.

Van Montfoort, M.C., et al.: Effects of ingestion of bicarbonate, citrate, lactate, and chloride on sprint running. *Med. Sci. Sports Exerc.*, 36:1239, 2004.

Varady, K.A., et al.: Plant sterols and endurance training combine to favorably alter plasma lipid profiles in previously sedentary hypercholesterolemic adults after 8 wk. *Am. J. Clin. Nutr.*, 80:1159, 2004.

Vierck, J.L., et al.: The effects of ergogenic compounds on myogenic satellite cells. *Med. Sci. Sports Exerc.*, 35:769, 2003.

Villareal, D.T., Holloszy, J.O.: Effect of DHEA on abdominal fat and insulin action in elderly women and men: a randomized controlled trial. *JAMA*, 292:2243, 2004.

Vincent, J.B.: The potential value and toxicity of chromium picolinate as a nutritional supplement, weight loss agent and muscle development agent. *Sports Med.*, 33:213, 2003.

Vistisen, B., et al.: Minor amounts of plasma medium-chain fatty acids and no improved time trial performance after consuming lipids. *J. Appl. Physiol.*, 95:2434, 2003.

Volek, J.S.: Influence of nutrition on responses to resistance training. *Med. Sci. Sports Exerc.*, 36:689, 2004.

Vuksan, V., et al.: American ginseng (Panex quinquefolius L.) attenuates postprandial glycemia in a time-dependent but not dose-dependent manner in healthy individuals. *Am. J. Clin. Nutr.*, 73:753, 2001.

Willoughby, D.S., Rosene, J.: Effects of oral creatine and resistance training on myogenic regulatory factor expression. *Med. Sci. Sports Exerc.*, 35:923, 2003.

Wiroth, J.B., et al.: Effects of oral creatine supplementation on maximal pedaling performance in older adults. *Eur. J. Appl. Physiol.*, 84:533, 2001.

Wolfe, R.R.: Regulation of muscle protein by amino acids. *J. Nutr.*, 132:3219S, 2002.

Yanovski, S.Z., Yanovski, J.A.: Drug therapy: obesity. *N. Engl. J. Med.*, 346:591, 2002.

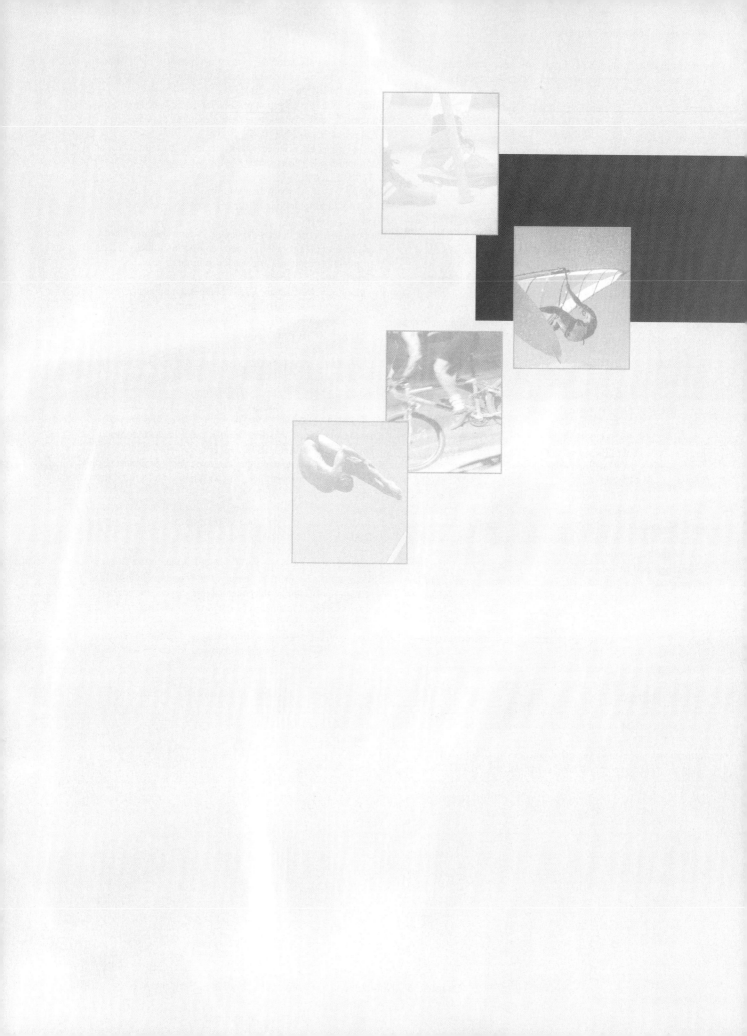

Section III

Energy Transfer

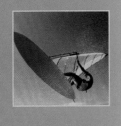

Biochemical reactions that do not consume oxygen generate considerable energy for short durations. This rapid energy generation becomes crucial in maintaining a high standard of performance in sprint activities and other bursts of all-out exercise. In contrast, longer duration (aerobic) exercise extracts energy more slowly from food catabolism through chemical reactions that require the continual use of oxygen. Gaining insight of how muscle tissue generates energy to sustain exercise, the sources that provide that energy, and the energy requirements of diverse physical activities enables planning of effective training to enhance exercise performance.

This section presents a broad overview of the fundamentals of human energy transfer during rest and exercise. We emphasize the means by which the body's cells extract chemical energy bound within food molecules and transfer it to a common compound that powers all forms of biologic work. The importance the food nutrients and processes of energy transfer to sustain physiologic function during light, moderate, and strenuous exercise is given special attention as are techniques to measure and evaluate the diverse human energy transfer capacities.

"I often say that when you can measure what you are speaking about, and express it in numbers, you know something about it; but when you cannot measure it, when you cannot express it in numbers, your knowledge is of a meagre and unsatisfactory kind."

—Lord Kelvin
(William Thomson, 1st Baron) (1824-1907)
English physicist and mathematician.

CHAPTER OBJECTIVES

- Describe the first law of thermodynamics related to energy balance and biologic work.

- Define the terms potential energy and kinetic energy and give examples of each.

- Give examples of exergonic and endergonic chemical processes within the body and indicate their importance.

- State the second law of thermodynamics and give a practical application.

- Identify and give examples of three forms of biologic work.

- Discuss the role of enzymes and coenzymes in bioenergetics.

- Identify the high-energy phosphates and discuss their contributions in powering biologic work.

- Outline the process of electron transport-oxidative phosphorylation.

- Explain oxygen's role in energy metabolism.

- Describe how anaerobic energy release occurs in cells.

- Describe lactate formation during progressively increasing exercise intensity.

- Outline the general pathways of the citric cycle during macronutrient catabolism.

- Contrast ATP yield from carbohydrate, fat, and protein catabolism.

- Explain the statement, "Fats burn in a carbohydrate flame."

CHAPTER OUTLINE

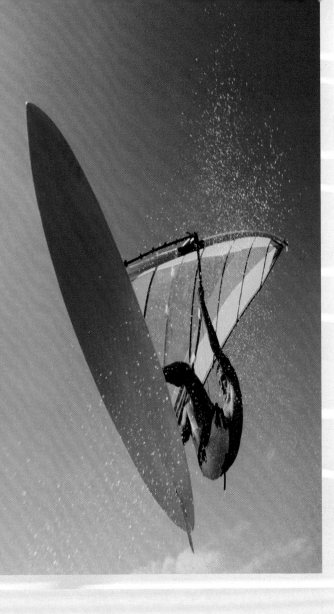

chapter 5

Fundamentals of Human Energy Transfer

The body's capacity to extract energy from food nutrients and transfer it to the contractile elements in skeletal muscle determines the capacity to swim, run, bicycle, and ski long distances at high intensity. Energy transfer occurs through thousands of complex chemical reactions that require the proper mixture of macro- and micronutrients continually fueled by oxygen. The term **aerobic** describes such oxygen-requiring energy reactions. In contrast, **anaerobic** chemical reactions generate energy rapidly for short durations without oxygen. Rapid energy transfer allows for a high standard of performance in maximal short-term sprinting in track and swimming, or repeated stop-and-go sports like soccer, basketball, lacrosse, water polo, volleyball, field hockey, and football. The following point requires emphasis: *The anaerobic and aerobic breakdown of ingested food nutrients provides the energy source for synthesizing the chemical fuel that powers all forms of biologic work.*

In this chapter, we present an overview of the different forms of energy and those factors affecting energy generation. We also discuss how the body obtains energy to power its diverse functions. A basic understanding of carbohydrate, fat, and protein catabolism and concurrent anaerobic and aerobic energy transfer forms the basis for much of the content of exercise physiology. Knowledge about human bioenergetics provides the practical basis for formulating sport-specific exercise training regimens, recommending activities for physical fitness and weight control, and advocating prudent dietary modifications for specific sport requirements. Understanding the impact of environmental stressors on the human organism requires knowledge of energy metabolism. Furthermore, evaluating the proposed benefits of the potpourri of alleged performance-enhancing drugs, compounds, foods, and procedures necessitates an understanding of how the body generates energy.

PART 1 •
Energy—The Capacity for Work

Extracting energy from the stored macronutrients and transferring it to the contractile proteins of skeletal muscle greatly influences exercise performance. Unlike the physical properties of matter, one cannot define energy in concrete terms of size, shape, or mass. Rather, the term energy suggests a dynamic state related to change; thus, the presence of energy emerges only when a change occurs. Within this context, energy relates to the performance of work (as work increases so does energy transfer) and the occurrence of change.

The **first law of thermodynamics** describes one of the most important principles related to biologic work. The basic tenet states that energy cannot be created or de-stroyed but, instead, transforms from one form to another without being depleted. In essence, this law describes the immutable principle of the **conservation of energy** that applies to both living and nonliving systems. In the body, chemical energy stored within the bonds of macronutrients does not immediately dissipate as heat during energy metabolism; instead, a large portion remains as chemical energy, which the musculoskeletal system then changes into mechanical energy (and then ultimately to heat energy). *The first law of thermodynamics dictates that the body does not produce, consume, or use up energy; rather, it transforms it from one form into another as physiologic systems undergo continual change.*

POTENTIAL AND KINETIC ENERGY

Potential energy and **kinetic energy** constitute the total energy of a system. **Figure 5.1** shows potential energy as energy of position, similar to a boulder tottering atop a cliff or water at the top of a hill before it flows downstream. In the example of flowing water, the energy change is proportional to the water's vertical drop (i.e., the greater the vertical drop, the greater the potential energy at the top). The waterwheel harnesses a portion of the energy from the falling water to produce useful work. In the case of the

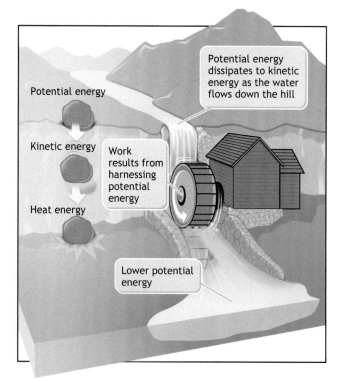

Figure 5.1. High-grade potential energy capable of performing work degrades to a useless form of kinetic energy. In the example of falling water, the water wheel harnesses potential energy to perform useful work. For the falling boulder, all of the potential energy dissipates to kinetic energy (heat) as the boulder crashes to the surface.

Box 5-1 • CLOSE UP

ATP—NATURE'S POWERFUL INGREDIENT

Animals and plants are as different as night and day, yet they share one important common biological trait; they each trap, store, and transfer energy through a complex series of chemical reactions that involve the compound adenosine triphosphate (ATP).

The history of the discovery of ATP reads like a mystery. It dates back to the 1860s in France and the work of Louis Pasteur, a leading scientist of the day. During one of his experiments with yeast, Pasteur proposed that this micro-organism's ability to degrade sugar to carbon dioxide and alcohol (ethanol) was strictly a living (Pasteur termed it "vitalistic") function of the yeast cell. He hypothesized that if the yeast cell died, the fermentation process would cease.

In 1897, the German chemist, Eduard Buchner (1860–1917), made a chance observation that proved Pasteur wrong. His discovery revolutionized the study of physiologic systems and represented the beginning of the modern science of **biochemistry**. Searching for therapeutic uses for protein, he concocted a thick paste of freshly grown yeast and sand in a large mortar and pressed out the yeast cell juice. The gummy liquid proved unstable and could not be preserved by techniques available at that time. One of the laboratory assistants suggested adding a large amount of sugar to the mixture—his wife used this technique to preserve fruit.

To everyone's surprise, what seemed like a silly solution worked; the nonliving juice from the yeast cells converted the sugar to carbon dioxide and alcohol (directly contradicting Pasteur's prevailing theorem). The epoch finding about non-cellular fermentation earned Professor Buchner the 1907 Nobel Prize in chemistry.

In 1905, British biochemists Arthur Harden and Australian biochemist William Young observed, as had their German predecessors, that the fermenting ability of yeast juice decreased gradually with time and could be restored only by adding fresh boiled yeast juice or blood serum. What revitalized the mixture? After prolonged research, inorganic phosphate, present in both liquids, was identified as the activating agent.

Other British scientists working with eventual Nobel Laureate Sir Arthur Harden (1929 Nobel Prize in Chemistry) and William Young also played important roles in the final discovery of ATP. For example, crude yeast juice pressed through a gelatin film yielded a filtrate free of protein. The filtrate and protein were completely inert. But when the filtrate and protein were recombined, vigorous fermentation began. They called this combination "zymase"; it consisted of the filtrate "cozymase" and the protein residue "apozymase." Many years passed before the two components were accurately analyzed and identified as containing "coenzyme" compounds. In addition, the apozymase consisted of many proteins, each a specific catalyst in the many reactions in sugar breakdown.

In 1929, a young German scientist, Karl Lohmann, working in Otto Meyerhoff's laboratory, studied the "energy" source responsible for cellular reactions involving yeast and sugar. Working with yeast juice, Lohmann found that an unstable substance in the cozymase filtrate was required to break down the sugar. This energizing substance contained the nitrogen-containing compound adenine linked to the sugar ribose and three phosphate groups. We now call this compound ATP. The potential energy stored in the "high-energy bonds" link the phosphate groups in the ATP molecule. The splitting of these phosphate bonds releases the energy for *all* biologic work.

The function of ATP is amazing for the variety of processes it powers in all living cells. This ubiquitous compound is found in microorganisms, plants, and animals ranging from nematodes to cockroaches and humans. Surprisingly, wherever ATP is found, it is always in the same structure, regardless of the organism's complexity.

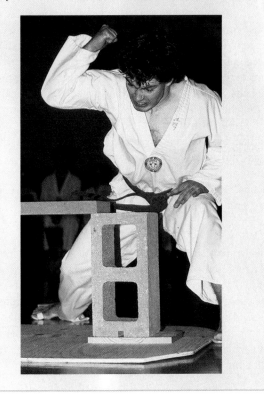

boulder, *all* potential energy transforms to kinetic energy and dissipates as useless heat as the boulder crashes to the ground.

Other examples of potential energy include bound energy within the internal structure of a battery, a stick of dynamite, or a macronutrient before release of its stored energy in metabolism. *Releasing potential energy transforms the basic ingredient into kinetic energy of motion.* In some cases, bound energy in one substance directly transfers to other substances to increase their potential energy. Energy transfers of this type provide the necessary energy for the body's chemical work of **biosynthesis**. In this process, specific building-block atoms of carbon, hydrogen, oxygen, and nitrogen become activated and join other atoms and molecules to synthesize important biologic compounds and tissues. Some newly created compounds provide structure as in bone or the lipid-containing plasma membrane that encloses each cell. Other synthesized compounds, such as adenosine triphosphate (ATP) and phosphocreatine (PCr), serve the cell's energy requirements.

ENERGY-RELEASING AND ENERGY-CONSERVING PROCESSES

The term **exergonic** describes any physical or chemical process that releases (frees up) energy to its surroundings. Such reactions represent "downhill" processes; they produce a decline in free energy—"useful" energy for biologic work that encompasses all of the energy-requiring, life-sustaining processes within cells. Chemical processes that store or absorb energy are termed **endergonic**; these reactions represent "uphill" processes and proceed with an increase in free energy for biologic work. In some instances, exergonic processes link or couple with endergonic reactions to transfer some energy to the endergonic process. In the body, such coupled reactions conserve a large portion of the chemical energy stored within the macronutrients in a usable form.

Changes in free energy occur when the bonds in the reactant molecules form new product molecules but with different bonding. The equation that expresses these changes, under conditions of constant temperature, pressure, and volume, takes the following form:

$$\Delta G = \Delta H - T\Delta S$$

The symbol Δ designates change. The change in free energy represents a keystone of chemical reactions. In exergonic reactions, ΔG is negative; the products contain *less* free energy than the reactants, with the energy differential released as heat. For example, when hydrogen unites with oxygen to form water, the union releases 68 kCal per mole (molecular weight of substance in g) of free energy in the following reaction:

$$H_2 + O \rightarrow H_2O - \Delta G\ 68\ kCal \cdot mol^{-1}$$

In the reverse endergonic reaction, ΔG remains positive because the product contains *more* free energy than the reactants. The infusion of 68 kCal of energy per mole of water causes the chemical bonds of the water molecule to split apart, freeing the original hydrogen and oxygen atoms. This "uphill" process of energy transfer provides the hydrogen and oxygen atoms with their original energy content to satisfy the principle of the first law of thermodynamics—the conservation of energy.

$$H_2 + O \leftarrow H_2O + \Delta G\ 68\ kCal \cdot mol^{-1}$$

Energy transfer in cells follows the same principles as in the waterfall–waterwheel example. Carbohydrate, lipid, and protein macronutrients possess considerable potential energy. The formation of product substances progressively reduces the nutrient molecule's original potential energy, with a corresponding increase in kinetic energy. Enzyme-regulated transfer systems harness or conserve a portion of this chemical energy in new compounds for use in biologic work. In essence, living cells serve as transducers with the capacity to extract and use chemical energy stored within a compound's atomic structure. Conversely, and equally important, they also bond atoms and molecules together, raising them to a higher level of potential energy.

The transfer of potential energy in any spontaneous process always proceeds in a direction that *decreases* the capacity to perform work. The tendency of potential energy to degrade to kinetic energy of motion with a lower capacity for work (i.e., increased **entropy**) reflects the **second law of thermodynamics**. A flashlight battery embodies this principle. The electrochemical energy stored within its cells slowly dissipates, even if the battery remains unused. The energy from sunlight also continually degrades to heat energy when light strikes and becomes absorbed by a surface. Food and other chemicals represent excellent stores of potential energy, yet this energy continually decreases as the compounds decompose through normal oxidative processes. Energy, like water, always runs downhill, so potential energy decreases. *Ultimately, all of the potential energy in a system degrades to the unusable form of kinetic or heat energy.*

INTERCONVERSIONS OF ENERGY

The total energy in an isolated system remains constant, so a decrease in one form of energy matches an equivalent increase in another form. During energy conversions, a loss of potential energy from one source often produces a temporary increase in the potential energy of another source. In this way, nature harnesses vast quantities of potential energy for useful purposes. Even under such favorable conditions, the net flow of energy in the biologic world still moves toward entropy, ultimately producing a loss of potential energy.

Figure 5.2 shows energy categorized into one of six forms: chemical, mechanical, heat, light, electric, and nuclear.

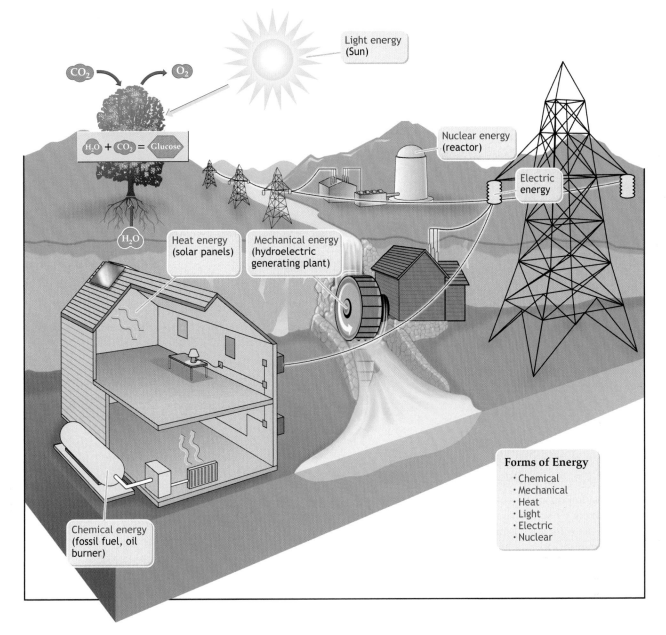

Figure 5.2. Interconversions of six forms of energy.

Examples of Energy Conversions

The conversion of energy from one form to another occurs readily in the inanimate and animate worlds. **Photosynthesis** and **respiration** represent the most fundamental examples of energy conversion in living cells.

Photosynthesis **Figure 5.3** depicts the dynamics of photosynthesis, an endergonic process powered by energy from sunlight. The pigment chlorophyll, which is within the leaf's cells large organelles, the chloroplasts, absorbs radiant (solar) energy to synthesize glucose from carbon dioxide and water, while oxygen flows to the environment. The plant also converts carbohydrates to lipids and proteins for storage as a future reserve for energy and growth. Animals then ingest plant nutrients to serve their own energy needs. *In essence, solar energy coupled with photosynthesis powers the animal world with food and oxygen.*

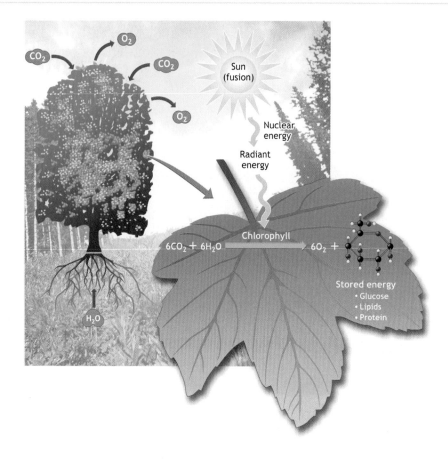

Figure 5.3. The endergonic process of photosynthesis in plants, algae, and some bacteria serves as the mechanism for synthesizing carbohydrates, lipids, and proteins. In this example, a glucose molecule forms from the union of carbon dioxide and water, with a positive free energy (useful energy) change ($+\Delta G$).

Cellular Respiration **Figure 5.4** shows that the reactions of respiration are the reverse of photosynthesis as the plant recovers its stored energy. During these exergonic reactions, the cells extract, in the presence of oxygen, the chemical energy stored in the carbohydrate, lipid, and protein molecules. For glucose, this releases 689 kCal per mole (180 g) oxidized. *A portion of the energy released during cellular respiration becomes conserved in other chemical compounds for use in energy-requiring processes; the remaining energy flows to the environment as heat.*

BIOLOGIC WORK IN HUMANS

Figure 5.4 also illustrates that biologic work takes one of three forms:

1. **Mechanical work** of muscle contraction
2. **Chemical work** that synthesizes cellular molecules
3. **Transport work** that concentrates various substances in the intracellular and extracellular fluids

Mechanical Work

The most obvious example of energy transformation occurs from mechanical work generated by muscle contraction and subsequent movement. The molecular motors in a muscle fiber's protein filaments directly convert chemical energy into the mechanical energy of movement. This does not represent the body's only form of mechanical work. In the cell nucleus, for example, contractile elements literally tug at the chromosomes to facilitate cell division.

Chemical Work

All cells perform chemical work for maintenance and growth. Continuous synthesis of cellular components takes place as other components break down. The extreme muscle tissue synthesis that occurs in response to chronic overload in resistance training vividly illustrates chemical work.

Transport Work

Cellular materials normally flow from an area of higher concentration to one of lower concentration. This passive process of **diffusion** does not require energy. However, to maintain proper physiologic functioning, certain chemicals require transport "uphill," against their normal concentration gradients from an area of lower to higher concentration. **Active transport** describes this energy-requiring process. Secretion and reabsorption in the kidney tubules use active transport mechanisms, as does neural tissue in establishing the proper electrochemical gradients about its plasma membranes. These "quiet" forms of biologic work require a continual expenditure of stored chemical energy.

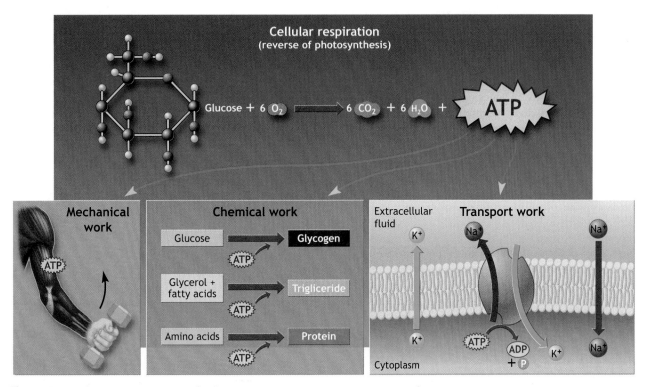

Figure 5.4. The exergonic process of cellular respiration. Exergonic reactions, such as the burning of gasoline or the oxidation of glucose, release potential energy. This results in a negative standard free energy change (i.e., reduction in total energy available for work; $-\Delta G$). In this illustration, cellular respiration harvests the potential energy in food to form ATP. Subsequently, the energy in ATP powers all forms of biologic work.

Questions & Notes

Describe the difference between kinetic and potential energy.

FACTORS AFFECTING BIOENERGETICS

The limits of exercise intensity ultimately depend on the rate that cells extract, conserve, and transfer the chemical energy in the food nutrients to the contractile filaments of skeletal muscle. *The sustained pace of the marathon runner at close to 90% of maximum aerobic capacity or the speed achieved by the sprinter in all-out exercise directly reflects the body's capacity to transfer chemical energy into mechanical work.* Enzymes and coenzymes significantly affect the rate of energy release during chemical reactions.

Complete the equation:

$H_2 + O \rightarrow$

Enzymes as Biological Catalysts

*An **enzyme**, a highly specific and large protein catalyst, accelerates the forward and reverse rates of chemical reactions within the body without being consumed or changed in the reaction.* Enzymes only govern reactions that would normally take place but at a much slower rate. Enzyme action takes place without altering the equilibrium constants and total energy released (free energy change or ΔG) in the reaction.

Enzymes possess the unique property of not being readily altered by the reactions they affect. Consequently, enzyme turnover in the body remains relatively low, and the specific enzymes are continually reused. A typical mitochondrion may contain up to 10 billion enzyme molecules, each carrying out millions of operations. During strenuous exercise, the rate of enzyme activity increases tremendously, as energy demands increase up to 100 times above resting levels. A single cell contains thousands of different enzymes, each with a specific function that

Give the major difference between photosynthesis and respiration.

catalyzes a distinct cellular reaction. For example, glucose breakdown to carbon dioxide and water requires 19 different chemical reactions, each catalyzed by its own specific enzyme. Enzymes contact precise locations on the surfaces of cell structures; they also operate within the structure itself. Many enzymes operate outside the cell—in the bloodstream, digestive mixture, or intestinal fluids.

Enzymes usually take the names of the functions they perform. The suffix *-ase* is usually appended to the enzyme whose prefix often indicates its mode of operation or the substance with which it interacts. For example, hydro*lase* adds water during hydrolysis reactions, prote*ase* interacts with protein, oxid*ase* adds oxygen to a substance, and ribonucle*ase* splits ribonucleic acid (RNA).

Reaction Rates   Enzymes do not all operate at the same rate; some operate slowly, and others operate much more rapidly. Consider the enzyme carbonic anhydrase, which catalyzes the hydration of carbon dioxide to form carbonic acid. Its maximum **turnover number**, which is the number of moles of substrate that react to form product per mole of enzyme per unit time, is 800,000. On the other hand, the turnover number for tryptophan synthetase, which catalyzes the final step in tryptophan synthesis, is 2. Enzymes often work cooperatively among their binding sites. While one substance "turns on" at a particular site, its neighbor "turns off" until the process completes. The operation then can reverse, with one enzyme becoming inactive and the other becoming active. pH and temperature dramatically affect enzyme activity. For some enzymes, peak activity requires relatively high acidity, while others function optimally on the alkaline side of neutrality.

Enzyme Mode of Action   How an enzyme interacts with its specific substrate represents a unique characteristic of an enzyme's three-dimensional globular protein structure. Interaction works much like a key fitting a lock. The enzyme "turns on" when its **active site** (usually a groove, cleft, or cavity on the protein's surface) joins in a "perfect fit" with the substrate's active site. Upon forming an **enzyme–substrate complex**, the splitting of chemical bonds forms a new product with new bonds, freeing the enzyme to act on additional substrate. This lock-and-key mechanism serves a protective function so only the correct enzyme activates a given substrate.

Coenzymes

Some enzymes remain totally dormant without activation by additional substances termed **coenzymes**. These complex nonprotein substances facilitate enzyme action by binding the substrate with its specific enzyme. Coenzymes then regenerate to assist in further similar reactions. The metallic ions iron and zinc play coenzyme roles, as do the B vitamins or their derivatives. Oxidation–reduction reactions use the B vitamins riboflavin and niacin, whereas other vitamins serve as transfer agents for groups of compounds in other metabolic processes. A coenzyme requires less specificity in its action than an enzyme because the coenzyme affects a number of different reactions. It either acts as a "cobinder" or serves as a temporary carrier of intermediary products in the reaction. For example, the coenzyme nicotinamide adenine dinucleotide (NAD^+) forms NADH in transporting hydrogen atoms and electrons that split from food fragments during energy metabolism.

SUMMARY

1. The first law of thermodynamics states that the body does not produce, consume, or use up energy; rather, it transforms it from one form into another as physiologic systems undergo continual change.

2. Potential energy and kinetic energy constitute the total energy of a system. Potential energy is the energy of position and/or form, while kinetic energy is the energy of motion. The release of potential energy transforms into kinetic energy of motion.

3. The term exergonic describes any physical or chemical process resulting in the release (freeing) of energy to its surroundings. Chemical processes that store or absorb energy are termed endergonic.

4. The second law of thermodynamics describes the tendency for potential energy to degrade to kinetic energy with a lower capacity to perform work.

5. The total energy in an isolated system remains constant; a decrease in one form of energy is matched by an equivalent increase in another form.

6. Biologic work takes one of three forms: mechanical work (work of muscle contraction); chemical work (synthesizing cellular molecules); and transport work (concentrating various substances in the intracellular and extracellular fluids).

7. An enzyme, a highly specific and large protein catalyst, accelerates the forward and reverse rates of chemical reactions within the body without being consumed or changed in the reaction.

8. Enzymes do not all operate at the same rate; some operate slowly, and others operate much more rapidly. Conditions of pH and temperature dramatically affect enzyme activity.

9. Coenzymes are nonprotein substances that facilitate enzyme action by binding the substrate with its specific enzyme.

THOUGHT QUESTIONS

1. Describe three examples of biologic processes involving energy transfer from one form to another.

2. From a metabolic perspective, why is the destruction of the rain forests throughout the world so bad for humans?

3. In terms of metabolism, why is body temperature maintained within a relatively narrow range?

PART 2 •
Phosphate-Bond Energy

The human body receives a continual supply of chemical energy to perform its many functions. Energy derived from food oxidation does not release suddenly at some kindling temperature because the body, unlike a mechanical engine, cannot use heat energy. Rather, complex, enzymatically controlled reactions within the relatively cool, watery medium of the cell extract the chemical energy trapped within the bonds of carbohydrate, fat, and protein molecules. This relatively slow extraction process reduces energy loss and enhances the efficiency of energy transformations. In this way, the body makes direct use of chemical energy for biologic work. In a sense, energy becomes available to the cells as needed. The body maintains a continuous energy supply through **adenosine triphosphate** or **ATP**, the special carrier for free energy.

ADENOSINE TRIPHOSPHATE: ENERGY CURRENCY

The energy in food does not transfer directly to cells for biologic work. Rather, the "macronutrient energy" releases and funnels through the energy-rich compound ATP to power cellular needs. **Figure 5.5** shows how an ATP molecule forms from a molecule of adenine and ribose (called adenosine), linked to three phosphate molecules. The bonds linking the two outermost phosphates, termed **high-energy bonds**, represent considerable stored energy.

A tight linkage (coupling) exists between the breakdown of the macronutrient energy molecules and ATP synthesis that "captures" a significant portion of the released energy. **Coupled reactions** occur in pairs; the breakdown of one compound provides energy for building another compound. To meet energy needs, ATP joins with water in the process of **hydrolysis**. This operation splits the outermost phosphate bond from the ATP molecule. The enzyme **adenosine triphosphatase** accelerates hydrolysis, forming a new compound **adenosine diphosphate** or **ADP**. These reactions, in turn, couple to other reactions that use the "freed" phosphate-bond chemical energy. The body uses ATP to transfer the energy produced during catabolic reactions to power reactions that synthesize new materials. In essence, this energy receiver–energy donor cycle represents the cells' two major energy-transforming activities:

Questions & Notes

Describe the major function of enzymes.

Give one example of an enzyme and one example of a coenzyme.

Enzyme –

Coenzyme –

Define hydrolysis.

In terms of energy use by the body, give the main difference between ATP and ADP.

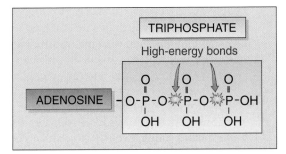

Figure 5.5. ATP, the energy currency of the cell. The starburst represents the high-energy bonds.

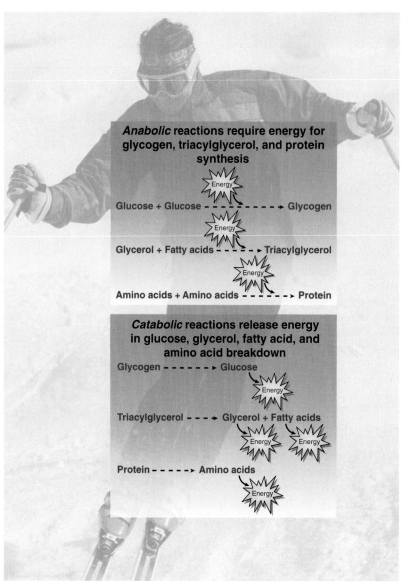

Anabolic reactions require energy for glycogen, triacylglycerol, and protein synthesis

Energy

Glucose + Glucose - - - - - - - - → Glycogen

Energy

Glycerol + Fatty acids - - - - - → Triacylglycerol

Energy

Amino acids + Amino acids - - - - - → Protein

Catabolic reactions release energy in glucose, glycerol, fatty acid, and amino acid breakdown

Glycogen - - - - - → Glucose

Energy

Triacylglycerol - - - → Glycerol + Fatty acids

Energy   Energy

Protein - - - - → Amino acids

Energy

Figure 5.6. Anabolic and catabolic reactions.

1. Form and conserve ATP from food's potential energy
2. Use energy extracted from ATP to power biologic work

Figure 5.6 illustrates examples of the anabolic and catabolic reactions that involve the coupled transfer of chemical energy. All of the energy released from catabolizing one compound does not dissipate as heat; rather, a portion becomes harvested and conserved within the chemical structure of the newly formed compound. ATP represents the common energy transfer "vehicle" in most coupled biologic reactions.

Anabolism requires energy for synthesizing new compounds. For example, many glucose molecules join together, much like the links in a chain of sausages, to form the larger more complex glycogen molecule; similarly, glycerol and fatty acids combine to make triacylglycerols, and amino acids link to form proteins. Each reaction starts with simple compounds and groups them as building blocks to form larger, more complex compounds.

Catabolic reactions release energy to form ATP. During this ATP process, adenosine triphosphatase catalyzes the reaction when ATP joins with water. For each mole of ATP degraded to ADP, the outermost phosphate bond splits and liberates approximately 7.3 kCal of **free energy**. This is the energy available for work.

$$ATP + H_2O \xrightarrow{\text{ATPase}} ADP + P_i - 7.3 \, kCal \, per \, mol$$

The free energy liberated in ATP hydrolysis reflects the energy difference between the reactant and end products. Because this reaction generates considerable energy, we refer to ATP as a **high-energy phosphate** compound. Some additional energy releases when another phosphate splits from ADP, but this infrequently occurs. In some reactions of biosynthesis, ATP donates its two terminal phosphates simultaneously to construct new cellular material. Adenosine monophosphate (AMP) becomes the new molecule with a single phosphate group.

The energy liberated during ATP breakdown directly transfers to other energy-requiring molecules. In muscle, this energy activates specific sites on the contractile elements causing muscle fibers to shorten. *Because energy from ATP powers all forms of biologic work, ATP constitutes the cell's "energy currency."* **Figure 5.7** illustrates the general role of ATP as energy currency.

The splitting of an ATP molecule takes place immediately and without oxygen. The cell's capability for ATP breakdown generates energy for rapid use; this would not occur if energy metabolism required oxygen at all times. Think of anaerobic energy release as a back-up power source that is called upon to deliver energy in excess of what can be generated aerobically. For this reason, any form of physical activity can take place immediately without instantaneously consuming oxygen; examples include sprinting for a bus, lifting a fork, driving a golf ball, spiking a volleyball, doing a pushup, or jumping up in the air. The well known practice of holding one's breath while sprint swimming provides a clear example of ATP splitting without reliance on atmospheric oxygen. Withholding air (oxygen), although not advisable, can be done during a 100-yard sprint on the track, lifting a barbell, a dash up several flights of stairs, or simply holding one's breath while rapidly flexing and extending the arms or fingers. In each case, energy metabolism proceeds uninterrupted because intramuscular anaerobic sources almost exclusively provide the energy to perform the activity.

ATP: A Limited Currency

A limited quantity of ATP serves as the energy currency for all cells. In fact, at any one time, the body stores only 80 to 100 g (3.5 oz) of ATP. This provides enough intramuscular stored energy for several seconds of explosive, all-out exercise. A limited quantity of "stored" ATP represents an additional advantage due to the molecule's heaviness. Biochemists estimate that a sedentary person each day uses an amount of ATP approximately equal to 75% of body mass. For an endurance athlete running a marathon race and generating 20 times the resting energy expenditure over 3 hours, total ATP usage could amount to 80 kg.

Because cells store only a small quantity of ATP, it must be resynthesized continually at its rate of use. This provides a biologically useful mechanism for regulating energy metabolism. By maintaining only a small amount of ATP, its relative concentration (and corresponding concentration of ADP) changes rapidly with any increase in a cell's energy demands. An ATP:ADP imbalance at the start of exercise immediately stimulates the breakdown of other stored energy-containing compounds to resynthesize ATP. As one might expect, increases in cellular en-

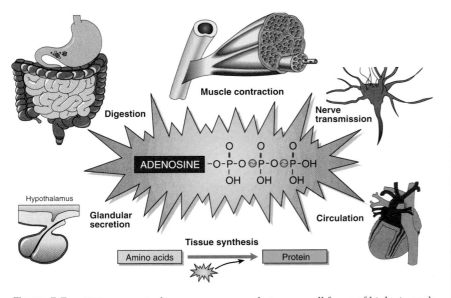

Figure 5.7. ATP represents the energy currency that powers all forms of biologic work.

ergy transfer depend on exercise intensity. Energy transfer increases about fourfold in the transition from sitting in a chair to walking. However, changing from a walk to an all-out sprint rapidly accelerates energy transfer rate about 120 times within active muscle. Generating significant energy output almost instantaneously demands ATP availability and a means for its rapid resynthesis.

PHOSPHOCREATINE: ENERGY RESERVOIR

Some energy for ATP resynthesis comes directly from the splitting (hydrolysis) of a phosphate from another intracellular high-energy phosphate compound—**phosphocreatine (PCr)** (also known as creatine phosphate or CP). PCr, similar to ATP, releases a large amount of energy when the bond splits between the creatine and phosphate molecules. The hydrolysis of PCr for energy begins at the onset of intense exercise, does not require oxygen, and reaches a maximum in about 8 to 12 seconds. Thus, PCr can be considered a "reservoir" of high-energy phosphate bonds. **Figure 5.8** illustrates the release and use of phosphate-bond energy in ATP and PCr. The term **high-energy phosphates** or **phosphagens** describes these two stored intramuscular compounds.

In both reactions, the arrows point in opposite directions to indicate reversible reactions. In other words, creatine (Cr) and inorganic phosphate (from ATP) can join again to reform PCr. This also holds true for ATP in which the union of ADP and P_i reforms ATP (see top part of figure). ATP resynthesis occurs if sufficient energy exists to rejoin an ADP molecule with one P_i molecule. The hydrolysis of PCr "fuels" this energy.

Cells store PCr in considerably larger quantities than ATP. Mobilization of PCr for energy takes place almost instantaneously and does not require oxygen. Interestingly, the concentration of ADP in the cell stimulates the activity level of **creatine kinase**, the enzyme that facilitates PCr

breakdown to Cr and ATP. This provides a crucial feedback mechanism for rapidly forming ATP from the high-energy phosphates. This latter reaction is known as the **creatine kinase reaction**.

The **adenylate kinase reaction** represents another single-enzyme–mediated reaction for ATP regeneration. The reaction uses two ADP molecules to produce one molecule of ATP and AMP as follows:

$$2\ ADP \xleftrightarrow{\text{adenylate kinase}} ATP + AMP$$

The creatine kinase and adenylate kinase reactions not only augment how well the muscles rapidly increase energy output (i.e., increase ATP availability), they also produce the molecular byproducts (AMP, P_i, ADP) that activate the initial stages of glycogen and glucose catabolism and the respiration pathways of the mitochondrion.

INTRAMUSCULAR HIGH-ENERGY PHOSPHATES

The energy released from ATP and PCr breakdown within muscle can sustain all-out running, cycling, or swimming for 5 to 8 seconds. In the 100-m sprint, for example, the body cannot maintain maximum speed for longer than this duration. During the last few seconds, runners actually slow down, with the winner slowing the least. From an energy perspective, the winner most effectively supplies and uses the limited but rapid supply of phosphate-bond energy.

In almost all sports, the energy transfer capacity of the ATP-PCr high-energy phosphates (**immediate energy system**) plays an important role in success or failure of some phase of performance. If all-out effort continues beyond about 8 seconds or if moderate exercise continues for much longer periods, ATP resynthesis requires an additional energy source. Without this additional ATP resynthesis, the "fuel" supply diminishes and high-intensity movement ceases. The foods we eat (and store) provide the energy to continually recharge cellular supplies of ATP and PCr.

Energy Source Important

Identifying the predominant source(s) of energy required for a particular sport or physical activity provides the basis for an effective exercise-training program. Football and baseball, for example, require a high-energy output for only brief periods. These performances rely almost exclusively on energy transfer from the intramuscular high-energy phosphates. Developing this rapid energy system becomes important when training to improve performance in movements of brief duration. Chapter 13 discusses specific training to optimize the power-output capacity of the different energy systems.

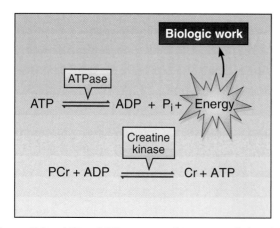

Figure 5.8.   ATP and PCr are anaerobic sources of phosphate-bond energy. The energy liberated from the hydrolysis (splitting) of PCr powers the union of ADP and P_i to reform ATP (the creatine kinase reaction).

Chemical Bonds Transfer Energy: Phosphorylation

Human energy dynamics involve transferring energy by chemical bonds. Bond splitting releases potential energy; energy conservation occurs by new bond formation. Some energy lost by one molecule transfers to the chemical structure of other molecules without appearing as heat. In the body, biologic work takes place when compounds relatively low in potential energy "juice-up" from the transfer of energy via high-energy phosphate bonds.

ATP serves as the ideal energy-transfer agent. In one respect, the phosphate bonds of ATP "trap" a large portion of the original food molecule's potential energy. ATP also readily transfers this energy to other compounds to raise them to a higher activation level. **Phosphorylation** refers to energy transfer through phosphate bonds.

CELLULAR OXIDATION

The energy for phosphorylation comes from **oxidation** ("biologic burning") of the carbohydrate, lipid, and protein macronutrients consumed in the diet. A molecule becomes **reduced** when it accepts electrons from an electron donor. In turn, the molecule that gives up the electron becomes **oxidized**.

Oxidation reactions (donating electrons) and **reduction reactions** (accepting electrons) remain coupled because every oxidation coincides with a reduction. *In essence, cellular oxidation–reduction constitutes the mechanism for energy metabolism.* The stored carbohydrate, fat, and protein molecules continually provide hydrogen atoms for this process. The complex but highly efficient **mitochondria**, the cell's "energy factories," contain carrier molecules that remove electrons from hydrogen (oxidation) and eventually pass them to oxygen (reduction). Synthesis of the high-energy phosphate ATP occurs during oxidation–reduction reactions.

Electron Transport

Figure 5.9 illustrates hydrogen oxidation and the accompanying electron transport to oxygen. During cellular oxidation, hydrogen atoms are not merely turned loose in the cell fluid. Rather, highly specific **dehydrogenase enzymes** catalyze hydrogen's release from the nutrient substrate. The coenzyme part of the dehydrogenase (usually the niacin-containing coenzyme, **nicotinamide adenine dinucleotide** or **NAD$^+$**) accepts pairs of electrons (energy) from hydrogen. While the substrate oxidizes and loses hydrogen (electrons), NAD$^+$ gains a hydrogen and

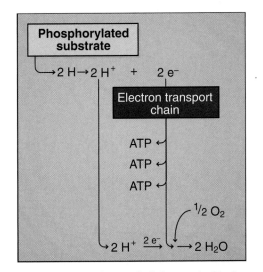

Figure 5.9. Oxidation (removal of electrons) of hydrogen and accompanying electron transport. In reduction, oxygen gains electrons and water forms.

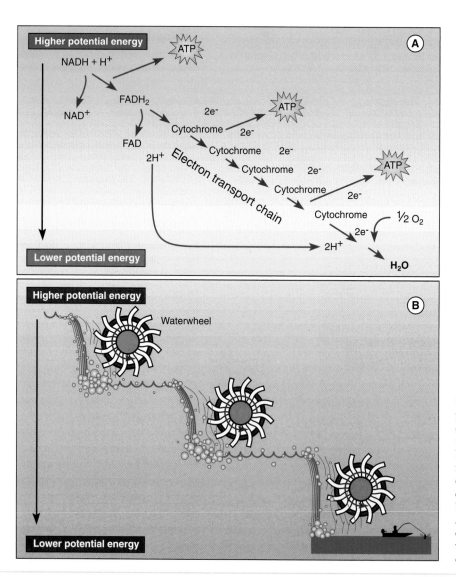

two electrons and reduces to NADH; the other hydrogen appears as H^+ in cell fluid.

The riboflavin-containing coenzyme **flavin adenine dinucleotide (FAD)** is the other important electron acceptor that oxidizes food fragments. FAD also catalyzes dehydrogenations and accepts pairs of electrons. Unlike NAD^+, however, FAD becomes $FADH_2$ by accepting both hydrogens. This distinct difference between NAD and FAD produces a different total number of ATP in the respiratory chain (see next section).

The NADH and $FADH_2$ formed in macronutrient breakdown represent energy-rich molecules because they carry electrons with a high-energy transfer potential. The cytochromes, a series of iron-protein electron carriers, then pass pairs of electrons carried by NADH and $FADH_2$ in "bucket brigade" fashion on the inner membranes of the mitochondria. The iron portion of each cytochrome exists in either its oxidized (ferric or Fe^{+++}) or reduced (ferrous or Fe^{++}) ionic state. By accepting an electron, the ferric portion of a specific cytochrome reduces to its ferrous form. In turn, ferrous iron donates its electron to the next cytochrome, and so on down the "bucket brigade." By shuttling between these two iron forms, the cytochromes transfer electrons to their ultimate destination where they reduce oxygen to form water. The NAD^+ and FAD then recycle for subsequent reuse in energy metabolism.

Electron transport by specific carrier molecules constitutes the **respiratory chain**, the final common pathway where electrons extracted from hydrogen pass to oxygen. *For each pair of hydrogen atoms, two electrons flow down the chain and reduce one atom of oxygen to form water.* Of the five specific cytochromes, only the last one, cytochrome oxidase (cytochrome aa₃ with a strong affinity for oxygen), discharges its electron directly to oxygen. **Figure 5.10A** shows the route for hydrogen oxidation, electron transport, and energy transfer in the respiratory chain. The respiratory chain releases free energy in relatively small amounts. In several of the electron transfers, energy conservation occurs by forming high-energy phosphate bonds.

Figure 5.10. Examples of harnessing potential energy. **A.** In the body. The electron transport chain removes electrons from hydrogens and ultimately delivers them to oxygen. In this oxidation-reduction process, much of the chemical energy stored within the hydrogen atom does not dissipate to kinetic energy. Rather, it becomes conserved in forming ATP. **B.** In industry. The captured energy from falling water drives the waterwheel, which in turn performs mechanical work.

Oxidative Phosphorylation

Oxidative phosphorylation refers to how ATP forms during electron transfer from NADH and $FADH_2$ to molecular oxygen. This crucial cellular metabolic process represents the cell's primary means for extracting and trapping chemical energy in the high-energy phosphates. *More than 90% of ATP synthesis takes place in the respiratory chain by oxidative reactions coupled with phosphorylation.*

Think of oxidative phosphorylation as a waterfall divided into several separate cascades by the waterwheels, which are located at different heights. Figure 5.10B depicts the waterwheels harnessing the energy of the falling water; similarly, electrochemical energy generated via electron transport in the respiratory chain becomes harnessed and transferred (or coupled) to ADP. The energy in NADH transfers to ADP to reform ATP at three distinct coupling sites during electron transport (Fig. 5.10A). Oxidation of hydrogen and subsequent phosphorylation occurs as follows:

$$NADH + H^+ + 3ADP + 3P_i + \frac{1}{2}O_2 \rightarrow NAD^+ + H_2O + 3ATP$$

Thus, three ATP form for each NADH plus H^+ oxidized. However, if $FADH_2$ originally donates hydrogen, only two molecules of ATP form for each hydrogen pair oxidized. This occurs because $FADH_2$ enters the respiratory chain at a lower energy level at a point beyond the site of the first ATP synthesis.

Efficiency of Electron Transport and Oxidative Phosphorylation

Each mole of ATP stores approximately 7 kCal of energy. Because 3 moles of ATP regenerate from oxidizing 1 mole of NADH, about 21 kCal (7 kCal per mole $\times$ 3) are conserved as chemical energy. A relative efficiency of 40% occurs for harnessing chemical energy via electron transport-oxidative phosphorylation because the oxidation of a mole of NADH liberates a total of 52 kCal (21 kCal $\div$ 52 kCal $\times$ 100). The remaining 60% of the energy dissipates from the body as heat. Considering that a steam engine transforms its fuel into useful energy at only about 30% efficiency, the value of 40% for the human body represents a remarkably high efficiency rate.

Role of Oxygen in Energy Metabolism

The continual resynthesis of ATP during coupled oxidative phosphorylation of the macronutrients has three prerequisites:

1. Availability of the reducing agents NADH or $FADH_2$
2. Presence of an oxidizing agent in the form of oxygen
3. Sufficient quantity of enzymes and metabolic machinery in the tissues to make the energy transfer reactions "go" at the appropriate rate

Satisfying these three conditions causes hydrogen and electrons to continually shuttle down the respiratory chain to molecular oxygen during food substrate catabolism. In strenuous exercise, inadequacy in oxygen delivery (prerequisite no. 2) or its rate of utilization (prerequisite no. 3) creates a relative imbalance between hydrogen release and oxygen's final acceptance of them. If either of these conditions occurs, electron flow down the respiratory chain "backs up," and hydrogens accumulate bound to NAD^+ and FAD. In essence, the temporarily "free" hydrogens require another molecule to bind with. In a subsequent section, we explain how lactate forms when the compound pyruvate temporarily binds these excess hydrogens (electrons); lactate formation allows electron transport-oxidative phosphorylation to proceed relatively unimpeded at the particular work intensity.

For aerobic metabolism, oxygen serves as the final electron acceptor in the respiratory chain and combines with hydrogen to form water during energy metabolism. Some might argue that the term aerobic metabolism is misleading because oxygen does not participate directly in ATP synthesis. Oxygen's presence at the "end of the line," however, largely determines one's capability for ATP production and ability to sustain high-intensity exercise. In this sense, the term aerobic seems justified.

Questions & Notes

Name the 2 specific coenzymes that catalyze hydrogen's release from nutrient substrates.

   1.

   2.

Fill-in:

For each pair of hydrogen atoms, _____ electrons flow down the respiratory chain and reduce _____ atoms of oxygen to form _____ .

Briefly describe oxidative phosphorylation.

Give the main function of oxygen in metabolism.

FOR YOUR INFORMATION

Free Radicals Formed During Aerobic Metabolism
The passage of electrons down the electron transport chain sometimes results in formation of free radicals, which are molecules that have an unpaired electron in their outer orbital making them highly reactive. These reactive, free radicals bind quickly to other molecules, resulting in potential damage to the combining molecule. Free radical formation in muscle, for example, might contribute to muscle fatigue or soreness or potential reduction in metabolic potential.

SUMMARY

1. Energy release occurs slowly in small amounts during complex, enzymatically controlled reactions, thus enabling more efficient energy transfer and conservation.

2. About 40% of the potential energy in food nutrients transfers to the high-energy compound ATP.

3. Splitting of ATP's terminal phosphate bond liberates free energy to power all biologic work.

4. ATP represents the body's energy currency, although its limited quantity amounts to only about 3.5 ounces.

5. Phosphocreatine (PCr) interacts with ADP to form ATP; this nonaerobic, high-energy reservoir replenishes ATP rapidly. Collectively, ATP and PCr are referred to as "high-energy phosphates."

6. Phosphorylation represents energy transfer in the form of energy-rich phosphate bonds. In this process, ADP and Cr continually recycle into ATP and PCr.

7. Cellular oxidation occurs on the inner lining of the mitochondrial membranes; it involves transferring electrons from NADH and $FADH_2$ to molecular oxygen. This releases and transfers chemical energy to form the union of ATP from ADP plus a phosphate ion.

8. During aerobic ATP resynthesis, oxygen (the final electron acceptor in the respiratory chain) combines with hydrogen to form water.

THOUGHT QUESTIONS

1. Based on the first law of thermodynamics, why is it imprecise to refer to energy "production" in the body?

2. Discuss the implications of the second law of thermodynamics for the measurement of energy expenditure.

3. Processing fat through the metabolic mill for energy requires some carbohydrate catabolism.

4. Aerobic breakdown of carbohydrate for energy occurs at about *twice* the rate as energy generated from fatty acid breakdown. Thus, depleting glycogen reserves significantly reduces exercise power output. In prolonged, high-intensity, aerobic exercise, such as marathon running, athletes often experience nutrient-related fatigue, a state associated with muscle and liver glycogen depletion.

PART 3 •
Energy Release From Food

The energy released in macronutrient breakdown serves one crucial purpose—to phosphorylate ADP to reform the energy-rich compound ATP (**Fig. 5.11**). Macronutrient catabolism favors generating phosphate-bond energy, yet the specific pathways of degradation differ depending on the nutrients metabolized. In the sections that follow, we show how ATP resynthesis occurs from extracting potential energy from food macronutrients.

ENERGY RELEASE FROM CARBOHYDRATE

Carbohydrates' primary function is to supply energy for cellular work. Our discussion of nutrient energy metabolism begins with carbohydrates for four reasons:

1. Carbohydrate represents the *only* macronutrient whose potential energy generates ATP anaerobically. This becomes important in vigorous exercise that requires rapid energy release above levels supplied by aerobic metabolic reactions.

2. During light and moderate aerobic exercise, carbohydrate supplies about one-half of the body's energy requirements.

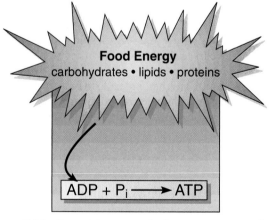

Figure 5.11 Potential energy in food powers ATP resynthesis.

The complete breakdown of one mole of glucose (180 g) to carbon dioxide and water yields a maximum of 686 kCal of chemical free energy available for work.

$$C_6H_{12}O_6 + 6O_2 \rightarrow 6CO_2 + 6H_2O + 686 \text{ kCal per mole}$$

In the body, glucose breakdown liberates the same quantity of energy, with a significant portion conserved as ATP. Synthesizing one mole of ATP from ADP and phosphate ion requires 7.3 kCal of energy. Therefore, coupling all of the energy from glucose oxidation to phosphorylation could theoretically form 94 moles of ATP per mole of glucose (686 kCal ÷ 7.3 kCal per mole = 94 moles). In the muscles, however, the phosphate bonds only conserve 38% or 263 kCal of energy, with the remainder dissipated as heat. This loss of energy represents the body's metabolic *inefficiency* for converting stored potential energy into useful energy. Consequently, glucose breakdown regenerates a net gain of 36 moles of ATP (net gain because 2 ATPs degrade to initiate glucose breakdown) per mole of glucose (263 kCal ÷ 7.3 kCal per mole = 36 ATP). An additional ATP forms if carbohydrate breakdown starts with glycogen. In the following sections, we describe ATP formation during energy transfer from carbohydrate, fat, and protein.

Anaerobic Versus Aerobic

Glucose degradation occurs in two stages. In stage 1, glucose breaks down rapidly into two molecules of pyruvate. Energy transfers occur without oxygen (anaerobic). In stage 2 of glucose catabolism, pyruvate degrades further to carbon dioxide and water. Energy transfer from these reactions requires electron transport and accompanying oxidative phosphorylation (aerobic).

Anaerobic Energy From Glucose: Glycolysis (Glucose Splitting)

The first stage of glucose degradation within cells involves a series of chemical reactions termed **glycolysis** (also termed the Embden-Meyerhoff pathway for its discoverers); **glycogenolysis** describes these reactions when they start with stored glycogen. These series of reactions, summarized in **Figure 5.12**, occur in the watery medium of the cell outside of the mitochondrion. In a way, glycolytic reactions represent a more primitive form of energy transfer that is well developed in amphibians, reptiles, fish, and marine mammals. In humans, the cells' limited capacity for glycolysis assumes a crucial role during physical activities that require maximal effort for up to 90 seconds in duration.

In the first reaction, ATP acts as a phosphate donor to phosphorylate glucose to **glucose 6-phosphate**. In most cells, this reaction "traps" the glucose molecule. In the presence of **glycogen synthase**, glucose can now link (become polymerized) with other glucose molecules to form glycogen. In energy metabolism, **glucose 6-phosphate** changes to **fructose 6-phosphate**. At this stage, no energy extraction occurs, yet energy incorporates into the original glucose molecule at the expense of one ATP molecule. In a sense, phosphorylation "primes the pump" for continued energy metabolism. The **fructose 6-phosphate** molecule gains an additional phosphate and changes to fructose 1, 6-diphosphate under control of **phosphofructokinase (PFK)**. The activity level of PFK probably places a limit on the rate of glycolysis during maximum-effort exercise. Fructose 1, 6-diphosphate then splits into two phosphorylated molecules with 3-carbon chains; these further decompose to **pyruvate** in five successive reactions.

Figure 5.13 shows an overview of the glucose-to-pyruvate sequence in terms of carbon atoms. Essentially, the 6-carbon glucose compound splits into two interchangeable 3-carbon compounds. This ultimately produces two 3-carbon pyruvate molecules and generates useful energy as ATP.

Questions & Notes

What is carbohydrate's major function in the body?

Complete the equation:

$C_6H_{12}O_6 + 6O_2 \rightarrow$

Give the number of kCals required to synthesize one mole of ATP from ADP and P_i.

Give the number of stages required for the complete breakdown of glucose in muscle.

Give the name of carbohydrate degradation when the starting substrate is stored glycogen.

_____ *describes the process of carbohydrate degradation when the starting substrate is stored glycogen.*

FOR YOUR INFORMATION

Carbohydrate Depletion Reduces Power Output

Carbohydrate depletion depresses work capacity (expressed as a percentage of maximum). Exercise capacity progressively decreases after 2 hours to 50% of the starting exercise intensity. Reduced power directly results from the slow rate of aerobic energy release from fat oxidation, which now becomes the major energy pathway.

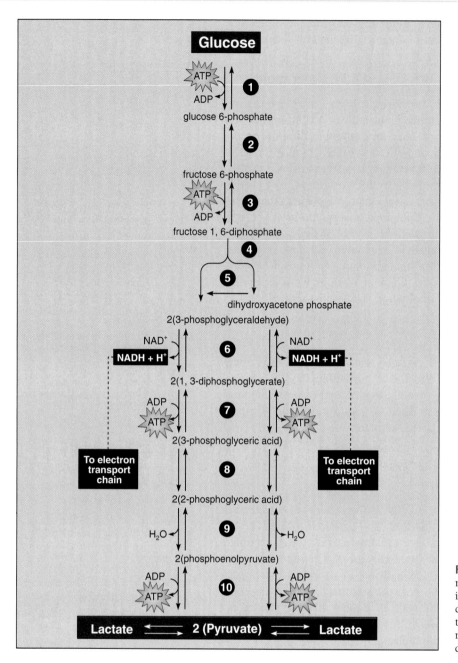

Figure 5.12. Glycolysis: Ten enzymatically controlled chemical reactions involve the anaerobic breakdown of glucose to two molecules of pyruvate. Lactate forms when NADH oxidation does not keep pace with its formation in glycolysis.

Substrate-Level Phosphorylation   Most of the energy generated in glycolysis does not resynthesize ATP but, instead, dissipates as heat. In reactions 7 and 10 in Figure 5.12, however, the energy released from the glucose intermediates stimulates the direct transfer of phosphate groups to ADPs, generating four molecules of ATP. Because two molecules of ATP were lost in the initial phosphorylation of the glucose molecule, glycolysis generates a *net gain* of two ATP molecules. Note that these specific energy transfers from substrate to ADP do not require molecular oxygen. Rather, energy directly transfers via phosphate bonds in the anaerobic reactions called **substrate-level phosphorylation**. Energy conservation during glycolysis operates at an efficiency of about 30%.

Glycolysis accounts only for about 5% of the total ATP generated during the glucose molecule's complete breakdown. However, due to the high concentration of glycolytic enzymes and the speed of the glycolytic reactions, significant energy for muscle action occurs rapidly during this process. The following represent examples of activities that rely heavily on ATP generated via glycolytic anaerobic reactions: sprinting at the end of the mile run, swimming all-out from start to finish in the 50- and 100-m swim, routines on gymnastics apparatus, and sprint-running races up to 200 meters. Anaerobic energy transfer from the macronutrients occurs *only* from carbohydrate breakdown during glycolytic reactions.

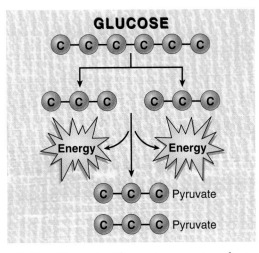

Figure 5.13. Glycolysis: Glucose-to-pyruvate pathway. A 6-carbon glucose splits into two 3-carbon compounds, which further degrade into two 3-carbon pyruvate molecules. Glucose splitting occurs under anaerobic conditions in the watery medium of the cell.

Questions & Notes

Give the efficiency of energy conservation during glycolysis.

Give the percentage of energy stored within ATP molecules compared to the total energy released during glycolysis.

Give 2 examples of activity that rely heavily on ATP generated via glycolytic anaerobic reactions.

1.

2.

The total (net and gross) number of ATP molecules generated in glycolysis is:

Net –

Gross –

Hydrogen Release in Glycolysis During glycolysis, two pairs of hydrogen atoms are stripped from the substrate (glucose), and their electrons are passed to NAD^+ to form NADH (see Fig. 5.12). Normally, if the respiratory chain processed these electrons directly, three molecules of ATP would generate for each molecule of NADH oxidized. The mitochondrion in skeletal muscle remains impermeable to NADH formed in the cytoplasm during glycolysis. Consequently, the electrons from extramitochondrial NADH shuttle indirectly into the mitochondria. In skeletal muscle, this route ends with electrons passing to FAD to form $FADH_2$ at a point below the first ATP formation (see Fig. 5.10A). Thus two, rather than three, ATP molecules form when the respiratory chain oxidizes cytoplasmic NADH. Because two molecules of NADH form in glycolysis, subsequent electron transport-oxidative phosphorylation aerobically generates four ATP molecules.

Lactate Formation Sufficient oxygen bathes the cells during light to moderate levels of energy metabolism. The hydrogens (electrons) stripped from the substrate and carried by NADH oxidize within the mitochondria to form water when they join with oxygen. In a biochemical sense, a "steady rate" exists because hydrogen oxidizes at about the same rate it becomes available. Biochemists frequently refer to this condition as **aerobic glycolysis**, with pyruvate as the end-product.

In strenuous exercise, when energy demands exceed either oxygen supply or utilization rate, the respiratory chain cannot process all of the hydrogen joined to NADH. Continued release of anaerobic energy in glycolysis depends on NAD^+ availability for oxidizing 3-phosphoglyceraldehyde (see reaction 6 in Fig. 5.12); otherwise, the rapid rate of glycolysis "grinds to a halt." In **anaerobic glycolysis**, NAD^+ "frees-up" as pairs of "excess" non-oxidized hydrogens combine temporarily with pyruvate to form lactate, catalyzed by the enzyme lactate dehydrogenase in the reversible reaction shown in **Figure 5.14**.

The temporary storage of hydrogen with pyruvate represents a unique aspect of energy metabolism because it provides a ready "storage bin" to temporarily bind the end products of anaerobic glycolysis. Once lactate forms within muscle, it diffuses rapidly into the blood for buffering and rapid removal from the site of energy metabolism. This allows glycolysis to continue supplying additional anaerobic energy for ATP resynthesis. However, this avenue for extra energy remains temporary; muscle and blood lactate levels increase, and ATP regeneration

FOR YOUR INFORMATION

Glucose not Retrievable from Fatty Acids
Cells can synthesize glucose from pyruvate and other 3-carbon compounds. However, glucose cannot form from the 2-carbon acetyl fragments of the β–oxidation of fatty acids. Consequently, fatty acids cannot readily provide energy for tissues that use glucose almost exclusively for fuel (e.g., brain and nerve tissues). Just about all dietary lipid occurs in triacylglycerol form. Triacylglycerol's glycerol component can yield glucose, but the glycerol molecule contains only 3 (6%) of the 57 carbon atoms in the molecule. Thus, fat from dietary sources or stored in adipocytes does not provide an adequate potential glucose source; about 95% of the fat molecule *cannot* be converted to glucose.

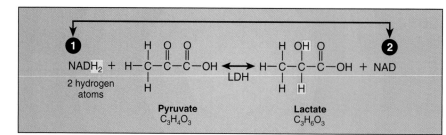

Figure 5.14. Lactate forms when excess hydrogens from NADH combine temporarily with pyruvate. This frees up NAD^+ to accept additional hydrogens generated in glycolysis. LDH = lactate dehydrogenase.

cannot keep pace with its utilization rate. Fatigue soon sets in, and exercise performance diminishes. Increased acidity probably mediates the fatigue process by inactivating various enzymes involved in energy transfer and diminishing some aspect of the muscle's contractile properties.

During rest, some lactate continually forms from the energy metabolism of red blood cells because these cells contain no mitochondria and must obtain their energy from anaerobic glycolysis. This lactate and the lactate that accumulates in intense exercise should not be viewed as a metabolic "waste product." To the contrary, it represents a valuable source of chemical energy. When sufficient oxygen once again becomes available during recovery or when exercise pace slows, NAD^+ scavenges hydrogens attached to lactate; these hydrogens subsequently oxidize to form ATP. In this regard, circulating blood lactate becomes an energy source because it readily reconverts to pyruvate for further catabolism. In addition, the liver's Cori cycle (**Fig. 5.15**) conserves the potential energy in lactate and pyruvate molecules by synthesizing their carbon skeletons to glucose and, subsequently, muscle glycogen (gluconeogenesis). This pathway progresses as follows:

Muscle glycogen → Glucose → Pyruvate →
Lactate (which travels to the liver) →
Glucose (which returns to muscle) →
Muscle glycogen

Aerobic Energy From Glucose: Citric Acid Cycle

The anaerobic reactions of glycolysis release only about 10% of the energy within the original glucose molecule; thus, extracting the remaining energy requires an additional metabolic pathway. This occurs when pyruvate irreversibly converts to acetyl–CoA, a form of acetic acid. Acetyl–CoA enters the second stage of carbohydrate breakdown known as the **citric acid cycle** (sometimes also termed Krebs cycle and tricarboxylic acid cycle).

Figure 5.16 shows the pyruvate-to-acetyl–CoA reactions. Each 3-carbon pyruvate molecule loses a carbon when it joins with a CoA molecule to form acetyl–CoA and carbon dioxide. The reaction from pyruvate proceeds in one direction only.

Figure 5.17 illustrates that the citric acid cycle within the mitochondria degrades the acetyl–CoA substrate to carbon dioxide and hydrogen atoms. Hydrogen atoms oxidize during electron transport-oxidative phosphorylation that regenerates ATP.

Figure 5.18 shows pyruvate preparing to enter the citric acid cycle by joining with the vitamin B-derivative coenzyme A (A stands for acetic acid) to form the 2-carbon compound acetyl–CoA. This process releases two hydrogens and transfers their electrons to NAD^+, forming one molecule of carbon dioxide as follows:

$$Pyruvate + NAD^+ + CoA \rightarrow Acetyl\text{–}CoA + CO_2 + NADH + H^+$$

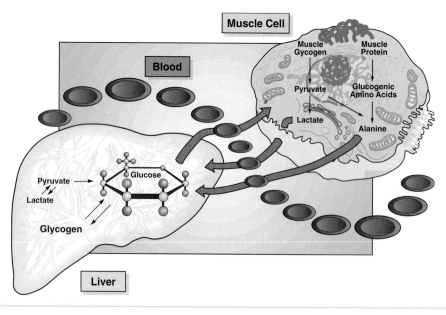

Figure 5.15. The Cori cycle in the liver synthesizes glucose from lactate released from active muscle. This gluconeogenic process maintains carbohydrate reserves.

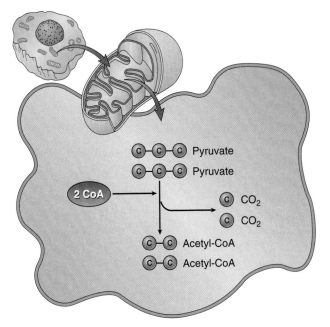

Figure 5.16. One-way reaction of pyruvate to acetyl–CoA. Two 3-carbon pyruvate molecules join with two coenzyme A molecules to form two 2-carbon acetyl–CoA molecules with 2 carbons lost as carbon dioxide.

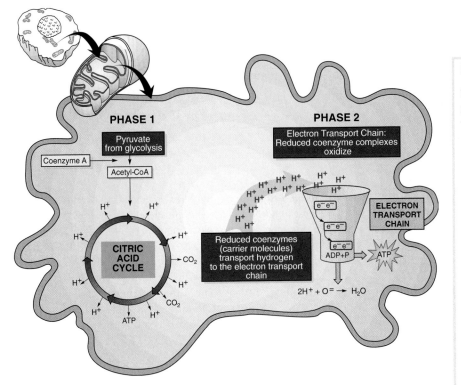

Figure 5.17. **Phase 1.** In the mitochondrion, citric acid cycle activity generates hydrogen atoms in acetyl–CoA breakdown. **Phase 2.** Significant ATP regenerates when hydrogens oxidize via the aerobic process of electron transport-oxidative phosphorylation (electron transport chain).

Questions & Notes

In what tissue does the Cori cycle function?

Name an end-product of the Cori cycle.

Give the major function of the citric acid cycle.

FOR YOUR INFORMATION

Fat-Burning Adaptations Within Skeletal Muscle with Aerobic Training

1. Facilitated rate of lipolysis and re-esterification within adipocytes
2. Capillary proliferation in trained muscle creates a greater total number and density of these microvessels
3. Improved free fatty acid transport through the plasma membrane of the muscle fiber
4. Augmented fatty acid transport within the muscle cell by carnitine and carnitine acyl transferase
5. Increased size and number of mitochondria
6. Increased quantity of enzymes involved in β–oxidation, critic acid cycle metabolism, and the electron-transport chain within specifically trained muscle fibers

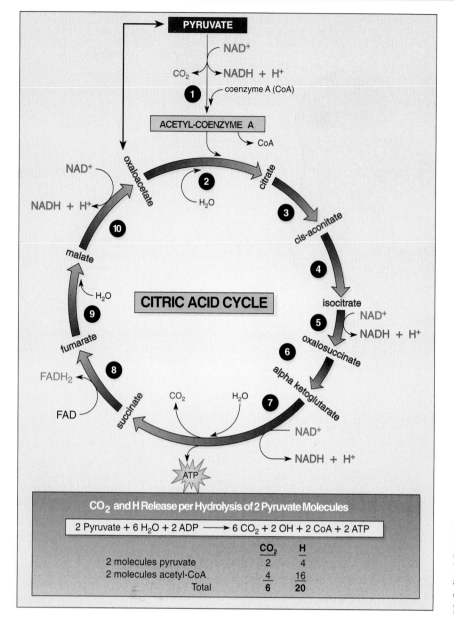

Figure 5.18. Release of H and CO_2 in the mitochondrion during breakdown of one pyruvate molecule. All values double when computing the net gain of H and CO_2 from pyruvate breakdown because glycolysis forms two molecules of pyruvate from one glucose molecule.

The acetyl portion of acetyl–CoA joins with oxaloacetate to form citrate (citric acid—the same 6-carbon compound found in citrus fruits) before proceeding through the citric acid cycle. The citric acid cycle continues to operate because it retains the original oxaloacetate molecule to join with a new acetyl fragment.

For each acetyl–CoA molecule entering the citric acid cycle, the substrate releases two carbon dioxide molecules and four pairs of hydrogen atoms. One molecule of ATP also regenerates directly by substrate-level phosphorylation from citric acid cycle reactions (see reaction 7 in Fig. 5.18). Note from the bottom of Figure 5.18 that four hydrogens release when acetyl–CoA forms from the two pyruvate molecules created in glycolysis, with an additional 16 hydrogens released in the citric acid cycle (acetyl–CoA hydrolysis). *Generating electrons for passage*

to the respiratory chain via NAD^+ and FAD represents the most important function of the citric acid cycle.

Oxygen does not participate directly in citric acid cycle reactions. However, the aerobic process of electron transport-oxidative phosphorylation transfers a considerable portion of the chemical energy in pyruvate to ADP. With adequate oxygen, including enzymes and substrate, NAD^+ and FAD regeneration takes place allowing citric acid cycle metabolism to proceed unimpeded.

Net Energy Transfer From Glucose Catabolism

Figure 5.19 summarizes the pathways for energy transfer during glucose breakdown in skeletal muscle. Two ATP

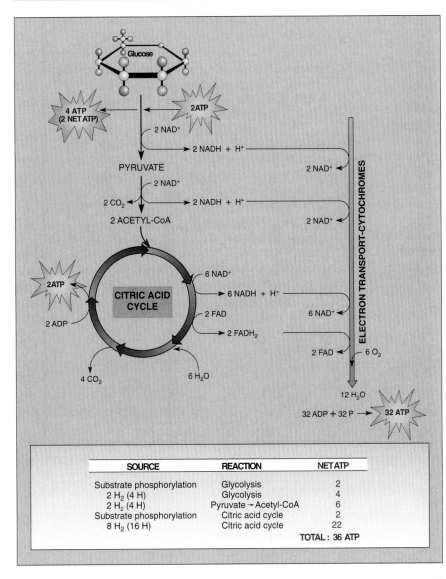

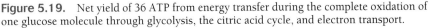

SOURCE	REACTION	NET ATP
Substrate phosphorylation	Glycolysis	2
2 H₂ (4 H)	Glycolysis	4
2 H₂ (4 H)	Pyruvate → Acetyl-CoA	6
Substrate phosphorylation	Citric acid cycle	2
8 H₂ (16 H)	Citric acid cycle	22
	TOTAL : 36 ATP	

Figure 5.19. Net yield of 36 ATP from energy transfer during the complete oxidation of one glucose molecule through glycolysis, the citric acid cycle, and electron transport.

molecules (net gain) form from substrate-level phosphorylation in glycolysis; similarly, two ATP molecules come from acetyl–CoA degradation in the citric acid cycle. The 24 released hydrogen atoms (and their subsequent oxidation) can be accounted for as follows:

1. Four extramitochondrial hydrogens (2 NADH) generated in glycolysis yield 4 ATP (6 ATP in heart, kidney, and liver)
2. Four hydrogens (2 NADH) released as pyruvate degrade to acetyl–CoA to yield 6 ATP
3. Twelve of the 16 hydrogens (6 NADH) released in the citric acid cycle yield 18 ATP
4. Four hydrogens joined to FAD (2 FADH₂) in the citric acid cycle yield 4 ATP

Thirty-eight ATP represent the total ATP yield from the complete breakdown of one glucose molecule. However, because 2 ATP initially phosphorylate glucose, 36 ATP molecules represent the *net ATP yield* from complete glucose breakdown in skeletal muscle. Four ATP molecules form directly from substrate-level phosphorylation (glycolysis and citric acid cycle). In contrast, 32 ATP molecules regenerate during oxidative phosphorylation. In Chapter 6, we explain the specifics of carbo-

Questions & Notes

True or False:

Oxygen directly participates in citric acid cycle reactions.

Give the net ATP yield from energy transfer during the complete oxidation of one glucose molecule.

Give the number of ATP generated via direct substrate phosphorylation.

FOR YOUR INFORMATION

Exercise Intensity and Duration Affect Fat Oxidation
On a relative basis, considerable fatty acid oxidation occurs during low-intensity exercise. For example, fat combustion almost totally powers exercise at 25% of aerobic capacity. Carbohydrate and fat contribute energy equally during moderate intensity exercise. Fat oxidation gradually increases as exercise extends to an hour or more and glycogen depletes. Toward the end of prolonged exercise (with glycogen reserves low), circulating free fatty acids supply nearly 80% of the total energy required.

FOR YOUR INFORMATION

Protein Breakdown Facilitates Water Loss
When protein provides energy, the body must eliminate the nitrogen-containing amine group (and other solutes produced from protein breakdown). This requires excretion of "obligatory" water because waste products from protein catabolism leave the body dissolved in fluid (urine). For this reason, excessive protein catabolism increases the body's fluid needs.

hydrate's role in energy release under anaerobic and aerobic exercise conditions.

ENERGY RELEASE FROM FAT

Stored fat represents the body's most plentiful source of potential energy. Relative to carbohydrate and protein, stored fat provides almost unlimited energy. The fuel reserves in an average young adult male represent between 60,000 and 100,000 kCal of energy from triacylglycerol in fat cells (adipocytes) and about 3000 kCal from intramuscular triacylglycerol stored in close proximity to muscle mitochondria. In contrast, the carbohydrate energy reserve only contributes about 2000 kCal.

Before energy release from fat, hydrolysis (**lipolysis**) splits the triacylglycerol molecule into glycerol and three water-insoluble fatty acid molecules. The enzyme *lipase* catalyzes triacylglycerol breakdown as follows:

$$\text{Triacylglycerol} + 3H_2O \xrightarrow{\text{Lipase}} \text{Glycerol} + 3 \text{ Fatty acids}$$

Adipocytes: Site of Fat Storage and Mobilization

All cells store some fat, but adipose tissue represents an active and major supplier of fatty acid molecules.

Adipocytes synthesize and store triglycerides. Triacylglycerol fat droplets occupy up to 95% of the adipocyte cell's volume. Once fatty acids diffuse from the adipocyte and enter the circulation, nearly all bind to plasma albumin for transport to diverse tissues as **free fatty acids (FFA)**. Fat utilization as an energy substrate varies closely with blood flow in the active tissue. As blood flow increases with exercise, adipose tissue releases more FFA to active muscle for energy metabolism. The activity level of **lipoprotein lipase (LPL)** facilitates the local cells' uptake of fatty acids for (1) energy use or (2) resynthesis (re-esterification) of stored triacylglycerol (in muscle and adipose tissue).

FFA do not exist as truly "free" entities. At the muscle site, FFA releases from the albumin–FFA complex to move across the plasma membrane. Once inside the muscle cell, FFA either esterify to form intracellular triacylglycerol or they bind with intramuscular proteins to enter the mitochondria for energy metabolism. Medium- and short-chain fatty acids do not depend on this carrier-mediated means of transport; most diffuse freely into the mitochondrion.

Breakdown of Glycerol and Fatty Acids

Figure 5.20 summarizes the pathways for the breakdown of the triacylglycerol molecule's glycerol and fatty acid components.

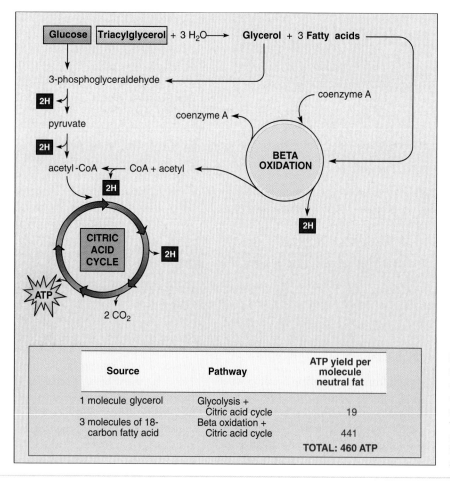

Source	Pathway	ATP yield per molecule neutral fat
1 molecule glycerol	Glycolysis + Citric acid cycle	19
3 molecules of 18-carbon fatty acid	Beta oxidation + Citric acid cycle	441
		TOTAL: 460 ATP

Figure 5.20. Breakdown of glycerol and fatty acid fragments of a triacylglycerol molecule. Glycerol enters the energy pathways of glycolysis. The fatty acid fragments enter the citric acid cycle via β–oxidation. The electron transport chain processes the released hydrogens from glycolysis, β–oxidation, and citric acid cycle metabolism to yield ATP.

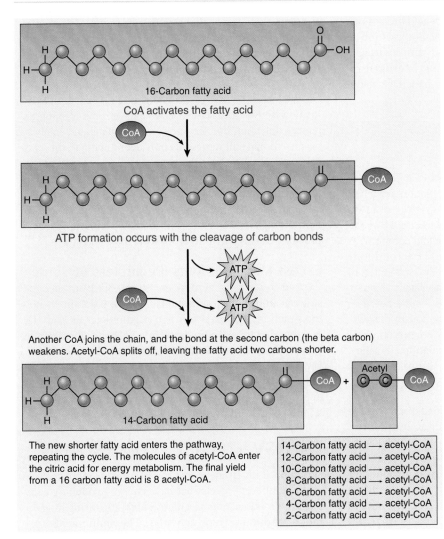

Figure 5.21. β–oxidation of a typical 16-carbon fatty acid. Fatty acids break down to 2-carbon fragments that combine with CoA to form acetyl–CoA.

Complete the equation:

$Triacylglycerol + 3\ H_2O \rightarrow$

Give the total ATP yield from the breakdown of one triacylglycerol (neural fat) molecule.

Give the major function of β-oxidation.

Under what condition does gluconeogenesis predominate?

Glycerol The anaerobic reactions of glycolysis accept glycerol as 3–phosphoglyceraldehyde, which then degrades to pyruvate to form ATP by substrate-level phosphorylation. Hydrogen atoms pass to NAD^+, and the citric acid cycle oxidizes pyruvate. The complete breakdown of the single glycerol molecule in a triacylglycerol synthesizes 19 ATP molecules. Glycerol also provides carbon skeletons for glucose synthesis. *The gluconeogenic role of glycerol becomes prominent when glycogen reserves deplete due to dietary restriction of carbohydrates or extended-duration exercise or intense training.*

Fatty Acids The fatty acid molecule transforms to acetyl–CoA in the mitochondrion during β–oxidation reactions (**Fig. 5.21**). This involves the successive release of 2-carbon acetyl fragments split from the fatty acid's long chain. ATP phosphorylates the reactions, water is added, hydrogens pass to NAD^+ and FAD, and acetyl-CoA forms when the acetyl fragment joins with coenzyme A. *This acetyl unit is the same one generated from glucose breakdown.* β–oxidation continues until the entire fatty acid molecule degrades to acetyl-CoAs that directly enter the citric acid cycle. Hydrogen released during fatty acid catabolism oxidizes

FOR YOUR INFORMATION

Excess Protein Accumulates Fat
Athletes and others who believe that taking protein supplements builds muscle beware. Extra protein consumed above the body's requirement (easily achieved with a well-balanced "normal" diet) ends up either catabolized for energy or converted to body fat! If an athlete wants to add fat, excessive protein intake achieves this end; this excess will not contribute to muscle tissue synthesis.

through the respiratory chain. Thus, fatty acid breakdown relates directly with oxygen uptake. For β–oxidation to proceed, oxygen must be present to join with hydrogen. Without oxygen (anaerobic conditions), hydrogen remains joined with NAD$^+$ and FAD and halts fat catabolism.

Total Energy Transfer From Fat Catabolism

For each 18-carbon fatty acid molecule, 147 molecules of ADP phosphorylate to ATP during β–oxidation and citric acid cycle metabolism. Because each triacylglycerol molecule contains three fatty acid molecules, 441 ATP molecules form from the triacylglycerol's fatty acid components (3 × 147 ATP). Also, 19 molecules of ATP form during glycerol breakdown, generating a total of 460 molecules of ATP for each triacylglycerol molecule catabolized. This represents a considerable energy yield because only a net of 36 ATP form during a glucose molecule's catabolism in skeletal muscle. The 40% efficiency of energy conservation for fatty acid oxidation duplicates glucose oxidation efficiency.

Fats Burn in a Carbohydrate Flame

Interestingly, fatty acid breakdown depends in part on a continual background level of carbohydrate breakdown. Recall that acetyl–CoA enters the citric acid cycle by combining with oxaloacetate to form citrate (see Fig. 5.18). Depleting carbohydrate decreases pyruvate production during glycolysis. Diminished pyruvate further reduces citric acid cycle intermediates, slowing citric acid cycle activity. Fatty acid degradation in the citric acid cycle depends on sufficient oxaloacetate availability to combine with the acetyl–CoA formed during β–oxidation (see Fig. 5.21). When carbohydrate level decreases, the oxaloacetate level may become inadequate, reducing fat catabolism. In this sense, *"fats burn in a carbohydrate flame."*

Metabolism Under Low-Carbohydrate Conditions Oxaloacetate converts to pyruvate (see Fig. 5.18; note two-way arrow), which can then be synthesized to glucose, when carbohydrates are inadequate (perhaps from fasting, prolonged exercise, or diabetes) and unavailable to combine with acetyl–CoA to form citrate. The liver converts the acetyl–CoA derived from the fatty acids into metabolites called *ketones*, or ketone bodies, which are strong acids. (Do not confuse ketones with keto acids, pyruvic acid, and other citric acid cycle intermediates.) The three major ketone bodies are acetoacetic acid, beta-hydroxybutryric acid, and acetone. Ketones are used as fuel primarily by muscles and, to a more limited extent, by tissues of the nervous system. If ketones are not catabolized, but instead accumulate in the central circulation, a condition called **ketosis** results. The high acidity of ketosis disrupts normal physiologic function, especially acid-base balance, which can ultimately be dangerous. Ketosis generally results more from an inadequate diet (as in

anorexia nervosa) or diabetes than from prolonged exercise, since muscle uses ketones as a fuel. During exercise, aerobically trained individuals use ketones more effectively than untrained individuals.

Slower Energy Release From Fat A rate limit exists for how active muscles use fatty acid. Aerobic training enhances this limit, but the rate of energy generated solely by fat breakdown still represents only about one-half the value achieved with carbohydrate as the chief aerobic energy source. Thus, depleting muscle glycogen decreases the intensity that a muscle can sustain aerobic power output. Just as the hypoglycemic condition coincides with a "central" or neural fatigue, exercising with depleted muscle glycogen probably causes "peripheral" or local muscle fatigue.

Excess Macronutrients (Regardless of Source) Convert to Fat Excess energy intake from any fuel source can be counterproductive. **Figure 5.22** shows how too much of any macronutrient accumulates as body fat. Surplus dietary carbohydrate first fills the glycogen reserves. Once these reserves fill, excess carbohydrate converts to triacylglycerols for storage in adipose tissue. Excess dietary fat calories move easily into the body's fat deposits. Once deaminated, the carbon residues of excess amino acids from protein readily convert to fat.

ENERGY RELEASE FROM PROTEIN

Figure 5.23 illustrates how protein supplies intermediates at three different levels that have energy-producing capabilities. Protein acts as an energy substrate during long duration, endurance-type activities. The amino acids (primarily the branched-chain amino acids leucine, isoleucine, valine, glutamine, and aspartic acid) first convert to a form that readily enters pathways for energy release. This conversion requires removing nitrogen from the amino acid molecule, a process known as deamination. The liver serves as the main site for deamination. However, skeletal muscle also contains enzymes that remove nitrogen from an amino acid and pass it to other compounds during transamination (removal of nitrogen; usually occurs when an amine group from a donor amino acid transfers to an acceptor acid from a new amino acid). In this way, the muscle directly uses for energy the carbon skeleton byproducts of donor amino acids. Enzyme levels for transamination favorably adapt to exercise training; this may further facilitate protein's use as an energy substrate. Only when an amino acid loses its nitrogen-containing amine group does the remaining compound (usually one of the citric acid cycle's reactive compounds) contribute to ATP formation. Some amino acids are glucogenic; when deaminated, they yield intermediate products for glucose synthesis via gluconeogenesis. In the liver, for example, pyruvate forms when alanine loses its amino group and gains a double-bond oxygen; this allows glucose synthesis from pyruvate. This **gluconeogenic** method is an important adjunct to the Cori cycle for providing

Box 5–2 • CLOSE UP

HOW TO ESTIMATE INDIVIDUAL PROTEIN REQUIREMENT

Total body protein remains constant when nitrogen intake from protein in food balances its excretion in feces, urine, and sweat. An imbalance in the body's nitrogen content provides (1) an accurate estimate of either protein's depletion or accumulation and (2) a measure of the adequacy of dietary protein intake. Evaluating nitrogen balance can estimate human protein requirements under various conditions, including intense exercise training.

The magnitude and direction of nitrogen balance in individuals engaged in exercise training depends on many factors including training status, quality and quantity of protein consumed, total energy intake, the body's glycogen levels, and intensity, duration, and type of exercise performed.

MEASURING NITROGEN BALANCE

Nitrogen Intake. Estimate protein intake (g) by carefully measuring total food consumed over a 24-hour period. Determine nitrogen quantity (g) by assuming protein contains 16% nitrogen. Then:

Total Nitrogen Intake, g = Total Protein

Intake, g × 0.16

Nitrogen Output. Researchers determine nitrogen output by collecting all of the nitrogen excreted over the same period that assessed nitrogen intake. This involves collecting nitrogen loss from urine, lungs, sweat, and feces. A simplified method estimates nitrogen output by measuring urinary urea nitrogen (UUN; plus 4 g to account for other sources of nitrogen loss):

Total Nitrogen Output = UUN + 4 g

EXAMPLE

Male: age, 22 y; total body mass, 75 kg; total energy intake (food diary), 2100 kCal; protein intake (food diary), 63 g; UUN (collection and analysis of urine output), 8 g.

$$\text{Nitrogen Balance} = \text{Nitrogen Intake, g}$$
$$- \text{Nitrogen Output, g}$$
$$= (63 \text{ g} \times 0.16)$$
$$- (8 \text{ g} + 4 \text{ g})$$
$$= -1.92 \text{ g}$$

This example shows that a daily negative nitrogen balance of −1.92 g occurred because protein catabolized in metabolism exceeded its replacement through dietary protein. To correct this deficiency and achieve nitrogen (protein) balance, the person would need to increase daily protein intake.

ESTIMATED DAILY PROTEIN NEEDS	
Condition	Protein Needs (g protein·kg body mass⁻¹)
Normal, healthy	0.8–1.0
Fever, fracture, infection	1.5–2.0
Protein depleted	1.5–2.0
Extensive burns	1.5–3.0
Intensive training	0.8–1.5

ESTIMATING INDIVIDUAL PROTEIN REQUIREMENTS

The table above estimates average protein needs under different conditions. For a healthy person who weighs 70 kg, the protein requirement equals 56 g.

$$0.8 \text{ g·kg}^{-1} \times 70 \text{ kg} = 56 \text{ g}$$

The same person with a chronic infection or in a protein-depleted state would require an upper-range estimate of 140 g of protein daily.

$$2.0 \text{ g·kg}^{-1} \times 70 \text{ kg} = 140 \text{ g}$$

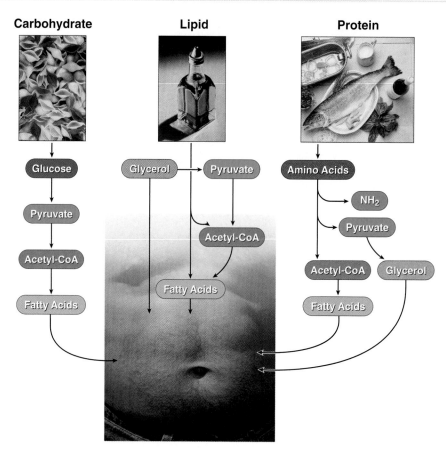

Figure 5.22.   Metabolic fate of macronutrient energy surplus.

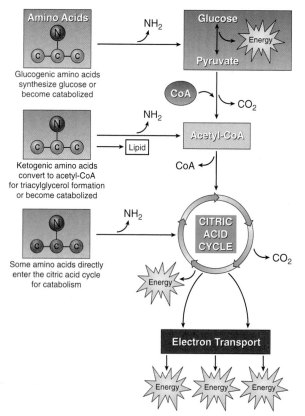

Figure 5.23.   Protein-to-energy pathways.

glucose during prolonged exercise that depletes glycogen reserves. Like fat and carbohydrate, certain amino acids are **ketogenic**; they cannot synthesize to glucose, but instead when consumed in excess, they synthesize to fat.

THE METABOLIC MILL

The "metabolic mill" illustrated in **Figure 5.24** depicts the citric acid cycle as the essential "connector" between macronutrient energy and the chemical energy of ATP. The citric acid cycle plays a much more important role than simply degrading pyruvate produced during glucose catabolism. Fragments from other organic compounds formed from fat and protein breakdown provide energy during citric acid cycle metabolism. Deaminated residues of excess amino acids enter the citric acid cycle at various intermediate stages. In contrast, the glycerol fragment of triacylglycerol catabolism gains entrance via the glycolytic pathway. Fatty acids become oxidized via β–oxidation to acetyl–CoA, which then enters the citric acid cycle directly.

In addition to its role in energy metabolism, the citric acid cycle serves as a metabolic hub to provide intermediates to synthesize nutrients for tissue maintenance and growth. For example, excess carbohydrates provide glycerol and acetyl fragments to synthesize triacylglycerol. Acetyl–CoA also functions as the starting point for synthesizing cholesterol and many hormones. In contrast,

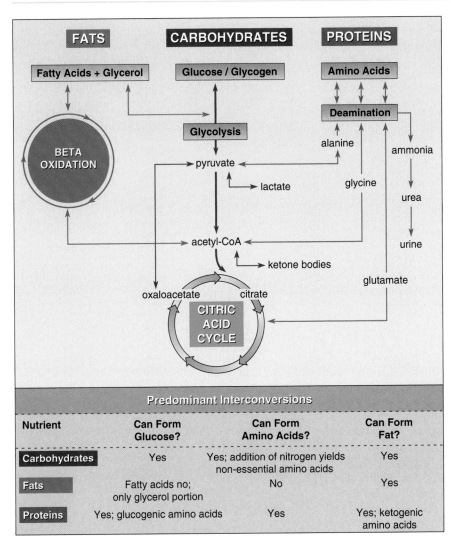

Figure 5.24. "Metabolic mill." Important interconversions between carbohydrates, fats, and proteins.

Table 5·1	Major Hormones and Their Role in Increasing (↑) or Decreasing (↓) Different Aspects of Macronutrient Metabolism During Exercise				
METABOLIC ACTIVITY	**GLUCAGON**	**EPINEPHRINE NOREPINEPHRINE**	**GROWTH HORMONE**	**CORTISOL**
Glycogenolysis (glycogen→glucose)	↑	↑	↑	↑
Glucose uptake/use	↓ (heavy exercise)	NA	↓	↓
Glycogenesis (glucose→glycogen)	↓	↓	↑	↑
Gluconeogenesis (making new glucose)	↑	↑	↑	↑
Lipolysis (FFA breakdown)	↑	↑	↑	↑
Lipogenesis (FFA formation)	↓	NA	↓	↓
Protein breakdown	NA	NA	NA	↑

NA, no major action; FFA, free fatty acid.

Box 5-3 • CLOSE UP

PH SPECIFICS

pH refers to a solution's concentration of protons or H^+. Solutions with relatively more OH^- than H^+ have a pH above 7.0 and are called basic or alkaline. Conversely, solutions with more H^+ than OH^- have a pH below 7.0 and are termed acidic. Chemically pure (distilled) water has a pH of 7.0 (neutral) with equal amounts of H^+ and OH^-. The pH scale, devised in 1909 by Danish chemist Sören Sörensen, ranges from +1.0 to +14.0.

An inverse relation exists between pH and the H^+ concentration ($[H^+]$). Because the pH scale is logarithmic, a one-unit change in pH corresponds to a tenfold change in $[H^+]$. For example, lemon juice and gastric juice (pH = 2.0) have 1000 times greater $[H^+]$ than black coffee (pH = 5.0), whereas hydrochloric acid (pH = 1.0) has approximately 1,000,000 times the $[H^+]$ of blood (pH = 7.4).

The pH of body fluids ranges from a low of 1.0 for the digestive acid hydrochloric acid to a slightly basic pH between 7.35 and 7.45 for arterial and venous blood (and most other body fluids). The term **alkalosis** refers to an increase in pH above the normal average of 7.4; this results directly from of a decrease in $[H^+]$ (increase in pH). Conversely, **acidosis** refers to an increase in $[H^+]$ (decrease in pH). The highly specific acid-base quality of various body fluids remains regulated within narrow limits because of the high sensitivity of metabolism to the $[H^+]$ of the reacting medium.

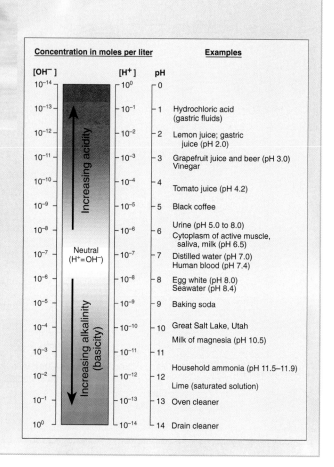

REGULATION OF ENERGY METABOLISM

Under normal conditions, electron transfer and subsequent energy release tightly couple to ADP phosphorylation. In general, without ADP availability for phosphorylation to ATP, electrons do not shuttle down the respiratory chain to combine with oxygen. Compounds that either inhibit or activate enzymes at key control points in the oxidative pathways modulate enzymatic regulatory control of glycolysis and the citric acid cycle. Each pathway has at least one enzyme considered "rate-limiting" because it controls the speed of that pathway's reac-

fatty acids do not contribute to glucose synthesis because pyruvate's conversion to acetyl–CoA does not reverse (notice the one-way arrow in Fig. 5.24). Many of the carbon compounds generated in citric acid cycle reactions provide the organic starting points for synthesizing nonessential amino acids. Amino acids with carbon skeletons resembling citric acid cycle intermediates after deamination synthesize to glucose.

tions. *By far, cellular ADP concentration exerts the greatest effect on the* **rate-limiting enzymes** *that control energy metabolism of the carbohydrate, fat, and protein macronutrients.* This control mechanism makes sense because any increase in ADP signals a need to supply energy to restore ATP levels. Conversely, high levels of cellular ATP signal a relatively low energy requirement and metabolic rate slows. From a broader perspective, ADP concentrations function as a cellular feedback mechanism to maintain a relative constancy (homeostasis) in the level of energy currency available for biologic work. Other rate-limiting modulators include cellular levels of phosphate, cyclic AMP, calcium, NAD^+, citrate, and pH.

Different hormones also play a critical role in regulating metabolism during rest and exercise. The five major hormones influencing metabolism during exercise include glucagon, epinephrine and norepinephrine, growth hormone (during intense exercise), and cortisol. **Table 5.1** displays the role of these hormones in different aspects of macronutrients metabolism. We discuss the different hormones and their regulatory functions more completely in Chapter 12.

SUMMARY

1. The complete breakdown of 1 mole of glucose liberates 689 kCal of energy. Of this total, ATP's bonds conserve about 263 kCal (38%), with the remainder dissipated as heat.

2. During glycolytic reactions in the cell's cytosol, a net of 2 ATP molecules form during anaerobic substrate-level phosphorylation.

3. In intense exercise, when hydrogen oxidation does not keep pace with its production, pyruvate temporarily binds hydrogen to form lactate.

4. In the mitochondrion, the second stage of carbohydrate breakdown converts pyruvate to acetyl–CoA. Acetyl–CoA then progresses through the citric acid cycle.

5. Hydrogen atoms released during glucose breakdown oxidize via the respiratory chain; the energy generated couples to ADP phosphorylation.

6. Oxidation of one glucose molecule in skeletal muscle yields a total of 36 ATP molecules (net gain).

7. Adipose tissue serves as an active and major supplier of fatty acid molecules.

8. The breakdown of a triacylglycerol molecule yields about 457 molecules of ATP. Fatty acid catabolism requires oxygen.

9. Protein can serve as an energy substrate. When deamination removes nitrogen from an amino acid molecule, the remaining carbon skeleton can enter metabolic pathways to produce ATP aerobically.

10. Numerous interconversions take place among the food nutrients. Fatty acids are an exception; they cannot be synthesized to glucose.

11. Fatty acids require a minimum level of carbohydrate breakdown for their continual catabolism for energy in the metabolic mill.

12. Cellular ADP concentration exerts the greatest effect on the rate-limiting enzymes that control energy metabolism.

THOUGHT QUESTIONS

1. How does aerobic and anaerobic energy metabolism affect optimal energy transfer capacity for a (1) 100-m sprinter, (2) 400-m hurdler, and (3) marathon runner?

2. How can elite marathoners run 26.2 miles at a 5-minute per mile pace, yet very few can run just one mile in 4 minutes?

3. In prolonged aerobic exercise like marathon running, explain why exercise capacity diminishes when glycogen reserves deplete, even though stored fat contains more than adequate energy reserves.

4. Is it important for weight lifters and sprinters to have a high capacity to consume oxygen? Explain.

5. From an exercise perspective, what are some advantages of having diverse sources of potential energy for synthesizing the cells' energy currency ATP?

SELECTED REFERENCES

Achten, J., Jeukendrup, A.E.: Optimizing fat oxidation through exercise and diet. *Nutrition*, 20(7–8):716, 2004.

Alberts, B., et al.: *Essential Cell Biology: An Introduction to the Molecular Biology of the Cell.* 2nd Ed. New York: Garland Publishers, 2003.

Åstrand, P.O., et al.: *Textbook of Work Physiology. Physiological Bases of Exercise.* 4th Ed. Champaign, IL: Human Kinetics, 2003.

Barnes, B.R., et al.: 5'-AMP-activated protein kinase regulates skeletal muscle glycogen content and ergogenics. *FASEB J.*, 19:773, 2005.

Berg, J.M., et al.: *Biochemistry*. 5th Ed. San Francisco: W.H. Freeman, 2002.

Binzoni, T.: Saturation of the lactate clearance mechanisms different from the "actate shuttle" determines the anaerobic threshold: prediction from the bioenergetic model. *J. Physiol. Anthropol. Appl. Human Sci.*, 24:175, 2005.

Brooks, G.A., et al.: *Exercise Physiology: Human Bioenergetics and its Applications.* 2nd Ed. Mountain View, CA: Mayfield, 2000.

Campbell, M.K., Farrell, S.O.: *Biochemistry.* 4th Ed. London: Thomson Brooks/Cole, 2003.

Campbell, P.N., et al.: *Biochemistry Illustrated.* 5th Ed. Philadelphia: Churchill Livingstone, 2005.

Carr, D.B., et al.: A reduced-fat diet and aerobic exercise in Japanese Americans with impaired glucose tolerance decreases intra-abdominal fat and improves insulin sensitivity but not beta-cell function. *Diabetes,* 54:340, 2005.

Fatouros, I.G., et al.: Oxidative stress responses in older men during endurance training and detraining. *Med. Sci. Sports Exerc.,* 36:2065, 2004.

Fox, S.I.: *Human Physiology.* 7th Ed. New York: McGraw-Hill, 2002.

Henderson, G.C., et al.: Pyruvate shuttling during rest and exercise before and after endurance training in men. *J. Appl. Physiol.,* 97:317, 2004.

Jeukendrup, A.E., Wallis, G.A.: Measurement of substrate oxidation during exercise by means of gas exchange measurements. *Int. J. Sports Med.,* 26 Suppl 1:S28, 2005.

Li, J., et al.: Interstitial ATP and norepinephrine concentrations in active muscle. *Circulation,* 111:2748, 2005.

Marieb, E.N.: *Essentials of Human Anatomy and Physiology.* 7th Ed. Menlo Park, CA: Pearson Education: Benjamin/Cummings, 2003.

Matthews, K., et al.: *Biochemistry.* 3rd Ed. Menlo Park, CA: Benjamin Cummings, 2000.

Nelson, D.L., Cox, M.M.: *Lehninger's Principles of Biochemistry.* 3rd Ed. New York, Worth Publishers, 2000.

Peres, S.B., et al.: Endurance exercise training increases insulin responsiveness in isolated adipocytes through IRS/PI3-kinase/Akt pathway. *J. Appl. Physiol.,* 98:1037, 2005.

Petibois, C., Deleris, G.: FT-IR spectrometry analysis of plasma fatty acyl moieties selective mobilization during endurance exercise. *Biopolymers,* 77:345, 2005.

Ricquier, D.: Respiration uncoupling and metabolism in the control of energy expenditure. *Proc. Nutr. Soc.,* 64:47, 2005.

Roberts, C.L., et al.: Pulmonary O2 uptake on-kinetics in rowing and cycle ergometer exercise. *Respir. Physiol. Neurobiol.,* 146:247, 2005.

Roepstorff, C., et al.: Regulation of oxidative enzyme activity and eukaryotic elongation factor 2 in human skeletal muscle: influence of gender and exercise. *Acta. Physiol. Scand.,* 184:215, 2005.

Tarnopolsky, M.: Protein requirements for endurance athletes. *Nutrition,* 20:662, 2004.

Tauler, P., et al.: Pre-exercise antioxidant enzyme activities determine the antioxidant enzyme erythrocyte response to exercise. *J. Sports Sci.,* 23:5, 2005.

van Loon, L.J.: Use of intramuscular triacylglycerol as a substrate source during exercise in humans. *J. Appl. Physiol.,* 97:1170, 2004.

Venables, M.C., et al.: Determinants of fat oxidation during exercise in healthy men and women: a cross-sectional study. *J. Appl. Physiol.,* 98:160, 2005.

Voet, D., Voet, J.G.: *Fundamentals of Biochemistry: Life at the Molecular Level.* 2nd Ed. New York: John Wiley, 2005.

Watson, J.D., Berry, A.: *DNA: The Secret of Life.* New York: Knopf, 2003.

CHAPTER OBJECTIVES

- Identify the body's three energy systems, and explain their relative contributions to exercise intensity and duration.

- Describe differences in blood lactate threshold between sedentary and aerobically trained individuals.

- Outline the time course for oxygen uptake during 10 minutes of moderate exercise.

- Draw a figure showing the relationship between oxygen uptake and exercise intensity during progressively increasing increments of exercise to maximum.

- Differentiate between the body's two types of muscle fibers.

- Explain differences in the pattern of recovery oxygen uptake from moderate and exhaustive exercise, and include factors that account for the EPOC from each exercise mode.

- Outline optimal recovery procedures from steady-rate and non–steady-rate exercise.

CHAPTER OUTLINE

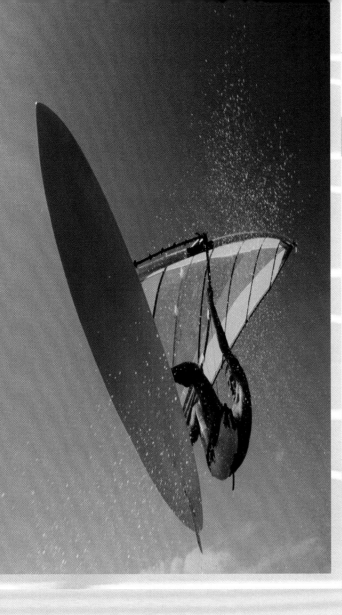

 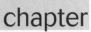

chapter 6

Human Energy Transfer During Exercise

Physical activity provides the greatest stimulus to energy metabolism. In sprint running and cycling, whole body energy output in world-class competitors exceeds 40 to 50 times their resting energy expenditure. In contrast, during less intense but sustained marathon running, energy requirements still exceed the resting level by 20 to 25 times. This chapter explains how the body's diverse energy systems interact to transfer energy during rest and different exercise intensities.

IMMEDIATE ENERGY: THE ATP–PCr SYSTEM

Performances of short duration and high intensity, such as the 100-m sprint, 25-m swim, smashing a tennis ball during the serve, or thrusting a heavy weight upwards, require an immediate and rapid energy supply. The high-energy phosphates adenosine triphosphate (ATP) and phosphocreatine (PCr) stored within muscles almost exclusively provide this energy.

Each kilogram of skeletal muscle stores approximately 5 millimoles (mmol) of ATP and 15 mmol of PCr. For a person with 30 kg of muscle mass, this amounts to between 570 and 690 mmol of phosphagens. If physical activity activates 20 kg of muscle, then stored phosphagen energy could power a brisk walk for 1 minute, a slow run for 20 to 30 seconds, or all-out sprint running and swimming for about 6 to 8 seconds. In the 100-m dash, for example, the body cannot maintain maximum speed for longer than this time, and the runner actually slows down towards the end of the race. *Thus, the quantity of intramuscular phosphagens significantly influences ability to generate "all-out" energy for brief durations.* The enzyme creatine kinase, which triggers PCr hydrolysis to resynthesize ATP, regulates the rate of phosphagen breakdown.

All movements use high-energy phosphates, although many rely almost exclusively on generating energy rapidly from this "energy system." For example, success in wrestling, weight lifting, routines in gymnastics, most field events, such as discus, shot put, pole vault, hammer, and javelin, and baseball and volleyball, require brief but all-out, maximal effort. For longer duration performance, the stored carbohydrate, fat, and protein macronutrients provide the necessary energy to recharge the pool of high-energy phosphates.

SHORT-TERM ENERGY: THE LACTIC ACID SYSTEM

The intramuscular phosphagens must continually resynthesize rapidly for strenuous exercise to continue beyond a brief period. During intense exercise, intramuscular stored glycogen provides the energy source to phosphorylate ADP during anaerobic glycogenolysis, forming lactate (see Chapter 5, Figs. 5.12 and 5.14).

With inadequate oxygen supply (or utilization) all of the hydrogens formed in glycolysis fail to oxidize; as a result, pyruvate converts to lactate (pyruvate + 2H → lactate). This enables the continuation of rapid ATP formation by anaerobic, substrate-level phosphorylation. Anaerobic energy for ATP resynthesis from glycolysis can be viewed as "reserve fuel" that activates when the oxygen demand/oxygen utilization ratio exceeds 1.0, as occurs during the last phase "sprint" of a 1-mile race. Anaerobic ATP production remains crucial during a 440-m run or 100-m swim or in **multiple-sprint sports** like ice hockey, field hockey, and soccer. These activities require rapid energy transfer that exceeds that supplied by stored phosphagens. If the intensity of "all-out" exercise decreases (thereby extending exercise duration), lactate buildup correspondingly decreases.

Blood Lactate Accumulation

Chapter 5 pointed out that some lactate continually forms even under resting conditions. However, lactate removal by heart muscle and nonactive skeletal muscle balances its production, yielding no net lactate build-up. Only when lactate removal does not match production does blood lactate accumulate. *Aerobic training produces cellular adaptations that increase rates of lactate removal, so accumulation occurs only at higher exercise intensities.* **Figure 6.1** illustrates the general relationship between oxygen uptake (expressed as a percentage of maximum) and blood lactate level during light, moderate, and strenuous exercise in endurance athletes and untrained individuals. During light and moderate exercise in both groups, aerobic metabolism adequately meets energy demands. Non-active tissues rapidly oxidize any lactate that forms. This permits blood lactate to remain fairly stable (i.e., no net blood lactate accumulates), even though oxygen uptake increases. In essence, ATP for muscular activity comes from energy-generating reactions that require the oxidation of hydrogen.

Blood lactate begins to increase exponentially at about 55% of the healthy, untrained person's maximal capacity for aerobic metabolism. The usual explanation for increased blood lactate in intense exercise assumes a relative tissue hypoxia (lack of oxygen). Even though there is poor experimental evidence demonstrating direct exercise-induced hypoxia within muscle, indirect measures support the notion of reduced cellular oxygen content. With lack of oxygen, anaerobic glycolysis partially meets the energy requirement, and hydrogen release begins to exceed its oxidation down the respiratory (electron transport) chain. At this point, lactate forms as the excess hydrogen produced during glycolysis passes to pyruvate (see Fig. 5.14). Lactate formation increases at progressively higher levels of exercise intensity when active muscle cannot meet the additional energy demands aerobically.

As Figure 6.1 illustrates, trained individuals show a similar pattern of blood lactate accumulation, except for the point where blood lactate sharply increases. The

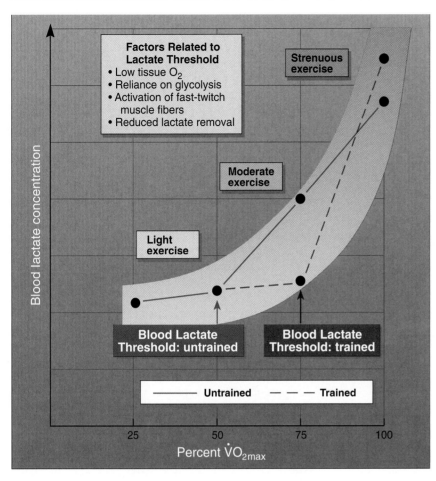

Figure 6.1 Blood lactate concentration at different levels of exercise expressed as a percentage of maximal oxygen uptake for endurance trained and untrained individuals.

Questions & Notes

Give the 2 compounds that comprise the high-energy phosphates.

   1.

   2.

Give 2 examples of sporting events that rely almost exclusively on the immediate energy system.

   1.

   2.

True or False:

Aerobic training produces cellular adaptations that increase rates of lactate removal.

Give the percentage of the maximal aerobic power where blood lactate begins to increase in healthy, untrained persons.

Fill-in:

The point of abrupt increase in blood lactate concentration during exercise of increasing intensity is known as the_____ _____ _____.

This value represents the percentage of $\dot{V}O_{2max}$ where blood lactate begins to increase in world-class endurance athletes.

point of abrupt increase in blood lactate, known as the **blood lactate threshold** (also termed **onset of blood lactate accumulation**, or **OBLA**), occurs at a higher percentage of an endurance athlete's aerobic power. This favorable metabolic response could result from genetic endowment (e.g., muscle fiber type distribution) and/or specific local muscle adaptations with training that favor less lactate formation and its more rapid removal rate. For example, endurance training significantly increases capillary density and mitochondria size and number. The concentrations of the various enzymes and transfer agents involved in aerobic metabolism also increase with training. Such alterations enhance the cell's capacity to generate ATP aerobically, particularly via fatty acid breakdown. These training adaptations also extend exercise intensity before the onset of blood lactate accumulation. For example, world-class endurance athletes sustain exercise intensities at 85% to 90% of their maximum capacity for aerobic metabolism before blood lactate accumulates.

The lactate formed in one part of an active muscle can be oxidized by other fibers in the same muscle or by less active neighboring muscle tissue. Lactate uptake by less active muscle fibers depresses blood lactate levels during light-to-moderate exercise and conserves blood glucose and muscle glycogen in prolonged work. The concept of the blood lactate threshold and its relation to endurance performance appears in Chapter 13.

FOR YOUR INFORMATION

Blood Lactate Threshold

Exercise intensity at the point of lactate buildup (blood lactate threshold) powerfully predicts aerobic exercise performance. The walking speed at which blood lactate began to build up in competitive race walkers predicted their race performance to within 0.6% of their actual race time.

Lactate-Producing Capacity

Capacity to generate high lactate levels during exercise enhances maximal power output for short durations. Because tissues continually use lactate during exercise, lactate accumulation can significantly underestimate total blood lactate production. Ability to generate a high lactate concentration in maximal exercise increases with specific sprint and power training; detraining subsequently decreases this advantage.

Well-trained "anaerobic" athletes who perform maximally for brief time periods generate 20% to 30% higher blood lactate levels than untrained individuals during similar exercise. To some extent, increased intramuscular glycogen stores with training contribute a greater amount of energy via anaerobic glycolysis. Enhanced lactate-producing capacity with sprint-type training also may result from improved motivation that often accompanies the trained state (i.e., trained persons "push" themselves harder) and an approximate 20% increase in glycolytic enzyme activity (particularly phosphofructokinase). However, these enzymatic changes do not match the impressive two- to threefold increase in aerobic enzymes induced by aerobic training.

Blood Lactate as an Energy Source

Chapter 5 pointed out how blood lactate serves as substrate for glucose retrieval (gluconeogenesis) and also as a direct fuel source for active muscle. Isotope tracer studies of muscle and other tissues reveal that lactate produced in fast-twitch muscle fibers can circulate to other fast-twitch or slow-twitch fibers for conversion to pyruvate. Pyruvate, in turn, converts to acetyl–CoA for entry to the citric acid cycle for aerobic energy metabolism. Such **lactate shuttling** between cells enables glycogenolysis in one cell to supply other cells with fuel for oxidation. *This makes muscle not only a major site of lactate production, but also a primary tissue for lactate removal via oxidation.*

A muscle oxidizes much of the lactate produced by it, without releasing lactate into the blood. The liver also accepts muscle-generated lactate from the bloodstream and synthesizes it to glucose through the Cori cycle's gluconeogenic reactions (Chapter 5). Glucose derived from lactate takes one of two routes: (1) it returns in the blood to skeletal muscle for energy metabolism or (2) it becomes synthesized to glycogen for storage. These uses of lactate make this anaerobic byproduct of intense exercise a valuable metabolic substrate and certainly not a waste product.

LONG-TERM ENERGY: THE AEROBIC SYSTEM

Although glycolysis releases anaerobic energy rapidly, only a relatively small total ATP yield results from this pathway. In contrast, aerobic metabolic reactions provide for the greatest portion of energy transfer, particularly when exercise duration extends longer than 2 to 3 minutes.

Oxygen Uptake During Exercise

The curve in **Figure 6.2** illustrates oxygen uptake during each minute of a slow jog continued at a steady pace for 20 minutes. The vertical Y-axis indicates the uptake of oxygen by the body (referred to as oxygen uptake or oxygen consumption); the horizontal X-axis displays exercise time. The abbreviation $\dot{V}O_2$ indicates oxygen uptake, where the **V** denotes the volume consumed; the dot placed above the $\dot{V}$ expresses oxygen uptake as a per minute value. Oxygen uptake during any minute can be determined easily by locating time on the X-axis and its corresponding point for oxygen uptake on the Y-axis. For example, after running 4 minutes, oxygen uptake equals approximately $17 \text{ mL·kg·min}^{-1}$.

From the graph, oxygen uptake increases rapidly during the first minutes of exercise and reaches a relative plateau between minutes 4 and 6. Oxygen uptake then remains relatively stable throughout the remainder of exercise. The flat portion or plateau of the oxygen uptake curve represents the **steady rate of aerobic metabolism**—a balance between energy required by the body and the rate of aerobic ATP production. Oxygen-consuming reactions supply the energy for steady-rate exercise; any lactate produced either oxidizes or reconverts to glucose in the liver, kidneys, and skeletal muscles. No net accumulation of blood lactate occurs under these steady-rate metabolic conditions.

Many Levels of Steady Rate For some individuals, lying in bed, working around the house, and playing an occasional round of golf represent the activity spectrum for steady-rate metabolism. A champion marathon runner, on the other hand, runs 26.2 miles in slightly more than 2 hours and can still maintain a steady rate of

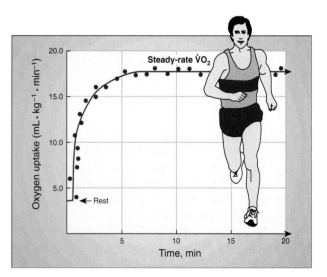

Figure 6.2 Time course of oxygen uptake during continuous jogging at a relatively slow pace. The dots along the curve represent measured values of oxygen uptake determined by open-circuit spirometry.

aerobic metabolism. This sub–5-minute-per-mile pace represents a magnificent physiologic–metabolic accomplishment. Maintenance of the required level of aerobic metabolism necessitates well-developed functional capacities to (1) deliver adequate oxygen to active muscles and (2) process oxygen within muscle cells for aerobic ATP production.

Oxygen Deficit   Note that the upward curve of oxygen uptake shown in Figure 6.2 does not increase instantaneously to a steady rate at the start of exercise. Instead, oxygen uptake remains considerably below the steady-rate level in the first minute of exercise, even though the exercise energy requirement remains essentially unchanged throughout the activity period. The temporary "lag" in oxygen uptake occurs because ATP provides the muscle's immediate energy requirement without the need for oxygen. Oxygen becomes important for ATP resynthesis in subsequent energy transfer reactions to serve as an electron acceptor to combine with the hydrogen produced during three biochemical cellular activities:

1. Glycolysis
2. β–oxidation of fatty acids
3. Citric acid cycle reactions

A deficit always exists in the oxygen uptake response to a new, higher steady-rate level, regardless of activity mode or exercise intensity.

The oxygen deficit quantitatively represents the difference between the total oxygen actually consumed during exercise and the amount that would have been consumed had a steady-rate, aerobic metabolism occurred immediately at the initiation of exercise. Energy provided during the deficit phase of exercise represents a predominance of anaerobic energy transfer. Stated in metabolic terms, the oxygen deficit represents the quantity of energy produced from stored intramuscular phosphagens plus energy contributed from rapid glycolytic reactions. This yields phosphate-bond energy until oxygen uptake and energy demands reach steady rate.

Figure 6.3 depicts the relationship between the size of the oxygen deficit and the energy contribution from the ATP-PCr and lactic acid energy systems. Exercise that generates about a 3- to 4-L oxygen deficit substantially depletes the intramuscular high-energy phosphates. Consequently, this intensity of exercise continues only on a "pay-as-you-go" basis; ATP must be replenished continually

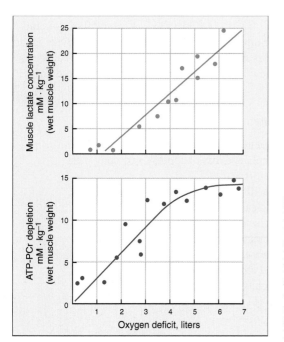

Figure 6.3 Muscle ATP and PCr depletion and muscle lactate concentration related to the oxygen deficit. (Adapted from Pernow, B., and Karlsson, J.: Muscle ATP, CP and lactate in submaximal and maximal exercise. In: *Muscle Metabolism During Exercise*. Pernow. B., and Saltin, B. (eds.). New York: Plenum Press, 1971.)

Give the percentage increase in blood lactate levels generated by anaerobic athletes compared to untrained individuals.

True or False:

Muscle is both a major lactate producer and a site for lactate removal via oxidation.

FOR YOUR INFORMATION

Lactic Acid and pH
Hydrogen ions (H^+) dissociating from lactic acid, rather than undissociated lactate (La^-), present the primary problem to the body. At normal pH levels, lactic acid almost completely dissociates immediately to H^+ and La^- ($C_3H_5O_3^-$). There are few problems if the amount of free H^+ does not exceed the body's ability to buffer them and maintain the pH at a relatively stable level. The pH decreases when excessive lactic acid (H^+) exceeds the body's immediate buffering capacity. Pain is perceived and performance decreases as the blood becomes more acidic.

FOR YOUR INFORMATION

Limited Duration of Steady-Rate Exercise
Theoretically, exercise could continue indefinitely when performed at a steady rate of aerobic metabolism. Factors other than motivation limit the duration of steady-rate work. These include loss of important body fluids in sweat and depletion of essential nutrients, especially blood glucose and glycogen stored in the liver and active muscles.

Box 6-1 • CLOSE UP

OVERTRAINING: TOO MUCH OF A GOOD THING

With intense and prolonged training, certain athletes experience **overtraining**, **staleness**, or **burnout**. The overtrained condition reflects more than just a short-term inability to train as hard as usual or a slight dip in competition-level performance; rather, it involves a more chronic fatigue experienced during exercise workouts and subsequent recovery periods. It associates with sustained poor exercise performance, frequent infections (particularly of the upper respiratory tract), and a general malaise and loss of interest in high-level training. Injuries also are more frequent in the overtrained state. Although the specific symptoms of overtraining are highly individualized, those outlined in the accompanying table represent the most common ones. Little is known about the etiology of this syndrome, although neuroendocrine alterations that affect the sympathetic nervous system, as well as alterations in immune function, probably are involved. These symptoms persist unless the athlete rests, with complete recovery requiring weeks or even months.

Carbohydrate's Possible Role in Overtraining. A gradual depletion of the body's carbohydrate reserves with repeated strenuous training may contribute to the over-training syndrome. In a classic pioneering study in the area, it was shown that after 3 successive days of running 16.1 km (10 miles), glycogen in the thigh muscle became nearly depleted. This occurred even though the runners' diets contained 40% to 60% of total calories as carbohydrates. In addition, glycogen use on the third day of the run averaged about 72% less than on day 1. The mechanism by which repeated occurrences of glycogen depletion may contribute to overtraining remains unclear.

Tapering Often Helps. Overtraining symptoms can range from mild to severe. They more often occur in highly motivated individuals, in instances where a large increase in training occurs abruptly and in situations where the overall training program does not include sufficient rest and recovery.

Overtraining symptoms often occur before season-ending competition. Therefore, to achieve peak performance, athletes should reduce training volume and significantly increase carbohydrate intake for at least several days before competition—a practice called **tapering**. The goal of tapering is to provide time for muscles to resynthesize glycogen to maximal levels and to allow them to heal from training-induced damage.

Overtraining Signs and Symptoms

Performance-Related Symptoms
- Consistent performance decline
- Persistent fatigue and sluggishness
- Excessive recovery required after competitive events
- Inconsistent performance

Physiological-Related Symptoms
- Decrease in maximum work capacity
- Frequent headaches or stomach aches
- Insomnia
- Persistent low-grade stiffness and muscle/joint soreness

- Frequent constipation or diarrhea
- Unexplained loss of appetite and body mass
- Amenorrhea
- Elevated resting heart rate on waking

Psychological-Related Symptoms
- Depression
- General apathy
- Decreased self-esteem
- Mood changes
- Difficulty concentrating
- Loss of competitive drive

through either glycolysis or the aerobic breakdown of carbohydrate, fat, and protein. Interestingly, lactate begins to increase in exercising muscle well before the phosphagens reach their lowest levels. This means that glycolysis contributes anaerobic energy early in vigorous exercise even before full utilization of the high-energy phosphates. *Energy for exercise does not merely result from a series of energy systems that "switch on" and "switch off" like a light switch. Rather, a muscle's energy supply represents a smooth transition between anaerobic and aerobic sources, with considerable overlap from one source of energy transfer to another.*

Oxygen Deficit in Trained and Untrained Individuals

Figure 6.4 shows the oxygen uptake response to submaximum cycle ergometer or treadmill exercise for a trained and untrained person. Similar values for steady-rate oxygen uptake during light and moderate exercise occur in trained and untrained individuals. The trained person, however, reaches the steady rate quicker; hence, this person has a smaller oxygen deficit for the same exercise duration compared with the untrained person. This indicates greater total oxygen consumed during exercise for the trained person, with a proportionately smaller anaerobic energy transfer component. A likely explanation for the differences in oxygen deficit between trained and untrained individuals relates to a more highly developed aerobic bioenergetic capacity of the trained person. An augmented aerobic power results from either improved central cardiovascular function and/or training-induced local adaptations that increase a muscle's capacity to generate ATP aerobically. These adaptations trigger an earlier onset of aerobic ATP production with less lactate formation for the trained person.

MAXIMAL OXYGEN UPTAKE

Figure 6.5 depicts the curve for oxygen uptake during a series of constant-speed runs up six hills, each progressively steeper than the next. In the laboratory, these "hills" are increasing treadmill elevations, raising the height of a step bench, providing greater resistance to pedaling a bicycle ergometer, or increasing the onward

Questions & Notes

List 2 symptoms of overtraining.

1.

2.

Define the term oxygen deficit.

For the same level of work production (duration and intensity of effort), does a trained or an untrained person record a greater oxygen deficit? Explain.

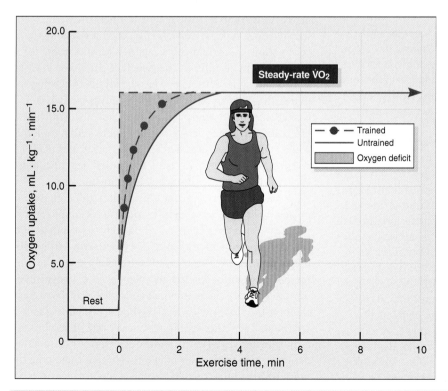

Figure 6.4 Oxygen uptake and oxygen deficit for trained and untrained individuals during submaximum cycle ergometer exercise. Both individuals reach the same steady-rate $\dot{V}O_2$, but the trained person reaches it at a faster rate, reducing the oxygen deficit.

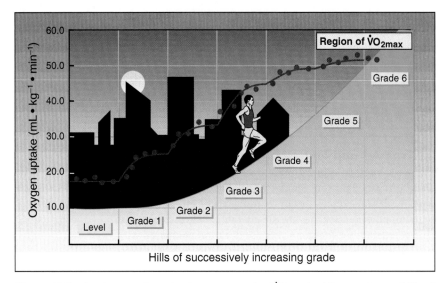

Figure 6.5 Attainment of maximal oxygen uptake ($\dot{V}O_{2max}$) while running up hills of increasing slope. This occurs in the region where a further increase in exercise intensity does not produce an additional and/or expected increase in oxygen uptake. The red dots represent measured values for oxygen uptake during the run up each hill.

rush of water while a swimmer maintains speed in a swim flume. Each successive hill (increase in exercise intensity) requires greater energy output and, thus, a greater demand for aerobic metabolism. Increases in oxygen uptake relate linearly and in direct proportion to exercise intensity during the climb up the first several hills. The runner maintains speed up the last two hills, yet oxygen uptake does not increase by the same magnitude as in the prior hills. In fact, oxygen uptake does not increase during the run up the last hill. *The maximal oxygen uptake ($\dot{V}O_{2max}$) describes the highest oxygen uptake achieved despite increases in exercise intensity.* The $\dot{V}O_{2max}$ holds great physiologic significance because of its dependence on the functional capacity and integration of the many biologic systems required for oxygen supply, transport, delivery, and use.

The $\dot{V}O_{2max}$ indicates an individual's capacity for aerobically resynthesizing ATP. Exercise performed above $\dot{V}O_{2max}$ can only take place by energy transfer predominantly from anaerobic glycolysis with subsequent lactate formation. A large build up of lactate, due to the additional anaerobic muscular effort, disrupts the already high rate of energy transfer for the aerobic resynthesis of ATP. To borrow an analogy from business economics: supply (aerobic resynthesis of ATP) does not meet demand (aerobic energy required for muscular effort). An aerobic energy supply-demand imbalance affects production (lactate accumulates) and compromises exercise performance.

Because of the importance of aerobic power in exercise physiology, subsequent chapters cover more detailed aspects of $\dot{V}O_{2max}$, including its measurement, physiologic significance, and role in endurance performance.

FAST-TWITCH AND SLOW-TWITCH MUSCLE FIBERS

Extracting about 20 to 40 mg of tissue (the size of a grain of rice; Fig. 6.6) during surgical biopsy gives exercise physiologists the means to study functional and structural characteristics of human skeletal muscle and its response to exercise. Two distinct types of muscle fiber exist in humans. A **fast-twitch (FT)**, **or type II**, fiber has two primary subdivisions, type IIa and type IIb, each possessing rapid contraction speed and high capacity for anaerobic ATP production in glycolysis. The type IIa fiber also possesses somewhat higher aerobic power. Type II fibers become active during change-of-pace and stop-and-go activities like basketball, soccer, and ice hockey. They also contribute increased force output when running or cycling up a hill while maintaining a constant speed or during all-out effort requiring rapid, powerful movements that depend almost exclusively on energy from anaerobic metabolism.

The second fiber-type, the **slow-twitch (ST)**, or **type I**, muscle fiber, generates energy primarily through aerobic pathways. This fiber possesses a relatively slow contraction speed compared with its fast-twitch counterpart. Its capacity to generate ATP aerobically intimately relates to numerous large mitochondria and high levels of enzymes required for aerobic metabolism, particularly fatty acid catabolism. Slow-twitch muscle fibers primarily sustain continuous activities requiring a steady rate of aerobic energy transfer. Fatigue in endurance exercise associates with glycogen depletion in the muscles' type I and type IIa muscle fibers. More than likely, the predominance of slow-

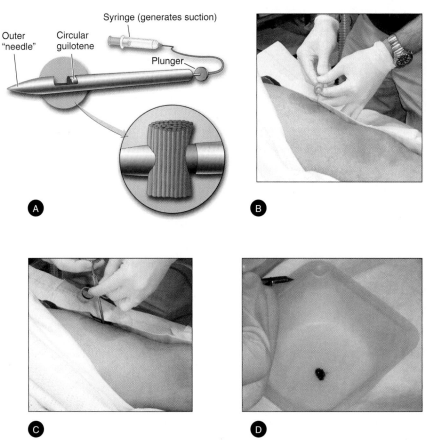

Figure 6.6   Muscle biopsy. **A.** Biopsy needle with attached suction device. The insert shows the inner guillotine portion of the needle. **B.** Anesthetizing thigh area with lidocaine prior to insertion of biopsy needle. **C.** Insertion of biopsy needle into thigh of subject. **D.** Piece of muscle taken from thigh. (From Professor Jeff Horowitz, University of Michigan, Division of Kinesiology.)

twitch muscle fibers greatly contributes to high blood lactate thresholds observed among elite endurance athletes.

The preceding discussion suggests that a muscle's predominant fiber type contributes significantly to success in certain sports or physical activities. Chapter 14 explores this idea more fully, including other considerations concerning metabolic, contractile, and fatigue characteristics of each fiber type.

ENERGY SPECTRUM OF EXERCISE

Figure 6.7 depicts the relative contributions of anaerobic and aerobic energy sources during various durations of maximal exercise. The data represent estimates from laboratory experiments of all-out treadmill running and stationary bicycling. They also can relate to other activities by drawing the appropriate time relationships. For example, a 100-m sprint run equates to any all-out activity lasting about 10 seconds, while an 800-m run lasts approximately 2 minutes. All-out exercise for 1 minute includes the 400-m dash in track, the 100-m swim, and multiple full-court presses during a basketball game.

Intensity and Duration Determine the Blend

The body's energy transfer systems should be viewed along a continuum of exercise bioenergetics. Anaerobic sources supply most of the energy for fast movements or

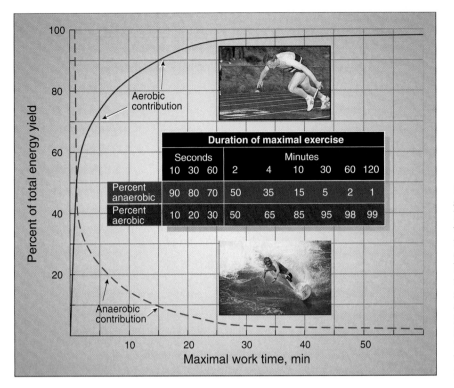

| Duration of maximal exercise | | | | | | | | |
| Seconds | | | Minutes | | | | | |
10	30	60	2	4	10	30	60	120
Percent anaerobic 90	80	70	50	35	15	5	2	1
Percent aerobic 10	20	30	50	65	85	95	98	99

Figure 6.7 Relative contribution of aerobic and anaerobic energy metabolism during maximal physical effort of various durations; 2 minutes of maximal effort requires about 50% of the energy from both aerobic and anaerobic processes. At a world-class 4-minute mile pace, aerobic metabolism supplies approximately 65% of the energy, with the remainder generated from anaerobic processes. (Adapted from Åstrand, P.O., and Rodahl, K.: *Textbook of Work Physiology.* New York: McGraw-Hill Book Company, 1977.)

during increased resistance to movement at a given speed. Also, when movement begins at either fast or slow speed (from performing a front handspring to starting a marathon run), the intramuscular phosphagens provide immediate anaerobic energy for the required muscle actions.

At the short-duration extreme of maximum effort, the intramuscular phosphagens ATP and PCr supply the major energy for the entire exercise. The ATP-PCr and lactic acid systems provide about one-half of the energy required for "best-effort" exercise lasting 2 minutes, whereas aerobic reactions provide the remainder. For top performance in all-out, 2-minute exercise, a person must possess a well-developed capacity for both aerobic and anaerobic metabolism. Intense exercise of intermediate duration performed for 5 to 10 minutes, like middle-distance running and swimming or stop-and-go sports like basketball and soccer, demands greater aerobic energy transfer. Longer duration marathon running, distance swimming and cycling, recreational jogging, cross-country skiing, and hiking and backpacking require a continual energy supply derived aerobically without reliance on lactate formation.

Intensity and duration determine the energy system and metabolic mixture that predominate during exercise. The aerobic system predominates in low-intensity exercise, with fat serving as the primary fuel source. The liver markedly increases its release of glucose to active muscle as exercise progresses from low to high intensity. Simultaneously, glycogen stored within muscle serves as the predominant carbohydrate energy source during the early stages of exercise and when exercise intensity increases. *During high-intensity aerobic exercise, the advan-*

tage of selective dependence on carbohydrate metabolism lies in its two times more rapid energy transfer capacity compared with fat and protein fuels. Compared with fat, carbohydrate also generates about 6% greater energy per unit of oxygen consumed. As exercise continues and muscle glycogen depletes, progressively more fat (intramuscular triacylglycerols and circulating FFA) enters the metabolic mixture for ATP production. In maximal anaerobic effort (reactions of glycolysis), carbohydrate becomes the sole contributor to the output of ATP.

A sound approach to exercise training analyzes an activity for its specific energy components and then establishes a training regimen to ensure optimal physiologic and metabolic adaptations. An improved capacity for energy transfer usually improves exercise performance.

Nutrient-Related Fatigue   Severe depletion of liver and muscle glycogen during intense aerobic exercise induces fatigue, despite sufficient oxygen availability to muscle and an almost unlimited energy supply from stored fat. Endurance athletes commonly refer to this extreme sensation of fatigue as "bonking" or hitting the wall. (The image of hitting the wall suggests an inability to continue exercising, which in reality does not occur, although pain exists in the active muscles, and exercise intensity decreases markedly.) Skeletal muscle does not contain the **phosphatase enzyme** (present in liver) that releases glucose from liver cells; thus, relatively inactive muscles retain all of their glycogen. Controversy exists as to why liver and muscle glycogen depletion during prolonged exercise reduces exercise capacity. Three factors are involved:

1. Central nervous system's use of blood glucose for energy
2. Muscle glycogen's role as a "primer" in fat catabolism
3. Significantly slower rate of energy release from fat compared with carbohydrate breakdown

OXYGEN UPTAKE DURING RECOVERY: THE SO-CALLED "OXYGEN DEBT"

Bodily processes do not immediately return to resting levels after exercise ceases. In light exercise (e.g., golf, archery, bowling), recovery to a resting condition takes place rapidly and often progresses unnoticed. With particularly intense physical activity (running full speed for 800-m or trying to swim 200-m as fast as possible), however, it takes considerable time for the body to return to resting levels. The difference in recovery from light and strenuous exercise relates largely to the specific metabolic and physiologic processes in each exercise mode.

A.V. Hill (1886–1977), the British Nobel physiologist (see Chapter 1), referred to oxygen uptake during recovery as the **oxygen debt**. Contemporary theory no longer uses this term. Instead, **recovery oxygen uptake** or **excess post-exercise oxygen consumption** (**EPOC**) defines the excess oxygen uptake above the resting level in recovery (i.e., the total oxygen consumed after exercise in excess of a pre-exercise baseline level).

Panel A in **Figure 6.8** shows that light exercise rapidly attains steady rate with a small oxygen deficit. Rapid recovery ensues from such exercise with an accompanying small EPOC. In moderate to intense aerobic exercise (Panel B), it takes longer to reach steady rate, and the oxygen deficit becomes considerably larger compared with light exercise. Oxygen uptake in recovery from this relatively strenuous aerobic exercise returns more slowly to the pre-exercise resting level. Recovery oxygen uptake initially declines rapidly (similar to recovery from light exercise) followed by a more gradual decline to the baseline. In both Panels A and B, computation of the oxygen deficit and EPOC uses the steady-rate oxygen uptake to represent the exercise oxygen (energy) requirement. During exhausting exercise, illustrated in Panel C, a steady rate of aerobic metabolism cannot be attained. This produces a large accumulation of blood lactate; it takes oxygen uptake considerable time to return to the pre-exercise level. It becomes nearly impossible to determine the true oxygen deficit in such exercise because no steady rate exists, and the energy requirement exceeds the individual's maximal oxygen uptake.

No matter how intense the exercise (walking, bowling, golf, snowboarding, wrestling, cross-country skiing, or sprint running), an oxygen uptake in excess of the resting value always exists when exercise stops. The shaded area under the recovery curve in Figure 6.8 indicates this quantity of oxygen; it equals the total oxygen consumed in recovery (until attaining the baseline level) minus the total oxygen that would normally be consumed at rest for an equivalent duration. An assumption underlying discussions of the physiologic meaning of EPOC holds that resting oxygen uptake remains essentially unchanged during exercise and recovery. This assumption may be incorrect, particularly following strenuous exercise.

The recovery curves in Figure 6.8 illustrate two fundamentals of oxygen uptake during recovery:

1. **Fast component:** In low-intensity, primarily aerobic exercise (with little increase in body temperature), about one-half the total EPOC takes place in 30 seconds; complete recovery requires several minutes.
2. **Slow component:** A second slower phase occurs in recovery from more strenuous exercise (often accompanied by considerable increases in blood lactate and body temperature). The slower phase of recovery, depending on exercise intensity and duration, may require 24 hours or more before re-establishing the pre-exercise oxygen uptake.

Questions & Notes

Give the 2 factors that determine the energy system and metabolic mixture that predominate during exercise.

1.

2.

Give the amount of time that the ATP–PCr and lactic acid system can power maximal, all-out exercise.

Compared to fat, carbohydrate generates about how much greater energy per unit of oxygen consumed?

Briefly explain the phenomenon known as "hitting the wall."

FOR YOUR INFORMATION

It's Difficult to Excel in All Sports
An understanding of the energy requirements of various physical activities partly explains why a world-record holder in the 1-mile run does not achieve similar success as a long-distance runner. Conversely, premier marathoners usually cannot run 1 mile in less than 4 minutes, yet they complete a 26-mile race averaging a 5-minute per mile pace.

Box 6–2 • CLOSE UP

HOW TO MEASURE WORK ON A TREADMILL, CYCLE ERGOMETER, AND STEP BENCH

An ergometer is an exercise apparatus that quantifies work and/or power output. The most common ergometers include treadmill, cycle and arm-crank ergometers, stair steppers, and rowers.

WORK

Work (W) represents application of force (F) through a distance (D):

$$W = F \times D$$

For example, for a body mass of 70 kg and vertical jump score of 0.5 m, work accomplished equals 35 kilogram-meters (kg-m) (70 kg $\times$ 0.5 m). The most common units of measurement to express work include: kilogram-meters (kg-m), foot-pounds (ft-lb), joules (J), Newton-meters (Nm), and kilocalories (kCal).

POWER

Power (P) represents W performed per unit time (T):

$$P = F \times D \div T$$

In the above example, if the person were to accomplish work in the vertical jump of 35 kg-m in 500 ms (0.500 s; 0.008 min), the power attained would equal 4375 kg-m·min^{-1}. The most common units of measurement for power are kg-m·min^{-1}, Watts (1 W = 6.12 kg-m·min^{-1}), and kCal·min^{-1}.

Calculation of Treadmill Work

The treadmill is a moving conveyor belt with variable angle of incline and speed. Work performed equals the product of the weight (mass) of the person (F) and the vertical distance achieved walking or running up the incline. Vertical distance equals the sine of the treadmill angle (theta or θ) multiplied by the distance traveled along the incline (treadmill speed $\times$ time).

$$W = \text{Body Mass (Force)} \times \text{Vertical Distance}$$

Example   For an angle θ of 8° (measured with an inclinometer or determined by knowing the percent grade of the treadmill), the sine of angle θ equals 0.1392 (see table). The vertical distance represents treadmill speed multiplied by exercise duration multiplied by sine θ. For example, vertical distance on the incline while walking at 5000 m·h^{-1} for 1 hour equals 696 m (5000 $\times$ 0.1392). If a person with a body mass of 50 kg walked on a treadmill at an incline of 8° (percent grade = approximately 14%) for 60 minutes at 5000 m·h^{-1}, work accomplished computes as:

$$\begin{aligned} W &= F \times \text{Vertical Distance (Sine } \theta \times D) \\ &= 50 \text{ kg} \times (0.1392 \times 5000 \text{ m}) \\ &= 34{,}800 \text{ kg-m} \end{aligned}$$

The value for power equals 34,800 kg-m ÷ 60 minutes or 580 kg-m·min^{-1}.

Ø (deg)	SINE Ø	TANGENT Ø	PERCENT GRADE
1	0.0175	0.0175	1.75
2	0.0349	0.0349	3.49
3	0.0523	0.0523	5.23
4	0.0698	0.0698	6.98
5	0.0872	0.0872	8.72
6	0.1045	0.1051	10.51
7	0.1219	0.1228	12.28
8	0.1392	0.1405	14.05
9	0.1564	0.1584	15.84
10	0.1736	0.1763	17.63
15	0.2588	0.2680	26.80
20	0.3420	0.3640	36.40

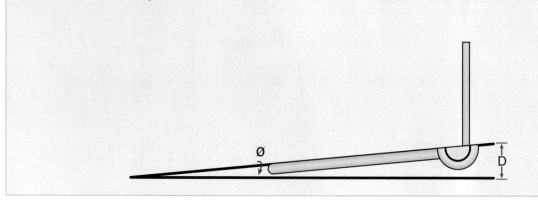

Box 6–2 • CLOSE UP *(Continued)*

Calculation of Cycle Ergometer Work

The typical mechanically braked cycle ergometer contains a flywheel with a belt around it connected by a small spring at one end and an adjustable tension lever at the other end. A pendulum balance indicates the resistance against the flywheel as it turns. Increasing the tension on the belt increases flywheel friction, which increases pedaling resistance. The force (flywheel friction) represents braking load in kg or kilopounds (kp = force acting on 1-kg mass at the normal acceleration of gravity). The distance traveled equals number of pedal revolutions times flywheel circumference.

Example A person pedaling a bicycle ergometer with a 6-m flywheel circumference at 60 rpm for 1 minute covers a distance (D) of 360 m each minute (6 m × 60). If the frictional resistance on the flywheel equals 2.5 kg, total work computes as:

$$W = F \times D$$
$$= \text{Frictional resistance} \times \text{Distance traveled}$$
$$= 2.5 \text{ kg} \times 360 \text{ m}$$
$$= 900 \text{ kg-m}$$

Power generated by the effort equals 900 kg-m in 1 min or 900 kg-m·min^{-1} (900 kg-m ÷ 1 min).

Calculation of Bench Stepping Work

Only the vertical (positive) work can be calculated in bench stepping. Distance (D) computes as bench height times the number of times the person steps; force (F) equals the person's body mass (kg).

Example If a 70-kg person steps on a bench 0.375 m high at a rate of 30 steps per minute for 10 minutes, total work computes as:

$$W = F \times D$$
$$= \text{Body Mass, kg} \times (\text{Vertical distance, m} \times \text{steps per min} \times 10 \text{ min})$$
$$= 70 \text{ kg} \times (0.375 \text{ m} \times 30 \times 10)$$
$$= 7875 \text{ kg-m}$$

Power generated during stepping equals 787 kg-m·min^{-1} (7875 kg-m ÷ 10 min).

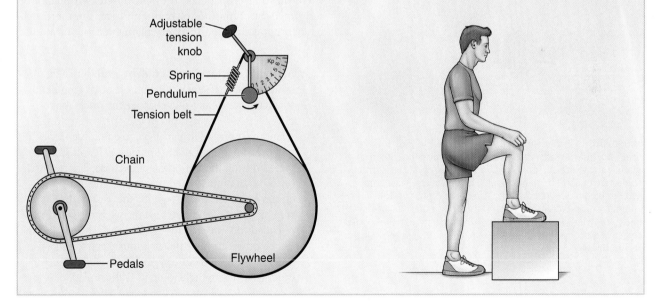

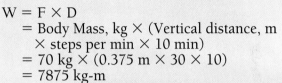

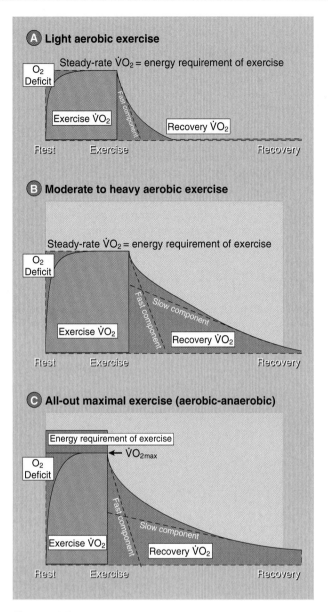

Figure 6.8 Oxygen uptake during exercise and recovery from (**A**) light steady-rate exercise, (**B**) moderate to heavy steady-rate exercise, and (**C**) exhaustive exercise with no steady rate of aerobic metabolism. The first phase (fast component) of recovery occurs rapidly; the second phase (slow component) progresses more slowly and may take considerable time to return to resting conditions. In exhaustive exercise, the oxygen requirement of exercise exceeds the measured exercise oxygen uptake.

Metabolic Dynamics of Recovery Oxygen Uptake

Traditional View: A.V. Hill's 1922 Oxygen Debt Theory
A.V. Hill first used the term "oxygen debt" in 1922, but Danish Nobel physiologist August Krogh (1874–1949; see Chapter 1) first reported the exponential decline in oxygen uptake after exercise. Hill and others discussed the dynamics of metabolism in ex-

ercise and recovery in financial-accounting terms. Based on his work with frogs, Hill likened the body's carbohydrate stores to energy "credits," and thus, expending stored credits during exercise would incur a "debt." The larger the energy "deficit" is (use of available stored energy credits), then the larger the energy debt. Recovery oxygen uptake, therefore, represented the added metabolic cost of repaying this debt and, hence, the term "oxygen debt."

Hill hypothesized that lactate accumulation during the anaerobic component of exercise represented the use of stored glycogen energy credits. Therefore, the subsequent oxygen debt served two purposes: (1) re-establish the original carbohydrate stores (credits) by resynthesizing approximately 80% of the lactate back to glycogen (gluconeogenesis via the Cori cycle) in the liver, and (2) catabolize the remaining lactate for energy through the pyruvate–citric acid cycle pathway. ATP generated by this latter pathway presumably powered glycogen resynthesis from the accumulated lactate. The **lactic acid theory of oxygen debt** frequently describes this early explanation of recovery oxygen uptake dynamics.

In 1933, following Hill's work, researchers at Harvard's famous Fatigue Laboratory (1927–1946; see Chapter 1) attempted to explain their observations that the initial fast component of the recovery oxygen uptake occurred before blood lactate decreased. In fact, they showed that an "oxygen debt" of almost 3 liters could incur without appreciably elevating blood lactate. To resolve these discrepancies, they proposed two phases of oxygen debt. This model explained the energetics of oxygen uptake during recovery from exercise for almost 60 years.

1. Alactic or **alactacid oxygen debt** (without lactate buildup): The alactacid portion of the oxygen debt (depicted for steady-rate exercise in panels A and B of Figure 6.8, or the rapid phase of recovery from strenuous exercise in panel C), restored the intramuscular high-energy phosphates ATP and PCr depleted during the last phase of exercise. The aerobic breakdown of the stored macronutrients during recovery provided the energy for this restoration. A small portion of the alactacid recovery oxygen uptake reloaded the muscles' myoglobin and hemoglobin in the blood returning from previously active tissues.
2. Lactic acid or **lactacid oxygen debt** (with lactate buildup): In keeping with A.V. Hill's explanation, the major portion of the lactacid oxygen debt represented reconversion of lactate to liver glycogen.

Testing Hill's Oxygen Debt Theory   Acceptance of Hill's explanation for the lactacid phase of the oxygen debt requires proof that the major portion of lactate produced in exercise actually resynthesizes to glycogen in recovery. This has never been proven. To the contrary, when researchers infuse radioactive-labeled lactate into rat muscle, more than 75% of it appears as radioactive carbon dioxide, and only 25% synthesized to glycogen. In experiments with humans, no substantial replenishment of glycogen occurred 10 minutes after strenuous exercise, even though blood lactate levels decreased significantly. Contrary to the traditional theory, the heart, liver, kidneys, and skeletal muscle use a major portion of blood lactate produced during exercise as an energy substrate during exercise and recovery.

Updated Theory to Explain EPOC

No doubt exists that the elevated aerobic metabolism in recovery helps restore the body's processes to pre-exercise conditions. Oxygen uptake following light and moderate exercise replenishes high-energy phosphates depleted in the preceding exercise sustaining the cost of a somewhat elevated overall level of physiologic function. In recovery from strenuous exercise, some oxygen resynthesizes a portion of lactate to glycogen. *However, a significant portion of recovery oxygen uptake supports physiologic functions actually taking place during recovery.* The considerably larger recovery oxygen uptake compared with oxygen deficit in high-intensity, exhaustive exercise results partly from an elevated body temperature. Core temperature frequently increases by about 3°C (5.4°F) during vigorous exercise and can remain elevated for several hours into recovery. This thermogenic "boost" directly stimulates metabolism and increases oxygen uptake during recovery.

In essence, all of the physiologic systems activated to meet the demands of muscular activity increase their need for oxygen during recovery. The recovery oxygen uptake reflects:

- Anaerobic metabolism of prior exercise
- Respiratory, circulatory, hormonal, ionic, and thermal disequilibriums caused by prior exercise

Implications of EPOC for Exercise and Recovery

Understanding the dynamics of recovery oxygen uptake provides a basis for optimizing recovery from strenuous physical activity. Blood lactate does not accumulate considerably with either steady-rate aerobic exercise or brief 5- to 10-second bouts of all-out effort powered by the intramuscular high-energy phosphates. Recovery proceeds rapidly (fast component), and exercise can begin again within a brief time. In contrast, anaerobic exercise powered mainly by glycolysis causes lactate buildup and significant disruption in physiologic processes and the internal environment. This requires considerably more time for complete recovery (slow component). It poses a problem in sports like basketball, hockey, soccer, tennis, and badminton because a performer pushed to a high level of anaerobic metabolism may not fully recover during brief rest periods, times outs, between points, or even half-time breaks.

Procedures for speeding recovery from exercise can classify as active or passive. **Active recovery** (often called "cooling-down" or "tapering-off") involves submaximum aerobic exercise performed immediately post exercise. Many believe that continued movement prevents muscle cramps and stiffness and facilitates the recovery process. In contrast, in **passive recovery**, a person usually lies down, assuming that complete inactivity reduces the resting energy requirements and "frees" oxygen for the recovery process. Modifications of active and passive recovery have included cold showers, massages, specific body positions, ice application, and ingesting cold fluids. Research findings have been equivocal about these recovery procedures.

Questions & Notes

Give the formula for computing work.

Name the 2 components of the recovery oxygen uptake curve.

1.

2.

Define the term EPOC.

FOR YOUR INFORMATION

Early Research about "Oxygen Debt"
Hill and other researchers of the time did not have a clear understanding of human bioenergetics. They frequently applied their knowledge of energy metabolism and lactate dynamics of amphibian and reptiles to observations on humans. In frogs, for example, most of the lactate formed in active muscle reconverts to glycogen, but this may not occur in humans.

FOR YOUR INFORMATION

Causes of Excess Postexercise Oxygen Consumption (EPOC) with Intense Exercise
1. Resynthesis of ATP and PCr
2. Resynthesis of blood lactate to glycogen (Cori cycle)
3. Oxidation of blood lactate in energy metabolism
4. Restoration of oxygen to blood, tissue fluids, and myoglobin
5. Thermogenic effects of elevated core temperature
6. Thermogenic effects of hormones, particularly the catecholamines epinephrine and norepinephrine
7. Increased pulmonary and circulatory dynamics and other elevated levels of physiologic function

Optimal Recovery From Steady-Rate Exercise

Most people can perform exercise below 55% to 60% of $\dot{V}O_{2max}$ in steady rate with little or no blood lactate accumulation. Recovery from such exercise resynthesizes high-energy phosphates, replenishes oxygen in the blood, body fluids, and muscle myoglobin, and supports the small energy cost to sustain an elevated circulation and ventilation. Passive procedures produce the most rapid recovery in such cases because exercise elevates total metabolism and delays recovery.

Optimal Recovery from Non–Steady-Rate Exercise

Lactate formation exceeds its rate of removal and blood lactate accumulates when exercise intensity exceeds the maximum steady-rate level. As work intensity increases, the level of lactate increases sharply, and the exerciser soon becomes exhausted. The precise mechanisms of fatigue during intense anaerobic exercise are not fully understood, but the blood lactate level indicates the relative strenuousness of exercise and reflects the adequacy of the recovery.

Active aerobic exercise in recovery accelerates lactate removal. The optimal level of exercise in recovery ranges between 30% and 45% of $\dot{V}O_{2max}$ for bicycle exercise and 55% and 60% of $\dot{V}O_{2max}$ when recovery involves treadmill running. The variation between these two forms of exercise probably results from the more localized nature of bicycling (i.e., more intense effort per unit muscle mass), which produces a lower lactate threshold compared with running.

Figure 6.9 illustrates blood lactate recovery patterns for trained men who performed 6 minutes of supermaximum bicycle exercise. Active recovery involved 40 minutes of continuous exercise at either 35% or 65% of $\dot{V}O_{2max}$. An exercise combination of 65% $\dot{V}O_{2max}$ performed for 7 minutes followed by 33 minutes at 35% $\dot{V}O_{2max}$ evaluated whether a higher intensity exercise interval early in recovery expedited blood lactate removal. Clearly, moderate aerobic exercise in recovery facilitated lactate removal compared with passive recovery. Combining higher intensity exercise followed by lower intensity exercise offered no greater benefit than a single exercise bout of moderate intensity. Recovery exercise above the lactate threshold might even prolong recovery by promoting lactate formation. In a practical sense, if left to their own choice, people voluntarily select their optimal intensity of recovery exercise for blood lactate removal.

Intermittent Exercise and Recovery: The Interval Training Approach One can exercise at an intensity that normally proves exhausting within 3 to 5 minutes using pre-established spacing of exercise and rest intervals. The utilization of exercise and rest intervals forms the basis of the **interval training** program. With this

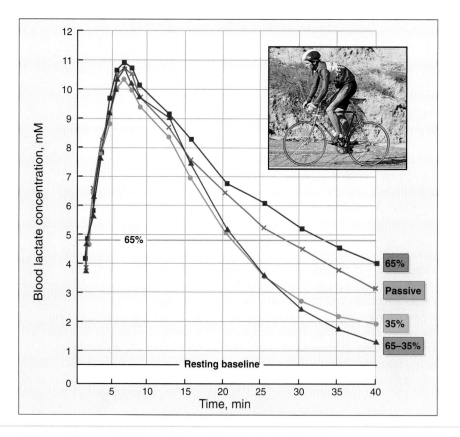

Figure 6.9 Blood lactate concentrations after maximal exercise during passive recovery and active exercise recoveries at 35% $\dot{V}O_{2max}$, 65% $\dot{V}O_{2max}$, and a combination of 35% and 65% of $\dot{V}O_{2max}$. The horizontal solid orange line indicates the level of blood lactate produced by exercise at 65% of $\dot{V}O_{2max}$ without previous exercise. (Adapted from Dodd, S., et al.: Blood lactate disappearance at various intensities of recovery exercise. *J. Appl. Physiol.*, 57:1462, 1984.)

approach, the exerciser applies various work-to-rest intervals using "supermaximum" effort to overload the specific systems of energy transfer. For example, with all-out exercise of up to 8 seconds in duration, intramuscular phosphagens provide the major portion of energy, with little demand on the glycolytic pathway. Rapid recovery ensues (fast component), and exercise can begin again after only a brief recovery. We discuss interval training further in Chapter 13.

SUMMARY

1. The major energy pathway for ATP production differs depending on exercise intensity and duration. Intense exercise of short duration (100-m dash, weight lifting) derives energy primarily from the intramuscular phosphagens ATP and PCr (immediate energy system). Intense exercise of longer duration (1 to 2 min) requires energy mainly from the anaerobic reactions of glycolysis (short-term energy system). The long-term aerobic system predominates as exercise progresses beyond several minutes in duration.

2. The steady-rate oxygen uptake represents a balance between exercise energy requirements and aerobic ATP resynthesis.

3. The oxygen deficit represents the difference between the exercise oxygen requirement and the actual oxygen consumed.

4. The maximum oxygen uptake or $\dot{V}O_{2max}$ represents quantitatively the maximum capacity for aerobic ATP resynthesis.

5. Humans possess different types of muscle fibers, each with unique metabolic and contractile properties. The two major fiber types include low glycolytic-high oxidative, slow-twitch fibers and low oxidative-high glycolytic, fast-twitch fibers.

6. Understanding the energy spectrum of exercise forms a sound basis for creating optimal training regimens.

7. Bodily processes do not immediately return to resting levels after exercise ceases. The difference in recovery from light and strenuous exercise relates largely to the specific metabolic and physiologic processes in each exercise.

8. Moderate exercise performed during recovery (active recovery) from strenuous physical activity facilitates recovery compared with passive procedures (inactive recovery). Active recovery performed below the point of blood lactate accumulation speeds lactate removal.

9. Proper spacing of exercise and rest intervals can optimize workouts geared to train a specific energy transfer system.

THOUGHT QUESTIONS

1. If the maximal oxygen uptake represents such an important measure of a person's capacity to resynthesize ATP aerobically, why does the person with the highest $\dot{V}O_{2max}$ not always achieve the best marathon run performance?

2. How does an understanding of the energy spectrum of exercise help formulate optimal training to improve specific exercise performance?

3. Why is it so unusual to find athletes who excel at both short- and long-distance running?

SELECTED REFERENCES

Aisbett, B., Le Rossignol, P.: Estimating the total energy demand for supra-maximal exercise using the VO2-power regression from an incremental exercise test. *J. Sci. Med. Sport*, 6:343, 2003.

Barnett, C., et al.: Muscle metabolism during sprint exercise in man: influence of sprint training. *J. Sci. Med. Sport*, 7:314, 2004.

Bendahan, D., et al.: ATP synthesis and proton handling in muscle during short periods of exercise and subsequent recovery. *J. Appl. Physiol.*, 94:239, 2003.

Beneke, R.: Methodological aspects of maximal lactate steady state-implications for performance testing. *Eur. J. Appl. Physiol.*, 89:95, 2003.

Berthoin, S., et al.: Plasma lactate and plasma volume recovery in adults and children following high-intensity exercises. *Acta. Paediatr.*, 92:283, 2003.

Borsheim, E., Bahr, R.: Effect of exercise intensity, duration and mode on post-exercise oxygen consumption. *Sports Med.*, 33:1037, 2003.

Bourdin, M., et al.: Laboratory blood lactate profile is suited to on water training monitoring in highly trained rowers. *J. Sports Med. Phys. Fitness*, 44:337, 2004.

Burnley, M., et al.: Effects of prior heavy exercise, prior sprint exercise and passive warming on oxygen uptake kinetics during heavy exercise in humans. *Eur. J. Appl. Physiol.*, 87:424, 2002.

Campbell-O'Sullivan, S.P., et al.: Low intensity exercise in humans accelerates mitochondrial ATP production and pulmonary oxygen kinetics during subsequent more intense exercise. *J. Physiol.*, 538:931, 2002.

Carter, H., et al.: Effect of prior exercise above and below critical power on exercise to exhaustion. *Med. Sci. Sports Exerc.*, 37:775, 2005.

Cleuziou, C., et al.: Dynamic responses of O2 uptake at the onset and end of exercise in trained subjects. *Can. J. Appl. Physiol.*, 28:630, 2003.

Crommett, A.D., Kinzey, S.J.: Excess postexercise oxygen consumption following acute aerobic and resistance exercise in women who are lean or obese. *J. Strength Cond. Res.*, 18:410, 2004.

DeLorey, D.S., et al.: Effect of age on O2 uptake kinetics and the adaptation of muscle deoxygenation at the onset of moderate-intensity cycling exercise. *J. Appl. Physiol.*, 97:165, 2004.

DeLorey, D.S., et al.: Effects of prior heavy-intensity exercise on pulmonary O2 uptake and muscle deoxygenation kinetics in young and older adult humans. *J. Appl. Physiol.*, 97:998, 2004.

DeLorey, D.S., et al.: Relationship between pulmonary O2 uptake kinetics and muscle deoxygenation during moderate-intensity exercise. *J. Appl. Physiol.*, 95:113, 2003.

Denadai, B.S., et al.: The relationship between onset of blood lactate accumulation, critical velocity, and maximal lactate steady state in soccer players. *J. Strength Cond. Res.*, 19:364, 2005.

Dorado, C., et al.: Effects of recovery mode on performance, O2 uptake, and O2 deficit during high-intensity intermittent exercise. *Can. J. Appl. Physiol.*, 29:227, 2004.

Duffield, R., et al.: Energy system contribution to 100-m and 200-m track running events. *J. Sci. Med. Sport*, 7:302, 2004.

Endo, M., et al.: Effects of priming exercise intensity on the dynamic linearity of the pulmonary VO2 response during heavy exercise. *Eur. J. Appl. Physiol.*, 91:545, 2004.

Ferguson, R.A., et al.: Effect of muscle temperature on rate of oxygen uptake during exercise in humans at different contraction frequencies. *J. Exp. Biol.*, 205:981, 2002.

Ferreira, L.F., et al.: Dynamics of skeletal muscle oxygenation during sequential bouts of moderate exercise. *Exp. Physiol.*, 90:393, 2005.

Gardner, A., et al.: A comparison of two methods for the calculation of accumulated oxygen deficit. *J. Sports Sci.*, 21:155, 2003.

Jubrias, S.A., et al.: Acidosis inhibits oxidative phosphorylation in contracting human skeletal muscle in vivo. *J. Physiol.*, 553:589, 2003.

Kang, J., et al.: Evaluation of physiological responses during recovery following three resistance exercise programs. *J. Strength Cond. Res.*, 19:305, 2005.

Koppo, K., Bouckaert, J.: Prior arm exercise speeds the VO2 kinetics during arm exercise above the heart level. *Med. Sci. Sports Exerc.*, 37:613, 2005.

Koppo, K., et al.: Influence of DCA on pulmonary VO2 kinetics during moderate-intensity cycle exercise. *Med. Sci. Sports Exerc.*, 36:1159, 2004.

Markovitz, G.H., et al.: On issues of confidence in determining the time constant for oxygen uptake kinetics. *Br. J. Sports Med.*, 38:553, 2004.

McCann, D.J., et al.: Phosphocreatine kinetics in humans during exercise and recovery. *Med. Sci. Sports Exerc.*, 27:378, 1995.

McMahon, S., Jenkins, D.: Factors affecting the rate of phosphocreatine resynthesis following intense exercise. *Sports Med.*, 32:761, 2002.

McMillan, K., et al.: Lactate threshold responses to a season of professional British youth soccer. *Br. J. Sports Med.*, 39:432, 2005.

Miller, B.F., et al.: Lactate and glucose interactions during rest and exercise in men: effect of exogenous lactate infusion. *J. Physiol.*, 544:963, 2002.

Ogata, H., Yano, T.: Kinetics of oxygen uptake during arm cranking with the legs inactive or exercising at moderate intensities. *Eur. J. Appl. Physiol.*, 94:17, 2005.

Ozyener, F., et al.: Negative accumulated oxygen deficit during heavy and very heavy intensity cycle ergometry in humans. *Eur. J. Appl. Physiol.*, 90:185, 2003.

Pringle, J.S., et al.: Effect of pedal rate on primary and slow-component oxygen uptake responses during heavy-cycle exercise. *J. Appl. Physiol.*, 94:1501, 2003.

Robergs, R., et al.: Influence of pre-exercise acidosis and alkalosis on the kinetics of acid-base recovery following intense exercise. *Int. J. Sport Nutr. Exerc. Metab.*, 15:59, 2005.

Ruby, B.C., et al.: Gender differences in glucose kinetics and substrate oxidation during exercise near the lactate threshold. *J. Appl. Physiol.*, 92:1125, 2002.

Sahlin, K., et al.: Prior heavy exercise eliminates $\dot{V}O_2$ slow component and reduces efficiency during submaximal exercise in humans. *J. Physiol.*, 564:765, 2005.

Scott, C.B., Kemp, R.B.: Direct and indirect calorimetry of lactate oxidation: implications for whole-body energy expenditure. *J. Sports Sci.*, 23:15, 2005.

Shepstone, T.N., et al.: Short-term high- vs. low-velocity isokinetic lengthening training results in greater hypertrophy of the elbow flexors in young men. *J. Appl. Physiol.*, 98:1768, 2005.

Smith, S.A., et al.: Use of phosphocreatine kinetics to determine the influence of creatine on muscle mitochondrial respiration: an in vivo 31P-MRS study of oral creatine ingestion. *J. Appl. Physiol.*, 96:2288, 2004.

Starritt, E.C., et al.: Effect of short-term training on mitochondrial ATP production rate in human skeletal muscle. *J. Appl. Physiol.*, 86:450, 1999.

Thornton, M.K., Potteiger, J.A.: Effects of resistance exercise bouts of different intensities but equal work on EPOC. *Med. Sci. Sports Exerc.*, 34:715, 2002.

Trimmer, J.K., et al.: Measurement of gluconeogenesis in exercising men by mass isotopomer distribution analysis. *J. Appl. Physiol.*, 93:233, 2002.

Van Hall, G., et al.: Leg and arm lactate and substrate kinetics during exercise. *Am. J. Physiol. Endocrinol. Metab.*, 284:E193, 2003.

Warburton, D.E., et al.: Effectiveness of high-intensity interval training for the rehabilitation of patients with coronary artery disease. *Am. J. Cardiol.*, 95:1080, 2005.

Whipp, B.J.: The slow component of O_2 uptake kinetics during heavy exercise. *Med. Sci. Sports Exerc.*, 26:1319, 1994.

Wilkerson, D.P., et al.: Effect of prior multiple-sprint exercise on pulmonary O_2 uptake kinetics following the onset of perimaximal exercise. *J. Appl. Physiol.*, 97:1227, 2004.

Wyatt, F.B.: Comparison of lactate and ventilatory threshold to maximal oxygen consumption: A meta-analysis. *J. Strength Cond. Res.*, 13:67, 1999.

Yano, T., et al.: Kinetics of CO2 excessive expiration in constant-load exercise. *J. Sports Med. Phys. Fitness*, 42:152, 2002.

Yano, T., et al.: Relationship in simulation between oxygen deficit and oxygen uptake in decrement-load exercise starting from low exercise intensity. *J. Physiol. Anthropol. Appl. Human Sci.*, 22:1, 2003.

Yoshida, T.: The rate of phosphocreatine hydrolysis and resynthesis in exercising muscle in humans using 31P-MRS. *J. Physiol. Anthropol. Appl. Human Sci.*, 21:247, 2002.

CHAPTER OUTLINE

CHAPTER OBJECTIVES

- Compare and contrast the concepts of measurement, evaluation, and prediction.

- Explain specificity and generality as they apply to exercise performance and physiologic function.

- Describe procedures to administer two practical "field tests" to evaluate power output capacity of the intramuscular high-energy phosphates (immediate energy system).

- Describe a commonly used test to evaluate the power output capacity of glycolysis (short-term energy system).

- Understand differences between direct and indirect calorimetry.

- Understand differences between open- and closed-circuit spirometry.

- Describe different systems used in open-circuit spirometry.

- Define the term respiratory quotient (RQ) including its use and importance.

- Explain factors that influence the RQ and respiratory exchange ratio.

- Define maximal oxygen uptake ($\dot{V}O_{2max}$), including its physiological significance.

- Define graded exercise stress test.

- List criteria that indicate when a person reaches "true" $\dot{V}O_{2max}$ and $\dot{V}O_{2peak}$ during a graded exercise test.

- Outline three commonly used treadmill protocols to assess $\dot{V}O_{2max}$.

- Explain how each of the following affects $\dot{V}O_{2max}$: (1) mode of exercise, (2) heredity, (3) state of training, (4) gender, (5) body composition, and (6) age.

- Describe procedures to administer a submaximal walking "field test" to predict $\dot{V}O_{2max}$.

- Outline the procedure for administering a step test to predict $\dot{V}O_{2max}$.

- List three assumptions when predicting $\dot{V}O_{2max}$ from submaximal exercise heart rate.

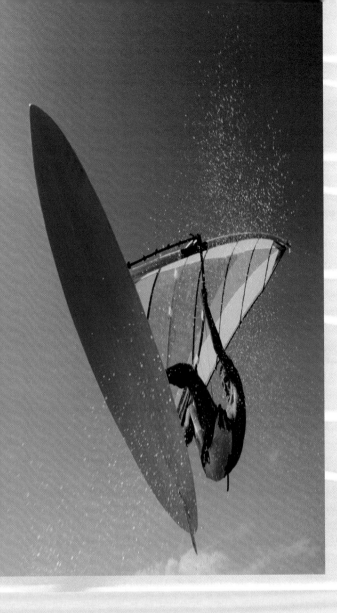

7

Measuring and Evaluating Human Energy-Generating Capacities During Exercise

Everybody possesses the capability for anaerobic and aerobic energy metabolism, although the *capacity* for each form of energy transfer varies considerably among individuals. These differences illustrate the concept of **individual differences** in metabolic capacity for exercise. A person's capacity for energy transfer (and for many other physiologic functions) does not exist as some general factor for all types of exercise but depends largely on the exercise mode used for training. A high maximal oxygen uptake ($\dot{V}O_{2max}$) in running, for example, does not necessarily ensure a similar $\dot{V}O_{2max}$ in swimming or rowing. The differences in $\dot{V}O_{2max}$ within an individual for different activities activating different muscle groups represents an example of **specificity of metabolic capacity**. In contrast, some individuals with high $\dot{V}O_{2max}$ in one form of exercise can also possess an above average aerobic power in other diverse activities. This illustrates the **generality of metabolic capacity**. *For the most part, more specificity exists than generality in metabolic and physiologic functions.* In this chapter, we discuss different tests (and their evaluation) of the capacity of the various energy transfer systems discussed in Chapter 6 with reference to measurement, specificity, and individual differences.

OVERVIEW OF ENERGY TRANSFER CAPACITY DURING EXERCISE

Figure 7.1 illustrates the **specificity–generality concept** of energy capacities. The non-overlapped areas represent specificity of physiologic function, and the overlapped areas represent generality of function. For each of the energy systems, specificity exceeds generality; rarely do individuals excel in markedly different activities (e.g.,

sprinting and long-distance running). While many world-class triathletes seem to possess "metabolically generalized" capacities for diverse aerobic activities, more than likely their performance results from long hours of highly specific training in *each* of the triathlon's three grueling events.

Based on the specificity principle, training for high aerobic power probably contributes little to one's capacity for anaerobic energy transfer and vice versa. *The effects of systematic exercise training remain highly specific for neurologic, physiologic, and metabolic responses.*

Figure 7.2 shows the involvement of the anaerobic and aerobic energy transfer systems for different durations of all-out exercise. At the initiation of either high- or low-speed movements, the intramuscular phosphagens, ATP and PCr, provide immediate and nonaerobic energy for muscle action. After the first few seconds of movement, the glycolytic energy system (initial phase of carbohydrate breakdown) provides an increasingly greater proportion of the total energy. Continuation of exercise, although at a lower intensity, places a progressively greater demand on aerobic metabolic pathways for ATP resynthesis.

Some activities require the capacity of more than one energy transfer system, whereas other activities rely predominately on a single system. In reality, all activities activate each energy system to some degree, depending on exercise intensity and duration. Of course, greater demand for anaerobic energy transfer occurs for higher intensity and shorter duration activities.

Measurement, Evaluation, and Prediction

Measurement, evaluation, and prediction are closely related processes. From a practical standpoint, **measurement** takes place when a test is administered and a score

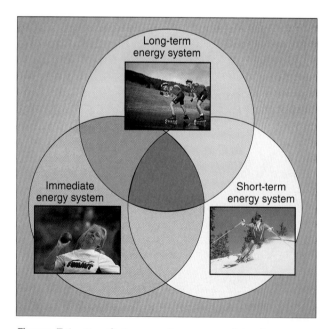

Figure 7.1 Specificity-generality concept of the three energy systems. The overlap of systems represents generality, and the remainder represents specificity.

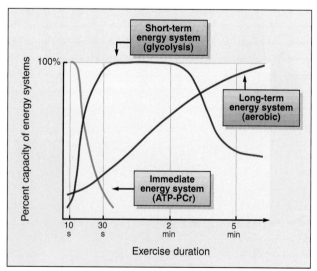

Figure 7.2 Three energy systems and their percentage contribution to total energy output during all-out exercise of different durations.

is obtained. If the test is quantitative, the score is a number; if the test is qualitative, the score may be a phrase or a word such as "excellent"; or it may be a number representing a phrase or word. Measurement is usually defined as *"the process of assigning a number to an attribute of a person or object."* By this definition, measurement is a quantitative and not a qualitative process.

Different tests require different procedures, depending on the exact attribute being measured. In some cases, measurements must be done in the laboratory, requiring different levels of sophistication and different levels of risk for the participant. Invasive tests, compared to non-invasive tests, involve diagnostic procedure requiring insertion of an instrument, device, or substance (like a contrast medium) into the body through the skin or body orifice.

The **evaluation** process involves interpretation of test scores. While the process of measurement is an objective nonjudgmental process, evaluation requires that judgments be made. For example, a $\dot{V}O_{2max}$ score obtained on a treadmill test to exhaustion can be evaluated (judged) relative to another individual's $\dot{V}O_{2max}$ score, and inferences can be made regarding each person's fitness or training status.

Testing different aspects of one's energy systems can be used for the following three purposes:

1. **Motivation:** provide insight into the power and capacity of one's physiology
2. **Diagnosis:** point out limitations or weaknesses of metabolic function
3. **Prescription:** once weaknesses have been diagnosed, it is possible to formulate a proper (exercise) prescription

Prediction uses test scores to estimate (predict) another function or attribute of the same individual. The strength of any prediction is based on the degree of relationship between the test scores and the estimated function. For example, $\dot{V}O_{2max}$ scores can predict endurance running performance in a 10-km race. An individual with a high $\dot{V}O_{2max}$ can be predicted to run a 10-km race faster than an individual with a lower $\dot{V}O_{2max}$ score.

PART 1 •
Measuring and Evaluating the Anaerobic Energy Systems

THE IMMEDIATE ENERGY SYSTEM

Two general approaches assess anaerobic power and capacity responses of individuals:

1. Measure changes in the chemical substances *used* (ATP and PCr levels) or *produced* (lactate) as a result of anaerobic metabolism.
2. Quantify the amount of external work performed or power generated during short-duration, high-intensity activity. This approach assumes that short-duration, high-intensity activity could not be done without anaerobic energy; therefore, measuring such work or power indirectly measures (predicts) anaerobic energy utilization.

PERFORMANCE TESTS OF ANAEROBIC POWER AND CAPACITY

Performance tests of anaerobic power and capacity that rely on maximal activation of the intramuscular ATP-PCr energy reserves have been developed as practical "field tests" to evaluate the **immediate energy system**. These maximal effort performances, referred to as power tests, evaluate the time-rate of doing work (i.e., work accomplished per unit of time). The following formula computes power output (P):

$$P = (F \times D) \div T$$

where **F** equals force generated, **D** equals distance through which the force moves, and **T** equals exercise duration. **Watts** represent a common expression of power; 1 watt equals 0.73756 ft-lb·s^{-1} or 6.12 kg-m·min^{-1}.

Stair-Sprinting Power Test

Researchers have measured immediate power output using a test that requires sprinting up a flight of stairs. **Figure 7.3** shows a subject running up a staircase as fast as possible taking three steps at a time. The external work performed equals the total vertical distance the body raises up the stairs; for six stairs, this distance usually equals about 1.05 m.

The power output for a 65-kg woman who traverses six steps in 0.52 seconds computes as follows:

$$F = 65 \text{ kg}; D = 1.05 \text{ m}; T = 0.52 \text{ s}$$
$$P = (65 \times 1.05) \div 0.52$$
$$= 131.3 \text{ kg-m·s}^{-1} \ (1287 \text{ watts})$$

Because body mass greatly influences the power-output score in stair-sprinting, a heavier person necessarily generates greater power at the same speed as a lighter person who covers the same vertical distance. Because of this influence of body mass, use caution in interpreting differences in stair-sprinting power scores and making inferences about individual differences in ATP-PCr energy capacity. *The test may be better suited to evaluate individuals of similar body mass or the same person before and after*

a specific training regimen designed to develop immediate anaerobic leg power.

Jumping Power Test

For years, physical fitness test batteries have included the jump-and-reach test (see Box 7-1, page 227) or a standing broad jump to evaluate anaerobic performance. The jump-and-reach test score equals the difference between a person's standing reach and the maximum jump-and-touch height. For the broad jump, the score represents the horizontal distance covered in a leap from a semi-crouched position. Although both tests purport to measure leg power, they probably do not achieve this goal. For one thing, with the jump tests, power generated in propelling the body from the crouched position occurs only in the time the feet contact the floor's surface. This brief period does not sufficiently evaluate a person's ATP and PCr power-output capacity.

Other Immediate Energy Power Tests

A 6- to 8-second performance involving all-out exercise measures a person's capacity for immediate power from the intramuscular high-energy phosphates (see Fig. 7.2). Examples of other similar tests include sprint running or cycling, shuttle runs, and more localized movements such as arm cranking or simulated stair climbing, rowing, or skiing. In the popular **Québec 10-second test** of leg cycling power, the subject performs two all-out, 10-second rides at a frictional resistance equal to 0.09 kg per kg of body mass, with 10 minutes of rest between exercise bouts. Exercise begins by pedaling as fast as possible as

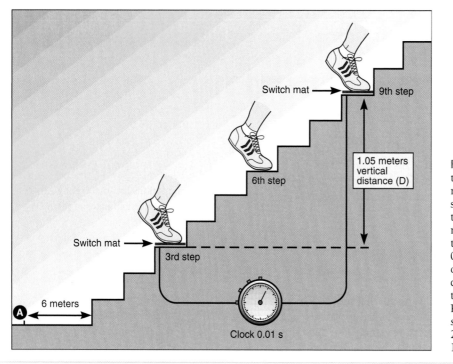

Switch mat → 9th step

1.05 meters vertical distance (D)

6th step

Switch mat → 3rd step

6 meters

Ⓐ

Clock 0.01 s

Figure 7.3 Stair-sprinting power test. The subject begins at point A and runs as fast as possible up a flight of stairs, taking three steps at a time. Electric switch mats placed on the steps record the time to cover the distance between stair 3 and stair 9 to the nearest 0.01 s. Power output equals the product of the subject's mass (F) and vertical distance covered (D), divided by the time (T). (Modified from Mathews, D. K., and Fox, E. L.: *The Physiological Basis of Physical Education and Athletics.* 2nd Ed. Philadelphia: W. B. Saunders, 1976.)

Box 7–1 · CLOSE UP

PREDICTING PEAK ANAEROBIC POWER OUTPUT USING A VERTICAL JUMP TEST

Peak anaerobic power output underlies success in many sport activities. The vertical jump test has become a widely used test to measure "explosive" peak anaerobic power.

VERTICAL JUMP TEST

The vertical jump measures the highest distance jumped from a semi-crouched position. The specific protocol for performing the test follows:

1. Establish standing reach height. The individual stands with the right shoulder adjacent to a wall with the feet flat on the floor before reaching up as high as possible to touch the wall with the middle finger. Measure the distance (cm) from the wall mark to the floor (Fig. 1).
2. Bend the knees to roughly a 90° angle, and place both arms back in a winged position.
3. Thrust forward and upward, touching as high as possible on the wall (Fig. 2); no leg movement is permitted prior to jumping.
4. Perform three trials of the jump test and use the highest score to represent the individual's "best" vertical jump height.
5. Compute vertical jump height as the difference between standing reach height and vertical jump height in centimeters.

PREDICT ANAEROBIC POWER OUTPUT

The following equation predicts **peak anaerobic power output** in watts (PAP_W) from vertical jump height in centimeters (VJ_{cm}) and body weight in kilograms (BW_{kg}). The equation applies to males and females:

$$PAP_W = (60.7 \times VJ_{cm}) + (45.3 \times BW_{kg}) - 2055$$

EXAMPLE

A 21-year-old male weighing 78 kg records a vertical jump height of 43 cm (standing reach height = 185 cm; vertical jump height = 228 cm); predict peak anaerobic power output in watts.

1. $PAP_W = (60.7 \times VJ_{cm}) + (45.3 \times BW_{kg}) - 2055$
2. $= (60.7 \times 43 \text{ cm}) + (45.3 \times 78 \text{ kg}) - 2055$
3. $= 4088.5 \text{ W}$

Applicability to Males and Females

For comparison purposes, average peak power output measured with this protocol averages 4620.2 W (SD = ±822.5 W) for males and 2993.7 W (SD = ±542.9 W) for females.

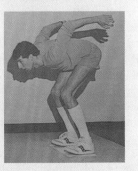

Figure 1

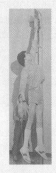

Figure 2

REFERENCE

1. Sayers, S., et al.: Cross-validation of three jump power equations. *Med. Sci. Sports Exerc.*, 31:572, 1999.

the friction load is applied and continues all-out for 10 seconds. Performance represents the average of the two tests reported in peak joules (or kCal) per kg of body mass and total joules (or kCal) per kg of body mass.

Relationships Among Anaerobic Power Tests

If the various power tests measure the same general anaerobic capacity, then one would assume individuals who rank high on one test would rank correspondingly high on a second or third test. Table 7.1 shows the interrelationships (expressed statistically as a correlation coefficient) among three tests that purport to measure immediate power output.

The relationships (ranging from poor [r = 0.31] to moderately strong [r = 0.88]) indicate some commonality between tests and suggest that each test is probably measuring a similar metabolic quality. Of practical significance, a fairly strong relationship exists between scores on the stair-sprinting power test and the 40-yard dash.

Several factors explain the low interrelationships among the other power output capacity test scores. First, a high degree of task specificity exists for human physical performance. This means that the best sprint runner may not necessarily be the best sprint swimmer, sprint cyclist, stair sprinter, repetitive volleyball leaper, or sprint arm-cranker. Even though the same metabolic reactions generate the energy to power each performance, energy transfer takes place within the specific muscles activated by the exercise. Furthermore, each specific test requires different neurologic skill components; the predominance of neuromuscular task specificity dictates that an individual will perform differently on each of the tests.

Power tests may be used to show changes in an athlete's performance with specific training. Such tests also serve as an excellent means for self-testing and motivation and often provide the actual movement-specific exercise for training the immediate energy system. Many football teams, for example, routinely use the 40-yard dash as a criterion to evaluate a player's speed. Although football requires many types of "speed," the 40-yard scores may provide useful information for player evaluation. Research needs to establish how 40-yard speed in a straight line relates to overall football ability for players at similar positions. A run test of shorter duration (10 to 20 yards) or one with frequent changes in direction may be equally or more important as a suitable performance measure.

THE SHORT-TERM ENERGY SYSTEM

Figure 7.2 showed that anaerobic reactions of glycolysis (short-term energy system) generate increasingly greater energy for ATP resynthesis when all-out exercise continues for longer than a few seconds. This does not mean that aerobic metabolism remains unimportant at this stage of exercise or that the oxygen-consuming reactions have not been "switched-on." To the contrary, Figure 7.2 reveals an increase in aerobic energy contribution very early in exercise. However, the energy requirement in relatively brief all-out exercise significantly exceeds energy generated by hydrogen's oxidation in the respiratory chain. This means that the anaerobic reactions of glycolysis predominate, presumably with large quantities of lactate accumulating within the active muscle and ultimately appearing in the blood.

No specific criteria exist to indicate when a person reaches a maximal anaerobic effort. In fact, one's level of self-motivation, including external factors in the test environment, likely influence test scores. *Researchers often use the blood lactate level to reveal the degree of activation of the short-term energy system.*

Physiologic Indicators of the Short-Term Energy System

Blood Lactate Levels Activation of the glycolytic energy pathway in maximal exercise results in a considerable accumulation of blood lactate. Blood lactate levels more than likely reflect the capacity of the short-term energy system.

Figure 7.4 presents data obtained from 10 college men who performed 10 all-out bicycle ergometer rides of different durations on the Katch test (see Performance Tests of Glycolytic Power, pages 229 and 230) on different days. The subjects included men involved in physical conditioning programs and varsity athletics. Unaware of the duration of each test, the men were urged to turn as many revolutions as possible. The researchers measured venous blood lactate before and immediately after each test and throughout recovery. The plotted points represent the average peak blood lactate values at the end of exercise for each test. Blood lactate levels increased directly with duration (and total work output) of all-out exercise. The highest blood lactates occurred at the end of 3 minutes of cycling, averaging about 130 mg in each 100 mL of blood (about 16 mmol).

Glycogen Depletion Because the short-term energy system largely depends on glycogen stored in specific

Table 7·1	Correlations among Tests Purported to Measure Power Output from the Immediate Energy System[a]		
VARIABLE	**JUMP & REACH**	**STAIR-SPRINTING**
40-yard dash	−0.48[b]	−0.88[b]
Jump and reach	—	−0.31

[a]From the Applied Physiology Laboratory, University of Michigan (N = 31 males).
[b]Negative correlations mean faster times (lower scores) associated with higher jumps or greater power output.

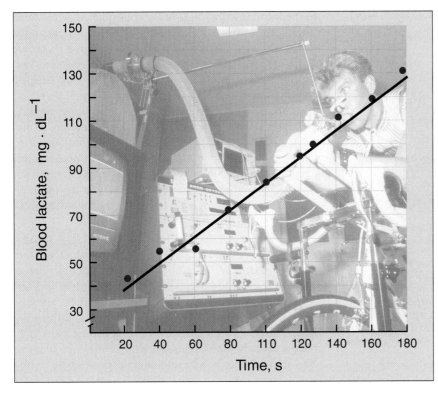

Figure 7.4 Pedaling a stationary bicycle ergometer at the highest possible power output increases blood lactate in direct proportion to the duration of exercise for up to 3 minutes. Each value represents the average of 10 subjects. (Data from the Applied Physiology Laboratory, University of Michigan.)

muscles activated by exercise, these muscles' pattern of glycogen depletion provides an indication of the contribution of glycolysis to exercise.

Figure 7.5 shows that the rate of glycogen depletion in the quadriceps femoris muscle during bicycle exercise closely parallels exercise intensity. With steady-rate exercise at about 30% of $\dot{V}O_{2max}$, a substantial reserve of muscle glycogen remains, even after cycling for 180 minutes. Because relatively light exercise relies mainly on a low level of aerobic metabolism, large quantities of fatty acids provide energy with only moderate use of stored glycogen. The most rapid and pronounced glycogen depletion occurs at the two heaviest workloads. This makes sense from a metabolic standpoint because glycogen provides the only stored nutrient for anaerobic ATP resynthesis. Thus, glycogen has high priority in the "metabolic mill" during strenuous exercise.

Performance Tests of Glycolytic Power

Activities that require substantial activation of the short-term energy system demand maximal work for up to 3 minutes. All-out runs and cycling exercise have usually tested anaerobic energy transfer capacity, although weight lifting (repetitive lifting of a certain percentage of maximum) and shuttle and agility runs have also been used. Because age, gender, skill, motivation, and body size affect maximal physical performance, selecting a suitable criterion test to develop normative standards for glycolytic energy capacity remains difficult. A test that maximally uses only leg muscles cannot adequately assess short-term anaerobic capacity for upper-body exercise such as rowing or swimming. *Considered within the framework of exercise specificity, the performance test must be similar to the activity or sport for which energy capacity is evaluated. In most cases, the actual activity serves as the test.*

In 1973, the **Katch test** used all-out leg cycling of short duration to estimate the power and capacity of the anaerobic energy systems. The frictional resistance

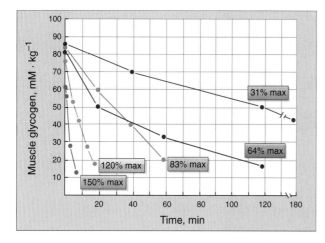

Figure 7.5 Glycogen depletion from the vastus lateralis portion of the quadriceps femoris muscle in bicycle exercise of different intensities and durations. Exercise at 31% of $\dot{V}O_{2max}$ (the lightest workload) caused some depletion of muscle glycogen, but the most rapid and largest depletion occurred with exercise that ranged from 83% to 150% of $\dot{V}O_{2max}$. (Adapted from Gollnick, P.D.: Selective glycogen depletion pattern in human muscle fibers after exercise of varying intensity and at varying pedaling rates. *J. Physiol.*, 241:45, 1974.)

against the bicycle's flywheel was preset at the high load of 6 kg for men and 5 kg for women. Subjects turned as many revolutions as possible in 40 seconds with pedal revolution rate recorded continuously. The peak power achieved represented **anaerobic power** (work per unit of time), and total work accomplished reflected **anaerobic capacity** (total work accomplished).

A subsequent modification of the Katch test, the **Wingate test**, involves 30 seconds of all-out exercise on either an arm-crank or leg-cycle ergometer. In this adaptation, the initial frictional resistance represents a function of the subject's body mass (0.075 kg of resistance per kg body mass), rather than a set value; the tester applies this resistance only after the subject overcomes the initial inertia and unloaded frictional resistance to pedaling (within about 3 seconds). Timing of the test then begins, with pedal revolutions counted continuously and usually reported every 5 seconds. **Peak power output** represents the highest mechanical power generated during any 3- to 5-second interval of the test; **average power output** equals the arithmetic average of total power generated during the 30-second test.

Anaerobic fatigue (percentage of decline in power relative to the peak value) provides an index of anaerobic endurance; it represents the maximal capacity for ATP production via a combination of intramuscular phosphagen breakdown and the reactions of glycolysis. **Anaerobic capacity** represents the total work accomplished over the 30-second exercise period (see Predicting Anaerobic Power and Capacity Using The Wingate Cycle Ergometer Test on page 232).

Interpretation of the Wingate test assumes that peak power output represents the energy-generating capacity

of the intramuscular high-energy phosphates, while total power output reflects anaerobic (glycolytic) capacity. Elite volleyball and ice hockey players have recorded some of the highest cycle ergometer power scores. The Wingate and Katch tests elicit reproducible performance scores with acceptable validity.

Figure 7.6 presents the relative contribution of each metabolic pathway during three different duration all-out cycle ergometer tests. Part A illustrates the findings as a percentage of total work output, and part B presents the data in estimated kilojoules (kJ) and kCal of energy (1 kJ = 4.2 kCal). Note the progressive change in the percentage contribution of each of the energy systems to the total work output as duration of effort increases.

Anaerobic Power Lower in Children Children perform poorer on tests of short-term anaerobic power compared with adolescents and young adults. Perhaps children's lower muscle glycogen concentrations and rates of glycogen utilization partly account for this difference. In addition, children have less lower leg muscle strength related to body mass compared with adults, which could also diminish anaerobic exercise performance.

Gender Differences in Anaerobic Performance

The significant difference in anaerobic power capacity between women and men cannot be fully explained by differences in body composition, physique, muscular strength, or neuromuscular factors. For example, supermaximal cycling exercise elicited a significantly higher peak oxygen deficit (a measure of anaerobic capacity) in men than in women per unit of fat-free leg volume. This difference persisted even though gender differences in active muscle mass had been considered. Similar observations occur for gender differences in anaerobic exercise capacity in children and adolescents.

The above findings suggest the possibility of a gender-related biologic difference in anaerobic exercise capacity. If this possibility proves correct, then physical testing that focuses on anaerobic exercise performance would further intensify performance differences between men and women to a greater degree than typically expected. Adjusting performance to body size or composition would not eliminate this effect. For physical testing in the occupational setting, justifiable concern exists that all-out anaerobic exercise testing exacerbates existing gender differences in performance scores; such testing adversely impacts females.

Factors Affecting Anaerobic Performance

Three factors influence individual differences in anaerobic performance.

1. **Specific Anaerobic Training:** Short-term supermaximal training produces higher levels of blood and muscle lactate and greater muscle glycogen depletion compared to untrained counterparts; better performances are usually associated with higher blood lactate

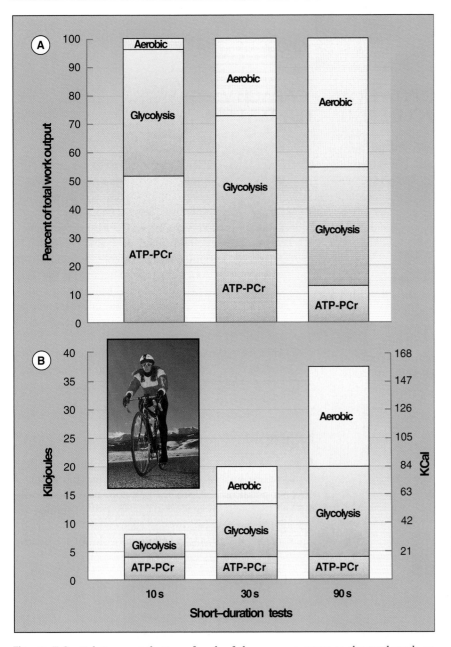

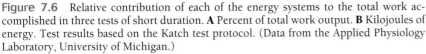

Figure 7.6 Relative contribution of each of the energy systems to the total work accomplished in three tests of short duration. **A** Percent of total work output. **B** Kilojoules of energy. Test results based on the Katch test protocol. (Data from the Applied Physiology Laboratory, University of Michigan.)

Questions & Notes

Give the duration of activity that requires substantial activation of the short-term energy system.

Give the duration and frictional resistance used in the popular Wingate test of anaerobic power and capacity.

Define what is meant by anaerobic fatigue in the Wingate test.

Give a reason why children usually record poorer results than adults on tests of short-term anaerobic power.

List 3 factors that influence anaerobic performance.

1.

2.

3.

levels, supporting the belief that training for brief, all-out exercise enhances the glycolytic system's capacity to generate energy.

2. **Buffering of Acid Metabolites:** Anaerobic training might enhance short-term energy transfer by increasing the body's buffering capacity (**alkaline reserve**) to enable greater lactate production; to date, no data show that trained individuals have a buffering capability within the range expected for healthy untrained people.

3. **Motivation:** Individuals with greater "pain tolerance," "toughness," or ability to "push" beyond the discomforts of fatiguing exercise have been shown to accomplish more anaerobic work. These people usually generate greater levels of blood lactate and glycogen depletion.

FOR YOUR INFORMATION

Benefits of Enhanced Alkaline Reserve
Pre-exercise altering of acid-base balance in the direction of alkalosis can temporarily but significantly enhance short-term, high-intensity exercise performance. Run times improve significantly by consuming a buffering solution of sodium bicarbonate before a high-intensity anaerobic effort. This effect is accompanied by higher blood lactate and extracellular H^+ concentrations, which indicate an increased anaerobic energy contribution.

Box 7–2 • CLOSE UP

PREDICTING ANAEROBIC POWER AND CAPACITY USING THE WINGATE CYCLE ERGOMETER TEST

The Wingate bicycle ergometer test represents the most popular test to assess anaerobic capacity. Developed at the Wingate Institute in Israel in the 1970s, test scores can reliably determine peak anaerobic power, anaerobic fatigue, and total anaerobic capacity.

THE TEST

A mechanically braked bicycle ergometer serves as the testing device. After warm-up (3–5 min), the subject begins pedaling as fast as possible without resistance. Within 3 seconds, a fixed resistance is applied to the flywheel; the subject continues to pedal "all out" for 30 seconds. An electrical or mechanical counter continuously records flywheel revolutions in 5-second intervals.

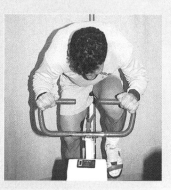

RESISTANCE

Flywheel resistance equals 0.075 kg per kg body mass. For a 70-kg person, the flywheel resistance would equal 5.25 kg (70 kg × 0.075). Higher resistances (1.0 to 1.3 kg × body mass) are often used to test power- and sprint-type athletes.

TEST SCORES

1. **Peak Power Output (PP):** The highest power output, observed during the first 5-second exercise interval, indicates the energy-generating capacity of the immediate energy system (intramuscular high-energy phosphates ATP and PCr). PP, expressed in watts (1 $W = 6.12$ kg-m·min^{-1}), computes as: Force × Distance (number of revolutions × distance per revolution) ÷ Time in minutes (5 s = 0.0833 min).

2. **Relative Peak Power Output (RPP):** Peak power output relative to body mass: PP ÷ Body mass, kg.

3. **Anaerobic Fatigue (AF):** Percentage decline in power output during the test; AF represents the total capacity to produce ATP via the immediate and short-term energy systems. AF computes as: Highest 5-second PP − Lowest 5-second PP ÷ Highest 5-second PP × 100.

4. **Anaerobic Capacity (AC):** Total work accomplished over 30 seconds; AC computes as the sum of each 5-second PP, or Force × Total distance in 30 seconds.

Example

A male weighing 73.3 kg (161.6 lb) performs the Wingate test on a Monark cycle ergometer (6.0 m traveled per pedal revolution) with an applied resistance of 5.5 kg (73.3 kg body mass × 0.075 = 5.497, rounded to 5.5 kg); pedal revolutions for each 5-second interval equal 12, 10, 8, 7, 6, and 5 (48 total revolutions in 30 s).

Calculations

1. Peak Power Output

$$PP = Force \times Distance \div Time$$
$$= 5.5 \times (12 \text{ rev} \times 6 \text{ m}) \div 0.0833$$
$$= 396 \div 0.0833$$
$$= 4753.9 \text{ kg-m·min}^{-1} \text{ or } 776.8 \text{ W}$$

2. Relative Peak Power Output

$$RPP = PP \div Body \text{ mass, kg}$$
$$= 776.8 \text{ W} \div 73.3 \text{ kg}$$
$$= 10.6 \text{ W·kg}^{-1}$$

Box 7–2 • CLOSE UP *(Continued)*

3. Anaerobic Fatigue

$$AF = \text{Highest PP} - \text{Lowest PP} \div \text{Highest PP} \times 100$$

[Highest PP = Force × Distance
  ÷ Time: 5.5 kg × (12 rev × 6 m)
  ÷ 0.0833 min = 4753.9 kg-m·min^{-1}
  or 776.8 W]

[Lowest PP = Force × Distance
  ÷ Time: 5.5 kg × (5 rev × 6 m)
  ÷ 0.0833 min = 1980.8 kg-m·min^{-1}
  or 323.7 W]

$$= 776.8 \text{ W} - 323.7 \text{ W} \div 776.8 \text{ W} \times 100$$
$$= 58.3\%$$

4. Anaerobic Capacity

$$AC = \text{Force} \times \text{Total Distance (in 30 s)}$$
$$= 5.5 \times [(12 \text{ rev} + 10 \text{ rev} + 8 \text{ rev}$$
$$+ 7 \text{ rev} + 6 \text{ rev} + 5 \text{ rev}) \times 6 \text{ m}]$$
$$= 1584 \text{ kg-m·min}^{-1} \text{ or } 258.8 \text{ W}$$

Percentile Data for Average and Peak Power for Active Young Adults

	AVERAGE POWER				PEAK POWER			
	MALE		FEMALE		MALE		FEMALE	
% RANK	W	WKG	W	WKG	W	WKG	W	WKG
90	662	8.24	470	7.31	822	10.89	560	9.02
80	618	8.01	419	6.95	777	10.39	527	8.83
70	600	7.91	410	6.77	757	10.20	505	8.53
60	577	7.59	391	6.59	721	9.80	480	8.14
50	565	7.44	381	6.39	689	9.22	449	7.65
40	548	7.14	367	6.15	671	8.92	432	6.96
30	530	7.00	353	6.03	656	8.53	399	6.86
20	496	6.59	336	5.71	618	8.24	376	6.57
10	471	5.98	306	5.25	570	7.06	353	5.98

W = watts; WKG = watts per kg body mass.
From Maud, P.J., and Schultz, B.B.: Norms for the Wingate anaerobic test with comparisons in another similar test. *Res. Q. Exerc. Sport*, 60:144, 1989.

SUMMARY

1. Measurement, evaluation, and prediction are closely related processes. From a practical standpoint, measurement takes place when a test is administered and a score is obtained.

2. The process of evaluation involves interpretation of test scores. Although the process of measurement is an objective nonjudgmental process, evaluation requires that judgments be made.

3. Prediction is a process whereby test scores are used to estimate (predict) another function or attribute of the same individual. The strength of any prediction is based on the degree of relationship between the test scores and the estimated function.

4. The concepts of individual differences and specificity help explain differences in capacity for anaerobic and aerobic power.

5. Individual differences refer to real differences among individuals, in contrast to variation in a physiologic response that characterizes the individual.

6. Specificity refers to a well-defined set of metabolic and physiologic responses that depend on a host of factors, including previous exercise training and method of evaluation.

7. The contribution of anaerobic and aerobic energy transfer depends largely on exercise intensity and duration. For sprint and strength-power activities,

primary energy transfer involves the immediate and short-term anaerobic energy systems. The long-term aerobic energy system becomes progressively more important in activities that last longer than 2 minutes.

8. Appropriate physiologic measurements and performance tests provide estimates of each energy system's capacity. Such testing evaluates a capacity at a particular time or reveals changes consequent to specific training programs.

9. The stair-sprinting test measures power output generated by the stored intramuscular high-energy phosphates. The 30-second, all-out Wingate test evaluates peak power and average power capacity from the glycolytic pathway. Interpretation of test results must consider the exercise specificity principle.

10. Training status, motivation, and acid–base regulation contribute to differences among individuals in the capacities of the immediate and short-term energy systems.

THOUGHT QUESTIONS

1. Significant specificity in physiologic function and exercise performance exists. How can one reconcile observations that certain individuals perform exceptionally well in many diverse physical activities (i.e., they appear to be "natural" athletes)?

2. How would you explain to an athlete the differences between the concepts of power and capacity? Give examples.

3. How would you react to the coach who says that "you can't train speed, it's a genetic gift"?

PART 2 •
Measuring and Evaluating the Aerobic Energy System

In this section, we describe techniques to measure activity of the aerobic energy system. These procedures form the basis for accurately quantifying differences among individuals in aerobic energy metabolism at rest and during physical activity.

DIRECT CALORIMETRY

All of the body's metabolic processes ultimately produce heat. Consequently, we can measure human energy metabolism by measuring heat production similarly to the method for determining the energy value of foods in the bomb calorimeter (see Figure 3.1, Chapter 3).

The **human calorimeter** illustrated in **Figure 7.7** consists of an airtight chamber where a person lives and works for extended periods. A known volume of water at a specified temperature circulates through a series of coils at the top of the chamber. Circulating water absorbs the heat produced and radiated by the individual. Insulation protects the entire chamber, so any change in water temperature relates directly to the individual's energy metabolism. Chemicals continually remove moisture and absorb carbon dioxide from the person's exhaled air. Oxygen added to the air recirculates through the chamber.

Professors W.O. Atwater (a chemist) and E.B. Rosa (a physicist) in the 1890s built and perfected the first human

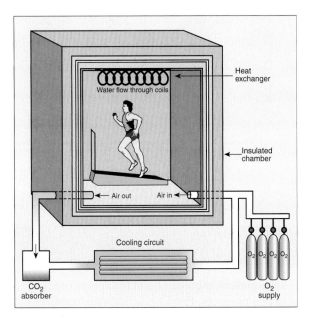

Figure 7.7 Directly measuring body's heat production in the human calorimeter.

calorimeter of major scientific importance at Wesleyan University (Connecticut). Their elegant human calorimetric experiments relating energy input to energy expenditure successfully verified the *law of the conservation of energy* and validated the relationship between direct and indirect calorimetry. The **Atwater-Rosa calorimeter** consisted of a small chamber where the subject lived, ate, slept, and exercised on a bicycle ergometer. Experiments lasted from several hours to 13 days; during some experiments, subjects cycled continuously for up to 16 hours, expending more than 10,000 kCal. The calorimeter's operation required 16 people working in teams of 8 for 12-hour shifts.

Direct measurement of heat production (**direct calorimetry**) in humans has considerable theoretical implications but limited practical application. Accurate measurements require considerable time, expense, and formidable engineering expertise. Thus, the direct calorimeter cannot determine energy expenditure for most sport, occupational, and recreational activities. In the 90 years since Atwater and Rosa published their papers on human calorimetry, other methodology evolved to infer energy expenditure indirectly from metabolic gas exchange.

INDIRECT CALORIMETRY

All energy-releasing reactions in the body ultimately depend on the use of oxygen Thus, by measuring a person's oxygen uptake, researchers obtain an indirect yet accurate estimate of energy expenditure. **Closed-circuit** and **open-circuit spirometry** represent the two methods of indirect calorimetry.

Closed-Circuit Spirometry

Figure 7.8 illustrates **closed-circuit spirometry** developed in the late 1800s and currently used in hospitals and research laboratories to estimate resting energy expenditure. The subject breathes 100% oxygen from a prefilled container (spirometer). The spirometer in this application is a "closed system" as the person rebreathes only the gas in the spirometer, and no outside air enters the system. A canister of soda lime (potassium hydroxide) placed in the breathing circuit absorbs the person's exhaled carbon dioxide. A drum attached to the

Questions & Notes

Briefly describe the major difference between direct and indirect calorimetry procedures.

Briefly describe the major difference between open- and closed-circuit spirometry procedures.

Give the percentage composition of oxygen, carbon dioxide, and nitrogen in ambient air.

Oxygen –

Carbon dioxide –

Nitrogen –

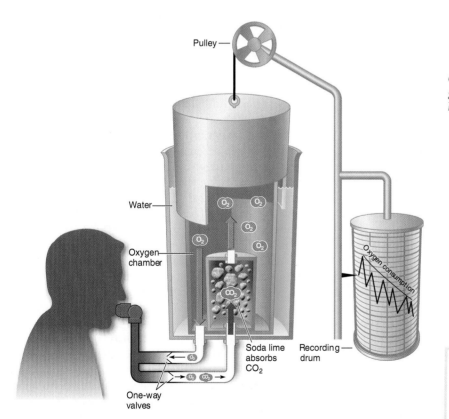

Figure 7.8   The closed-circuit method uses a spirometer prefilled with 100% oxygen. As the subject rebreathes from the spirometer, soda lime removes the expired air's carbon dioxide. The difference between the initial and final volumes of oxygen in the calibrated spirometer indicates oxygen consumption during the measurement interval.

FOR YOUR INFORMATION

Calorimetry Versus Spirometry
Calorimetry represents the measurement of heat energy liberated or absorbed in metabolic processes, whereas spirometry is an indirect calorimetry method for estimating heat production.

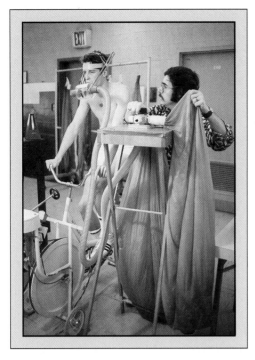

Figure 7.9 Oxygen uptake measurement by open-circuit spirometry (bag technique) during stationary cycle ergometer exercise.

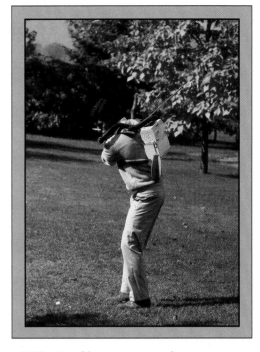

Figure 7.10 Portable spirometer used to measure oxygen uptake by the open-circuit method during golf.

spirometer revolves at a known speed and records the difference between the initial and final volumes of oxygen in the calibrated spirometer, thus indicating the oxygen uptake ($\dot{V}O_2$) during the measurement interval.

This system is not suitable for use during exercise where subject movement is required and large volumes of air are exchanged.

Open-Circuit Spirometry

Open-circuit spirometry represents the most widely used technique to measure oxygen uptake during exercise. A subject inhales ambient air with a constant composition of 20.93% oxygen, 0.03% carbon dioxide, and 79.04% nitrogen. The nitrogen fraction also includes a small quantity of inert gases. Changes in oxygen and carbon dioxide percentages in expired air compared with inspired ambient air indirectly reflect the ongoing process of energy metabolism. Thus, analysis of two factors—volume of air breathed during a specified time period and composition of exhaled air—measures oxygen uptake.

Three common open-circuit, indirect calorimetric procedures measure oxygen uptake during physical activity: (1) bag technique, (2) portable spirometry, and (3) computerized instrumentation.

Bag Technique   Figure 7.9 depicts the **bag technique**. In this example, a subject rides a stationary bicycle ergometer wearing headgear containing a two-way, high-velocity, low-resistance breathing valve. Ambient air passes through one side of the valve and expels out the other

side. The expired air then passes into either large canvas or plastic bags or rubber meteorologic balloons, or directly through a gas meter, which continually measures air volume. A small sample of the expired air is analyzed for oxygen and carbon dioxide composition and subsequent calculations of $\dot{V}O_2$ and calories.

Portable Spirometry   German scientists in the early 1940s perfected a lightweight, portable system to indirectly determine the energy expended during physical activity. The activities included war-related operations, such as traveling over different terrain with full battle gear, operating transportation vehicles including tanks and aircraft, and simulating tasks that soldiers would encounter during actual combat. The subject (in this example, shown striking a golf ball) carries the 3-kg box-shaped apparatus on the back like a backpack (**Fig. 7.10**). Ambient air passes through a two-way valve, and expired air exits through a gas meter. The meter measures total expired air volume and collects a small gas sample (aliquot) for later analysis of oxygen and carbon dioxide content and subsequent determination of $\dot{V}O_2$ and energy expenditure.

Computerized Instrumentation   With advances in computer and microprocessor technology, the exercise scientist can now accurately and rapidly measure aerobic energy expenditure in many different environments under varied conditions. Computer chips interface with a system to continuously sample the subject's expired air, a flow-measuring device to record air volume breathed, and oxygen and carbon dioxide analyzers to measure the expired gas mixture's composition.

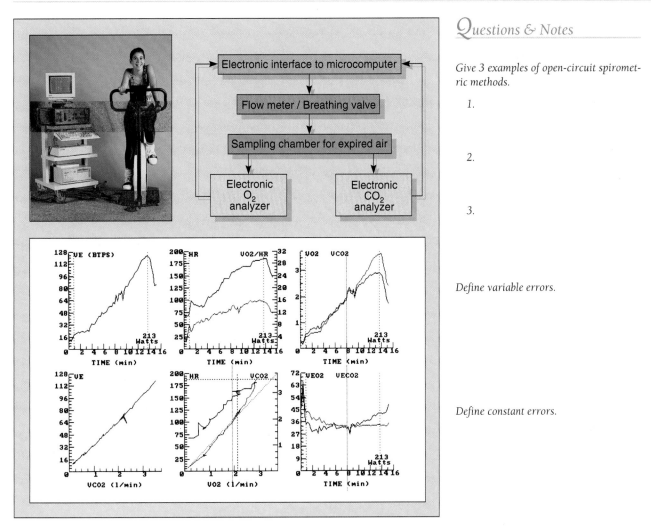

Give 3 examples of open-circuit spirometric methods.

1.

2.

3.

Define variable errors.

Define constant errors.

Give an average energy equivalent for 1 L oxygen.

Figure 7.11 Computer systems approach to the collection, analysis, and rapid display of physiologic and metabolic data. (Photos courtesy of AEI Technologies, Pittsburgh, PA.)

The computer performs the metabolic calculations based on electronic signals it receives from each instrument. A printed or graphic display of the data appears during each measurement period. More advanced systems include automated blood pressure, heart rate, and temperature monitors, and preset instructions to regulate speed, duration, and workload of a treadmill, bicycle ergometer, stepper, rower, swim flume, or other exercise apparatus. **Figure 7.11** depicts an example of a stationary **computerized metabolic collection system**. These computerized systems make it possible to collect vast amounts of data on a breath-by-breath basis. Miniature, portable metabolic data collection systems are now available that can literally fit in the palm of your hand. These portable, wireless systems are used during a broad range of exercise, sport, and occupational activities. In conjunction with telemetry, data appear in "real time" on a host or network computer or the Internet. In the not too distant future, a fully functional metabolic measurement system that can be worn on the wrist will be available at a cost no more expensive than a wireless telephone with embedded video camera!

Give the formula for computing RQ.

Calibration Required

Regardless of the apparent sophistication of a particular automated system, the output data reflect the accuracy of the measuring device. Therefore, accuracy and validity of measurement devices require careful and frequent calibration using established reference

Box 7–3 • CLOSE UP

HOW TO CALIBRATE AN INSTRUMENT

Most measuring instruments exhibit two types of errors, variable error and constant error.

Variable errors are unpredictable and produce inconsistent scores (i.e., scores fluctuate randomly in both positive and negative directions). Variable errors are most often influenced by (1) instrument reading errors, (2) effects of uncontrolled environmental influences (temperature or barometric pressure), and (3) variable functioning inherent to the instrument's operation.

Constant errors include systematic errors that either add or subtract a consistent amount to the resulting score. Many scientific instruments exhibit a consistent drift of the zero so that it always reads consistently several units higher (or lower) than an established, criterion value.

CALCULATING ERRORS

Suppose you want to calibrate a new ventilation meter (**NM**) that can record expired air volumes ($\dot{V}_E$) in $L \cdot min^{-1}$ during rest and up to maximum ventilation (e.g., 7 to 120 $L \cdot min^{-1}$). Calculating constant and variable errors involves comparing volumes obtained using the new meter (**NM**) versus volumes obtained using a criterion device (instrument known to yield correct values). In this example, a Tissot gasometer (**TG**) (see Fig. 1) serves as the criterion device for assessing gas volume.

To calibrate the **NM** a subject breathes in ambient air through a two-way respiratory value and the expired air passes into the **NM** and then into the **TG**, connected in series with low-resistance corrugated tubing (**Fig. 1**).

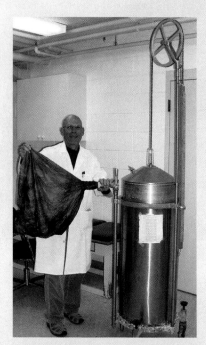

Figure 1 Tissot gasometer (water filled and weight balanced spirometer) capable of measuring up to 125 liters of gas. The contents of a meteorological balloon containing expired air are being transferred to the gasometer for precise measurement.

Minute ventilation volumes are measured for 8 minutes under the following conditions: rest, and light, moderate, and intense exercise. **Table 1** presents the $\dot{V}_E$ ($L \cdot min^{-1}$) for **NM** and **TG** and the difference between the two during the light exercise condition.

Table 1	Ventilation Data for the New Meter (NM) and Criterion Tissot Gasometer (TG)		
Minute	Tissot (TG) Volume, $L \cdot min^{-1}$	New Meter (NM) Volume, $L \cdot min^{-1}$	TG − NM Volume, $L \cdot min^{-1}$
1	29.6	35.9	−6.2
2	33.8	38.5	−4.7
3	31.2	36.3	−5.1
4	31.2	34.7	−3.5
5	30.6	36.9	−6.3
6	40.5	43.0	−2.5
7	39.5	45.9	−6.4
8	27.5	33.8	−6.3
	$\bar{X}$ = 32.99	$\bar{X}$ = 38.13	$\bar{X}_{diff}$ = −5.13
	SD = 4.37	SD = 3.95	SD = 1.38

Box 7–3 • CLOSE UP *(Continued)*

Constant Error

The mean absolute difference between the two methods (-5.13 L·min^{-1}; last column, Table 1) represents the constant error (i.e., the **NM**, on average, consistently records 5.13 L·min^{-1} higher than the criterion **TG**). The constant error can be subtracted from each **NM** recording to more closely approximate **TG** values. The constant error is sometimes referred to as a **calibration factor**.

Variable Error

The standard deviation of the differences ($\pm$ 1.38 L·min^{-1}; last column, Table 1) represents the variable error of the **NM**. Expressed as a percentage of the mean criterion gas volume [(1.38 L·min^{-1} $\div$ 32.99 L·min^{-1}) $\times$ 100], the variable error represents $\pm$ 4.2% of the actual gas volume. Since the variable error represents a random inconsistency in recording an accurate volume, it cannot be added or subtracted to more closely approximate the "true" **TG** volume; it will have to be determined whether this magnitude of variable error for the NM is small enough to warrant its use.

ERRORS AT DIFFERENT VOLUMES

The previous example illustrates constant and variable error for a volume averaging about 30 L·min^{-1}. The same procedures are performed at different expiratory volumes to determine whether errors (constant and variable) change in relation to the size of the volume breathed into the meter. **Table 2** presents data for constant and variable errors for six ventilation volume ranges. (The data from Table 1 are included in this table.)

In this example, note that the constant error remains stable throughout the different volume ranges. This is not the case with the variable error. A plot of the variable errors (L·min$_{-1}$) as a function of the mean criterion volume (L·min$_{-1}$) in **Figure 2** reveals that the new meter becomes progressively more inconsistent. It reaches $\pm$ 12.3% (12.8 $\div$ 104.1 $\times$ 100) of the criterion at the highest ventilation rate.

INTERPRETATION

While constant errors can be corrected (or accounted for), variable errors cannot. It becomes necessary to calculate the effects of a particular variable error before concluding if its magnitude reaches unacceptable levels. For example, a $\dot{V}_E$ variable error of $\pm$ 2% to 4% by itself would not be considered large, but when used for calculating oxygen consumption, it may represent an unacceptable level of error. This is the case at the highest ventilatory rates, where the calibration data show the new meter resulting in large and inconsistent errors. Therefore, this meter should not be used for determining ventilatory volume for the purposes of determining oxygen uptake.

Variable Errors

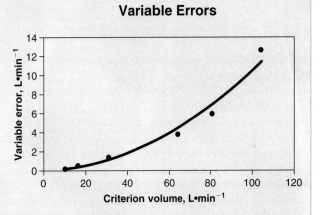

Figure 2 Plot of variables errors (L·min^{-1}) versus criterion volume. At the highest rate, the variable error of 12.8 L·min^{-1} amounts to 12.3% of the criterion volume (see Table 2).

Table 2	Constant and Variable Errors for Six Ventilation Ranges			
Ventilation Range, L·min^{-1}	**Mean Criterion Volume, L·min^{-1}**	**Constant Error, L·min^{-1}**	**Variable Error, L·min^{-1}**	**Variable Error, % Criterion**
8–15	12.3	−5.0	0.113	0.92
15–25	18.4	−5.10	0.52	2.8
30–40	32.9	−5.13	1.38	4.2
50–75	65.2	−5.10	3.85	5.9
75–100	81.7	−5.0	6.05	7.4
+100	104.1	−5.2	12.80	12.3

standards. Metabolic measurements require frequent calibration of the meter that measures the volume breathed and the oxygen and carbon dioxide analyzers. Most laboratories have criterion instruments used for calibration purposes. The accompanying Close Up details an example of how to calibrate a new ventilation meter (see page 238).

DIRECT VERSUS INDIRECT CALORIMETRY

Energy metabolism studied simultaneously using direct and indirect calorimetry provides convincing evidence for the validity of the indirect method. At the turn of the century, the two calorimetric methods were compared by Atwater and Rosa for 40 days with three men who lived in calorimeters similar to the one shown in Figure 7.7. Their daily caloric outputs averaged 2723 kCal when measured directly by heat production and 2717 kCal when computed indirectly using closed-circuit measures of oxygen uptake. Other experiments with animals and humans based on moderate exercise also demonstrated close agreement between direct and indirect methods; in most instances, the difference averaged less than ± 1%. In the Atwater and Rosa calorimetry experiments, the ± 0.2% method error represents a remarkable achievement, given that these experiments used hand-made instruments.

Caloric Transformation for Oxygen

Bomb calorimeter studies show that approximately 4.82 kCal release when a blend of carbohydrate, lipid, and protein burns in one liter of oxygen. Even with large variations in the metabolic mixture, this **caloric value for oxygen** varies only slightly (within ± 2% to 4%).

An energy–oxygen equivalent of 5.0 kCal per liter provides a convenient yardstick to transpose any aerobic physical activity to a caloric (energy) frame of reference. Indirect calorimetry through oxygen uptake measurement provides the basis for quantifying the caloric cost of most physical activities.

RESPIRATORY QUOTIENT (RQ)

Complete oxidation of a molecule's carbon and hydrogen atoms to carbon dioxide and water end-products requires different amounts of oxygen due to inherent chemical differences in carbohydrate, lipid, and protein composition. Consequently, the substrate metabolized determines the quantity of carbon dioxide produced in relation to oxygen consumed. The **respiratory quotient (RQ)** refers to the following ratio of metabolic gas exchange:

$$RQ = CO_2 \text{ produced} \div O_2 \text{ consumed}$$

The RQ helps to approximate the nutrient mixture catabolized for energy during rest and aerobic exercise. Also, because the caloric equivalent for oxygen differs somewhat depending on the nutrients oxidized, precisely determining the body's heat production (kCal) requires information about oxygen uptake and RQ.

RQ for Carbohydrate

All of the oxygen consumed in carbohydrate combustion oxidizes the carbon in the carbohydrate molecule to carbon dioxide. This is because the ratio of hydrogen to oxygen atoms in carbohydrates always exists in the same ratio (2:1) as in water. The complete oxidation of one glucose molecule requires six oxygen molecules and produces six molecules of carbon dioxide and water as follows:

$$C_6H_{12}O_6 + 6\,O_2 \rightarrow 6\,CO_2 + 6\,H_2O$$

Gas exchange during glucose oxidation produces an equal number of CO_2 molecules to O_2 molecules consumed; therefore, RQ for carbohydrate equals 1.00:

$$RQ = 6CO_2 \div 6O_2 = 1.00$$

RQ for Lipid

The chemical composition of lipids differs from carbohydrates because lipids contain considerably fewer oxygen atoms in proportion to carbon and hydrogen atoms. Consequently, lipid catabolism for energy requires considerably more oxygen in relation to carbon dioxide production. Palmitic acid, a typical fatty acid, oxidizes to carbon dioxide and water, producing 16 carbon dioxide molecules for every 23 oxygen molecules consumed. The following equation summarizes this exchange to compute RQ:

$$C_{16}H_{32}O_2 + 23O_2 \rightarrow 16CO_2 + 16H_2O$$
$$RQ = 16CO_2 \div 23O_2 = 0.696$$

Generally, a value of 0.70 represents the RQ for lipid, ranging between 0.69 and 0.73, depending on the oxidized fatty acid's carbon chain length.

RQ for Protein

Proteins do not simply oxidize to carbon dioxide and water during energy metabolism in the body. Rather, the liver first deaminates (removes nitrogen) the amino acid molecule; then the body excretes the nitrogen and sulfur fragments in the urine, sweat, and feces. The remaining "keto acid" fragment oxidizes to carbon dioxide and water to provide energy for biologic work. Short-chain keto acids require more oxygen in relation to carbon dioxide produced to achieve complete combustion. For example, the protein albumin oxidizes as follows:

$$C_{72}H_{112}N_2O_{22}S + 77O_2 \rightarrow 63CO_2$$
$$+ 38H_2O + SO_3 + 9CO(NH_2)_2$$
$$RQ = 63CO_2 \div 77O_2 = 0.818$$

The general value 0.82 characterizes the RQ for protein.

| Table 7·2 | Thermal Equivalents of Oxygen for the Non-Protein Respiratory Quotient, Including Percent kCal and Grams Derived From Carbohydrate and Fat | | | | |

NON-PROTEIN RQ	KCAL PER LITER O_2 UPTAKE	PERCENTAGE KCAL DERIVED FROM		GRAMS PER LITER O_2 UPTAKE	
		CARBOHYDRATE	FAT	CARBOHYDRATE	FAT
0.707	4.686	0.0	100.0	0.000	.496
.71	4.690	1.1	98.9	.012	.491
.72	4.702	4.8	95.2	.051	.476
.73	4.714	8.4	91.6	.900	.460
.74	4.727	12.0	88.0	.130	.444
.75	4.739	15.6	84.4	.170	.428
.76	4.750	19.2	80.8	.211	.412
.77	4.764	22.8	77.2	.250	.396
.78	4.776	26.3	73.7	.290	.380
.79	4.788	29.9	70.1	.330	.363
.80	4.801	33.4	66.6	.371	.347
.81	4.813	36.9	63.1	.413	.330
.82	4.825	40.3	59.7	.454	.313
.83	4.838	43.8	56.2	.537	.297
.84	4.850	47.2	52.8	.579	.280
.85	4.862	50.7	49.3	.579	.263
.86	4.875	54.1	45.9	.621	.247
.87	4.887	57.5	42.5	.663	.230
.88	4.887	60.8	39.2	.705	.213
.89	4.911	64.2	35.8	.749	.195
.90	4.924	67.5	32.5	.791	.178
.91	4.936	70.8	29.2	.834	.160
.92	4.948	74.1	25.9	.877	.143
.93	4.961	77.4	22.6	.921	.125
.94	4.973	80.7	19.3	.964	.108
.95	4.985	84.0	16.0	1.008	.090
.96	4.998	87.2	12.8	1.052	.072
.97	5.010	90.4	9.6	1.097	.054
.98	5.022	93.6	6.4	1.142	.036
.99	5.035	96.8	3.2	1.186	.018
1.00	5.047	100.0	0	1.231	.000

From Zuntz, N.: Ueber die Bedeutung der verschiedenen Nährstoffe als Erzeuger der Muskelkraft. *Arch. Gesamte Physiol.*, Bonn, Ger.: LXXXIII, 557–571, 1901. *Pflügers Arch. Physiol.*, 83:557, 1901.

RQ for a Mixed Diet

During activities ranging from complete bed rest to mild aerobic exercise (walking or slow jogging), the RQ seldom reflects the oxidation of pure carbohydrate or pure fat. Instead, metabolizing a mixture of nutrients occurs with an RQ intermediate between 0.70 and 1.00. *For most purposes, we assume an RQ of 0.82 from the metabolism of a mixture of 40% carbohydrate and 60% fat, applying the caloric equivalent of 4.825 kCal per liter of oxygen for the energy transformation.* Using 4.825 kCal, the maximum error possible in estimating energy metabolism from steady-rate oxygen uptake equals about 4%.

Table 7.2 presents the energy expenditure per liter of oxygen uptake for different **non-protein RQ** values, including corresponding percentages and grams of carbohydrate and fat used for energy. *The non-protein RQ value assumes that the metabolic mixture comprises only carbohydrate and fat.* Interpret the table as follows:

Suppose oxygen uptake during 30 minutes of aerobic exercise averages 3.22 L·min^{-1} with CO_2 production of 2.78 L·min^{-1}. The RQ, computed as $\dot{V}CO_2 \div \dot{V}O_2$ (2.78 ÷ 3.22), equals 0.86. From Table 7.2, this RQ value (left column) corresponds to an energy equivalent of 4.875 kCal per liter of oxygen uptake, or an exercise energy output of 15.7 kCal·min^{-1} (3.22 L O_2·min^{-1} × 4.875 kCal). Based on a non-protein RQ, 54.1% of the calories come from the combustion of carbohydrate and 45.9% come from fat. The

FOR YOUR INFORMATION

RQ Versus RER

The RER (respiratory exchange ratio: ratio of the amount of CO_2 produced to the amount of O_2 consumed) reflects what is happening on a total body level, whereas the RQ (ratio of CO_2 produced to O_2 consumed) represents the gas exchange from substrate metabolism on the cellular level.

Box 7–4 · CLOSE UP

PREDICTING $\dot{V}O_{2max}$ USING A WALKING TEST

A walking test devised in the 1980s for use on large groups predicts $\dot{V}O_{2max}$ (L·min^{-1}) from the following variables (see Equation 1): body weight (W) in pounds; age (A) in years; gender (G): 0 = female, 1 = male; time (T1) for the 1-mile track walk expressed as minutes and hundredths of a minute; and peak heart rate (HR$_{peak}$) in beats·min^{-1} at the end of the last one-quarter mile (measured as a 15-s pulse immediately after the walk × 4 to convert to b·min^{-1}). The test consisted of having individuals walk 1 mile as fast as possible without jogging or running.

For most individuals, $\dot{V}O_{2max}$ ranged within ± 0.335 L·min^{-1} (± 4.4 mL·kg^{-1}·min^{-1}) of actual $\dot{V}O_{2max}$. This prediction method applies to a broad segment of the general population (ages 30 to 69 y).

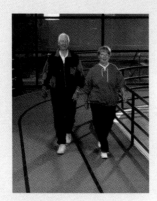

EQUATIONS

Equation 1

Predicts $\dot{V}O_{2max}$ in L·min^{-1}:

$$\dot{V}O_{2max} = 6.9652 + (0.0091 \times W)$$
$$- (0.0257 \times A)$$
$$+ (0.5955 \times G) - (0.224 \times T1)$$
$$- (0.0115 \times HR_{peak})$$

Equation 2

Predicts $\dot{V}O_{2max}$ in mL·kg^{-1}·min^{-1}:

$$\dot{V}O_{2max} = 132.853 - (0.0769 \times W)$$
$$- (0.3877 \times A) + (6.315 \times G)$$
$$- (3.2649 \times T1)$$
$$- (0.1565 \times HR_{peak})$$

Example

Predict $\dot{V}O_{2max}$ (mL·kg^{-1}·min^{-1}) from the following data: gender, female; age, 30 years; body weight, 155.5 lb; T1, 13.56 min; HR$_{peak}$, 145 b·min^{-1}.

Substituting the above values in equation 2:

$$\dot{V}O_{2max} = 132.853 - (0.0769 \times 155.5)$$
$$- (0.3877 \times 30.0) + (6.315 \times 0)$$
$$- (3.2649 \times 13.56)$$
$$- (0.1565 \times 145)$$
$$= 132.853 - (11.96) - (11.63)$$
$$+ (0) - (44.27) - (22.69)$$
$$= 42.3 \text{ mL·kg}^{-1}\text{·min}^{-1}$$

REFERENCE

Kline, G., et al.: Estimation of $\dot{V}O_{2max}$ from a one-mile track walk, gender, age, and body weight. *Med. Sci. Sports Exerc.*, 19:253, 1987.

total calories expended during the 30-minute exercise period equal 471 kCal (15.7 kCal·min^{-1} × 30).

RESPIRATORY EXCHANGE RATIO (R)

Application of the RQ requires the assumption that the O_2 and CO_2 exchange measured at the lungs reflects the actual gas exchange from nutrient metabolism on the cellular level. This assumption is reasonably valid for rest and during steady-rate (mild-to-moderate) aerobic exercise conditions with no lactate accumulation. However, factors can alter the exchange of oxygen and carbon dioxide in the lungs so that the gas exchange ratio no longer reflects *only* the substrate mixture in cellular energy metabolism. For example, carbon dioxide elimination increases during hyperventilation because breathing increases to disproportionately high levels in relation to the actual metabolic demands. By overbreathing, the normal level of

CO_2 in the blood decreases because the gas "blows off" in expired air. A corresponding increase in oxygen uptake does not accompany additional CO_2 elimination. Consequently, the exchange ratio often exceeds 1.00. *Respiratory physiologists refer to the ratio of carbon dioxide produced to oxygen consumed under such conditions as the* **respiratory exchange ratio** (**R** or **RER**). This ratio computes in exactly the same manner as RQ. An increase in the respiratory exchange ratio above 1.00 cannot be attributed to foodstuff oxidation.

Exhaustive exercise presents another situation where R usually increases above 1.00. Sodium bicarbonate in the blood buffers or "neutralizes" the lactate generated during anaerobic metabolism to maintain proper acid-base balance in the reaction:

$$HLa + NaHCO_3 \rightarrow NaLa + H_2CO_3 \rightarrow H_2O + CO_2 \rightarrow Lungs$$

Lactate buffering produces the weaker carbonic acid. In the pulmonary capillaries, carbonic acid breaks down to its components, carbon dioxide and water, allowing carbon dioxide to readily exit through the lungs. The R increases above 1.00 because buffering adds "extra" CO_2 to expired air above the quantity normally released during cellular energy metabolism.

Relatively low R values can occur after exhaustive exercise when carbon dioxide remains in body fluids to replenish bicarbonate that buffered the accumulating lactate. This action reduces expired carbon dioxide without affecting oxygen uptake, causing the R to go below 0.70.

THE MAXIMAL OXYGEN UPTAKE ($\dot{V}O_{2MAX}$)

The $\dot{V}O_{2max}$ (aerobic power) represents the greatest amount of oxygen a person can use to produce ATP aerobically on a per minute basis. This usually occurs during high-intensity, endurance-type exercise. The data in **Figure 7.12** illustrate that persons who engage in sports that require sustained, high-intensity exercise possess large aerobic energy transfer capacity.

Men and women who compete in distance running, swimming, bicycling, and cross-country skiing record the highest maximal oxygen uptakes. *These athletes have nearly twice the aerobic capacity as sedentary individuals.* This does not mean that only $\dot{V}O_{2max}$ determines endurance exercise capacity. Other factors, particularly those at the muscle level, such as capillary density, enzymes, and muscle fiber type, strongly influence capacity to sustain exercise at a high percentage of $\dot{V}O_{2max}$ (i.e., achieve a high blood lactate threshold). However, the $\dot{V}O_{2max}$ provides useful information about long-term energy system capacity. Furthermore, attainment of $\dot{V}O_{2max}$ requires integration of the ventilatory, cardiovascular, and neuromuscular systems; this gives significant physiologic "meaning" to this metabolic measure. *In essence, $\dot{V}O_{2max}$ represents a fundamental measure in exercise physiology and serves as a standard to compare performance estimates of aerobic capacity and endurance fitness.*

Tests for $\dot{V}O_{2max}$ use exercise tasks that activate large muscle groups with sufficient intensity and duration to engage maximal aerobic energy transfer. Typical exercise includes treadmill walking or running, bench stepping, or cycling, tethered and flume swimming and swim-bench ergometry, and simulated rowing, skiing, in-line skating, stair-climbing, ice skating, and arm-crank exercise. Considerable research effort has been directed toward the (1) development and standardization of tests for $\dot{V}O_{2max}$ and (2) establishment of norms related to age, gender, state of training, and body composition.

Criteria for $\dot{V}O_{2max}$

A leveling-off or peaking-over in oxygen uptake during increasing exercise intensity (**Fig. 7.13**) *signifies attainment of maximum capacity for aerobic metabolism (i.e., a "true" $\dot{V}O_{2max}$).* When this accepted criterion is not met or local muscle fatigue in the arms or legs rather than central circulatory dynamics limits test performance, the term **peak oxygen uptake** ($\dot{V}O_{2peak}$) usually describes the highest oxygen uptake value during the test.

Questions & Notes

Give the "general" RQ values for the 3 major macronutrients.

Carbohydrate –

Lipid –

Protein –

Give the difference between RER and the RQ.

Give the kCal per L O_2 uptake for a non-protein RQ = 0.86.

True or False:

An increase in the R above 1.00 directly reflects the mixture of micronutrients oxidized for energy.

Name the product produced from lactate buffering.

Give the R value typically observed after exhaustive exercise.

FOR YOUR INFORMATION

kCal Equivalent for 1 Liter Oxygen
Assuming the combustion of a mixed diet, a rounded value of 5.0 kCal per liter of oxygen consumed designates the appropriate conversion factor for estimating energy expenditure under steady-rate conditions of aerobic metabolism.

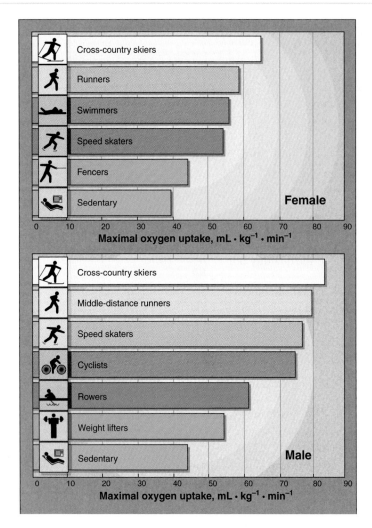

Figure 7.12 Maximal oxygen uptake of male and female Olympic-caliber athletes in different sport categories compared to healthy sedentary subjects. (Adapted from Saltin, B., and Åstrand, P.O.: Maximal oxygen uptake in athletes. *J. Appl. Physiol.*, 23:3523, 1967.)

The data in Figure 7.13 reflect oxygen uptake with progressive increases in treadmill exercise intensity; the test terminates when the subject decides to stop even when prodded to continue. For the average oxygen uptake values of 18 subjects plotted in this figure, the highest oxygen uptake occurred before subjects attained their maximum exercise level. This peaking-over criterion substantiates attainment of a true $\dot{V}O_{2max}$.

In many instances, a peaking-over or slight decrease in oxygen uptake does not occur as exercise intensity increases. Often, the highest oxygen uptake occurs during the last minute of exercise without the plateau criterion for $\dot{V}O_{2max}$. Thus, additional criteria for establishing $\dot{V}O_{2max}$ (more precisely $\dot{V}O_{2peak}$) have been suggested based on metabolic and physiologic responses. These include:

- Failure for oxygen uptake versus exercise intensity to increase by some value usually expected from previous observations with the particular test ($\dot{V}O_{2max}$ criterion).
- Blood lactate levels that reach at least 70 or 80 mg per 100 mL of blood or about 8 to 10 mmol (ensures the subject has significantly exceeded the lactate threshold with a near-maximal exercise effort; $\dot{V}O_{2peak}$ criterion).
- Attainment of near age-predicted maximum heart rate, or a respiratory exchange ratio (R) in excess of 1.00 (indicates that subject exercised at close to maximum intensity; $\dot{V}O_{2peak}$ criterion).

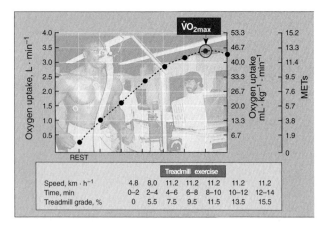

Figure 7.13 Peaking over in oxygen uptake with increasing intensity of treadmill exercise. Each point represents the average oxygen uptake of 18 sedentary males. The point at which oxygen uptake fails to increase the expected amount or even decreases slightly with increasing exercise intensity represents the $\dot{V}O_{2max}$. (Data from the Applied Physiology Laboratory, University of Michigan.)

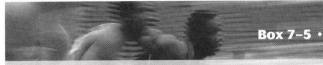

Box 7–5 • CLOSE UP

PREDICTING $\dot{V}O_{2MAX}$ USING A STEP TEST

Recovery heart rate from a standardized stepping exercise can classify people on cardiovascular fitness and $\dot{V}O_{2max}$ with a reasonable degree of accuracy.

THE TEST

Individuals step to a four-step cadence ("up-up-down-down") on a bench 16 1/4 inches high (height of standard gymnasium bleachers). Women perform 22 complete step-ups per minute to a metronome set at 88 beats per minute; men use 24 step-ups per minute at a metronome setting of 96 beats per minute.

Stepping begins after a brief demonstration and practice period. Following stepping, the person remains standing while another person measures pulse rate (carotid or radial artery) for a 15-second period, 5 to 20 seconds into recovery. Fifteen-second recovery heart rate converts to beats per minute (15-s HR × 4), which converts to a percentile ranking for predicted $\dot{V}O_{2max}$ (see table).

Equations

The following equations predict $\dot{V}O_{2max}$ ($mL \cdot kg^{-1} \cdot min^{-1}$) from step-test heart rate recovery for men and women ages 18 to 24 years:

Men: $\dot{V}O_{2max} = 111.33$
$$- (0.42 \times \text{step-test pulse rate, } b \cdot min^{-1})$$

Women: $\dot{V}O_{2max} = 65.81$
$$- (0.1847 \times \text{step-test pulse rate, } b \cdot min^{-1})$$

The "Predicted $\dot{V}O_{2max}$" columns of the table present the $\dot{V}O_{2max}$ values for men and women from different recovery heart rate scores.

Percentile Ranking for Recovery Heart Rate and Predicted $\dot{V}O_{2max}$ ($mL \cdot kg^{-1} \cdot min^{-1}$) for Male and Female College Students

PERCENTILE	RECOVERY HR FEMALES	PREDICTED $\dot{V}O_{2max}$	RECOVERY HR MALES	PREDICTED $\dot{V}O_{2max}$
100	128	42.2	120	60.9
95	140	40.0	124	59.3
90	148	38.5	128	57.6
85	152	37.7	136	54.2
80	156	37.0	140	52.5
75	158	36.6	144	50.9
70	160	36.3	148	49.2
65	162	35.9	149	48.8
60	163	35.7	152	47.5
55	164	35.5	154	46.7
50	166	35.1	156	45.8
45	168	34.8	160	44.1
40	170	34.4	162	43.3
35	171	34.2	164	42.5
30	172	34.0	166	41.6
25	176	33.3	168	40.8
20	180	32.6	172	39.1
15	182	32.2	176	37.4
10	184	31.8	178	36.6
5	196	29.6	184	34.1

From McArdle, W.D., et al.: Percentile norms for a valid step test in college women. *Res. Q.*, 44:498, 1973; McArdle, W.D., et al.: Reliability and interrelationships between maximal oxygen uptake, physical work capacity, and step test scores in college women. *Med. Sci. Sports.*, 4:182, 1972.

Tests of Aerobic Power

There are different standardized tests to measure $\dot{V}O_{2max}$. Such tests remain independent of muscle strength, speed, body size, and skill, with the exception of specialized swimming, rowing, and ice skating tests.

The $\dot{V}O_{2max}$ test may require a continuous 3- to 5-minute "supermaximal" effort, but it usually consists of increments in exercise intensity (referred to as a **graded exercise test** or **GXT**) until the subject stops. Some researchers have imprecisely termed the end point "exhaustion," but it should be kept in mind that the subject terminates the test for a variety of reasons, and exhaustion is only one possible reason. A variety of psychologic or motivational factors can influence this decision, rather than true physiologic exhaustion. It can take considerable urging and encouragement to get subjects to the criterion point for $\dot{V}O_{2max}$. Children and adults encounter particular difficulty if they have had little prior experience performing strenuous exercise with its associated central (cardiorespiratory) and peripheral (local muscular) discomforts. *Attaining a plateau in oxygen uptake during the* $\dot{V}O_{2max}$ *test requires high motivation and a large anaerobic component because of the maximal exercise requirement.*

Comparisons Among $\dot{V}O_{2max}$ Tests

Two types of $\dot{V}O_{2max}$ tests are typically used:

1. **Continuous Test** — no rest among exercise increments
2. **Discontinuous Test** — several minutes of rest between exercise increments

The data in **Table 7.3** show a systematic comparison of $\dot{V}O_{2max}$ scores measured by six common continuous and discontinuous treadmill and bicycle procedures.

Although only a small 8-mL difference occurred in $\dot{V}O_{2max}$ between continuous and discontinuous bicycle tests, $\dot{V}O_{2max}$ averaged 6.4% to 11.2% below values on the treadmill. The largest difference among any of the three treadmill tests equaled only 1.2%. The walking test, on the other hand, elicited $\dot{V}O_{2max}$ scores about 7% above values achieved on the bicycle but 5% less than the average for the three run tests.

Subjects reported intense local discomfort in the thigh muscles during intense exercise on both the continuous and discontinuous bicycle tests. In walking, subjects reported discomfort in the lower back and calf muscles, particularly at higher treadmill elevations. The running tests produced little local discomfort, yet subjects experienced a general fatigue usually categorized as feeling "winded." For ease of administration testing *healthy* subjects, we recommend a continuous treadmill run. Total time to administer the test averaged a little over 12 minutes, whereas the discontinuous running test averaged about 65 minutes. Subjects seemed to "tolerate" the continuous test well and preferred the shorter test time. In fact, $\dot{V}O_{2max}$ can be achieved with a continuous exercise protocol where exercise intensity increases progressively in 15-second intervals. With such an approach, total test time for either bicycle or treadmill exercise averages only about 5 minutes.

Commonly Used Treadmill Protocols

Figure 7.14 summarizes six commonly used treadmill protocols to assess aerobic capacity in healthy individuals and patients with cardiovascular disease. Features common to each test include manipulation of exercise duration and treadmill speed and grade. The Harbor treadmill test (example F), referred to as a **ramp test**, is unique because treadmill grade increases every minute up to 10 minutes by a constant amount that ranges from 1% to 4% depending on the subject's fitness. This quick procedure linearly increases oxygen uptake to the maximum level. Healthy individuals and monitored cardiac patients tolerate the protocol without problems.

Manipulating Test Protocol to Increase $\dot{V}O_{2max}$

When a person completes a maximal oxygen uptake test, one assumes the tester has made every attempt to "push" the subject to the near-limits of performance. This effort includes verbal encouragement from laboratory staff and peers or a monetary incentive. If the test meets the usual criteria, one assumes the test score represents the subject's "true" $\dot{V}O_{2max}$.

In one study, 44 sedentary and trained men and women performed a continuous treadmill $\dot{V}O_{2max}$ test to the point where they refused to continue exercising ("exhaustion"). They recovered for 2 minutes and then performed a second $\dot{V}O_{2max}$ test. During active recovery from test 1, the

Table 7·3	Average Maximal Oxygen Uptakes for 15 College Students During Continuous (cont.) and Discontinuous (discont.) Tests on the Bicycle and Treadmill					
VARIABLE	**BIKE DISCONT.**	**BIKE, CONT.**	**TREADMILL, DISCONT. WALK-RUN**	**TREADMILL, CONT. WALK**	**TREADMILL, DISCONT. RUN**	**TREADMILL, CONT. RUN**
$\dot{V}O_{2max}$, mL·min^{-1}	3691 ± 453	3683 ± 448	4145 ± 401	3944 ± 395	4157 ± 445	4109 ± 424
$\dot{V}O_{2max}$, mL·kg^{-1}·min^{-1}	50.0 ± 6.9	49.9 ± 7.0	56.6 ± 7.3	56.6 ± 7.6	55.5 ± 7.6	55.5 ± 6.8

Values are means ± standard deviation. Adapted from McArdle, W. D., et al.: Comparison of continuous and discontinuous treadmill and bicycle tests for max $\dot{V}O_2$. *Med. Sci Sport.*, 5:156, 1973.

Box 7–6 · CLOSE UP

PREDICTING $\dot{V}O_{2MAX}$ DURING PREGNANCY USING SUBMAXIMUM OXYGEN UPTAKE AND HEART RATE

Authorities recommend physical activity during pregnancy. Most agree that such exercise should be guided by an individualized exercise prescription because of concerns about fetal safety. An exercise prescription typically specifies intensity, duration, and frequency of physical activity. Exercise intensity is usually expressed as a percentage of the maximal oxygen uptake ($\%\dot{V}O_{2max}$) and is obtained from equations relating heart rate (HR) to $\%\dot{V}O_{2max}$. Determining $\dot{V}O_{2max}$ requires that subjects exercise to near-exhaustion. Consequently, prediction of $\dot{V}O_{2max}$ from submaximal exercise data is a more prudent approach during pregnancy.

PREDICTING $\dot{V}O_{2MAX}$ DURING PREGNANCY

The technique to predict $\dot{V}O_{2max}$ during pregnancy involves having individuals perform a 3-stage, submaximum cycle ergometer test. Oxygen uptake ($\dot{V}O_2$) and HR are measured at the last exercise stage to predict $\dot{V}O_{2max}$ using regression analyses.

SUBMAXIMUM CYCLE ERGOMETER TEST

Subject rests for 10 minutes and then performs a 3-stage, 6 minutes per stage, cycle ergometer test:

1. Stage 1: 0 watts (W) (unloaded cycling)
2. Stage 2: 30 W (184 kg-m·min^{-1})
3. Stage 3: 60 W (367 kg-m·min^{-1})

Measure $\dot{V}O_2$ in L·min^{-1} and HR in b·min^{-1} during the final 3 minutes of the last stage, and use the average values in the following regression equation to predict $\%\dot{V}O_{2max}$ in L·min^{-1}:

Predicted $\%\dot{V}O_{2max}$

$$= (0.634 \times HR\ [b{\cdot}min^{-1}]) - 30.79$$

Predict $\dot{V}O_{2max}$ (L·min^{-1}) from the following equation using the predicted $\%\dot{V}O_{2max}$ and observed $\dot{V}O_2$ (L·min^{-1}) during the last exercise stage:

Predicted $\dot{V}O_{2max}$

$$= \dot{V}O_2 \div Predicted\ \%\dot{V}O_{2max} \times 100$$

EXAMPLE

A 26-year-old female, who is 20 weeks pregnant and weighs 70.4 kg (pre-pregnancy weight = 59.8 kg) performs a 3-level cycle ergometer test (zero, 30 W, 60 W); each load is performed for 6 minutes. Heart rate and $\dot{V}O_2$ are recorded during the final 3 minutes of the last work stage: HR (b·min^{-1}) = 155; $\dot{V}O_2$ (L·min^{-1}) = 1.80.

1. Compute Predicted $\%\dot{V}O_{2max}$.

Predicted $\%\dot{V}O2max$

$$= (0.634 \times HR\ [b{\cdot}min-1]) - 30.79$$
$$= (0.634 \times 155) - 30.79$$
$$= 67.5\%$$

2. Compute Predicted $\dot{V}O_{2max}$.

Predicted $\dot{V}O2max$

$$= \dot{V}O_2 \div Predicted\ \%\dot{V}O_{2max} \times 100$$
$$= 1.80 \div 67.5 \times 100$$
$$= 2.67\ L{\cdot}min^{-1}\ (37.9\ mL{\cdot}kg^{-1}{\cdot}min^{-1})$$

REFERENCE

Sady, S.P., et al.: Prediction of $\dot{V}O_{2max}$ during cycle exercise in pregnant women. *J. Appl. Physiol.* 65:657, 1988.

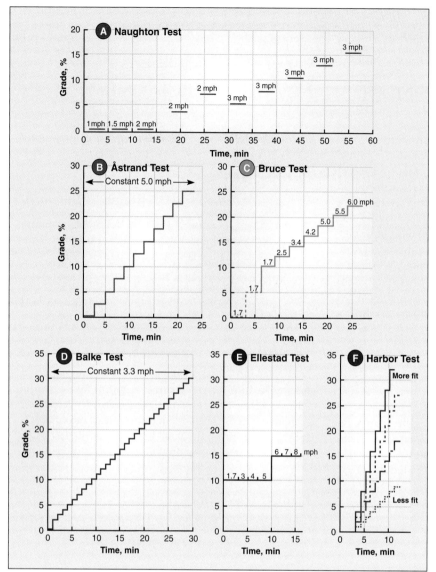

Figure 7.14 Six commonly used treadmill procedures. **A.** Naughton test. Three-minute exercise periods of increasing intensity alternating with 3 minutes of rest. The exercise periods vary in grade and speed. **B.** Åstrand test. Speed remains constant at 5 mph. After 3 minutes at 0% grade, grade increases 2.5% every 2 minutes. **C.** Bruce test. Grade and/or speed change every 3 minutes. Healthy subjects do not perform grades 0% and 5%. **D.** Balke test. After 1 minute at 0% grade and 1 minute at 2% grade, grade increases 1% per minute (all at a speed of 3.3 mph). **E.** Ellestad test. The initial grade is 10%, the later grade 15%, while the speed increases every 2 or 3 minutes. **F.** Harbor test. After 3 minutes of walking at a comfortable speed, grade increases at a constant preselected amount each minute (1%, 2%, 3%, or 4%), so the subject reaches $\dot{V}O_{2max}$ in approximately 10 minutes. (From Wasserman, K., et al.: *Principles of Exercise Testing and Interpretation.* 3rd Ed. Baltimore: Lippincott Williams & Wilkins, 1999.)

researchers lowered the treadmill grade at least 2.5% below the final grade of the previous test and reduced running speed from 11.0 $km \cdot h^{-1}$ to 9.0 $km \cdot h^{-1}$ for the trained subjects and from 9.0 $km \cdot h^{-1}$ to 6.0 $km \cdot h^{-1}$ for the sedentary subjects. After 2 minutes, treadmill speed increased to the test 1 speed for 30 seconds, at which time percent grade increased to the final grade achieved in test 1. Treadmill grade increased every 2 minutes thereafter until the subject once again terminated the test. Subjects received strong verbal encouragement, particularly during the last minutes of exercise during both tests.

The $\dot{V}O_{2max}$ scores averaged 1.4% higher on the second test. The statistically significant difference of 48 mL (0.7 $mL \cdot kg^{-1} \cdot min^{-1}$ for a typical subject), although small, was almost double the difference that is typically measured between the two final oxygen uptake readings on either continuous or discontinuous tests. A "booster" test after a normally administered aerobic capacity test can increase the final oxygen uptake, illustrating the need to pay careful attention to $\dot{V}O_{2max}$ administrative techniques.

Factors Affecting Maximal Oxygen Uptake

Many factors influence $\dot{V}O_{2max}$; the most important include exercise mode and the person's training state, heredity, gender, body composition, and age.

Exercise Mode *Variations in $\dot{V}O_{2max}$ during different modes of exercise reflect the quantity of muscle mass activated.* In experiments that measured $\dot{V}O_{2max}$ on the same subjects during diverse exercise, treadmill exercise produced the highest values. Bench-stepping generates $\dot{V}O_{2max}$ scores nearly identical to treadmill values and significantly higher than bicycle ergometer values. With arm-crank exercise, a person's aerobic capacity reaches only about 70% of treadmill $\dot{V}O_{2max}$.

For skilled but untrained swimmers, $\dot{V}O_{2max}$ during swimming falls about 20% below treadmill values. A definite test specificity exists in this form of exercise because trained collegiate swimmers achieved $\dot{V}O_{2max}$ values swimming that were only 11% below treadmill values; some elite competitive swimmers equal or even exceed their treadmill $\dot{V}O_{2max}$ scores during a swimming test for aerobic capacity. Similarly, a distinct exercise and training specificity occurs among competitive racewalkers who achieve oxygen uptakes during walking that equal $\dot{V}O_{2max}$ values during treadmill running. If competitive cyclists pedal at their fast rate in competition, they also achieve $\dot{V}O_{2max}$ values equivalent to treadmill scores.

The treadmill represents the laboratory apparatus of choice for determining $\dot{V}O_{2max}$ in healthy subjects. The treadmill easily quantifies and regulates exercise intensity. Compared with other forms of exercise, subjects achieve one or more of the criteria for establishing $\dot{V}O_{2max}$ or $\dot{V}O_{2peak}$ more easily on the treadmill. Bench stepping or bicycle exercise serve as suitable alternatives under non-laboratory "field" conditions.

Heredity   A question that is frequently raised concerns the relative contribution of natural endowment to physiologic function and exercise performance. For example, to what extent does heredity determine the extremely high aerobic capacities of endurance athletes? Although answers remain incomplete, some researchers have focused on the question of how genetic variability accounts for differences among individuals in physiologic and metabolic capacity.

Early studies on this topic were conducted on 15 pairs of identical twins (same heredity since they came from the same fertilized egg) and 15 pairs of fraternal twins (did not differ from ordinary siblings because they result from separate fertilization of two eggs) raised in the same city by parents with similar socioeconomic backgrounds. The researchers concluded that heredity alone accounted for up to 93% of the observed differences in $\dot{V}O_{2max}$. Subsequent investigations of larger groups of brothers, fraternal twins, and identical twins indicate a significant but much smaller effect of inherited factors on aerobic capacity and endurance performance.

Current estimates of the genetic effect ascribe about 20% to 30% for $\dot{V}O_{2max}$, 50% for maximum heart rate, and 70% for physical working capacity. Future research will someday determine the exact upper limit of genetic determination, but present data show that inherited factors contribute *significantly* to physiologic functional capacity and exercise performance. A large genotype-dependency also exists for the potential to improve aerobic and anaerobic power and the adaptations of most muscle enzymes to training. In other words, members of the same twin-pair show the same response to exercise training.

Training State   Maximal oxygen uptake must be evaluated relative to the person's state of training at the time of measurement. Aerobic capacity with training improves between 6% and 20%, although increases have been reported as high as 50% above pretraining levels. The largest $\dot{V}O_{2max}$ improvement occurs among the most sedentary individuals.

Gender $\dot{V}O_{2max}$ $(mL \cdot kg^{-1} \cdot min^{-1})$ *for women typically average 15% to 30% below scores for men.* Even among trained athletes, the difference ranges between 10% and 20%. Such differences increase considerably when expressing $\dot{V}O_{2max}$ as an absolute value $(L \cdot min^{-1})$ rather than relative to body mass $(mL \cdot kg^{-1} \cdot min^{-1})$. Among world class male and female cross-country skiers, a 43% lower $\dot{V}O_{2max}$ for women (6.54 vs. 3.75 $L \cdot min^{-1}$) decreased to 15% (83.8 vs. 71.2 $mL \cdot kg^{-1} \cdot min^{-1}$) when using the athletes' body mass in the $\dot{V}O_{2max}$ ratio expression.

The apparent gender difference in $\dot{V}O_{2max}$ has been attributed to differences in body composition and the blood's hemoglobin concentration. Untrained young adult women possess about 25% body fat, whereas the corresponding value for men averages 15%. Although trained athletes have a lower body fat percentage, trained women still possess significantly more body fat than male counterparts. Thus, the male generates more total aerobic energy simply because he possesses a relatively large muscle mass and less fat than the female.

$Questions$ & $Notes$

State the major criterion for achieving $\dot{V}O_{2max}$ during graded exercise testing.

Name the 2 types of $\dot{V}O_{2max}$ tests.

1.

2.

Name 3 different GXT tests.

1.

2.

3.

Name 5 factors that affect $\dot{V}O_{2max}$.

1.

2.

3.

4.

5.

Briefly explain why different modes of exercise elicit different $\dot{V}O_{2max}$ values.

Give the average percentage different in $\dot{V}O_{2max}$ between untrained men and women.

Probably due to higher levels of testosterone, men also show a 10% to 14% greater concentration of hemoglobin than women. This difference in the blood's oxygen-carrying capacity enables males to circulate more oxygen during exercise, thus giving them an edge in aerobic capacity.

Differences in normal physical activity level between an "average" male and "average" female provide a possible explanation. Perhaps less opportunity exists for women to become as physically active as men due to social structure and constraints. Even among prepubertal children, boys exhibit a higher level of physical activity in daily life.

Despite these possible limitations, the aerobic capacity of physically active females exceeds that of sedentary males. For example, female cross-country skiers have $\dot{V}O_{2max}$ scores 40% higher than untrained males of the same age.

Body Composition   *Differences in body mass explain roughly 70% of the differences in $\dot{V}O_{2max}$ (L·min^{-1}) among individuals.* Thus, meaningful comparisons of $\dot{V}O_{2max}$ (particularly when expressed in L·min^{-1}) become difficult among individuals who differ in body size or body composition. This has led to the common practice of expressing oxygen uptake in terms by body surface area, body mass (BM), fat-free body mass (FFM), or even limb volume (i.e., dividing the $\dot{V}O_{2max}$ scores by FFM or BM) in the hope that $\dot{V}O_{2max}$ will be expressed independent of the respective divisor.

Table 7.4 presents typical oxygen uptake values for an untrained man and woman who differ considerably in body mass. The percentage difference in $\dot{V}O_{2max}$ between these individuals, when expressed in L·min^{-1}, amounts to 43%. The woman still exhibits about a 20% lower value when expressing $\dot{V}O_{2max}$ related to body mass (mL·kg^{-1}·min^{-1}); when divided by FFM, the difference is reduced to 9%.

Similar findings also occur for $\dot{V}O_{2peak}$ for men and women during arm-cranking exercise. Adjusting the arm-crank $\dot{V}O_{2peak}$ for variations in arm and shoulder size equalized values between the men and women. This suggests that gender differences in aerobic capacity largely reflect the size of the contracting muscle mass. Such observations foster the argument that no gender difference exists in the capacity of active muscle mass to generate ATP aerobically. On the other hand, simply dividing $\dot{V}O_{2max}$ or $\dot{V}O_{2peak}$ by some measure of body composition does not automatically "adjust" for observable gender differences. Researchers still must determine whether real differences exist (i.e., biologic in origin) or whether factors other than inherited characteristics (environmental-sociological factors) influence the difference between men and women.

Current research suggests a portion of the gender difference in aerobic capacity may be biologically inherent and unalterable. This does not mean that aerobic capacity cannot be significantly improved by training. Rather, it may be inappropriate to expect "sex-free" differences in aerobic capacity.

Age   Changes in $\dot{V}O_{2max}$ relate to chronological age. Although limitations exist in drawing inferences from cross-sectional studies of different people at different ages, the available data provide insight into the possible effects of aging on physiologic function.

Absolute Values   **Figure 7.15** shows that maximal oxygen uptake (L·min^{-1}) increases dramatically during the growth years. Longitudinal studies (measuring the same individual over a prolonged period) of children's $\dot{V}O_{2max}$ show that absolute values increase from about 1.0 L·min^{-1} at age 6 years to 3.2 L·min^{-1} at 16 years. $\dot{V}O_{2max}$ in girls peaks at about age 14 years and declines thereafter. At age 14, the differences in $\dot{V}O_{2max}$ (L·min^{-1}) between boys and girls is approximately 25%, with the spread reaching 50% by age 16 years.

Relative Values   When expressed relative to body mass, the $\dot{V}O_{2max}$ remains constant at about 53 mL·kg^{-1}·min^{-1} between the ages of 6 and 16 years for boys. In contrast, relative $\dot{V}O_{2max}$ in girls gradually decreases from 52.0 mL·kg^{-1}·min^{-1} at age 6 to 40.5 mL·kg^{-1}·min^{-1} at age 16 years. Greater accumulation of body fat in females provides the most common explanation for this discrepancy.

Beyond age 25, $\dot{V}O_{2max}$ declines steadily at about 1% per year, so that by age 55, it averages 27% below values reported for 20 year olds. Although active adults retain a relatively high $\dot{V}O_{2max}$ at all ages (Fig. 7.15, inset graph), their aerobic power still declines with advancing years. However, research continues to show that one's habitual level of physical activity through middle age determines changes in $\dot{V}O_{2max}$ to a greater extent than chronological age per se.

Table 7·4	Different Ways of Expressing Oxygen Uptake		
VARIABLE	**FEMALE**	**MALE**	**% DIFFERENCE[a]**
$\dot{V}O_{2max}$, L·min^{-1}	2.00	3.50	−43
$\dot{V}O_{2max}$, mL·min^{-1}	40.0	50.0	−20
$\dot{V}O_{2max}$, mL·kg FFM^{-1}·min^{-1}	53.3	58.8	−9.0
Body mass, kg	50	70	−29
Percent body fat	25	15	+67
Fat-free body mass (FFM), kg	37.5	59.5	−37

[a]Female versus male.

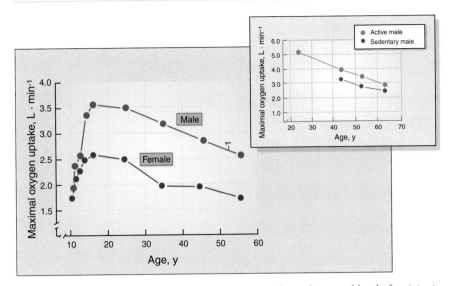

Figure 7.15 General trend for maximal oxygen uptake with age and level of activity in males and females.

What type of test is the most popular for predicting $\dot{V}O_{2max}$?

Give 2 reasons that prediction of $\dot{V}O_{2max}$ should be approached with caution.

1.

2.

List 2 factors that affect endurance walking-running other than $\dot{V}O_{2max}$.

1.

2.

MAXIMAL OXYGEN UPTAKE PREDICTIONS

Directly measuring $\dot{V}O_{2max}$ requires an extensive laboratory, specialized equipment, and considerable motivation on the subject's part to perform "all out." As such, $\dot{V}O_{2max}$ tests do not lend themselves to measuring large groups of untrained subjects outside of the laboratory. In addition, maximal exercise can be hazardous to adults who have not received proper medical clearance or who are tested without appropriate safeguards or supervision (refer to Chapter 18).

In view of these considerations, alternative tests have been devised to predict $\dot{V}O_{2max}$ from submaximal performances (*see different examples throughout this chapter*). The most popular $\dot{V}O_{2max}$ predictions use walking and running endurance performance. Easily administered, these tests can be used with large groups without the need of a laboratory setting. Endurance running tests assume that maximal oxygen uptake largely determines the distance one can run in a specified time (greater than 5 or 6 min). The first of the endurance running tests required subjects to run-walk as far as possible in 15 minutes, and a 1968 revision of the test shortened the duration to 12 minutes or 1.5 miles.

Findings from many research studies suggest that the prediction of aerobic capacity should be approached with caution when using walking and running performance. Establishing a consistent level of motivation and effective pacing becomes critical for inexperienced subjects. Some individuals may run too fast early in the run and, thus, must slow down or even stop as the test progresses. Other individuals may begin too slowly and continue this way, so their final run score reflects inappropriate pacing or motivation, rather than physiologic and metabolic capacity.

In addition, endurance walking-running performance results from factors other than $\dot{V}O_{2max}$. Body mass and body fatness, running economy (which continually improves during childhood), and one's percentage of aerobic capacity sustainable without blood lactate buildup (blood lactate threshold) all contribute to the final $\dot{V}O_{2max}$ predicted score.

Heart Rate Predictions of $\dot{V}O_{2max}$

Common tests to predict $\dot{V}O_{2max}$ from exercise or postexercise heart rate use a standardized regimen of submaximal exercise on a bicycle ergometer, motorized treadmill, or step test. Such tests make use of the essentially linear (straight-line)

Box 7-7 • CLOSE UP

PREDICTING $\dot{V}O_{2max}$ USING AGE FOR SEDENTARY, PHYSICALLY ACTIVE, AND ENDURANCE-TRAINED INDIVIDUALS

Estimates from cross-sectional data indicate $\dot{V}O_{2max}$ declines approximately 0.4 mL·kg^{-1}·min^{-1} each year for most individuals (4.0 mL·kg^{-1}·min^{-1} each decade; **Table 1**). This may be an overestimate because a clear difference exists in the rate of decline with aging between sedentary versus highly trained individuals. Sedentary individuals may have nearly two-fold faster rates of decline in $\dot{V}O_{2max}$ as they age. Heredity undoubtedly plays an important role, as does the well-documented decrement in muscle mass with age. The normal decline in aerobic power may follow a two-component curve; one portion of the curve represents a faster rate of decline in sedentary adults from age 20 to 30 years compared to adults who are more physically active; thereafter, a slower rate of decline occurs for both groups. Thus, for both active and sedentary persons, it is possible to predict $\dot{V}O_{2max}$ from age estimates.

EQUATIONS

Table 2 presents different equations to predict $\dot{V}O_{2max}$ using age as the predictor variable.

Table 1	Rate of $\dot{V}O_{2max}$ Decline per Decade	
FITNESS LEVEL	**RATE OF DECLINE (mL·kg^{-1}·min^{-1})**	**RATE OF DECLINE (%)**
Sedentary	4.0	9.0
Moderately Active	4.0	7.7
Endurance Trained	3.0	5.0

Table 2	Equations to Predict $\dot{V}O_{2max}$ (mL·kg^{-1}·min^{-1}) From Age	
GROUP	**EQUATION**	**CORRELATION**
1. Sedentary[a]	Predicted $\dot{V}O_{2max}$ = 54.2 − 0.40 (age, y)	r = 0.88
2. Moderately Active[b]	Predicted $\dot{V}O_{2max}$ = 61.4 − 0.39 (age, y)	r = 0.80
3. Endurance Trained[c]	Predicted $\dot{V}O_{2max}$ = 77.2 − 0.46 (age, y)	r = 0.89
4. Alternate equations (independent of relative fitness status)		
Males: Predicted $\dot{V}O_{2max}$ = 59.48 − 0.46 (age, y)		
Females: Predicted $\dot{V}O_{2max}$ = 53.7 − 0.537 (age, y)		

[a]No physical activity.
[b]Occasional physical activity, about 2 d·wk^{-1}.
[c]Physical activity = 3 d·wk^{-1} for at least 1 full year.

Box 7–7 • CLOSE UP *(Continued)*

Example 1 – Endurance Trained Male, Age 55 y (Equation 3, Table 2)

Predicted $\dot{V}O_{2max}$ = 77.2 − 0.46 (age, y)

$= 77.2 − 0.46\ (55)$

$= 51.7\ mL\cdot kg^{-1}\cdot min^{-1}$

Example 2 – Active Female, Age 21 y (Equation 2, Table 2)

Predicted $\dot{V}O_{2max}$ = 61.4 − 0.39 (age, y)

$= 61.4 − 0.39\ (21)$

$= 53.2\ mL\cdot kg^{-1}\cdot min^{-1}$

Example 3 – 23-Y-Old Female of Unknown Fitness Status (Equation 4, Table 2)

Predicted $\dot{V}O_{2max}$ = 53.7 − 0.537 (age, y)

$= 53.7 − 0.537$

$= 53.2\ mL\cdot kg^{-1}\cdot min^{-1}$

REFERENCES

1. Wilson, T.M., and Seals, D.R.: Meta-analysis of the age-associated decline in maximal aerobic capacity in men: Relation to habitual aerobic status. *Med. Sci. Sports Exerc.,* 31:S385, 1995.

2. Jackson, A.S., et al.: Changes in aerobic power of women age 20–64 y. *Med. Sci. Sports Exerc.,* 28:884, 1996.

relationship between heart rate and oxygen uptake for various intensities of light to moderately heavy exercise. The slope of this line (rate of HR increase per unit of $\dot{V}O_2$ increase) reflects the individual's aerobic power. $\dot{V}O_{2max}$ is estimated by drawing a best-fit straight line through several submaximum points that relate heart rate and oxygen uptake (or exercise intensity) and then extending this line to an assumed maximum heart rate for the person's age.

Figure 7.16 applies this **extrapolation procedure** for a trained and untrained subject. Four submaximal measures during bicycle exercise provided the data points to draw the heart rate–oxygen uptake (HR–$\dot{V}O_2$) line. Each person's HR–$\dot{V}O_2$ line tends to be linear, but the slope of the individual lines can differ considerably, largely because of variations in the amount of blood the heart pumps with each beat (stroke volume). A person with relatively high aerobic power can accomplish more intense exercise and achieves a higher oxygen uptake before reaching their HR_{max} than a less "fit" person. The person with the lowest heart rate increase tends to have the highest exercise capacity and largest $\dot{V}O_{2max}$. The data in Figure 7.16 predict $\dot{V}O_{2max}$ by extrapolating the HR–$\dot{V}O_2$ line to a heart rate of 195 b·min^{-1} (the assumed maximum heart rate for these college-age subjects).

The following four assumptions limit the accuracy of predicting $\dot{V}O_{2max}$ from submaximal exercise heart rate:

1. **Linearity of the HR–$\dot{V}O_2$ (exercise intensity) relationship.** Various intensities of light to moderately heavy exercise meet this assumption. For some subjects, the HR–$\dot{V}O_2$ line curves or asymptotes at the heavier work loads in a direction that indicates a larger than expected increase in oxygen uptake per unit increase in heart rate. Oxygen uptake increases more than predicted through linear extrapolation of the HR–$\dot{V}O_2$ line, thus *underestimating* the $\dot{V}O_{2max}$.

Box 7–8 • CLOSE UP

PREDICTING V̇O$_{2MAX}$ USING AVERAGE RUNNING SPEED (KM·H^{-1}) DURING DIFFERENT RACING DISTANCES

Different performance tests, such as maximal endurance "racing" runs on a track, have been devised and validated for predicting V̇O$_{2max}$. Generally, these tests are practical, inexpensive, less time-consuming than laboratory tests, easy to administer for large groups, and accurate (for predictive purposes) when properly conducted. The endurance run distances usually are 1 mile or greater.

To convert km race distance to kilometers per hour (km·h^{-1}):

1. multiply km distance by 60
2. divide race time in min:s expressed in decimal form (i.e., seconds divided by 60 to convert to decimal minutes)

To convert a 5-km run in 18 min, 25 s (18:25) to km·h^{-1}:

km·h^{-1} = (5 km × 60) ÷ 18.42
km·h^{-1} = 16.29

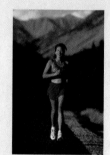

PREDICTION EQUATIONS FOR MAXIMAL SPEED RUNS

Prediction equations to predict V̇O$_{2max}$ from ability to run a given distance in kilometers (km) at maximal speed are presented in **Table 1**.

These equations assume the person tested runs the distance at maximum speed. The average running speed computes in kilometers per hour, km·h^{-1}, and the (appropriate) equation used to calculate the V̇O$_{2max}$ is expressed in METs. [One MET equals the resting oxygen consumption of 3.5 mL·kg^{-1}·min^{-1}; to convert METs to V̇O$_{2max}$ multiply the number of METs by 3.5 mL·kg^{-1}·min^{-1}.]

EXAMPLE 1

A person completes a 5-km race in 18 min, 25 s; predict the V̇O$_{2max}$ (mL·kg^{-1}·min^{-1}).

1. Compute km·h^{-1}

$$18 \text{ min, } 25 \text{ s} = 18.42 \text{ min}$$
$$\text{km·h}^{-1} = (5 \text{ km} \times 60) \div 18.42 \text{ km·h}^{-1}$$
$$= 16.29$$

2. METs [from Table 1] = 3.1747 + (0.9139 × km·h^{-1})

$$\text{METs} = 3.1747 + (0.9139 \times 16.29)$$
$$= 3.1747 + 14.887$$
$$= 18.1 \text{ (rounded up)}$$

Table 1	Prediction of Exercise MET Level From Average Running Speed for Different Racing Distances
RACE DISTANCE	**EQUATION TO PREDICT V̇O$_{2MAX}$ FROM METS**
1.5 km	METs = 2.4388 + (0.8343 × km·h^{-1})
1.6093 km (1 mile)	METs = 2.5043 + (0.8400 × km·h^{-1})
3 km	METs = 2.9266 + (0.8900 × km·h^{-1})
5 km	METs = 3.1747 + (0.9139 × km·h^{-1})
10 km	METs = 4.7226 + (0.8698 × km·h^{-1})
42.195 km (marathon)	METs = 6.9021 + (0.8246 × km·h^{-1})

km·h^{-1} = average racing speed in competition in kilometers per hour [multiply km distance by 60; divide by race time in min:s expressed in decimal form].
1 MET = 3.5 mL·kg^{-1}·min^{-1}; multiply MET value obtained by 3.5 mL·kg^{-1}·min^{-1} value to obtain V̇O$_{2max}$.

Box 7–8 •   CLOSE UP (Continued)

3. $\dot{V}O_{2max}$ $(mL \cdot kg^{-1} \cdot min^{-1})$ = 18.1 METs × 3.5 $mL \cdot kg^{-1} \cdot min^{-1}$

$$\dot{V}O_{2max}\ (mL \cdot kg^{-1} \cdot min^{-1}) = 63.35$$

EXAMPLE 2

A person completes a 10-km race in 59 min, 30 s; predict the $\dot{V}O_{2max}$ $(mL \cdot kg^{-1} \cdot min^{-1})$.

1. Compute $km \cdot h^{-1}$

$$59\ min,\ 30\ s = 59.5\ min$$
$$km \cdot h^{-1} = (10\ km \times 60) \div 59.5$$
$$= 10.08$$

2. METs = 4.7226 + (0.8698 × $km \cdot h^{-1}$) [from Table 1]

$$METs = 3.1747 + (0.8698 \times 10.08)$$
$$= 3.1747 + 8.698$$
$$= 11.87$$

3. $\dot{V}O_{2max}$ $(mL \cdot kg^{-1} \cdot min^{-1})$ = 11.87 METs × 3.5 $mL \cdot kg^{-1} \cdot min^{-1}$

$$\dot{V}O_{2max}\ (mL \cdot kg^{-1} \cdot min^{-1}) = 41.55$$

Table 2 presents calculations from the equations in Table 1 showing equivalent relationships between $\dot{V}O_{2max}$ and running performances for races ranging from 1.5 km to 42.2 km (standard marathon distance). Note that running a 6:01 mile results in the same predicted $\dot{V}O_{2max}$ (56 $mL \cdot kg^{-1} \cdot min^{-1}$) as running the 5 km in 21:23 or the 10 km in 46:17, and a marathon in 3:49:28.

Table 2   Equivalent Performance Times for Different Distances

$\dot{V}O_{2max}$ $mL \cdot kg^{-1} \cdot min^{-1}$	METs	PERFORMANCE TIME FOR DIFFERENT DISTANCES (hours:minutes:seconds)				
		1.5 km	1 mile	5 km	10 km	42.2 km
28	8	13:30	14:46	56:49	2:39:14	31:41:25
31.5	9	11:27	12:29	47:04	2:02:00	16:35:05
35	10	9:56	10:49	40:10	1:38:53	11:13:52
38.5	11	8:46	9:33	35:02	1:23:08	8:29:26
42	12	7:51	8:33	31:04	1:11:43	6:49:30
45.5	13	7:07	7:44	27:54	1:03:03	5:42:21
49	14	6:30	7:03	25:20	56:15	4:54:07
52.5	15	5:59	6:29	23:11	50:47	4:17:48
56	16	5:32	6:01	21:23	46:17	3:49:28
59.5	17	5:09	5:36	19:50	42:30	3:26:44
63	18	4:50	5:14	18:30	39:33	3:08:06
66.5	19	4:32	4:55	17:20	36:33	2:52:34
70	20	4:17	4:38	16:18	34:10	2:39:23
73.5	21	4:03	4:23	15:23	32:12	2:28:05
77	22	3:50	4:09	14:34	30:12	2:18:16
80.5	23	3:39	3:57	13:50	28:33	2:09:41
84	24	3:29	3:46	13:10	27:04	2:02:06
87.5	25	3:20	3:36	12:34	25:44	1:55:21

REFERENCE

Tokmakidis, S.P., et al.: New approaches to predict $\dot{V}O_{2max}$ and endurance from running performance. *J. Sports Med.*, 27:401, 1987.

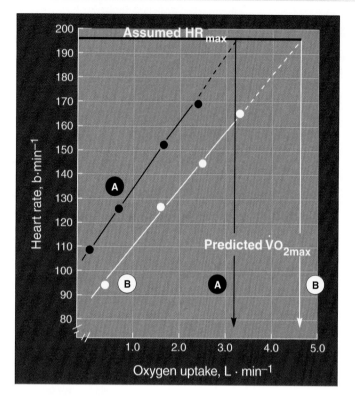

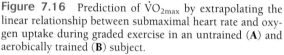

Figure 7.16 Prediction of $\dot{V}O_{2max}$ by extrapolating the linear relationship between submaximal heart rate and oxygen uptake during graded exercise in an untrained (**A**) and aerobically trained (**B**) subject.

2. **Similar maximum heart rates for all subjects.** The standard deviation for the average maximum heart rate for individuals of the same age ($HR_{max} = 220$ minus age, y) equals ± 10 b·min^{-1}. The $\dot{V}O_{2max}$ of a 25-year-old person with a maximum heart rate of 185 b·min^{-1} would be *overestimated* if the HR–$\dot{V}O_2$ line extrapolated to an assumed maximum heart rate for this age group of 195 b·min^{-1}. The opposite would occur if this subject's maximum heart rate equaled 210 b·min^{-1}. HR_{max} also decreases with age. Without considering the age effect, older subjects would consistently be *overestimated* by assuming a maximum heart rate of 195 b·min^{-1}. This represents the appropriate estimation for 25 year olds.

3. **Assumed constant exercise economy.** The predicted $\dot{V}O_{2max}$ can vary because of variability in exercise economy when estimating submaximal oxygen uptake from exercise level. A subject with low economy (submaximal $\dot{V}O_2$ higher than assumed) is *underestimated* for $\dot{V}O_{2max}$ because heart rate increases from added oxygen cost of uneconomical exercise. The opposite occurs for a person with high exercise economy. The variation among individuals in oxygen uptake during walking, stepping, or cycling does not usually exceed $\pm 6\%$. However, seemingly small modifications in test procedures profoundly affect the metabolic cost of exercise. Allowing individuals to support themselves with treadmill handrails can reduce exercise oxygen cost by 30%. Failure to maintain cadence on a bicycle ergometer or step test can dramatically alter the oxygen requirement.

4. **Day-to-day variation in exercise heart rate.** Even under highly standardized conditions, an individual's submaximal heart rate varies by about ± 5 beats per minute with day-to-day testing at the same exercise intensity. This variation in exercise heart rate represents an additional source of error.

Considering these four limitations, $\dot{V}O_{2max}$ predicted from submaximal heart rate generally falls within 10 to 20% of the person's actual $\dot{V}O_{2max}$. Clearly, this represents too large an error for research purposes. These tests are better suited for screening and classification of aerobic fitness.

A Word of Caution About Predictions

All predictions involve error. The error is referred to as the **standard error of estimate (SEE)** and is computed from the original equation that generated the prediction. Errors of estimate are expressed in units of the predicted variable or as a percentage. For example, say the $\dot{V}O_{2max}$ (mL·kg^{-1}·min^{-1}) prediction from a walking test equals 55 mL·kg^{-1}·min^{-1}, and the SEE of the predicted score equals ± 10 mL·kg^{-1}·min^{-1}. This means that, in reality, the actual $\dot{V}O_{2max}$ probably (68% likelihood) ranges within ± 10 mL·kg^{-1}·min^{-1} of the predicted value (in this case, between 45 and 65 mL·kg^{-1}·min^{-1}). This example represents a relatively large error ($\pm 18.2\%$ of the actual value).

Obviously, a larger prediction error creates a less than useful predicted score because the true score falls within a broad range of possible values. Without knowing the magnitude of the error, one cannot judge the usefulness of the predicted score. Whenever predictions are made, one must interpret the predicted score in light of the magnitude of the prediction error. With a small error, prediction of $\dot{V}O_{2max}$ proves useful in appropriate situations where direct measurement is not feasible.

SUMMARY

1. Direct and indirect calorimetry determine the body's rate of energy expenditure. Direct calorimetry measures the actual heat production in an insulated calorimeter. Indirect calorimetry infers energy expenditure from oxygen uptake and carbon dioxide production using closed-circuit or open-circuit spirometry.

2. All energy-releasing reactions in the body ultimately depend on oxygen use. By measuring a person's oxygen uptake during steady-rate exercise, researchers obtain an indirect yet accurate estimate of energy expenditure.

3. Portable spirometry, bag technique, and computerized instrumentation represent three common open-circuit, indirect calorimetric procedures to measure oxygen uptake during physical activity.

4. The complete oxidation of each nutrient requires a different quantity of oxygen uptake compared with carbon dioxide production. The ratio of carbon dioxide produced to oxygen consumed (the respiratory quotient or RQ) provides important information about the nutrient mixture catabolized for energy. The RQ averages 1.00 for carbohydrate, 0.70 for fat, and 0.82 for protein.

5. For each RQ value, a corresponding caloric value exists for one liter of oxygen consumed. The RQ-kCal relationship determines energy expenditure during exercise with a high degree of accuracy.

6. During strenuous exercise, RQ does not represent specific substrate use because of nonmetabolic production of carbon dioxide in lactate buffering (which spuriously increases the $CO_2 \div O_2$ ratio).

7. The respiratory exchange ratio (R) reflects the pulmonary exchange of carbon dioxide and oxygen under various physiologic and metabolic conditions; R does not fully mirror the macronutrient mixture catabolized for energy.

8. Maximal oxygen uptake ($\dot{V}O_{2max}$) provides reliable and important information on the power of the long-term aerobic energy system, including the functional capacity of various physiologic support systems.

9. A leveling-off or peaking-over in oxygen uptake during increasing exercise intensity signifies attainment of maximum capacity for aerobic metabolism (i.e., a "true" $\dot{V}O_{2max}$). When this accepted criterion is not met or local muscle fatigue in the arms or legs rather than central circulatory dynamics limits test performance, the term "peak oxygen uptake" ($\dot{V}O_{2peak}$) usually describes the highest oxygen uptake value.

10. There are different standardized tests to measure $\dot{V}O_{2max}$. Such tests remain independent of muscle strength, speed, body size, and skill, with the exception of specialized swimming, rowing, and ice skating tests.

11. The $\dot{V}O_{2max}$ test may require a continuous 3- to 5-minute "supermaximal" effort, but it usually consists of increments in exercise intensity (referred to as a graded exercise test or GXT).

12. Two types of $\dot{V}O_{2max}$ tests are typically used: (1) continuous test, with no rest between exercise increments; and (2) discontinuous test, with several minutes of rest between exercise increments.

13. Many factors influence $\dot{V}O_{2max}$; the most important include exercise mode, the person's training state, heredity, gender, body composition, and age.

14. Differences in body mass explain roughly 70% of the differences in $\dot{V}O_{2max}$ ($L \cdot min^{-1}$) among individuals.

15. Changes in $\dot{V}O_{2max}$ relate to chronological age.

16. Tests to predict $\dot{V}O_{2max}$ from submaximal physiologic and performance data can be useful for classification purposes. The validity of prediction equations relies on the following assumptions: linearity of the HR–$\dot{V}O_2$ line, similar maximal heart rate for individuals of the same age, a constant exercise economy, and a relatively small day-to-day variation in exercise heart rate.

17. Field methods to predict $\dot{V}O_{2max}$ provide useful information for screening purposes in the absence of the direct measurement of aerobic capacity.

THOUGHT QUESTION

Explain how oxygen uptake translates to heat production during exercise.

SELECTED REFERENCES

Aisbett, B., et al.: The influence of pacing during 6-minute supra-maximal cycle ergometer performance. *J. Sci. Med. Sport*, 6:187, 2003.

Amann, M., et al.: An evaluation of the predictive validity and reliability of ventilatory threshold. *Med. Sci. Sports Exerc.*, 36:1716, 2004.

Ansley, L., et al.: Anticipatory pacing strategies during supramaximal exercise lasting longer than 30 s. *Med. Sci. Sports Exerc.*, 36:309, 2004.

Atwater, W.O., and Rosa, E.B.: Description of a new respiration calorimeter and experiments on the conservation of energy in the human body. Bulletin No. 63, Washington, D.C., U.S. Department of Agriculture, Office of Experiment Stations, Government Printing Office, 1899.

Balmer, J., et al.: Mechanically braked Wingate powers: agreement between SRM, corrected and conventional methods of measurement. *J. Sports Sci.*, 22:661, 2004.

Bar-Or, O.: The Wingate anaerobic test: An update on methodology, reliability, and validity. *Sports Med.*, 4: 381, 1987.

Bentley, D.J., McNaughton, L.R.: Comparison of W(peak), VO2(peak) and the ventilation threshold from two different incremental exercise tests: relationship to endurance performance. *J. Sci. Med. Sport*, 6:422, 2003.

Berthon, P., Fellmann, N.: General review of maximal aerobic velocity measurement at laboratory. Proposition of a new simplified protocol for maximal aerobic velocity assessment. *J. Sports Med. Phys. Fitness*, 42:257, 2002.

Binzoni, T.: Saturation of the lactate clearance mechanisms different from the "lactate shuttle" determines the anaerobic threshold: prediction from the bioenergetic model. *J. Physiol. Anthropol. Appl. Human Sci.*, 24:175, 2005.

Blain, G., et al.: Assessment of ventilatory thresholds during graded and maximal exercise test using time varying analysis of respiratory sinus arrhythmia. *Br. J. Sports Med.*, 39:448, 2005.

Bosquet, L., et al.: Methods to determine aerobic endurance. *Sports Med.*, 32:675, 2002.

Bouchard, C., et al.: Familial resemblance for VO_{2max} in the sedentary state: The Heritage family study. *Med. Sci. Sports Exerc.*, 30:252, 1998.

Brooks, G.A.: Intra- and extra-cellular lactate shuttles. *Med. Sci. Sports Exerc.*, 32:790, 2000.

Buckley, J.P., et al.: Reliability and validity of measures taken during the Chester step test to predict aerobic power and to prescribe aerobic exercise. *Br. J. Sports Med.*, 38:197, 2004.

Buresh, R., Berg, K.: Scaling oxygen uptake to body size and several practical applications. *J. Strength Cond. Res.*, 16:46, 2002.

Cain, S. M.: Mechanisms which control VO_2 near VO_{2max}: An overview. *Med. Sci. Sports Exerc.*, 27:60, 1995.

Canavan, P.K., Vescovi, J.D.: Evaluation of power prediction equations: peak vertical jumping power in women. *Med. Sci. Sports Exerc.*, 36:1589, 2004.

Carlock, J.M., et al.: The relationship between vertical jump

power estimates and weightlifting ability: a field-test approach. *J. Strength Cond. Res.*, 18:534, 2004.

Cooper, K.: Correlation between field and treadmill testing as a means for assessing maximal oxygen intake. *JAMA*, 203:201, 1968.

Cooper, S.M., et al.: A simple multistage field test for the prediction of anaerobic capacity in female games players. *Br. J. Sports Med.*, 38:784, 2004.

Donovan, C.M., Pagliassotti, M.J.: Quantitative assessment of pathways for lactate disposal in skeletal muscle fiber types. *Med. Sci. Sports Exerc.*, 32:772, 2000.

Dulloo, A.G., et al.: A low-budget and easy-to-operate room respirometer for measuring daily energy expenditure in man. *Am. J. Clin. Nutr.*, 48:1367, 1988.

Duncan, G.E., et al.: Applicability of VO_{2max} criteria: discontinuous versus continuous protocols. *Med. Sci. Sports Exerc.*, 29:273, 1997.

Gayagay, G., et al.: Elite endurance athletes and the ACE I allele—the rose of genes in athletic performance. *Hum. Genet.*, 103:48, 1998.

Giacomoni, M., et al.: Influence of the menstrual cycle phase and menstrual symptoms on maximal anaerobic performance. *Med. Sci. Sports Exerc.*, 32:486, 2000.

Gladden, L.B.: Muscle as a consumer of lactate. *Med. Sci. Sports Exerc.*, 32:764, 2000.

Gladden, L.B.: The role of skeletal muscle in lactate exchange during exercise: introduction. *Med. Sci. Sports Exerc.*, 32:753, 2000.

Hagberg, J.M., et al.: Specific genetic markers of endurance performance and VO_{2max}. *Exerc. Sport Sci. Rev.*, 29:15, 2001.

Haldane, J.S., and Priestley, J.G.: *Respiration*. New York: Oxford University Press, 1935.

Hiilloskorpi, H.K., et al.: Use of heart rate to predict energy expenditure from low to high activity levels. *Int. J. Sports Med.*, 24:332, 2003.

Hochachka, P.W., Burelle, Y.: Control of maximum metabolic rate in humans: dependence on performance phenotypes. *Mol. Cell. Biochem.*, 256:95, 2004.

Jéquier, E., and Schutz, Y.: Long-term measurements of energy expenditure in humans using a respiration chamber. *Am. J. Clin. Nutr.*, 38:989, 1983.

Katch, V. L., et al.: Optimal test characteristics for maximal anaerobic work on the bicycle ergometer. *Res. Q.*, 48:319, 1977.

Keytel, L.R., et al.: Prediction of energy expenditure from heart rate monitoring during submaximal exercise. *J. Sports Sci.*, 23:289, 2005.

Kotzamanidis, C., et al.: The effect of a combined high-intensity strength and speed training program on the running and jumping ability of soccer players. *J. Strength Cond. Res.*, 19:369, 2005.

Krustrup, P., et al.: The yo-yo intermittent recovery test: physiological response, reliability, and validity. *Med. Sci. Sports Exerc.*, 35:697, 2003.

Margaria, R., et al.: Measurement of muscular power (anaerobic) in man. *J. Appl. Physiol.*, 21:1662, 1966.

Markovic, G., et al.: Reliability and factorial validity of squat and countermovement jump tests. *J. Strength Cond. Res.*, 18:551, 2004.

Mastrangelo, M.A., et al.: Predicting anaerobic capabilities in 11–13-year-old boys. *J. Strength Cond. Res.*, 18:72, 2004.

McArdle, W.D., et al.: Specificity of run training on $\dot{V}O_{2max}$ and heart rate changes during running and swimming. *Med. Sci. Sports*, 10:16, 1978.

McLester, J.R., et al.: Effects of standing vs. seated posture on repeated Wingate performance. *J. Strength Cond. Res.*, 18:816, 2004.

McMurray, R.G., et al.: Predicted maximal aerobic power in youth is related to age, gender, and ethnicity. *Med. Sci. Sports Exerc.*, 34:145, 2002.

Moore, A., Murphy, A.: Development of an anaerobic capacity test for field sport athletes. *J. Sci. Med. Sport*, 6:275, 2003.

Porszasz, J., et al.: A treadmill ramp protocol using simultaneous changes in speed and grade. *Med. Sci. Sports Exerc.*, 35:1596, 2003.

Proctor, D.N., Joyner, M.J.: Skeletal muscle mass and the reduction of VO2max in trained older subjects. *J. Appl. Physiol.*, 82:1411, 1997.

Ravussin, E., et al.: Determinants of 24-hour energy expenditure in man: Methods and results using a respiratory chamber. *J. Clin. Invest.*, 78:1568, 1986.

Rumpler, W., et al.: Repeatability of 24-hour energy expenditure measurements in humans by indirect calorimetry. *Am. J. Clin. Nutr.*, 51:147, 1990.

Saunders, P.U., et al.: Factors affecting running economy in trained distance runners. *Sports Med.*, 34:465, 2004.

Scholander, P.F.: Analyzer for accurate estimation of respiratory gases in one-half cubic centimeter samples. *J. Biol. Chem.*, 167:235, 1947.

Sharp, M.A., et al.: Comparison of the physical fitness of men and women entering the U.S. Army: 1978–1998. *Med. Sci. Sports Exerc.*, 34:356, 2002.

Souissi, N., et al.: Circadian rhythms in two types of anaerobic cycle leg exercise: force-velocity and 30-s Wingate tests. *Int. J. Sports Med.*, 25:14, 2004.

Speakman, J.R.: The history and theory of the doubly labeled water technique. *Am. J. Clin. Nutr.*, 68(Suppl):932S, 1998.

Spencer, M.R., Gastin, P.B.: Energy system contribution during 200-m to 1500-m running in highly trained athletes. *Med. Sci. Sports Exerc.*, 33:157, 2001.

Spriet, L.L., et al.: An enzymatic approach to lactate production in human skeletal muscle during exercise. *Med. Sci. Sports Exerc.*, 32:756, 2000.

Tiainen, K., et al.: Heritability of maximal isometric muscle strength in older female twins. *J. Appl. Physiol.*, 96:173, 2004.

Uth, N., et al.: Estimation of $\dot{V}O_{2max}$ from the ratio between HR_{max} and HR_{rest}—the heart rate ratio method. *Eur. J. Appl. Physiol.*, 91:111, 2004.

Wagner, P.D.: New ideas on limitations to $\dot{V}O_{2max}$. *Exer. Sport Sci. Rev.*, 1:10, 2000.

Wasserman, K., et al.: *Principles of Exercise Testing and Interpretation* 3rd Ed. Baltimore: Lippincott Williams & Wilkins, 1999.

Weibel, E.R., et al.: Allometric scaling of maximal metabolic rate in mammals: muscle aerobic capacity as determinant factor. *Respir. Physiol. Neurobiol.*, 140:115, 2004.

Weltman, A., et al.: The lactate threshold and endurance performance. *Adv. Sports Med. Fitness*, 2:91, 1989.

Wilmore, J.H., et al.: An automated system for assessing metabolic and respiratory function during exercise. *J. Appl. Physiol.*, 40:619, 1976.

Zajac, A., et al.: The diagnostic value of the 10- and 30-second Wingate test for competitive athletes. *J. Strength Cond. Res.*, 13:16, 1999.

CHAPTER OBJECTIVES

- Define basal metabolic rate, indicating factors that affect it.
- Explain the effect of body weight on the energy cost of different forms of physical activity.
- Identify factors that contribute to the total daily energy expenditure.
- Outline different classification systems for rating the strenuousness of physical activity.
- Describe two means to predict resting daily energy expenditure.
- Explain the concept of exercise efficiency and exercise economy.
- List factors that affect the energy cost of walking and running.
- Identify factors that contribute to the lower exercise economy of swimming compared with running.

CHAPTER OUTLINE

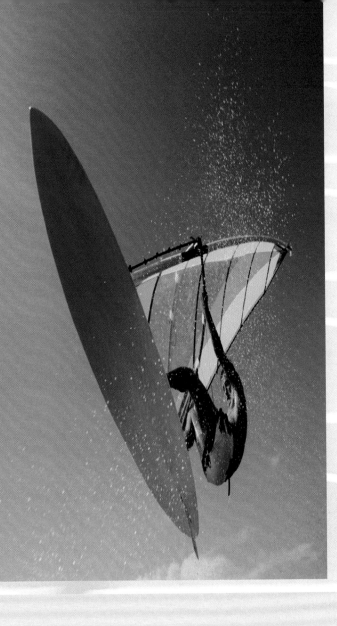

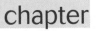

chapter 8

Energy Expenditure During Rest and Physical Activity

PART 1 •
Energy Expenditure at Rest

Three factors determine total daily energy expenditure (**Fig. 8.1**):

1. Resting metabolic rate, which includes basal and sleeping conditions plus the added cost of arousal
2. Thermogenic influence of food consumed
3. Energy expended during physical activity and recovery

ENERGY EXPENDITURE AT REST: BASAL METABOLIC RATE

For each individual, a minimum energy requirement sustains the body's functions in the waking state. Measuring oxygen uptake under the following three standardized conditions quantifies this requirement called the **basal metabolic rate** (**BMR**):

1. No food consumed for at least 12 hours before measurement; the **postabsorptive state** describes this condition
2. No undue muscular exertion for at least 12 hours before measurement
3. Measured after the person has been lying quietly for 30 to 60 minutes in a dimly lit, temperature-controlled (thermoneutral) room

Maintaining controlled conditions provides a method to study the relationships among energy expenditure and

body size, gender, and age. The BMR also establishes an important energy baseline for implementing a prudent program of weight control by food restraint, exercise, or both. In most instances, basal values measured in the laboratory remain only marginally lower than values for resting metabolic rate measured under less strict conditions, e.g., 3 to 4 hours after a light meal without physical activity. *In these discussions, we use the terms basal and resting metabolism interchangeably.*

INFLUENCE OF BODY SIZE ON RESTING METABOLISM

Body surface area frequently provides a common denominator for expressing basal metabolism.

Figure 8.2 shows that BMR (expressed as kCal per body surface area per hour, or $kCal \cdot m^{-2} \cdot h^{-1}$) averages 5% to 10% lower in females compared with males at all ages. A female's larger percentage body fat and smaller muscle mass in relation to body size helps explain her lower metabolic rate per unit surface area. From ages 20 to 40 years, average values for BMR equal 38 kCal per squared meter (m^2) of body surface per hour ($kCal \cdot m^{-2} \cdot h^{-1}$) for men, and 36 $kCal \cdot m^{-2} \cdot h^{-1}$ for women. For a more precise estimate of BMR, the actual average value for a specific age can be read directly from the curves. By using the value for heat production (BMR) in Figure 8.2 combined with the appropriate surface area value, a person's resting metabolic rate ($kCal \cdot min^{-1}$) can be estimated and converted to a total daily resting requirement.

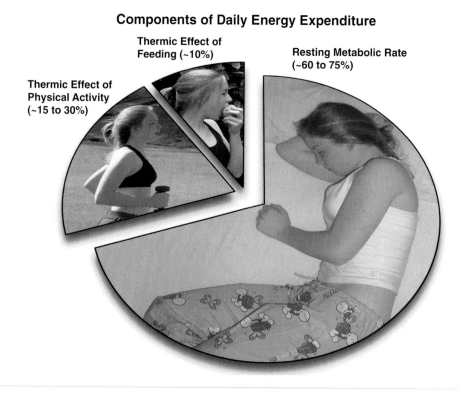

Components of Daily Energy Expenditure

Thermic Effect of Feeding (~10%)

Resting Metabolic Rate (~60 to 75%)

Thermic Effect of Physical Activity (~15 to 30%)

Figure 8.1 Components of daily energy expenditure.

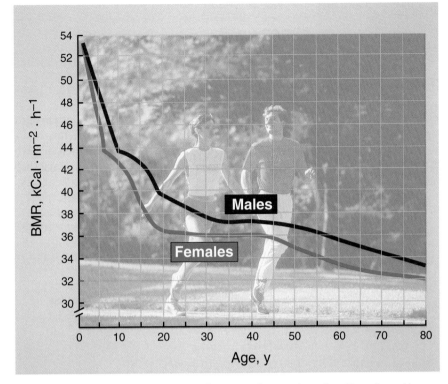

Figure 8.2 Basal metabolic rate as a function of age and gender. (Data from Altman, P.L., and Dittmer, D.: *Metabolism*. Bethesda, MD: Federation of American Societies for Experimental Biology, 1968.)

Questions & Notes

Give 2 of the standardized conditions for measuring BMR.

1.

2.

Describe the general trend of the relationship between BMR and age.

Give the units of measurements for the BMR.

ESTIMATING RESTING DAILY ENERGY EXPENDITURE

To estimate an individual's **resting daily energy expenditure**, multiply the appropriate average BMR value in Figure 8.2 by body surface area (see Box 8-1, *Calculating and Interpreting Body Surface Area* on page 264). Then multiply this hourly value by 24 to obtain a 24-hour estimate.

For a 55-year-old woman, for example, the estimated BMR equals 34 $kCal \cdot m^{-2} \cdot h^{-1}$. If her surface area were 1.40 m^{-2}, the hourly energy expenditure would equal 47.6 kCal (34 × 1.40 m^2). On a 24-hour basis, this amounts to a basal energy expenditure of 1142 kCal (47.6 × 24).

FACTORS AFFECTING TOTAL DAILY ENERGY EXPENDITURE

The important factors affecting **total daily energy expenditure** (**TDEE**) include physical activity, dietary-induced thermogenesis, and climate. Pregnancy also affects TDEE through its effect on the energy cost of many forms of physical activity.

Physical Activity

Physical activity profoundly affects human energy expenditure. World-class athletes nearly double their daily caloric outputs with 3 or 4 hours of hard training. Most people can sustain metabolic rates that average 10 times the resting value during "big muscle" exercises, such as fast walking, running, cycling, and swimming. *Physical activity generally accounts for between 15% and 30% of TDEE.*

FOR YOUR INFORMATION

Regular Exercise Slows a Decrease in Metabolism With Age
Increases in body fat and decreases in fat-free body mass (FFM) largely explain the 2% decline in BMR per decade through adulthood. Regular physical activity blunts the decrease in BMR. In addition, an accompanying 8% increase in resting metabolism occurred when 50- to 65-year-old men increased their FFM with heavy resistance training. These findings indicate that endurance and resistance exercise training offsets the decrease in resting metabolism usually observed with aging.

Box 8-1 • CLOSE UP

CALCULATING AND INTERPRETING BODY SURFACE AREA

Body surface area (BSA) refers to the body's external area usually expressed in square meters (m^2). Aside from using BSA to express basal metabolic rate and lung function measures, BSA sometimes serves as the frame of reference for equating different size individuals for energy expenditure. The early measurements of BSA involved wrapping the whole body with gauze and then determining gauze area (total area, m^2 = length, m × width, m). Subsequent research showed that it is possible to accurately predict BSA from stature and body mass.

CALCULATIONS

Stature in m and body mass in kg predict BSA in m^2 as follows:

$$BSA = 0.20247 \times Stature^{0.725} \times Body\ mass^{0.425}$$

Example

Male: stature, 1.778 m (177.8 cm; 70 in); body mass, 75 kg (165.3 lb)

$$BSA = 0.20247 \times 1.778^{0.725} \times 75^{0.425}$$
$$= 0.20247 \times 1.51775 \times 6.2647$$
$$= 1.925\ m^2$$

The accompanying nomogram provides a method to readily compute BSA based on stature and body mass. Locate stature on Scale I and body mass on Scale II. Connect the two points with a straight edge. The intersection at Scale III gives surface area in m^2. For example, if stature equals 185 cm and body mass equals 75 kg, BSA (Scale III) equals 1.98 m^2.

Scale I Stature		Scale III Surface area	Scale II Body mass	
in	cm	m^2	lb	kg
6'8"		2.9	340	160
6'6"	200	2.8	320	150
		2.7	300	140
6'4"	190	2.6	280	130
6'2"		2.5		
		2.4	260	120
6'0"	180	2.3	240	110
5'10"		2.2		105
5'8"	170	2.1	220	100
				95
5'6"		2.0	200	90
5'4"	165	1.9	190	85
	160		180	80
5'2"	155	1.8	170	75
		1.7	160	70
5'0"	150	1.6	150	
4'10"	145		140	65
4'8"	140	1.5	130	60
		1.4	120	55
4'6"	135		110	50
4'4"	130	1.3	100	45
4'2"	125	1.2	90	40
4'0"	120	1.1	80	35
3'10"	115	1.0	70	30
3'8"	110	0.9	60	
3'6"	105			25
3'4"	100	0.8	50	
3'2"	95	0.7		20
3'0"	90		40	
	85	0.6 0.58		15

Nomogram to estimate body surface area from stature and mass. (Reprinted from "Clinical Spirometry," as prepared by Boothby and Sandiford of the Mayo Clinic, courtesy of Warren E. Collins Inc., Braintree, MA.)

Dietary-Induced Thermogenesis

Consuming food increases energy metabolism from the energy-requiring processes of digesting, absorbing, and assimilating nutrients. **Dietary-induced thermogenesis (DIT**; also termed **thermic effect of food [TEF]**) typically reaches maximum within 1 hour after eating, depending on food quantity and type. The magnitude of DIT ranges between 10% and 35% of the ingested food energy. A meal of pure protein, for example, elicits a thermic effect often equaling 25% of the meal's total energy content.

All too often, advertisements have touted the high thermic effect of protein consumption to promote a high-protein diet for weight loss. Advocates maintain that fewer calories ultimately become available to the body compared with a lipid- or carbohydrate-rich meal of similar caloric value. This point has some validity, but other factors must be considered in formulating a prudent weight loss program. These include the potentially harmful strain on kidney and liver function induced by excessive dietary protein or the cholesterol-stimulating effects of the large amount of saturated fatty acids usually contained in high-protein (meat) foods. Well-balanced nutrition requires a blend of macronutrients with appropriate quantities of vitamins and minerals. When combining exercise with food restriction for weight loss, carbohydrate (not protein) intake provides energy for exercise and conserves lean tissue often lost through dieting.

Individuals with poor control over body weight often have a depressed thermic response to eating, an effect most likely related to a genetic predisposition. This undoubtedly contributes to considerable body fat accumulation over a period of years. If a person's lifestyle includes regular moderate physical activity, then the thermogenic effect represents only a small portion of TDEE. Also, exercising after eating augments an individual's normal thermic response to food intake. This supports the wisdom of "going for a brisk walk" following a meal.

Climate

Environmental factors influence resting metabolic rate. The resting metabolism of people living in tropical climates, for example, averages 5% to 20% higher than counterparts in more temperate regions. Exercise performed in hot weather also imposes a small additional metabolic load, causing about a 5% elevation in oxygen uptake compared with the same work performed in a thermoneutral environment. This increase in metabolism comes from a direct thermogenic effect of elevated core temperature, plus additional energy required for sweat-gland activity and altered circulatory dynamics.

Cold environments also can increase energy metabolism, depending on a person's body fat content and thermal quality of clothing. During extreme cold stress, resting metabolism can triple because shivering generates heat to maintain a stable core temperature. The effects of cold stress during exercise become most evident in cold water from difficulty maintaining a stable core temperature in this hostile environment.

Pregnancy

Maternal cardiovascular dynamics follow normal response patterns. Moderate exercise presents no greater physiologic stress to the mother than those imposed by the additional weight gain and possible encumbrance of fetal tissue. Pregnancy does not compromise the absolute value for aerobic capacity ($L \cdot min^{-1}$). *As pregnancy progresses, increases in maternal body weight add significantly to exercise effort during weight-bearing activities like walking, jogging, and stair climbing and may reduce the economy of effort. Pregnancy, particularly in the later stages, also increases pulmonary ventilation at a given submaximal exercise intensity. Progesterone increases sensitivity of the respiratory center to carbon dioxide and directly stimulates maternal hyperventilation.*

List 3 factors that affect total daily energy expenditure.

1.

2.

3.

Give the percentage range that physical activity comprises of the total daily energy expenditure.

Give the formula for predicting body surface area.

Calculate the body surface area for a female who weighs 50 kg with a stature of 160 cm.

True or False:

Moderate exercise during pregnancy provides a considerable physiologic stress to the mother because of the greatly increased metabolic and physiologic demands of the developing fetus.

Do extremes of temperature increase or decrease metabolic rate?

Box 8-2 • CLOSE UP

PREDICTING RESTING DAILY ENERGY EXPENDITURE (RDEE) FROM FAT-FREE BODY MASS (FFM) AND FROM BODY MASS, STATURE, AND AGE

PREDICTION FROM FAT-FREE BODY MASS

The following generalized equation, applicable to men and women, predicts RDEE (kCal·24 h^{-1}) over a broad range of FFM to an accuracy of ± 5%:

$$RDEE = 370 + 21.6 \times FFM, kg$$

Example

Calculate RDEE for a person weighing 90.9 kg (200 lb) with 21% body fat (estimated using one of the several indirect procedures described in Chapter 16), fat mass of 19.1 kg (90.9 kg × 0.21), and FFM (90.9 kg − 19.1 kg) of 71.8 kg (158 lb).

$$RDEE = 370 + 21.6 \times 71.8$$
$$= 1921 \text{ kCal}$$

Estimation of RDEE (kCal ·24h^{-1}) Based on Fat-Free Body Mass (kg)

FFM	RDEE	FFM	RDEE	FFM	RDEE	FFM	RDEE	FFM	RDEE	FFM	RDEE
44	1320	55	1558	66	1796	77	2033	88	2271	99	2508
45	1342	56	1580	67	1817	78	2055	89	2292	100	2530
46	1364	57	1601	68	1839	79	2076	90	2314	101	2552
47	1385	58	1623	69	1860	80	2098	91	2336	102	2573
48	1407	59	1644	70	1882	81	2120	92	2357	103	2595
49	1428	60	1666	71	1904	82	2141	93	2379	104	2616
50	1450	61	1688	72	1925	83	2163	94	2400	105	2638
51	1472	62	1709	73	1947	84	2184	95	2422	106	2660
52	1493	63	1731	74	1968	85	2206	96	2444	107	2681
53	1515	64	1752	75	1990	86	2228	97	2465	108	2703
54	1536	65	1774	76	2012	87	2249	98	2487	109	2724

From Cunningham, J.J.: Body composition and resting metabolic rate: The myth of feminine metabolism. *Am. J. Clin. Nutr.*, 36:721, 1982.

PREDICTION FROM BODY MASS (BM), STATURE (S), AND AGE (A)

Body mass (BM), stature (S in cm), and age (A in y) also successfully predict RDEE.

Equations

Women: RDEE = 655 + (9.6 × BM) + (1.85 × S) − (4.7 × A)
Men: RDEE = 66.0 + (13.7 × BM) + (5.0 × S) − (6.8 × A)

Examples

Woman: BM = 62.7 kg; S = 172.5 cm; A = 22.4 y.

$$RDEE = 655 + (9.6 \times 62.7)$$
$$+ (1.85 \times 172.5) - (4.7 \times 22.4)$$
$$= 655 + 601.92 + 319.13 - 105.28$$
$$= 1471 \text{ kCal}$$

Man: BM = 80 kg; S = 189.0 cm; A = 30 y.

$$RDEE = 66.0 + (13.7 \times 80) + (5.0 \times 189.0)$$
$$- (6.8 \times 30.0)$$
$$= 66.0 + 1096 + 945 - 204$$
$$= 1903 \text{ kCal}$$

REFERENCE

Harris, J.A., and Benedict, F.G.: A biometric study of basal metabolism in man. Publ. No. 279. Washington, DC: Carnegie Institute, 1919.

SUMMARY

1. Basal metabolic rate (BMR) reflects the minimum energy required for vital functions in the waking state. BMR relates inversely to age and gender, averaging 5% to 10% lower in women compared to men. Fat-free body mass (FFM) and percentage body fat largely account for the age and gender differences in BMR.

2. Total daily energy expenditure (TDEE) represents the sum of energy required in basal and resting metabolism, thermogenic influences (particularly the thermic effect of food), and energy generated in physical activity.

3. Body mass, stature, and age, or estimates of FFM mass provide for accurate estimates of resting daily energy expenditure.

4. Physical activity, dietary-induced thermogenesis, environmental factors, and pregnancy significantly affect TDEE.

5. Dietary-induced thermogenesis refers to the increase in energy metabolism attributable to digestion, absorption, and assimilation of food nutrients.

6. Exposure to hot and cold environments cause a small increase in TDEE.

THOUGHT QUESTIONS

1. Discuss the factors contributing to total energy expenditure. Explain which factor contributes the most.

2. Discuss the notion that for some individuals "a calorie really is not a calorie" in terms of energy storage.

3. What would be the ideal exercise prescription to optimize increases in energy expenditure?

PART 2 •
Energy Expenditure During Physical Activity

An understanding of resting energy metabolism provides an important frame of reference to appreciate the potential of humans to increase daily energy output. According to numerous surveys, *physical inactivity* (e.g., watching television, lounging around the home, and other sedentary activities) accounts for about one-third of a person's waking hours. This means that regular physical activity can significantly boost the TDEE of large numbers of men and women. Actualizing this potential depends on the intensity, duration, and type of physical activity performed.

Researchers have measured the energy expended during diverse activities like brushing teeth, house cleaning, mowing the lawn, walking the dog, driving a car, playing ping-pong, bowling, dancing, swimming, rock climbing, and physical activity during space flight. Consider an activity such as rowing continuously at 30 strokes a minute for 30 minutes. How can we determine the number of calories "burned" during the 30 minutes? If the amount of oxygen consumed averaged 2.0 L·min^{-1} during each minute of rowing, then in 30 minutes the rower would consume 60 liters of oxygen. A reasonably accurate estimate of the energy expended in rowing can be made because 1 liter of oxygen generates about 5 kCal of energy. In this example, the rower expends 300 kCal (60 L × 5 kCal) during the exercise. This value represents the **gross energy expenditure** for the exercise period.

The 300 kCal of energy cannot all be attributed solely to rowing because this value also includes the resting requirement during the 30-minute row. The rower's body surface area of 2.04 m^2, estimated from the nomogram in *Calculating and Interpreting Body Surface Area* (body mass = 81.8 kg; stature = 183 cm), multiplied by the average BMR for gender (38 kCal·m^{-2}·h^{-1} × 2.04 m^2) gives the

Questions & Notes

If the V̇O$_2$ averages 2.5 L•min^{-1} during skiing, how many kCal would be expended during 45 minutes?

What assumption did you have to make to answer the question above?

Compute the RDEE for a male with a FFM of 65 kg.

resting metabolism per hour, which is approximately 78 kCal per hour or 39 kCal "burned" over 30 minutes. Based on these computations, the **net energy expenditure** attributable solely to rowing equals gross energy expenditure (300 kCal) minus the requirement for rest (39 kCal), or approximately 261 kCal.

TDEE is estimated by determining the time spent in daily activities (using a diary) and determining the activities' corresponding energy requirement. Listings of energy expenditure for a wide range of physical activities can be found on the web at different sites (try the following site: *http://www.caloriesperhour.com/index_burn.html*).

ENERGY COST OF RECREATIONAL AND SPORT ACTIVITIES

Table 8.1 illustrates the energy cost among diverse recreational and sport activities. Notice, for example, that volleyball requires about 3.6 kCal per minute (216 kCal per hour) for a person weighing 71 kg (157 lb). The same person expends more than twice this energy, or 546 kCal per hour, swimming the front crawl. Viewed somewhat differently, 25 minutes spent swimming expends about the same number of calories as playing 1-hour of recreational volleyball. If the pace of the swim increases or volleyball becomes more intense, energy expenditure increases proportionately.

Effect of Body Mass   Body size plays an important contributing role in exercise energy requirements. **Figure 8.3** illustrates that heavier people expend more energy to perform the same activity than people who weigh less. This occurs because the energy expended during **weight-bearing exercise** increases directly with the body mass transported. *Such a strong relationship exists that one can predict energy expenditure during walking or running from body mass with almost as much accuracy as measuring oxygen uptake under controlled laboratory conditions.* In non–weight-bearing or **weight-supported exercise** (e.g.,

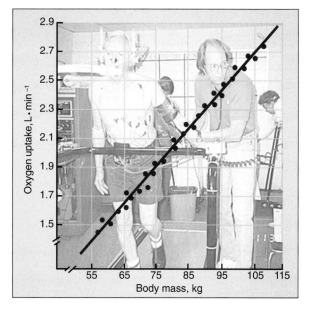

Figure 8.3   Relationship between body mass and oxygen uptake measured during submaximal, brisk treadmill walking. (From Applied Physiology Laboratory, Queens College, Flushing, NY.) Photo courtesy of Dr. Jay Graves, University of Utah.

stationary cycling), little relationship exists between body mass and exercise energy cost.

From a practical standpoint, walking and other weight-bearing exercises requires a substantial calorie burn for heavier people. Notice in Table 8.1 that playing tennis or volleyball requires considerably greater energy expenditure for a person weighing 83 kg than for someone who is 20 kg lighter. Expressing caloric cost of weight-bearing exercise in relation to body mass, as kCal per kilogram of body mass per minute ($kCal \cdot kg^{-1} \cdot min^{-1}$), greatly reduces the difference in energy expenditure among individuals of different body weights. However, the absolute cost of the exercise ($kCal \cdot min^{-1}$) remains greater for the heavier person.

Table 8·1	Gross Energy Cost for Selected Recreational and Sports Activities in Relation to Body Mass[a]											
ACTIVITY	**kg** **lb**	**50** **110**	**53** **117**	**56** **123**	**59** **130**	**62** **137**	**65** **143**	**68** **150**	**71** **157**	**74** **163**	**77** **170**	**80** **176**	**83** **183**
Volleyball		2.5	2.7	2.8	3.0	3.1	3.3	3.4	3.6	3.7	3.9	4.0	4.2
Aerobic dancing		6.7	7.1	7.5	7.9	8.3	8.7	9.2	9.6	10.0	10.4	10.8	11.2
Cycling, leisure		5.0	5.3	5.6	5.9	6.2	6.5	6.8	7.1	7.4	7.7	8.0	8.3
Tennis		5.5	5.8	6.1	6.4	6.8	7.1	7.4	7.7	8.1	8.4	8.7	9.0
Swimming, slow crawl		6.4	6.8	7.2	7.6	7.9	8.3	8.7	9.1	9.5	9.9	10.2	10.6
Touch football		6.6	7.0	7.4	7.8	8.2	8.6	9.0	9.4	9.8	10.2	10.6	11.0
Running, 8-min mile		10.8	11.3	11.9	12.5	13.11	3.6	14.2	14.8	15.4	16.0	16.5	17.1
Skiing, uphill racing		13.7	14.5	15.3	16.2	17.0	17.8	18.6	19.5	20.3	21.1	21.9	22.7

[a] Data from Katch F., Katch, V.L., and McArdle, W.D.: *Calorie Expenditure Charts.* Ann Arbor, MI: Fitness Technologies Press, 1996.

Note: Energy expenditure computes as the number of minutes of participation multiplied by the kCal value in the appropriate body weight column. For example, the kCal cost of 1 hour of tennis for a person weighing 150 pounds equals 444 kCal (7.4 kCal × 60 min).

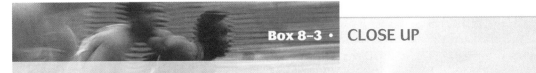

Box 8–3 • CLOSE UP

THE HALDANE TRANSFORMATION TO CALCULATE OXYGEN UPTAKE

Measurement of oxygen uptake ($\dot{V}O_2$) using open-circuit spirometry provides fundamental data in exercise physiology. The open-circuit method assumes that the body neither produces nor retains gaseous nitrogen during the measurement period (i.e., the quantity of nitrogen remains equal in the inspired and expired air). Under this assumption, there is no need to collect and analyze *both* inspired and expired air volumes during measurements of oxygen consumption and carbon dioxide production. The following equation, known as the **Haldane transformation**, describes the mathematical expression of the relationship between inspired and expired air volumes based on an assumed constancy for gaseous nitrogen.

$$\dot{V}_I = \dot{V}_E \times F_E N_2 \div F_I N_2$$

where $\dot{V}_I$ equals air volume inspired, $\dot{V}_E$ equals air volume expired, and $F_E N_2$ and $F_I N_2$ equal the fractional concentrations of nitrogen in the expired and inspired air, respectively. Because the fractional concentrations for inspired oxygen ($F_I O_2$), carbon dioxide ($F_I CO_2$), and nitrogen ($F_I N_2$) are known, only $\dot{V}_E$ (or $\dot{V}_I$) and the expired air concentrations of CO_2 ($F_E CO_2$) and O_2 ($F_E O_2$) are required to calculate $\dot{V}O_2$, assuming no net production or retention of N_2.

$$\dot{V}O_2 = \dot{V}_E \times (F_E N_2/F_I N_2) \times F_I O_2 - \dot{V}_E \times F_E O_2$$

In this formula, $F_E N_2$ equals:

$$1.00 - (F_E O_2 + F_E CO_2)$$

Comparisons of $\dot{V}O_2$ calculated from only expired ventilation (applying the Haldane transformation) versus $\dot{V}O_2$ calculated using measured inspired and expired ventilations at different exercise intensities are needed to study net nitrogen retention or production.

The data in the figure show the experimental results in which six subjects completed treadmill exercise by walking on the level at 4 mph; a 5-minute jog followed at 6 mph, followed again by a 5-minute run at 7.5 mph. Oxygen uptake was continuously monitored using open-circuit spirometry and measures of inspired and expired pulmonary ventilations. Measurements also included barometric pressure, inspired and expired gas temperatures, relative humidity, and $F_E O_2$, $F_E CO_2$, $F_I O_2$, and $F_I CO_2$.

The figure plots $\dot{V}O_2$ estimated using only expired $\dot{V}_E$ (Y-axis) versus actual $\dot{V}O_2$ calculated from both $\dot{V}_I$ and $\dot{V}_E$ (X-axis).

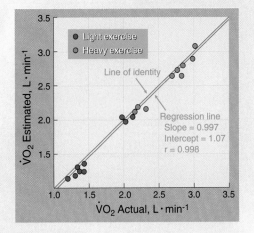

The solid line represents the line of identity; if all data points fall on this line, then perfect association exists between the two $\dot{V}O_2$ estimates. The slope of the regression line relating the two $\dot{V}O_2$ estimates deviated only 0.003 unit from unity, and the intercept approximates zero. This indicates an impressively close relationship between the actual oxygen uptake and that predicted by the Haldane transformation. The largest difference between the actual and estimated $\dot{V}O_2$ values equaled 230 mL, an error of 7.3%. The average difference of 0.8% for all subjects occurred within the instrument's measurement error. For the nitrogen data, a difference of 1.6% occurred between the minute volume of nitrogen inspired and expired for any subject at any exercise level; 11 of 17 subject-work rates exhibited less than a ± 1% difference. The largest difference, 1099 mL $N_2 \cdot min^{-1}$, occurred during heavy exercise (2.1% difference).

These findings justify the continued use of the Haldane transformation to calculate $\dot{V}O_2$ during exercise. Although production and/or retention of N_2 can occur, it has little effect on the $\dot{V}O_2$ computation.

REFERENCE

Wilmore, J.H., and Costill, D.L.: Adequacy of the Haldane transformation in the computation of exercise $\dot{V}O_2$ in man. *J. Appl. Physiol.*, 35:85, 1973.

Table 8·2	Average Rates of Energy Expenditure for Men and Women Living in the United States[a]					
	AGE (y)	BODY MASS		STATURE		ENERGY EXPENDITURE
		(kg)	(lb)	(cm)	(in)	(kCal)
Males	15–18	66	145	176	69	3000
	19–24	72	160	177	70	2900
	25–50	79	174	176	70	2900
	51+	77	170	173	68	2300
Females	15–18	55	120	163	64	2200
	19–24	58	128	164	65	2200
	25–50	63	138	163	64	2200
	50+	65	143	160	63	1900

ACTIVITY	AVERAGE TIME SPENT DURING THE DAY TIME (H)
Sleeping and lying down	8
Sitting	6
Standing	6
Walking	2
Recreational activity	2

Data from Food and Nutrition Board, National Research Council: *Recommended Dietary Allowances*, revised. Washington, DC, National Academy of Sciences, 1989.
[a] The information in this table was designed for the maintenance of practically all healthy people in the United States.

AVERAGE DAILY RATES OF ENERGY EXPENDITURE

A committee of the United States Food and Nutrition Board proposed various norms to represent average rates of energy expenditure for men and women in the United States. These values apply to people with occupations considered between sedentary and active and who participate in some recreational activities (i.e., weekend swimming, golf, and tennis). **Table 8.2** shows that between 2900 and 3000 kCal for males and 2200 kCal for females between the ages of 15 and 50 years represent the average daily energy expenditures. As shown in the lower part of the table, the typical person spends about 75% of the day in sedentary activities. This predominance of physical *inactivity* has prompted some sociologists to refer to the modern-day American as *homosedentarius*. This descriptor is supported by compelling evidence that at least 60% of American adults do not get enough physical activity to provide health benefits. In fact, more than 25% of adults receive no additional physical activity at all in their leisure time. Physical activity decreases with age, and sufficient activity becomes less common among women than men, and among those with lower incomes and less education. Unfortunately, nearly one-half of youths aged 12 to 21 years are not vigorously active on a regular basis. Moreover, physical activity declines substantially during adolescence.

CLASSIFICATION OF WORK BY ENERGY EXPENDITURE

All of us at one time or another have performed some type of physical work we would classify as exceedingly "difficult." This includes walking up a long flight of stairs, shoveling a snow-filled driveway, sprinting to catch a bus, loading and unloading furniture on a truck, digging trenches, skiing or snow-shoeing through a snowstorm, or running in soft beach sand. Two factors affect how researchers rate the difficulty of a particular task: (1) *duration of activity* and (2) *intensity of effort*. Both factors can vary considerably. Running a 26-mile marathon at various speeds illustrates this point. One runner runs at maximum pace and completes the race in a little more than 2 hours. Another runner of similar fitness selects a slower, more "leisurely" pace and completes the run in 3 hours. In these examples, the intensity of exercise differentiates the performance. In another situation, two people run at the same speed, but one runs twice as long as the other. Here, exercise duration differentiates performance.

MET

Oxygen uptake and kCal commonly express differences in exercise intensity. As an alternative, a convenient way to express exercise intensity would be to classify physical effort as multiples of resting energy expenditure, with a unitless measure. To this end, scientists have developed the concept of **METs**, an acronym derived from the term *Metabolic EquivalenT*. One **MET** represents an adult's average, seated, resting oxygen consumption or energy expenditure—about 250 mL $O_2 \cdot min^{-1}$, 3.5 mL $O_2 \cdot kg^{-1} \cdot min^{-1}$, 1 $kCal \cdot kg^{-1} \cdot h^{-1}$, or 0.017 $kCal \cdot kg^{-1} \cdot min^{-1}$ (1 $kCal \cdot kg^{-1} \cdot h^{-1} \div 60$ $min \cdot h^{-1} = 0.017$). Using this as frame of reference, a 2-MET activity requires twice the resting metabolism, or about 500 mL of oxygen per minute; a 3-MET intensity level would require three times as much energy expended at rest, and so on.

The MET provides a convenient way to rate exercise intensity with respect to a resting baseline (i.e., multiples of resting energy expenditure). Conversion from MET to $kCal \cdot min^{-1}$ necessitates knowledge of body mass and use of the following conversion: 1.0 $kCal \cdot kg^{-1} \cdot h^{-1} = 1$ MET. For example, if a person weighing 70 kg bicycled at 10 mph, which is listed as a 10-MET activity, the corresponding kCal expenditure calculates as follows:

$$10.0 \text{ METs} = 10.0 \text{ kCal} \cdot kg^{-1} \cdot h^{-1} \times 70 \text{ kg} \div 60 \text{ min}$$
$$= 700 \text{ kCal} \div 60 \text{ min}$$
$$= 11.7 \text{ kCal} \cdot min^{-1}$$

Table 8.3 presents a five-level classification scheme of physical activity based on energy expenditure and corresponding MET levels for untrained men and women.

Heart Rate to Estimate Energy Expenditure

For each person, heart rate and oxygen uptake relate linearly throughout a broad range of aerobic exercise intensities. By knowing this precise relationship, exercise heart rate provides an estimate of oxygen uptake (and thus energy expenditure) during physical activity. This approach has served as a substitute when oxygen uptake cannot be measured during the actual activity.

Figure 8.4 presents data for two members of a nationally ranked women's basketball team during a laboratory treadmill running test. Heart rate for each woman increased linearly with exercise intensity—a proportionate increase in heart rate accompanied each increase in oxygen uptake. However, a similar heart rate for each athlete does not correspond to the same level of oxygen uptake be-

Questions & Notes

Describe the difference between gross and net energy expenditure.

Compute the gross energy expenditure for a 62 kg person who plays touch football for 25 minutes.

List 2 factors that determine the strenuousness of a particular exercise task.

1.

2.

Define the term MET.

Compute the kCal•min^{-1} for a 54 kg person who exercises at a 10-MET level.

Table 8·3	Five-Level Classification of Physical Activity Based on Exercise Intensity			
	ENERGY EXPENDITURE[a]			
	MEN			
LEVEL	**kCal·min^{-1}**	**L·min^{-1}**	**mL·kg^{-1}·min^{-1}**	**METs**
Light	2.0–4.9	0.40–0.99	6.1–15.2	1.6–3.9
Moderate	5.0–7.4	1.00–1.49	15.3–22.9	4.0–5.9
Heavy	7.5–9.9	1.50–1.99	23.0–30.6	6.0–7.9
Very heavy	10.0–12.4	2.00–2.49	30.7–38.3	8.0–9.9
Unduly heavy	12.5–	2.50–	38.4–	10.0–
	WOMEN			
	kCal·min^{-1}	**L·min^{-1}**	**mL·kg^{-1}·min^{-1}**	**METs**
Light	1.5–3.4	0.30–0.69	5.4–12.5	1.2–2.7
Moderate	3.5–5.4	0.70–1.09	12.6–19.8	2.8–4.3
Heavy	5.5–7.4	1.10–1.49	19.9–27.1	4.4–5.9
Very heavy	7.5–9.4	1.50–1.89	27.2–34.4	6.0–7.5
Unduly heavy	9.5–	1.90–	34.5–	7.6–

[a] $L \cdot min^{-1}$ based on 5 kCal per liter of oxygen; $ml \cdot kg^{-1} \cdot min^{-1}$ based on 65-kg man and 55-kg woman; one MET equals average resting oxygen uptake of 3.5 $mL \cdot kg^{-1} \cdot min^{-1}$.

FOR YOUR INFORMATION

A Considerable Energy Output

During a marathon, elite athletes generate a steady-rate energy expenditure of about 25 kCal per minute for the duration of the run. Among elite rowers, a 5- to 7-minute competition generates about 36 kCal per minute!

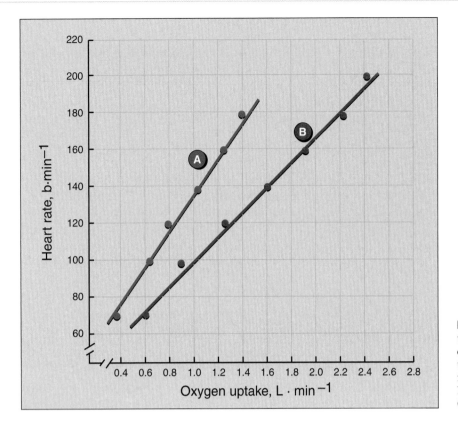

Figure 8.4 Linear relationship between heart rate and oxygen uptake during graded exercise on a treadmill in two collegiate basketball players of different aerobic fitness levels. Data from Laboratory of Applied Physiology, Queens College, NY.

cause the slope (rate of change) of the **HR–$\dot{V}O_2$ line** differs considerably between the women. For a given increase in oxygen uptake, the heart rate of subject B increases less than for subject A. For player A, an exercise heart rate of 140 b·min^{-1} corresponds to an oxygen uptake of 1.08 L·min^{-1}. The same heart rate for player B corresponds to an oxygen uptake of 1.60 L·min^{-1}.

A major consideration when using heart rate to estimate oxygen uptake lies in the similarity between the laboratory assessment of the HR–$\dot{V}O_2$ line and the specific "in vivo" field activity applied to this relationship. It should be noted that factors other than oxygen uptake influence heart rate response to exercise. These include environmental temperature, emotional state, previous food intake, body position, muscle groups exercised, continuous or discontinuous nature of the exercise, and whether the muscles act statically or more dynamically. During aerobic dance, for example, significantly higher heart rates occur while dancing at a specific oxygen uptake than at the same oxygen uptake while walking or running on a treadmill. Arm exercise, or when muscles act statically in a straining-type exercise, produces consistently higher heart rates compared with dynamic leg exercise at any submaximum oxygen uptake. Consequently, applying heart rates during upper-body or static exercise to a HR–$\dot{V}O_2$ line established during running or cycling *overpredicts* the criterion oxygen uptake.

SUMMARY

1. Energy expenditure can be expressed in gross or net terms. Gross (total) values include the resting energy requirement, whereas net energy expenditure reflects the energy cost of the activity excluding the value for resting metabolism over an equivalent time period.

2. Daily rates of energy expenditure classify different occupations and sports professions. Within any classification, variability exists from energy expended in recreational and/or on-the-job pursuits. Heavier individuals expend more energy in most physical activities than lighter counterparts.

3. Average daily energy expenditure ranges between 2900 to 3000 kCal for males and 2200 kCal for females aged 15 to 50 years. Large individual differences in physical activity level affect daily energy expenditure.

4. Different classification systems rate the strenuousness of physical activities. These include ratings based on energy cost expressed in kCal·min^{-1}, oxygen requirement in L·min^{-1}, or multiples of the resting metabolic rate (METs).

5. Exercise heart rate can estimate energy expenditure during physical activity from an individual's heart

rate–oxygen uptake (HR–$\dot{V}O_2$) line determined in the laboratory. Researchers then apply the heart rates during recreational, sport, or occupational activity to the HR–$\dot{V}O_2$ line to estimate exercise oxygen uptake.

6. Because of the diverse factors that influence heart rate independent of the oxygen consumption, estimates of energy cost from heart rate response is limited to only select types of physical activities.

THOUGHT QUESTIONS

1. What circumstances would cause a particular exercise task to be rated "strenuous" in intensity by one person but only "moderate" by another?

2. Discuss limitations of using exercise heart rate to estimate the energy cost of vigorous resistance training based on an HR–$\dot{V}O_2$ line determined from treadmill walking.

PART 3 •
Energy Expenditure During Walking, Running, and Swimming

Total energy expended each day largely depends on the type, intensity, and duration of physical activity. The following sections detail the energy expenditure of three popular endurance activities: walking, running, and swimming. These activities play an important role for weight control, physical conditioning, and cardiac rehabilitation.

ECONOMY AND EFFICIENCY OF ENERGY EXPENDITURE

Three factors determine, to a large extent, success in aerobic endurance performance:

1. Aerobic power ($\dot{V}O_{2max}$)
2. Ability to sustain effort at a large percentage of $\dot{V}O_{2max}$
3. Efficiency of energy use and/or economy of movement

Exercise physiologists correctly consider a high $\dot{V}O_{2max}$ as prerequisite for success in endurance activities. However, among long-distance runners with nearly identical aerobic powers (as often occurs at the highest levels of competition), other factor(s) often explain success in competition. For example, a performance edge would clearly exist for an athlete able to run at a higher percentage of $\dot{V}O_{2max}$ than competitors. Similarly, the runner who maintains a given pace with relatively low energy expenditure maintains a competitive advantage.

Efficiency of Energy Use

When an individual exercises, the actual energy expenditure related to external work represents only a portion of the total energy utilized. The remainder appears as heat. **Mechanical efficiency (ME)** indicates the percentage of the total chemical energy expended (denominator) that contributes to the external work output (numerator). Within this context:

$$ME(\%) = \frac{Work\ Output}{Energy\ Expended} \times 100$$

Force, acting through a vertical distance (F × D) and usually recorded as foot-pounds (ft-lb) or kilogram-meters (kg-m), indicates the external work accomplished

Questions & Notes

Briefly describe the HR–$\dot{V}O_2$ line.

List the 2 factors that determine efficiency of energy expenditure.

1.

2.

List 3 factors that determine aerobic endurance performance.

1.

2.

3.

(work output). External work output is routinely determined during cycle ergometry or other exercises that require lifting the body mass like stair climbing or bench stepping. In horizontal walking or running, work output cannot be computed because (technically) external work does not take place. Reciprocal leg and arm movements negate each other, and the body achieves no net gain in vertical distance. If a person walks or runs up a grade, the work component can be estimated from body mass and vertical distance (lift) achieved during the exercise period (see *How to Measure Work on a Treadmill, Cycle Ergometer, and Step Bench,* page 214). Work output converts to kCal using the following standard conversions:

1. 1 kCal = 426.8 kg-m
2. 1 kCal = 3087.4 ft–lb
3. 1 kCal = 1.5593×10^{-3} hp·h^{-1}
4. 1 watt = 0.01433 kCal·min^{-1}
5. 1 watt = 6.12 kg-m·min^{-1}

Steady-rate oxygen uptake during exercise infers the energy input portion of the efficiency equation (denominator). To obtain common units, the oxygen uptake converts to energy units (1.0 L O_2 = 5.0 kCal; see Table 7.2 for precise calorific transformations based on the nonprotein RQ).

Three terms express efficiency: (1) gross, (2) net, and (3) delta. Each expression calculates differently, and each exhibits a particular advantage. Each method assumes a submaximal steady-rate condition and requires that both work output and energy expenditure be expressed in the same units, typically kCal. Applying the different calculation methods to the same exercise modality yields varying results for ME, ranging from 8% to 25% using gross calculations, 10% to 30% using net calculations, and 24% to 35% using delta calculations.

Gross Mechanical Efficiency

Gross ME, the most frequently calculated type of efficiency, applies when values for specific rates of work and speed are of interest. It also is used in nutritional studies where energy expenditures over long time periods are of interest. Gross efficiency computations use the total oxygen uptake during the exercise.

For example, suppose a 15-minute ride on a stationary bicycle generated 13,300 kg-m of work or 31.2 kCal (13,300 kg-m ÷ 426.8 kCal per kg-m). The oxygen consumed performing the work totaled 25 L with an RQ of 0.88. An RQ of 0.88 indicates that each liter of oxygen uptake generates an energy equivalent of 4.9 kCal (see Table 7.2). Thus, the exercise expended 122.5 kCal (25 L × 4.9 kCal). Mechanical efficiency (%) computes as follows:

$$ME(\%) = \frac{Work\ Output}{Energy\ Expended} \times 100$$

$$= \frac{31.2\ kCal}{122.5\ kCal} \times 100$$

$$= 25.5\%$$

As with all machines, the human body's efficiency for producing mechanical work falls considerably below 100%. The energy required to overcome internal and external friction becomes the biggest factor affecting ME. Overcoming friction represents essentially wasted energy because it accomplishes no external work; consequently, work input always exceeds work output. The ME of human locomotion in walking, running, and cycling ranges between 20% and 30%.

Net Mechanical Efficiency

Net ME involves subtracting the resting energy expenditure from the total energy expended during exercise. This indicates the efficiency of the work per se, unaffected by differences in resting energy expenditure.

Net ME calculates as follows:

$$Net\ ME(\%) = \frac{Work\ Output}{Energy\ Expended\ Above\ Rest} \times 100$$

Resting energy output is determined for the same time duration as the work output.

In the previous example for gross ME, if the resting oxygen uptake equaled 250 mL·min^{-1} (0.25 L·min^{-1}) and RQ equaled 0.91 (4.936 kCal·L $O_2$$^{-1}$; 0.250 L·min^{-1} × 4.936 = 1.234 kCal·min^{-1}), net ME computes as:

$$Net\ ME(\%) = \frac{Work\ Output}{Energy\ Expended\ Above\ Rest} \times 100$$

$$= \frac{31.2\ kCal}{122.5\ kCal - (1.234\ kCal \cdot min^{-1} \times 15\ min)}$$

$$\times 100$$

$$= 30\%$$

Delta Efficiency

Delta efficiency calculates as the relative energy cost of performing an additional increment of work. That is, the ratio of the difference between work output at two levels of work output to the difference in energy expenditure determined for the two levels of work output.

Delta (Δ) Efficiency

$$= \frac{\begin{array}{c} Difference\ in\ Work\ Output \\ Between\ Two\ Exercise\ Levels \end{array}}{\begin{array}{c} Difference\ in\ Energy\ Expended \\ Between\ Two\ Exercise\ Levels \end{array}} \times 100$$

For example, suppose an individual cycles at 100 watts for 5 minutes (100 W = 1.433 kCal·min^{-1}) at a steady-rate oxygen uptake of 1.70 L·min^{-1} with an RQ of 0.83 (4.838 kCal·L $O_2$$^{-1}$). This corresponds to an energy expenditure of 8.23 kCal·min^{-1}. The person then completes another 5 minutes at 200 watts (200 W = 2.866 kCal·min^{-1}) at a steady-rate oxygen uptake of 2.80 L·min^{-1} with an RQ of 0.90 (4.924 kCal·L $O_2$$^{-1}$). This results in an energy expenditure of 13.8 kCal·min^{-1}. Delta efficiency computes as:

Delta (Δ) Efficiency

$$= \frac{\text{Difference in Work Output Between Two Exercise Levels}}{\text{Difference in Energy Expended Between Two Exercise Levels}} \times 100$$

$$= \frac{\begin{array}{c} 2.866 \ kCal\cdot min^{-1} \\ - \ 1.433 \ kCal\cdot min^{-1} \end{array}}{\begin{array}{c} 13.79 \ kCal\cdot min^{-1} \\ - \ 8.23 \ kCal\cdot min^{-1} \end{array}} \times 100$$

$$= \frac{1.433 \ kCal\cdot min^{-1}}{5.56 \ kCal\cdot min^{-1}} \times 100$$

$$= 25.8\%$$

Delta efficiency becomes the calculation of choice when assessing efficiency of treadmill exercise since it is impossible to determine work output accurately during horizontal movement.

Factors Influencing Exercise Efficiency

Seven factors influence exercise efficiency:

1. **Work rate:** Efficiency generally decreases as work rate increases because the relationship between energy expenditure and work rate is curvilinear rather than linear. Thus, as work rate increases, total energy expenditure increases disproportionately to work output, resulting in a lowered mechanical efficiency.

2. **Movement speed:** An optimum speed of movement exists for any given work rate for every individual. Generally, the optimum movement speed increases as power output increases (i.e., higher power outputs require greater movement speed for optimum efficiency). Any deviation from the optimal movement speed decreases efficiency. Low efficiencies at slow speeds most likely result from inertia (increased energy expended to overcome internal starting and stopping), whereas an efficiency decline at high speeds might result from increases in muscular friction and resulting increases in internal work and energy expenditure.

3. **Extrinsic factors:** Improvements in equipment design have increased efficiency in many physical activities. For example, changes in shoe design (lighter/softer) permit running at given speed with a lower energy expenditure, thus increasing efficiency of movement; changes in clothing (lighter more absorbent fabrics) have produced a similar effect.

4. **Muscle fiber composition:** Activation of slow-twitch muscle fibers produces greater efficiency than the same work accomplished by fast-twitch fibers (slow-twitch fibers require less ATP per unit work compared to fast-twitch fibers). Thus, individuals with a higher percentage of slow-twitch muscle fibers display increased mechanical efficiency.

5. **Fitness level:** More fit individuals perform a given task at a higher efficiency because of decreased energy expenditure for non–exercise-related functions like temperature regulation, increased circulation, and waste removal.

6. **Body composition:** Fatter individuals perform a given exercise task (particularly weight-bearing exercises like walking and running) at a lower efficiency. This results from an increased energy cost of transporting the extra body fat.

7. **Technique:** Improved technique produces fewer extraneous body movements, resulting in a lower energy expenditure and hence higher efficiency. The golf swing is a prime example. Millions of men and women expend considerable "energy" trying to hit the ball where they want it to go—most of the time with less than perfect execution. In contrast, the golf pro expends seemingly little

Questions & Notes

Give the formula for gross mechanical efficiency.

Complete the following conversions:

1 kCal = ___ kg-m

1 kCal = ___ ft-lb

1 watt = _____ kCal•min^{-1}

1 watt = _____ kg-min•min^{-1}

Compute the mechanical efficiency for a 10-minute ride on a bicycle ergometer that generates 28 kCal of energy; oxygen uptake totaled 20 L with an RQ of 0.88.

Give the formula for net mechanical efficiency.

Give the formula for delta efficiency.

Define economy of movement.

"energy" in coordinating the legs, hips, shoulders, and arms to strike the ball some 250–300 yards on a perfect trajectory. There is no question that perfectly practicing the swing hundreds of thousands of times "grooves" the movement so it seemingly becomes effortless—coupled with precise timing and coordination patterns—to reliably and consistently strike the ball with just the right amount of force and spin to make it land near the intended target. Like a well-tuned machine, the pro's golf swing accomplishes the task with great muscular efficiency. A recreational player, while striving for the perfection of the pro, falls short of the efficiency (mechanics and technique) to achieve the desired result. In this case, the efficiency of movement (with greater energy required to execute the precise muscular movements) remains less than for the pro golfer.

ECONOMY OF MOVEMENT

The concept of exercise economy can also be viewed as the relationship between energy input and energy output. For **economy of human movement**, the quantity of energy to perform a particular task relative to performance quality represents an important concern. In a sense, many of us assess economy by visually comparing the ease of movement of highly trained athletes. It does not require a trained eye to discriminate the ease of effort in comparisons of elite swimmers, skiers, dancers, gymnasts, and divers with less proficient counterparts who seem to expend considerable "wasted energy" to perform the same tasks. Anyone who has learned a new sport recalls the difficulties encountered performing basic movements that, with practice, became automatic and seemingly "effortless."

Exercise Oxygen Uptake Reflects Economy

A common method to assess differences between individuals in economy of movement evaluates the steady-rate oxygen uptake during a specific exercise at a set power output or speed. This approach only applies to steady-rate exercise where oxygen uptake closely mirrors energy expenditure. *For example, at a given submaximum speed of running, cycling, or swimming, an individual with greater movement economy consumes less oxygen.* Economy takes on importance during longer-duration exercise, where the athlete's aerobic capacity and the oxygen requirements of the task determine success. *All else being equal, a training adjustment that improves economy of effort directly translates to improved exercise performance.* **Figure 8.5** relates running economy to endurance performance in elite athletes of comparable aerobic fitness. Clearly, athletes with greater running economies (lower oxygen uptake at the same running pace) achieve better performance.

No single biomechanical factor accounts for individual differences in running economy. Significant variation in

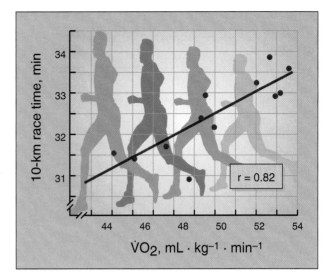

Figure 8.5 Relationship between submaximum $\dot{V}O_2$ at 16.1 $km \cdot h^{-1}$ and 10-km race time in elite male runners of comparable aerobic capacity.

economy at a particular running speed occurs even among trained runners. In general, improved running economy results from years of arduous run training. Short-term training that emphasizes only the "proper techniques" of running (e.g., arm movements and body alignment) probably does not improve running economy. However, distance runners who lack an economical stride-length pattern benefit from a short-term program of audio-visual feedback that focuses on optimizing stride length.

ECONOMY DURING WALKING

For most individuals, the most common form of exercise, walking, represents the major type of physical activity that falls outside the realm of sedentary living. **Figure 8.6** displays the curvilinear relationship between energy expenditure versus walking at slow and fast speeds. A linear relationship exists between walking speeds of 3.0 and 5.0 $km \cdot h^{-1}$ (1.9 to 3.1 mph) and oxygen uptake; at faster speeds, walking becomes less economical, and the relationship curves upward to indicate a disproportionate increase in energy cost related to walking speed. In general, the **crossover velocity** (note intersection of two straight lines) at which running becomes more economical than walking appears to be about 6.5 $km \cdot h^{-1}$ (4.0 mph).

Competition Walking

The energy expenditure of Olympic-caliber walkers has been studied at various speeds while walking and running on a treadmill. Their walking speeds in competition average a remarkable 13.0 $km \cdot h^{-1}$ (11.5 to 14.8 $km \cdot h^{-1}$ or 7.1 to 9.2 mph) over distances ranging from 1.6 to 50 km. [The world record for the 20-km walk (12.6 mile) of 1:17:21 (Jefferson Perez, 2003, ECU) equals a speed of

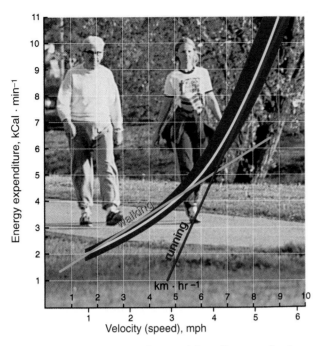

Figure 8.6 Energy expenditures while walking on a level surface at different speeds. The line represents a compilation of values reported in the literature.

Questions & Notes

List 3 factors that influence exercise economy.

   1.

   2.

   3.

Give the velocity (speed) where running becomes more economical than walking for most individuals.

Predict the energy expenditure (kCal•min⁻¹) for a 54-kg person who walks at 3.0 mph (4.83 km•h⁻¹) for 60 minutes.

15.51 km·h^{-1} (9.64 mph)]. The crossover velocity where running becomes more economical than walking for these competitive race-walkers occurs at about 8.0 km·h^{-1} (4.97 mph). The oxygen uptake of race-walkers during treadmill walking at competition speeds averages only slightly lower than the highest oxygen uptake measured for these athletes during treadmill running. Also, a linear relationship existed between oxygen uptake and walking at speeds above 8 km·h^{-1}, but the slope of the line was *twice* as steep compared with running at the same speeds. The athletes could walk at velocities up to 16 km·h^{-1} (9.94 mph) and attain oxygen uptakes as high as those while running; the economy of walking faster than 8 km·h^{-1} averaged one-half of running at similar speeds.

True or False:

Energy cost almost doubles walking in sand compared with walking in soft snow.

Effects of Body Mass

Body mass can predict energy expenditure with reasonable accuracy at horizontal walking speeds ranging from 3.2 to 6.4 km·h^{-1} (2.0 to 4.0 mph) for people of diverse body size and composition. The predicted values for energy expenditure during walking listed in **Table 8.4** fall within ± 15% of the actual energy expen-

Table 8•4	Prediction of Energy Expenditure (kCal·min^{-1}) From Speed of Level Walking and Body Mass							
		BODY MASS						
SPEED		kg	36	45	54	64	73	82	91
mph	**km·h^{-1}**	**lb**	**80**	**100**	**120**	**140**	**160**	**180**	**200**
2.0	3.22		1.9	2.2	2.6	2.9	3.2	3.5	3.8
2.5	4.02		2.3	2.7	3.1	3.5	3.8	4.2	4.5
3.0	4.83		2.7	3.1	3.6	4.0	4.4	4.8	5.3
3.5	5.63		3.1	3.6	4.2	4.6	5.0	5.4	6.1
4.0	6.44		3.5	4.1	4.7	5.2	5.8	6.4	7.0

How to use the chart: A 54-kg (120-lb) person who walks at 3.0 mph (4.83 km·h^{-1}) expends 3.6 kCal·min^{-1}. This person would expend 216 kCal during a 60-min walk (3.6 × 60).

FOR YOUR INFORMATION

Exercise Economy and Muscle Fiber Type
Muscle fiber type affects economy of cycling effort. During submaximal cycling, the exercise economies of trained cyclists varied up to 15%. Differences in muscle fiber types in the active muscles accounted for an important component of this variation. Cyclists exhibiting the most economical cycling pattern possessed the greater percentage of slow-twitch (Type I) muscle fibers in their legs. This suggests that the Type I fiber acts with greater mechanical efficiency than the faster-acting Type II fiber.

Box 8-4 • CLOSE UP

PREDICTING ENERGY EXPENDITURE DURING TREADMILL WALKING AND RUNNING

A linear relationship exists between oxygen uptake (energy expenditure) and walking speeds between 3.0 and 5.0 km·h^{-1} (1.9 and 3.1 mph) and running at speeds faster than 8.0 km·h^{-1} (5 to 10 mph). Adding the resting oxygen uptake to the oxygen requirements of the horizontal and vertical components of the walk or run makes it possible to estimate total (gross) exercise oxygen uptake ($\dot{V}O_2$) and energy expenditure.

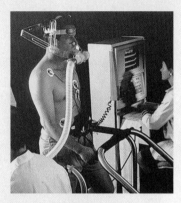

BASIC EQUATION

$\dot{V}O_2$ (mL·kg^{-1}·min^{-1}) = Resting component (1 MET; 3.5 mL O$_2$·kg^{-1}·min^{-1}) + Horizontal component (speed, m·min^{-1} × oxygen cost of horizontal movement) + Vertical component (percent grade × speed, m·min^{-1} × oxygen cost of vertical movement).

[To convert mph to m·min^{-1}, multiply by 26.82; to convert m·min^{-1} to mph, multiply by 0.03728.]

1. Walking: Oxygen cost of the horizontal component of movement equals 0.1 mL·kg^{-1}·min^{-1}, and 1.8 mL·kg^{-1}·min^{-1} for the vertical component.
2. Running: Oxygen cost of the horizontal component of movement equals 0.2 mL·kg^{-1}·min^{-1}, and 0.9 mL·kg^{-1}·min^{-1} for the vertical component.

PREDICTING ENERGY COST OF TREADMILL WALKING

Problem

A 55-kg person walks on a treadmill at 2.8 mph (2.8 × 26.82 = 75 m·min^{-1}) up a 4% grade. Calculate: (1) $\dot{V}O_2$ (mL·kg^{-1}·min^{-1}), (2) METs, and (3) energy expenditure (kCal·min^{-1}). [Note: express % grade as a decimal value; i.e., 4% grade = 0.04]

Solution

1. $\dot{V}O_2$ (mL·kg^{-1}·min^{-1}) = Resting component + Horizontal component + Vertical component

$\dot{V}O_2$ = Resting $\dot{V}O_2$ (mL·kg^{-1}·min^{-1})
   + [speed (m·min^{-1})
   × 0.1 mL·kg^{-1}·min^{-1}]
   + [% grade × speed (m·min^{-1})
   × 1.8 mL·kg^{-1}·min^{-1}]
 = 3.5 + (75 × 0.1)
   + (0.04 × 75 × 1.8)
 = 3.5 + 7.5 + 5.4
 = 16.4 mL·kg^{-1}·min^{-1}

2. METs = $\dot{V}O_2$ (mL·kg^{-1}·min^{-1})
   ÷ 3.5 mL·kg^{-1}·min^{-1}
 = 16.4 ÷ 3.5
 = 4.7

3. kCal·min^{-1} = $\dot{V}O_2$ (mL·kg^{-1}·min^{-1})
   × Body mass (kg)
   × 5.05 kCal·L^{-1}
 = 16.4 mL·kg^{-1}·min^{-1}
   × 55 kg
   × 5.05 kCal·L^{-1}
 = 0.902 L·m^{-1}
   × 5.05 kCal·L^{-1}
 = 4.6

PREDICTING ENERGY COST OF TREADMILL RUNNING

Problem

A 55-kg person runs on a treadmill at 5.4 mph (5.4 × 26.82 = 145 m·min^{-1}) up a 6% grade. Calculate: (1) $\dot{V}O_2$ in mL·kg^{-1}·min^{-1}, (2) METs, and (3) energy expenditure (kCal·min^{-1}).

Box 8–4 • CLOSE UP *(Continued)*

Solution

1. $\dot{V}O_2$ (mL·kg^{-1}·min^{-1}) = Resting component + Horizontal component + Vertical component

$\dot{V}O_2$ = Resting $\dot{V}O_2$ (mL·kg^{-1}·min^{-1})
+ [speed (m·min^{-1})
× 0.2 mL·kg^{-1}·min^{-1}]
+ [% grade × speed (m·min^{-1})
× 0.9 mL·kg^{-1}·min^{-1}]
= 3.5 + (145 × 0.2)
+ (0.06 × 145 × 0.9)
= 3.5 + 29.0 + 7.83
= 40.3 mL·kg^{-1}·min^{-1}

2. METs = $\dot{V}O_2$ (mL·kg^{-1}·min^{-1})
÷ 3.5 mL·kg^{-1}·min^{-1}
= 40.3 ÷ 3.5
= 11.5

3. kCal·min^{-1} = $\dot{V}O_2$ (mL·kg^{-1}·min^{-1})
× Body mass (kg)
× 5.05 kCal·L^{-1}
= 40.3 mL·kg^{-1}·min^{-1}
× 55 kg × 5.05 kCal·L^{-1}
= 2.22 L·min^{-1}
× 5.05 kCal·L^{-1}
= 11.2

diture for men and women of different body weights up to 91 kg (200 lb). On a daily basis, the estimated energy expended while walking would only be in error by about 50 to 100 kCal, assuming the person walks 2 hours daily. Extrapolations can be made for heavier individuals but with some loss in accuracy.

Effects of Terrain and Walking Surface

Table 8.5 summarizes the influence of terrain and surface on the energy cost of walking. Similar economies exist for level walking on a grass track or paved surface. Not surprisingly, the energy cost almost doubles walking in sand compared with walking on a hard surface; in soft snow, the metabolic cost increases 3-fold compared with treadmill walking. A brisk walk along a beach or in freshly fallen snow provides excellent exercise for programs designed to "burn up" calories or improve physiologic fitness.

Effects of Footwear

It requires considerably more energy to carry added weight on the feet or ankles than to carry similar weight attached to the torso. For example, for a weight equal to 1.4% of body mass placed on the ankles, the energy cost of walking increases an average of 8%, or nearly 6 times more than with the same weight carried on the torso. In a practical sense, the energy cost of locomotion during walking and running significantly increases when wearing boots compared with running shoes. Simply adding an additional 100 g to each shoe increases oxygen uptake by 1% during moderate running. The implication of these findings seems clear for the design of running shoes, hiking and climbing boots, and work boots traditionally required in mining, forestry, fire fighting, and the military; small changes in shoe weight produce large changes in economy of locomotion (energy expenditure). The cushioning properties of shoes also affect movement economy. A softer-soled running shoe reduced the oxygen cost of running at moderate speed by about 2.4% compared with a similar shoe with a firmer cushioning system, even though the softer-soled shoes weighed an additional 31 g. The preceding observations about terrain, footwear, and economy of locomotion

Questions & Notes

Which muscle fiber, type I or type II, acts with greater mechanical efficiency?

True or False:

It requires more energy to carry added weight in the hands or on the torso than to carry a similar weight on the feet or ankles.

Give the basic equation to predict energy expenditure during treadmill walking or running up an incline.

Table 8·5	Effect of Different Terrain on the Energy Expenditure of Walking Between 5.2 and 5.6 km·h^{-1}	
TERRAIN[a]		**CORRECTION FACTOR**[b]
Paved road (similar to grass track)		0.0
Plowed field		1.5
Hard snow		1.6
Sand dune		1.8

[a] First entry from Passmore, R., and Dumin, J.V.G.A.: Human energy expenditure. *Physiol. Rev.*, 35:801, 1955. Last three entries from Givoni, B., and Goldman, R.F.: Predicting metabolic energy cost. *J. Appl. Physiol.*, 30:429, 1971.

[b] The correction factor represents a multiple of the energy expenditure for walking on a paved road or grass track. For example, the energy cost of walking in a plowed field averages 1.5 times the cost of walking on the paved road.

indicate that, at the extreme, one could dramatically elevate energy cost by walking in soft sand at rapid speed wearing heavy work boots and ankle weights. Of course, another more prudent approach would involve unweighted race-walking or running on a firm surface.

Use of Hand-Held and Ankle Weights

The impact force on the legs during running equals about 3 times body mass, whereas the amount of leg shock with walking reaches only about 30% of this value.

Ankle weights increase the energy cost of walking to values usually observed for running. This benefits people who want to use only walking as a relatively low-impact training modality, yet require intensities of effort higher than at normal walking speeds. Hand-held weights also increase the energy cost of walking, particularly when arm movements accentuate a pumping action. However, this procedure may disproportionately elevate systolic blood pressure, due perhaps to increased intramuscular tension with gripping the weight. For individuals with hypertension or coronary heart disease, an unnecessarily "induced" elevated blood pressure would contraindicate the use of hand-held weights. For these individuals, increasing running speed (or distance) offers a more desirable alternative to increase energy expenditure than hand or ankle weights.

ENERGY EXPENDITURE DURING RUNNING

Terrain, weather, training goals, and the performer's fitness level influence the speed of running. There are two ways to quantify energy expenditure for running:

1. During performance of the actual activity

2. On a treadmill in the laboratory, with precise control over running speed and grade

Jogging and running represent qualitative terms related to speed of locomotion. This difference relates largely to the relative aerobic energy demands required in raising and lowering the body's center of gravity and accelerating and decelerating the limbs during the run. At identical running speeds, a highly conditioned distance runner runs at a lower percentage of aerobic capacity than an untrained runner, even though the oxygen uptake during the run may be similar for both people. The demarcation between jogging and running depends on the participant's fitness; a jog for one person represents a run for another.

Independent of fitness, it becomes more economical from an energy standpoint to discontinue walking and begin to jog or run at speeds greater than about 6.5 km·h^{-1} (4.0 mph) (Fig. 8.6).

Economy of Running

The data in Figure 8.6 also illustrate an important principle in relation to running speed (e.g., >5 mph or 8 km·h^{-1}) and energy expenditure. Oxygen uptake relates linearly to running speed; thus, the same total caloric cost results when running a given distance at a steady-rate oxygen uptake at a fast or slow pace. In simple terms, if one runs a mile at a 10-mph pace (16.1 km·h^{-1}), it requires about twice as much energy per minute as a 5-mph pace (8 km·h^{-1}). The runner finishes the mile in 6 minutes, whereas running at the slower speed requires twice the time, or 12 minutes. Consequently, about the same **net** energy cost for the mile exists regardless of the pace ($\pm$ 10%).

For horizontal running, net energy cost (i.e., excluding the resting requirement) per kilogram of body mass per kilometer traveled averages approximately 1 kCal or 1 kCal·kg^{-1}· km^{-1}. For an individual who weighs 78 kg, the net energy requirement for running 1 km equals about 78 kCal, regardless of running speed. Expressed as oxygen uptake, this amounts to 15.6 liters of oxygen consumed per kilometer (1 L O$_2$ = 5 kCal).

Energy Cost Values

Table 8.6 presents values for net energy expended during running for 1 hour at various speeds. The table expresses running speed as kilometers per hour, miles per hour, and number of minutes required to complete 1 mile at a given running speed. The boldface values represent net calories expended to run 1 mile for a person of a given body mass; this energy requirement remains independent of running speed. For example, for a person who weighs 62 kg, running a 26.2-mile marathon requires about 2600 net kCal whether the run takes just over 2 hours or 4 hours.

The energy cost per mile increases proportionately with the runner's body mass (refer to column 3). This observation certainly supports the role of weight-bearing

Table 8·6	Net Energy Expenditure Per Hour for Horizontal Running in Relation to Velocity and Body Mass[a,b]								

	km·h^{-1}	8	9	10	11	12	13	14	15	16
	mph	4.97	5.60	6.20	6.84	7.46	8.08	8.70	9.32	9.94
Body Mass	**min per mile**	12:00	10:43	9:41	8:46	8:02	7:26	6:54	6:26	6:02
kg **lb**	**kCal per mile**									
50 110	80	400	450	500	550	600	650	700	750	800
54 119	86	432	486	540	594	648	702	756	810	864
58 128	93	464	522	580	638	696	754	812	870	928
62 137	99	496	558	620	682	744	806	868	930	992
66 146	106	528	594	660	726	792	858	924	990	1056
70 154	112	560	630	700	770	840	910	980	1050	1120
74 163	118	592	666	740	814	888	962	1036	1110	1184
78 172	125	624	702	780	858	936	1014	1092	1170	1248
82 181	131	656	738	820	902	984	1066	1148	1230	1312
86 190	138	688	774	860	946	1032	1118	1204	1290	1376
90 199	144	720	810	900	990	1080	1170	1260	1350	1440
94 207	150	752	846	940	1034	1128	1222	1316	1410	1504
98 216	157	784	882	980	1078	1176	1274	1372	1470	1568
102 225	163	816	918	1020	1122	1224	1326	1428	1530	1632
106 234	170	848	954	1060	1166	1272	1378	1484	1590	1696

[a] Interpret the table as follows: For a 50-kg person, the *net* energy expenditure for running for 1 hour at 8 km·h^{-1} (4.97 mph) equals 400 kCal; this speed represents a 12-minute per mile pace. Thus, 5 miles would be run in 1 hour and 400 kCal would be expended. If the pace increased to 12 km·h^{-1} (7.46 mph), 600 kCal would be expended during the 1-hour run.
[b] Running speeds expressed as kilometers per hour (km·h^{-1}), miles per hour (mph), and minutes required to complete each mile (min per mile). The values in **boldface type** equal *net* calories (resting energy expenditure subtracted) expended to run 1 mile for a given body mass, independent of running speed.

exercise as a caloric stress for overweight individuals who want to increase energy expenditure for weight loss. For example, a 102-kg person who jogs 5 miles daily at any comfortable pace expends 163 kCal for each mile completed, or a total of 815 kCal for the 5-mile run. Increasing or decreasing the speed (within the broad range of steady-rate paces) simply alters the length of the exercise period; it has little effect on total *net* energy expended through exercise.

Stride Length, Stride Frequency, and Running Speed

Running speed can increase in three ways:

1. Increase the number of steps each minute (stride frequency)
2. Increase the distance between steps (stride length)
3. Increase stride length and stride frequency

Although the third option may seem the obvious way to increase running speed, several experiments provide objective data concerning this question.

In 1944, researchers studied the stride pattern for the Danish champion in the 5- and 10-km running events. At a running speed of 9.3 km·h^{-1} (5.8 mph), this athlete's stride frequency equaled 160 per minute with a corresponding stride length of 97 cm (38.2 in). When running speed increased 91% to 17.8 km·h^{-1} (11.1 mph), stride frequency increased only 10% to 176 per minute, whereas an 83% increase to 168 cm occurred in stride length. These data illustrate that running speed increases predominantly by lengthening stride. Only at faster speeds does stride frequency become important.

Optimum Stride Length An optimum combination of stride length and frequency exists for running at a particular constant speed. The optimum combination depends largely on the person's "style" of running and cannot be deter-

FOR YOUR INFORMATION

Calories Add Up With Regular Exercise
For distance runners who train up to 100 miles a week, or slightly less than the distance of four marathons at close to competitive speeds, the weekly caloric expenditure from exercise averages about 10,000 kCal. For the serious marathon runner who trains year-round, the total energy expended in training for 4 years before an Olympic competition exceeds two million calories—the caloric equivalent of 555 pounds of body fat. This more than likely contributes to the low levels of body fat (3% to 5% of body mass for men; 12% to 17% for women) possessed by these athletes.

mined from objective body measurements. Running speed chosen by the person incorporates the most economical stride length. Lengthening the stride above the optimum increases oxygen uptake more than a shorter-than-optimum stride length. Urging a runner who shows signs of fatigue to "lengthen your stride" to maintain speed produces counterproductive results for oxygen cost (exercise economy).

Well-trained runners run at a stride length "selected" through years of training. This produces the most economical running performance, in keeping with the concept that the body naturally attempts to achieve a level of "minimum effort." No "best" style exists to characterize elite runners. Instead, individual differences in body size, inertia of limb segments, and anatomic development interact to vary one's stride.

Effects of Air Resistance

Anyone who has run into a headwind knows it requires more energy to maintain a given pace compared with running in calm weather or with the wind at one's back. Three factors influence how air resistance affects energy cost of running:

1. Air density
2. Runner's projected surface area
3. Square of headwind velocity

Depending on running speed, overcoming air resistance accounts for 3% to 9% of the total energy requirement of running in calm weather. Running into a headwind creates an additional energy expense. In one study, for example, running at 15.9 km·h^{-1} (9.9 mph) in calm conditions produced an oxygen uptake of 2.92 L·min^{-1}. This increased by 5.5% to 3.09 L·min^{-1} against a 16-km·h^{-1} (9.9 mph) headwind and to 4.1 L·min^{-1} while running against the strongest wind (41 mph); running into the strongest wind represents a 40% additional expenditure of energy to maintain running velocity.

Some may argue that the negative effects of running into a headwind counterbalance on one's return with the tailwind. This does not occur because the energy cost of cutting through a headwind exceeds the reduction in exercise oxygen uptake with an equivalent wind velocity at one's back. Wind tunnel tests show that running performance increases by wearing form-fitting clothing; even trimming one's hair improves aerodynamics and reduces wind resistance effects by up to 6%. In competitive cycling, manufacturers continually modify clothing and helmets (including the rider's body position on the bicycle and frame design) to reduce the effects of air resistance on energy cost.

At altitude, wind velocity affects energy expenditure less than at sea level due to reduced air density at higher elevations. Speed skaters experience a lower oxygen requirement while skating at a particular speed at altitude compared to sea level. Overcoming air resistance at alti-

tude only becomes important at the faster skating speeds. In all likelihood, an altitude effect also applies to competitive cycling, where the impeding effect of air resistance becomes considerable at the high speeds achieved by these athletes.

Drafting To counter the negative effects of air resistance and headwind on energy cost, athletes use "**drafting**" by following directly behind a competitor. For example, running 1 meter behind another runner at a speed of 21.6 km·h^{-1} (13.4 mph) decreases the total energy expenditure by about 7%. Drafting at this speed could save about 1 second for each 400 m covered during a race. The beneficial aerodynamic effect of drafting on the economy of effort also has been observed for cross-country skiing, speed skating, and cycling. About 90% of the power generated when cycling at 40 km·h^{-1} (24.9 mph) on a calm day goes to overcoming air resistance. At this speed, energy expenditure decreases between 26% and 38% when a competitor follows closely behind another cyclist.

Treadmill Versus Track Running

Researchers use the treadmill almost exclusively to evaluate the physiology of running in the laboratory. A question concerns the association between treadmill running and running performance on a track or road race. For example, does it require the same energy to run a given speed or distance on a treadmill and a track in calm weather? To answer this question, researchers studied eight distance runners on both a treadmill and track at three submaximum speeds of 10.8, 12.6, and 15.6 km·h^{-1} (6.7, 7.8, and 9.7 mph). They also studied the athletes during a graded exercise test to determine possible differences between treadmill and track running on submaximal and maximal oxygen uptake.

From a practical standpoint, no measurable differences occurred in aerobic requirements of submaximal running (up to 17.2 km·h^{-1}) on the treadmill or track or between the $\dot{V}O_{2max}$ measured in both forms of exercise under similar environmental conditions. The possibility exists, however, that at the faster running speeds of endurance competition, air resistance could negatively impact outdoor running performance and oxygen cost may significantly exceed that of "stationary" treadmill running at the same speed.

Marathon Running

As of January 2005, the world marathon record is 2 h:04 min:55 s (set on September 28, 2003). The average speed of less than 5 minutes per mile represents an outstanding achievement in human performance. Not only does this pace require a steady-rate aerobic metabolism that greatly exceeds the aerobic capacity of the average male college student, it also represents about 85% of the marathoners' $\dot{V}O_{2max}$ maintained for just over 2 hours. Aerobic capacity

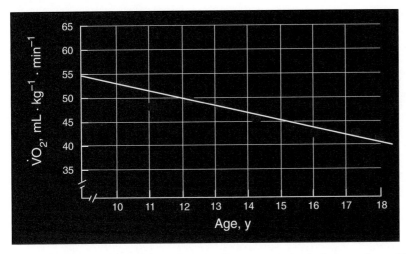

Figure 8.7 Effects of growth on submaximal oxygen uptake during running at 12.1 km·h^{-1}. (Adapted from Daniels, J., et al.: Differences and changes in $\dot{V}O_2$ among runners 10 to 18 years of age. *Med. Sci. Sports,* 10:200, 1978.)

of these athletes averages about 4.4 L·min^{-1} or between 70 and 84 mL·kg^{-1}·min^{-1}. This rate of energy expenditure results in a total caloric expenditure of about 2400 kCal for the marathon alone, excluding any elevated energy expenditure during recovery that can persist for up to 24 to 48 hours.

Running Economy: Children and Adults, Trained and Untrained

Boys and girls are less economical runners than adults; they require between 20% and 30% more oxygen per unit of body mass to run at a given speed. A larger ratio of surface area to body mass, greater stride frequency, shorter stride lengths, and anthropometric and biomechanical factors contribute to children's inferior movement economy.

The age-related decreases in steady-rate oxygen uptake at a given speed shown in **Figure 8.7** indicate that running economy improves steadily from ages 10 to 18 years. This partly explains the relatively poor performance of young children in distance running and their progressive improvement throughout adolescence. Improved endurance occurs even though aerobic capacity relative to body mass (mL O$_2$·kg^{-1}·min^{-1}) remains relatively constant during this time.

At a particular speed, elite endurance runners run at a lower oxygen uptake than less trained or less successful counterparts of similar age. This holds for 8- to 11-year-old cross-country runners and adult marathoners. Elite distance athletes, as a group, run with 5% to 10% greater economy than well-trained middle-distance runners.

ENERGY EXPENDITURE DURING SWIMMING

Swimming differs in several important respects from walking or running. For one thing, swimmers must expend energy to maintain buoyancy while, at the same time, generate horizontal movement using the arms and legs, either in combination or separately. Other differences include the energy requirements for overcoming drag forces that impede the movement of an object through a water medium. The amount of drag depends on the characteristics of the medium and the object's size, shape, and velocity. *These factors all contribute to a significantly lower economy in swimming compared with running. More specifically, it requires about four times more energy to swim a given distance than to run the same distance.*

Questions & Notes

Give the impact force on the legs during running.

Give the increase in energy expenditure walking in hard snow compared with walking on a hard, paved road.

List the 3 ways to increase running speed.

1.

2.

3.

Give the major factor that determines optimum stride length and frequency.

List 2 factors that determine how air resistance affects the energy cost of running.

1.

2.

Does "drafting" increase or decrease energy cost of running? If yes, by about how much?

Are boys and girls more or less economical runners than adults of similar fitness status?

What factors contribute to the lower economy of effort in swimming compared to running?

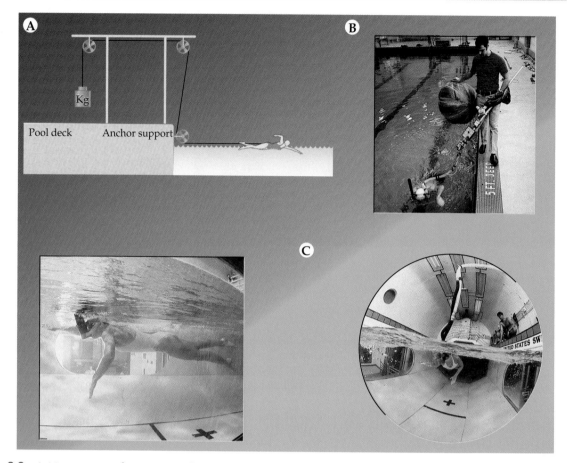

Figure 8.8 **A.** Measurement of energy expenditure during tethered swimming. **B.** Open-circuit spirometry (bag technique) to measure oxygen consumption during front-crawl swimming. **C.** Swimming treadmill. An environmental chamber surrounding the swimming treadmill controls atmospheric pressure (and other environmental conditions) during swimming. Using the swimming treadmill, researchers conduct physiologic and biomechanical experiments during swimming that simulate actual performance conditions. The underwater viewing area provides a convenient means for directly observing swimming performance related to stroke mechanics. (Schematic and photos of swimming treadmill courtesy of the United States Swimming International Center for Aquatic Research, Colorado Springs, CO.)

Methods of Measurement

Energy expenditure has been computed from oxygen uptake measured by open-circuit spirometry during swimming (**Fig. 8.8**). In studies conducted in the pool, the researcher walks alongside the swimmer while carrying the portable gas collection equipment (Fig. 8.8B). In another form of swimming exercise illustrated in Figure 8.8A, the subject remains stationary and attached ("tethered") to a cable and pulley system by a belt worn around the waist. Periodically increasing the amount of weight attached to the cable forces the swimmer to exert more effort to keep from being pulled backward.

Figure 8.8C shows a subject swimming in a flume or "swim-mill." Water circulates, and its velocity can vary from a slow swimming speed to a near-record pace for a free-style sprint. Also, water temperature in the 38,000-L swim-mill can be regulated between 10 and 40°C. Windows on the side of the flume beneath the water's surface enable photographic analysis of stroke mechanics. Skilled swimmers achieve essentially identical aerobic capacity values when measured by either tethered, free, or flume swimming. This

means that each mode measurement evaluates the functional capacity of the aerobic system during swimming.

Energy Cost and Drag

Three components comprise the total drag force that impedes a swimmer's forward movement:

1. **Wave drag** caused by waves that build up in front of and form hollows behind the swimmer moving through the water. This component of drag only becomes a significant factor at fast speeds.
2. **Skin friction drag** produced as the water slides over the skin's surface. Removal of body hair reduces drag to slightly decrease the energy cost and physiologic demands during swimming.
3. **Viscous pressure drag** contributes substantially to counter the propulsive efforts of the swimmer at slow velocities. It results from the separation of the thin sheet of water (boundary layer) adjacent to the swimmer. The pressure differential created in front of and behind the swimmer represents viscous pressure drag. Highly skilled swimmers who "streamline" their

stroke reduce this component of total drag. Streamlining with improved stroke mechanics reduces the separation region by moving the separation point closer to the trailing edge of the water. This also occurs when an oar slices through the water with the blade parallel rather than perpendicular to water flow.

Differences in total drag force between swimmers can make the difference between winning and losing, particularly in longer distance races. Wet suits worn during the swim portion of a triathlon can reduce body drag by 14%. Improved swimming economy largely explains the significantly faster swim times of athletes who wear wet suits. As in running, cross-country skiing, and cycling, drafting in ocean swimming (following closely behind the wake of a lead swimmer) reduces energy expenditure. This enables an endurance swimmer to conserve energy and possibly improve performance toward the end of competition.

Energy Cost, Swimming Velocity, and Skill

Elite swimmers swim a particular stroke at a given velocity at a lower oxygen uptake than either less elite or recreational swimmers. Elite swimmers swim a given speed with a lower oxygen uptake than the untrained yet skilled swimmers. For different swimming strokes in terms of energy expenditure, swimming the breast-stroke "costs" the most at any speed, followed by the backstroke. The front crawl represented the least "expensive" (calorie-wise) among the three strokes.

Effects of Buoyancy: Men Versus Women

Women of all ages possess, on average, more total body fat than men. Because fat floats and muscle and bone sink, the average woman gains a hydrodynamic lift and floats more easily than the average male. This difference in buoyancy can explain women's greater swimming economy compared to men. For example, women swim a given distance at a lower energy cost than men; expressed another way, women achieve a higher swimming velocity than men for the same level of energy expenditure.

The distribution of body fat towards the periphery in women causes their legs to float higher in the water, making them more horizontal or "streamlined," whereas men's leaner legs tend to swing down in the water. Lowering the legs to a deeper position increases body drag and thus reduces swimming economy. The potential hydrodynamic benefits enjoyed by women become noteworthy in longer distances where swimming economy and body insulation take on added importance. For example, the woman's record for swimming the 21-mile English Channel from England to France equals 7 h:40 min. The men's record equals 7 h:17 min, a difference of only 5.2%. In several instances, as displayed in **Table 8.7**, women actually swim faster than men. In fact, the first woman to swim the Channel (1926) swam 35% faster than the first male who completed the swim (1875).

Questions & Notes

List 3 components of swimming drag.

1.

2.

3.

About how much can wet suits reduce swimming drag?

True or False:

Elite swimmers swim a given distance with a higher $\dot{V}O_2$.

True or False:

Women have higher buoyancy than men.

Table 8·7	Comparisons of English Channel World Record Swimming Times Between Males and Females		

ENGLISH CHANNEL RECORDS (HR:MIN): MALE VS. FEMALE

Record	Male	Female	% Difference (male:female)
First attempt–one way	21:45 (1875)	14:39 (1926)	34.9
Fastest–one way	07:17 (1994)	7:40 (1978)	−5.26
Youngest–one way	11:54 (11 y, 11 mo; 1988)	15:28 (12 y, 11 mo; 1983)	−29.9
Oldest–one way	18:37 (67 y; 1987)	12:32 (57 y; 1999)	32.69
Fastest–2 way	16:10 (1987)	17:14 (1991)	−6.6
Fastest–3 way	28:21 (1987)	34:40 (1990)	−22.2

Note that for two records (first attempt, oldest) females bettered the male record by more than 30%.

SUMMARY

1. Mechanical efficiency represents the percentage of total chemical energy expended that contributes to external work, with the remainder representing lost heat.

2. Exercise economy can be viewed as the relationship between energy input and energy output. A common method to assess differences between individuals in economy of movement evaluates oxygen uptake while the subject exercises at a set power output or speed.

3. Walking speed relates linearly to oxygen uptake between speeds of 1.9 and 3.1 mph; at speeds faster than 4.0 mph, walking becomes less economical.

4. Walking surface impacts energy expenditure; walking on sand requires about twice the energy expenditure as walking on hard surfaces. The energy cost of such weight-bearing exercise becomes proportionally larger for heavier people.

5. Hand-held and ankle weights increase the energy cost of walking to values usually observed for running. This benefits those wanting to use only walking as a low-impact form of exercise training.

6. It becomes more economical from an energy standpoint to jog-run rather than to walk at speeds that exceed 8 km·h^{-1} (5 mph). The difference between jogging and running depends on the fitness level of the participant; a jog for one person may represent a run for another.

7. Total energy cost for running a given distance remains independent of running speed. For horizontal running, the net energy expenditure averages about 1 kCal·kg^{-1}·km^{-1}.

8. Shortening running stride and increasing stride frequency to maintain a constant running speed requires less energy than lengthening the stride and reducing stride frequency. An individual subconsciously "selects" the combination of stride length and frequency that favors optimal economy.

9. Overcoming air resistance accounts for 3% to 9% of the total energy cost of running in calm weather. This percentage increases by the square of the wind velocity as the runner attempts to maintain pace while running into a headwind.

10. Running directly behind a competitor, a favorable aerodynamic technique called "drafting," counters the negative effect of air resistance and headwind on the energy cost of running.

11. It requires the same amount of energy to run a given distance or speed on a treadmill as on a track under identical environmental conditions.

12. Children run at a given speed with less economy compared with adults because they require between 20% and 30% more oxygen per unit of body mass. This relatively lower running economy accounts for the poor endurance performance of children compared with adults with similar aerobic capacity.

13. It takes about four times more energy to swim than to run the same distance. In contrast to running, a swimmer must expend considerable energy to maintain buoyancy and overcome the various drag forces that impede movement.

14. Elite swimmers expend fewer calories to swim a given stroke at any velocity.

15. Significant gender differences exist for body drag, economy, and net oxygen uptake during swimming. Women swim a given distance at about 30% lower energy cost than men.

THOUGHT QUESTIONS

1. A 60-kg (132-lb) elite marathoner who trains year-round expends about 4000 kCal daily over a 4-year training period before Olympic competition. Assuming body mass remains unchanged and 70% of daily caloric intake comes from carbohydrate and 1.4 g per kg body mass comes from protein, compute the runner's total 4-year calorie intake and total grams consumed from carbohydrate and protein.

2. How would you respond to this question: "Why do children who run in 10-km races never seem to perform as well as adults?"

3. Most people assume they expend more total calories if they run a given distance faster. Explain why this is not true. In what way does correcting this misunderstanding contribute to a recommendation for the use of exercise for weight loss?

4. An elite 120-lb runner claims that she consistently consumes 12,000 kCal daily simply to maintain body weight owing to the strenuousness of her training. Using examples of exercise energy expenditures, discuss whether this level of intake could reflect a plausible regular energy intake requirement.

SELECTED REFERENCES

ACSM's Guidelines for Exercise Testing and Prescription. 7th Ed. Baltimore: Lippincott Williams & Wilkins, 2006.

ACSM's Resource Manual for Guidelines for Exercise Testing and Prescription. 5th Ed. Baltimore: Lippincott Williams & Wilkins, 2006.

Alexander, R.M.: Physiology: enhanced: walking made simple. *Science,* 308:58, 2005.

Alfonzo-Gonzalez, G., et al.: Estimation of daily energy needs with the FAO/WHO/UNU 1985 procedures in adults: comparison to whole-body indirect calorimetry measurements. *Eur. J. Clin. Nutr.,* 58:1125, 2004.

Barbosa, T.M., et al.: Energy cost and intracyclic variation of the velocity of the centre of mass in butterfly stroke. *Eur. J. Appl. Physiol.,* 93:519, 2005.

Bertram, J.E.: Constrained optimization in human walking: cost minimization and gait plasticity. *J. Exp. Biol.,* 208:979, 2005.

Blanc, S., et al.: Energy requirements in the eighth decade of life. *Am. J. Clin. Nutr.,* 79:303, 2004.

Butte, N.F., et al.: Energy requirements of women of reproductive age. *Am. J. Clin. Nutr.,* 77:630, 2003.

Byrne, N.M., et al.: The metabolic equivalent: One size does not fit all. *J. Appl. Physiol.,* 2005.

Chasan-Taber, L., et al.: Development and validation of a pregnancy physical activity questionnaire. *Med. Sci. Sports Exerc.,* 36:1750, 2004.

Chatard, J-C, et al.: Drafting distance in swimming. *Med. Sci. Sports Exerc.,* 35:1176, 2003.

Coyle, E.F.: Improved muscular efficiency displayed as Tour de France champion matures. *J. Appl. Physiol.,* 98:2191, 2005.

Crouter, S.E., et al.: Accuracy of polar S410 heart rate monitor to estimate energy cost of exercise. *Med. Sci. Sports Exerc.,* 36:1433, 2004.

da Rocha, E.E., et al.: Can measured resting energy expenditure be estimated by formulae in daily clinical nutrition practice? *Curr. Opin. Clin. Nutr. Metab. Care,* 8:319, 2005.

Das, S.K., et al.: Energy expenditure is very high in extremely obese women. *J. Nutr.,* 134:1412, 2004.

DeLany, J.P., et al.: Energy expenditure in African American and white boys and girls in a 2-y follow-up of the Baton Rouge Children's Study. *Am. J. Clin. Nutr.,* 79:268, 2004.

Delextrat, A., et al.: Drafting during swimming improves efficiency during subsequent cycling. *Med. Sci. Sports Exerc.,* 35:1612, 2003.

Dennis, S.C., Noakes, T.D.: Advantages of a smaller body mass in humans when distance-running in warm, humid conditions. *Eur. J. Appl. Physiol.,* 79:280, 1999.

Doke, J., et al.: Mechanics and energetics of swinging the human leg. *J. Exp. Biol.,* 208:439, 2005.

Donahoo, W.T., et al.: Variability in energy expenditure and its components. *Curr. Opin. Clin. Nutr. Metab. Care,* 7:599, 2004.

Duffield, R., et al.: Energy system contribution to 100-m and 200-m track running events. *J. Sci. Med. Sport,* 7:302, 2004.

Entin, P.L., Coffin, L.: Physiological basis for recommendations regarding exercise during pregnancy at high altitude. *High Alt. Med. Biol.,* 5:321, 2004.

Farshchi, H.R., et al.: Decreased thermic effect of food after an irregular compared with a regular meal pattern in healthy lean women. *Int. J. Obes. Relat. Metab. Disord.,* 28:653, 2004.

Flodmark, C.E.: Calculation of resting energy expenditure in obese children. *Acta. Paediatr.,* 93:727, 2004.

Garet, M., et al.: Estimating relative physical workload using heart rate monitoring: a validation by whole-body indirect calorimetry. *Eur. J. Appl. Physiol.,* 94:46, 2005.

Gottschall, J.S., Kram, R.: Ground reaction forces during downhill and uphill running. *J. Biomech.,* 38:445, 2005.

Hall, C., et al.: Energy expenditure of walking and running: comparison with prediction equations. *Med. Sci. Sports Exerc.,* 36:2128, 2004.

Hausswirth, C., et al.: Effects of cycling alone or in a sheltered position on subsequent running performance during a triathlon. *Med. Sci. Sports Exerc.,* 31:599, 1999.

Hiilloskorpi, H.K., et al.: Use of heart rate to predict energy expenditure from low to high activity levels. *Int. J. Sports Med.,* 24:332, 2003.

Hoyt, R.W., et al.: Total energy expenditure estimated using foot-ground contact pedometry. *Diabetes Technol. Ther.,* 6:71, 2004.

Hukshorn, C.J., Saris, W.H.: Leptin and energy expenditure. *Curr. Opin. Clin. Nutr. Metab. Care,* 7:629, 2004.

Keytel, L.R., et al.: Prediction of energy expenditure from heart rate monitoring during submaximal exercise. *J. Sports Sci.,* 23:289, 2005.

Kien, C.L., Ugrasbul, F.: Prediction of daily energy expenditure during a feeding trial using measurements of resting energy expenditure, fat-free mass, or Harris-Benedict equations. *Am. J. Clin. Nutr.,* 80:876, 2004.

Kram, R. Muscular force or work: what determines the metabolic energy cost of running? *Exer. Sport Sci. Rev.,* 28:138, 2000.

Kyrölälinen, H., et al.: Interrelationships between muscle structure, muscle strength, and running economy. *Med. Sci. Sports Exerc.,* 35:45, 2003.

Larsson, L., Lindqvist, P.G.: Low-impact exercise during

pregnancyóa study of safety. *Acta. Obstet. Gynecol. Scand.*, 84:34, 2005.

Lin, P.H., et al.: Estimation of energy requirements in a controlled feeding trial. *Am. J. Clin. Nutr.*, 77:639, 2003.

Malison, E.R., et al.: Running performance in middle-school runners. *J. Sports Med. Phys. Fitness*, 44:383, 2004.

Morgan, D.W., et al.: Longitudinal stratification of gait economy in young boys and girls: the locomotion energy and growth study. *Eur. J. Appl. Physiol.*, 91:30, 2004.

Morgan, D.W., et al.: Prediction of the aerobic demand of walking in children. *Med. Sci. Sports Exerc.*, 34:2097, 2002.

Pendergast, D., et al.: Energy balance of human locomotion in water. *Eur. J. Appl. Physiol.*, 90:377, 2003.

Pendergast, D., et al.: The influence of drag on human locomotion in water. *Undersea Hyperb. Med.*, 32:45, 2005.

Pendergast, D.R., et al.: Evaluation of fins used in underwater swimming. *Undersea Hyperb. Med.*, 30:57, 2003.

Pontzer, H.: A new model predicting locomotor cost from limb length via force production. *J. Exp. Biol.*, 208:1513, 2005.

Porcari, J.: Pump up your walk. *ACSM Health Fitness J.*, 3(1):25, 1999.

Ramirez-Marrero, F.A., et al.: Comparison of methods to estimate physical activity and energy expenditure in African American children. *Int. J. Sports Med.*, 26:363, 2005.

Royer T.D., Martin, P.E.: Manipulations of leg mass and moment of inertia: effects on energy cost of walking. *Med. Sci. Sports Exerc.*, 37:649, 2005.

Saunders, P.U., et al.: Reliability and variability of running economy in elite distance runners. *Med. Sci. Sports Exerc.*, 36:1972, 2004.

Scott, C.B., Devore, R.: Diet-induced thermogenesis: variations among three isocaloric meal-replacement shakes. *Nutrition*, 21:874, 2005.

Semih, S.Y., Feluni, T.: A comparison of the endurance training responses to road and sand running in high school and college students. *J. Strength Cond. Res.*, 12:79, 1998.

Slawinski, J.S., Billat, V.L.: Difference in mechanical and energy cost between highly, well, and nontrained runners. *Med. Sci. Sports Exerc.*, 36:1440, 2004.

Spadano, J.L., et al.: Energy cost of physical activities in 12-y-old girls: MET values and the influence of body weight. *Int. J. Obes. Relat. Metab. Disord.*, 27:1528, 2003.

Speakman, J.R.: Body size, energy metabolism and lifespan. *J. Exp. Biol.*, 208:1717, 2005.

Tharion, W.J., et al.: Energy requirements of military personnel. *Appetite*, 44:47, 2005.

Vasconcellos, M.T., Anjos, L.A.: A simplified method for assessing physical activity level values for a country or study population. *Eur. J. Clin. Nutr.*, 57:1025, 2003.

Vercruyssen, F., et al.: Cadence selection affects metabolic responses during cycling and subsequent running time to fatigue. *Br. J. Sports Med.*, 39:267, 2005.

Weissgerber, T.L., et al.: The role of regular physical activity in preeclampsia prevention. *Med. Sci. Sports Exerc.*, 36:2024, 2004.

Westerterp-Plantenga, M.S.: Fat intake and energy-balance effects. *Physiol. Behav.*, 83:579, 2004.

Westerterp-Plantenga, M.S.: The significance of protein in food intake and body weight regulation. *Curr. Opin. Clin. Nutr. Metab. Care*, 6:635, 2003.

Weyand, P.G., Bundle, M.W.: Energetics of high-speed running: integrating classical theory and contemporary observations. *Am. J. Physiol. Regul. Integr. Comp. Physiol.*, 288:R956, 2005.

Zamparo, P., et al.: An energy balance of front crawl. *Eur. J. Appl. Physiol.*, 94:134, 2005.

Section IV

The Physiologic Support Systems

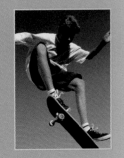

Most sport, recreational, and occupational activities require a moderately intense yet sustained energy release. The aerobic breakdown of carbohydrates, fats, and proteins generates this energy from ADP phosphorylation to ATP. Without a steady rate between oxidative phosphorylation and the energy requirements of physical activity, an anaerobic-aerobic energy imbalance develops, lactate accumulates, tissue acidity increases, and fatigue quickly ensues. Two factors limit an individual's ability to sustain a high level of exercise intensity without undue fatigue:

1. Capacity for oxygen delivery to active muscle cells
2. Capacity of active muscle cells to generate ATP aerobically

Understanding the role of the ventilatory, circulatory, muscular, and endocrine systems during exercise explains the broad range of individual differences in exercise capacity. Knowing the energy requirements of exercise and the corresponding physiologic adjustments necessary to meet these requirements helps formulate an effective physical fitness program and properly evaluate physiologic and fitness status before and during such a program.

All the problems of the world could be settled easily if men were only willing to think. The trouble is that men very often resort to all sorts of devices in order not to think, because thinking is such hard work.

—THOMAS J. WATSON
(IBM HEAD)

CHAPTER OBJECTIVES

- Diagram the ventilatory system, and show the glottis, larynx, trachea, bronchi, bronchioles, and alveoli.

- Describe the dynamics of inspiration and expiration during rest and exercise.

- Describe the "Valsalva maneuver" and its physiologic consequences.

- Define minute ventilation, alveolar minute ventilation, ventilation-perfusion ratio, and anatomic and physiologic dead spaces.

- Explain the "Bohr effect" and its benefit during physical activity.

- List and quantify three means for carbon dioxide transport in blood.

- Identify major factors that regulate pulmonary ventilation during rest and exercise.

- Describe how hyperventilation extends breath-holding time but can have dangerous consequences in sport diving.

- Graph relationships among pulmonary ventilation, blood lactate concentrations, and oxygen uptake during incremental exercise. Indicate the demarcation points for the lactate threshold and onset of blood lactate accumulation.

- Explain what triggers exercise-induced asthma, and identify factors that affect its severity.

CHAPTER OUTLINE

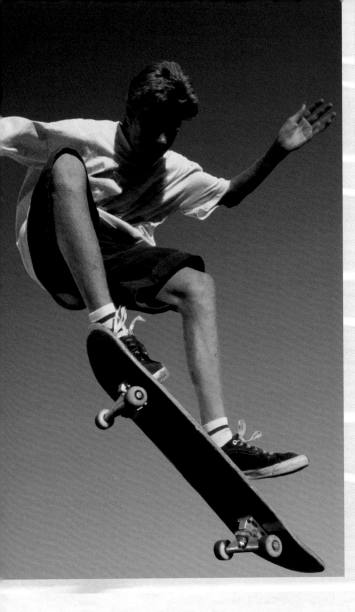

The Pulmonary System and Exercise

PART 1 •
Pulmonary Structure and Function

If oxygen supply depended only on diffusion through the skin, it would be impossible to support the basal energy requirement, let alone the 4- to 6-liter oxygen uptake each minute to sustain a world-class 5-minute per mile marathon pace. The remarkably effective **ventilatory system** meets the body's needs for gas exchange. This system, depicted in **Figure 9.1**, regulates the gaseous state of our "external" environment for aerating fluids of the "internal" environment during rest and exercise. The major functions of the ventilatory system include:

1. Supply oxygen required in metabolism
2. Eliminate carbon dioxide produced in metabolism
3. Regulate hydrogen ion concentration [H$^+$] to maintain acid-base balance

ANATOMY OF VENTILATION

The term **pulmonary ventilation** describes how ambient atmospheric air moves into and exchanges with air in the lungs. A distance of about 0.3 m (1 ft) separates ambient air just outside the nose and mouth from the blood flowing through the lungs. Air entering the nose and mouth flows into the conductive portion of the ventilatory system. Here, it adjusts to body temperature and is filtered and almost completely humidified as it passes through the trachea. The trachea, a short 1-inch diameter tube that extends from the larynx, divides into two tubes of smaller diameter called bronchi. The bronchi serve as primary conduits within the right and left lungs. They further subdivide into numerous bronchioles that conduct inspired air through a narrow route until eventually mixing with the air in the **alveoli**, the terminal branches of the respiratory tract.

Lungs

The lungs provide the surface between blood and the external environment. Lung volume varies between 4 and 6 liters (amount of air in a basketball) and provides an exceptionally large moist surface. The lungs of an average-sized person weigh about 1 kg, yet if spread out, they would cover a surface of 60 to 80 m^2, about 35 times the external surface of the person, and almost one-half the size of a tennis court or an entire badminton court. This represents a considerable interface for aeration of blood because, during any 1 second of maximal exercise, no more than 1 pint of blood flows in the lung tissue's web-like, intricate, and interlaced network of blood vessels.

Alveoli

Lung tissue contains more than 600 million alveoli. These elastic, thin-walled, membranous sacs provide the vital surface for gas exchange between the lungs and blood. Alveolar tissue has the largest blood supply of any organ in the body. Millions of thin-walled capillaries and alveoli

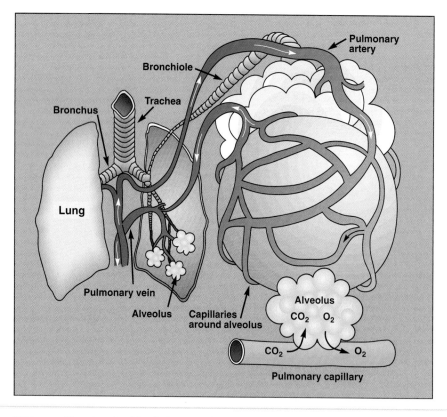

Figure 9.1. Overview of the ventilatory system showing the respiratory passages, alveoli, and gas exchange function in an alveolus.

Box 9–1 · CLOSE UP

COMMON SYMBOLS USED BY PULMONARY PHYSIOLOGISTS

PULMONARY VENTILATION		EXTERNAL RESPIRATION		INTERNAL RESPIRATION	
$\dot{V}_E =$	Minute ventilation	$\dot{V}_A =$	Alveolar ventilation	a-v$O_{2diff} =$	Quantity of oxygen carried in the arteries minus the amount carried in the veins
$V_d =$	Dead space	$P_{A}O_2 =$	Partial pressure of oxygen in the alveoli		
$V_T =$	Tidal volume				
$F =$	Breathing frequency	$PaO_2 =$	Partial pressure of oxygen in arterial blood	$PaO_2 =$	Partial pressure of oxygen in arterial blood
$V_d/V_T =$	Ratio of dead space to tidal volume	(A-a)$PO_{2diff} =$	Oxygen or PO_2 pressure gradient between the alveoli and arteries	$PaCO_2 =$	Partial pressure of carbon dioxide in arterial blood
				$PvCO_2 =$	Partial pressure of carbon dioxide in venous blood
		$SaO_{2\%} =$	Percent saturation of arterial blood with oxygen	$SvO_{2\%} =$	Percent saturation of venous blood with oxygen
		$P_{A}CO_2 =$	Partial pressure of carbon dioxide in the alveoli	$PvO_2 =$	Partial pressure of oxygen in venous blood

lie side by side, with air moving on one side and blood on the other. The capillaries form a dense, mesh-like cover that almost encircles the entire outside of each alveolus (**Fig. 9.2A**). This web becomes so dense that blood flows as a sheet over each alveolus. Once blood reaches the pulmonary capillaries, only a single cell barrier, the **respiratory membrane**, separates blood from air in the alveolus (Fig. 9.2B). This thin tissue-blood barrier permits rapid diffusion between alveolar and blood gases.

During rest, approximately 250 mL of oxygen *leave* the alveoli each minute and enter the blood, and about 200 mL of carbon dioxide diffuse *into* the alveoli. When trained endurance athletes perform intense exercise, about 20 times the resting oxygen uptake transfers across the respiratory membrane into the blood each minute. The primary function of pulmonary ventilation during rest and exercise attempts to maintain relatively constant and favorable concentrations of oxygen and carbon dioxide in the alveolar chambers. This ensures effective alveolar gaseous exchange before the blood exits the lungs for transit throughout the body.

Mechanics of Ventilation

Figure 9.3 illustrates the physical principle underlying breathing dynamics. The example shows two balloons connected to a jar whose glass bottom has been replaced by a thin rubber membrane. When the membrane lowers, the jar's volume increases, and air pressure within the jar becomes less than air pressure outside the jar. Consequently, air rushes into the balloons, and they inflate. Conversely, if the elastic membrane recoils, the pressure within the jar temporarily increases, and air rushes out. Considerable air exchange occurs within the balloons as the distance and rate of descent and ascent of the rubber membrane increases.

The lungs are not merely suspended in the chest cavity as depicted with the balloons and jar. Rather, the difference in pressure within the lungs and the lung-chest wall interface causes the lungs to adhere to the chest wall interior and literally follow its every movement. Any change in thoracic cavity volume thus produces a corresponding change in lung volume. Skeletal muscle action during inspiration and expiration alters thoracic dimensions to change lung volume.

Questions & Notes

Define pulmonary ventilation.

List 2 functions of the ventilatory system.

1.

2.

This amount of oxygen leaves the alveoli and enters the blood each minute during rest.

This amount of carbon dioxide leaves the alveoli and enters the blood each minute at rest.

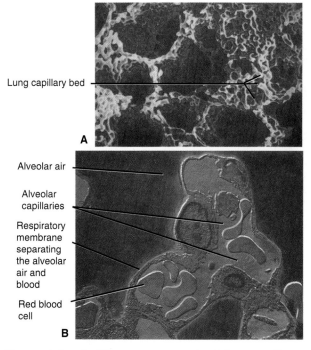

Figure 9.2. **A.** Electron micrograph of lung capillaries (×1300). Note the extremely dense capillary bed; the dark areas represent the alveolar chambers. **B.** Electron micrograph of a pulmonary capillary (×6000). Note the extremely thin respiratory membrane layer separating alveolar air from red blood cells. (Courtesy of Dr. R.L. Malvin, University of Michigan.)

Inspiration

The **diaphragm**, a large, dome-shaped sheet of muscle, serves the same purpose as the jar's rubber membrane in Figure 9.3. The diaphragm muscle makes an airtight separation between the abdominal and thoracic cavities. During inspiration, the diaphragm contracts, flattens out, and moves downward up to 10 cm toward the abdominal cavity. This enlarges and elongates the chest cavity. The air in the lungs then expands, reducing its pressure (referred to as **intrapulmonic pressure**) to about 5 mm Hg below atmospheric pressure. *The pressure differential between the lungs and ambient air literally sucks air in through the nose and mouth and inflates the lungs.* The degree of lung filling depends on two factors:

1. Magnitude of inspiratory movements
2. Pressure gradient between air inside and air outside the lung

Inspiration concludes when thoracic cavity expansion ceases and intrapulmonic pressure increases to equal atmospheric pressure.

During exercise, the scaleni and external intercostal muscles between the ribs contract. This causes the ribs to rotate and lift up and away from the body—an action similar to the movement of the handle lifted up and away from the side of the bucket at the right in Figure 9.3. Air moves into the lungs when chest cavity volume increases from three factors: (1) descent of the diaphragm, (2) upward lift of the ribs, and (3) outward thrust of the sternum.

Expiration

Expiration, a predominantly passive process, occurs as air moves out of the lungs from the recoil of stretched lung tissue and relaxation of the inspiratory muscles. This causes the sternum and ribs to swing down, while the diaphragm moves toward the thoracic cavity. These movements decrease chest cavity volume and compress alveolar gas; this forces it out through the respiratory tract to the atmosphere. During ventilation in moderate to intense exercise, the internal intercostal muscles and abdominal muscles act powerfully on the ribs and abdominal cavity to produce a rapid and greater depth of exhalation. Greater involvement of the pulmonary musculature during progressively intense exercise causes larger pressure differentials and concomitant increases in air movement.

LUNG VOLUMES AND CAPACITIES

Figure 9.4 presents a typical lung volume tracing with average values for men and women while they breathe from a calibrated recording spirometer, shown in **Figure 9.5**. The spirometer is also used for closed circuit measurements of oxygen uptake (see Chapter 8).

Two types of measurements, static and dynamic, provide information about lung volume dimensions and capacities. **Static lung volume** tests evaluate the *dimensional component* for air movement within the pulmonary tract and impose no time limitation on the subject. In contrast, **dynamic lung volume** measures evaluate the *power component* of pulmonary performance during different phases of the ventilatory excursion.

Static Lung Volumes

During static lung function measurement, the spirometer bell falls and rises with each inhalation and exhalation to provide a record of the ventilatory volume and breathing rate. **Tidal volume (TV)** describes air moved during either the inspiratory or expiratory phase of each breathing cycle. For healthy men and women, TV under resting conditions ranges between 0.4 and 1.0 L of air per breath.

After recording several representative TVs, the subject breathes in normally and then inspires maximally. An additional volume of about 2.5 to 3.5 L above TV air represents the reserve for inhalation, termed the **inspiratory reserve volume (IRV)**. The normal breathing pattern begins once again following the IRV. After a normal exhalation, the subject continues to exhale and forces as much air as possible from the lungs. This additional volume, the **expiratory reserve volume (ERV)**, ranges between 1.0 and 1.5 L for an average-size man (10% to 20% lower for a woman). During exercise, TV increases considerably because of encroachment on IRV and ERV, but particularly IRV.

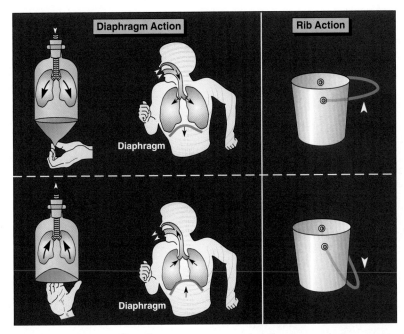

Diaphragm Action

Rib Action

Diaphragm

Diaphragm

Figure 9.3. Mechanics of breathing. During inspiration, the chest cavity increases in size because the ribs rise and the muscular diaphragm lowers. During exhalation, the ribs swing down and the diaphragm returns to a relaxed position. This reduces thoracic cavity volume, and air rushes out. The movement of the jar's rubber bottom causes air to enter and leave the two balloons, simulating the diaphragm's action. The movement of the bucket handle simulates rib action.

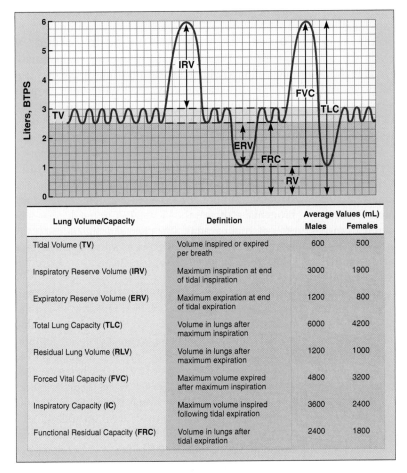

Lung Volume/Capacity	Definition	Average Values (mL)	
		Males	Females
Tidal Volume (**TV**)	Volume inspired or expired per breath	600	500
Inspiratory Reserve Volume (**IRV**)	Maximum inspiration at end of tidal inspiration	3000	1900
Expiratory Reserve Volume (**ERV**)	Maximum expiration at end of tidal expiration	1200	800
Total Lung Capacity (**TLC**)	Volume in lungs after maximum inspiration	6000	4200
Residual Lung Volume (**RLV**)	Volume in lungs after maximum expiration	1200	1000
Forced Vital Capacity (**FVC**)	Maximum volume expired after maximum inspiration	4800	3200
Inspiratory Capacity (**IC**)	Maximum volume inspired following tidal expiration	3600	2400
Functional Residual Capacity (**FRC**)	Volume in lungs after tidal expiration	2400	1800

Figure 9.4. Static measures of lung volume and capacity.

Questions & Notes

List 2 factors that determine lung filling.

1.

2.

Briefly explain the difference between static and dynamic lung volumes.

Give an average tidal volume for men and women.

Men:

Women:

Give an average vital capacity for men and women.

Men:

Women:

Give an average residual lung volume for men and women.

Men:

Women:

FOR YOUR INFORMATION

Body Position Facilitates Breathing
Athletes frequently bend forward from the waist to facilitate breathing after intense exercise. This body position serves two purposes:

1. Facilitates blood flow to the heart
2. Minimizes antagonistic effects of gravity on respiratory movements

---

Chapter 9   The Pulmonary System and Exercise   •   297

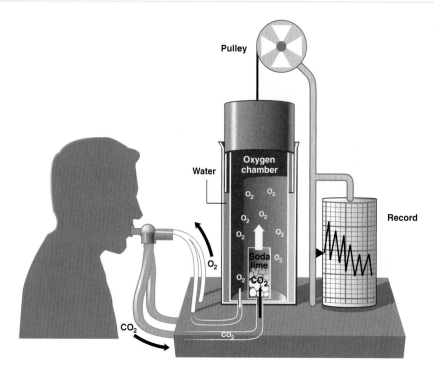

Figure 9.5. Closed-circuit spirometer.

Forced vital capacity (FVC) represents the total air volume moved in one breath from full inspiration to maximum expiration, or vice versa. FVC varies considerably with body size and body position during the measurement; values usually average 4 to 5 L in healthy young men and 3 to 4 L in healthy young women. FVCs of 6 to 7 L are not uncommon for tall individuals, and a value of 7.6 L has been reported for a professional football player and 8.1 L for an Olympic gold medalist in cross-country skiing. Some athletes' large lung volumes probably reflect genetic influences because exercise training does not change appreciably static lung volumes.

Residual Lung Volume
Following a maximal exhalation, a volume of air remains in the lungs that cannot be exhaled. This volume, the **residual lung volume (RLV)**, averages between 1.0 and 1.2 L for young adult women and 1.2 and 1.6 L for men.

Aging changes the various lung volumes due to decreases in lung tissue elasticity and a decline in pulmonary muscle power. These two factors probably do not entirely result from aging per se but result more from the effects of a sedentary lifestyle as one grows older. For example, endurance training in older athletes slows the normal decline in lung function (see Chapter 18). *Sedentary living, rather than true aging, most likely accounts for the largest changes in lung volumes and pulmonary function.*

Dynamic Lung Volumes

Dynamic measures of pulmonary ventilation depend on the *volume* of air moved and the *speed* of air movement.

Airflow speed depends on the pulmonary airways' resistance to the smooth flow of air and resistance offered by the chest and lung tissue to changes in shape during breathing.

Forced Expiratory Volume-to-Forced Vital Capacity Ratio
Normal values for vital capacity can occur in severe lung disease if no time limit exists to expel air. For this reason, a dynamic lung function measure, such as the **percentage of FVC expelled in 1 second ($FEV_{1.0}$)**, serves a more useful diagnostic purpose than static measures. *Forced expiratory volume-to-forced vital capacity ratio ($FEV_{1.0}/FVC$) reflects expiratory power and overall resistance to air movement in the lungs.* Normally, the $FEV_{1.0}/FVC$ averages about 85%. With severe obstructive pulmonary disease (e.g., emphysema and/or bronchial asthma), the $FEV_{1.0}/FVC$ often decreases below 40% of vital capacity. *The clinical demarcation for airway obstruction represents the point at which a person can expel less than 70% of the FVC in 1 second.*

Maximum Voluntary Ventilation
Another dynamic assessment of ventilatory capacity requires rapid, deep breathing for 15 seconds. Extrapolation of this 15-second volume to the volume breathed for 1 minute represents the **maximum voluntary ventilation (MVV)**. For healthy, young men, the MVV ranges between 140 and 180 $L \cdot min^{-1}$. The average for women equals 80 to 120 $L \cdot min^{-1}$. Male members of the United States Nordic Ski Team averaged 192 $L \cdot min^{-1}$, with an individual high MVV of 239 $L \cdot min^{-1}$. Patients with obstructive lung disease achieve only about 40% of the MVV predicted normal for their age and stature. Specific pulmonary therapy benefits these patients because training the muscles used in

Box 9–2 • CLOSE UP

PREDICTING PULMONARY FUNCTION VARIABLES FROM STATURE AND AGE

Pulmonary function variables do not directly relate to measures of physical fitness in healthy individuals, but their measurement often forms part of a standard medical/health/fitness exam, particularly for individuals at risk for limited pulmonary function (e.g., chronic cigarette smokers, asthmatics). Measurement of diverse components of pulmonary dimension and lung function with a water-filled spirometer or electronic spirometer (see Fig. 9.5) provide the framework to discuss pulmonary dynamics during rest and exercise. Proper evaluation of measured values for pulmonary function requires comparison to norms from the clinical literature. Pulmonary function variables associate closely with stature and age; these two variables predict the lung function value expected to be average (normal) for a particular individual.

EXAMPLES

Predictions use cm for stature (ST) and years for age (A).

Data

Man: Age, 22 y; Stature, 182.9 cm (72 in)
Woman: Age, 22 y; Stature, 165.1 cm (65 in)

Woman

1. Forced vital capacity (FVC)

$$FVC, L = (0.0414 \times ST) - (0.0232 \times A)$$
$$- 2.20$$
$$= 6.835 - 0.5104 - 2.20$$
$$= 4.12 \, L$$

2. Forced expiratory volume in 1 second ($FEV_{1.0}$)

$$FEV_{1.0}, L = (0.0268 \times ST) - (0.0251 \times A)$$
$$- 0.38$$
$$= 4.425 - 0.5522 - 0.38$$
$$= 3.49 \, L$$

3. Percentage forced vital capacity in 1 second ($FEV_{1.0}/FVC$)

$$FEV_{1.0}/FVC, \% = (-0.2145 \times ST)$$
$$- (0.1523 \times A) + 124.5$$
$$= -35.41 - 3.35 + 124.5$$
$$= 85.7\%$$

4. Maximum voluntary ventilation (MVV)

$$MMV, L \cdot min^{-1} = 40 \times FEV_{1.0}$$
$$= 40 \times 3.49 \, (from \, eq. \, 2)$$
$$= 139.6 \, L \cdot min^{-1}$$

Man

1. Forced vital capacity (FVC)

$$FVC, L = (0.0774 \times ST) - (0.0212 \times A)$$
$$- 7.75$$
$$= 14.156 - 0.4664 - 7.75$$
$$= 5.49 \, L$$

2. Forced expiratory volume in 1 second ($FEV_{1.0}$)

$$FEV_{1.0}, L = (0.0566 \times ST) - (0.0233 \times A)$$
$$- 0.491$$
$$= 10.35 - 0.5126 - 4.91$$
$$= 4.93 \, L$$

3. Percentage forced vital capacity in 1 second ($FEV_{1.0}/FVC$)

$$FEV_{1.0}/FVC, \% = (-0.1314 \times ST)$$
$$- (0.1490 \times A) + 110.2$$
$$= -24.03 - 3.35 + 110.2$$
$$= 82.8\%$$

4. Maximum voluntary ventilation (MVV)

$$MMV, L \cdot min^{-1} = 40 \times FEV_{1.0}$$
$$= 40 \times 4.93 \, (from \, eq. \, 2)$$
$$= 197.2 \, L \cdot min^{-1}$$

REFERENCES

1. Miller, A.: *Pulmonary Function Tests in Clinical and Occupational Disease.* Philadelphia: Grune & Stratton, 1986.

2. Wasserman, K., et al.: *Principles of Exercise Testing.* Baltimore: Lippincott Williams & Wilkins, 1999.

breathing increases the strength and endurance of the respiratory muscles and enhances MVV.

PULMONARY VENTILATION

Minute Ventilation

During quiet breathing at rest, an adult's breathing rate averages 12 breaths per minute, and tidal volume averages about 0.5 L of air per breath. Under these conditions, the volume of air breathed each minute, termed **minute ventilation**, equals 6 L.

$$\text{Minute ventilation } (\dot{V}_E) = \text{Breathing rate}$$
$$\times \text{ Tidal volume}$$
$$6.0 \text{ L·min}^{-1} = 12 \times 0.5 \text{ L}$$

An increase in depth or rate of breathing or both increases minute ventilation. During maximal exercise, the breathing rate of healthy young adults increases to 35 to 45 breaths per minute, while elite athletes often achieve 60 to 70 breaths per minute. In addition, tidal volume commonly increases to 2.0 L and greater during intense exercise. This causes exercise minute ventilation in adults to readily reach 100 L or about 17 times the resting value. In well-trained male endurance athletes, ventilation can increase to 160 L·min^{-1} during maximal exercise, with several studies of elite endurance athletes reporting ventilation volumes exceeding 200 L·min^{-1}. *Even with these large minute ventilations, tidal volume rarely exceeds 55% to 65% of vital capacity.*

Alveolar Ventilation

Alveolar ventilation refers to the portion of minute ventilation that mixes with the air in the alveolar chambers. A portion of each breath inspired does not enter the alveoli and does not engage in gaseous exchange with blood. The air that fills the nose, mouth, trachea, and other nondiffusible conducting portions of the respiratory tract constitutes the **anatomic dead space**. In healthy people, this volume equals 150 to 200 mL, or about 30% of the resting tidal volume. Almost equivalent composition exists between dead-space air and ambient air, except for dead-space air's full saturation with water vapor.

Because of dead-space volume, approximately 350 mL of the 500 mL of ambient air inspired in each tidal volume at rest mixes with existing alveolar air. This does not mean that only 350 mL of air enters and leaves the alveoli with each breath. To the contrary, if tidal volume equals 500 mL, then 500 mL of air enters the alveoli but only 350 mL represents fresh air (about one-seventh of the total air in the alveoli). This relatively small, seemingly inefficient alveolar ventilation prevents drastic changes in alveolar air composition. This ensures a consistency in arterial blood gases throughout the breathing cycle.

Table 9.1 shows that minute ventilation does not always reflect the actual alveolar ventilation. In the first example of shallow breathing, tidal volume decreases to 150 mL, yet a 6-L minute ventilation occurs when the breathing rate increases to 40 breaths per minute. The same 6-L minute volume can be achieved by decreasing the breathing rate to 12 breaths per minute and increasing tidal volume to 500 mL. Doubling tidal volume and reducing ventilatory rate by half, as in the example of deep breathing, again produces a 6-L minute ventilation. Each ventilatory adjustment drastically affects alveolar ventilation. In the example of shallow breathing, dead-space air represents the entire air volume moved (no alveolar ventilation has taken place). The other examples involve deeper breathing; thus, a larger portion of each breath mixes with existing alveolar air. *Alveolar ventilation, not dead-space ventilation, determines gaseous concentrations at the alveolar-capillary membrane.*

Physiologic Dead Space

Some alveoli may not function adequately in gas exchange due to underperfusion of blood or inadequate ventilation relative to alveolar surface area. The term **physiologic dead space** describes that portion of the alveolar volume with poor tissue regional perfusion (or inadequate ventilation). **Figure 9.6** illustrates that only a negligible physiologic dead space exists in the healthy lung.

Physiologic dead space can increase to 50% of resting tidal volume. This occurs because of two factors: (1) inadequate perfusion during hemorrhage or blockage of the pulmonary circulation from an embolism or blood clot, or (2) inadequate alveolar ventilation in chronic pulmonary

Table 9·1	Relationships Among Tidal Volume, Breathing Rate, and Minute and Alveolar Minute Ventilation						
CONDITION	TIDAL VOLUME (mL)	×	BREATHING RATE (breaths·min^{-1})	=	MINUTE VENTILATION (mL·min^{-1})	− DEAD SPACE VENTILATION (mL·min^{-1})	= ALVEOLAR VENTILATION (mL·min^{-1})
Shallow breathing	150		40		6000	(150 mL × 40)	0
Normal breathing	5000		12		6000	(150 mL × 12)	4200
Deep breathing	1000		6		6000	(150 mL × 6)	5100

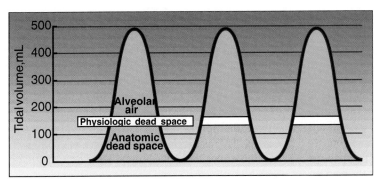

Figure 9.6. Distribution of tidal volume in the lungs of a healthy subject at rest. Tidal volume includes about 350 mL of ambient air that mixes with alveolar air, 150 mL of air in the larger air passages (anatomic dead space), and a small portion of air distributed to either poorly ventilated or poorly perfused alveoli (physiologic dead space).

disease. *Adequate gas exchange and aeration of blood are impossible when the lung's total dead space exceeds 60% of lung volume.*

Depth Versus Rate

Adjustments in breathing rate and depth maintain alveolar ventilation as exercise intensity increases. In moderate exercise, trained endurance athletes maintain adequate alveolar ventilation by increasing tidal volume and only minimally by increasing breathing rate. With deeper breathing, alveolar ventilation usually increases from 70% of minute ventilation at rest to over 85% of the total ventilation in exercise. *This increase occurs because deeper breathing causes a greater percentage of the incoming tidal volume to enter the alveoli.*

Figure 9.7 shows that increasing tidal volume in exercise results largely from encroachment on inspiratory reserve volume, with an accompanying but smaller decrease in end-expiratory level. As exercise intensity increases, tidal volume plateaus at about 60% of vital capacity; further increases in minute ventilation result from an increase in breathing rate. These ventilatory adjustments occur unconsciously; each individual develops a "style" of breathing by blending breathing rate and tidal vol-

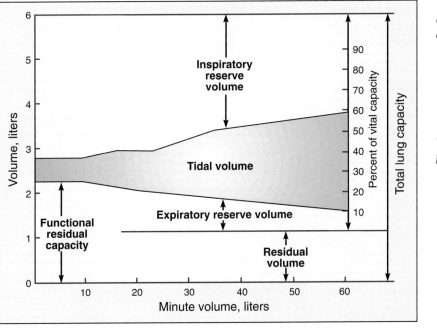

Figure 9.7. Tidal volume and subdivisions of pulmonary air during rest and exercise.

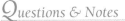

Questions & Notes

Give the average $FEV_{1.0}$/FVC for healthy adults.

Fill-in:

    TV rarely exceeds _____% to _____% of vital capacity.

Give the normal range for the anatomic dead space (volume) for healthy adults.

Compute $\dot{V}_E$ for an individual with a tidal volume of 0.6 L and a breathing rate of 15 breaths per minute.

Give an average value for physiologic dead space.

Why do novice exercisers sometimes experience dyspnea during exercise?

ume so alveolar ventilation matches alveolar perfusion. *Conscious attempts to modify breathing during running and other general physical activities do not benefit exercise performance. In most instances, conscious manipulation of breathing detracts from the exquisitely regulated ventilatory adjustments to exercise.* During rest and exercise, each individual should breathe in the manner that seems most natural. Most individuals performing rhythmical exercises, such as walking, running, cycling, and rowing, naturally synchronize breathing frequency with limb movements. This breathing pattern, termed **entrainment**, reduces the energy cost of the activity.

DISRUPTIONS IN NORMAL BREATHING PATTERNS

Breathing patterns during exercise generally progress in an effective and highly economical manner, yet some pulmonary responses negatively impact exercise performance.

Dyspnea

Dyspnea refers to shortness of breath or subjective distress in breathing. The sense of the inability to breathe during exercise, particularly in novice exercisers, usually accompanies elevated arterial carbon dioxide and [H$^+$]. Both chemicals excite the inspiratory center to increase breathing rate and depth. Failure to adequately regulate arterial carbon dioxide and [H$^+$] most likely relates to low aerobic fitness levels and a poorly conditioned ventilatory musculature. The strong neural drive to breathe during exercise causes poorly conditioned respiratory muscles to fatigue, disrupting normal plasma levels of carbon dioxide and [H$^+$]. This accelerates the pattern of shallow, ineffective breathing, and the individual senses an inability to breathe sufficient air.

Hyperventilation

Hyperventilation refers to an increase in pulmonary ventilation that exceeds the oxygen needs of metabolism. This "overbreathing" quickly lowers normal alveolar carbon dioxide concentration, which causes excess carbon dioxide to leave body fluids via the expired air. An accompanying decrease in [H$^+$] increases plasma pH. Several seconds of hyperventilation generally produces lightheadedness; prolonged hyperventilation can lead to unconsciousness from excessive carbon dioxide unloading from the blood (see page 314).

SUMMARY

1. The lungs provide a large interface between the body's internal fluid environment and the gaseous external environment. No more than 1 pint of blood flows in the pulmonary capillaries during any 1 second for most individuals.

2. Pulmonary ventilation adjustments maintain favorable concentrations of alveolar oxygen and carbon dioxide to ensure adequate aeration of lung blood flow.

3. Pulmonary airflow depends on small pressure differences between ambient air and air within the lungs. The action of muscles that alter the dimensions of the thoracic cavity produces these pressure differences.

4. Lung volumes vary with age, gender, and body size, and stature; they should be evaluated only in relation to norms based on these variables.

5. Tidal volume increases during exercise by encroachment on inspiratory and expiratory reserve volumes.

6. When a person breathes to vital capacity, air remains in the lungs at maximal exhalation. This residual lung volume allows for an uninterrupted exchange of gas during the breathing cycle.

7. Forced expiratory volume in 1 second and maximum voluntary ventilation provide a dynamic assessment of the ability to sustain high airflow levels and serve as excellent screening tests to detect lung disease.

8. Minute ventilation equals breathing rate times tidal volume. It averages about 6 L at rest. In maximum exercise, increases in breathing rate and tidal volume produce minute ventilations as high as 200 L in large, endurance-trained individuals.

9. Alveolar ventilation represents the portion of minute ventilation entering the alveoli for gaseous exchange with the blood.

10. Healthy people exhibit their own unique breathing styles during rest and exercise. Conscious attempts to modify breathing pattern during aerobic exercise confer no physiologic or performance benefits.

11. Disruptions in normal breathing patterns during exercise include dyspnea (shortness of breath), hyperventilation (overbreathing), and a Valsalva maneuver (forcefully trying to exhale against a closed glottis).

Box 9–3 •   CLOSE UP

THE VALSALVA MANEUVER CAN IMPEDE BLOOD FLOW RETURN TO THE HEART

With quiet breathing, pressure within the airways and alveoli (**intrapulmonic pressure**) decreases by only about 3 to 5 mm Hg below atmospheric pressure during the inspiratory cycle, while exhalation produces a similar pressure increase (**A**). Closing the glottis following a full inspiration and then activating the expiratory muscles causes the compressive forces of exhalation to increase considerably (**B**). Maximal exhalation force against a closed glottis can increase pressure within the thoracic cavity (**intrathoracic pressure**) by more than 150 mm Hg above atmospheric pressure, with somewhat higher pressures within the abdominal cavity. A **Valsalva maneuver** describes this forced exhalation against a closed glottis. This ventilatory maneuver occurs commonly in weightlifting and other activities requiring a rapid, maximum application of force for short duration. The fixation of the abdominal and thoracic cavities with this Valsalva optimizes the force-generating capacity of the chest musculature.

Physiologic Consequences

With the onset of a Valsalva maneuver (in straining-type exercises; see figure), blood pressure briefly rises abruptly as elevated intrathoracic pressure forces blood from the heart into the arterial system (**C**). Simultaneously, the inferior vena cava compresses because pressure within the thoracic and abdominal cavities exceeds the relatively low pressures within the venous system. This significantly reduces blood flow into the heart (venous return). Reduced venous return and subsequent *fall* in arterial blood pressure diminishes the brain's blood supply, producing dizziness, "spots before the eyes," and even fainting. Normal blood flow re-establishes (with perhaps even an "overshoot") once the glottis opens and intrathoracic pressure decreases.

THOUGHT QUESTIONS

1. Advise a track athlete trying to change her breathing pattern in the hope of becoming a more economical runner.

2. How might regular resistance and aerobic exercise training blunt the typical decline in lung function with advancing age?

3. After straining to "squeeze out" a maximum lift in the standing press, the person states: "I feel slightly dizzy and see spots before my eyes." Provide a plausible physiologic explanation. What can be done to prevent this from happening?

PART 2 •
Gas Exchange

Oxygen supply depends on the oxygen concentration in ambient air and its pressure. Ambient air composition remains relatively constant: 20.93% oxygen, 79.04% nitrogen (including small quantities of inert gases that behave physiologically like nitrogen), 0.03% carbon dioxide, and usually small quantities of water vapor. The gas molecules move quickly and exert a pressure against any surface they contact. At sea level, the pressure of air's gas molecules raises a column of mercury to an average height of 760 mm (29.9 in). This barometric reading varies somewhat with changing weather conditions and decreases predictably at increased altitude.

RESPIRED GASES: CONCENTRATIONS AND PARTIAL PRESSURES

Gas concentration should not be confused with gas pressure:

- Gas concentration reflects the amount of gas in a given volume—determined by the product of the gas' partial pressure and solubility.
- Gas pressure represents the force exerted by the gas molecules against the surfaces they encounter.
- A mixture's total pressure equals the sum of the **partial pressures** of the individual gases.

Partial pressure computes as:

Partial Pressure = Percentage concentration

× Total pressure of gas mixture

Ambient Air

Table 9.2 presents the percentages, partial pressures, and volumes of the specific gases in 1 liter of dry, ambient air at sea level. The partial pressure (the letter P before the gas symbol denotes partial pressure) of oxygen equals 20.93% of the total 760 mm Hg pressure exerted by the air mixture, or 159 mm Hg (0.2093 × 760 mm Hg); the random movement of the minute quantity of

carbon dioxide exerts a pressure of only 0.2 mm Hg (0.0003 × 760 mm Hg), while nitrogen molecules exert a pressure that raises the mercury in a manometer about 600 mm Hg (0.7904 × 760 mm Hg). For sea level ambient air: P_{O_2} = 159 mm Hg; P_{CO_2} = 0.2 mm Hg; and P_{N_2} = 600 mm Hg.

Tracheal Air

Air entering the nose and mouth passes down the respiratory tract; it completely saturates with water vapor, which slightly dilutes the inspired air mixture. At body temperature, the pressure of water molecules in humidified air equals 47 mm Hg; this leaves 713 mm Hg (760 − 47) as the total pressure exerted by the inspired dry air molecules at sea level. This decreases the effective P_{O_2} in tracheal air by about 10 mm Hg from its dry ambient value of 159 mm Hg to 149 mm Hg (0.2093 × [760 − 47 mm Hg]). Humidification has little effect on inspired P_{CO_2} because of carbon dioxide's near negligible concentration in inspired air.

Alveolar Air

Alveolar air composition differs considerably from the incoming breath of ambient air because carbon dioxide continually enters the alveoli from the blood, whereas oxygen leaves the lungs for transport throughout the body. **Table 9.3** shows that moist alveolar air contains approximately 14.5% oxygen, 5.5% carbon dioxide, and 80.0% nitrogen.

After subtracting vapor pressure in moist alveolar gas, the average alveolar P_{O_2} equals 103 mm Hg (0.145 × [760 − 47 mm Hg]) and P_{CO_2} equals 39 mm Hg (0.055 × [760 − 47 mm Hg]). These values represent the average pressures exerted by oxygen and carbon dioxide molecules against the alveolar side of the respiratory membrane. They do not exist as physiologic constants but vary slightly with the phase of the ventilatory cycle and adequacy of ventilation in different lung segments.

MOVEMENT OF GAS IN AIR AND FLUIDS

Knowledge of how gases act in air and fluids allows us to understand the mechanism for gas movement between the

Table 9•2	Percentages, Partial Pressures, and Volumes of Gases in 1 Liter of Dry Ambient Air at Sea Level		
GAS	**PERCENTAGE**	**PARTIAL PRESSURE (at 760 mm Hg)**	**VOLUME OF GAS (mL·L^{-1})**
Oxygen	20.93	159 mm Hg	209.3
Carbon dioxide	0.03	0.2 mm Hg	0.4
Nitrogen	79.04[a]	600 mm Hg	790.3

[a] Includes 0.93% argon and other trace rare gases.

Table 9·3	Percentages, Partial Pressures, and Volumes of Gases in 1 Liter of Moist Alveolar Air at Sea Level (37°C)		
GAS	**PERCENTAGE**	**PARTIAL PRESSURE (at 760 − 47 mm Hg)**	**VOLUME OF GAS (mL·L⁻¹)**
Oxygen	14.5	103 mm Hg	145
Carbon dioxide	5.5	39 mm Hg	55
Nitrogen	80.0	571 mm Hg	800
Water vapor		47 mm Hg	

external environment and the body's tissues. In accord with **Henry's law**, the amount of a gas dissolved in a fluid depends on two factors:

1. Pressure differential between the gas above the fluid and dissolved in it
2. Solubility of the gas in the fluid

Pressure Differential

Figure 9.8 shows three examples of gas movement between air and fluid. Oxygen molecules continually strike the water surface in each of the three chambers. The pure water in container A contains no oxygen, so a large number of oxygen molecules dissolve in water. Some oxygen molecules also leave the water because the dissolved molecules move continuously in random motion. In chamber B, the pressure gradient between air and water still favors oxygen's net movement (diffusion) into the fluid from the gaseous state, but the quantity of additional oxygen dissolving in the fluid remains less than in chamber A. Eventually, the pressures for gas movement attain equilibrium, and the number of molecules entering and leaving the fluid equalize (chamber C). Conversely, if the pressure of dissolved oxygen molecules exceeds the air's oxygen pressure, oxygen leaves the fluid until it attains a new pressure equilibrium. These examples illustrate that the net diffusion of a gas occurs only when a *difference* exists in gas pressure. A specific gas' partial pressure gradient represents the driving force for its diffusion. Similarly, the concentration gradient provides the driving force for diffusion of nongaseous molecules (like glucose, sodium, and calcium).

Solubility

Gas solubility reflects the quantity of a gas dissolved in fluid at a particular pressure. A gas with greater solubility has a higher concentration at a specific pressure. For two different gases at identical pressure differentials, the solubility of each gas determines the number of molecules moving into or out of a fluid. *For*

Questions & Notes

The ambient air percentages for oxygen, carbon dioxide, and nitrogen are:

O_2 –

CO_2 –

N_2 –

Give the formula for computing partial pressure.

What determines gas concentration?

Alveolar's air concentration for oxygen and carbon dioxide at rest is:

O_2 –

CO_2 –

Give the PO_2 in ambient air at sea level.

FOR YOUR INFORMATION

The Gas Laws
The four laws governing gas behavior include:
1. **Boyle's Law:** If temperature remains constant, the pressure of a gas varies inversely with its volume.
2. **Gay–Lussac's Law:** If gas volume remains constant, its pressure increases in direct proportion to its absolute temperature.
3. **Law of Partial Pressures:** In a mixture of gases, each gas exerts a partial pressure, proportional to its concentration.
4. **Henry's Law:** If temperature remains constant, the quantity of a gas dissolved in a liquid varies in direct proportion to its partial pressure.

FOR YOUR INFORMATION

Gas Exchange Occurs Rapidly
Diffusion in a healthy lung occurs so rapidly that blood gas and alveolar gas equilibrate in less than 1 second, equal to the midpoint of the blood's transit through the pulmonary vasculature.

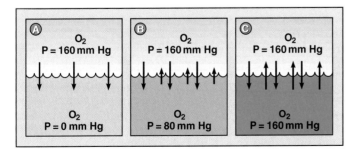

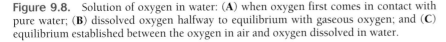

Figure 9.8. Solution of oxygen in water: (**A**) when oxygen first comes in contact with pure water; (**B**) dissolved oxygen halfway to equilibrium with gaseous oxygen; and (**C**) equilibrium established between the oxygen in air and oxygen dissolved in water.

Box 9–4 •   CLOSE UP

EXERCISE-INDUCED ASTHMA (EIA)

Asthma, a chronic obstructive pulmonary disease, affects 20.3 million Americans, with 6.3 million children under age 18 years report having asthma (see insert table for more statistics [*http://www.cdc.gov/nchs/fastats/asthma .htm*]). A high fitness level does not confer immunity from this ailment. Hyperirritability of the pulmonary airways, usually manifested by coughing, wheezing, and shortness of breath, characterizes an asthmatic condition.

Asthma Statistics

- 70% of people with asthma also suffer from allergies.
- More than 5,000 deaths from asthma annually.
- Direct health care costs for asthma in the United States total more than $8.1 billion annually; indirect costs (lost productivity) add another $4.6 billion, for a total of $12.7 billion.
- More than 14 million school days are missed annually due to asthma.
- Reduced productivity due to loss of school days represents the largest single indirect cost related to asthma in children, approaching $1.5 billion.
- Asthma accounts for approximately 14.5 million missed work days annually.
- Asthma is 26% more prevalent in African American children than in white children.
- 40% of children who have asthmatic parents will develop asthma.

With exercise, catecholamines released from the sympathetic nervous system produce a relaxation effect on smooth muscle that lines the pulmonary airways. Everyone experiences initial bronchodilation with exercise. For the asthmatic, however, bronchospasm and excessive mucus secretion follow normal bronchodilation. An acute episode of airway obstruction often appears 10 minutes after exercise; recovery usually occurs spontaneously within 30 to 90 minutes. One technique for diagnosing EIA uses progressive increments of exercise on a treadmill or bicycle ergometer. During a 10- to 20-minute recovery after each exercise bout, a spirometer evaluates $FEV_{1.0}$ / FVC. A 15% reduction in pre-exercise values confirms the diagnosis of EIA.

Sensitivity to Thermal Gradients

An attractive theory to explain EIA relates to the rate and magnitude of alterations in pulmonary heat exchange as ventilation increases in exercise. As the incoming breath of air moves down the pulmonary pathways, heat and water transfer from the respiratory tract as air warms and humidifies. This form of "air-conditioning" cools and dries the respiratory mucosa; an abrupt airway rewarming occurs during recovery. The thermal gradient from cooling and subsequent rewarming (and loss of water from mucosal tissue) stimulates the release of proinflammatory chemical mediators that cause bronchospasm.

Environment Makes a Difference

Exercising in a humid environment, regardless of ambient air temperature, diminishes the EIA response. This is perplexing because conventional belief maintains that a dry climate best suits the asthmatic. In fact, inhaling ambient air fully saturated with water vapor in exercising patients often abolishes the bronchospastic response. This also explains why asthmatics tolerate walking or jogging on a warm, humid day or swimming in an indoor pool, whereas outdoor winter sports usually trigger an asthmatic attack. An asthmatic should perform 15 to 30 minutes of continuous warm-up because it initiates a "refractory period" that minimizes the severity of a bronchoconstrictive response during subsequent, more intense exercise.

Hopefully, researchers will soon be able to better understand additional factors related to EIA. Physicians would then be able to "prescribe" an optimum environment and exercise intensity so asthmatics could benefit physically and psychologically from regular exercise. Currently, medications offer considerable relief from bronchoconstriction for individuals who want to exercise on a regular basis without affecting their performance. Exercise training cannot "cure" the asthmatic condition, but it can increase airway reserve and reduce the work of breathing during physical activity.

Minimize Exercise-Induced Asthma

- Choose appropriate type and duration of exercise
- Use adequate pre-exercise warm-up
- Reduce respiratory heat and water loss as much as possible
- Use medical therapy (if necessary)

---

each unit of pressure favoring diffusion, approximately 25 times more carbon dioxide than oxygen moves into (or from) a fluid.

GAS EXCHANGE IN THE BODY

The exchange of gases between the lungs and blood and their movement at the tissue level takes place passively by diffusion. **Figure 9.9** illustrates the pressure gradients favoring gas transfer in the body.

Gas Exchange in the Lungs

The first step in oxygen transport involves the transfer of oxygen from the alveoli into the blood. Three factors account for the dilution of oxygen in inspired air as it passes into the alveolar chambers:

1. Water vapor saturates relatively dry inspired air
2. Oxygen continually leaves alveolar air
3. Carbon dioxide continually enters alveolar air

Considering these three factors, alveolar P_{O_2} averages about 100 mm Hg, a value considerably below the 159 mm Hg in dry ambient air. Despite this reduced P_{O_2}, the pressure of oxygen molecules in alveolar air still averages about 60 mm Hg higher than the P_{O_2} in venous blood that enters pulmonary capillaries. This allows oxygen to diffuse through the alveolar membrane into the blood. Carbon dioxide exists under slightly greater pressure in returning venous blood than in the alveoli, causing carbon dioxide to diffuse from the blood to the lungs. Although only a small pressure gradient of 6 mm Hg exists for carbon dioxide diffusion compared with oxygen, adequate carbon dioxide transfer occurs rapidly because of carbon dioxide's high solubility. Nitrogen, an inert gas in metabolism, remains essentially unchanged in alveolar-capillary gas.

Questions & Notes

Give 2 ways oxygen transports in blood.

  1.

  2.

At an alveolar PO$_2$ of 100 mm Hg, the amount of oxygen dissolved in each 100 mL of blood plasma equals _____.

Complete the follow:

  O$_2$ carrying capacity =

  Percentage saturation =

Name the vertical and horizontal axes for the oxyhemoglobin dissociation curve.

  Vertical axis –

  Horizontal axis –

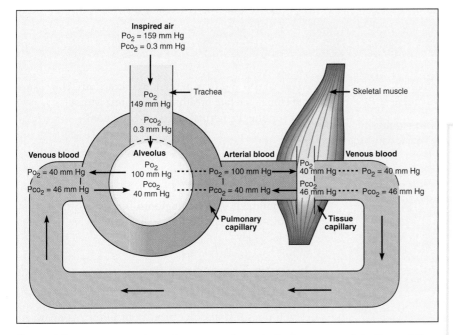

Figure 9.9.   Pressure gradients for gas transfer in the body at rest, and the P_{O_2} and P_{CO_2} of ambient, tracheal, and alveolar air and these gas pressures in venous and arterial blood and muscle. Gases always diffuse at the alveolar-capillary and tissue-capillary membranes from an area of higher partial pressure to lower partial pressure.

FOR YOUR INFORMATION

Stitch in the Side

During intense exercise, individuals frequently experience a severe, sharp pain in the lower, lateral aspects of the chest (thoracic) wall. This pain, called a "stitch in the side," has no universally accepted explanation nor has it been possible to duplicate its occurrence in the laboratory. Because it usually occurs during adjustment to new metabolic demands and occurs most frequently in the untrained, it seems reasonable to speculate insufficient blood flow (ischemia) to either the diaphragm or intercostals muscles as the cause.

Gas Exchange in Tissues

In the tissues, where energy metabolism consumes oxygen at a rate almost equal to carbon dioxide production, gas pressures differ considerably from arterial blood (see Fig. 9.9). At rest, the average P_{O_2} within the muscle rarely drops below 40 mm Hg, while intracellular P_{CO_2} averages about 46 mm Hg. In contrast, vigorous exercise reduces the pressure of oxygen molecules in active muscle tissue to 3 mm Hg, whereas carbon dioxide pressure approaches 90 mm Hg. The large pressure differential between gases in plasma and tissues establishes the gradient for diffusion—oxygen leaves capillary blood and diffuses toward metabolizing cells, while carbon dioxide flows from the cell into the blood. Blood then enters the veins and returns to the heart for delivery to the lungs. Diffusion rapidly begins when venous blood enters the lung's dense capillary network.

SUMMARY

1. The partial pressure of a specific gas in a gas mixture varies proportionally to its concentration in the mixture and the total pressure exerted by the mixture.

2. Pressure and solubility determine the quantity of gas that dissolves in a fluid. Because of carbon dioxide's 25 times greater solubility than oxygen in plasma, more carbon dioxide molecules move down relatively small pressure gradients in body fluids.

3. Gas molecules diffuse in the lungs and tissues down their concentration gradients from higher concentration (higher pressure) to lower concentration (lower pressure).

4. Alveolar ventilation adjusts during intense exercise so the composition of alveolar gas remains similar to resting conditions. Alveolar and arterial oxygen pressures equal about 100 mm Hg, while carbon dioxide pressure remains at 40 mm Hg.

5. Compared to alveolar gas, venous blood contains oxygen at lower pressure than carbon dioxide; this makes oxygen diffuse into the blood and carbon dioxide diffuse into the lungs.

6. Diffusion gradients in the tissues favor oxygen movement from the capillaries to the tissues and carbon dioxide movement from the cells to the blood. Exercise expands these gradients, making oxygen and carbon dioxide diffuse rapidly.

7. Exercise-induced asthma (EIA) represents a relatively common obstructive lung disorder associated with the rate and magnitude of airway cooling (and drying) and subsequent rewarming. Breathing humidified air during exercise often eliminates EIA.

THOUGHT QUESTIONS

1. Discuss the driving forces for the exchange of respiratory gases in the lungs and active muscles.

2. One technique during "natural" childbirth requires the woman to breathe rapidly to effectively "work with" the normal ebb and flow of uterine contractions. How can a person accelerate breathing rate at rest without disrupting the normal alveolar ventilation?

PART 3 •
Oxygen and Carbon Dioxide Transport

OXYGEN TRANSPORT IN THE BLOOD

The blood transports oxygen in two ways:

1. **In physical solution**—dissolved in the fluid portion of the blood

2. **Combined with hemoglobin**—in loose combination with the iron-protein hemoglobin molecule in the red blood cell

Oxygen Transport in Physical Solution

Oxygen does not dissolve readily in fluids. At an alveolar P_{O_2} of 100 mm Hg, only about 0.3 mL of gaseous oxygen dissolves in the plasma of each 100 mL of blood (3 mL·L^{-1}). Because the average adult's total blood volume equals about 5 liters, 15 mL of oxygen dissolves for transport in the fluid portion of the blood ($3 \text{ mL} \cdot \text{L}^{-1} \times 5 = 15 \text{ mL}$). This amount of oxygen would sustain life for only about 4 seconds. Viewed from a different perspective, the body would need to circulate 80 liters of blood each minute just to supply the resting oxygen requirements if oxygen were transported only in physical solution.

Despite its limited quantity, oxygen transported in physical solution serves a vital physiologic function. Dissolved oxygen establishes the P_{O_2} of the blood and tissue fluids to help regulate breathing and determines the magnitude that hemoglobin loads with oxygen in the lungs and unloads it in the tissues.

Oxygen Combined With Hemoglobin

The blood of many animal species contains a metallic compound to augment its oxygen-carrying capacity. In humans, the iron-containing protein pigment hemoglobin constitutes the main component of the body's 25 trillion red blood cells. *Hemoglobin increases the blood's oxygen-carrying capacity 65 to 70 times above that normally dissolved in plasma.* For each liter of blood, hemoglobin temporarily "captures" about 197 mL of oxygen. Each of the four iron atoms in a hemoglobin (Hb) molecule loosely binds one molecule of oxygen to form oxyhemoglobin in the reversible **oxygenation reaction**:

$$\text{Hb} + 4 \text{ O}_2 \rightarrow \text{Hb}_4\text{O}_8$$

This reaction requires no enzymes; it progresses without a change in the valance of Fe^{++}, as occurs in the more permanent process of oxidation. *The partial pressure of oxygen in solution solely determines the oxygenation of hemoglobin to oxyhemoglobin.*

Oxygen-Carrying Capacity of Hemoglobin
In men, each 100 mL of blood contains approximately 15 to 16 g of Hb. The value averages 5% to 10% less for women, or about 14 g per 100 mL of blood. The gender difference in Hb concentration contributes to the lower aerobic capacity of women, even after adjusting statistically for gender-related differences in body mass and body fat.

Each gram of Hb can combine loosely with 1.34 mL of oxygen. Thus, the oxygen-carrying capacity of the blood from its Hb concentration computes as follows:

$$\text{Oxygen-carrying capacity} = \text{Hb (g} \cdot 100 \text{ mL blood}^{-1})$$
$$\times \text{ Oxygen capacity of Hb}$$

If the blood's Hb concentration equals 15 g, then approximately 20 mL of oxygen (15 g per 100 mL $\times$ 1.34 mL = 20.1) combine with the Hb in each 100 mL of blood if Hb achieved full oxygen saturation (i.e., if all Hb existed as Hb_4O_8).

P_{O_2} and Hemoglobin Saturation
The discussion of the blood's oxygen-carrying capacity assumes that Hb achieves full saturation with oxygen when exposed to alveolar gas. **Figure 9.10A** shows the relationship between percentage saturation of Hb (left vertical axis) at various P_{O_2}s under normal resting physiologic conditions (arterial pH 7.4, 37°C) and the effects of changes in pH and temperature (insert figures) on Hb's affinity for oxygen. Percentage saturation of Hb computes as follows:

$$\text{Percentage saturation} = (\text{Total O}_2 \text{ combined with Hb} \div$$
$$\text{Oxygen carrying capacity of Hb}) \times 100$$

This curve, termed the **oxyhemoglobin dissociation curve**, also quantifies the amount of oxygen carried in each 100 mL of blood in relation to plasma P_{O_2} (right vertical axis, Fig. 9.10A). For example, at a P_{O_2} of 90 mm Hg (95% Hb saturation), the normal complement of Hb in 100 mL of blood carries about 19 mL of oxygen; at a P_{O_2} of 40 mm Hg (75% Hb saturation), the oxygen quantity decreases to about

Questions & Notes

The alveolar-capillary oxygen partial pressure equals _____ mm Hg.

Give the amount of hemoglobin in each 100 mL of blood for normal men and women.

Men –

Women –

Briefly describe the oxygen transport cascade.

At what P_{O_2} does percentage saturation of hemoglobin begin to dramatically decrease?

Give the average P_{O_2} in most cell fluids under resting conditions.

Complete the equation:

$HbO_2 \rightarrow$

Briefly describe the Bohr effect.

FOR YOUR INFORMATION

Second Wind
Second wind, experienced as a changeover from dyspnea (labored breathing, shortness of breath) to eupnea (normal breathing) as exercise progresses, probably reflects a change in skeletal muscular efficiency brought about by respiratory adjustments to a new workload. Second wind may also relate to the adjustments brought about by increasing muscle temperature and adjustments in sweat output associated with a new level of energy expenditure.

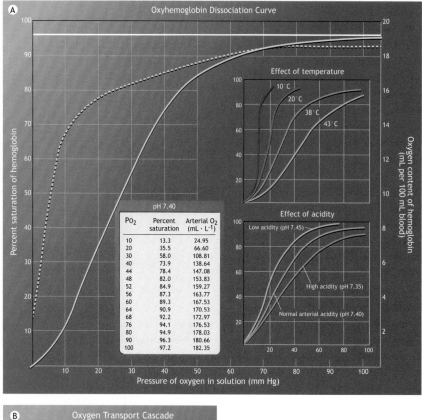

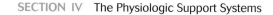

Figure 9.10. **A.** The oxyhemoglobin dissociation curve. The lines indicate the percent saturation of hemoglobin (*solid yellow line*) and myoglobin (*dashed yellow line*) in relation to oxygen pressure. The *right ordinate* shows the quantity of oxygen carried in each 100 mL of blood under normal conditions. The *inset curves within the figure* illustrate the effects of temperature and acidity in altering hemoglobin's affinity for oxygen (Bohr effect). *Inset box* presents oxyhemoglobin percentage saturation and arterial blood's oxygen-carrying capacity for different P_{O_2} values with hemoglobin concentration of 14 g·100 mL blood^{-1}. The *white horizontal line at the top of the graph* indicates percentage saturation of hemoglobin at the average sea-level alveolar P_{O_2} of 100 mm Hg. **B.** Partial pressures as oxygen moves from ambient air at sea level to the mitochondria of maximally active muscle tissue (oxygen transport cascade).

15 mL, and the oxygen quantity is only slightly more than 2 mL at a P_{O_2} of 10 mm Hg. These values indicate that, at relatively low oxygen partial pressures at the capillary-tissue membrane, oxygen readily dissociates (unloads) from Hb for use by the cell. Figure 9.10B also shows the partial pressure gradients as oxygen moves from ambient air at sea level into the mitochondria. The "**oxygen transport cascade**" describes the downward steps in oxygen partial pressures from ambient air at sea level to the mitochondria of maximally active muscle, with the progressively lowering of P_{O_2} facilitating the unloading of oxygen.

P_{O_2} in the Lungs

At the alveolar-capillary P_{O_2} of 100 mm Hg, Hb remains 98% saturated with oxygen; under these conditions, the Hb in each 100 mL of blood contains about 19.7 mL of oxygen. Any addi-

tional increase in alveolar P_{O_2} contributes little to how much oxygen combines with Hb. Each 100 mL of plasma in arterial blood contains about 0.3 mL of oxygen in physical solution. For healthy individuals who breathe ambient air at sea level, 100 mL of arterial blood carries 20.0 mL of oxygen (19.7 mL bound to Hb and 0.3 mL dissolved in plasma).

Careful examination of Figure 9.10A shows that Hb saturation changes little until oxygen pressure decreases to about 60 mm Hg. This relatively flat upper portion of the oxyhemoglobin dissociation curve provides a margin of safety to ensure near full loading of Hb despite relatively large decreases in alveolar P_{O_2}. Alveolar P_{O_2} reduction to 75 mm Hg (as occurs in certain lung diseases or when one travels to moderate altitude) only decreases arterial Hb saturation by about 6%. In contrast, when P_{O_2} drops below 60 mm Hg, a sharp decrease occurs in how much oxygen combines with Hb.

Tissue PO_2

The PO_2 in the cell fluids at rest averages 40 mm Hg. Thus, dissolved oxygen in arterial plasma (PO_2 = 100 mm Hg) readily diffuses across the capillary membrane through tissue fluids into cells. This reduces plasma PO_2 below that in the red blood cells, causing Hb to release its oxygen (HbO_2 → Hb + O_2). The oxygen then moves from the blood cells through the capillary membrane into the tissues.

At the tissue-capillary PO_2 of 40 mm Hg at rest, Hb holds about 75% of its total capacity for oxygen (see solid line, Fig. 9.10A). Therefore, each 100 mL of blood leaving the resting tissues carries only 15 mL of oxygen; nearly 5 mL has been released to the cells for energy metabolism. The **arteriovenous-oxygen difference (a-v O$_2$ difference)** describes this difference in oxygen content between arterial and venous blood (expressed in mL per 100 mL blood).

The a-v O_2 difference in most tissues at rest averages 5 mL. The large quantity of oxygen still remaining with Hb provides an "automatic" reserve for cells to immediately obtain oxygen should oxygen demands suddenly increase. As the cell's need for oxygen increases with any exercise above rest, tissue PO_2 rapidly decreases. This forces Hb to release greater quantities of oxygen to meet the metabolic requirements. In vigorous exercise, tissue PO_2 decreases to about 15 mm Hg, and Hb retains only about 5 mL of oxygen. This expands the tissue a-v O_2 difference to 15 mL of oxygen per 100 mL of blood. When active muscles' PO_2 decreases to about 3 mm Hg during exhaustive exercise, Hb releases virtually all of its remaining oxygen to the active tissues. Even without any increase in local blood flow, the amount of oxygen released to active muscle increases almost three times above that supplied at rest, simply by a more complete unloading of Hb.

Bohr Effect

The insert figures in Figure 9.10 show that increases in acidity ([H$^+$] and CO$_2$) and temperature cause the oxyhemoglobin dissociation curve to shift downward and to the right (enhanced unloading), particularly in the PO_2 range of 20 to 50 mm Hg. This phenomenon, known as the **Bohr effect** (named after its discoverer Danish physiologist Christian Bohr, 1855–1911), results from alterations in hemoglobin's molecular structure.

The existence of the Bohr effect becomes particularly important in vigorous exercise because increased metabolic heat and acidity in active tissues augments oxygen release. For example, at a PO_2 of 20 mm Hg and normal body temperature (37°C), percentage saturation of Hb with oxygen equals 35%. At the same PO_2, but with body temperature increased to 43°C (a temperature often recorded at the end of a marathon run), Hb's percentage saturation decreases to about 23%. This means that more oxygen unloads from Hb for use in cellular metabolism. Similar effects take place with increased acidity during intense exercise. The lack of a negligible Bohr effect in pulmonary capillary blood at normal alveolar PO_2 means that Hb becomes fully loaded with oxygen as blood passes through the lungs, even during maximal exercise.

The compound **2,3-diphosphoglycerate (2,3-DPG)**, the anaerobic metabolite produced in red blood cells during glycolysis, also affects Hb's affinity for oxygen. 2,3-DPG facilitates oxygen dissociation by combining with subunits of Hb to reduce its affinity for oxygen. Individuals with cardiopulmonary disease and high-altitude inhabitants have increased levels of this metabolic intermediate. Elevated 2,3-DPG for these individuals represents a compensatory adjustment that facilitates oxygen release to the cell. In general, adaptations in 2,3-DPG occur relatively slowly compared with the immediate Bohr effect from increased tissue temperature, acidity, and carbon dioxide.

Myoglobin and Muscle Oxygen Storage

Skeletal and cardiac muscle contain the iron-protein compound **myoglobin**. Myoglobin, like Hb, combines reversibly with oxygen; however, each myoglobin molecule contains only one iron atom in contrast to Hb, which contains

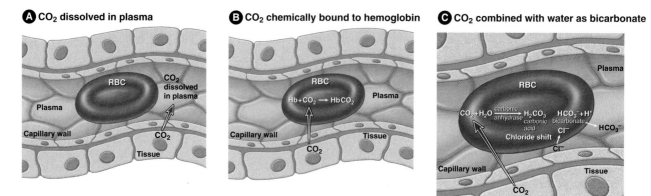

A CO_2 dissolved in plasma   **B** CO_2 chemically bound to hemoglobin   **C** CO_2 combined with water as bicarbonate

Figure 9.11.   Carbon dioxide transport in blood. **A.** Physically dissolved in blood plasma. **B.** Chemically bound to hemoglobin (Hb). **C.** Combined with water as bicarbonate.

four atoms. Myoglobin adds additional oxygen to the muscle in the following reaction:

$$MbO_2 \rightarrow MbO_2$$

Myoglobin facilitates oxygen transfer to the mitochondria, notably at the start of exercise and during intense exercise when cellular P_{O_2} decreases considerably. Figure 9.10A reveals that the dissociation curve for myoglobin (dashed yellow line) forms a rectangular hyperbola, not the s-shaped curve for Hb. This makes myoglobin bind and retain oxygen at low pressures much more readily than Hb. During rest and moderate exercise (when cellular P_{O_2} remains relatively high), myoglobin remains highly saturated with oxygen. At a P_{O_2} of 40 mm Hg, for example, myoglobin retains 85% of its oxygen. MbO_2 releases its greatest quantity of oxygen when tissue P_{O_2} decreases to less than 10 mm Hg. Unlike Hb, myoglobin does not exhibit a Bohr effect.

CARBON DIOXIDE TRANSPORT IN BLOOD

Once carbon dioxide forms in cells, diffusion and transport to the lungs in venous blood provides its only means for "escape." **Figure 9.11 (A, B, and C)** illustrates that blood transports carbon dioxide to the lungs in three ways:

1. In physical solution in plasma (7%–10%)
2. In loose combination with Hb (20%)
3. Combined with water as bicarbonate (70%)

Carbon Dioxide in Solution

Plasma transports 7% to 10% of carbon dioxide produced in energy metabolism as free carbon dioxide in physical solution (Fig. 9.11A). The random movement of this relatively small quantity of dissolved carbon dioxide molecules establishes the P_{CO_2} of the blood.

Carbon Dioxide as Carbamino Compounds

About 20% of carbon dioxide reacts directly with the amino acid molecules of blood proteins to form carbamino compounds (Fig. 9.11B). The globin portion of Hb carries a significant amount of carbon dioxide in the blood as follows:

$$\underset{\text{Hemoglobin}}{CO_2 + \quad HbNH} \rightarrow \underset{\text{Carbaminohemoglobin}}{HbNHCOOH}$$

Formation of carbamino compounds reverses in the lungs as plasma P_{CO_2} decreases. This moves carbon dioxide into solution for diffusion into the alveoli. Concurrently, Hb's oxygenation reduces its capacity to bind carbon dioxide. The interaction between oxygen loading and carbon dioxide release, termed the **Haldane effect**, facilitates carbon dioxide removal from the lungs.

Carbon Dioxide as Bicarbonate

The major portion (70%) of carbon dioxide in solution combines with water to form carbonic acid (Fig. 9.11C).

$$CO_2 + H_2O \leftrightarrow H_2CO_3{}^-$$

Because of the relatively slow rate of this reaction, relatively little carbon dioxide would transport in this form without **carbonic anhydrase**, a zinc-containing enzyme within red blood cells. This catalyst accelerates the interaction of carbon dioxide and water about 5000 times.

In the Tissues   Once carbonic acid forms in the tissues, most of it ionizes to hydrogen ions (H^+) and bicarbonate ions ($HCO_3{}^-$) as follows:

$$CO_2 + H_2O \xrightarrow{\text{Carbonic anhydrase}} H_2CO_3 \rightarrow H^+ + HCO_3{}^-$$

The protein portion of the Hb molecule then buffers the H^+ to maintain blood pH within narrow limits. Because of bicarbonate's high solubility, it diffuses from the red blood cell into the plasma in exchange for a chloride ion (Cl^-), which then moves into the blood cell to maintain ionic equilibrium. The term **"chloride shift"** describes this exchange of Cl^- for HCO^-; it accounts for the higher Cl^- content of the erythrocytes in venous blood compared with arterial blood.

In the Lungs   As tissue P_{CO_2} increases, carbonic acid forms rapidly. Conversely, in the lungs, carbon dioxide diffuses from the plasma into the alveoli; this lowers plasma P_{CO_2} and disturbs the equilibrium between carbonic acid and the formation of bicarbonate ions. The H^+ and HCO_3^- recombine to form carbonic acid. In turn, carbon dioxide and water reform, allowing carbon dioxide to exit through the lungs as follows:

$$H^+ + HCO_3^- \rightarrow H_2CO_3 \xrightarrow{\text{Carbonic anhydrase}} CO_2 + H_2O$$

Plasma bicarbonate concentration decreases in the pulmonary capillaries, permitting the Cl^- to move from the red blood cell back into plasma.

SUMMARY

1. Hemoglobin (Hb), the iron-protein pigment in red blood cells, increases oxygen-carrying capacity of whole blood about 65 times compared with the amount dissolved in physical solution in plasma.

2. The small quantity of oxygen dissolved in plasma exerts molecular movement and establishes the blood's P_{O_2}. Plasma P_{O_2} determines the loading of Hb at the lungs (oxygenation) and its unloading at the tissues (deoxygenation).

3. The blood's oxygen transport capacity changes only slightly with normal variations in Hb content. Gender differences in Hb concentration contribute to the lower aerobic capacity of women, even after adjusting for gender-related differences in body mass and body fat.

4. The s-shaped nature of the oxyhemoglobin dissociation curve dictates that Hb-oxygen saturation changes little until P_{O_2} decreases below 60 mm Hg. Because such low P_{O_2}s occur in the tissues, oxygen releases rapidly from capillary blood and flows into the cells to meet metabolic demands.

5. About 25% of the blood's total oxygen releases to the tissues at rest; the remaining 75% returns "unused" to the heart in the venous blood. This relatively small arteriovenous oxygen difference indicates that blood maintains an oxygen reserve if metabolic demands suddenly increase.

6. Increases in acidity, temperature, and carbon dioxide concentration alter hemoglobin's molecular structure, reducing its effectiveness to hold oxygen (Bohr effect). Because exercise accentuates these factors, oxygen release to tissues becomes further facilitated.

7. Myoglobin stores "extra" oxygen in skeletal and cardiac muscle. Myoglobin releases its oxygen only at a low P_{O_2}, thus facilitating oxygen transfer to the mitochondria during strenuous exercise.

8. About 7% of carbon dioxide dissolves as free carbon dioxide in plasma to establish the blood's P_{CO_2}.

9. About 20% of the body's carbon dioxide combines with blood proteins (including Hb) to form carbamino compounds.

10. Approximately 70% of carbon dioxide combines with water to form bicarbonate. This reaction reverses in the lungs, allowing carbon dioxide to leave the blood and move into the alveoli.

THOUGHT QUESTIONS

1. Discuss whether it would be advantageous for runners to breathe 100% oxygen immediately before running a marathon to "load-up" on oxygen.

2. Why do minute amounts of impurities like CO_2 and CO in a breathing mixture exert profound physiologic effects?

PART 4 •
Regulation of Pulmonary Ventilation

VENTILATORY CONTROL DURING REST

The body exquisitely regulates the rate and depth of breathing in response to metabolic needs. During all exercise intensities in healthy individuals, arterial pressures for oxygen, carbon dioxide, and pH remain essentially at resting values. Neural information from higher centers in the brain, from the lungs, and from mechanical and chemical sensors throughout the body regulates pulmonary ventilation. The gaseous and chemical state of the blood that bathes the brain (medulla) and the aortic and carotid chemoreceptors also affect alveolar ventilation. **Figure 9.12** lists the primary factors in ventilatory control.

Neural Factors

The normal respiratory cycle comes from inherent, automatic activity of inspiratory neurons whose cell bodies reside in the **medial medulla.** The lungs inflate because neurons activate the diaphragm and intercostal muscles. The inspiratory neurons cease firing from their own self-limitation and from inhibitory influence from the medulla's expiratory neurons. Inflation of lung tissue stimulates stretch receptors in the bronchioles that inhibit inspiration and stimulate expiration.

Exhalation begins by the passive recoil of the stretched lung tissue and raised ribs when the inspiratory muscles relax. Activation of expiratory neurons and associated muscles that further facilitate expiration synchronizes with this passive phase. As expiration proceeds, the inspiratory center is released once again from inhibition and progressively becomes more active.

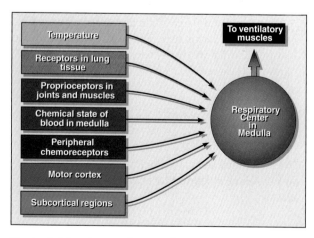

Figure 9.12. Primary factors affecting medullary control of pulmonary ventilation.

Humoral Factors

The chemical state of the blood largely regulates pulmonary ventilation at rest. Variations in arterial P_{O_2}, P_{CO_2}, acidity, and temperature activate sensitive neural units in the medulla and arterial system, so ventilation adjusts to maintain arterial blood chemistry within narrow limits.

Plasma P_{O_2} and Chemoreceptors Inhaling a gas mixture of 80% oxygen increases alveolar P_{O_2} and reduces minute ventilation by about 20%. Conversely, reducing inspired oxygen concentration increases minute ventilation, particularly if alveolar P_{O_2} falls below 60 mm Hg. Recall that, at 60 mm Hg, Hb's oxygen saturation dramatically decreases. The point at which decreasing arterial P_{O_2} stimulates ventilation has been termed the **hypoxic threshold**; it usually occurs at an arterial P_{O_2} between 60 and 70 mm Hg.

Sensitivity to reduced arterial oxygen pressure (arterial hypoxia) results from stimulation of small structures located outside the central nervous system called **chemoreceptors**. **Figure 9.13** shows these specialized neurons in the arch of the aorta (**aortic bodies**) and at the branching of the carotid arteries in the neck (**carotid bodies**). The carotid bodies, about 5 mm in diameter, maintain a strategic position to monitor arterial blood status just before it perfuses brain tissues. Nerves from the carotid and aortic bodies activate the brain's respiratory neurons.

Peripheral chemoreceptors provide an "early warning system" to alert against reduced oxygen pressure. These structures also stimulate ventilation in response to increased carbon dioxide, temperature, and acidity, a decrease in blood pressure, and perhaps a decline in circulating potassium.

Plasma P_{CO_2} and H^+ Concentration *Carbon dioxide pressure in arterial plasma provides the most important respiratory stimulus at rest.* Small increases in the P_{CO_2} of inspired air stimulate the medulla and peripheral chemoreceptors to initiate large increases in minute ventilation. For example, resting ventilation almost doubles when inspired P_{CO_2} increases to just 1.7 mm Hg (0.22% CO_2 in inspired air).

Molecular carbon dioxide does not entirely account for its effect on ventilatory control. Recall that carbonic acid formed from the union of carbon dioxide and water rapidly dissociates to bicarbonate ions and hydrogen ions. The increase in $[H^+]$, which varies directly with the blood's CO_2 content in the cerebrospinal fluid bathing the respiratory areas, stimulates inspiratory activity. The resulting increase in ventilation eliminates carbon dioxide, which lowers arterial $[H^+]$.

Hyperventilation and Breath-Holding

If a person breath-holds after a normal exhalation, it takes about 40 seconds before breathing commences. This urge

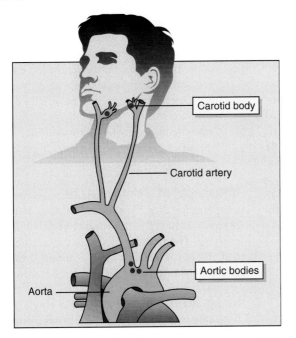

Figure 9.13. Aortic and carotid cell bodies (sensitive to a reduced plasma P_{O_2}) located in the aortic arch and bifurcation of carotid arteries. These peripheral receptors defend against arterial hypoxia.

to breathe results mainly from the stimulating effects of increased arterial P_{CO_2} and $[H^+]$, and not from a decreased arterial P_{CO_2}. *The "break point" for breath-holding corresponds to an increase in arterial P_{CO_2} to about 50 mm Hg.*

If this same person consciously increased alveolar ventilation above the normal level before breath-holding, the composition of alveolar air becomes more like ambient air. Alveolar P_{CO_2} with hyperventilation may decrease to 15 mm Hg, creating a considerable diffusion gradient for carbon dioxide run-off from venous blood that enters the pulmonary capillaries. Consequently, a larger than normal amount of carbon dioxide leaves the blood, decreasing arterial P_{CO_2} below normal levels. Reduced arterial P_{CO_2} extends the breath-hold until the arterial P_{CO_2} and/or $[H^+]$ increase to a level that stimulates ventilation.

Swimmers and sport divers hyperventilate and breath-hold to improve physical performance. In sprint swimming, it is biomechanically undesirable to roll the body and turn the head during the stroke's breathing phase. These swimmers hyperventilate on the starting blocks to prolong breath-hold time during the swim. The snorkel diver hyperventilates to extend breath-hold time, but often with tragic results. As the length and depth of the dive increase, the oxygen content of the blood can fall to critically low values before arterial P_{CO_2} increases to stimulate breathing and signal the need to ascend to the surface. Reduced arterial P_{O_2} can cause loss of consciousness before the diver reaches the surface.

VENTILATORY CONTROL DURING EXERCISE

Chemical Factors

Chemical stimuli cannot fully explain the increased ventilation (**hyperpnea**) during physical activity. For example, manipulating arterial P_{O_2}, P_{CO_2}, and acidity does not increase minute ventilation nearly as much as vigorous exercise.

Arterial P_{O_2} in exercise does not decrease to the point that stimulates ventilation by chemoreceptor activation. In fact, large breathing volumes in vigorous exercise actually increase alveolar (and arterial) P_{O_2} above the average resting

Name 2 neurogenic factors that regulate pulmonary ventilation.

   1.

   2.

Give the major effect of cigarette smoking on peripheral airway resistance.

Give the P_{O_2} that corresponds to the break point for breath-holding.

Why do some swimmers hyperventilate on the blocks?

True or False:

Arterial P_{O_2} in exercise increases to stimulate ventilation by chemoreceptor activation.

FOR YOUR INFORMATION

Less Breathing During Swimming
Lower ventilatory equivalents from restrictive breathing occur at all levels of energy expenditure during prone swimming. Depressed ventilation may hinder gas exchange during maximal swimming and contribute to the lower $\dot{V}O_{2max}$ with swimming compared with running.

value of 100 mm Hg. **Figure 9.14** illustrates the dynamics of venous and alveolar P_{CO_2} and alveolar P_{O_2} related to oxygen uptake in men during a graded exercise test. During light and moderate exercise ($\dot{V}O_2$ = <2000 mL·min^{-1}), pulmonary ventilation closely couples to oxygen uptake and carbon dioxide production in a manner that maintains alveolar P_{O_2} at about 100 mm Hg and P_{CO_2} at 40 mm Hg. Increases in acidity (and subsequent increases in CO_2 and $[H^+]$) in strenuous exercise provide an additional ventilatory stimulus that reduces alveolar P_{CO_2} to below 40 mm Hg and sometimes to as low as 25 mm Hg. This eliminates carbon dioxide and decreases arterial P_{CO_2}. Concurrently, augmented ventilation slightly increases alveolar P_{O_2} to facilitate oxygen loading.

Nonchemical Factors

Ventilation increases so rapidly when exercise begins that it occurs almost within the first ventilatory cycle. A plateau lasting about 20 seconds follows this abrupt increase in ventilation; thereafter, minute ventilation gradually increases and approaches a steady level in relation to the demands for metabolic gas exchange. When exercise stops, ventilation decreases rapidly to a point about 40% of the final exercise value and then slowly returns to resting levels. The rapidity of the ventilatory response at the onset and cessation of exercise shows that input other than from changes in arterial P_{CO_2} and $[H^+]$ mediate these components of exercise (and recovery) hyperpnea.

Neurogenic Factors

Cortical and peripheral factors regulate pulmonary ventilation in exercise.

- **Cortical Influence:** Neural outflow from regions of the motor cortex during exercise and cortical activation in anticipation of exercise stimulate respiratory neurons in the medulla. Cortical outflow acting in concert with the demands of exercise abruptly increases ventilation when exercise begins
- **Peripheral Influence:** Sensory input from joints, tendons, and muscles adjust ventilation during exercise. The specific peripheral receptors remain unknown, but experiments involving passive limb movements, electrical muscle stimulation, and voluntary exercise with the muscle's blood flow occluded support the existence of **mechanoreceptors** in peripheral tissues that produce reflex hyperpnea

Influence of Temperature   An increase in body temperature directly excites neurons of the respiratory center and likely helps control ventilation in prolonged exercise. The rapidity of ventilatory changes at the onset and end of exercise, however, cannot be explained by the relatively *slow* changes in core temperature.

Integrated Regulation   *No single factor controls breathing in exercise; rather, it depends on the combined and perhaps simultaneous effects of several chemical and neural stimuli* (**Fig. 9.15**). The current model suggests the following scenario for ventilatory control during exercise:

1. Neurogenic stimuli from the cerebral cortex (**central command**) and active limbs cause the initial, abrupt increase in breathing when exercise begins (termed **phase I ventilation**).
2. After a short (about 20-s) plateau, minute ventilation gradually increases to a steady level that adequately meets the demands for metabolic gas exchange (**phase II ventilation**). Central command input plus factors intrinsic to medullary control system neurons and peripheral stimuli from chemoreceptors and mechanoreceptors contribute to the control of this phase of ventilation.
3. The final phase of control (**phase III ventilation**) involves "fine tuning" of ventilation through peripheral sensory feedback mechanism (e.g., temperature, CO_2, and $[H^+]$).

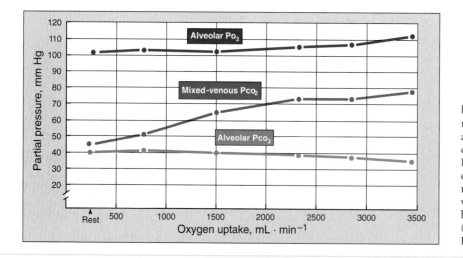

Figure 9.14. Values for P_{CO_2} in mixed-venous blood entering the lungs, and alveolar P_{O_2} and P_{CO_2} related to oxygen uptake during graded exercise. Despite increased metabolism with exercise, alveolar P_{O_2} and P_{CO_2} remain near resting levels. Increases in mixed-venous P_{CO_2} result from increased carbon dioxide production in metabolism. (Data from the Laboratory of Applied Physiology, Queens College.)

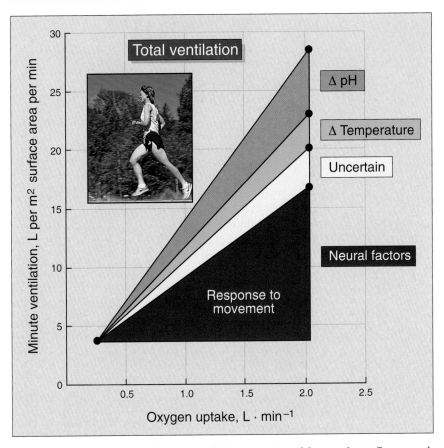

Figure 9.15. Generalized illustration of the composite of factors that influence pulmonary ventilation in exercise. The different colors estimate the contribution of changes in acidity (pH), temperature, and the effects of neurogenic stimuli from cerebral regions and/or joints and muscles. The yellow-shaded wedge represents ventilatory change not quantitatively accounted for by the other three factors. (From Lambertson, C.J.: Interactions of physical, chemical, and nervous factors in respiratory control. In: *Medical Physiology*. Mountcastle, V.B. (ed.). St. Louis: C.V. Mosby Co., 1974.)

FOR YOUR INFORMATION

Perhaps a "Weak Link" Among the Elite

The ventilatory system of elite endurance athletes, whose cardiovascular and muscular systems attain exceptional development, may be taxed maximally or even lag behind the functional capacity of other components of the "aerobic system" during strenuous exercise. This could compromise the complete aeration of blood, producing less than optimal exercise performance.

FOR YOUR INFORMATION

Cigarette Smoke Constricts Airways

The increase in peripheral airway resistance (and subsequent increased oxygen cost of breathing) with cigarette smoking results mainly from a vagal reflex (possibly triggered from sensory stimulation by minute particles in smoke) and partially from nicotine's stimulation of parasympathetic nerves.

SUMMARY

1. Inherent activity of neurons in the medulla controls the normal respiratory cycle. Neural circuits that relay information from higher brain centers, the lungs themselves, and other sensors throughout the body modulate medullary activity.

2. Arterial P_{CO_2} and acidity $[H^+]$ act directly on the respiratory center or modify its activity reflexly through chemoreceptors to control alveolar ventilation at rest.

3. Peripheral chemoreceptor activation stimulates breathing when arterial P_{O_2} decreases during high-altitude ascent or in severe pulmonary disease.

4. Hyperventilation lowers arterial P_{CO_2} and $[H^+]$. This prolongs breath-hold time until carbon dioxide and acidity increase to levels that stimulate breathing.

5. Extended breath-hold by hyperventilation should not be practiced during underwater swimming because it could produce deadly consequences.

6. Nonchemical regulatory factors augment ventilatory adjustments to exercise. These include cortical activation in anticipation of exercise, and outflow from the motor cortex when exercise begins; peripheral sensory input from mechanoreceptors in joints and muscles; and elevation in body temperature.

7. Neural and chemical factors that operate either singularly or in combination effectively regulate exercise alveolar ventilation. Each factor adjusts a particular phase of the ventilatory response to exercise.

THOUGHT QUESTION

Outline the mechanism by which hyperventilation extends breath-hold duration. Why is hyperventilation ill-advised in breath-hold diving?

Pulmonary Ventilation During Exercise

PULMONARY VENTILATION AND ENERGY DEMANDS

Physical activity increases oxygen uptake and carbon dioxide production more than any other physiologic stress. Large amounts of oxygen diffuse from the alveoli into the blood returning to the lungs during exercise. Conversely, considerable carbon dioxide moves from the blood into the alveoli. Concurrently, increases in pulmonary ventilation maintain stable alveolar gas concentrations, so oxygen and carbon dioxide exchange proceeds unimpeded. **Figure 9.16** illustrates the relationship between minute ventilation and oxygen uptake through the range of steady-rate and non–steady-rate exercise levels up to $\dot{V}O_{2max}$.

Ventilation in Steady-Rate Exercise

During light and moderate exercise ($\dot{V}O_2 < 2.5$ L·min^{-1} in this example), pulmonary ventilation increases linearly in men with oxygen uptake; ventilation mainly increases by increases in tidal volume.

The **ventilatory equivalent for oxygen** ($\dot{V}_E/\dot{V}O_2$) represents the ratio of minute ventilation to oxygen uptake. This index indicates breathing economy because it reflects the quantity of air breathed per amount of oxygen consumed. Healthy young adults usually maintain $\dot{V}_E/\dot{V}O_2$ at about 25 (i.e., 25 L air breathed per L oxygen consumed) during submaximal exercise up to about 55% of $\dot{V}O_{2max}$. Higher ventilatory equivalents occur in children, averaging about 32 in 6-year olds. Despite individual differences in the ventilatory equivalent for oxgen of healthy children and adults during steady-rate exercise, complete aeration of blood takes place because of two factors:

1. Alveolar PO_2 and PCO_2 remain at near-resting values
2. Transit time for blood flowing through the pulmonary capillaries proceeds slowly enough to permit complete gas exchange

During steady-rate exercise, the **ventilatory equivalent for carbon dioxide** ($\dot{V}_E/\dot{V}CO_2$) also remains relatively constant because pulmonary ventilation eliminates the carbon dioxide produced during cellular respiration.

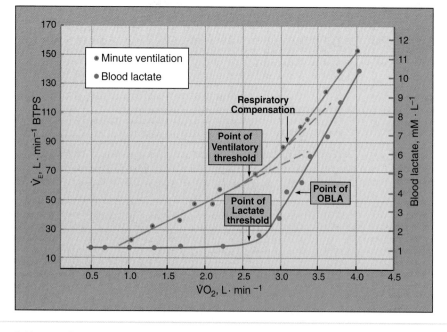

Figure 9.16. Pulmonary ventilation, blood lactate, and oxygen uptake during graded exercise to maximum. The dashed lines extrapolate the linear relationship between $\dot{V}_E$ and $\dot{V}O_2$ during submaximal exercise. The lactate threshold indicates the oxygen uptake (or work intensity) at which blood lactate begins to increase above the resting value. It is detected at the point where the relation between $\dot{V}_E$ and $\dot{V}O_2$ deviates from linearity. (OBLA represents the point of lactate increase above a 4 mM·L^{-1} baseline.) Respiratory compensation indicates a further increase in pulmonary ventilation to counter the falling pH in intense anaerobic exercise.

Ventilation in Non–Steady-Rate Exercise

Ventilatory Threshold   Note in Figure 9.16 that, as exercise oxygen uptake increases, minute ventilation eventually increases disproportionately to the increase in oxygen uptake. This increases the ventilatory equivalent above the steady-rate exercise value; it may reach as high as 35 or 40 in maximal exercise. The point at which pulmonary ventilation increases disproportionately with oxygen uptake during graded exercise has been termed **ventilatory threshold (VT)**. At this exercise intensity, pulmonary ventilation no longer links tightly to oxygen demand at the cellular level. Rather, the "excess" ventilation relates directly to carbon dioxide's increased output from the buffering of lactate that begins to accumulate from anaerobic metabolism.

Recall that sodium bicarbonate in the blood buffers the lactate generated during anaerobic metabolism in the following reaction:

$$Lactate + NaHCO_3 \rightarrow Na\ lactate + H_2CO_3 \rightarrow H_2O + CO_2$$

Excess, non-metabolic carbon dioxide liberated in this buffering reaction stimulates pulmonary ventilation that disproportionately increases $\dot{V}_E/\dot{V}O_2$. The respiratory exchange ratio ($\dot{V}CO_2/\dot{V}O_2$) exceeds 1.00 when additional carbon dioxide is exhaled due to acid buffering.

The term **anaerobic threshold** originally defined the abrupt increase in ventilatory equivalent caused by non-metabolic carbon dioxide production due to lactate

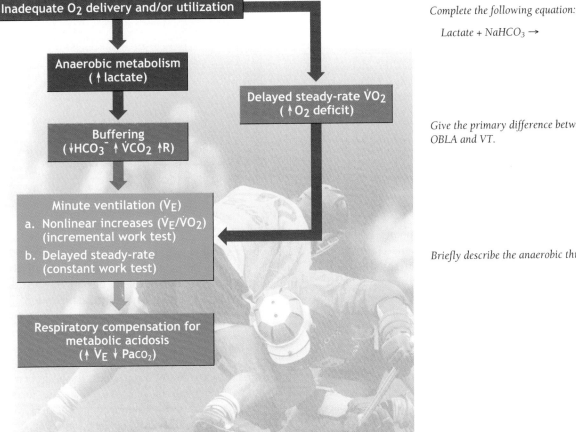

Figure 9.17.   Factors that relate to pulmonary gas exchange dynamics for detecting the lactate threshold.

Box 9–5 • **CLOSE UP**

CAN VENTILATION LIMIT AEROBIC POWER IN ENDURANCE ATHLETES?

For endurance athletes, the pulmonary system may lag behind their exceptional cardiovascular and aerobic muscular adaptations to training. The potential for inequality in alveolar ventilation relative to pulmonary capillary blood flow (i.e., impaired ventilation perfusion ratio) during high-intensity exercise may compromise arterial saturation and oxygen transport capacity—a condition termed **exercise-induced arterial hypoxemia (EIH)**. EIH among trained individuals remains variable. It sometimes occurs at exercise levels as low as 40% $\dot{V}O_{2max}$ at sea level and mild and moderate altitudes. When some highly trained endurance athletes exercise at near $\dot{V}O_{2max}$ ($\sim$ 65 mL·kg^{-1}·min^{-1}; see figure), pressure differentials between alveolar (PAO_2) and arterial oxygen (PaO_2) widen to more than 30 mm Hg. This causes arterial oxygen saturation to fall below 90%, with a corresponding arterial PO_2 below 75 mm Hg. This indicates that some elite aerobic athletes cannot achieve complete aeration of the blood in the pulmonary capillaries in high-intensity exercise; arterial desaturation becomes more apparent as exercise duration progresses.

Alterations in pulmonary structure at the alveolar–capillary interface probably do not produce EIH. Possible functionally based causes for arterial desaturation include:

1. Inequality in ventilation-perfusion ratio within the lungs or specific portions of the lungs

2. Shunting of blood between venous and arterial circulations, thus bypassing areas for diffusion

3. Failure to achieve end-capillary equilibrium between alveolar oxygen pressure and pressure of oxygen in blood perfusing the pulmonary capillaries; interstitial pulmonary edema or rapid blood flow in endurance athletes through a relatively normal-sized pulmonary capillary volume could produce this diffusion limitation

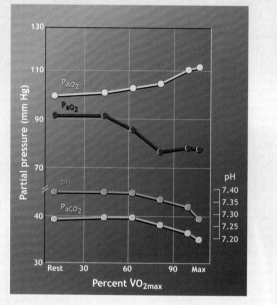

buffering. Some researchers believed this point signaled the body's shift to anaerobic metabolism (lactate formation). The researchers proposed the anaerobic threshold as a noninvasive ventilatory measure of the onset of anaerobiosis. Subsequent research has shown that the ratios of $\dot{V}_E/\dot{V}O_2$ or $\dot{V}CO_2/\dot{V}O_2$ do not necessarily link in a *causal* manner with lactate production (or accumulation) in exercise. Even if the association between ventilatory dynamics and cellular metabolic events is noncausal, useful information can be obtained about exercise performance by applying these indirect procedures. **Figure 9.17** outlines underlying factors that relate to anaerobic threshold detected from pulmonary gas exchange dynamics during graded exercise.

Onset of Blood Lactate Accumulation   Steady-rate exercise indicates that oxygen supply and utilization satisfy the energy requirements of muscular effort. When this occurs, lactate production does not exceed its removal, and blood lactate does not accumulate. Figure 9.16 illus-

trates that exercise intensity or oxygen uptake where blood lactate begins to increase above a baseline level of about 4 mM·L^{-1} indicates the point of **onset of blood lactate accumulation (OBLA)**. OBLA normally occurs between 55% and 65% of $\dot{V}O_{2max}$ in healthy, untrained subjects and often equals more than 80% $\dot{V}O_{2max}$ in highly trained endurance athletes.

Causes of OBLA   The exact cause of the OBLA remains controversial. Many believe it represents the point of muscle hypoxia (inadequate oxygen) and, therefore, anaerobiosis. Muscle lactate accumulation does not necessarily coincide with hypoxia because lactate forms even in the presence of adequate muscle oxygenation. The OBLA, however, does imply an imbalance between the rate of blood lactate appearance and disappearance. This imbalance may not result from muscle hypoxia, but rather, it may result from a decreased lactate clearance in total or increased lactate production only in specific muscle fibers. Practitioners should interpret cautiously the specific metabolic significance of the OBLA and its possible relationship to tissue hypoxia.

OBLA and Endurance Performance   The point of OBLA often increases with aerobic training, without an accompanying increase in $\dot{V}O_{2max}$. This suggests that separate factors influence OBLA and $\dot{V}O_{2max}$. Traditionally, exercise physiologists have applied $\dot{V}O_{2max}$ as the main yardstick to gauge capacity for endurance exercise. This measure generally relates to long-duration exercise performance but does not fully explain all aspects of success. Experienced distance athletes generally compete at an exercise intensity slightly above the point of OBLA. Exercise intensity at the OBLA has emerged as a consistent and powerful predictor of aerobic exercise performance. *Changes in endurance performance with training often relate more closely to training-induced changes in the exercise level for OBLA than to $\dot{V}O_{2max}$ changes.*

DOES VENTILATION LIMIT AEROBIC CAPACITY FOR THE AVERAGE PERSON?

With inadequate breathing capacity, the line relating pulmonary ventilation and oxygen uptake in Figure 9.16 would not curve upward (increase in ventilatory equivalent) during heavy exercise; instead, it would level-off or slope downward to the right to reflect a decrease in ventilatory equivalent. Such a response would indicate a *failure* for ventilation to keep pace with increasing oxygen demands; in this case, a person truly would "run out of wind." Actually, a healthy individual tends to overbreathe in relation to oxygen uptake with increasing exercise intensity. Figure 9.14 demonstrated that the ventilatory adjustment to strenuous exercise decreases alveolar P_{CO_2} concomitant with small increases in alveolar P_{O_2}. Arterial P_{O_2} and Hb oxygen saturation remain at near-resting values during intense exercise for most individuals. This means that pulmonary function does not represent the "weak link" in the oxygen transport system of healthy individuals with average to moderately high aerobic capacities.

Work of Breathing

Two major factors determine the energy requirements of breathing:

1. Compliance of the lungs and thorax
2. Resistance of the airways to the smooth flow of air

Lung and thorax **compliance** refers to how "easily" these tissues stretch. The radius of the bronchi primarily establishes resistance to airflow. More specifically, airflow resistance varies inversely with a vessel's radius raised to the fourth power in accordance with Poiseuille's law. Reducing airway radius by one-half causes airway resistance to increase 16 times. Normally, bronchi and bronchiole dimensions do not impede smooth air flow, so breathing requires relatively little energy. In some lung diseases, airways constrict and/or lung tissues themselves lose compliance; this imposes considerable resistance to airflow. Trying to breathe through a drinking straw gives some indication of breathing difficulties encountered by the person with severe obstructive lung disease.

A healthy person rarely senses the breathing effort, even during moderate exercise. In contrast, respiratory disease often makes the work of breathing during exercise an exhausting physical task. For patients with **chronic obstructive pulmonary disease** (COPD; e.g., asthma, emphysema), the breathing effort at rest can reach three times that of healthy individuals. In severe pulmonary disease, breathing's energy requirement may easily reach 40% of the total exercise oxygen uptake. This obviously encroaches on the oxygen available to the active, nonrespiratory muscles, and seriously limits the exercise capacity of these patients.

Figure 9.18 shows the relationship in healthy subjects between pulmonary ventilation and oxygen uptake during rest and submaximal exercise, and its division

Questions & Notes

Briefly discuss whether ventilation limits the aerobic capacity of normal individuals.

Do physiologic changes with endurance training relate more to improvement in the exercise level for OBLA than to improvement in VO_{2max}?

List 2 factors that determine the energy requirements of breathing.

1.

2.

Briefly describe the relationship between pulmonary ventilation and oxygen uptake during rest and various levels of submaximal exercise.

What percentage of the total oxygen uptake is due to the oxygen cost of breathing in moderate and intense exercise?

Moderate exercise –

Intense exercise –

Name 3 air pollutants that may affect health and exercise performance.

FOR YOUR INFORMATION

Even the Fit Have Asthma
Champions are not immune from asthma. One of the most famous examples is 1984 Olympic marathon champion Joan Benoit Samuelson who experienced breathing problems during several races in 1991 that led to the discovery of her asthmatic condition. Despite breathing difficulties during the 1991 New York Marathon, she finished with a time of 2 h:33 min:40 s!

Box 9–6 • CLOSE UP

AIR POLLUTION, LUNG FUNCTION, AND EXERCISE

Air pollution has become such a pervasive problem across the country that there are virtually no places left unaffected. Exercise increases exposure to air pollutants for two reasons:

1. Exercise considerably increases the total volume of air breathed
2. Breathing through the mouth during exercise bypasses the nose's filtering system

Polluted air contains compounds from the combustion of fossil fuels and automobile emissions. They include oxides of sulfur and nitrogen, carbon monoxide, particulates, lead, and ozone. These substances may produce acute effects on health and exercise performance.

SPECIFIC POLLUTANTS

Ozone

Ozone, a colorless gas, constitutes up to 95% of smog. It is produced by sunlight action on nitrogen oxides and hydrocarbons from automobile emissions. Concentrations are highest in the afternoons on sunny days with little wind. Symptoms of ozone exposure include chest tightness, eye irritation, sore throat, wheezing, coughing, shortness of breath, and headache. These symptoms indicate a decline in lung function and the ability of lung tissue to transport oxygen to the bloodstream. People vary in sensitivity to ozone. Limited studies to date suggest that impaired performance may begin with ozone levels at 0.12 parts per million (ppm) and is very likely at 0.20 ppm for most athletes.

Sulfur Dioxide

Sulfur dioxide, produced by the combustion of sulfur-containing fuels (coal and oil), affects asthmatics more than other people. Symptoms worsen in cold air, but pretreatment with inhaled bronchodilators (albuterol) or allergy modifiers (cromolyn) lessens the airflow restriction.

Nitrogen Dioxide

Nitrogen dioxide (NO_2) from fuel combustion and cigarette smoking is a precursor to ozone and reacts with water to form nitrous acid. It causes the brown color and pungent odor of smog. The health standard is set at 0.05 ppm averaged over a year. Exercise studies done at 0.5 to 1.0 ppm, mimicking high levels of outdoor pollution, reported only slight changes in lung function. Researchers have so far concluded that nitrogen dioxide does not pose a danger for outdoor exercise.

Other Particulates

Polluted air can also contain a variety of particulates. These are visible as soot, dust, or smoke. It also con-

Air Pollutants Known to Impair Exercise Performance

POLLUTANT	UPPER HEALTHY LIMIT[a]	EFFECTS
Carbon dioxide (CO_2)	NA	Hyperventilation, acid-base imbalance, headaches
Carbon monoxide (CO)	9 ppm	Greater affinity for hemoglobin than oxygen
Nitrogen dioxide (NO_2)	0.05 ppm	Irritates lung tissue
Ozone (O_3)	0.12 ppm	Decreases lung function, headaches
Sulfuric Acid (H_2SO_4)	NA	Upper respiratory tract irritant
Sulfur dioxide (SO_2)	0.14 ppm	Increases exercise-induced bronchospasm
Other particulates		Aggravates asthma symptoms

[a] From the National Average Air Quality Standards of the USA; ppm = parts per million; NA = not applicable.

Box 9–6 • **CLOSE UP** *(Continued)*

tains airborne pollens, molds, sulfuric acid, and lead. Asthmatics appear more sensitive to particulates; non-asthmatics increase mucus production and may cough but experience no significant short-term impairment of lung function. Long-term exposure, however, is difficult to research, and its effects are generally not known.

Carbon Monoxide

Carbon monoxide (CO) is a colorless, odorless gas produced by automobiles and cigarette smoking. It enters the body through the lungs, but unlike ozone, it does not directly affect this tissue. CO quickly enters the bloodstream and binds to hemoglobin in red blood cells, replacing the oxygen normally carried. This effect reduces the amount of oxygen available to the body.

The heart and brain are most sensitive to lowered oxygen levels. Exposure to cigarette smoke, even sidestream (second-hand) smoke, increases carbon monoxide levels. Symptoms of exposure include headache and chest pain in individuals with heart disease. It takes several hours after exposure for CO concentration to decline and symptoms to lessen.

THE AIR QUALITY INDEX (AQI)

The AQI provides an index for reporting daily air quality in terms of its cleanliness. The AQI also focuses on health effects a person may experience within a few hours or days after breathing polluted air. The Environmental Protection Agency (EPA) calculates the AQI for five major air pollutants regulated by the Clean Air Act: ground-level ozone, particle pollution (also known as particulate matter), carbon monoxide, sulfur dioxide, and nitrogen dioxide. For each of these pollutants, the EPA has established national air quality standards to protect public health. Think of the AQI as a yardstick that runs from 0 to 500. The higher the AQI value, the greater the level of air pollution with concomitant health concerns. For example, an AQI value of 50 represents good air quality with little potential to affect public health, while an AQI value over 300 represents hazardous air quality.

An AQI value of 100 generally corresponds to the national air quality standard for the pollutant, which represents the EPA level set to protect public health. Think of AQI values below 100 as satisfactory. When AQI values are above 100, air quality is considered unhealthy—first for certain sensitive groups, then for everyone at higher AQI values.

Air Quality Index (AQI)	Levels of Health Concern	Colors
When the AQI is in this range	...air quality conditions are	...as symbolized by this color
0 to 50	Good	Green
51 to 100	Moderate	Yellow
101 to 150	Unhealthy for Sensitive Groups	Orange
151 to 200	Unhealthy	Red
201 to 300	Very Unhealthy	Purple
301 to 500	Hazardous	Maroon

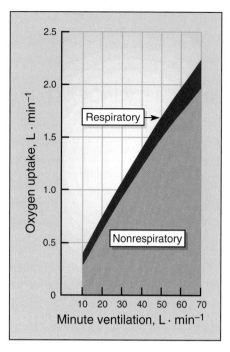

Figure 9.18. Relationship between oxygen uptake and pulmonary ventilation and the respiratory and nonrespiratory oxygen cost components during submaximal exercise in healthy subjects. (From Levison, H., and Cherniack, R.: Ventilatory cost of exercise in chronic obstructive pulmonary disease. *J. Appl. Physiol.*, 25:21, 1968.)

into respiratory and nonrespiratory components. At rest and in light exercise, the relatively small oxygen requirement of breathing averages between 1.9 and 3.1 mL of oxygen per liter of air breathed, or about 4% of the total energy expenditure. As the rate and depth of breathing increase during exercise, the energy cost of breathing increases to about 4 mL of oxygen per liter of ventilation. It can increase to 9 mL of oxygen in maximal exercise when pulmonary ventilation exceeds 100 L·min^{-1}. *At these exercise intensities, the oxygen cost of breathing represents between 10% and 20% of the total oxygen uptake.*

Exercise and Cigarette Smoking

Since the initial 1964 release of the *Surgeon General's Report on Smoking and Health*, numerous review articles have concluded that a causal link exists between smoking and lung cancer, chronic bronchitis and emphysema, cardiovascular disease, and cancers of the lip, larynx, esophagus, and urinary bladder. However, little research has related cigarette smoking habits to exercise performance, even though most endurance athletes avoid cigarettes for fear of hindering performance from what they consider "loss of wind." The chronic cigarette smoker exhibits decreases in dynamic lung function, which, in severe cases, manifests as obstructive lung disorders. Such pathologic processes usually take years to develop. Teenage and young adult smokers rarely exhibit chronic lung function deterioration of a magnitude to significantly impair exercise performance. Because of increased fitness, the young, fit smoker often believes he or she is immune from smoking's crippling effects.

Other, more acute effects of cigarette smoking adversely affect exercise capacity. For example, airway resistance at rest can increase threefold in chronic smokers and nonsmokers after 15 puffs on a cigarette during a 5-minute period. Added resistance to breathing lasts an average of 35 minutes, with only minor negative effects in light exercise where the oxygen cost of breathing remains small. In vigorous exercise, however, the residual effect of smoking on airway resistance proves detrimental because the additional cost of breathing becomes physiologically significant. In one study of habitual cigarette smokers who exercised at 80% of $\dot{V}O_{2max}$, the energy requirement of breathing averaged 14% of the exercise oxygen uptake after smoking but averaged only 9% in the "nonsmoking" trials. Also, exercise heart rates averaged 5% to 7% lower after 1 day of smoking abstinence; all subjects reported they felt better exercising in the nonsmoking condition. Almost complete reversibility of the increased oxygen cost of breathing with smoking can occur in chronic smokers with only 1 day of abstinence. *Thus, athletes who cannot conquer the smoking habit should at least stop 24 hours before competition.*

SUMMARY

1. Pulmonary ventilation increases linearly with oxygen uptake during light and moderate exercise. The ventilatory equivalent at these exercise intensities averages 20 to 25 liters of air breathed per liter of oxygen consumed.

2. In non–steady-rate exercise, pulmonary ventilation increases disproportionately with increases in oxygen uptake, and the ventilatory equivalent may reach 35 or 40.

3. The eventual sharp upswing in pulmonary ventilation related to oxygen uptake during incremental exercise

indicates the point of onset of blood lactate accumulation (OBLA).

4. OBLA effectively predicts endurance performance and can be measured without significant metabolic acidosis or cardiovascular strain.

5. Breathing normally requires a relatively small oxygen cost even during exercise. In respiratory disease, the work of breathing becomes excessive, and exercise alveolar ventilation often becomes inadequate.

6. Pulmonary ventilation does not limit optimal alveolar gas exchange in healthy individuals who perform maximal exercise.

7. Airway resistance increases significantly after cigarette smoking. The added oxygen cost of breathing can impair high-intensity, aerobic exercise performance. Reversibility of these effects occurs with 1 day of cigarette smoking abstinence.

THOUGHT QUESTIONS

1. How would the relationship change between $\dot{V}_E/\dot{V}O_2$ under the following conditions: (1) aging person who remains sedentary versus aging person who performs regular aerobic exercises; (2) transition from adolescence to young adulthood; and (3) person training for American football?

2. Present arguments to justify that pulmonary ventilation does not limit aerobic exercise performance for most healthy people.

3. In what ways are the terms lactate threshold and onset of blood lactate accumulation biochemically more precise than the term anaerobic threshold?

SELECTED REFERENCES

Abu-Hasan, M., et al.: Exercise-induced dyspnea in children and adolescents: if not asthma then what? *Ann. Allergy Asthma Immunol.*, 94:366, 2005.

Agostoni, P., et al.: Exercise-induced pulmonary edema in heart failure. *Circulation*, 25;108:2666, 2003.

Ascensao, A.A., et al.: Cardiac mitochondrial respiratory function and oxidative stress: the role of exercise. *Int. J. Sports Med.*, 26:258, 2005.

Baldari, C., et al.: Lactate removal during active recovery related to the individual anaerobic and ventilatory thresholds in soccer players. *Eur. J. Appl. Physiol.*, 93:224, 2004.

Bassett D.R. Jr., Howley, E.T.: Limiting factors for maximum oxygen uptake and determinants of endurance performance. *Med. Sci. Sports Exerc.*, 32:270, 2000.

Bernaards, C.M., et al.: A longitudinal study in smoking in relationship top fitness and heart rate response. *Med. Sci. Sports Exerc.*, 35:793, 2003.

Boulet, L.P., et al.: Lower airway inflammatory responses to high-intensity training in athletes. *Clin. Invest. Med.*, 28:15, 2005.

Broekhuizen, R., et al.: Polyunsaturated fatty acids improve exercise capacity in chronic obstructive pulmonary disease. *Thorax*, 60:376, 2005.

Chung, Y., et al.: Control of respiration and bioenergetics during muscle contraction. *Am. J. Physiol. Cell. Physiol.*, 288:C730, 2005.

Dantas De Luca, R., et al.: The lactate minimum test protocol provides valid measures of cycle ergometer VO₂peak. *J. Sports Med. Phys. Fitness*, 4:279, 2003.

Day, J.R., et al.: The maximally attainable VO₂ during exercise in humans: the peak vs. maximum issue. *J. Appl. Physiol.*, 95:1901, 2003.

Dekerle, J., et al.: Maximal lactate steady state, respiratory compensation threshold and critical power. *Eur. J. Appl. Physiol.*, 89:281, 2003.

Dempsey, J.A.: Crossing the apnoeic threshold: causes and consequences. *Exp. Physiol.*, 90:13, 2005.

Gonzalez, J., et al.: A chest wall restrictor to study effects on pulmonary function and exercise. 2. The energetics of restrictive breathing. *Respiration*, 66:188, 1999.

Hansen, J.E., et al.: Reproducibility of cardiopulmonary exercise measurements in patients with pulmonary arterial hypertension. *Chest*, 126:816, 2004.

Hashizume, K., et al.: Effects of abstinence from cigarette smoking on the cardiorespiratory capacity. *Med. Sci. Sports Exerc.*, 32:386, 2000.

Haverkamp, H.C., Dempsey, J.A.: On the normal variability of gas exchange efficiency during exercise: does sex matter? *J. Physiol.*, 557:345, 2004.

Jack, S., et al.: Behavioral influences and physiological indices of ventilatory control in subjects with idiopathic hyperventilation. *Behav. Modif.*, 27:637, 2003.

Jack, S., et al.: Ventilatory responses to inhaled carbon dioxide, hypoxia, and exercise in idiopathic hyperventilation. *Am. J. Respir. Crit. Care Med.*, 170:118, 2004.

Kelly, G.E., et al.: Models for estimating the change-point in gas exchange data. *Physiol. Meas.*, 25:1425, 2004.

Kowalchuk, J.M., et al.: The effect of resistive breathing on leg muscle oxygenation using near-infrared spectroscopy during exercise in men. *Exp. Physiol.*, 87:601, 2002.

Laplaud, D., Menier, R.: Reproducibility of the instant of equality of pulmonary gas exchange and its physiological significance. *J. Sports Med. Phys. Fitness*, 43:437, 2003.

Lau, A.C., et al.: Altered exercise gas exchange as related to microalbuminuria in type 2 diabetic patients. *Chest*, 125:1292, 2004.

Lucas, S.R., Platts-Mills, T.A.: Physical activity and exercise in asthma: relevance to etiology and treatment. *J. Allergy Clin. Immunol.*, 115:928, 2005.

Luo, Y.M., Moxham, J.: Measurement of neural respiratory drive in patients with COPD. *Respir. Physiol. Neurobiol.*, 15;146:165, 2005.

Mahler, D.A., et al.: Responsiveness of continuous ratings of dyspnea during exercise in patients with COPD. *Med. Sci. Sports Exerc.*, 37:529, 2005.

Miller, J.D., et al.: Skeletal muscle pump versus respiratory muscle pump: modulation of venous return from the locomotor limb in humans. *J. Physiol.*, 563:925, 2005.

Ozcelik, O., Kelestimur, H.: Effects of acute hypoxia on the determination of anaerobic threshold using the heart rate-work rate relationships during incremental exercise tests. *Physiol. Res.*, 53:45, 2004.

Puente-Maestu, L., et al.: Effects of training on the tolerance to high-intensity exercise in patients with severe COPD. *Respiration*, 70:367, 2003.

Richardson, R.S., et al.: Skeletal muscle intracellular PO_2 assessed by myoglobin desaturation: response to graded exercise. *J. Appl. Physiol.*, 91:2679, 2001.

Ricquier, D.: Respiration uncoupling and metabolism in the control of energy expenditure. *Proc. Nutr. Soc.*, 64:47, 2005.

Smith, C.A., et al.: The essential role of carotid body chemoreceptors in sleep apnea. *Can. J. Physiol. Pharmacol.*, 81:774, 2003.

Smith, C.A., et al.: Ventilatory responsiveness to CO_2 above & below eupnea: relative importance of peripheral chemoreception. *Adv. Exp. Med. Biol.*, 551:65, 2004.

Svedahl, K., MacIntosh, B.R.: Anaerobic threshold: the concept and methods of measurement. *Can. J. Appl. Physiol.*, 28:299, 2003.

Van Schuylenbergh, R., et al.: Correlations between lactate and ventilatory thresholds and the maximal lactate steady state in elite cyclists. *Int. J. Sports Med.*, 25:403, 2004.

Wagner, P.D.: Why doesn't exercise grow the lungs when other factors do? *Exerc. Sport Sci. Rev.*, 33:3, 2005.

Wasserman, K.: Anaerobic threshold and cardiovascular function. *Monaldi Arch. Chest Dis.*, 58:1, 2002.

Wasserman, K., et al.: *Principles of Exercise Testing and Interpretation.* 3rd Ed. Baltimore: Lippincott Williams & Wilkins, 1999.

Winter, B., Whipp, B.J.: Immediate effects of bilateral carotid body resection on total respiratory resistance and compliance in humans. *Adv. Exp. Med. Biol.*, 551:15, 2004.

Yasunobu, Y., et al.: End-tidal PCO_2 abnormality and exercise limitation in patients with primary pulmonary hypertension. *Chest*, 127:1637, 2005.

CHAPTER OBJECTIVES

- List important functions of the cardiovascular system.

- Describe how to use the auscultatory method to measure blood pressure, and give average values for systolic and diastolic blood pressure during rest and moderate aerobic exercise.

- Describe the blood pressure response during (1) resistance exercise, (2) upper-body exercise, and (3) exercise in the inverted position.

- State potential benefits of aerobic exercise for treating moderate hypertension.

- Identify intrinsic and extrinsic factors that regulate heart rate during rest and exercise.

- Identify neural and local metabolic factors that regulate blood flow during rest and exercise.

- Compare average values of cardiac output during rest and maximal exercise for an endurance-trained athlete and sedentary person.

- Explain three physiologic mechanisms that affect the heart's stroke volume.

- Describe the relationship between maximal cardiac output and maximal oxygen uptake among individuals with varied aerobic fitness levels.

CHAPTER OUTLINE

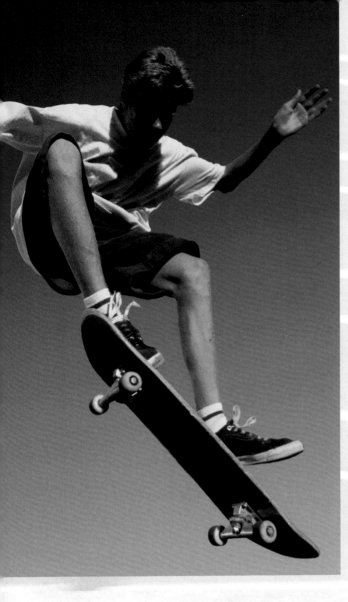

The Cardiovascular System and Exercise

The Greek physician Galen (Chapter 1) theorized that blood flowed like the tides of the sea, surging and abating into arteries, then away from the heart and back again. In Galen's view, fluid carried with it "humors," good and evil that determined well-being. If a person became ill, the standard practice required "blood-letting" to drain off the diseased humors and restore health. This theory prevailed until the seventeenth century when physician William Harvey (Chapter 1) proposed a different scenario. Experimenting with frogs, cats, and dogs, Harvey demonstrated the existence of valves in the heart that provided for a one-way flow of blood through the body, a finding incompatible with Galen's "ebb-and-flow" view. In a set of ingenious experiments, Harvey measured the volume of the heart's chambers and counted the number of times the heart contracted in 1 hour. He concluded that if the heart emptied only one-half its volume with each beat, the body's total blood volume would be pumped in minutes. This finding led Harvey to hypothesize that blood moved (circulated) within a closed system in a circular, unidirectional pattern throughout the body. Harvey, of course, was correct; the heart pumps the entire blood volume, approximately 5 liters, in 1 minute. Harvey's experiments changed medical science forever, yet it would take nearly 200 more years for his ideas to play important roles in physiology and medicine.

From Harvey's early experiments to sophisticated research at the dawn of the twenty-first century, we know that the highly efficient ventilatory system described in Chapter 9 complements a rapid transport and delivery system comprised of blood, the heart, and more than 60,000 miles of blood vessels that integrate the body as a unit. The circulatory system serves five important functions during physical activity:

1. Delivers oxygen to active tissues
2. Aerates blood returned to the lungs
3. Transports heat, a byproduct of cellular metabolism, from the body's core to the skin
4. Delivers fuel nutrients to active tissues
5. Transports hormones, the body's chemical messengers

PART 1 •
The Cardiovascular System

COMPONENTS OF THE CARDIOVASCULAR SYSTEM

The cardiovascular system consists of an interconnected, continuous vascular circuit containing a pump (heart), a high-pressure distribution system (arteries), exchange vessels (capillaries), and a low-pressure collection and return system (veins). **Figure 10.1** presents a schematic view of this system.

Heart

The heart provides the force to propel blood throughout the vascular circuit. This four-chambered organ, a fist-sized pump, beats at rest an average of 70 b·min^{-1}, 100,800 times a day, and 36.8 million times a year. Even for a person of average fitness, maximum output of blood from this remarkable organ exceeds fluid output from a household faucet turned wide open.

The heart muscle (**myocardium**) consists of striated muscle similar to skeletal muscle. Unlike skeletal muscle, the individual fibers interconnect in latticework fashion. As a result, stimulation (depolarization) of one myocardial cell spreads an action potential throughout the myocardium causing the heart to function as a unit. **Figure 10.2** details the heart as a pump. Functionally, the heart consists of two separate pumps: the *left heart pump* receives blood from the body and pumps it to the lungs for aeration (**pulmonary circulation**), and the *right heart pump* accepts oxygenated blood from the lungs and pumps it throughout the body (**systemic circulation**).

The hollow chambers of the right heart pump perform two important functions:

1. Receive blood returning from all parts of the body
2. Pump blood to the lungs for aeration via the pulmonary circulation

The chambers of left heart pump also perform two important functions:

1. Receive oxygenated blood from the lungs
2. Pump blood into the thick-walled, muscular aorta for distribution throughout the body via the systemic circulation

A thick, solid muscular wall (septum) separates the left and right sides of the heart. The **atrioventricular (AV) valves** situated within the heart direct the one-way flow of blood from the right atrium to the right ventricle (**tricuspid valve**) and from the left atrium to the left ventricle (**mitral valve** or **bicuspid valve**). The **semilunar valves** located in the arterial wall just outside the heart prevent blood from flowing back (regurgitation) into the heart between ventricular contractions.

The relatively thin-walled, sac-like atrial chambers receive and store blood returning from the lungs and body during ventricular contraction. About 70% of the blood returning to the atria flows directly into the ventricles before the atria contract. Simultaneous contraction of both atria forces the remaining blood into the respective ventricles directly below. Almost immediately after atrial contraction, the ventricles contract and force blood into the arterial systems.

Arteries

The arteries are the high-pressure tubing that conducts oxygen-rich blood to the tissues. **Figure 10.3** shows the arteries composed of layers of connective tissue and

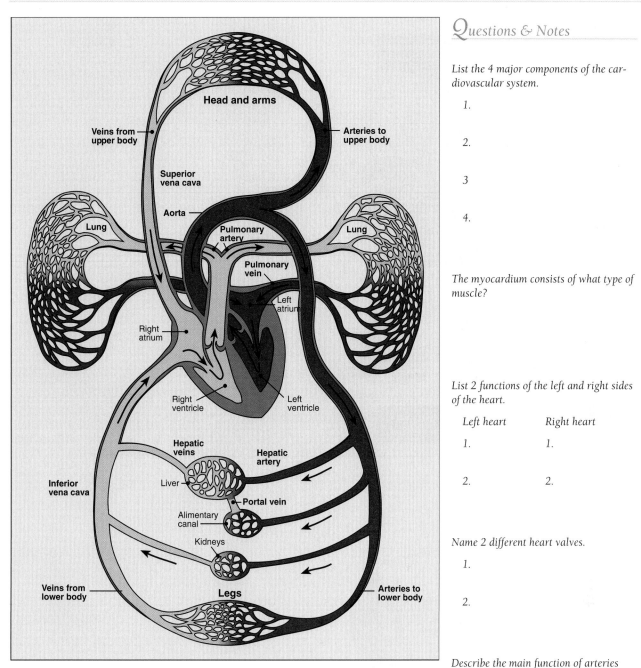

Figure 10.1   Schematic view of the cardiovascular system consisting of the heart and the pulmonary and systemic vascular circuits. The darker red shading shows oxygen-rich arterial blood, whereas deoxygenated venous blood appears somewhat paler. In the pulmonary circuit, the situation reverses, and oxygenated blood returns to the heart via the right and left pulmonary veins.

smooth muscle. Because of their thickness, no gaseous exchange takes place between arterial blood and surrounding tissues. Blood pumped from the left ventricle into the highly muscular yet elastic aorta circulates throughout the body via a network of arteries and **arterioles**, or smaller arterial branches. *Arteriole walls contain circular layers of smooth muscle that either constrict or relax to regulate peripheral blood flow.* The redistribution function of arterioles becomes important during exercise because blood diverts to working muscles from areas that can temporarily compromise their blood supply.

Questions & Notes

List the 4 major components of the cardiovascular system.

1.

2.

3

4.

The myocardium consists of what type of muscle?

List 2 functions of the left and right sides of the heart.

Left heart   Right heart

1.   1.

2.   2.

Name 2 different heart valves.

1.

2.

Describe the main function of arteries and arterioles.

Describe the major differences between the "right heart pump" and the "left heart pump."

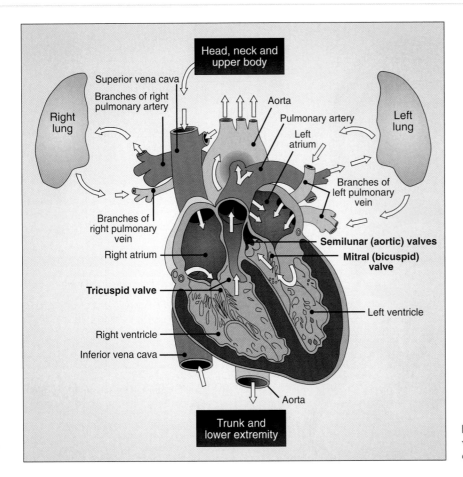

Figure 10.2 The heart's valves provide for the one-way flow of blood indicated by the yellow arrows.

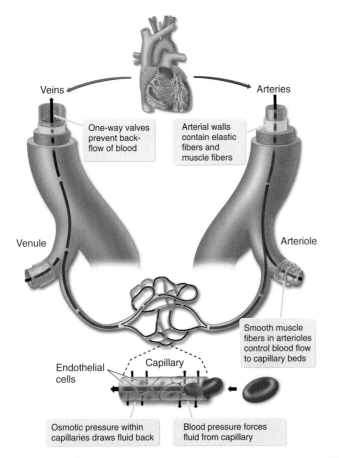

Figure 10.3 The structure of the walls of the various blood vessels. A single layer of endothelial cells lines each vessel. Fibrous tissue, wrapped in several layers of smooth muscle, surrounds the arterial walls. A single layer of muscle cells sheathes the arterioles; capillaries consist of only one layer of endothelial cells. In the venule, fibrous tissue encases the endothelial cells; veins also possess a layer of smooth muscle. A vessel's resistance to flow depends on its diameter. Decreasing vessel diameter by one-half increases resistance 16-fold.

Capillaries

The arterioles continue to branch and form smaller and less muscular vessels called metarterioles. These tiny vessels merge into **capillaries** (see bottom of Fig. 10.3), a network of microscopic blood vessels so thin they provide only enough room for blood cells to squeeze through in single file. Capillaries contain about 5% of the total blood volume at any time. Gases, nutrients, and waste products rapidly transfer across the thin, porous, capillary walls. A ring of smooth muscle (**precapillary sphincter**) encircles the capillary at its origin to control the vessel's internal diameter. This sphincter provides a local means for regulating capillary blood flow within a specific tissue to meet metabolic requirements that change rapidly and dramatically in exercise.

Capillary branching increases the total cross-sectional area of the microcirculation 800 times more than the 1-inch diameter aorta. Because blood flow velocity relates inversely to the vasculature's total cross section, velocity progressively decreases as blood moves toward and into the capillaries.

Veins

The vascular system maintains continuity of blood flow as capillaries feed deoxygenated blood at almost a trickle into the small veins or **venules** (Fig. 10.3). Blood flow then increases slightly because the venous system's cross-sectional area becomes less than for capillaries. The lower body's smaller veins eventually empty into the largest vein, the **inferior vena cava**, which travels through the abdominal and thoracic cavities toward the heart. Venous blood draining the head, neck, and shoulder regions empties into the **superior vena cava** and moves downward to join the inferior vena cava at heart level. The mixture of blood from the upper and lower body then enters the **right atrium** and descends into the **right ventricle** for delivery through the pulmonary artery to the lungs. Gas exchange takes place in the lungs' alveolar-capillary network; here, the pulmonary veins return oxygenated blood to the left heart pump, where the journey through the body resumes.

Venous Return A unique characteristic of veins solves a potential problem related to the low pressure of venous blood. **Figure 10.4** shows that thin, membranous, flap-like valves spaced at short intervals within the vein permit one-way blood flow back to the heart. Veins compress because of low venous blood pressure, muscular contractions, or minor pressure changes within the chest cavity during breathing. Alternate venous compression and relaxation, combined with the one-way action of valves, provides a "milking" effect similar to the action of the heart. Venous compression imparts considerable energy for blood flow, whereas "diastole" (relaxation) allows vessels to refill as blood moves toward the heart. Without valves, blood would stagnate or pool (as it sometimes does) in extremity veins, and people would faint every time they stood up because of reduced blood flow to the brain.

A Significant Blood Reservoir The veins do not merely function as passive conduits. At rest, the venous system normally contains about 65% of total blood volume; hence, veins serve as capacitance vessels or blood reservoirs. A slight increase in tension (tone) by the vein's smooth muscle layer alters the diameter of the venous tree. A generalized increase in **venous tone** rapidly redistributes blood from peripheral veins toward the central blood volume returning to the heart. *In this manner, the venous system plays an important role as an **active** blood reservoir to either retard or enhance blood flow to the systemic circulation.*

Varicose Veins Sometimes valves within a vein become defective and do not maintain one-way blood flow. This condition of **varicose veins** usually occurs in superficial veins of the lower extremities from the force of gravity that retards

For Your Information

Determinants of Blood Pressure
Arterial blood pressure affects arterial blood flow per minute (cardiac output) and peripheral vascular resistance to blood flow in the following relationships:

Blood pressure

= Cardiac output

× Total peripheral resistance

Total peripheral resistance

= Blood pressure

÷ Cardiac output

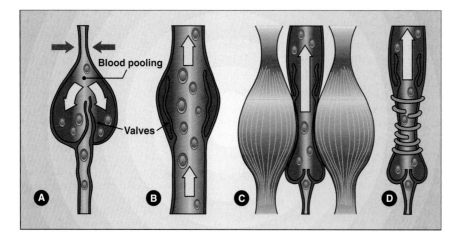

Figure 10.4 The valves in veins (**A**) prevent the backflow of blood but do not hinder the (**B**) normal one-way flow of blood. (**C**) Contraction of nearby active muscle or (**D**) constriction of smooth muscle bands within veins propels blood through the venous circuit.

blood flow in an upright posture. As blood accumulates, these veins distend excessively and become painful, often impairing circulation from surrounding areas. In severe cases, the venous wall becomes inflamed and degenerates, a condition called **phlebitis**, which often requires surgical removal of the damaged vessel.

Individuals with varicose veins should avoid excessive straining exercises like heavy resistance training. During sustained, non-rhythmic muscle actions, the muscle and ventilatory "pumps" do not contribute to venous return. Increased abdominal pressure with straining also impedes blood flow return. These factors cause blood to pool (temporarily stagnate) in the veins of the lower body which could aggravate existing varicose veins. Whether regular aerobic exercise prevents the occurrence of varicose veins remains unknown. Rhythmic physical activity could minimize complications because dynamic muscle actions continually propel peripheral blood toward the heart.

Venous Pooling   The fact that people faint when forced to maintain an upright posture without movement (e.g., standing at attention for a prolonged period) demonstrates the importance of muscle contractions to venous return. Also, changing from a lying to a standing position affects the dynamics of venous return and triggers physiologic responses. Heart rate and blood pressure stabilize during bed rest. If a person suddenly rises and remains erect, an uninterrupted column of blood exists from heart level to the toes, creating a hydrostatic force of 80 to 100 mm Hg. Swelling (edema) occurs from pooling of blood in the lower extremities and creates "back pressure" that forces fluid from the capillary bed into surrounding tissues. Concurrently, impaired venous return decreases blood pressure; at the same time, heart rate accelerates and venous tone increases to counter the hypotensive condition. Maintaining an upright position without movement leads to dizziness and eventual fainting from insufficient cerebral blood supply. Resuming a horizontal or head-down position restores circulation and consciousness.

Active Cool-Down   The potential for venous pooling justifies continued slow jogging or walking immediately following strenuous exercise. "Cooling down" with rhythmic exercise facilitates blood flow through the vascular circuit (including the heart) during recovery. An "active recovery" of light to moderate exercise also speeds lactate removal from the blood. Pressurized suits worn by test pilots and special support stockings also retard hydrostatic shifts of blood to veins of the lower extremities in the upright position. A similar supportive effect occurs in upright exercise in a swimming pool because the water's external support facilitates venous return.

BLOOD PRESSURE

A surge of blood enters the aorta with each contraction of the left ventricle, distending the vessel and creating pressure within it. The stretch and subsequent recoil of the aortic wall propagates as a wave through the entire arterial system. The pressure wave readily appears as a pulse in the following areas: the superficial radial artery on the thumb side of the wrist, the temporal artery (on the side of the head at the temple), and carotid artery along the side of the trachea. In healthy persons, pulse rate equals heart rate.

Rest

The highest pressure generated by left ventricular contraction (**systole**) to move blood through a healthy, resilient arterial system at rest usually reaches 120 mm Hg. As the heart relaxes (**diastole**) and aortic valves close, the natural elastic recoil of the aorta and other arteries provides a continuous head of pressure to move blood into the periphery until the next surge from ventricular systole. During the cardiac cycle's diastole, arterial blood pressure decreases to 70 to 80 mm Hg. Arteries "hardened" by mineral and fatty deposits within their walls or arteries with excessive peripheral resistance to blood flow from kidney malfunction induce systolic pressures as high as 300 mm Hg and diastolic pressures above 120 mm Hg.

High blood pressure (**hypertension**) imposes a chronic strain on normal cardiovascular function. If left untreated, severe hypertension leads to congestive heart failure as the heart muscle weakens, unable to maintain its normal pumping ability. Degenerating, brittle vessels can obstruct blood flow, or can burst, cutting off vital blood flow to brain tissue and precipitating a stroke.

During Exercise

Rhythmic Exercise   During rhythmic muscular activities like brisk walking, hiking, jogging, swimming, and bicycling, dilation of the active muscles' blood vessels increases the vascular area for blood flow. The alternate, rhythmic contraction and relaxation of skeletal muscles forces blood through the vessels and returns it to the heart. Increased blood flow during moderate exercise increases systolic pressure in the first few minutes; it then levels off, usually between 140 and 160 mm Hg. Diastolic pressure remains relatively unchanged.

Figure 10.5 illustrates the relationship between blood pressure during exercise of progressively increasing intensity and the quantity of blood ejected into the arterial circuit each minute (cardiac output). Various indices of arterial blood pressure increase linearly with cardiac output, with the largest increases occurring during cardiac systole. Diastolic pressure increases only about 12% during the full range of exercise intensities. Exercise-trained and sedentary subjects show similar responses. However, systolic blood pressure often increases to 200 mm Hg during maximum exercise in healthy endurance athletes because of these athletes' large cardiac outputs.

Resistance Exercise   Straining-type exercise (e.g., heavy resistance exercise, shoveling wet snow) increases blood pressure dramatically because sustained muscular force compresses peripheral arterioles, considerably increasing resist-

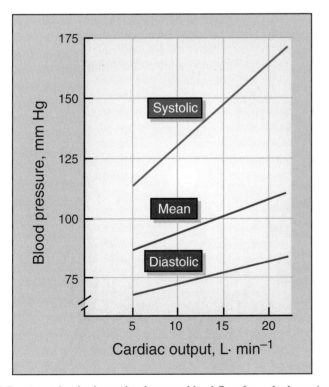

Figure 10.5   Generalized relationship between blood flow from the heart (cardiac output) and systemic arterial pressures measured at the brachial artery during exercise. Mean arterial blood pressure represents the average force exerted by the blood against the arterial walls during the entire cardiac cycle. It equals slightly less than the arithmetic average of the systolic and diastolic pressures because the heart remains in diastole longer than in systole.

Questions & Notes

Give a normal blood pressure at rest.

Systolic –

Diastolic –

Systolic blood pressure estimates what physiologic factor?

Describe the relationship between systolic blood pressure and cardiac output during exercise of increasing intensity.

What happens to blood pressure during resistance exercise?

FOR YOUR INFORMATION

Hypertension and Race
African-Americans have twice the incidence of high blood pressure as white counterparts and nearly seven times the rate of severe hypertension. The fact that African-Americans in the United States have a much greater incidence of hypertension than blacks in Africa compounds the issue of race and hypertension. Ongoing research focuses on diet, stress, cigarette smoking, and other lifestyle and environmental factors that trigger this chronic blood pressure response in genetically susceptible blacks. (*http://www.ash-us.org/*)

Box 10–1 • CLOSE UP

HOW TO MEASURE BLOOD PRESSURE

Blood pressure represents the force (pressure) exerted by blood against the arterial walls during a cardiac cycle. Systolic blood pressure, the higher of the two pressure measurements, occurs during ventricular contraction (systole) as the heart propels 70 to 100 mL of blood into the aorta. After systole, the ventricles relax (diastole), the arteries recoil, and arterial pressure continually declines as blood flows into the periphery and the heart refills with blood. The lowest pressure reached during ventricular relaxation represents diastolic blood pressure. Normal systolic blood pressure in an adult varies between 110 and 130 mm Hg, and diastolic pressure varies between 60 and 85 mm Hg. Elevated systolic or diastolic blood pressure (termed Stage 1 hypertension) is defined as a resting systolic blood pressure of 139 mm Hg or greater and diastolic pressure 90 mm Hg and above. The accompanying table (next page) lists the latest guidelines for adults for the classification and management of hypertension.

Pulse pressure reflects the difference between systolic and diastolic pressures.

MEASUREMENT PROCEDURES

Blood pressure is measured indirectly by **auscultation** (listening to sounds; described in 1902 by Russian physician N.S. Korotkoff; 1874–1920), which uses a stethoscope and sphygmomanometer, consisting of a blood pressure cuff and an aneroid or mercury column pressure gauge.

1. Subject sits in a quiet room with the upper arm exposed.
2. Subject bends the arm to bring the elbow to heart level.
3. Locate the brachial artery at the inner side of the upper arm, approximately 1 inch above the bend in the elbow.
4. Take the free end of the cuff and gently slide it through the metal loop (or wrap over exposed velcro) and flap it back over so the cuff wraps around the upper arm at heart level. Align the arrows on the cuff with the brachial artery. Secure the velcro parts of the cuff. The sphygmomanometer cuff should fit snugly (but not tight) to obtain accurate readings. Use appropriate-sized cuffs for children and the obese.
5. Place the stethoscope bell below the antecubital space over the brachial artery.
6. The cuff should now have the connecting tube (from the sphygmomanometer bulb and gauge) exiting the cuff towards the arm.
7. Before inflating the cuff, make sure the air release valve remains closed (turn the knob clockwise).

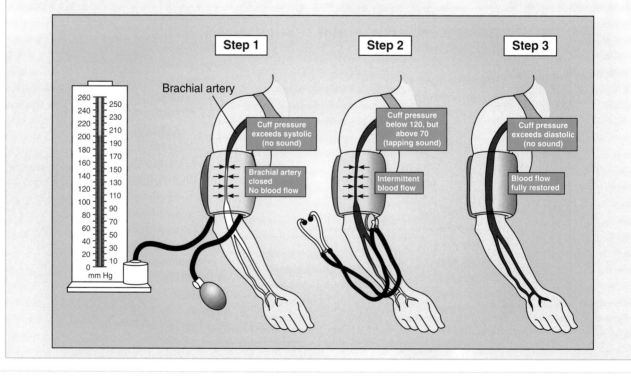

Box 10-1 • CLOSE UP *(Continued)*

8. Inflate the cuff with quick, even pumps to about 180 mm Hg.
9. Gradually release cuff pressure (about 3 mm per s) by slowly opening the air release knob (counter-clockwise turn), noting the first sound that results from turbulence from the rush of blood as the formerly closed artery briefly opens during the highest pressure in the cardiac cycle. *This represents systolic blood pressure.*

10. Continue to reduce the pressure, noting when the sound becomes muffled (*4th phase diastolic pressure*) and when the sound disappears (*5th phase diastolic pressure*). Clinicians usually record the 5th phase as diastolic blood pressure.
11. If the measured pressure exceeds 140/90 mm Hg, allow a 10-minute rest and repeat the procedure.

Blood Pressure Classification and Management for Adults

BP CLASSIFICATION	SBP* MMHG	DBP* MMHG	WITHOUT LIFESTYLE MODIFICATON	WITHOUT COMPELLING INDICATION	WITH COMPELLING INDICATION**
Normal	<120	and <80	Encourage		
Prehypertension	120–139	or 80–89	Yes	No drugs indicated	Drug(s) for compelling indications
Stage 1 Hypertension	140–159	or 90–99	Yes	Thiazide-type diuretics for most. May consider ACEI, ARB, BB, CCB, or combination	Drug(s) for compelling indications.** Other antihypertensive drugs (diuretics, ACEI, ARB, BB, CCB) as needed.
Stage 2 Hypertension	≥160	or ≥100	Yes	Two-drug combination for most*** (usually thiazide-type diuretic and ACEI or ARB or BB or CCB)	

DBP = diastolic blood pressure; SBP = systolic blood pressure.
*Treatment determined by highest BP category.
**Compelling indications include individuals with heart failure, postmyocardial infarction, high coronary disease risk and diabetes.
***Initial combined therapy should be used cautiously for those at risk for orthostatic hypotension; treat patients with chronic kidney disease or diabetes to BP goal of <130/80 mmHg.
ACEI = angiotensin converting enzyme inhibitor; ARB = angiotensin receptor blocker; BB = beta blocker; CCB = calcium channel blocker.
From: Seventh report of the joint committee on prevention, detection, evaluation, and treatment of high blood pressure (JNCV): US Department of Health and Human Services. National Institutes of Health, National Heart, Lung, and Blood Institute. National High Blood Pressure Education Program. NIH Publication No. 03-5233, May, 2003.

ance to blood flow. The heart's additional workload from acute elevations in blood pressure increases risk for individuals with existing hypertension or coronary heart disease. In such cases, rhythmic forms of moderate physical activity provide less risk and greater health benefits. **Figure 10.6** shows blood pressure responses during rhythmic aerobic exercise and heavy resistance movements that engage small and large amounts of muscle mass.

Upper-Body Exercise Exercise at a given percentage of $\dot{V}O_{2max}$ increases systolic and diastolic blood pressures substantially more in rhythmic arm (upper-body) compared with rhythmic leg (lower-body) exercise. The smaller arm muscle mass and vasculature offer greater resistance to blood flow than the larger and more vascularized lower-body regions. This means that blood flow to the arms

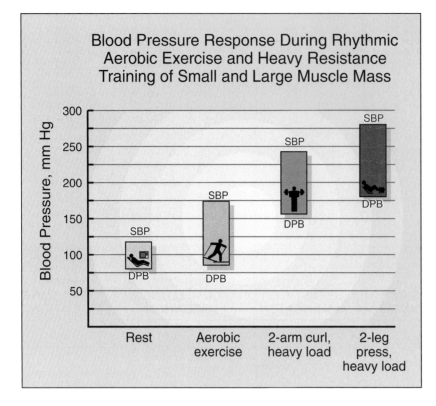

Figure 10.6 Blood pressure response during rhythmic aerobic exercise and heavy resistance training of a small (arms) and large (legs) muscle mass. The top of each bar represents systolic blood pressure; the bottom represents diastolic blood pressure.

during exercise requires a much larger systolic pressure head and accompanying increase in myocardial workload and vascular strain. For individuals with cardiovascular dysfunction, more prudent exercise involves larger muscle groups (walking, running, bicycling, stair climbing) rather than unregulated exercises of a limited muscle mass (shoveling, overhead hammering, or even arm-crank ergometry).

In Recovery

After a bout of sustained light- to moderate-intensity exercise, systolic blood pressure temporarily decreases below pre-exercise levels for up to 12 hours in normal and hypertensive subjects. Pooling of blood in the visceral organs and lower limbs during recovery reduces central blood volume, which contributes to lower blood pressure. The **hypotensive recovery response** further supports exercise as an important non-pharmacologic hypertension therapy. A potentially effective approach spreads several bouts of moderate physical activity throughout the day.

HEART'S BLOOD SUPPLY

Over 7000 gallons of blood flow from the heart each day, but none of its oxygen or nutrients pass directly to the myocardium from the heart's chambers. The myocardium maintains its own elaborate circulatory system. **Figure 10.7** illustrates these vessels as a visible, crown-like network, the **coronary circulation**, that arises from the top portion of the heart.

The openings for the left and right coronary arteries emerge from the aorta just above the semilunar valves where oxygenated blood leaves the left ventricle. The arteries then curl around the heart's surface; the **right coronary artery** supplies predominantly the right atrium and ventricle, whereas the greatest blood volume flows in the **left coronary artery** to the left atrium and ventricle, and a small portion of the right ventricle. These vessels divide to eventually form a dense capillary network within the myocardium. Blood leaves the tissues of the left ventricle through the coronary sinus; blood from the right ventricle exits through the anterior cardiac veins and empties directly into the right atrium.

Myocardial Oxygen Utilization

Oxygen utilization by the heart muscle remains high in relation to its blood flow. At rest, the myocardium extracts 70% to 80% of the oxygen from the blood flowing in the coronary vessels. In contrast, most other tissues use only about 25% of the blood's available oxygen. Because near-maximal oxygen extraction occurs in the myocardium at rest, increases in coronary blood flow provide the primary means to meet myocardial oxygen demands in exercise. In vigorous exercise, coronary blood flow increases four to six times above the resting level because of elevated myocardial metabolism and increased aortic pressure.

Anterior view

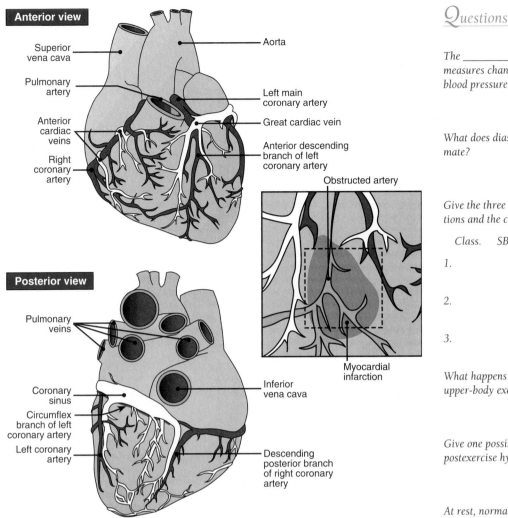

Superior vena cava

Pulmonary artery

Anterior cardiac veins

Right coronary artery

Aorta

Left main coronary artery

Great cardiac vein

Anterior descending branch of left coronary artery

Obstructed artery

Myocardial infarction

Posterior view

Pulmonary veins

Coronary sinus

Circumflex branch of left coronary artery

Left coronary artery

Inferior vena cava

Descending posterior branch of right coronary artery

Figure 10.7   Anterior and posterior views of the coronary circulation, with arteries shaded dark and veins unshaded. Inset figure illustrates a myocardial infarction resulting from the blockage (occlusion) of a coronary vessel.

Profuse myocardial vascularization supplies each muscle fiber with at least one capillary. Adequate oxygenation becomes so crucial that impairment in coronary blood flow triggers chest discomfort and pain, a condition termed **angina pectoris**. The pain increases during exercise when myocardial oxygen demand rises considerably and supply remains limited. A blood clot (**thrombus**) lodged in one of the coronary vessels can severely impair normal heart function. This form of "heart attack" (**termed myocardial infarction**) often injures the myocardium; severe damage to this muscle can result in death.

Rate-Pressure Product: An Estimate of Myocardial Work   Three important mechanical factors determine myocardial oxygen uptake:

1. Tension development within the myocardium
2. Myocardial contractility
3. Heart rate

When each of these factors increases during exercise, myocardial blood flow adjusts to balance oxygen supply with demand. The product of systolic blood pres-

Questions & Notes

The _____ method measures changes in sound to estimate blood pressure.

What does diastolic blood pressure estimate?

Give the three blood pressure classifications and the cut-off values for each:

   Class.   *SBP Cut-off*   *DBP Cut-off*

1.

2.

3.

What happens to blood pressure during upper-body exercise?

Give one possible explanation for the postexercise hypotensive response.

At rest, normal blood flow to the myocardium represents approximately _____ percent of total cardiac output.

At rest, how much oxygen is extracted from the coronary blood flow?

List 2 factors that increase coronary blood flow during vigorous exercise.

  1.

  2.

Write the equation for the rate-pressure product.

What is RPP related to?

sure (SBP; measured at the brachial artery) and heart rate (HR) provides a convenient estimate of myocardial workload (oxygen uptake). This index of *relative* cardiac work, called the **double product** or **rate-pressure product (RPP)**, closely reflects directly measured myocardial oxygen uptake and coronary blood flow in healthy subjects over a range of exercise intensities. RPP computes as:

$$RPP = SBP \times HR$$

Exercise studies of people with coronary heart disease have linked the RPP to the onset of angina and/or electrocardiographic abnormalities. RPP has also assessed various clinical, surgical, and exercise interventions for their effects on cardiac performance. The reductions in exercise heart rate and systolic blood pressure at a specific level of submaximal effort with endurance training improve cardiac patients' exercise capacity because of the reduced myocardial oxygen requirement. In addition, aerobic training increases the RPP of patients before they experience the onset of heart disease symptoms. In nine patients who were followed over 7 years of exercise training, RPP increased 11.5% before ischemic abnormalities appeared. These important findings provide indirect evidence for a training-induced improvement in myocardial oxygenation, perhaps from greater coronary vascularization, reduced obstruction, or a combination of both factors. Typical values for RPP range from 6000 at rest (HR = 50 b·min^{-1}; SBP = 120 mm Hg) to 40,000 during intense exercise (HR = 200 b·min^{-1}; SBP = 200 mm Hg). Changes in heart rate and blood pressure contribute equally to a change in RPP.

Heart's Energy Supply

The heart relies almost exclusively on aerobic energy metabolism. Myocardial fibers contain the greatest mitochondrial concentration of all tissues, with exceptional capacity for long-chain fatty acid catabolism as a primary fuel for ATP resynthesis. Glucose and the lactate formed in skeletal muscle during anaerobic glycolysis also provide energy for proper myocardial functioning. In essence, the heart uses whatever energy substrate it "sees" on a physiologic level. After a meal, for example, glucose becomes the preferred energy substrate. When lactate efflux from skeletal muscle into blood increases during heavy exercise, the heart derives as much as 50% of its total energy by oxidizing circulating lactate. During prolonged submaximal exercise, myocardial free fatty acid catabolism increases to nearly 70% of the heart's total energy requirement.

SUMMARY

1. The heart functions as two separate pumps: one pump receives blood from the body and pumps it to the lungs for aeration (pulmonary circulation); the other pump accepts oxygenated blood from the lungs and pumps it throughout the body (systemic circulation).

2. Pressure changes during the cardiac cycle act on the heart's valves to provide one-way blood flow through the vascular circuit.

3. The dense capillary network provides a large, effective surface for exchange between blood and tissues. These microscopic vessels adjust blood flow in response to the tissue's metabolic activity.

4. Vein compression and relaxation through muscle actions impart considerable energy for venous return. "Muscle-pump" action justifies use of active recovery from vigorous exercise.

5. Nerves and hormones constrict or stiffen the smooth muscle layer in venous walls. Alterations in venous tone profoundly affect redistribution of total blood volume.

6. Systolic pressure represents the highest pressure generated during the cardiac cycle; diastolic pressure describes the lowest pressure before the next ventricular contraction.

7. Hypertension imposes a chronic stress on cardiovascular function. Regular aerobic training modestly reduces systolic and diastolic blood pressures during rest and submaximal exercise.

8. During graded exercise, systolic blood pressure increases in proportion to oxygen uptake and cardiac output, whereas diastolic pressure remains unchanged or increases slightly. The same relative exercise intensity (%$\dot{V}O_{2max}$) produces a larger blood pressure response with upper-body compared with lower-body exercise.

9. During recovery from light and moderate exercise, blood pressure falls below pre-exercise levels (hypotensive response) and remains lower for up to 12 hours.

10. Peak systolic and diastolic blood pressures mirror the hypertensive state during standard resistance exercises. Inordinately high blood pressure (and rate-pressure product) in such exercise poses a risk to individuals with hypertension and coronary heart disease.

11. Regular resistance exercise training blunts the hypertensive response to straining-type exercise.

12. At rest, the myocardium extracts about 80% of the oxygen from coronary blood flow. Consequently, increased myocardial oxygen demands in exercise

depend on proportionate increases in coronary blood flow.

13. Impaired coronary blood flow causes chest discomfort and pain (angina pectoris); blockage of a coronary artery (myocardial infarction) can irreversibly damage the myocardium.

14. The product of heart rate and systolic blood pressure (rate-pressure product) estimates relative myocardial

workload. Clinicians use this index to study exercise-training effects on cardiac performance in heart disease patients.

15. Glucose, fatty acids, and lactate represent the heart's main substrates for energy metabolism. Percent utilization varies with nutritional status and with exercise intensity and duration.

THOUGHT QUESTION

What advantage does a "closed" circulatory system provide to the physically active individual?

PART 2 •
Cardiovascular Regulation and Integration

At rest in a comfortable environment, the skin receives 250 mL (5%) of the 5 L of blood pumped from the heart each minute. In contrast, 20% of the total cardiac output flows to the body's surface for heat dissipation with exercise in a hot, humid environment. The rapid redistribution ("shunting") of blood to meet metabolic and physiologic requirements (with appropriate maintenance of blood pressure) requires a closed circulatory system with both central and local control of pump output and vascular dimensions.

HEART RATE REGULATION

Cardiac muscle possesses intrinsic rhythmicity. Without external stimuli, the adult heart would beat steadily between 50 and 80 times each minute. Within the body, nerves that directly supply the myocardium and chemicals within the blood rapidly alter heart rate. Extrinsic control of cardiac function causes the heart to speed up in "anticipation," even before exercise begins. To a large extent, extrinsic regulation can adjust heart rate to as slow as 40 b·min^{-1} at rest and in some endurance athletes and as fast as 215–220 b·min^{-1} during maximum exercise.

Intrinsic Regulation

A mass of specialized muscle tissue, the **sinoatrial (S-A) node**, lies within the posterior wall of the right atrium. The S-A node spontaneously depolarizes and repolarizes to provide an "innate" stimulus to the heart. For this reason, the term "**pacemaker**" describes the S-A node. **Figure 10.8** shows the normal route for transmitting the electrical impulse across the myocardium.

Heart's Electrical Impulse

Rhythms originating at the S-A node spread across the atria to another small knot of tissue, the **atrioventricular (A-V) node**. This node delays the impulse about 0.10 seconds to provide sufficient time for the atria to contract and force blood into the ventricles. The A-V node gives rise to the **A-V bundle (bundle of His)**, which speeds the impulse rapidly through the ventricles over specialized con-

Questions & Notes

Name the heart's "pacemaker" and indicate its role.

Trace the route of the electrical impulse from the SA node into the ventricles.

Name the area where the electrical impulse originates in a healthy heart.

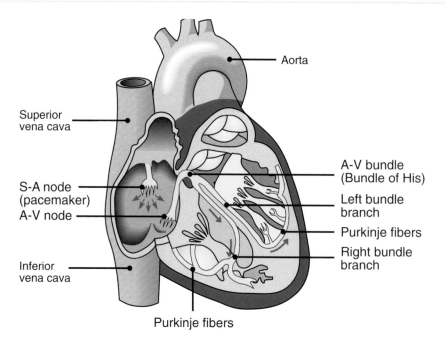

Figure 10.8 Normal route for excitation and conduction of the cardiac impulse. This impulse originates at the S-A node, travels to the A-V node, and then flows throughout the ventricular mass.

ducting fibers called the **Purkinje system**. Purkinje fibers form distinct branches that penetrate the right and left ventricles. Each ventricular cell becomes stimulated within 0.06 seconds from passage of the impulse into the ventricles; this causes simultaneous contraction of both ventricles. Cardiac impulse transmission progresses as follows:

S-A node → Atria → A-V node →

   A-V bundle (Purkinje fibers) → Ventricles

Electrocardiogram

The electrical activity generated by the myocardium creates an electrical field throughout the body. Because salty body fluid conducts electricity well, electrodes placed on the skin's surface detect the sequence of electrical events during each cardiac cycle. The **electrocardiogram (ECG)** provides a graphic record of voltage changes during the heart's electrical activity. Figure 10.9 illustrates a normal ECG with important sequences of major myocardial electrical activity.

The ECG provides a means to monitor heart rate during exercise. Radiotelemetry allows ECG transmission while a person freely performs diverse physical activities including football, weightlifting, basketball, ice hockey, dancing, and even swimming. Electrocardiography can uncover abnormalities in heart function related to cardiac rhythm, electrical conduction, myocardial oxygen supply, and actual tissue damage (see Close Up: *How to Place Electrodes for Bipolar and 12-Lead ECG Recordings*, on page 359).

Extrinsic Regulation

Neural impulses override the inherent myocardial rhythmicity. The signals originate in the cardiovascular center in the medulla and travel through the sympathetic and parasympathetic components of the autonomic nervous system.

Sympathetic Influence   Stimulation of the sympathetic cardioaccelerator nerves releases the **catecholamines** epinephrine and norepinephrine. These neural hormones increase myocardial contractility and accelerate S-A node depolarization to increase heart rate, a response termed **tachycardia**. Epinephrine, released from the medullary portion of the adrenal glands in response to general sympathetic activation, also produces a similar though slower-acting effect on cardiac function.

Parasympathetic Influence   Acetylcholine, the parasympathetic nervous system hormone, retards the sinus discharge rate to slow the heart. This response, termed **bradycardia**, comes from the **vagus nerve** whose cell bodies originate in the cardioinhibitory portion of the medulla. Vagal stimulation does not affect myocardial contractility. **Table 10.1** summarizes the effects of the autonomic nervous system on cardiovascular function.

Vascular smooth muscles also contract and relax in response to chemical substances released by endothelium tissue (cells comprising the inner lining of the blood vessels). Relaxing factors include nitric oxide (NO), the most potent factor. NO, released from endothelial cells in large arteries that supply muscle, appears particularly important in supplying the muscles with adequate blood during exercise. NO is released by the endothelium in response to pulsatile blood flow and blood vessel wall stress, both of which increase during exercise. Other relaxing factors include protacyclin and endothelium-derived hyperpolarizing factor. Contracting factors include endothelin and vasoconstrictor protaglandins.

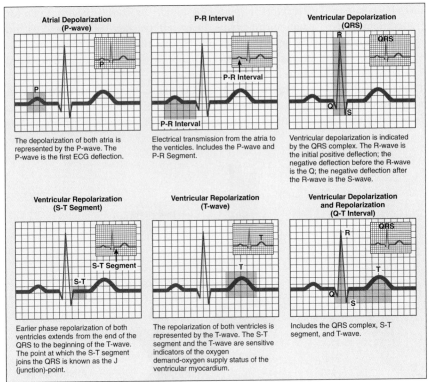

Atrial Depolarization (P-wave)

The depolarization of both atria is represented by the P-wave. The P-wave is the first ECG deflection.

P-R Interval

Electrical transmission from the atria to the ventricles. Includes the P-wave and P-R Segment.

Ventricular Depolarization (QRS)

Ventricular depolarization is indicated by the QRS complex. The R-wave is the initial positive deflection; the negative deflection before the R-wave is the Q; the negative deflection after the R-wave is the S-wave.

Ventricular Repolarization (S-T Segment)

Earlier phase repolarization of both ventricles extends from the end of the QRS to the beginning of the T-wave. The point at which the S-T segment joins the QRS is known as the J (junction)-point.

Ventricular Repolarization (T-wave)

The repolarization of both ventricles is represented by the T-wave. The S-T segment and the T-wave are sensitive indicators of the oxygen demand-oxygen supply status of the ventricular myocardium.

Ventricular Depolarization and Repolarization (Q-T Interval)

Includes the QRS complex, S-T segment, and T-wave.

Figure 10.9 Different phases of the normal electrocardiogram (ECG) from atrial depolarization (upper left) to repolarization of the ventricles (lower three figures).

Draw and label a typical ECG tracing.

List 2 uses for the ECG.

1.

2.

What is the function of catecholamines?

Endurance training creates an imbalance between sympathetic accelerator and parasympathetic depressor activity to favor greater vagal (parasympathetic) dominance. The effect occurs primarily from increased parasympathetic activity, with some decrease in sympathetic discharge. Training may also decrease the S-A node's intrinsic firing rate. These adaptations account for the significant bradycardia frequently observed among highly conditioned endurance athletes or sedentary individuals who undertake aerobic training.

Cortical Influence   Impulses originating in the brain's higher somatomotor **central command system** pass via small afferent nerves to directly modulate the activity of the cardiovascular center in the **ventrolateral medulla**. This provides the coordinated and rapid response of the heart and blood vessels to optimize tissue perfusion and maintain central blood pressure in relation to motor cortex involvement. The central command exerts its effect not only during exercise but also at rest and in the pre-exercise period. Thus, variation in emotional state can significantly affect cardiovascular responses, often obscuring "true" resting values for heart rate

Under what condition are you more likely to experience tachycardia?

Table 10·1	The Autonomic Nervous System and Cardiovascular Function

SYMPATHETIC INFLUENCE	PARASYMPATHETIC INFLUENCE
• Increase heart rate	• Decrease heart rate
• Increase myocardial contraction force	• Decrease myocardial contraction force
• Dilate coronary blood vessels	• Constrict coronary blood vessels
• Constrict pulmonary blood vessels	• Dilate pulmonary blood vessels
• Dilate muscle and skin blood vessels	• Constrict muscle and skin blood vessels
• Constrict blood vessels in abdomen, muscle, skin, and kidney	• Dilate blood vessels in abdomen, muscle, skin, and kidney

FOR YOUR INFORMATION

Heart's Rest Period
The heart's relatively long depolarization period requires about 0.30 seconds before the myocardium can receive another impulse and contract again. This "rest" or refractory period provides sufficient time for ventricular filling between beats.

and blood pressure. Cortical input also causes heart rate to rise rapidly in anticipation of exercise. The combined effects of an increase in sympathetic discharge and reduction of vagal tone produce the **anticipatory heart rate**.

The heart "turns on" for exercise from four sources: (1) increased sympathetic activity, (2) decreased parasympathetic activity, combined with (3) input from the brain's central command, and (4) feedback information from activation of receptors in joints and muscles as exercise begins. *Even for non-sprint events, heart rate reaches 180 b·min^{-1} within 30 seconds of 1- and 2-mile runs. Further heart rate increases progress gradually, with plateaus attained several times during the runs.

Figure 10.10 depicts major factors controlling heart rate and myocardial contractility. The medulla receives continual input about blood pressure from baroreceptors

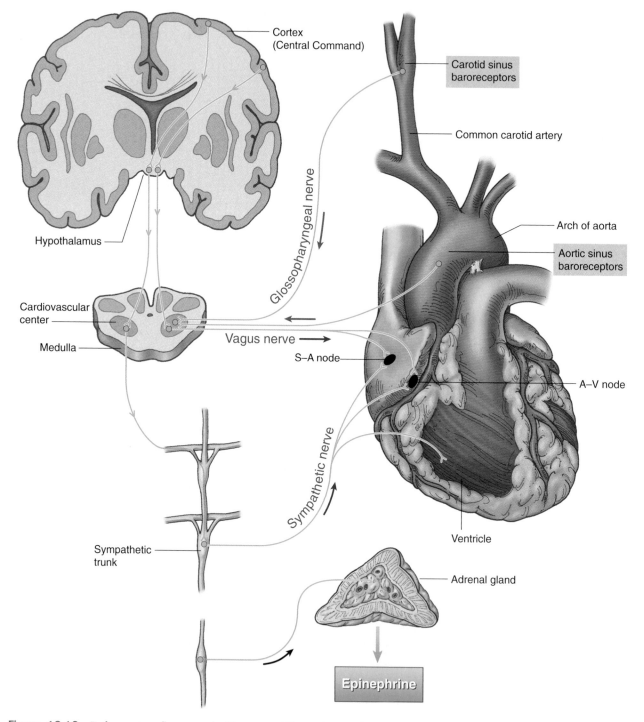

Figure 10.10   Pathways in reflex control of heart rate. The cardiovascular center in the medulla receives input from (1) baroreceptors in the carotid sinus and aortic arch and (2) cortical stimulation (central command). Efferent pathways from the medulla activate the heart by the vagus (parasympathetic) and sympathetic nerves.

within the carotid arteries and aorta. The medulla also acts as an integrating and coordinating center, receiving stimuli from the cortex and peripheral tissues, and routing an appropriate response to the heart and blood vessels.

Peripheral Input   The cardiovascular center in the medulla receives sensory input from mechanical receptors (**mechanoreceptors**) and chemical receptors (chemoreceptors) in blood vessels, joints, and muscles. Stimuli from these peripheral receptors monitor the state of active muscle; they modify either vagal or sympathetic outflow to create an appropriate cardiovascular response. Reflex neural input from active muscle, termed the **exercise pressor reflex**, in conjunction with output originating in the brain's higher motor areas, assess the nature and intensity of exercise and the quantity of muscle recruited. Input from mechanoreceptors provides particularly important feedback for the central nervous system's regulation of blood flow and blood pressure during dynamic exercise. Receptors in the aortic arch and carotid sinus respond to changes in arterial blood pressure. As blood pressure increases, the stretch of arterial vessels activates these **baroreceptors**, which reflexly slows heart rate and dilates peripheral vasculature. This lowers blood pressure toward normal levels. Exercise overrides this particular feedback mechanism because both heart rate and blood pressure increase. Baroreceptors likely prevent abnormally high blood pressure levels in exercise.

Carotid Artery Palpation   For healthy adults and cardiac patients, **carotid artery palpation** has little effect on heart rate during rest, exercise, and recovery. Certain vascular diseases, however, affect carotid sinus sensitivity. Under these conditions, strong external pressure against the carotid artery slows heart rate, probably from direct stimulation of carotid artery baroreceptors.

Accurate heart rate measurement provides the basis for establishing "target heart rates" during exercise training. If heart rate measurement consistently underestimated actual values, the person would exercise at higher levels than prescribed, which is certainly an undesirable effect when prescribing exercise for cardiac patients. An excellent substitute method involves determining pulse rate at the radial or temporal arteries (see Close Up: *Assessing Heart Rate by Palpation and Auscultation Methods*, page 346) because palpation at these sites does not change heart rate.

Arrhythmias

The exquisite regulation of heart rate by intrinsic and extrinsic mechanisms generally progresses unnoticed and without adverse consequence. However, electrocardiographic and heart rate irregularities do occur and can herald significant myocardial disease. The term **arrhythmia** describes heart rhythm irregularities.

Heart Rate Irregularities   Interruption of regular heart rate pattern often occurs as extra beats (**extrasystoles**). Parts of the atria can become prematurely electrically active and depolarize spontaneously prior to S-A node excitation, a condition called **premature atrial contraction** or **PAC**. Premature excitation of ventricles (**premature ventricular contraction** or **PVC**) also occurs during the interval between two regular beats. Occasional extrasystoles appear during rest and usually progress unnoticed. Psychological stress, anxiety, and caffeine consumption can trigger extrasystoles, probably from the effects of catecholamines on the rate of change of the S-A node's membrane potential. Removal of such stimuli usually re-establishes normal heart rhythm. If this fails, medication blocking norepinephrine's action on the beta-receptors of atrial cells (**beta-blockers**) effectively treats this condition. Atrial arrhythmias do not compromise the heart's pumping ability (recall that atrial contraction contributes little to ventricular filling). A potentially dangerous situation arises when PACs link successively to create **atrial fibrillation**.

Questions & Notes

Name the cardiovascular control center that regulates the output of blood from the heart.

What autonomic neural fibers stimulate atria and ventricles?

Atria:

Ventricles:

Name the two catecholamines.

1.

2.

What is another name for the sympathetic constrictor fibers?

Cholinergic nerve fibers release _____.

FOR YOUR INFORMATION

ECG or EKG?

The electrocardiogram (ECG) sometimes appears abbreviated as EKG. The "K" comes from the German spelling of the word electrocardiograph. In 1895, Dutch physiologist Wilhelm Einthoven (1860–1927), the 1924 Noble Prize winner in physiology or medicine for his pioneering work in myocardial electrophysiology, made the first tracings of the heart's electrical activity. He used his invention of a 500-pound string galvanometer (thin quartz wire in a magnetic field) to record the heart's electrical activity.

Box 10–2 • CLOSE UP

ASSESSING HEART RATE BY PALPATION AND AUSCULTATION METHODS

The rate of the cardiac cycle (heart rate or HR) provides a fundamental tool to set exercise intensity and assess changes from exercise training. Four methods can measure heart rate: (1) by ear (auscultation), (2) by touch (palpation), (3) with a heart rate monitor, or (4) using an ECG recorder (electrical). The auscultation and palpation methods are practical and useful.

FACTORS THAT AFFECT HEART RATE

1. Drugs and medications: many drugs and drug-containing compounds like coffee (caffeine) and tobacco increase HR
2. Muscular activity: any muscular activity (even activation of postural muscles during standing) increases HR
3. Dietary status: HR increases with food consumption
4. Environment: noise, temperature extremes, and air pollution can increase HR

HEART RATE BY THE AUSCULTATION METHOD

The auscultation method uses a stethoscope to amplify and direct sound waves, thus bringing the ear of the listener closer to the sound source (heart).

Using the stethoscope

1. With the ear tips of the stethoscope pointing forward, insert them directly down each ear canal.
2. Gently tap the diaphragm of the stethoscope to be sure you can hear the sound adequately.
3. Position the stethoscope just below the left breast (pectoralis major muscle) over the third intercostal space to the left of the sternum.

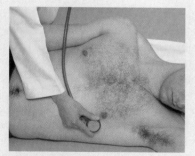

(Reprinted with permission from Bickely, L. S.: *Bate's Guide to Physical Examination and History Taking.* 8th Ed. Philadelphia: Lippincott Williams & Wilkins, 2003.

4. Hold the diaphragm of the stethoscope firmly against the skin (not over clothing).

Auscultation of the heartbeat at rest with a stethoscope is often more difficult than during exercise because heart sounds are less pronounced during rest.

HEART RATE BY PALPATION

Heart rate measurement by palpation is the most practical of the four methods. Palpation feels a pulse or vibration with the finger or hand. The pulse wave generated by the pumping of blood through the arteries appears over the radial or carotid arteries. Use the tip of the middle and index fingers; do not use the thumb because it has a pulse of its own and may confound results. Press lightly with the fingers to avoid obstructing blood flow.

An **apical beat** (vibration pulse) generated by the left ventricle hitting the chest wall near the left fifth rib becomes prominent immediately following exercise in lean individuals. Position the entire hand over the left side of the chest at heart level to palpate an apical beat.

Location for Palpation Method

The four common palpation sites include:

1. *Brachial artery*: anteromedial aspect of the arm below the belly of the biceps brachii, 2 to 3 cm (1 in) above the antecubital fossa
2. *Carotid artery*: just lateral to the larynx (do not apply excessive pressure at this site because it may trigger a reflex that slows HR)
3. *Radial artery*: anterolateral aspect of the wrist directly in line with the base of the thumb
4. *Temporal artery*: at the temple, around the hairline of the head

COUNTING HEART RATE

Record HR as a rate per minute (e.g., 150 b·min^{-1}). Two common methods for counting HR include the timed heart rate method and the thirty-beat heart rate method.

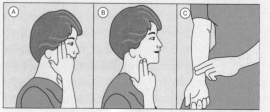

Three typical locations for palpating pulse: (A) temporal; (B) carotid; (C) radial arteries.

Box 10–2 • CLOSE UP *(Continued)*

Timed Heart Rate Method

This method counts the number of pulses in a specific amount of time. Usually, pulse counts are taken for 6, 10, or 15 seconds. If palpating the pulse for 6 seconds, multiply by 10 to express as a per-minute rate; for a 10-second palpation, multiply by 6; and if palpating for 15 seconds, multiply the pulse count by 4. Table 1 presents the HR conversion for each of the above 6-, 10-, or 15-second multiplications. Obviously, the 6-second count produces the least accurate pulse count.

| Table 1 | Heart Rate (bpm) Conversion. Find the Number of Pulse Counts for 6, 10, or 15 Seconds; Read Across for the bpm | | | | |

6-S COUNT	PER MIN RATE	10-S COUNT	PER MIN RATE	15-S COUNT	PER MIN RATE
4	40	7	42	10	40
5	50	8	48	11	44
6	60	9	54	12	48
7	70	10	60	13	52
8	80	11	66	14	56
9	90	12	72	15	60
10	100	13	78	16	64
11	110	14	84	17	68
12	120	15	90	18	72
13	130	16	96	19	76
14	140	17	102	20	80
15	150	18	108	21	84
16	160	19	114	22	88
17	170	20	120	23	92
18	180	21	126	24	96
19	190	22	132	25	100
20	200	23	138	26	104
21	210	24	144	27	108
22	220	25	150	28	112
		26	156	29	116
		27	162	30	120
		28	168	31	124
		29	174	32	128
		30	180	33	132
		31	186	34	136
		32	192	35	140
		33	198	36	144
		34	204	37	148
		35	210	38	152
		36	216	39	156
		37	222	40	160
				41	164
				42	168
				43	172
				44	176
				45	180
				46	184
				47	188
				48	192
				49	196
				50	200
				51	204
				52	208
				53	212
				54	216
				55	220

Box 10–2 • CLOSE UP *(Continued)*

Thirty-Beat Heart Rate Method

This method counts the time for 30 pulse beats to occur. Count the first beat as "zero" and simultaneously begin to record the time to count 30-pulse beats. The computational formula for computing HR in beats per min (bpm) follows:

$$HR \text{ (bpm)} = 30 \text{ b} \div \text{time (s)} \times 60 \text{ s} \div 1 \text{ min}$$

For example, if 30 beats (b) occur in 20 seconds:

$$
\begin{aligned}
HR \text{ (bpm)} &= 30 \text{ b} \div \text{time (s)} \times 60 \text{ s} \div 1 \text{ min} \\
&= 30 \text{ b} \div 20 \text{ s} \times 60 \text{ s} \div 1 \text{ min} \\
&= 1.5 \times 60 \\
&= 90 \text{ bpm}
\end{aligned}
$$

Table 2 presents a conversion chart for the above method, with HR rounded to the nearest whole number. Find the time for recording 30 beats and the corresponding heart rate (bpm).

Table 2	Conversion Chart for 30-Beat Heart Rate Method				
TIME FOR 30 BEATS, S	**HR, BPM**	**TIME FOR 30 BEATS, S**	**HR, BPM**	**TIME FOR 30 BEATS, S**	**HR, BPM**
8	225	21	86	34	53
9	200	22	82	35	51
10	180	23	78	36	50
11	164	24	75	37	49
12	150	25	72	38	47
13	138	26	69	39	46
14	129	27	67	40	45
15	120	28	64	41	44
16	113	29	62	42	43
17	106	30	60	43	42
18	100	31	58	44	41
19	95	32	56	45	40
20	90	33	55		

REFERENCE

http://sprojects.mmi.mcgill.ca/heart/egcyhome.html. The Online Journal of Cardiology.

Ventricular fibrillation is the most serious cardiac arrhythmia. With this condition, foci of stimulation continually affect different parts of the ventricle, rather than the normal single stimulus from the A-V node. *Portions of the ventricle contract in an uncoordinated manner with repetitive PVCs, thus hindering the ventricle's ability to pump blood. Cardiac output and blood pressure decrease, and the person rapidly loses consciousness.*

Resuscitation takes two forms: (1) re-establish normal heart pumping action to restore blood pressure and blood flow and (2) halt fibrillation and re-establish normal electrical rhythm. **Cardiopulmonary resuscitation (CPR)** mechanically simulates the heart's pumping action and often reverses fibrillation. If this fails, a defibrillator applies a strong burst of electric current across the entire myocardium. This depolarizes the heart, which can initiate normal rhythm from the S-A node upon repolarization. All exercise specialists need to be CPR certified (and re-certified each year). The American Red Cross maintains CPR testing and certification programs for all interested persons (*http://www.redcross.org/; http://depts. washington.edu/learncpr/*).

BLOOD DISTRIBUTION

Exercise Effects

Increased energy expenditure requires rapid readjustments in blood flow that affect the entire cardiovascular system. For example, nerves and local metabolic conditions act on the smooth muscle bands of arteriole walls, causing them to alter their internal diameter almost instantaneously. Concurrently, neural stimulation of venous capacitance vessels causes them to "stiffen," moving blood from peripheral veins into the central circulation.

During exercise, the vascular portion of active muscles increases through dilation of local arterioles; at the same time, other vessels constrict to "shut down" blood flow to tissues that can temporarily compromise blood supply. Kidney function vividly illustrates regulatory capacity for adjusting regional blood flow. Renal circulation at rest normally averages 1100 mL·min^{-1} or about 20% of cardiac output. In maximal exercise, renal blood flow decreases to 250 mL·min^{-1}, which represents only 1% of a 25-L exercise cardiac output.

Blood Flow Regulation

Pressure differentials and resistances determine fluid movement through a vessel. Resistance varies directly with the length of the vessel and inversely with its diameter; greater driving force increases flow, while increased resistance impedes it. The following equation expresses the interaction between pressure, resistance, and fluid flow:

$$\text{Flow} = \text{Pressure} \div \text{Resistance}$$

Three factors determine resistance to blood flow:

1. Viscosity or blood thickness
2. Length of conducting tube
3. Radius of blood vessel

The following equation, referred to as **Poiseuille's law**, expresses the general relationship between pressure differential (gradient), resistance, and flow in a cylindrical vessel:

$$\text{Flow} = \text{Pressure gradient} \times \text{Vessel radius}^4 \div \text{Vessel length}$$
$$\times \text{Fluid viscosity}$$

Blood viscosity and transport vessel length remain relatively constant in the body. Consequently, blood vessel radius represents the most important factor affecting blood flow. *Resistance to flow changes with vessel radius raised to the fourth power.* Reducing a vessel's radius by one-half decreases flow by a factor of 16; conversely, doubling the radius increases volume 16-fold. This means that a relatively small degree of vasoconstriction or vasodilation dramatically alters regional blood flow.

Local Factors

One of every 30 to 40 capillaries actually remains open in muscle tissue at rest. Thus, opening of large numbers of "dormant" capillaries with exercise serves three important functions:

1. Increases muscle blood flow
2. Only a small increase in velocity accompanies an increase in blood-flow volume
3. Increases effective surface for gas and nutrient exchange between blood and individual muscle fibers

A decrease in tissue oxygen supply stimulates local vasodilation in skeletal and cardiac muscle. Local increases in temperature, carbon dioxide, acidity, adenosine, nitric oxide, and magnesium and potassium ions also enhance regional blood flow. These **autoregulatory mechanisms** for blood flow make sense physiologically because they reflect elevated tissue metabolism and increased oxygen need. Rapid, local vasodilation provides the most effective, immediate step for increasing a tissue's oxygen supply.

Neural Factors

Central vascular control via sympathetic and, to a minor degree, parasympathetic portions of the autonomic nervous system overrides vasoregulation afforded by local factors. For example, muscles contain small sensory nerve fibers highly sensitive to chemical substances released in active muscle during exercise. Stimulation of these fibers provides input to the central nervous system to bring about appropriate cardiovascular responses. With central regulation, blood flow in one area cannot dominate when a concurrent oxygen need exists in other, more "needy" tissues.

Sympathetic nerve fibers end in the muscular layers of small arteries, arterioles, and precapillary sphincters. Norepinephrine acts as a general vasoconstrictor released at certain sympathetic nerve endings (**adrenergic fibers**). Other sympathetic neurons in skeletal and heart muscle release acetylcholine; these **cholinergic fibers** dilate the blood vessel. Continual sympathetic constrictor neuron activity maintains a relative state of vasoconstriction termed **vasomotor tone**. Dilation of blood vessels regulated by adrenergic neurons results more from reduced vasomotor tone than increased sympathetic or parasympathetic dilator fiber activity. Powerful local vasodilation induced by metabolic byproducts also maintains blood flow in active tissue.

Hormonal Factors

Sympathetic nerves terminate in the medullary portion of the adrenal glands. With sympathetic activation, this glandular tissue releases large quantities of epinephrine and a small amount of norepinephrine into the blood. These hormones cause a general constrictor response *except* in blood vessels of the heart and skeletal muscles. Adrenal hormones provide relatively minor control of regional blood flow during exercise compared with the more rapid and powerful local sympathetic neural drive.

INTEGRATED RESPONSE IN EXERCISE

Table 10.2 summarizes the integrated chemical, neural, and hormonal adjustments immediately before and during exercise.

At the start of exercise (or even slightly before exercise begins), nerve centers above the medullary region initiate cardiovascular activity. The adjustments increase the rate and pumping strength of the heart and alter regional blood flow in direct proportion to exercise intensity. As exercise continues and becomes more intense, sympathetic cholinergic outflow plus local metabolic factors (acting on chemosensitive nerves and directly on blood vessels) dilate resistance vessels in the active musculature. Reduced peripheral resistance permits muscle tissue to accommodate greater blood flow. Constrictor adjustments in less active tissues maintain adequate perfusion pressure despite dilation of the muscle's vasculature. Vasoconstriction in non-active areas also promotes blood redistribution to meet specific tissues' metabolic requirements during exercise.

Table 10·2	Summary of Integrated Chemical, Neural, and Hormonal Adjustments Prior to and During Exercise	
CONDITION	**ACTIVATOR**	**RESPONSE**
Pre-exercise "anticipatory" response	Activation of motor cortex and higher areas of brain causes increase in sympathetic outflow and reciprocal inhibition of parasympathetic activity	Acceleration of heart rate; increased myocardial contractility; vasodilation in skeletal and heart muscle (cholinergic fibers); vasoconstriction in other areas, especially skin, gut, spleen, liver, and kidneys (adrenergic fibers); increase in arterial blood pressure
Exercise	Continued sympathetic cholinergic outflow; alterations in local metabolic conditions due to hypoxia ($\downarrow$ph, $\uparrow$Pco$_2$, $\uparrow$ADP, $\uparrow$Mg^{++}, $\uparrow$Ca^{++}, $\uparrow$NO, $\uparrow$temperature)	Further dilation of muscle vasculature
	Continued sympathetic adrenergic outflow in conjunction with epinephrine and norepinephrine from the adrenal medulla	Concomitant constriction of vasculature in inactive tissues to maintain adequate perfusion pressure throughout the arterial system
		Venous vessels stiffen to reduce their capacity
		Venoconstriction facilitates venous return and maintains the central blood volume

Factors that affect venous return play an equally important role as those regulating arterial flow. Muscle and ventilatory pump action and stiffening of veins through neural stimulation propel blood into the central circulation and toward the right ventricle. This balances cardiac output and venous return.

SUMMARY

1. The cardiovascular system rapidly regulates heart rate and distributes blood while maintaining blood pressure in response to the metabolic and physiologic demands of increased physical activity.

2. The cardiac impulse originates at the S-A node. It then travels across the atria to the A-V node; after a brief delay, it spreads rapidly across the large ventricular mass. With a normal conduction pattern, atria and ventricles contract effectively to provide the impetus for blood flow.

3. The electrocardiogram displays a record of the sequence of myocardial electrical events during a cardiac cycle.

4. The majority of heart rhythm irregularities (arrhythmias) involve extra beats (extrasystoles). Atrial arrhythmias generally do not compromise the heart's pumping ability. Ventricular fibrillation, the most serious arrhythmia, results from repetitive, spontaneous discharge of portions of the ventricular mass.

5. The sympathetic catecholamines epinephrine and norepinephrine accelerate heart rate and increase myocardial contractility. Acetylcholine, a parasympathetic neurotransmitter, slows heart rate via the vagus nerve.

6. Increases in temperature, carbon dioxide, acidity, adenosine, nitric oxide, and magnesium and potassium ions provide potent stimuli to autoregulate blood flow in active tissues. Of these, nitric oxide occupies a role of considerable importance as a "relaxer" of arteriole smooth muscle.

7. The heart "turns on" in transition from rest to exercise from increased sympathetic and decreased parasympathetic activity.

8. Neural and hormonal extrinsic factors modify the heart's inherent rhythmicity. The heart can accelerate rapidly in anticipation of exercise and increase to more than 200 b·min^{-1} in maximum exercise.

9. Carotid artery palpation accurately measures heart rate during and immediately after exercise. In certain medical conditions, pressure against the carotid artery reflexly slows the heart, which underestimates the heart rate during exercise.

10. Cortical stimulation immediately prior to and during the initial stages of physical activity accounts for a substantial part of the heart rate adjustment to exercise.

11. Regulation of blood flow occurs when nerves, hormones, and local metabolic factors alter the internal diameter of smooth muscle bands in blood vessels. Vasoconstriction occurs when adrenergic sympathetic fibers release norepinephrine; cholinergic sympathetic neurons secrete acetylcholine that triggers vasodilation.

THOUGHT QUESTIONS

1. Give a physiologic rationale for biofeedback and relaxation techniques to treat hypertension and stress-related disorders.

2. If heart transplantation surgically removes all nerves to the myocardium, explain why heart rate increases for these patients during exercise.

3. The Romans executed criminals by tying their arms and legs to a cross mounted in the vertical position. Discuss the physiologic responses that would cause death under these circumstances.

PART 3 •
Cardiovascular Dynamics During Exercise

CARDIAC OUTPUT

Cardiac output provides the most significant indicator of the circulatory system's functional capacity to meet the demands for physical activity. As with any pump, the rate of pumping (**heart rate**) and quantity of blood ejected with each stroke (**stroke volume**) determine the heart's output of blood:

$$\text{Cardiac output} = \text{Heart rate} \times \text{Stroke volume}$$

The relationship between cardiac output, oxygen uptake, and difference between the oxygen content of arterial and mixed-venous blood (**a-v̄O_2 difference**) embodies the principle discovered by German physiologist Adolph Fick (1829–1901) in 1870.

$$\text{Cardiac output, mL}\cdot\text{min}^{-1} = [\dot{V}O_2, \text{mL}\cdot\text{min}^{-1}$$
$$\div \text{ a-v̄}O_2 \text{ diff, mL}\cdot\text{dL blood}^{-1}] \times 100$$

RESTING CARDIAC OUTPUT: UNTRAINED VERSUS TRAINED

Each minute, the left ventricle ejects the entire 5-L blood volume of an average-sized adult male. This value pertains to most individuals, but stroke volume and heart rate vary considerably depending on cardiovascular fitness status. A heart rate of about 70 b·min^{-1} sustains the average adult's 5-L resting cardiac output. Substituting this heart rate value in the cardiac output equation (cardiac output = stroke volume × heart rate; stroke volume = cardiac output ÷ heart rate), yields a calculated stroke volume of 71 mL per beat.

Resting heart rate for an endurance athlete averages close to 50 b·min^{-1}. Because the athlete's resting cardiac output also averages 5 L·min^{-1}, blood circulates with a proportionately larger stroke volume of 100 mL per beat (5000 mL ÷ 50). Stroke volumes for women usually average 25% below values for men with equivalent training. The smaller body size of the average woman chiefly accounts for this "sex difference."

The following table summarizes average values for cardiac output, heart rate, and stroke volume for endurance-trained and untrained men at rest:

	Cardiac Output L·min^{-1}	Heart Rate, b·min^{-1}	Stroke Volume, mL·b^{-1}
Untrained	5000	70	71
Trained	5000	50	100

The underlying mechanisms for the heart rate and stroke volume differences between trained and untrained individuals remain unclear. Does the bradycardia that accompanies increased aerobic fitness "cause" a larger stroke volume, or vice versa, because the myocardium becomes strengthened and internal ventricular dimensions increase with training? These two factors probably interact as aerobic fitness improves as follows:

1. Increased vagal tone slows the heart, allowing more time for ventricular filling
2. Enlarged ventricular volume and a more powerful myocardium eject a larger volume of blood with each systole

EXERCISE CARDIAC OUTPUT: UNTRAINED VERSUS TRAINED

Blood flow from the heart increases in direct proportion to exercise intensity. From rest to steady-rate exercise, cardiac output increases rapidly, followed by a more gradual increase until it plateaus as blood flow matches exercise metabolic requirements.

In sedentary, college-age men, cardiac output in maximal aerobic exercise increases about four times the resting level to an average maximum of 22 L of blood per minute. Maximum heart rate for these young adults averages 195 b·min^{-1}. Consequently, stroke volume averages 113 mL of blood per beat during exercise (22,000 mL ÷ 195). In contrast, world-class endurance athletes generate maximum cardiac outputs of 35 L·min^{-1}, with a similar or slightly lower maximum heart rate than untrained counterparts. The difference between maximum cardiac output of both individuals relates *solely* to differences in stroke volume. The cardiac output of a Nordic Olympic medal winner in cross-country skiing increased eight times above rest to 40 L·min^{-1} during a maximum exercise test. The accompanying stroke volume averaged 210 mL per beat, which is twice the typical maximum volume of blood pumped per beat by a healthy, sedentary person of the same age. The following table summarizes average values for cardiac output, heart rate, and stroke volume of endurance-trained and untrained men during maximal exercise:

	Cardiac Output L·min^{-1}	Heart Rate, b·min^{-1}	Stroke Volume, mL·b^{-1}
Untrained	22,000	195	113
Trained	35,000	195	179

EXERCISE STROKE VOLUME

Figure 10.11 relates stroke volume and percentage $\dot{V}O_{2max}$ (to better equate exercise intensity among subjects) for eight healthy, college-age men during graded exercise on a cycle ergometer. Stroke volume increases progressively

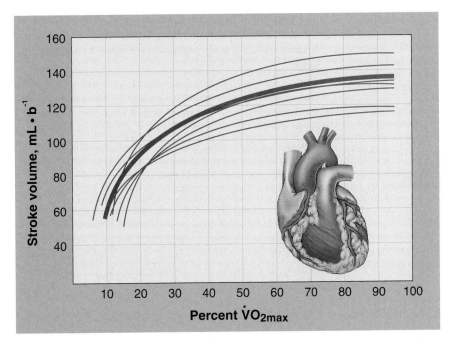

Figure 10.11   Stroke volume (mL·b^{-1}) related to increasing exercise intensity (percent $\dot{V}O_{2max}$) for 8 male subjects. (Data from the Applied Physiology Laboratory, University of Michigan.)

with exercise to about 50% $\dot{V}O_{2max}$ and then gradually levels off until termination of exercise. For several subjects, stroke volume decreased slightly at near-maximal exercise intensities.

Stroke Volume and $\dot{V}O_{2max}$

Table 10.3 shows the importance of stroke volume in differentiating people with high and low $\dot{V}O_{2max}$. The subjects represented three groups: (1) patients with mitral stenosis, a valvular disease that causes inadequate emptying of the left ventricle, (2) healthy but sedentary men, and (3) athletes. Differences in $\dot{V}O_{2max}$ among the groups closely paralleled differences in maximal stroke volume. Aerobic capacity and maximum stroke volume of mitral stenosis patients averaged one-half the values of sedentary subjects. This close linkage also emerged in comparisons between healthy subjects; a 60% larger stroke volume in athletes compared with sedentary men paralleled the 62% larger $\dot{V}O_{2max}$. All groups showed fairly similar maximum heart rates; thus, stroke volume differences accounted for the variations in maximum cardiac output and $\dot{V}O_{2max}$ among groups.

Table 10·3	Maximal Values for Oxygen Uptake ($\dot{V}O_{2max}$), Heart Rate (HR_{max}), Stroke Volume (SV_{max}), and Cardiac Output ($\dot{Q}_{max}$) in Three Groups Having Low, Normal, and High Aerobic Capacities			
GROUP	$\dot{V}O_{2max}$ (L · min^{-1})	HR_{max} (B · min^{-1})	SV_{max} (ML · B^{-1})	$\dot{Q}_{max}$ (L · min^{-1})
Mitral stenosis	1.6	190	50	9.5
Sedentary	3.2	200	100	20.0
Athlete	5.2	190	160	30.4

Modified from Rowell, L.B.: Circulation. *Med. Sci. Sports*, 1:15, 1969.

Questions & Notes

Cardiac output = _____ ×
_____ .

Blood flow from the heart increases in direct proportion to exercise _____.

Give typical cardiac output values for untrained versus trained during rest and maximal exercise.

	Trained	Untrained
Rest	_____	_____
Maximal Exercise	_____	_____

Draw and label the relationship between stroke volume and percent $\dot{V}O_{2max}$.

Name the 3 physiologic mechanisms that increase the heart's stoke volume during exercise.

1.

2.

3.

Stroke Volume Increases

Three physiologic mechanisms increase the heart's stroke volume during exercise. The first, intrinsic to the myocardium, involves enhanced cardiac filling in diastole, followed by a more forceful systolic contraction. Neurohormonal influence governs the second mechanism, which involves normal ventricular filling with a subsequent forceful ejection and emptying during systole. The third mechanism for increased stroke volume entails training adaptations that expand blood volume and reduce resistance to blood flow in peripheral tissues.

Greater Systolic Emptying Versus Enhanced Diastolic Filling   Greater ventricular filling in diastole during the cardiac cycle occurs through any factor that increases venous return (**preload**) or slows heart rate. An increase in end-diastolic volume stretches myocardial fibers, causing a powerful ejection stroke as the heart contracts. This expels the normal stroke volume plus the additional blood that entered the ventricles and stretched the myocardium.

German physiologist Otto Frank (1865–1944) and British colleague Ernest H. Starling's (1866–1927) experiments with animals in the early 1900s first described relationships between muscle force and resting fiber length. Improved contractility of a stretched muscle (within a limited range) probably relates to a more optimum arrangement of intracellular myofilaments as the muscle stretches. **Frank-Starling's law of the heart** describes this phenomenon applied to the myocardium.

For many years, physiologists taught the Frank-Starling mechanism as the main cause for all increases in stroke volume during exercise. They believed that enhanced venous return in exercise caused greater cardiac filling, which stretched the ventricles in diastole to produce a more forceful ejection. In all likelihood, this pattern describes the stroke volume response in transition from rest to exercise or when a person moves from the upright to recumbent position. Enhanced diastolic filling probably also occurs in activities like swimming, where the body's horizontal position optimizes venous return and myocardial preload.

Body position affects circulatory dynamics. Cardiac output and stroke volume reach the highest and most stable levels in the horizontal position. *Near-maximal stroke volume occurs at rest in the horizontal position and increases only slightly during exercise.* In contrast, gravity's effect in the upright position counters venous return and lowers stroke volume. This postural effect becomes prominent when comparing circulatory dynamics at rest in the upright and supine positions. As upright exercise intensity increases, stroke volume also increases to approach the maximum value in the supine position.

In most forms of upright exercise, the heart does not fill to an extent that increases cardiac volume to values observed in the recumbent position. The increase in stroke volume during exercise likely results from the *combined effects* of enhanced diastolic filling and more complete systolic emptying. In both recumbent and upright positions, the heart's stroke volume increases in exercise despite resistance to flow from increased systolic pressure (**afterload**).

At rest in the upright position, 40% to 50% of the total end-diastolic blood volume remains in the left ventricle after systole; this **residual volume of the heart** amounts to 50 to 70 mL of blood. The sympathetic hormones epinephrine and norepinephrine enhance myocardial stroke power and systolic emptying during exercise; this reduces the heart's residual blood volume.

More than likely, endurance training also increases compliance of the left ventricle (reduced cardiac stiffness) to facilitate its ability to accept blood in the diastolic phase of the cardiac cycle. Whether endurance training enhances the myocardium's *innate* contractile state remains unclear. If this adaptation does occur, it too would contribute to a larger stroke volume.

Cardiovascular Drift: Reduced Stroke Volume and Increased Heart Rate During Prolonged Exercise   Submaximal exercise for more than 15 minutes, particularly in the heat, produces progressive water loss through sweating and a fluid shift from plasma to tissues. A rise in core temperature also causes redistribution of blood to the periphery for body cooling. At the same time, the progressive fall in plasma volume decreases central venous cardiac filling pressure (preload), which reduces stroke volume. A reduced stroke volume initiates a compensatory heart rate increase to maintain a nearly constant cardiac output as exercise progresses. The term **cardiovascular drift** describes this gradual time-dependent downward "drift" in several cardiovascular responses, most notably stroke volume (with concomitant heart rate increase), during prolonged steady-rate exercise. Under these circumstances, a person usually must exercise at a lower intensity than if cardiovascular drift did not occur.

One explanation for cardiovascular drift suggests that a stroke volume decline during prolonged exercise in a thermoneutral environment relates to an increased exercise heart rate (and not increased cutaneous blood flow, as hypothesized by some researchers). More than likely, the progressive increase in exercise heart rate with cardiovascular drift decreases end-diastolic volume, subsequently reducing the heart's stroke volume.

EXERCISE HEART RATE

Graded Exercise

Figure 10.12 depicts the relationship between heart rate and oxygen uptake during increasing intensity exercise (graded exercise) to maximum for endurance trained individuals and sedentary counterparts. Heart rate for the untrained person accelerates relatively rapidly with increasing exercise demands; a much smaller heart rate increase occurs for the trained person. Thus, the trained person achieves a higher level of exercise oxygen uptake

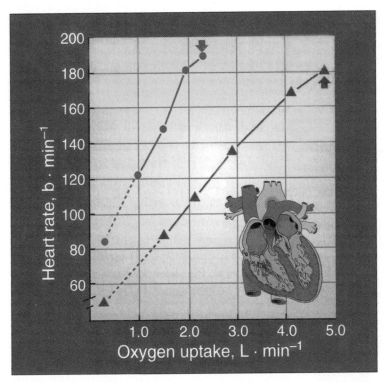

Figure 10.12   Heart rate in relation to oxygen uptake during exercise in trained individuals (▲) and sedentary counterparts (•). (Adapted from Saltin, B.: Physiological effects of physical conditioning. *Med. Sci. Sports*, 1:50, 1969.)

at a particular submaximal heart rate than a sedentary person. Maximum heart rate and the heart rate–oxygen uptake relationship remain fairly consistent for a particular individual from day to day, although the slope of the relationship decreases considerable with aerobic training.

Submaximum Exercise

Heart rate increases rapidly and levels off within several minutes during submaximum steady-rate exercise. A subsequent increase in exercise intensity increases heart rate to a new plateau as the body attempts to match the cardiovascular response to the metabolic demands. Each increment in exercise intensity requires progressively more time to achieve heart rate stabilization.

CARDIAC OUTPUT DISTRIBUTION

Blood flow to specific tissues increases in proportion to their metabolic activities.

Rest

Figure 10.13A shows the approximate distribution of a 5-L cardiac output at rest. More than one-fourth of the cardiac output flows to the liver, one-fifth flows to kidney and muscles, and the remainder diverts to the heart, skin, brain, and other tissues.

During Exercise

Figure 10.13B illustrates the distribution of cardiac output to various tissues during intense aerobic exercise. *Regional blood flow varies considerably depending on environmental conditions, level of fatigue, and exercise mode, yet active muscles receive a disproportionately large portion of the cardiac output in exercise.* Each 100 g

Questions & Notes

Briefly describe Frank-Starling's law of the heart.

This body position produces near-maximal values for stroke volume at rest.

The residual volume of the heart at rest in the upright position averages _____ mL.

What is meant by cardiovascular drift?

Give one explanation for cardiovascular drift.

Explain why a trained person has a lower heart rate than an untrained person when both exercise at the same submaximal oxygen uptake.

For Your Information

The Amazing Heart
Here's a straightforward calculation with an amazing answer about the heart.
"How many cars with 20-gallon capacity gas tanks would 60 years of resting cardiac output fill-up?" (Hint: Use an average resting cardiac output of 5 L·min^{-1}.)

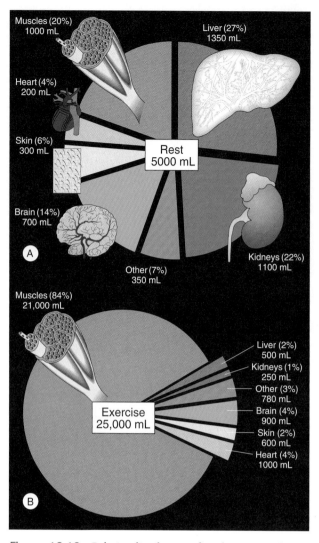

Figure 10.13   Relative distribution of cardiac output during rest (**A**) and strenuous endurance exercise (**B**). The numbers in parentheses indicate percent of total cardiac output. Despite its large mass, muscle tissue receives about the same amount of blood as the much smaller kidneys at rest. In strenuous exercise, however, nearly 85% of the total cardiac output diverts to active muscles.

of muscle receives 4 to 7 mL of blood per minute during rest. Muscle blood flow increases steadily during exercise to reach a maximum of between 50 to 75 mL per 100 g of active muscle tissue.

Blood Flow Redistribution   The increase in muscle blood flow with exercise comes largely from increased cardiac output. Due to neural and hormonal vascular regulation, including local metabolic conditions within muscles, additional blood moves through active muscles from areas that temporarily tolerate a reduction in normal blood flow. Shunting of blood away from specific tissues occurs primarily in intense exercise. Blood flow to the skin increases during light and moderate exercise, so metabolic heat generated in muscle can dissipate at the skin's surface. During intense, short-duration exercise,

cutaneous blood flow becomes reduced even when exercising in a hot environment.

In some tissues, blood flow during exercise decreases as much as four-fifths of the flow at rest. The kidneys and splanchnic tissues use only 10% to 25% of the oxygen available in their blood supply at rest. Consequently, these tissues tolerate a considerably reduced blood flow before oxygen demand exceeds supply and compromises organ function. With reduced blood flow, increased oxygen extraction from available blood maintains a tissue's oxygen needs. Visceral organs can tolerate substantially reduced blood flow for more than an hour during intense exercise. This "frees" as much as 600 mL of oxygen each minute for use by active musculature.

Blood Flow to the Heart and Brain   The myocardium and brain tissues cannot compromise their blood supplies. At rest, the myocardium normally uses 75% of the oxygen in the blood flowing through the coronary circulation. With such a limited "margin of safety," increased coronary blood flow primarily meets the heart's oxygen demands. Cerebral blood flow increases up to 30% with exercise compared with rest; the largest portion of any "extra" blood probably moves to areas related to motor functions.

CARDIAC OUTPUT AND OXYGEN TRANSPORT

Rest

Each 100 mL (deciliter or dL) of arterial blood normally carries approximately 20 mL of oxygen or 200 mL of oxygen per liter of blood at sea level conditions (see Chapter 9). Trained and untrained adults circulate 5 L of blood each minute at rest, so potentially 1000 mL of oxygen becomes available during 1 minute (5 L blood × 200 mL O_2). Resting oxygen uptake averages only about 250 mL·min^{-1}; this means 750 mL of oxygen returns "unused" to the heart. This does not represent an unnecessary waste of cardiac output. To the contrary, extra oxygen in the blood above the resting needs maintains oxygen in reserve—a margin of safety for immediate use should the need arise.

During Exercise

A person with a maximum heart rate of 200 b·min^{-1} and a stroke volume of 80 mL per beat generates a maximum cardiac output of 16 L (200 × 0.080 L). Even during maximum exercise, hemoglobin remains fully saturated with oxygen, so each liter of arterial blood carries about 200 mL of oxygen. Consequently, 3200 mL of oxygen circulate each minute via a 16-L cardiac output (16 L × 200 mL O_2). If the body extracted all of the oxygen delivered in a 16-L cardiac output, $\dot{V}O_{2max}$ would equal 3200 mL. This represents the theoretical upper limit for this person because the oxygen needs of tissues like the brain do not increase greatly with exercise, yet they require an uninterrupted blood supply.

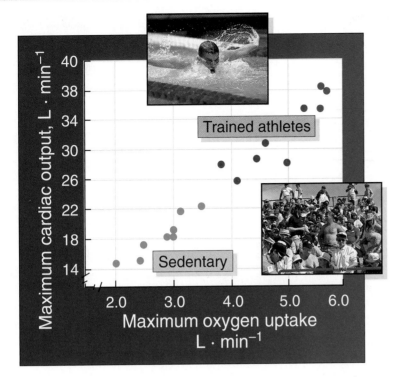

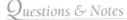

Questions & Notes

How much oxygen is transported in each liter of a healthy person's blood?

For a cardiac output of 5 L·min⁻¹, how much total oxygen moves through the body each minute?

Figure 10.14 Relationship between maximal cardiac output and maximal oxygen uptake in trained and untrained individuals. Maximal cardiac output relates to $\dot{V}O_{2max}$ in a ratio of about 6:1. (Swimmer photo courtesy of Jim Richardson, University of Michigan.)

Describe the relationship between $\dot{V}O_{2max}$ and maximum cardiac output.

An increase in maximum cardiac output directly improves a person's capacity to circulate oxygen. If the heart's stroke volume increased from 80 to 200 mL while maximum heart rate remained unchanged at 200 b·min⁻¹, maximum cardiac output would dramatically increase to 40 L·min⁻¹. This means that the amount of oxygen circulated in maximum exercise each minute increases approximately 2.5 times from 3200 to 8000 mL (40 L × 200 mL O_2).

Maximum Cardiac Output and $\dot{V}O_{2max}$

Figure 10.14 displays the relationship between maximum cardiac output and $\dot{V}O_{2max}$ and includes values representative of sedentary individuals and elite endurance athletes. An unmistakable relationship emerges. A low aerobic capacity links closely to a low maximum cardiac output, whereas a 30- to 40-L cardiac output always accompanies the ability to generate a 5- or 6-L $\dot{V}O_{2max}$.

Give one reason why females have a larger cardiac output compared to males at the same absolute sub-maximum $\dot{V}O_2$.

Cardiac Output Differences Among Men and Women and Children

Cardiac output and oxygen consumption remain linearly related during graded exercise for boys and girls and men and women. However, teenage and adult females generally exercise at any level of submaximal oxygen consumption with a 5% to 10% larger cardiac output than males. Any apparent gender difference in submaximal cardiac output most likely results from the 10% lower hemoglobin concentration in women than in men. A proportionate increase in submaximal cardiac output compensates for this small decrease in the blood's oxygen-carrying capacity.

Higher heart rates in children than in adults during submaximal treadmill and cycle ergometer exercise do not fully compensate for their smaller stroke volume. This produces a smaller cardiac output for children at a given submaximal exercise oxygen consumption. Consequently, the a-v̄O_2 difference expands to satisfy the oxygen requirements. The biologic significance of this difference in central

List 2 mechanisms for how oxygen supply leads to an increase in oxygen uptake capacity.

1.

2.

circulatory function between children and adults remains unclear. Comparisons of cardiac responses (stroke volume, aortic peak blood flow velocity, and systolic ejection time) between prepubertal children and adults fail to demonstrate any age-related exercise impairment.

EXTRACTION OF OXYGEN: THE a-v̄O₂ DIFFERENCE

If blood flow were the only means for increasing a tissue's oxygen supply, cardiac output would need to increase from 5 L·min⁻¹ at rest to 100 L in maximum exercise to achieve a 20-fold increase in oxygen uptake (an oxygen uptake increase common among endurance athletes). Fortunately, intense exercise does not require such a large cardiac output because hemoglobin releases its considerable "extra" oxygen from blood perfusing active tissues.

Two mechanisms for oxygen supply increase a person's oxygen uptake capacity:

1. Increased tissue blood flow
2. Use of the relatively large quantity of oxygen that remains unused by tissues at rest (i.e., expand the a-v̄O₂ difference)

The following rearrangement of the Fick equation summarizes the important relationship between maximum cardiac output, maximum a-v̄O₂ difference, and $\dot{V}O_{2max}$:

$$\dot{V}O_{2max} = \text{Max cardiac output}$$
$$\times \text{ Max a-}\bar{v}O_2 \text{ difference}$$

a-v̄O₂ Difference During Rest and Exercise

Figure 10.15 shows a representative pattern for changes in a-v̄O₂ difference from rest to maximum exercise for physically active men. A similar pattern emerges for women except that the arterial oxygen content averages 5% to 10% lower due to lower hemoglobin concentrations. The figure includes values for the oxygen content of arterial blood and mixed-venous blood during different exercise intensities. Arterial blood oxygen content varies little from its value of 20 mL·dL⁻¹ at rest throughout the full exercise intensity range. In contrast, mixed-venous oxygen content varies between 12 and 15 mL·dL⁻¹ at rest to a low of 2 to 4 mL·dL⁻¹ during maximum exercise. The difference between arterial and mixed-venous blood oxygen content at any time (a-v̄O₂ difference) represents oxygen extraction from blood as it circulates through the body's tissues. At rest, for example, a-v̄O₂ difference equals 5 mL of oxygen, or only 25% of the blood's oxygen content (5 mL ÷ 20 mL × 100); 75% of the oxygen returns "unused" to the heart bound to hemoglobin.

The progressive expansion of the a-v̄O₂ difference to at least three times the resting value occurs from a reduced venous oxygen content, which, in maximal exercise, approaches 20 mL in the active muscle (all oxygen ex-

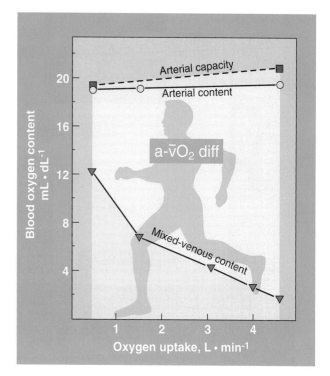

Figure 10.15 Changes in a-v̄O₂ difference from rest to maximal exercise in physically active men.

tracted). The oxygen content of a true mixed-venous sample from the pulmonary artery rarely falls below 2 to 4 mL·dL⁻¹ because blood returning from active tissues mixes with oxygen-rich venous blood from metabolically less active regions.

Figure 10.15 also indicates that the capacity of each dL of arterial blood to carry oxygen actually increases during exercise. This results from an increased concentration of red blood cells (hemoconcentration) from the progressive movement of fluid from the plasma to the interstitial space because of two factors:

1. Increases in capillary hydrostatic pressure as blood pressure rises
2. Metabolic byproducts of exercise metabolism create an osmotic pressure that draws fluid from the plasma into tissue spaces

FACTORS AFFECTING EXERCISE a-v̄O₂ DIFFERENCE

Central and peripheral factors interact to increase oxygen extraction in active tissue during exercise. Diverting a large portion of the cardiac output to active muscles influences the magnitude of the a-v̄O₂ difference in maximal exercise. As mentioned previously, some tissues temporarily compromise blood supply during exercise by redistributing blood to make more oxygen available for muscle metabolism. Exercise training facilitates redirection of the central circulation to active muscle.

Increases in skeletal muscle microcirculation also increase tissue oxygen extraction. Muscle biopsy specimens

Box 10–3 •

HOW TO PLACE ELECTRODES FOR BIPOLAR AND 12-LEAD ECG RECORDINGS

The electrocardiogram (ECG) represents a composite record of the heart's electrical events during a cardiac cycle. These events provide a means to monitor heart rate during different physical activities and exercise stress testing. The ECG can detect contraindications to exercise including previous myocardial infarction, ischemic S-T segment changes, conduction defects, and left ventricular enlargement (hypertrophy). A valid ECG tracing requires proper electrode placement. The term **ECG lead** indicates the specific placement of *a pair* of electrodes on the body that transmits the electrical signal to a recorder. The record of electrical differences across diverse ECG leads creates the composite electrical "picture" of myocardial activity.

SKIN PREPARATION

Proper skin preparation reduces extraneous electrical "noise" (interference and skeletal muscle artifact). Abrade the skin with fine sandpaper or commercially available pads and alcohol to remove surface epidermis and oil; the skin should appear red, slightly irritated, dry, and clean.

BIPOLAR (3-ELECTRODE) CONFIGURATION

The left figure shows the typical electrode placement for a bipolar configuration. This positioning provides less sensitivity for diagnostic testing but proves useful for routine ECG monitoring in functional exercise testing and radiotelemetry of the ECG during physical activity. The ground (green or black) electrode attaches over the sternum, the positive (red) electrode attaches on the left side of the chest in the V_5 position (level of the 5th intercostal space adjacent to the midaxillary line), and the positive (white) electrode attaches on the right side of the chest, just below the nipple at the level of the 5th intercostal space. Placement of the positive electrode can be altered to optimize the recording (e.g., 3rd and 4th intercostal spaces, anterior portion of the right shoulder, or near the clavicle). Correct electrode placement can be remembered as follows: *white to right, green to ground, red to left.*

MODIFIED 12-LEAD (10-ELECTRODE TORSO-MOUNTED) CONFIGURATION FOR EXERCISE STRESS TESTING

The standard 12-lead ECG consists of three limb leads, three augmented unipolar leads, and six chest leads. For improved exercise ECG recordings, electrodes mounted on the torso (abdominal level) replace the conventional ankle (leg) and wrist electrodes. This "torso-mounted limb lead system" (right figure) reduces electrical artifact introduced by limb movement during exercise.

Electrode Positioning in the Modified 10-Electrode, Torso-Mounted System

1. RL (right leg): just above right iliac crest on midaxillary line
2. LL (left leg): just above left iliac crest on midaxillary line
3. RA (right arm): just below right clavicle medial to deltoid muscle
4. LA (left arm): just below left clavicle medial to deltoid muscle
5. V_1: on right sternal border in 4th intercostal space
6. V_2: on left sternal border in 4th intercostal space
7. V_3: at midpoint of a straight line between V_2 and V_4
8. V_4: on midclavicular line in 5th intercostal space
9. V_5: on anterior axillary line and horizontal to V_4
10. V_6: on midaxillary line and horizontal to V_4 and V_5

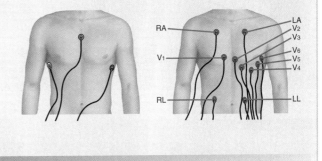

REFERENCE

Phibbs, B., and Buckels, L.: Comparative yields of ECG leads in multistage stress testing. *Am. Heart J.*, 90:275, 1985.

from the quadriceps femoris show a relatively large ratio of capillaries to muscle fibers in individuals who exhibit large a-v̄O₂ differences in intense exercise. An increase in the capillary to fiber ratio reflects a positive adaptation that enlarges the interface for nutrient and gas exchange during exercise. Individual muscle cells' ability to generate energy aerobically represents another important factor governing oxygen extraction capacity. A training-induced increase in the size and number of mitochondria and greater aerobic enzyme activity also improve a muscle's metabolic capacity in exercise.

CARDIOVASCULAR ADJUSTMENTS TO UPPER-BODY EXERCISE

The highest oxygen uptake during upper-body exercise generally averages between 70% to 80% of the $\dot{V}O_{2max}$ in bicycle and treadmill exercise. Similarly, maximal heart rate and pulmonary ventilation remain lower in arm exercise. The relatively smaller muscle mass of the upper body largely accounts for these physiologic differences. The lower maximal heart rate in exercise that activates a smaller muscle mass most likely results from the following:

1. Reduced output stimulation from the motor cortex central command to the cardiovascular center in the medulla (less feedforward stimulation)
2. Reduced feedback stimulation to the medulla from the smaller active musculature

In submaximal exercise, the metabolic and cardiovascular response pattern reverses. **Figure 10.16** shows that any level of submaximal power output produces a higher oxygen uptake with arm compared with leg exercise. This difference remains small during light exercise but becomes progressively larger as intensity of effort increases. Lower economy of effort in arm-crank exercise probably results from static muscle actions that do not produce external work but consume extra oxygen. In addition, extra musculature activated to stabilize the torso during most forms of arm exercise adds to the oxygen requirement. Upper-body exercise also produces greater physiologic strain (heart rate, blood pressure, pulmonary ventilation, and perception of physical effort) for any level of oxygen uptake (or percentage of maximal oxygen uptake) than primarily lower-body leg exercise.

Understanding differences in physiologic response between upper- and lower-body exercise enables the clinician to formulate prudent exercise programs using both exercise modes. A standard exercise load produces greater metabolic and physiologic strain with the arms, so exercise prescriptions based on running and bicycling *cannot* be applied to upper-body exercise. Also, $\dot{V}O_{2max}$ for arm exercises does not strongly relate to leg exercise $\dot{V}O_{2max}$; thus, one cannot predict accurately one's aerobic capacity for arm exercise from a test using the legs, and vice versa. *This further substantiates the concept of aerobic fitness specificity.*

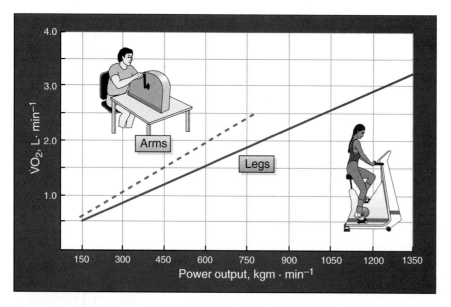

Figure 10.16 Arm (upper-body) exercise requires a greater oxygen uptake compared with leg (lower-body) exercise at any power output throughout the comparison range. The largest differences occur during intense exercise. Average data for men and women. (From Laboratory of Applied Physiology, Queens College, NY.)

SUMMARY

1. Cardiac output reflects the functional capacity of the circulatory system. Heart rate and stroke volume determine the heart's output capacity in the following relationship: Cardiac output = Heart rate × Stroke volume.

2. Cardiac output increases in proportion to exercise intensity from about 5 L·min⁻¹ at rest to an exercise maximum of 20 to 25 L·min⁻¹ in untrained college-age men and to 35 to 40 L·min⁻¹ in elite male endurance athletes.

3. Differences in maximum cardiac output primarily relate to individual differences in the heart's maximum stroke volume.

4. During upright exercise, stroke volume increases during the transition from rest to moderate exercise, reaching maximum at about 50% $\dot{V}O_{2max}$. Thereafter, increases in heart rate increase cardiac output.

5. Stroke volume increases in upright exercise generally result from interactions between greater ventricular filling during diastole and more complete emptying during systole. Sympathetic hormones that augment myocardial force generated during systole increase stroke volume.

6. Training adaptations that expand blood volume and reduce resistance to blood flow in peripheral tissues also contribute to an enhanced stroke volume.

7. Heart rate and oxygen uptake relate linearly throughout the major portion of the exercise range in trained and untrained individuals. Endurance training shifts the heart rate–oxygen uptake line to the right because of an improved stroke volume.

8. Local metabolism generally determines blood flow in specific tissues; it causes substantial diversion of cardiac output to active muscles during exercise. Kidneys and splanchnic regions temporarily compromise their blood supplies to reroute blood to active muscles.

9. Maximum cardiac output and maximum a-$\bar{v}O_2$ difference determine $\dot{V}O_{2max}$ in the following relationship: $\dot{V}O_{2max}$ = maximum cardiac output × maximum a-$\bar{v}O_2$ difference.

10. Large cardiac outputs clearly differentiate endurance athletes from untrained counterparts. Training also expands the maximum a-$\bar{v}O_2$ difference.

THOUGHT QUESTIONS

1. Moderate increases in hemoglobin concentration increase $\dot{V}O_{2max}$ during maximal exercise at sea level. This effect supports the contention that what component of the cardiac output equation limits maximal oxygen consumption? Discuss.

2. How would factors that influence the a-$\bar{v}O_2$ difference in maximal exercise explain the specificity of $\dot{V}O_{2max}$ improvement with different modes of aerobic training?

SELECTED REFERENCES

ACSM position stand: Exercise and hypertension. *Med. Sci. Sports Exerc.*, March, 2004.

Barauna, V.G., et al.: Cardiovascular adaptations in rats submitted to a resistance-training model. *Clin. Exp. Pharmacol. Physiol.*, 32:249, 2005.

Bolad, I., Delafontaine, P.: Endothelial dysfunction: its role in hypertensive coronary disease. *Curr. Opin. Cardiol.*, 20:270, 2005.

Carter, J.B., et al.: The effect of age and gender on heart rate variability after endurance training. *Med. Sci. Sports Exerc.*, 35:1333, 2003.

Cooke, W.H., Carter, J.R.: Strength training does not affect vagal-cardiac control or cardiovagal baroreflex sensitivity in young healthy subjects. *Eur. J. Appl. Physiol.*, 93:719, 2005.

Coyle, E.F., González-Alonso, J.: Cardiovascular drift during prolonged exercise: new perspectives. *Exer. Sport Sci. Rev.*, 28:88, 2001.

DeVan, A.E., et al.: Acute effects of resistance exercise on arterial compliance. *J. Appl. Physiol.*, 98:2287, 2005.

Dibrezzo, R., et al.: Exercise intervention designed to improve strength and dynamic balance among community-dwelling older adults. *J. Aging Phys. Act.*, 13:198, 2005.

Farias, M. 3rd, et al.: Plasma ATP during exercise: possible role in regulation of coronary blood flow. *Am. J. Physiol. Heart Circ. Physiol.*, 288:H1586, 2005.

Harvey, P.J., et al.: Hemodynamic after-effects of acute dynamic exercise in sedentary normotensive postmenopausal women. *J. Hypertens.*, 23:285, 2005.

Hwu, C.M., et al.: Physical inactivity is an important lifestyle determinant of insulin resistance in hypertensive patients. *Blood Press.*, 13:355, 2004.

Izquierdo, M., et al.: Effects of combined resistance and cardiovascular training on strength, power, muscle cross-sectional area, and endurance markers in middle-aged men. *Eur. J. Appl. Physiol.*, 94:70, 2005.

Ketelhut, G., et al.: Regular exercise as an effective approach in antihypertensive therapy. *Med. Sci. Sports Exerc.*, 36:4, 2004.

Krediet, C.T., et al.: Syncope during exercise, documented with continuous blood pressure monitoring during ergometer testing. *Clin. Auton. Res.*, 15:59, 2005.

Kurbel, S., et al.: Can arteries of skeletal muscles act as a circulatory bottleneck during heavy exercise? *Med. Hypotheses*, 64:367, 2005.

Kurl, S., et al.: Cardiac power during exercise and the risk of stroke in men. *Stroke*, 36:820, 2005.

Laszlo, G.: Respiratory measurements of cardiac output: from elegant idea to useful test. *J. Appl. Physiol.*, 96:428, 2004.

Lockwood, J.M., et al.: Postexercise hypotension is not explained by a prostaglandin-dependent peripheral vasodilation. *J. Appl. Physiol.*, 98 447, 2005.

Lucas, J.W., et al.: Summary health statistics for U.S. adults: National Health Interview Survey, 2001. *Vital Health Stat. 10*, 218:1, 2004.

MacDonnell, S.M., et al.: Improved myocardial beta-adrenergic responsiveness and signaling with exercise training in hypertension. *Circulation*, 111:3420, 2005.

Maeda, S., et al.: Resistance exercise training reduces plasma endothelin-1 concentration in healthy young humans. *J. Cardiovasc. Pharmacol.*, 44:S443, 2004.

Mortensen, S.P., et al.: Limitations to systemic and locomotor limb muscle oxygen delivery and uptake during maximal exercise in humans. *J. Physiol.*, 566:273, 2005.

Nottin, S., et al.: Central and peripheral cardiovascular adaptations during maximal cycle exercise in boys and men. *Med. Sci. Sports Exerc.*, 34:456, 2002.

Pricher, M.P., et al.: Regional hemdodynamics during postesercise hypotension. I. Splanchnic and renal circulations. *J. Appl. Physiol.*, 97:2065, 2004.

Rakobowchuk, M., et al.: Effect of whole body resistance training on arterial compliance in young men. *Exp. Physiol.*, 90:645, 2005.

Rowell, L.B., et al.: Integration of cardiovascular control systems in dynamic exercises. In: *Handbook of Physiology*. Rowell, LB, and Shepard J. (eds.). New York: Oxford University Press, 1996.

Rowell, L.B.: *Human Cardiovascular Control*. Cary, NC: Oxford University Press, 1994.

Rowland, T., et al.: Cardiac responses to exercise in normal children: a synthesis. *Med. Sci. Sports Exerc.*, 32:253, 2000.

Sagiv, M., et al.: Left ventricular function at peak all-out anaerobic exercise in older men. *Gerontology*, 51:122, 2005.

Sun, X.G., et al.: Comparison of exercise cardiac output by the Fick prinicple using oxygen and carbon dioxide. *Chest*, 118:631, 2000.

Swank, A.M., et al.: Echocardiographic evaluation of stress test for determining safety of participation in strength training. *J. Strength Cond. Res.*, 19:389, 2005.

Thomas, S.N., et al.: Cerebral blood flow during submaximal and maximal dynamic exercise in humans. *J. Appl. Physiol.*, 67:744, 1989.

Tune, J.D., et al.: Matching coronary blood flow to myocardial oxygen consumption. *J. Appl. Physiol.*, 97:404, 2004.

Wingo, J.E., et al.: Cardiovascular drift is related to reduced maximal oxygen uptake during heat stress. *Med. Sci. Sports Exerc.*, 37:248, 2005.

Young, D.R., et al.: Physical activity, cardiorespiratory fitness, and their relationship to cardiovascular risk factors in African Americans and non-African Americans with above-optimal blood pressure. *J. Comm. Health*, 30:107, 2005.

CHAPTER OBJECTIVES

- Identify the major structural components of the central nervous system that control human movement.

- Diagram the anterior motoneuron, and discuss its role in human movement.

- Draw and label the basic components of a reflex arc.

- Define (1) motor unit, (2) neuromuscular junction, (3) autonomic nervous system, (4) excitatory postsynaptic potential, (5) inhibitory postsynaptic potential.

- Explain factors associated with neuromuscular fatigue.

- Describe the function of muscle spindles and Golgi tendon organs.

- Draw and label a skeletal muscle fiber's ultrastructural components.

- Describe the sequence of chemical and mechanical events during skeletal muscle contraction and relaxation.

- Contrast slow-twitch and fast-twitch (including subdivisions) muscle fiber characteristics.

- Outline muscle fiber-type distribution patterns among diverse groups of elite athletes.

- Explain how exercise training modifies muscle fibers and fiber types.

CHAPTER OUTLINE

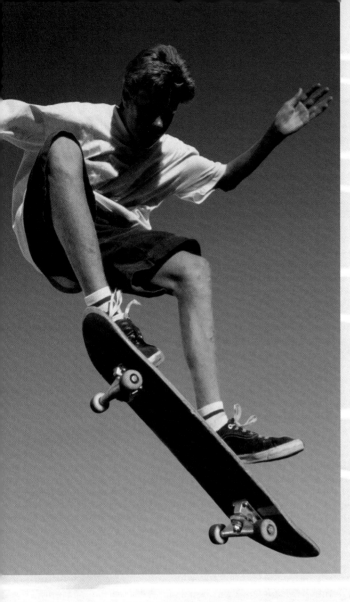

chapter 11

The Neuromuscular System and Exercise

PART 1 •
Neural Control of Human Movement

Similarities exist between a modern computer and the human body's neuromuscular circuitry. Not surprisingly, the integrative and organizational complexity of the human nervous system far exceeds any computer. In response to changing internal and external stimuli, interactive neural control mechanisms selectively process bits of sensory input. Movements requiring little force or complex movements requiring great force depend on the coordinated reception and integration of sensory neural input to transmit signals to effector organs, the muscles.

This chapter describes the neural control of human movement that includes:

1. Structural organization of the neuromotor system, with emphasis on the central and peripheral nervous systems
2. Neuromuscular transmission
3. Sensory input for muscular activity
4. Motor unit type, function, and activation

NEUROMOTOR SYSTEM ORGANIZATION

The human nervous system consists of two major parts: (1) the **central nervous system** (CNS), which includes the brain and spinal cord, and (2) the **peripheral nervous system** (PNS) comprised of cranial and spinal nerves. **Figure 11.1** presents an overview of the human nervous system.

Central Nervous System – The Brain

Figure 11.2A illustrates the brain's six main areas:

1. Medulla oblongata
2. Pons
3. Midbrain
4. Cerebellum
5. Diencephalon
6. Telencephalon

Each of the 12 cranial nerves originates in one of these anatomic areas. Figure 11.2B views the brain from the top (superior view). The longitudinal fissure runs down the midline and separates the brain's right and left sides (hemispheres). Below the fissure, a large tract of nerve fibers (corpus callosum, not shown) connects the two hemispheres. The outer portion of the brain, the **cerebral cortex** or **gray matter** (because nerve fibers lack a white myelin coating), consists of a series of folded convolutions. The bottom panel (Figure 11.2C) depicts the four lobes of the cerebral cortex (**occipital**, **parietal**, **temporal**, and **frontal**) and the sensory and motor areas and cerebellum.

The bony skull and a composite of four tough membranes (meninges), which contain a jelly-like, cushioning substance, surround the brain to protect it from injury.

Central Nervous System – The Spinal Cord

Figure 11.3A depicts the spinal cord (about 45 cm long and 1 cm in diameter) encased by 33 vertebrae (7 cervical, 12 thoracic, 5 lumbar, 5 sacral, and 4 coccygeal). The 12 pairs of peripheral nerves (grouped into cervical, thoracic, lumbar, and sacral sections according to their location along the spine) exit the cord through a small hole (foramen) at the juncture between each pair of vertebrae (Fig. 11.3C).

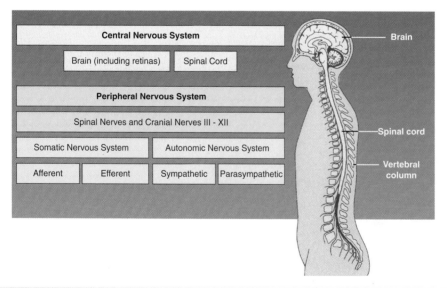

Figure 11.1 Central and peripheral divisions of the human nervous system.

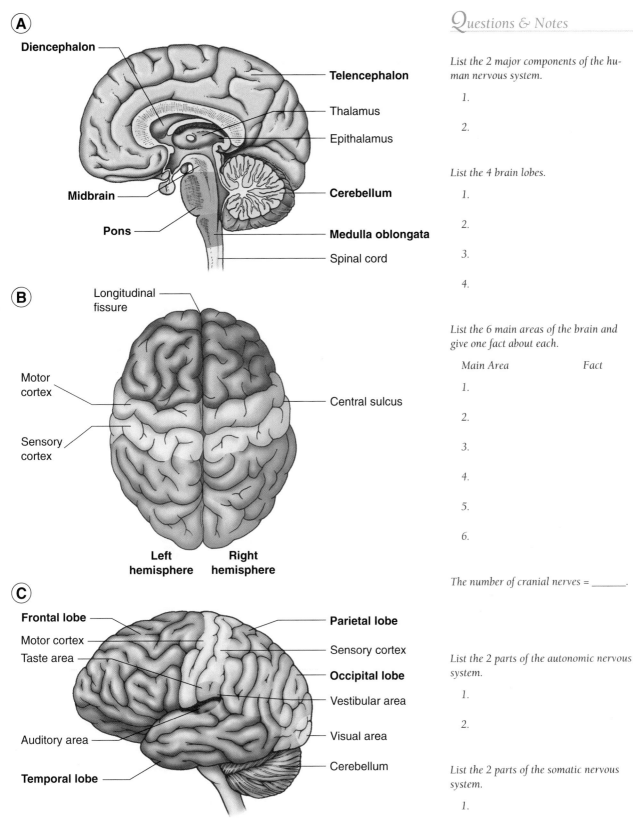

A

Diencephalon

Telencephalon

Thalamus

Epithalamus

Midbrain

Cerebellum

Pons

Medulla oblongata

Spinal cord

B

Longitudinal fissure

Motor cortex

Central sulcus

Sensory cortex

Left hemisphere   Right hemisphere

C

Frontal lobe

Parietal lobe

Motor cortex

Sensory cortex

Taste area

Occipital lobe

Vestibular area

Visual area

Auditory area

Cerebellum

Temporal lobe

Figure 11.2 **(A)** Principal six divisions of the brain, lateral view. **(B)** Superior view of the brain. **(C)** Four lobes of the cerebral cortex.

Questions & Notes

List the 2 major components of the human nervous system.

1.

2.

List the 4 brain lobes.

1.

2.

3.

4.

List the 6 main areas of the brain and give one fact about each.

Main Area   Fact

1.

2.

3.

4.

5.

6.

The number of cranial nerves = _____.

List the 2 parts of the autonomic nervous system.

1.

2.

List the 2 parts of the somatic nervous system.

1.

2.

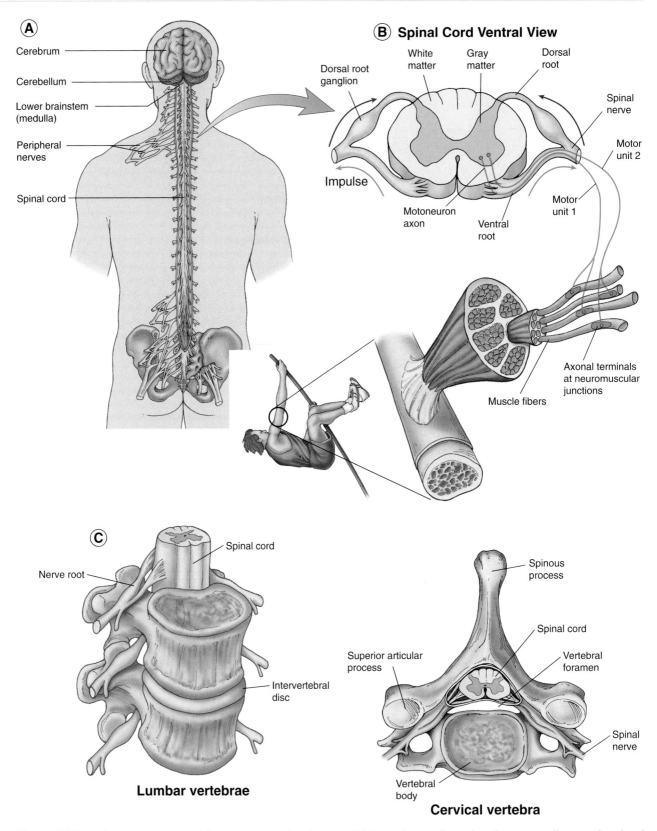

(A)

Cerebrum

Cerebellum

Lower brainstem
(medulla)

Peripheral
nerves

Spinal cord

(B) **Spinal Cord Ventral View**

Dorsal root
ganglion

White
matter

Gray
matter

Dorsal
root

Spinal
nerve

Motor
unit 2

Impulse

Motor
unit 1

Motoneuron
axon

Ventral
root

Axonal terminals
at neuromuscular
junctions

Muscle fibers

(C)

Nerve root

Spinal cord

Spinous
process

Superior articular
process

Spinal cord

Vertebral
foramen

Intervertebral
disc

Spinal
nerve

Vertebral
body

Lumbar vertebrae

Cervical vertebra

Figure 11.3 **(A)** Human spinal cord showing the peripheral nerves. **(B)** Ventral view of spinal cord section to illustrate dorsal and ventral root neural pathways and nerve impulse direction. **(C)** Junction of two lumbar vertebral bodies and a cross-section through one cervical vertebra.

This unique anatomical design allows extreme vertebral movement without affecting spinal nerves. **Intervertebral discs** separate adjacent vertebrae and under normal circumstances provide a cushioning surface. Unfortunately, a disc can bulge into the space occupied by that segment's spinal nerve, compressing it and causing pain in an area the nerve innervates (e.g., lower back or leg). This unfortunate cascade of events can cause loss of motor control. If the condition persists (with significant muscle weakness), surgical repair or removal of the offending disc often relieves the pressure and pain.

When viewed in cross section (Fig. 11.3B), the spinal cord shows its H-shaped core of gray matter. The limbs of this core, the ventral (anterior) and dorsal (posterior) horns, contain principally three types of nerves:

1. Interneurons
2. Sensory neurons
3. Motoneurons (motor neurons)

Motor (efferent) neurons exit the cord via the ventral root to supply extrafusal and intrafusal skeletal muscle fibers. **Sensory (afferent) neurons** enter the spinal cord via the dorsal root. An area of white matter containing ascending and descending nerve tracts within the cord itself surrounds the gray core. The ascending nerve tracts within the spinal cord transmit sensory information from peripheral sensory receptors to the brain. Tracts of nerve tissue descend from the brain and terminate at neurons in the spinal cord. One tract of neurons, the **pyramidal tract**, transmits impulses downward through the spinal cord. By direct routes and interconnecting spinal cord neurons, these nerves eventually excite motoneurons that control skeletal muscles. **Extrapyramidal tract** nerves originate in the brain stem and connect at all levels of the spinal cord. These neurons control posture; they provide a continual background level of neuromuscular tone, in contrast to discrete movements stimulated by the pyramidal tract nerves.

Brain Neurotransmitters

Nerves communicate by releasing at their terminal ends chemical messengers (**neurotransmitters**) that diffuse across the junction (**synapse**) between one nerve end and the cell body of another nerve. The neurotransmitter combines with a specific receptor molecule on the postsynaptic membrane to facilitate depolarization or, in some instances, hyperpolarization. Many of the neurons of the central nervous system, particularly in the brain, release and/or respond to these neurotransmitters. Important brain neurotransmitters include:

- **Monoamines:** Modified amino acids include epinephrine, norepinephrine, serotonin, histamine, and dopamine.
- **Neuropeptides:** Short chains of amino acids include arginine, vasopressin, and angiotensin II (also act as hormones [see Chapter 12]). Enkephalins and endorphins (sometimes called opioid neurotransmitters) represent other neuropeptides that produce a general sense of well-being. Release of endogenous opioid neurotransmitters with exercise contributes to the exercise "high."
- **Nitric Oxide (NO):** Neurons in the central nervous system and other cell types contain NO receptors that modulate blood pressure and local blood flow.

Peripheral Nervous System

The **peripheral nervous system** consists of 31 pairs of spinal nerves (8 cervical, 12 thoracic, 5 lumbar, 5 sacral, and 1 coccygeal) and 12 pairs of cranial nerves. Numbers identify these nerves (e.g., C-1, first nerve from cervical region). Careful experiments have tracked their exact location of the spinal nerves and mapped the muscles they innervate. Injury to a specific spinal cord area produces predictable neurologic consequences. For example, quadriplegia almost always results from damage to the upper thoracic vertebra and corresponding descending nerve tract. The peripheral nervous system includes afferent nerves that relay sensory information from muscles, joints, skin, and bones *toward* the brain and ef-

Questions & Notes

Give the primary function of intervertebral discs.

List the 3 types of neurons in the human nervous system.

1.

2.

3.

Give the main function of the extrapyramidal tract nerves.

Name 3 important human brain neurotransmitters.

1.

2.

3.

Give the main physiologic function of nitric oxide.

List the number of pairs of spinal nerves for the following regions of the spinal cord.

Cervical:

Thoracic:

Lumbar:

Sacral:

Coccygeal:

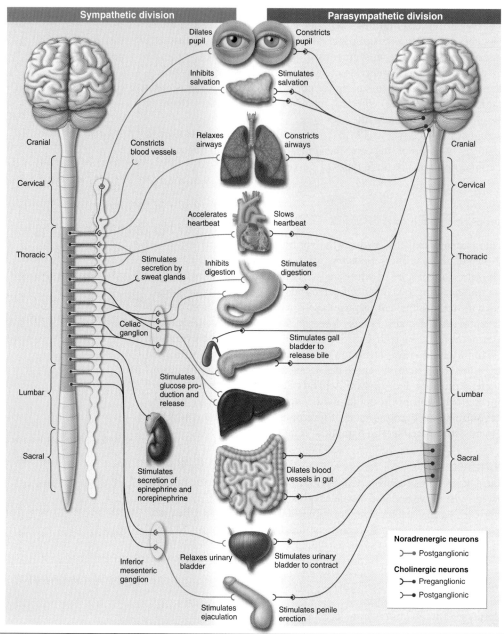

Comparison of effects of sympathetic and parasympathetic activation on end organs		
End organ	**Sympathetic effects**	**Parasympathetic effects**
Skeletal muscle	Increase blood flow	Decrease blood flow
Ventilation	Increase	Decrease
Sweat glands	Increase perspiration	No effect
Heart	Increase force and contraction rate	Decrease force and contraction rate
GI tract motility	Decrease	Increase
Eyes	Dilate pupils	Constrict pupils
Secretion of digestive juices	Decrease	Increase
Blood pressure	Increase mean pressure	Decrease mean pressure
Airways	Increase diameter	Decrease diameter

Figure 11.4   The sympathetic and parasympathetic divisions of the autonomic nervous system: comparisons of effects of activation of each. The preganglionic inputs of both divisions use acetylcholine (Ach; colored red) as neurotransmitter. The postganglionic parasympathetic innervation of the visceral organs also uses Ach, but postganglionic sympathetic innervation uses norepinephrine (NE; colored blue), with the exception of innervation of the sweat glands, which use Ach. The adrenal medulla receives preganglionic sympathetic innervation and secretes epinephrine into the bloodstream when activated. In general, sympathetic stimulation produces catabolic effects that prepare the body to "fight" or "flee," while parasympathetic stimulation produces anabolic responses that promote normal function and conserve energy. (Modified from Bear, M. F., et al.: *Neuroscience: Exploring the Brain.* 2nd Ed. Baltimore: Lippincott Williams & Wilkins, 2000.)

ferent nerves that transmit information *away* from the brain to glands and muscles. The somatic and autonomic nervous systems consist of efferent neurons.

Somatic Nervous System

The **somatic nervous system** innervates skeletal muscle (voluntary muscle). Somatic efferent nerve firing excites muscle activation, whereas autonomic nerve firing discussed in the next section can excite or inhibit activation.

Autonomic Nervous System

Efferent nerves of the autonomic nervous system activate the viscera and other tissues on the subconscious level. Autonomic nerves innervate smooth muscle (involuntary muscle) in the intestines, sweat and salivary glands, myocardium, and some endocrine glands. The heart and intestines display automatic excitability, but one can exert conscious control over these tissues under some circumstances. For example, individuals who practice yoga or meditation can modify their heart rate and regional blood flow on command. In hypnosis (from Greek "sleep"), a state of heightened awareness and focused concentration can manipulate pain perception, access repressed material, and "re-program" some behaviors. Some champion weight lifters apply hypnosis prior to attempting heavy lifts to focus all their muscular efforts on the lift without the possible distraction of discomfort in attempting the lift (just prior to the lift as muscles tense and prepare for an all-out effort). This self-induced "trance" blocks out superfluous neural input that might hinder a maximal effort.

Conscious modulation of aspects of the autonomic nervous system offers alternative treatment in medicine (e.g., control of hypertension and stress-related disorders through biofeedback techniques) and applies to certain sports. Competitors in archery and other target-shooting events consciously modify cardiovascular and respiratory patterns so normal breathing and pulse rate temporarily "stop" during the crucial steadying phase of performance.

The autonomic nervous system functions as a unit to maintain constancy in the internal environment; two distinct divisions exist: **sympathetic** and **parasympathetic** (**Fig. 11.4**). Sympathetic nerve fibers mediate excitation, whereas parasympathetic activation inhibits excitation (except for vagal parasympathetic excitation of gastrointestinal motility and tone, and secretion of insulin by the pancreas). In contrast to the somatic nervous system, some cell bodies (ganglia) of sympathetic and parasympathetic neurons exist outside the central nervous system.

Sympathetic Nervous System

Sympathetic nerve fibers supply the heart, smooth muscle, sweat glands, and viscera. These neurons exit the spinal cord and enter a series of ganglia near the cord (**sympathetic chain**). The nerves terminate relatively far from the target organ in adrenergic endings that release norepinephrine (**adrenergic fibers**). Excitation of the sympathetic nervous system occurs during fight-or-flight situations that require whole-body arousal for emergencies. Autonomic sympathetic stimulation accelerates breathing and heart rate instantaneously; the pupils dilate; and blood flows from the skin to deeper tissues in anticipation of a perceived challenge.

Parasympathetic Nervous System

Parasympathetic nerve fibers leave the brain stem and sacral segments of the spinal cord to supply the thorax, abdomen, and pelvic regions. Parasympathetic nerve endings release acetylcholine (**cholinergic fibers**). The postganglionic parasympathetic nerve fibers, located close to the organs they innervate, produce effects *opposite* of sympathetic fibers. For example, parasympathetic neural stimulation via the vagus nerve slows heart rate, whereas sympathetic stimulation accelerates heart rate.

Most organs receive sympathetic and parasympathetic stimulation. Both systems maintain a constant degree of activation (neural tone); depending on physiologic need, one system becomes more active while the other simultaneously becomes inhibited. Dual innervation of this type permits a finer level of control at

Somatic efferent nerve firing always produces what effect?

Indicate the areas of the body innervated by the sympathetic and parasympathetic nervous system.

   Sympathetic:

   Parasympathetic:

Parasympathetic nerve endings release _____.

Sympathetic nerve endings release _____.

Excitation of the sympathetic nervous system occurs during _____ *or* _____ *situations.*

Parasympathetic neural stimulation via the vagus nerves _____ *heart rate.*

Sympathetic neural stimulation _____ *heart rate and* _____ *myocardial contractility.*

the end organs. This can be likened to hot and cold faucets being open at the same time; minor adjustment in both faucets rapidly and precisely changes temperature compared with alternately turning each of the faucets on or off.

Autonomic Reflex Arc

Figure 11.5 illustrates a typical neural arrangement for a monosynaptic **reflex arc** in the spinal cord. Sensory input (a knee tap and the subsequent excitation of muscle spindles within the quadriceps muscle) initiates transmission of afferent impulses to the spinal cord via the sensory (dorsal) root. This, in turn, stimulates the anterior motoneuron to the quadricep femoris to contract and extend the lower leg (counteracting the initial stretch). In a polysynaptic reflex arc, the nerves synapse in the cord through interneurons that distribute information to various cord levels. The impulse then passes over the motor root pathway through anterior motoneurons to the effector organ.

Another example of a simple reflex arc occurs when a person accidentally touches a hot object. Stimulation of pain receptors in the fingers fires sensory information over afferent fibers to the spinal cord to activate efferent motor fibers to remove the hand from the hot object. Concurrently, the signal transmits via interneurons up the cord to the sensory area in the brain that actually "*feels*" the pain. The various operational levels for sensory input, processing, and motor output, including the reflex action just described, explain how the hand withdraws from the hot object *before* the person perceives pain. Reflex actions in the spinal cord and other subconscious areas of the central nervous system control many muscle functions. These reflex actions even operate for people who have had their spinal cords severed above the level required for the reflex.

Complex Reflexes

Complex spinal reflexes that involve multiple synapses and muscle groups also exist. Consider the situation of stepping on a tack with the left foot. Almost simultaneously as the tack pierces the skin, the right leg straightens to remove weight from the injured foot, which lifts off the ground. **Figure 11.6** illustrates the neural and motor pathways activated in this complex action, termed the **crossed-extensor reflex**, in the following sequence:

Patella Tendon Reflex

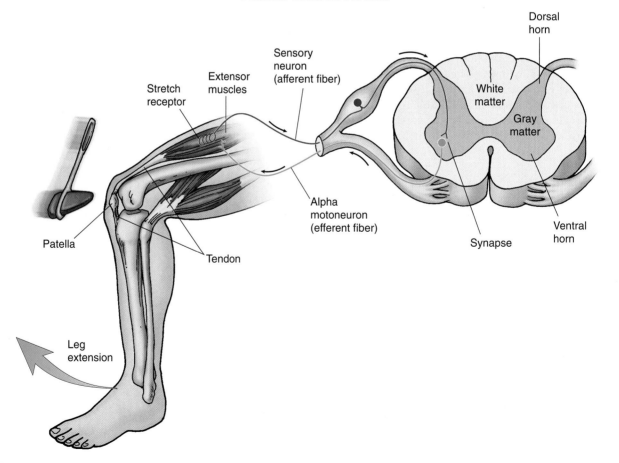

Figure 11.5 Patella tendon reflex (knee-jerk reflex) represents the simplest autonomic reflex arc involving only one synapse (monosynaptic). The gray matter contains neuron cell bodies; the white matter carries longitudinal columns of nerve fibers. Stimulation of a single alpha motoneuron can affect up to 3000 muscle fibers. The diagram shows only one side of the spinal nerve complex.

Crossed-Extensor Reflex

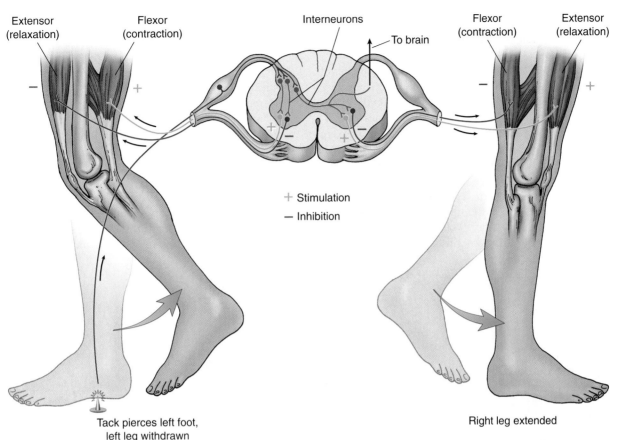

Figure 11.6   Crossed-extensor reflex in both legs represents a more complex reflex with multiple synapses and muscle groups.

1. The tack stimulates pain receptors in the skin. The receptors transmit the message to the spinal cord via the sensory nerve.
2. Sensory neurons branch to each side of the cord to activate interneurons in the gray matter.
3. Interneurons synapse with motoneurons, innervating both flexor and extensor muscles in each leg.
4. Inhibition and stimulation of appropriate leg flexor and extensor muscles cause concurrent rapid extension of the uninjured limb and flexion (removal) of the injured limb.
5. Interneuron connections simultaneously activate neural pathways to transmit information to appropriate sensory areas of the brain where the pain is "felt."

Learned Reflexes   The knee-jerk and crossed-extensor reflexes occur automatically and require no learning. Practice facilitates other more complex reflex patterns such as most sports performances or occupational tasks. Consider a trained office worker who types 90 words a minute. At an average of five letters per word, this requires six to eight keystrokes per second. For this person, the sight of a word to type initiates a series of rapid hand and finger movements requiring little conscious effort. A beginning typist, in contrast, proceeds slowly; thought must be given to the position of each key and proper execution of wrist and finger movements. As neuromuscular pathways become "ingrained" through hours of proper or meaningful practice, the typing movements progressively become reflex actions as the beginner approaches expert status. Perfecting a particular sports skill, no matter how simple it may appear (swinging a baseball bat to

Questions & Notes

Draw and label a typical autonomic reflex arc in the spinal cord.

contact a "fast" pitch, or shaping a golf shot right or left to fly over a bunker to land on the green), requires hundreds or even thousands of practice hours to *engrain* the movement until it becomes automatic.

Nerve Supply to Muscle   The terminal branches of one neuron innervate at least one of the body's approximately 250 million muscle fibers. About 420,000 motor nerves exist, yet a single nerve usually supplies numerous individual muscle fibers. *The ratio of muscle fibers to nerve generally relates to a muscle's particular movement function.* The delicate, precise movement of the eye muscles, for example, requires one neuron to control fewer than 10 muscle fibers. For less complex movements of the large leg muscles, a motoneuron may innervate as many as 3000 muscle fibers. The next sections review how information processed in the central nervous system activates specific muscles to cause an appropriate motor response.

MOTOR UNIT ANATOMY

The motor unit, comprised of an anterior motoneuron and the specific muscle fibers it innervates, represents the functional unit of movement. A motor nerve can innervate many muscle fibers because the terminal end of an axon forms numerous branches. A muscle fiber, in contrast, receives stimulation from only one nerve fiber.

Anterior Motoneuron

Figure 11.7 shows an **anterior motoneuron** that consists of a cell body, axon, and dendrites. The cell's unique design enables it to transmit electrochemical impulses from the

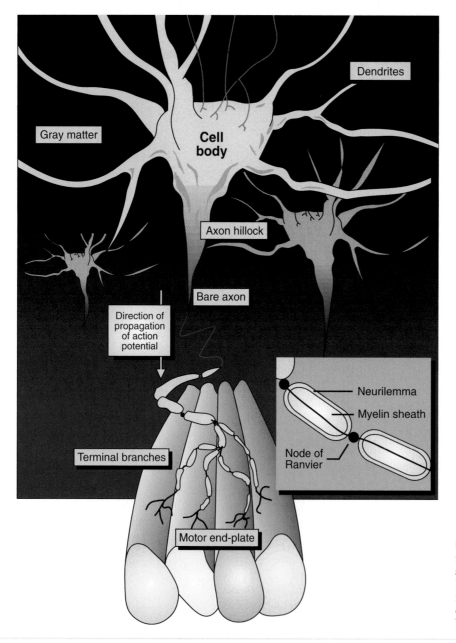

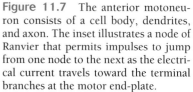

Figure 11.7   The anterior motoneuron consists of a cell body, dendrites, and axon. The inset illustrates a node of Ranvier that permits impulses to jump from one node to the next as the electrical current travels toward the terminal branches at the motor end-plate.

spinal cord to muscle. The **cell body**, located within the spinal cord's gray matter, houses the *control center*—the structures involved in replicating and transmitting the genetic code. The **axon** extends from the cord and delivers an impulse to the muscle fibers it innervates. Short neural branches called **dendrites** receive impulses through numerous spinal cord connections and conduct them toward the cell body.

Nerve cells conduct impulses *in one direction only* down the axon away from the stimulation point. As the axon approaches the muscle, it branches with each terminal branch to innervate a single muscle fiber. A whole muscle contains numerous motor units, each with a single motoneuron and its complement of muscle fibers. All of a motor unit's muscle fibers do not cluster within the muscle, but rather disperse over subregions of the muscle with other motor unit fibers. Consequently, the force generated by a motor unit distributes over a larger tissue area to reduce localized mechanical stress.

A lipid-protein membrane, the **myelin sheath**, encircles the axon of nerve fibers that are either long in length or large in diameter. In the peripheral nervous system, specialized **Schwann cells** encase the bare axon and then spiral around it. Myelin forms a large part of this sheath and insulates the axon. A thinner membrane, the **neurilemma**, covers the myelin sheath. **Nodes of Ranvier** interrupt the Schwann cells and myelin every 1 or 2 mm along the axon's length. Whereas the myelin sheath insulates the axon to ion flow, the nodes of Ranvier permit axon depolarization along axon segments. The alternating sequence of myelin sheath and node of Ranvier allows impulses to "jump" from node to node as electrical current travels toward the terminal branches at the motor end-plate. Nerve conduction in this manner accounts for the higher transmission velocity in myelinated compared with unmyelinated fibers.

Neuromuscular Junction (Motor End-Plate)

The **neuromuscular junction** (or **motor end-plate**) provides the interface between the end of a myelinated motoneuron and a muscle fiber (**Fig. 11.8**). It func-

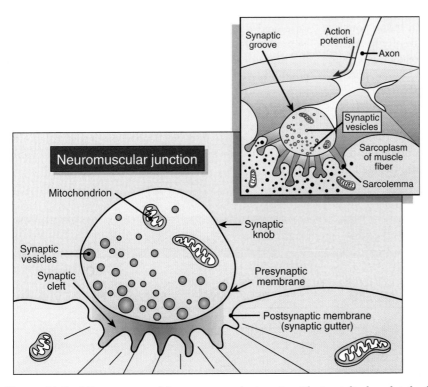

Figure 11.8   Microanatomy of the neuromuscular junction. The inset displays details of presynaptic and postsynaptic contact areas between the motoneuron and the muscle fiber it innervates.

tions to transmit the nerve impulse to muscle fibers. For each muscle fiber, usually one neuromuscular junction exists.

The terminal portion of the axon forms several smaller axon branches whose endings, the presynaptic terminals, lie close to but not in contact with the muscle fiber's plasma membrane (**sarcolemma**). The region of the postsynaptic membrane (**synaptic gutter**) contains infoldings that increase its surface area. Between the synaptic gutter and the presynaptic terminal of the axon lies the **synaptic cleft**, the region where neural impulse transmission occurs.

Excitation   *Excitation normally occurs only at the neuromuscular junction.* The neurotransmitter **acetylcholine** provides the chemical stimulus to change an electrical neural impulse into a chemical stimulus at the motor endplate. Acetylcholine, released from small, sac-like vesicles within the terminal axon, increases the postsynaptic membrane's permeability to sodium and potassium ions. This spreads the impulse over the entire muscle fiber as a wave of depolarization. As depolarization progresses, the muscle fiber's contractile machinery primes for its major function—contraction.

The enzyme **cholinesterase**, concentrated at the borders of the synaptic cleft, degrades acetylcholine within 5 milliseconds of its release from the synaptic vesicles. This action rapidly repolarizes the postsynaptic membrane. The axon resynthesizes acetylcholine from acetic acid and choline (byproducts of cholinesterase action) so the entire process can begin again with the arrival of another nerve impulse.

Facilitation   A motoneuron generates an action potential when its microvoltage decreases sufficiently to reach its threshold for excitation. **Excitatory postsynaptic potential (EPSP)** describes the change in membrane potential (increase in positive charges inside the cell) at the junction between two neurons. *The EPSP hypopolarizes the neuron, making it easier to fire.* With a subthreshold EPSP, the neuron does not discharge, but its resting membrane potential still lowers, temporarily increasing its tendency to fire. A neuron fires when many subthreshold ex-

citatory impulses arrive in rapid succession, a condition termed **temporal summation**. **Spatial summation** describes the simultaneous stimulation of different presynaptic terminals on the same neuron. The "summing" of each excitatory effect often initiates an action potential.

Removing inhibitory neural influences becomes important under certain exercise conditions. In all-out strength and power activities, disinhibition and maximal activation of all motoneurons required for a movement enhances performance. *Effective disinhibition fully activates muscle groups during maximal lifting; an effect that accounts for the rapid, highly specific strength increases early in a resistance training program.* Enhanced neuromuscular activation accounts for significant improvements in muscular strength without concomitant increases in muscle size. Central nervous system excitation (also called "neuronal facilitation") explains why intense concentration (psyching) can augment maximal strength and power performances.

Inhibition   Some presynaptic terminals generate inhibitory impulses by releasing chemicals that increase postsynaptic membrane permeability to potassium and chloride ions. The efflux of positively charged potassium ions (or influx of negatively charged chloride ions) increases the membrane's resting electrical potential to create an **inhibitory postsynaptic potential (IPSP)**. *The IPSP hyperpolarizes the neuron, making it more difficult to fire.* No action potential generates when a motoneuron encounters excitatory and inhibitory influences or encounters a large IPSP. For example, one can usually override (inhibit) the reflex to pull the hand away when removing a splinter.

The neurotransmitter amino acids gamma-aminobutyric acid (GABA) and glycine exert inhibitory effects. Neural inhibition serves protective functions and reduces the input of unwanted stimuli to produce smooth, purposeful responses.

MOTOR UNIT PHYSIOLOGY

Three physiologic and mechanical properties categorize motor units and the muscle fibers they innervate (**Table 11.1**):

Table 11•1	Characteristics and Correspondence Between Motor Units and Muscle Fiber Types				
MOTOR UNIT DESIGNATION	**FORCE PRODUCTION**	**CONTRACTION SPEED**	**FATIGUE RESISTANCE**	**SAG[a]**	**MOTOR UNIT MUSCLE FIBER TYPE**
Fast Fatigable (FF)	High	Fast	Low	Yes	Fast Glycolytic (FG)
Fast Fatigue-Resistant (FR)	Moderate	Fast	High	Yes	Fast Oxidative-Glycolytic (FOG)
Slow (S)	Low	Slow	High	No	Slow Oxidative (SO)

[a] Under repetitive stimuli, some motor units respond smoothly with a systematic increase in tension, while others first increase tension and then decrease or "sag" slightly in response to the same tetanic stimulus. These sag characteristics can classify the different motor units. Only the slow (S) motor units do not exhibit sag, which probably relates more to their lower force-generating capabilities than their fatigue characteristics.
Modified from Lieber, R.L.: *Skeletal Muscle Structure, Function, and Plasticity.* Baltimore: Lippincott Williams & Wilkins, 2002.

1. Twitch (speed of contraction) characteristics
2. Tension-generating (force) characteristics
3. Neuromuscular fatigability

Twitch Characteristics

Motor units with the capacity for low force production show slow contraction velocities yet resist fatigue; motor units that generate higher tension contract rapidly but fatigue early. **Figure 11.9** illustrates these characteristics for the following three motor unit categories:

1. Fast-twitch, high-force, and fast-fatigue (type IIb)
2. Fast-twitch, moderate-force, and fatigue-resistant (type IIa)
3. Slow-twitch, low-tension, and fatigue-resistant (type I)

Relatively large motoneurons with fast conduction velocities innervate between 300 to 500 fast-twitch muscle fibers. These fast-fatigable (FF) and fast-fatigue–resistant (FR) units reach greater peak tension and develop it faster than slow-twitch (S) motor units innervated by small motoneurons with slow conduction velocities. However, slow-twitch motor units exhibit less fatigue than fast-twitch units. Specific exercise training modifies the fatigue characteristics of motor

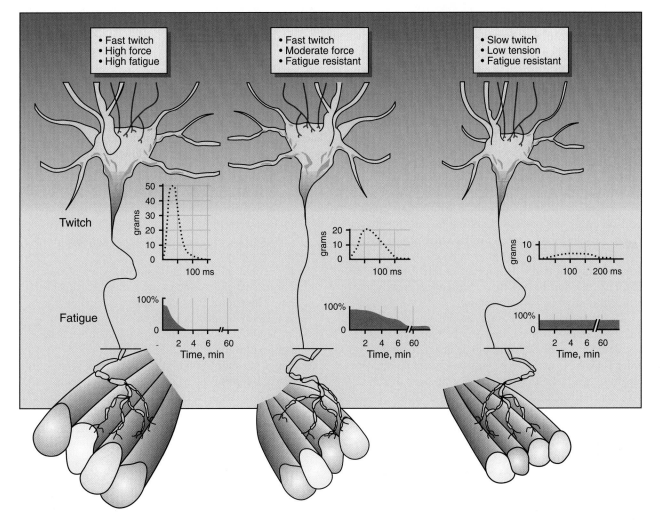

Figure 11.9   Speed, force, and fatigue characteristics of motor units. Fast-twitch motoneurons fire rapidly with short bursts; slow-twitch motoneurons fire slowly but continuously. (Modified from Edington, D.W., and Edgerton, V.R.: *The Biology of Physical Activity.* Boston: Houghton-Mifflin, 1976.)

units. For example, with prolonged aerobic training, some fast-twitch units become almost as fatigue resistant as their slow-twitch counterparts.

Tension-Generating Characteristics

All-or-None Principle If a stimulus triggers an action potential in the motoneuron, all of the accompanying muscle fibers contract synchronously. A single motor unit cannot generate strong and weak contractions; either the impulse elicits a contraction or it does not. Once the neuron fires and the impulse reaches the neuromuscular junction, the muscle cells always contract (to the fullest extent) in accord with the **all-or-none principle**.

Gradation of Force The force of muscle action varies from slight to maximal in one of two ways:

1. Increasing the *number* of motor units recruited
2. Increasing the *frequency* of motor unit discharge

Activation of all motor units in a muscle generates considerable force compared with activating only a few units. Total tension also increases if repetitive stimuli reach a muscle before it relaxes. Blending recruitment of motor units and their firing rate permits a wide variety of graded muscle actions. The golf swing provides a good example of force gradation. Tension in hands, arms, and legs continually adjusts during the backswing, swing initiation and acceleration, club-ball contact, and follow-through. The seemingly simple task of writing with a pen involves a myriad of complex, coordinated, and diverse neuromuscular forces and actions.

Motor Unit Recruitment Low force muscle actions activate only a few motor units, whereas higher force actions progressively enlist more units. **Motor unit recruitment** describes the process of adding motor units to increase muscle force. Motoneurons with progressively larger axons become recruited as muscle force increases. This response, termed the **size principle**, provides an anatomic basis for the orderly recruitment of specific motor units to produce a smooth action.

All of a muscle's motor units do not fire at the same time. For example, when lifting a barbell, specific muscles contract to move the limb and weight at a particular speed under a given magnitude of tension development. One can lift a relatively light weight at a number of speeds. With heavier weight, the speed options decrease considerably. *From the standpoint of neural control, slow-twitch and fast-twitch motor units become selectively recruited and modulated in their firing pattern to produce the desired response.*

In accordance with the size principle, slow-twitch motor units with low activation thresholds become selectively recruited during light-to-moderate effort. Activation of more powerful, higher threshold, fast-twitch units progresses as force requirements increase. Sustained, submaximal jogging, cycling, cross-country skiing on a level grade, and lifting a light weight at slow speed involve selective recruitment of slow-twitch motor units. With rapid, powerful movements, like sprint running or swimming, the fast-twitch fibers become activated, particularly type IIb fibers. A runner or bicyclist who ascends a hill or maintains a constant pace over varied terrain activates fast-twitch units.

The differential control of the motor unit firing pattern distinguishes specific athletic groups and skilled from unskilled performers. Weightlifters, for example, demonstrate a synchronous pattern of motor-unit firing (i.e., many motor units recruited simultaneously during lifting). Endurance athletes generally exhibit an asynchronous firing pattern (i.e., some motor units fire while others recover). The synchronous firing of fast-twitch fibers certainly aids the weightlifter in generating rapid force. Conversely, asynchronous firing of slow-twitch, fatigue-resistant motor units provides a built-in recuperative period to enable the endurance athlete to continue with reduced fatigue.

Neuromuscular Fatigue Resistance to fatigue (the decline in muscle tension with repeated stimulation) represents another important quality distinguishing differences in motor units. Fatigue can result from disruption in the chain of events among any of the following four components of the neuromotor system (in order of hierarchy):

1. Central nervous system
2. Peripheral nervous system
3. Neuromuscular junction
4. Muscle fiber

Factors associated with a decrease in the muscle's force-generating capacity include the following four factors:

1. Exercise-induced alterations in levels of central nervous system transmitters in various brain regions, along with the neuromodulators ammonia and cytokines secreted by immune cells, probably alter one's psychic or perceptual state to cause deterioration in ability to exercise.
2. Reductions in muscle glycogen and blood glucose produce fatigue during prolonged, submaximal exercise. This "nutrient-related fatigue" occurs despite availability of sufficient oxygen and fatty acid substrate for ATP regeneration through aerobic metabolic pathways.
3. Fatigue in short-term maximal exercise reflects insufficient oxygen availability and/or utilization, increased lactate accumulation, and an increase in $[H^+]$ within active muscle fibers. Extreme reliance on anaerobic metabolism ultimately: (a) inhibits the contractile mechanism; (b) depletes intramuscular high-energy phosphates; (c) impairs energy transfer via glycolysis from reduced activity of key enzymes; (d) disturbs the tubular system for transmitting the impulse throughout the cell; and (e) creates ionic imbalances. For example, disruption of intracellular Ca^{++} alters myofilament activity and impairs muscular performance.

4. Fatigue at the neuromuscular junction causes failure of the action potential to cross from the motoneuron to the muscle fiber. The mechanism for this aspect of neural fatigue remains unknown.

PROPRIOCEPTORS IN MUSCLES, JOINTS, AND TENDONS

Muscles, joints, and tendons contain specialized sensory receptors sensitive to stretch, tension, and pressure. These end organs, called **proprioceptors**, rapidly relay information about muscular dynamics, limb position, and movement (i.e., kinesthesia and proprioception) to conscious and subconscious portions of the central nervous system. Proprioception allows continual monitoring of the progress of any movement or sequence of movements and serves as the basis for modifying subsequent motor patterns.

Muscle Spindles

Muscle spindles provide sensory information about changes in a muscle fiber's length and tension. They primarily respond to muscle stretch through reflex action and initiate a stronger muscle action to reduce the stretch.

Figure 11.10 illustrates the fusiform-shaped spindle attached in parallel to regular muscle fibers (**extrafusal fibers**). Consequently, any elongation of the muscle stretches the spindle. The number of spindles per gram of muscle varies depending on the muscle group. More spindles exist in muscles that routinely perform complex movements. The spindle contains two types of specialized fibers with contractile capabilities called **intrafusal fibers**.

Two afferent (sensory) and one efferent (motor) nerve fibers service the spindles. The motor spindles consist of thin gamma efferent fibers that innervate the contractile, striated ends of intrafusal fibers. These fibers, activated by higher brain centers, maintain the spindle at peak operation at all muscle lengths.

Stretch Reflex   The regulation of movement and posture depends on how well a muscle spindle detects, responds to, and controls changes in extrafusal muscle fiber length. Neural input continuously bombards postural muscles to maintain their readiness to respond to voluntary movements and provide continual force to counter gravity's pull and maintain upright posture. To this end, the stretch reflex provides a fundamental controlling mechanism for neuromuscular regulation. The stretch reflex has three main components:

1. Muscle spindle that responds to stretch
2. Afferent nerve fibers that carry sensory impulses from the muscle spindle to the spinal cord
3. Efferent motoneuron that activates the stretched muscle fibers

Figure 11.11 illustrates the neural pathways involved in the stretch reflex. In part A, the biceps muscle shortens to maintain the bony lever at a 90° angle while holding a 1-kg book. Suddenly increasing the book's weight threefold (part B) stretches the muscle, causing the spindles' sensory endings to direct impulses through the dorsal root to the spinal cord to activate the motoneuron. The returning motor impulses (part C) contract the muscle more forcefully, returning the limb to its original non-stretched position.

The reflex concurrently activates interneurons in the spinal cord to facilitate an appropriate "whole body" movement response. Excitatory impulses activate synergistic muscles that support the desired movement, while inhibitory impulses flow to neurons of muscles antagonistic to the movement. In this way, the stretch reflex acts as a self-regulating, compensating mechanism; it enables the muscle to adjust automatically to differences in load (and length) without immediately processing information through higher centers of the central nervous system.

Questions & Notes

List 3 physiologic and mechanical properties that categorize motor units.

1.

2.

3.

List 2 factors that contribute to the ability to vary the force of muscular action.

1.

2.

Describe the major factor that distinguishes a skilled from an unskilled individual.

List 4 factors to explain muscular fatigue during exercise.

1.

2.

3.

4.

FOR YOUR INFORMATION

Camillo Golgi

Camillo Golgi (1843–1926), an Italian neurohistochemist, discovered the minute tendon organs that now bear his name in 1878 using a silver nitrate stain described in his masterful text, *On the Fine Anatomy of the Nervous System.* Golgi received the Nobel Prize in physiology or medicine in 1906 with Santiago Ramón y Cajal (1852–1934) for their insightful contributions about the structures of the nervous system.

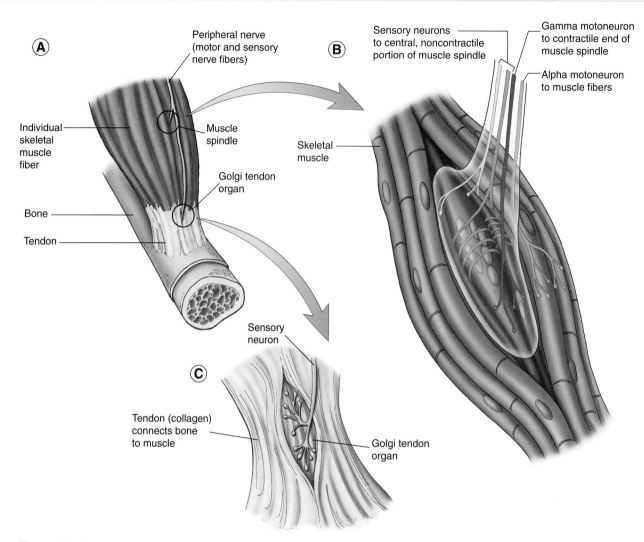

Figure 11.10 (**A**) General location of muscle spindles and Golgi tendon end organs. (**B**) Muscle spindle surrounded by skeletal muscle fibers. Two types of sensory neurons innervate the spindle's central portion: (1) fast-adapting neurons with spiral endings, and (2) slow-adapting neurons with branched endings. Gamma motoneurons innervate the contractile ends of muscle spindle cells, and alpha motoneurons activate skeletal muscle cells. (**C**) Slow-adapting sensory neurons innervate Golgi tendon organs (see Fig. 11.12).

Golgi Tendon Organs

Golgi tendon organs connect in series to as many as 25 extrafusal fibers in contrast to muscle spindles that lie parallel to extrafusal muscle fibers. The tiny sensory receptors, also located in ligaments of joints, primarily detect differences in muscle tension rather than length. **Figure 11.12** shows that Golgi tendon organs respond as a feedback monitor to discharge impulses when muscle shortens or stretches.

When activated by excessive muscle tension or stretch, Golgi receptors rapidly conduct signals to cause reflex inhibition of the muscles they supply. This occurs because of an overriding influence of inhibitory spinal interneurons on the motoneurons supplying muscle. With extreme tension or stretch, the sensor's discharge increases to further depress motoneuron activity and reduce tension in muscle fibers. Ultimately, the Golgi tendon organs protect muscle and its connective tissue harness from injury induced by excessive load.

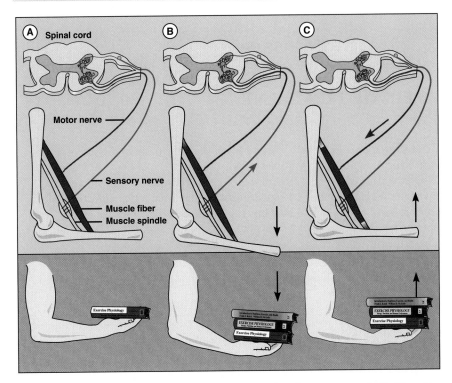

Figure 11.11 Schematic representation of the stretch reflex. Because spindle fibers (intrafusal fibers) run parallel to skeletal muscle (extrafusal) fibers, spindle fibers stretch (and fire) when extrafusal fibers stretch. Activation of the spindle's sensory receptors reflexly stimulates alpha motoneurons. Contraction of extrafusal fibers removes stretch from the intrafusal fibers and silences the spindle afferents. The diagram illustrates how the stretch reflex acts as a self-regulating mechanism to maintain relative constancy of limb position.

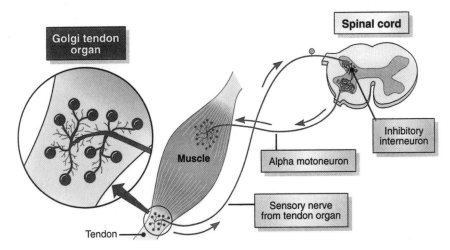

Figure 11.12 The Golgi tendon organ. Excessive tension or stretch on a muscle activates the tendon's Golgi receptors, which brings about a reflex inhibition of the muscles they supply. In this way, the Golgi tendon organ functions as a protective sensory mechanism to detect and subsequently inhibit undue strain within the muscle-tendon structure.

Questions & Notes

List the 3 variables monitored by proprioceptors:

1.

2.

3.

What is the major function of a muscle spindle?

Give 3 facts about the structural organization of muscle spindles.

1.

2.

3.

List 2 types of spindle nerve fibers.

1.

2.

List the 3 main components of the stretch reflex.

1.

2.

3.

Describe the major function of Golgi tendon organs.

Box 11–1 · CLOSE UP

PROVIDING PRUDENT, IMMEDIATE TREATMENT FOR SOFT-TISSUE INJURIES

The most common injuries during general fitness programs include sprains (overstretching or tearing of ligamentous tissue) and strains (overstretching or tearing of muscle or tendinous tissues). The extent of tissue damage depends on the magnitude of the unusual force and duration of its application. Strains and sprains are classified as first, second, or third degree. The prudent, immediate treatment of soft-tissue injury reduces further damage prior to medical treatment.

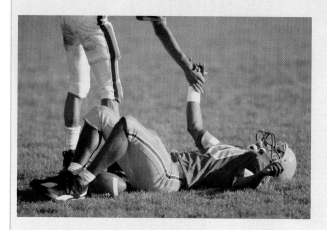

INJURY CLASSIFICATION

1. **First degree, mild injury.** Does not compromise the ligament or tendon. Physical activity can usually begin again within one week. Some localized tenderness and swelling within the muscle or connective tissue may occur, accompanied by reduced normal range of motion.
2. **Second degree, moderate injury.** Involves a tear of a ligamentous or muscle section, impairing function. Joint laxity becomes noticeable under stress; significant swelling and discoloration may occur, with in-

creased pain through the range of motion of the affected joint area.
3. **Third degree, severe injury.** Complete tear or rupture of the ligament/tendon at either end of its attachment, accompanied by joint instability. Extreme swelling, spasms, with persistent pain occur.

INJURY TREATMENT

The five-letter acronym **PRICE** (Protection, Rest, Ice, Compression, Elevation) describes the preferred immediate treatment sequence for soft-tissue injury.

1. **Protection:** Isolate the injured area to protect it from further damage.
2. **Rest:** Restrict further activity/use of the injured area.
3. **Ice:** Apply ice immediately to the injured area and continue application for 24 to 72 hours depending on injury severity. Surround the area with an ice pack secured with elastic wrap. Ice causes vasoconstriction, reducing internal bleeding and swelling (fluid seepage into surrounding tissues). Ice also reduces pain. The standard ice application interval lasts 15 to 20 minutes, with reapplication hourly or when pain persists. Ice or compression at bedtime is unnecessary unless the pain interferes with sleep. If the injury involves a contusion (bruise) to a muscle belly, mildly stretch the muscle before applying ice; if possible, maintain the stretched position for the duration of ice application.
4. **Compression:** Compression should be firm but not tight; the wrap should begin distal to the injury and proceed toward the injured area.
5. **Elevation:** Raise the injured area above heart level to minimize gravity's hydrostatic effect on venous pooling and fluid efflux into injured tissues. Elevate the limb when practical. During sleep, elevate the injured limb with blankets or pillows.

SUMMARY

1. Central nervous system neural control mechanisms finely regulate human movement. In response to internal and external stimuli, bits of sensory input are automatically and rapidly routed, organized, and retransmitted to the effector organs, the muscles.

2. The cerebellum, the major comparing, evaluating, and integrating center, fine tunes muscular activity.

3. The spinal cord and other subconscious areas of the central nervous system control numerous muscular functions.

4. The reflex arc processes and initiates automatic (subconscious) muscular movements and responses.

5. The number of muscle fibers in a motor unit depends on the muscle's movement function. Intricate movement patterns require a relatively small fiber-to-neuron ratio, whereas for gross movements, a single neuron may innervate several thousand muscle fibers.

6. The anterior motoneuron (cell body, axon, and dendrites) transmits the electrochemical neural impulse from the spinal cord to the muscle. Dendrites receive impulses and conduct them toward the cell body; the axon transmits the impulse in one direction only (down the axon to the muscle).

7. The neuromuscular junction provides the interfaces between the motoneuron and its muscle fibers. Acetylcholine release at this junction activates the muscle.

8. Excitatory and inhibitory impulses continually bombard synaptic junctions between neurons. These alter a neuron's threshold for excitation by increasing or decreasing its tendency to fire. In all-out, high-power exercise, a large degree of disinhibition benefits performance because it maximally activates a muscle's motor units.

9. Gradation of muscle force results from an interaction of factors that regulate the number and type of motor units recruited and their frequency of discharge. In accordance with the size principle, light exercise predominantly recruits slow-twitch motor units followed by activation of fast-twitch units when force output requirements increase.

10. Alterations in motor unit recruitment and firing pattern explain a large portion of strength improvement with resistance training, particularly during the first few training sessions when muscles "learn" the intricacies of highly specific neuromuscular interactions.

11. Sensory receptors in muscles, tendons, and joints relay information about muscular dynamics and limb movement to specific portions of the central nervous system. This provides crucial sensory feedback information to the central nervous system to optimize movement economy and prevent injury.

THOUGHT QUESTIONS

1. Discuss why fatigue may not relate to purely muscular factors.

2. Discuss factors to explain why some individuals are "faster learners" of certain tasks.

3. How might drugs that mimic neurotransmitters affect physiologic response and performance in maximal exercise?

PART 2 •
Muscular System: Organization and Activation

Skeletal muscles transform the chemical energy in ATP into the mechanical energy of motion. Part 2 presents the architectural organization of skeletal muscle and focuses on its gross and microscopic structure. The discussion includes the sequence of chemical and mechanical events in muscular contraction and relaxation and the differences in muscle fiber characteristics among elite performers in different sports.

COMPARISON OF SKELETAL, CARDIAC, AND SMOOTH MUSCLE

Humans possess three types of muscle (cardiac, smooth, and skeletal) and each exhibits functional and anatomical differences. Cardiac muscle, as the name implies, occurs only in the heart. It shares several common features with skeletal muscle; both appear striated under microscopic examination and contract in a similar manner. Smooth muscle lacks a striated appearance but shares cardiac muscle's characteristic of non-conscious regulation. **Table 11.2** contrasts the structural and functional characteristics of the three types of muscle.

GROSS STRUCTURE OF SKELETAL MUSCLE

Each of the more than 430 voluntary muscles in the body contains various wrappings of fibrous connective tissue. **Figure 11.13** shows a muscle cross section that consists of thousands of cylindrical cells called fibers. These long, slender multinucleated fibers (whose number largely becomes fixed by the second trimester of fetal development) lie parallel to one another, with the force of contraction occurring along the fiber's long axis.

A fine layer of connective tissue, the **endomysium**, wraps each fiber and separates it from neighboring fibers. Another layer of connective tissue, the **perimysium**, surrounds a bundle of up to 150 fibers to form a **fasciculus**. The **epimysium** surrounds the entire muscle with a fascia of fibrous connective tissue. This protective sheath tapers at its distal end as it blends into and joins the intramuscular tissue sheaths to form the dense, strong connective tissue of **tendons**. Tendons connect each end of the muscle to the **periosteum**, the outermost covering of the skeleton.

The force of muscle action transmits directly from the muscle's connective tissue harness to the tendons at their bony points of attachment.

Beneath the endomysium and surrounding each muscle fiber lays the **sarcolemma**, a thin, elastic membrane that encloses the fiber's cellular contents. The sarcoplasm, the cell's aqueous protoplasm, contains contractile proteins, enzymes, energy compounds, nuclei, and specialized cellular organelles. The sarcoplasm includes an extensive interconnecting network of tubular channels and vesicles called the **sarcoplasmic reticulum**. This highly specialized, intricate support system provides the cell with structural integrity; it also helps to activate and support the muscle fiber.

Chemical Composition

Skeletal muscle contains about 75% water and 20% protein, with the remaining 5% comprising inorganic salts and high-energy phosphates, urea, lactate, calcium, magnesium, and phosphorus; enzymes and pigments; sodium, potassium, and chloride ions; and amino acids, fats, and carbohydrates.

Blood Supply

Intense dynamic exercise often requires an oxygen uptake of 4000 mL·min^{-1} and higher, and the oxygen consumed by active muscle increases at least 70 times above its resting level to about 3400 mL·min^{-1}. To accommodate the increased oxygen requirement, the local vascular bed redirects blood flow through active tissues. In continuous, rhythmic running, swimming, and cycling, muscle blood flow fluctuates; it decreases during the shortening action and increases during muscle relaxation. Alternating contraction and re-

Table 11·2 Characteristics of the Three Types of Human Muscle			
	TYPE OF MUSCLE		
CHARACTERISTICS	**SKELETAL**	**CARDIAC**	**SMOOTH**
Location	Attached to bones	Heart only	Part of blood vessel structure: surrounds many internal hollow organs
Function	Movement	Pumps blood	Constricts blood vessels; moves contents of internal organs
Anatomical description	Large cylindrical, multinucleated cells arranged in parallel	Quadrangular cells	Small, spindle-shaped cells with long axis oriented in the same direction
Striated	Yes	Yes	No
Initiation of action potential	By neuron only	Spontaneous (pacemaker cells)	Spontaneous
Duration of electrical activity	Short (1–2 ms)	Long (~200 ms)	Very long, slow (~300 ms)
Energy source	Anaerobic, Aerobic	Aerobic	Aerobic
Energy efficiency	Low	Moderate	High
Fatigue resistance	Low to high	Low	Very low
Rate of shortening	Fast	Moderate	Very slow
Duration of action	As brief as 100 ms; prolonged tetanus	Short (~300 ms); summation and tetanus not possible	Very long; may be sustained indefinitely

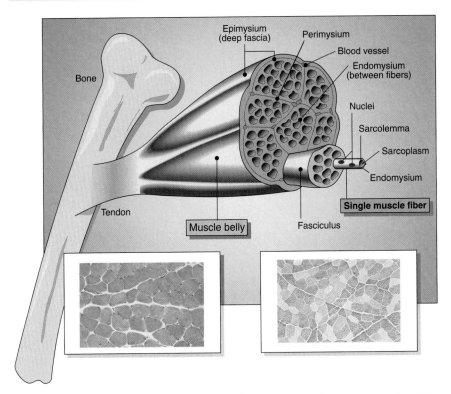

Figure 11.13   Cross section of an intact muscle and its connective tissue wrappings. The inset displays transverse sections of striated muscle where different staining procedures identify different muscle fiber types. (Inset photos from Sobotta, J., and Hammersen, F.: *Histology. Color Atlas of Microscopic Anatomy.* 3rd Ed. Baltimore: Urban & Schwarzenberg, 1992.)

What does the five-letter acronym PRICE refer to?

Draw and label the cross section of a muscle.

laxation provides a "milking action" to facilitate blood flow through the muscles back to the heart. Concurrently, the rapid dilation of previously dormant capillaries within muscle increases the effective surface for nutrient and gaseous exchange.

Straining-type activities present a somewhat different picture. When a muscle contracts to about 60% of its force-generating capacity, blood flow within the muscle diminishes from elevated intramuscular pressure. The muscle's compressive force with a maximal isometric action literally retards blood flow. As a result, the breakdown of stored intramuscular phosphagens and anaerobic glycolytic reactions provide the energy to sustain muscular effort.

Muscle Capillarization   The capillary microcirculation removes heat and metabolic byproducts from active tissues. Aerobic training enhances these functions by increasing skeletal muscle capillary density up to 40%.

SKELETAL MUSCLE ULTRASTRUCTURE

Electron microscopy, x-ray diffraction, and histochemical staining techniques have revealed the ultrastructure of skeletal muscle. **Figure 11.14** shows the different levels of subcellular organization within a muscle fiber.

Each muscle fiber contains smaller functional units that lie parallel to the fiber's long axis. The **myofibrils**, approximately 1 μ in diameter, contain even smaller subunits (called **myofilaments**) that also run parallel to the myofibril's long axis. The myofilaments consist mainly of two proteins, **actin** and **myosin**, that constitute about 84% of the myofibrillar complex.

The Sarcomere

At low magnification under a light microscope, the alternating light and dark bands along the length of the skeletal muscle fiber appear **striated**. **Figure 11.15**

The stable skeletal part to which the muscle attaches is the _____; the distal attachment of the muscle to the moving bone is the _____.

Why is the sarcoplasmic reticulum important?

Indicate the percentage composition of skeletal muscle for the following:

Water:

Protein:

Other:

The capillarization of skeletal muscle is about _____% greater in endurance athletes than untrained counterparts.

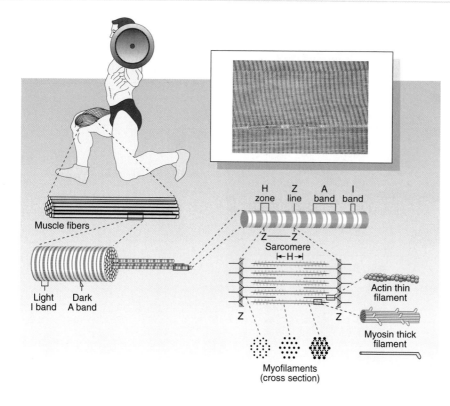

Figure 11.14 Microscopic organization of skeletal muscle (microscope magnification, approximately times 205,000). Muscle fibers comprise the contractile component of whole muscle; these fibers contain myofibrils (composed of actin and myosin protein filaments). The inset displays skeletal muscle fibers with prominent cross-striations.

illustrates the structural details of this cross-striation pattern within a myofibril.

The **I band** shows up as the lighter area, while the darker zone is the **A band**. The **Z line** bisects the I band and adheres to the sarcolemma to stabilize the entire structure. *The sarcomere, the repeating unit between two Z lines, comprises the functional unit of the muscle cell.* The actin and myosin filaments within a sarcomere provide the mechanical mechanism for muscle action.

The position of the sarcomere's thin actin and thicker myosin proteins overlaps the two filaments. The center of the A band contains the **H zone**, a region of lower optical density because of the absence of actin filaments in this region. The **M line** bisects the central portion of the H zone and delineates the sarcomere's center. The M line contains

the protein structures that support the arrangement of myosin filaments.

Actin-Myosin Orientation

Figure 11.16 illustrates actin-myosin orientation within a sarcomere at resting length. Six thin actin filaments, each about 50 angstroms (Å; 1 Å = 100-millionths of a cm) in diameter and 1 μ long, surround a thicker myosin filament (150 Å in diameter and 1.5 μ long). This forms an impressive muscular substructure. For example, a 1 μ-diameter myofibril contains about 450 thick filaments in the center of the sarcomere and 900 thin filaments at each end. Consequently, a single muscle fiber 100 μ in diameter and 1 cm long contains about 8000 myofibrils, each

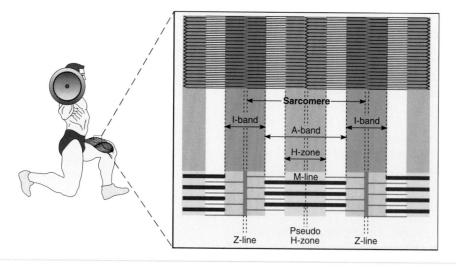

Figure 11.15 Structural orientation of myofilaments in a sarcomere. The Z line borders the sarcomere at both ends.

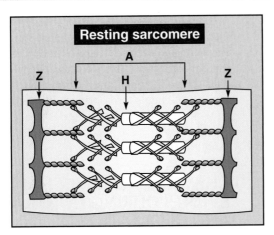

Figure 11.16   Ultrastructure of actin-myosin orientation within a resting sarcomere.

Questions & Notes

Diagram the microscopic anatomy of a muscle sarcomere. Identify actin and myosin filaments, I and A bands, Z line, and H zone.

with 4500 sarcomeres. In a single muscle fiber, this translates to a total of 16 billion thick and 64 billion thin filaments in a single muscle fiber.

Figure 11.17 details the spatial orientation of various proteins that form the contractile filaments. Projections, or **crossbridges**, spiral around the myosin filament in the region where the actin and myosin filaments overlap. Crossbridges repeat at intervals of 450 Å along the filament. Their globular, lollipop-like heads extend perpendicularly to interact with the thinner actin strands; this creates the structural and functional link between myofilaments.

Tropomyosin and **troponin**, the two most important constituents of the actin helix structure, regulate the make-and-break contacts between myofilaments during muscle action. Tropomyosin distributes along the length of the actin filament in a groove formed by the double helix. It inhibits actin and myosin interaction (coupling) and prevents their permanent bonding. Troponin, embedded at fairly regular intervals along the actin strands, exhibits a high affinity for calcium ions (Ca^{++}), which play a crucial role in muscle function and fatigue. The action of Ca^{++} and troponin triggers myofibrils to interact and slide past each other. Once

Which cellular component gives the muscle fiber its striated appearance?

Name the functional unit of the muscle fiber.

Name the sarcomere's 2 contractile proteins.

1.

2.

What is the structural link between thin and thick myofilaments?

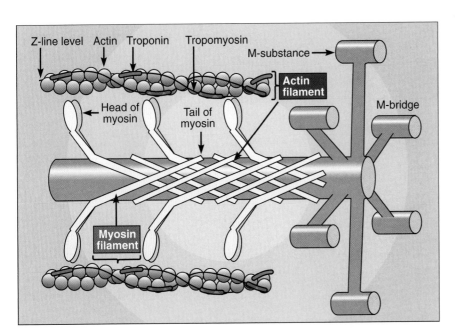

Figure 11.17   Details of the thick and thin protein filaments, including tropomyosin, troponin, and the M line. The globular heads of myosin contain the enzyme myosin ATPase; these active heads free energy from ATP to power contraction.

fiber activation occurs, troponin molecules change to tug on the tropomyosin protein strand, moving the tropomyosin deeper into the groove between the two actin strands. This uncovers actin's active molecular sites and allows muscle action to proceed.

The *M* line consists of transverse and longitudinally oriented proteins that maintain proper orientation of the thick filament within a sarcomere. Figure 11.17 shows that the perpendicular oriented M-bridges connect with six adjacent thick (myosin) filaments in a hexagonal pattern.

Intracellular Tubule Systems

Figure 11.18 illustrates the tubule system within a muscle fiber. The sarcoplasmic reticulum's extensive network of interconnecting tubular channels runs parallel to the myofibrils. The lateral end of each tubule terminates in a sac-like vesicle that stores Ca^{++}. Another network of tubules, the transverse-tubule system (or **T-tubule system**), runs perpendicular to the myofibril. The T tubules lie between the lateral-most portion of two sarcoplasmic channels; the vesicles of these structures abut the T tubule. The repeating pattern of two vesicles and T tubules in the region of each Z line forms a **triad**. Each sarcomere contains two triads; this pattern repeats regularly throughout the myofibril's length.

The T tubules pass through the fiber and open externally from the inside of the muscle cell. *The triad and T-tubule system function as a microtransportation or plumbing network for spreading the action potential (wave of depolarization) from the fiber's outer membrane inward to the deeper regions of the cell.* The triad sacs release Ca^{++} during depolarization; this diffuses a short distance to activate the actin filaments. Contraction begins when the myosin filaments' crossbridges interact with the active sites on actin filaments. When electrical excitation ceases, cytoplasmic free Ca^{++} concentration decreases and the muscle relaxes.

CHEMICAL AND MECHANICAL EVENTS DURING CONTRACTION AND RELAXATION
Sliding-Filament Theory

*The sliding-filament theory (http://muscle.ucsd.edu/musintro/Bridge.shtml) proposes that muscle fibers shorten or lengthen because thick and thin myofilaments slide past each other without the filaments themselves changing length. The myosin crossbridges, which cyclically attach, rotate, and detach from the actin filaments with energy from ATP hydrolysis, provide the **molecular motor** to drive fiber shortening.* Muscle contraction changes the relative size of the sarcomere's various zones and bands. Figure 11.19 illustrates that the thin actin myofilaments slide past the myosin myofilaments and move into the region of the A band during contraction and move out in relaxation.

The major structural rearrangement during contraction occurs in the I band region. The I band decreases

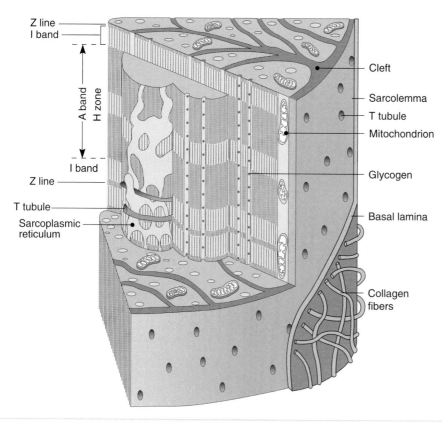

Figure 11.18 Three-dimensional view of the sarcoplasmic reticulum and T-tubule system within the muscle fiber.

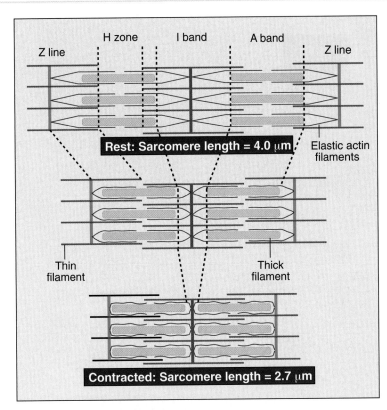

In which muscle band region does major structural rearrangement take place during muscle action.

Give the structure that provides the mechanical power stroke for actin and myosin filiaments to slide past each other.

Figure 11.19   Structural rearrangement of actin and myosin filaments at resting muscle length and during contraction (1 μm = 0.000001 m).

markedly in size as the Z bands become pulled toward each sarcomere's center. No change occurs in A band width, although the H zone can disappear when the actin filaments contact at the center of the sarcomere. An isometric muscle action generates force, while the fiber's length remains relatively unchanged. In this situation, the relative spacing of I and A bands remains constant, allowing the same molecular groups to repeatedly interact with each other. The A band widens when a muscle generates force while lengthening in an eccentric action.

Write the formula for the dissociation of actomyosin.

Mechanical Action of Crossbridges

The globular head of the myosin crossbridge provides the mechanical power stroke for actin and myosin filaments to slide past each other. **Figure 11.20** shows the oscillating to-and-fro action of the crossbridges, which move similar to the action of oars in water. But unlike oars, the crossbridges do not all move synchronously. During muscle activation, each crossbridge undergoes repeated but independent cycles of attachment and detachment to actin. Because a single crossbridge moves only a short distance, crossbridges must attach, produce movement, and detach thousands of times to shorten the sarcomere. Only about 50% of the crossbridges contact the actin filaments at any instant to form the contractile protein complex **actomyosin**; the remaining crossbridges maintain some other position in their vibrating cycle.

Name the substance that provides energy for crossbridge movement.

The right side of Figure 11.20 illustrates that each crossbridge action contributes only a small longitudinal displacement to the filaments' total sliding action. This process has been likened to climbing a rope, with the arms and legs representing the crossbridges. Climbing occurs by first reaching with the arms, then grabbing, pulling, contacting with the legs, and breaking arm contact, and then repeating this cycle throughout the climb.

Link Between Actin, Myosin, and ATP   Interaction and movement of the protein filaments during a muscle action require that the myosin cross-

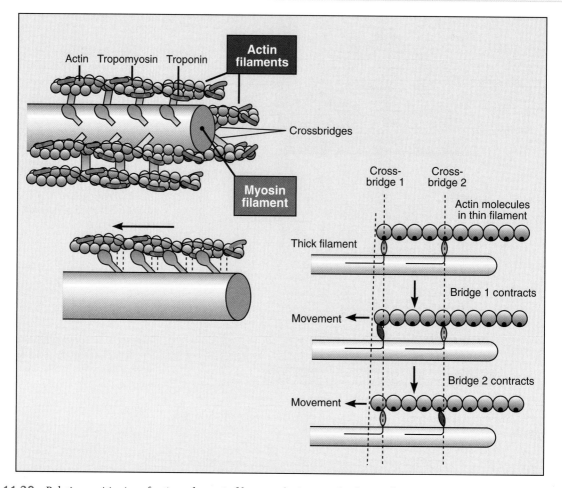

Figure 11.20   Relative positioning of actin and myosin filaments during crossbridge oscillation. The action of each bridge produces a small movement. For clarity, we omitted one of the actin strands from the left-hand portion of the figure.

bridges continually oscillate by combining, detaching, and recombining to new sites along the actin strands (or the same sites in a static action). When an ATP molecule joins the actomyosin complex, it detaches the myosin crossbridges from the actin filament. This reaction permits the myosin crossbridge to resume its original state so it can again bind to a new active actin site. The dissociation of actomyosin occurs in the following chemical reaction:

$$Actomyosin + ATP \rightarrow Actin + Myosin\text{-}ATP$$

ATP serves an important function in muscle action. *Splitting the terminal phosphate from ATP provides energy for crossbridge movement.* One of the reacting sites on the globular head of the myosin crossbridge binds to a reactive site on actin. The other myosin active site acts as the enzyme myofibrillar adenosine triphosphatase (**myosin-ATPase**) that splits ATP to release its energy. ATP splits relatively slowly if myosin and actin remain apart; when joined, the ATP hydrolysis rate increases tremendously. Energy released from ATP changes the shape of the globular head of the myosin crossbridge so it interacts and oscillates with the appropriate actin molecule.

Excitation-Contraction Coupling

Excitation-contraction coupling provides the physiologic mechanism whereby an electrical discharge at the muscle initiates the chemical events that cause activation.

An inactive muscle's Ca^{++} concentration remains relatively low. When stimulated to contract, the arrival of the action potential at the transverse tubules releases Ca^{++} from the lateral sacs of the sarcoplasmic reticulum, dramatically increasing intracellular Ca^{++} levels. The rapid binding of Ca^{++} to troponin in the actin filaments releases troponin's inhibition of actin-myosin interaction. In a sense, the muscle "turns on" for action.

Myosin-ATPase splits ATP when the active sites of actin and myosin join together. Energy transfer from ATP breakdown moves the myosin crossbridges, allowing the muscle to generate tension.

$$Actin + Myosin\ ATPase \rightarrow Actomyosin\ ATPase$$

The crossbridges uncouple from actin when ATP binds to the myosin bridge. Coupling and uncoupling continue as long as Ca^{++} concentration remains at a level sufficient to inhibit the troponin-tropomyosin system. Discontinuing the nerve stimulus to the muscle moves Ca^{++} back into the lateral sacs of the sarcoplasmic reticulum. This restores the inhibitory effect of troponin-tropomyosin; the presence of ATP maintains actin and myosin separation.

$$\text{Actomyosin-ATPase} \rightarrow \text{Actomyosin} + \text{ADP} + \text{Pi} + \text{Energy}$$

Figure 11.21 illustrates the interaction among actin and myosin filaments, Ca^{++}, and ATP in relaxed and contracted muscle fibers. In essence, the magnitude and duration of contraction relates directly to the presence of calcium. Contraction ceases (and relaxation begins) when calcium moves back into the sarcoplasmic reticulum, allowing the troponin-tropomyosin complex to inhibit myosin and actin interaction.

Relaxation

Following muscle action, active transport mechanisms pump Ca^{++} into the sarcoplasmic reticulum, concentrating Ca^{++} in the lateral vesicles. Calcium retrieval from the myofilament proteins "turns off" the active sites on the actin filament. Deactivation of troponin-tropomyosin prevents mechanical linkage between myosin crossbridges and actin filaments. This reduces myosin ATPase activity, so ATP hydrolysis ceases. Relaxation ends when the actin and myosin filaments return to their original state.

Sequence of Events in Muscle Excitation-Contraction

Nine important steps describe muscle activation and relaxation:

1. Initiation of an action potential by the anterior motoneuron. The impulse spreads over the muscle fiber's surface as the sarcolemma depolarizes.
2. The muscle's action potential depolarizes the transverse tubules at the sarcomere's A-I junction.

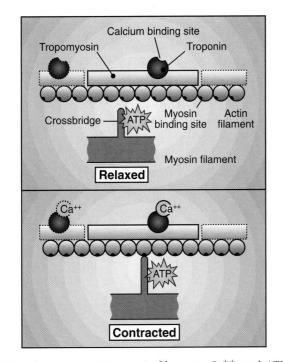

Figure 11.21   Interaction among actin-myosin filaments, Ca^{++}, and ATP in relaxed and contracted muscle. In the relaxed state, troponin and tropomyosin interact; actin prevents coupling of a myosin crossbridge to actin. During contraction, the crossbridge couples with actin because Ca^{++} binds with troponin-tropomyosin.

3. Depolarization of the transverse tubules releases Ca^{++} from the lateral sacs of the sarcoplasmic reticulum.

4. Ca^{++} binds to troponin-tropomyosin in the actin filaments. This releases the inhibition that prevents actin from combining with myosin.

5. Actin combines with myosin ATP. Actin also activates myosin ATPase, which then splits ATP. Energy from ATP hydrolysis powers the movement of the myosin crossbridges.

6. Binding of ATP to the myosin crossbridge breaks the actin-myosin bond and allows the crossbridge to separate from actin. This creates relative movement (sliding) of the thick and thin filaments, and the muscle shortens.

7. Crossbridge activation continues as long as Ca^{++} concentration remains high enough (due to membrane depolarization) to inhibit the troponin-tropomyosin system.

8. Ca^{++} concentration rapidly decreases when muscle stimulation ceases, and active transport pumps Ca^{++} back into the lateral sacs of the sarcoplasmic reticulum.

9. Ca^{++} removal restores the inhibitory action of troponin-tropomyosin. In the presence of ATP, actin and myosin remain in a dissociated, relaxed state.

MUSCLE FIBER TYPE

As discussed in Part 1, human skeletal muscle does not consist of a homogeneous group of fibers with similar metabolic and functional properties. *Two* distinct fiber types have emerged for classification by their *contractile* and *metabolic* characteristics: fast twitch and slow twitch. **Table 11.3** lists characteristics of these fiber types and subdivisions.

Measurement of Muscle Fiber Types

One of the first methods classified muscle fiber types by histochemical staining, placing fibers into one of three categories based on stain shading (from dark to light, with an intermediate shade). Another method using gel electrophoresis identifies specific types of myosin found in the muscle (called myosin isoforms). Slow-contracting (**type I**) fibers stain dark and have myosin isoforms with low ATPase activity; these fibers shorten at a slow rate. In comparison, fast fibers (**type II**) contain myosin isoforms with high ATPase activity that promote a rapid breakdown of ATP for the energy requirements for high-speed muscle shortening.

Other classification schemes for **muscle fiber typing** utilize fiber structure, biochemistry, function, and contractility. Complications inherent with muscle fiber typing include the inability to generalize from a single, small sample from one muscle to the entire body musculature. Fiber types tend to layer within a muscle. Thus, a small sample of muscle secured from a single area may not represent the biopsied muscle's total fiber population. The multiple criteria for classifying and characterizing human muscle depicted in Table 11.3 may be a more appropriate classification strategy than applying only one criterion.

Table 11·3   Classification of Skeletal Muscle Fiber Types

| | FIBER TYPES | | |
| | FAST-TWITCH | | SLOW-TWITCH |
CHARACTERISTIC	**TYPE IIB**	**TYPE IIA**	**TYPE I**
Electrical activity patterns	Phasic; high frequency		Tonic; low frequency
Morphology	FTb	FTa	ST
Color	White	White/red	Red
Fiber diameter	Large	Intermediate	Small
Capillaries/mm^2	Low	Intermediate	High
Mitochondrial volume	Low	Intermediate	High
Histochemistry and	IIB	IIA	I
biochemistry	FG	FOG	SO
Myosin ATPase	High	High	Low
Calcium capacity	High	Medium/high	Low
Glycolytic capacity	High	High	Low
Oxidative capacity	Low	Medium/high	High
Function and	FF	FR	S
contractility	FT	FT	ST
Speed of action	Fast	Fast	Slow
Speed of relaxation	Fast	Fast	Slow
Fatigue resistance	High	Moderate/high	Low
Force capacity	High	Intermediate	Low

FT = fast-twitch; FG = fast, glycolytic; FOG = fast, oxidative, glycolytic; SO = slow, oxidative; FF = fast-contracting, fast-fatigue; FR = fast-contracting, fatigue-resistant; S = slow-contracting.
From Kraus, W.: Skeletal muscle adaptation to chronic low-frequency motor nerve stimulation. *Exerc. Sport Sci. Rev.*, 22:313, 1994.

Fast-Twitch Muscle Fibers

Fast-twitch muscle fibers exhibit the following characteristics:

1. Rapidly transmit action potentials
2. High activity level of myosin ATPase
3. Rapid rate of calcium release and uptake by the sarcoplasmic reticulum
4. Generate rapid crossbridge turnover

These four qualities relate to how well a fast-twitch fiber rapidly transfers energy for quick, forceful muscle actions. Recall that myosin-ATPase splits ATP to provide energy for muscle action. The fast-twitch fiber's intrinsic speed of contraction and tension development averages two to three times the speed of fibers classified as slow-twitch.

Fast-twitch fibers rely on a well-developed, short-term glycolytic system for energy transfer. They have been labeled FG fibers to signify fast glycogenolytic capabilities. Short-term, high-power output activities and other forceful muscular actions that depend almost entirely on anaerobic metabolism for energy activate fast-twitch fibers. Stop-and-go or change-of-pace sports (basketball, soccer, rugby, lacrosse, field hockey) also require rapid energy from anaerobic pathways in fast-twitch fibers.

Fast-Twitch Subdivisions   Fast-twitch fiber subdivisions exist in humans. The type IIa fiber combines a fast contraction speed with a moderately well-developed capacity for aerobic energy transfer (high level of the aerobic enzyme succinic dehydrogenase [SDH]) and anaerobic energy transfer (high level of the anaerobic enzyme phosphofructokinase [PFK]). The term **fast-oxidative-glycolytic (FOG)** also describes these fibers. Another subdivision, the type IIb fiber (considered the true **fast-glycolytic [FG] fiber**), possesses the greatest potential for anaerobic energy transfer.

Slow-Twitch Muscle Fibers

Slow-twitch muscle fibers generate energy for ATP resynthesis predominantly by aerobic energy transfer. They possess a low activity level of myosin ATPase, a slow speed of contraction, and a glycolytic capacity less well developed than fast-twitch counterparts (Table 11.3). Slow-twitch fibers contain relatively large and numerous mitochondria and iron-containing cytochromes of the electron transport chain (which contribute to their red appearance). A high concentration of mitochondrial enzymes supports the enhanced aerobic metabolic machinery. Consequently, slow-twitch fibers resist fatigue and power prolonged aerobic exercise. These fibers are labeled **slow-oxidative (SO) fibers**, which describes their slow contraction speed and predominant reliance on oxidative metabolism.

Studies of muscle glycogen depletion patterns indicate that slow-twitch muscle fibers almost exclusively power prolonged, moderate exercise. Even after exercising for 12 hours, the limited but still available glycogen exists in the unused fast-twitch fibers. Differences in oxidative capacity of the two fiber types also determine blood flow capacity through muscle tissues during exercise; slow-twitch fibers receive considerably more blood than fast-twitch counterparts. Exercise at near-maximum aerobic and anaerobic levels, as in middle-distance running, swimming, or multiple-sprint sports (field hockey, lacrosse, basketball, ice hockey, soccer), activates both muscle fiber types.

Muscle Fiber Type Differences Among Athletic Groups

Several interesting observations emerge concerning muscle fiber type variation among individuals and sport categories and possible influence of specific exercise training on fiber composition and metabolic capacity. On average, sedentary chil-

Questions & Notes

List 3 characteristics of FT muscle fibers.
   1.

   2.

   3.

List 2 subdivisions of FT muscle fibers.
   1.

   2.

FOR YOUR INFORMATION

Rigor Mortis
Soon after death, the muscles become stiff and rigid, a condition termed *rigor mortis*. This occurs because the muscle cells no longer contain ATP. Without ATP, the myosin crossbridges and actin remain attached, so the muscle does not return to a relaxed state.

FOR YOUR INFORMATION

Muscle Fiber Training Specificity
Why do some highly trained athletes who switch to a sport requiring different muscle groups feel essentially untrained for the new activity? The answer is fairly straightforward: only the specific fibers used in training adapt metabolically and physiologically to the specific exercise regimen. Thus, swimmers or canoeists do not necessarily transfer their upper-body "fitness" to a running sport unless they specifically train the muscles required for that sport.

Box 11–2 • CLOSE UP

PROPRIOCEPTIVE NEUROMUSCULAR FACILITATION (PNF) STRETCHING

Static stretching involves a slow and sustained action to increase the range of motion (ROM) of a joint. Advantages of static stretching include:

- Decreased possibility of exceeding the normal ROM
- Lower energy expenditure
- Reduced potential for specific muscle soreness

Static stretching techniques include passive (relaxation of all voluntary and reflex muscular resistance followed by passive assistance from another person or device during voluntary movement), active assistive (involves assistance from another person as the segment moves through its normal ROM), active (a muscle or joint actively moves through its ROM), and proprioceptive neuromuscular facilitation (PNF; an inverse stretch reflex induces relaxation in a muscle prior to its being stretched, allowing for increased stretch).

Proprioceptive Neuromuscular Facilitation Stretching

PNF stretching increases ROM by augmenting prior muscle relaxation through spinal reflex mechanisms using one of two techniques:

1. **Contract-relax stretch** (hold-relax stretch). This stretching technique involves a prior isometric action of the muscle group to be stretched, followed by a slow, static stretch (relaxation phase).

2. **Contract-relax-contract stretch** (hold-relax-contract stretch), also referred to as the **contract-relax with agonist contraction (CRAC)** technique. This approach involves an isometric action of the muscle group to be stretched; the relax stretching phase is accompanied by a submaximal action of the opposing (agonist) muscle group.

Both PNF techniques use **reciprocal inhibition**; the isometric action of the antagonists (muscle group being stretched) induces a reflex facilitation and contraction of the agonist. This suppresses the contractile activity in the antagonist muscle during the slow, static stretch phase. Inhibition allows for an increased stretch of the antagonist muscle and connective tissue harness. The CRAC technique supposedly induces additional inhibitory input to the antagonist through reciprocal inhibition, allowing for greater stretch of the antagonist.

Performing PNF Stretches

1. Stretch the target muscle group by moving the joint to the end of its ROM (Figure 1A).
2. Isometrically contract the prestretched muscle group against an immovable resistance (e.g., partner) for 5 to 6 seconds.
3. Relax the contracted muscle group as the partner stretches the muscle group to a new, increased ROM (Figure 1B). With CRAC, the opposing muscle group (agonist) contracts submaximally for 5 to 6 seconds to facilitate relaxation and produce further stretching of the muscle group.

---

dren and adults possess about 50% slow-twitch fibers. The percentage of fast-twitch fibers probably distributes equally between subdivisions. However, fiber-type distribution varies considerably among individuals. Generally, one's muscle fiber-type distribution remains consistent for the body's major muscle groups.

Elite athletes possess distinct patterns of fiber distribution. Successful endurance athletes, for example, possess a predominance of slow-twitch fibers in the muscles routinely activated in their sport; the fast-twitch muscle fiber predominates for sprint athletes. **Figure 11.22** illustrates sport-specific tendencies for muscle fiber type among top Nordic competitors from different sports. Distance runners and cross-country skiers with the highest aerobic and endurance capacities possess the greatest percentages of slow-twitch fibers, often as high as 90%. In contrast, weightlifters, ice-hockey players, and sprinters tend to

have more fast-twitch fibers and a relatively lower $\dot{V}O_{2max}$. As might be expected, male and female middle-distance specialists show approximately equal percentages of the two muscle fiber types. Equal fiber-type distribution also exists for throwers, jumpers, and high jumpers (power athletes).

Relatively clear-cut distinctions between performance and muscle fiber composition emerge only for elite athletes who have achieved prominence in a specific sport category. Regardless of performance status, muscle fiber composition does not exclusively determine success. Within groups of trained or untrained individuals, knowledge of a person's predominant fiber type provides limited value in predicting performance outcome. Achievement depends on a blending of many physiologic, biochemical, neurologic, and biomechanical support systems, and not simply on a single factor like muscle fiber type.

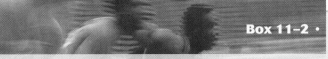

Box 11–2 •   CLOSE UP *(Continued)*

PNF Example   To stretch the hamstring muscles, the individual lies on the floor with the arms extended to the side (Fig. 1A). The person contracts the hamstrings muscle isometrically as the partner offers resistance to

horizontal extension (Fig. 1A). Following the isometric action, the partner stretches the hamstrings to new increased ROM (Fig. 1B).

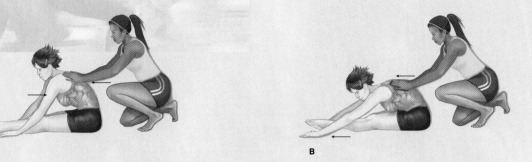

A   B

Figure 1   Proprioceptive neuromuscular facilitation (PNF) stretching technique: **(A)** isometric phase; **(B)** stretching phase.

Guidelines for Proper Stretching Using PNF

1. Determine the appropriate posture or position to ensure proper position and alignment prior to the stretch.
2. Emphasize proper breathing. Inhale through the nose and exhale during the stretch through pursed lips, with the eyes closed to increase concentration and awareness of the stretch.
3. Hold end-points progressively for 30 to 90 seconds, followed by another deep breath.

4. Exhale and feel the muscle being stretched and relaxed to achieve further ROM.
5. Do *not* bounce or spring while stretching.
6. Do *not* force a stretch while breath-holding.
7. Increasing stretching range during exhalation encourages full-body relaxation.
8. Slowly reposition from the stretch posture and allow muscles to recover to their natural resting length.

REFERENCES

Sady, S.P., et al.: Flexibility training: Ballistic, static or proprioceptive neuromuscular facilitation? *Arch. Phys. Med. Rehabil.,* 63:261, 1982.

http://www.thestretchinghandbook/archives/pnf-stretching.htm

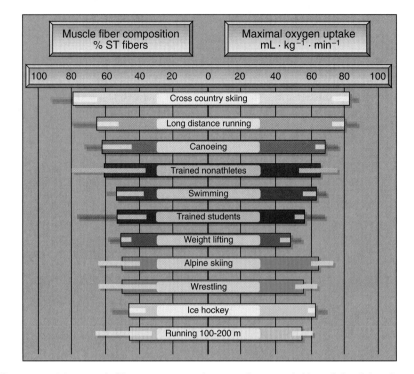

Figure 11.22   Muscle fiber composition (percent slow-twitch fibers, left side) and maximal oxygen uptake (right side) in athletes representing different sports. The outer, lightly shaded bars denote the range. (From Bergh, U., et al.: Maximal oxygen uptake and muscle fiber types in trained and untrained humans. *Med. Sci. Sports,* 10:151, 1978.)

SUMMARY

1. Various wrappings of connective tissue that encase skeletal muscle eventually blend into and join the tendinous attachment to bone. With this harness, muscles act on the bony levers to transform chemical energy of ATP into mechanical energy and motion.

2. Skeletal muscle contains approximately 75% water and 20% protein, with the remaining 5% containing inorganic salts, enzymes, minerals, pigments, fats, proteins, and carbohydrates.

3. Vigorous aerobic exercise increases the active muscle's oxygen uptake nearly 70 times above its resting level. Aerobic training augments a muscle's oxygen supply by increasing capillary density up to 40%.

4. The sarcomere contains the contractile proteins actin and myosin—the muscle fiber's functional unit. An average-sized muscle fiber contains about 4500 sarcomeres and a total of 16 billion thick (myosin) and 64 billion thin (actin) filaments. The actin and myosin filaments within the sarcomere provide the mechanical mechanism for muscle action.

5. Crossbridge projections link thin and thick contractile filaments. The globular head of the myosin crossbridge provides the mechanical power stroke for actin and myosin filaments to slide past each other.

6. Tropomyosin and troponin, two myofibrillar proteins, regulate the make-and-break contacts between filaments during muscle action. Tropomyosin inhibits actin and myosin interaction; troponin with calcium triggers the myofibrils to interact and slide past each other.

7. The triad and T-tubule microtransportation system network spreads the action potential from the fiber's outer membrane inward to deeper cell regions. Contraction occurs when calcium activates actin, attaching the myosin crossbridges to active sites on the actin filaments. Relaxation occurs when calcium concentration decreases.

8. The sliding-filament theory proposes that a muscle fiber shortens or lengthens because its protein filaments slide past each other without changing length. Excitation-contraction coupling initiates an electrical discharge that triggers the chemical events for contraction.

9. Two types of muscle fibers are classified according to their contractile and metabolic characteristics: (1)

fast-twitch fibers (type II), which predominantly generate energy anaerobically for quick, powerful contractions; and (2) slow-twitch fibers (type I), which contract at relatively slow speeds and generate energy for ATP resynthesis largely by aerobic metabolism.

10. Muscle fiber type distribution differs in individuals. Genetic code largely determines a person's predominant fiber type.

11. Specific exercise training improves the metabolic capacity of each fiber type.

THOUGHT QUESTIONS

1. Show how knowledge about neuromuscular exercise physiology can enhance an athlete's (1) muscular strength and power, and (2) sports skill performance.

2. In terms of neuromuscular physiology, discuss the validity of the adage, "Practice makes perfect."

3. Discuss the meaning of *molecular motor* to describe how the myofilament crossbridges contribute to muscle fiber action.

SELECTED REFERENCES

Antonio, J., and Gonyea, W.J.: Skeletal muscle fiber hyperplasia. *Med. Sci. Sports Exerc.,* 25:1333, 1993.

Armstrong, R.B.: Muscle fiber recruitment patterns and their metabolic correlates. In: *Exercise, Nutrition, and Energy Metabolism.* Horton, E.S., and Terjung, R.L. (eds.). New York: Macmillan, 1988.

Asmussen, E.: Muscle fatigue. *Med. Sci. Sports Exerc.,* 25:412, 1993.

Asp, S., et al.: Muscle glycogen accumulation after a marathon: Roles of fiber type and pro- and macroglycogen. *J. Appl. Physiol.,* 86:474, 1999.

Baldwin, J., et al.: Muscle IMP accumulation during fatiguing submaximal exercise in endurance trained and untrained men. *Am. J. Physiol.,* 277:R295, 1999.

Barash, I.A., et al.: Rapid muscle-specific gene expression changes after a single bout of eccentric contractions in the mouse. *Am. J. Physiol. Cell. Physiol.,* 286:C355, 2004.

Basmajian, J.V., and Deluca, C.J.: *Muscles Alive. Their Functions Revealed by Electromyography.* 5th Ed. Baltimore: Williams & Wilkins, 1985.

Berggren, J.R., et al.: Glucose uptake in muscle cell cultures from endurance-trained men. *Med. Sci. Sports Exerc.,* 37:579, 2005.

Billeter, R., and Hoppler, H.: Muscular basis of strength. In: *Strength and Power in Sport.* Komi, P. (ed.). London: Blackwell Scientific Publications, 1992.

Boe, S.G., et al.: Decomposition-based quantitative electromyography: effect of force on motor unit potentials and motor unit number estimates. *Muscle Nerve,* 31:365, 2005.

Burelle, Y., Hochachka, P.W.: Endurance training induces muscle-specific changes in mitochondrial function in skinned muscle fibers. *J. Appl. Physiol.,* 92:2429, 2002.

Carins, S.P., et al.: Role of extracellular [Ca^{2+}] in fatigue of isolated mammalian skeletal muscle. *J. Appl. Physiol.,* 84:1395, 1998.

Carlson, C.J., et al.: Skeletal muscle myostatin mRNA expression is fiber-type specific and increases during hindlimb unloading. *Am. J. Physiol.,* 277:R601, 1999.

Carrasco, D.I., et al.: Effect of concentric and eccentric muscle actions on muscle sympathetic nerve activity. *J. Appl. Physiol.,* 86:558, 1999.

Davis, J.M., and Bailey, S.P.: Possible mechanisms of central nervous system fatigue during exercise. *Med. Sci. Sports Exerc.,* 29:45, 1997.

Dawson, B., et al.: Changes in performance, muscle metabolites, enzymes and fiber types after short sprint training. *Eur. J. Appl. Physiol.,* 78:163, 1998.

Demirel, H.A., et al.: Exercise induced alterations in skeletal muscle myosin heavy chain phenotype: Dose-response relationship. *J. Appl. Physiol.,* 86:1002, 1999.

Farina, D., et al.: Spike-triggered average torque and muscle fiber conduction velocity of low-threshold motor units following submaximal endurance contractions. *J. Appl. Physiol.,* 98:1495, 2005.

Fowles, J.R., Green, H.J.: Coexistence of potentiation and low-frequency fatigue during voluntary exercise in human skeletal muscle. *Can. J. Physiol. Pharmacol.,* 81:1092, 2003.

Gordon, T., et al.: The resilience of the size principle in the organization of motor unit properties in normal and reinnervated adult skeletal muscles. *Can. J. Physiol. Pharmacol.,* 82:645, 2004.

Gosmanov, A.R., et al.: ATP-sensitive potassium channels mediate hyperosmotic stimulation of NKCC in slow-twitch muscle. *Am. J. Physiol. Cell Physiol.,* 286:C586, 2004.

Green, H., et al.: Regulation of fiber size, oxidative potential, and capillarization in human muscle by resistance exercise. *Am. J. Physiol.*, 276:R591, 1999.

Green, H.J., et al.: Adaptations in human muscle sarcoplasmic reticulum to prolonged submaximal training. *J. Appl. Physiol.*, 94:2034, 2003.

Green, H.J., et al.: Malleability of human skeletal muscle Na+-K+-ATPase pump with short-term training. *J. Appl. Physiol.*, 97:143, 2004.

Green, H.J., et al.: Reversal of muscle fatigue during 16-h of heavy intermittent cycle exercise. *J. Appl. Physiol.*, 97:2166, 2004.

Green, H.J.: Membrane excitability, weakness, and fatigue. *Can. J. Appl. Physiol.*, 29:291, 2004.

Gregory, C.M., Bickel, C.S.: Recruitment patterns in human skeletal muscle during electrical stimulation. *Phys. Ther.*, 85:358, 2005.

Heckmann, C.J., et al.: Persistent inward currents in motoneuron dendrites: implications for motor output. *Muscle Nerve*, 31:135, 2005.

Hochachka, P.W.: *Muscles as Molecular and Metabolic Machines.* Boca Raton, FL: CRC Press, 1994.

Hogan, M.D., et al.: Increased [lactate] in working dog muscle reduces tension development independent of pH. *Med. Sci. Sports Exerc.*, 27:371, 1995.

Holloszy, J.O., and Coyle, E.F.: Adaptations of skeletal muscle to endurance training and their metabolic consequences. *J. Appl. Physiol.*, 56:831, 1984.

Huey, K.A., et al.: Inactivity-induced modulation of Hsp20 and Hsp25 content in rat hindlimb muscles. *Muscle Nerve*, 30:95, 2004.

Kadi, F., et al.: Cellular adaptation of the trapezius muscle in strength-trained athletes. *Histochem. Cell Biol.*, 111:189, 1999.

Keenan, K.G., et al.: Influence of amplitude cancellation on the simulated surface electromyogram. *J. Appl. Physiol.*, 98:120, 2005.

Kernell, D.: Principles of force gradation in skeletal muscles. *Neural Plast.*, 10:69, 2003.

Kraus, W.E., et al.: Skeletal muscle adaptation to chronic low-frequency motor nerve stimulation. *Exerc. Sport Sci. Rev.*, 22:313, 1994.

Lambert, E.V., et al.: Complex systems model of fatigue: integrative homoeostatic control of peripheral physiological systems during exercise in humans. *Br. J. Sports Med.*, 39:52, 2005.

Lewis, S.F., and Fulco, C.S.: A new approach to studying muscle fatigue and factors affecting performance during dynamic exercise in humans. *Exerc. Sport Sci. Rev.*, 26:91, 1998.

Lieber, R.L., et al.: Biomechanical properties of the brachioradialis muscle: Implications for surgical tendon transfer. *J. Hand Surg. [Am].*, 30:273, 2005.

Lieber, R.L.: *Skeletal Muscle Structure and Function: Implications for Rehabilitation and Sports Medicine.* Baltimore: Williams & Wilkins, 1992.

Lieber, R.L., et al.: Structural and functional changes in spastic skeletal muscle. *Muscle Nerve*, 29:615, 2004.

Lutz, G.J., and Lieber, R.L.: Skeletal muscle myosin II structure and function. *Exerc. Sport Sci. Rev.*, 27:63, 1999.

MacLaren, C.P., et al: A review of metabolic and physiological factors in fatigue. In: *Exercise and Sport Sciences Reviews.* Vol. 17. Pandolf, K.B. (ed.). Baltimore: Williams & Wilkins, 1989.

Masuda, K., et al.: Changes in surface EMG parameters during static and dynamic fatiguing contractions. *J. Electromyogr. Kinesiol.*, 9:39, 1999.

McAinch, A.J., et al.: Dietary regulation of fat oxidative gene expression in different skeletal muscle fiber types. *Obes. Res.*, 11:1471, 2003.

McDonough, P., et al.: Recovery of microvascular PO2 during the exercise off-transient in muscles of different fiber type. *J. Appl. Physiol.*, 96:1039, 2004.

Moritz, C.T., et al.: Discharge rate variability influences the variation in force fluctuations across the working range of a hand muscle. *J. Neurophysiol.*, 93:2449, 2005.

Mottram, C.J., et al.: Motor-unit activity differs with load type during a fatiguing contraction. *J. Neurophysiol.*, 93:1381, 2005.

Nichols, T.R., et al.: Rapid spinal mechanisms of motor coordination. *Exerc. Sport Sci. Rev.*, 27:255, 1999.

Noakes, T.D., et al.: From catastrophe to complexity: a novel model of integrative central neural regulation of effort and fatigue during exercise in humans: summary and conclusions. *Br. J. Sports Med.*, 39:120, 2005.

Otten, E.: Concepts and models of functional architecture in skeletal muscle. In: *Exercise and Sport Sciences Reviews.* Vol. 16. Pandolf, K.B. (ed.). New York: Macmillan, 1988.

Patel, T.J., and Lieber, R.L.: Force transmission in skeletal muscle: From actomyosin to external tendons. *Exer. Sport Sci. Rev.*, 25:321, 1997.

Putman, C.T., et al.: Satellite cell content and myosin isoforms in low-frequency-stimulated fast muscle of hypothyroid rat. *J. Appl. Physiol.*, 86:40, 1999.

Roy, R.R., et al.: Modulation of myonuclear number in functionally overloaded and exercised rat plantaris fibers. *J. Appl. Physiol.*, 87:634, 1999.

Schunk, K., et al.: Contributions of dynamic phosphorus-31 magnetic resonance spectroscopy to the analysis of muscle fiber distribution. *Invest. Radiol.*, 34:348, 1999.

Seals, D.R., and Victor, R.G.: Regulation of muscle sympathetic nerve activity during exercise in humans. In: *Exercise and Sport Sciences Reviews.* Vol. 19. Holloszy, J.O. (ed.). Baltimore: Williams & Wilkins, 1991.

Sweeney, L.J., et al.: An introductory biology lab that uses enzyme histochemistry to teach students about skeletal muscle fiber types. *Adv. Physiol. Educ.*, 28:23, 2004.

Tarpenning, K.M., et al.: Endurance training delays age of decline in leg strength and muscle morphology. *Med. Sci. Sports Exerc.*, 36:74, 2004.

Tikkanen, H.O., et al.: Significance of skeletal muscle properties on fitness, long-term physical training and serum lipids. *Atherosclerosis*, 142:367, 1999.

Tupling, A.R., et al.: Paradoxical effects of prior activity on human sarcoplasmic reticulum Ca2+-ATPase response to exercise. *J. Appl. Physiol.*, 95:138, 2003.

Westad, C., Westgaard, R.H.: The influence of contraction amplitude and firing history on spike-triggered averaged trapezius motor unit potentials. *J. Physiol.*, 562:965, 2005.

Weston, A.R., et al.: African runners exhibit greater fatigue resistance, lower lactate accumulation, and higher oxidative enzyme activity. *J. Appl. Physiol.*, 86:915, 1999.

Wickham, J.B., and Brown, J.M.: Muscles within muscles: The neuromotor control of intra-muscular segments. *Eur. J. Appl. Physiol.*, 78:219, 1998.

Williams, J.H.: Contractile apparatus and sarcoplasmic reticulum function: Effects of fatigue, recovery, and elevated Ca^{2+}. *J. Appl. Physiol.*, 83:444, 1997.

Zanoteli, E., et al.: Deficiency of muscle alpha-actinin-3 is compatible with high muscle performance. *J. Mol. Neurosci.*, 20:39, 2003.

Zawadowska, B., et al.: Characteristics of myosin profile in human vastus lateralis muscle in relation to training background. *Folia. Histochem. Cytobiol.*, 42:181, 2004.

Zhou, P., Rymer, W.Z.: An evaluation of the utility and limitations of counting motor unit action potentials in the surface electromyogram. *J. Neural. Eng.*, 1:238, 2004.

CHAPTER OBJECTIVES

- Draw the location of the major endocrine glands within an outline of the human body.

- Describe how hormones alter cellular reaction rates of specific target cells.

- Describe how hormonal, humoral, and neural factors stimulate endocrine glands.

- List the hormones secreted by the anterior and posterior pituitary glands, and describe how exercise affects these secretions.

- List the thyroid gland hormones, their functions, and response to exercise.

- List the hormones of the adrenal medulla and adrenal cortex, their functions, and their response to exercise.

- List the hormones of the pancreas' alpha and beta cells, their functions, and their response to exercise.

- Define type 1 and type 2 diabetes mellitus, and give three differences between these two diabetes subdivisions.

- List five risk factors for type 2 diabetes.

- Outline the benefits of regular physical activity for a type 2 diabetic.

- Explain the general effects of exercise training on endocrine function.

CHAPTER OUTLINE

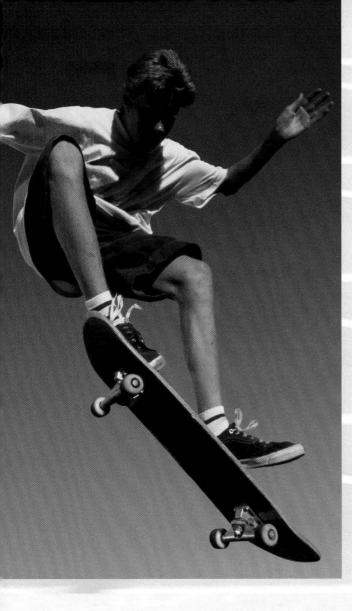

Hormones, Exercise, and Training

Like most branches of science, endocrinology has no discrete discovery date. In fact, most endocrine glands were first "identified" by early hunters and cooks or by the medical anatomists of antiquity and the Renaissance.

The writings of medieval and Renaissance physicians first described several unknown disorders such as diabetes, goiter, cretinism, dwarfism, and gigantism that we now know are caused by endocrine malfunction. Before the latter half of the 19th century, physicians and biologists formulated the concept of special human "internal secretions" with profound powers. By the end of the 18th century, direct connections were made between certain physical traits with too little or too much of different internal secretions. In 1849, British physician-scientist Thomas Addison (1793–1860) contributed to the scientific literature information about the endocrine system through studies of patients with diseased glands. Also in 1849, the German physician A. A. Berthold conducted one of the first formal endocrinology experiments. Berthold's experiments involved the removal of the testes from roosters and subsequent observation that the birds immediately became less aggressive without a sex drive. When the testes were surgically replaced, the normally aggressive male behavior resumed. Berthold concluded that the testes were not connected to nerves so they must have secreted a substance into the blood that affected the entire body.

We now know that hormones affect almost every aspect of human function. They regulate growth, metabolism, and reproduction, with heightened acute and chronic response to physical and psychological stress. Hormones maintain internal homeostasis by modulating electrolyte and acid-base balance and adjusting energy metabolism to power biologic work.

The endocrine system works in tandem with the nervous system to provide hormonal secretions throughout the body. The hormones produced within endocrine glands serve as "chemical messengers" in the bloodstream, while the nervous system serves as the "electrical" system. The nervous system works instantaneously with short-lived results, but endocrine system hormones act slower and often with longer-lasting results.

Approximately 10% of the world's population will suffer from some type of endocrine system malfunction—hyperthyroidism, hypothyroidism, diabetes, and hypoglycemia.

This chapter reviews aspects of the endocrine system, including its functions during rest and physical activity and response to exercise training.

ENDOCRINE SYSTEM OVERVIEW

Figure 12.1 shows the location of the major endocrine organs: the pituitary, thyroid, parathyroid, adrenal, pineal, and thymus glands. Several organs contain discrete areas of endocrine tissue that also produce hormones. These include the pancreas, gonads (ovaries and testes), and hypothalamus (also a major organ of the nervous system).

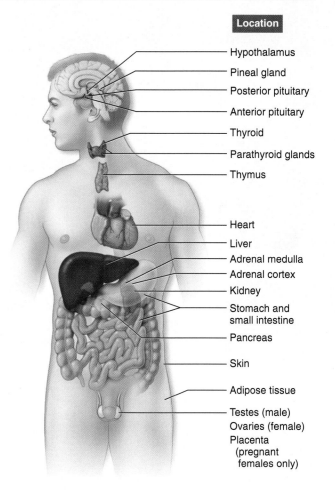

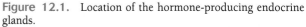

Location

- Hypothalamus
- Pineal gland
- Posterior pituitary
- Anterior pituitary
- Thyroid
- Parathyroid glands
- Thymus
- Heart
- Liver
- Adrenal medulla
- Adrenal cortex
- Kidney
- Stomach and small intestine
- Pancreas
- Skin
- Adipose tissue
- Testes (male) Ovaries (female) Placenta (pregnant females only)

Figure 12.1. Location of the hormone-producing endocrine glands.

Table 12.1 lists the different endocrine glands and nonglandular endocrine cells and their major hormonal secretions, target tissue(s), and main bodily effects.

ENDOCRINE SYSTEM ORGANIZATION

Three components characterize the endocrine system:

1. Host gland
2. Hormones
3. Target (receptor) cells or organs

Glands are classified as either endocrine, exocrine, or both. **Endocrine glands** secrete hormones; they lack ducts (ductless) but discharge their substances directly into the extracellular space around the gland. Hormones then diffuse into the blood for transport throughout the body. Similar to neuromuscular responses, hormone secretion adjusts rapidly to changing bodily functions. For this reason, many hormone secretions occur in a pulsatile manner rather than at a constant rate.

Exocrine glands (sweat glands and upper digestive tract glands) contain secretory ducts that lead directly to

Table 12·1			Endocrine Organs and Their Secretions		
Location	**Gland or Cell**	**Chemical Type**	**Hormone**	**Target**	**Main Effect**
Adipose tissue	Cells	Peptide	Leptin; adiponectin (resistin)	Hypothalamus, other tissues	Food intake, metabolism, reproduction
Adrenal cortex	Gland	Steroid	Mineralocorticoids (aldosterone)	Kidney	Stimulates Na^+ reabsorption and K^+ secretion
			Glucocorticoids (cortisol; corticosterone)	Many tissues	Promotes protein and fat catabolism; raises blood glucose levels; adapts body to stress
			Androgens (androstenedione; dehydroepiandro-sterone [DHEA]; estrone)	Many tissues	Promotes sex drive
Adrenal medulla	Gland	Amine	Epinephrine, norepinephrine	Many tissues	Facilitates sympathetic activity; increases cardiac output; regulates blood vessels; increases glycogen catabolism and fatty acid release
Gastrointestinal tract (stomach and small intestine)	Cells	Peptide	Gastrin; cholecystokinin (CCK); secretin; glucose-dependent insulinotropic peptide (GIP)	GI tract and pancreas	Assist digestion and absorption of nutrients; regulates gastrointestinal motility
Heart	Cells	Peptide	Atrial natriuretic peptide (ANP)	Kidney tubules	Inhibits sodium reabsorption
Hypothalamus	Clusters of neurons	Peptide	Trophic hormones (releasing and release-inhibiting hormones: corticotrophin-releasing hormone [CHR]; thyrotrophin-releasing hormone [TRH]; growth hormone-releasing hormone [GHRH]; gonadrotrophin-releasing hormone [GnRH])	Anterior pituitary	Release or inhibit anterior pituitary hormones
Kidney	Cells	Peptide Steroid	Erythropoietin (EPO) 1,25 Dihydroxy-vitamin D_3 (calciferol)	Bone marrow Intestine	Red blood cell production Increase calcium absorption
Liver	Cells	Peptide	Angiotensinogen	Adrenal cortex, blood vessels, brain	Aldosterone secretion; increase blood pressure
			Insulin-like growth factors (IGF-1)	Many tissues	Growth
Muscle	Cells	Peptide	Insulin-like growth factors (IGF-1, IGF-II); myogenic regulatory factors (MRFs)	Many tissues	Growth

(continued)

Table 12•1 *(Continued)*

Location	Gland or Cell	Chemical Type	Hormone	Target	Main Effect
Pancreas	Gland	Peptide	Insulin	Many tissues	Lowers blood glucose levels; promotes protein, lipid, and glycogen synthesis
			Glucagon	Many tissues	Raises blood glucose levels; promotes glycogenolysis and gluconeogenesis
			Somatostatin (SS)	Many tissues	Inhibits secretion of pancreatic hormones; regulates digestion and absorption of nutrients by GI system
Parathyroid	Gland	Peptide	Parathyroid hormone (PTH)	Bone, kidney	Promotes Ca^{++} release from bone, Ca^{++} absorption by intestine and Ca^{++} reabsorption by kidney; raises blood Ca^{++} levels; stimulates vitamin D_3 synthesis
Pineal gland	Gland	Amine	Melatonin	Unknown	Controls circadian rhythms
Pituitary-anterior	Gland	Peptides	Growth hormone (GH)	Many tissues	Growth; stimulates bone and soft tissue growth; regulates protein, lipid, and CHO metabolism
			Adrenocorticotropic hormone (ACTH)	Adrenal cortex	Stimulates glucocorticoid secretion
			Thyroid-stimulating hormone (TSH)	Thyroid gland	Stimulates secretion of thyroid hormones
			Prolactin	Breast	Milk secretion
			Follicle-stimulating hormone (FSH)	Gonads	Females: stimulates growth and development of ovarian follicles and estrogen secretion; Males: sperm production by testis
			Luteinizing hormone (LH)	Gonads	Females: stimulates ovulation, secretion of estrogen and progesterone; Males: testosterone secretion by testis
Pituitary-posterior	Extension of hypothalamic neurons	Peptide	Oxytocin (OT)	Breast and uterus	Females: stimulates uterine contractions and milk ejection by mammary glands; Males: unknown function
			Antidiuretic hormone (ADH or vasopressin)	Kidney	Decreases urine output by kidneys; promotes blood vessel (arterioles) constriction

(continued)

Table 12•1 *(Continued)*

Location	Gland or Cell	Chemical Type	Hormone	Target	Main Effect
Placenta (pregnant female)	Gland	Steroid	Estrogens and progesterone	Many tissues	Fetal and maternal development
		Peptide	Chorionic somatomammotropin (CS)		Metabolism
			Chorionic gonadotropin (CG)		Hormone secretion
Skin	Cells	Steroid	Vitamin D_3	Intermediate form of hormone	Precursor of 1,25 dihydroxy-vitamin D_3
Ovaries (female)	Glands	Steroid	Estrogens (estradiol)	Many tissues	Egg production; secondary sex characteristics
			Progestins (progesterone)	Uterus	Promotes endometrial growth to prepare uterus for pregnancy
Testes (male)	Glands	Peptide	Ovarian inhibin	Anterior pituitary	Inhibit FSH secretion
		Steroid	Androgen	Many tissues	Sperm production; secondary sex characteristics
		Peptide	Inhibin	Anterior pituitary	Inhibit FSH secretion
Thymus	Gland	Peptide	Thymosin, thymopoietin	Lymphocytes	Stimulates proliferation and function of T lymphocytes
Thyroid	Gland	Iodinated amines	Triiodothyronine (T_3); thyroxine (T_4)	Many tissues	Increases metabolic rate; normal physical development
		Peptide	Calcitonin (CT)	Bone	Promotes calcium deposition in bone; lowers blood calcium levels

the specific compartment or surface that requires the hormone. The nervous system controls almost all exocrine glands.

What Makes a Chemical a Hormone?

The term hormone was coined from the Greek verb meaning "to excite or arouse." An accepted operational definition describes a hormone as "*a chemical secreted by a cell or group of cells into the blood for transport to a distant target, where it exerts its effect at low concentrations.*" Recent findings suggest that this may be too broad a definition because many different non-hormone substances also function as chemical messengers.

Must Hormones Be Transported to Distant Targets?   Physiologists have recently questioned whether a chemical must be transported to distant targets to classify as a hormone. For example, the different hypothalamic regulating hormones, the trophic chemical messengers (releasing and release-inhibiting chemicals) and the different "growth factors" (IGF-1), seem to lack widespread distribution in the circulation, yet they meet the other qualifications for hormone classification.

Hormones Exert Their Effect at Low Concentrations   With the discovery of new signal molecules and receptors, the boundary between hormone

Questions & Notes

List 3 components that characterize the endocrine system.

1.

2.

3.

FOR YOUR INFORMATION

Small but Crucial

Endocrine glands are small compared with other organs of the body; combined, they weigh only about 0.5 kg. Endocrine hormone secretions occur in minute amounts, measured in micrograms (μg; 10^{-6} g), nanograms (ng; 10^{-9} g), and picograms (pg; 10^{-12} g).

and non-hormone molecules becomes blurred, particularly with respect to their physiologically effective concentrations. While some hormones act at concentrations in the nanomolar (10^{-9} M) to picomolar (10^{-12} M) range, other chemicals transported in the blood exist in higher concentrations before an effect occurs. For example, cytokines, a group of regulatory peptides that control cell development, differentiation, and the immune response, act on target cells at a much higher concentration than a typical hormone. Erythropoietin, the molecule that controls red blood cell synthesis, classifies as a hormone but functionally behaves as a cytokine.

Hormones Bind to Receptors   All hormones bind to target cell receptors and initiate biochemical responses. This characteristic varies from one hormone to another and from one tissue to another. Some hormones act on multiple tissues in different ways or have no effect at different times. Insulin, for example, exhibits varied effects depending on the target tissue; in muscle and adipose cells, insulin alters glucose and protein transport and enzymes for glucose metabolism. In the liver, insulin modulates enzyme activity without directly affecting glucose and protein transport, and in brain tissues, glucose metabolism does not require insulin.

Hormone Classification

Hormones are typically classified according to several different systems: their sources, their receptor type, or, their chemical structure (the most common classification scheme). Three different structures exist: (1) peptide hormones composed of linked amino acids, (2) steroid hormones derived from cholesterol and amine hormones, and (3) hormones derived from a single type of amino acid.

Table 12.2 compares the storage, synthesis, release mechanism, transport medium, receptor location and receptor-ligand binding, and target organ response of the peptide, steroid, and amine hormones.

Peptide Hormones   Peptide hormones range from small peptides of only three amino acids to large proteins and glycoproteins. These hormones are water-soluble and, thus, dissolve easily for transport in the body's extracellular fluids. The half-life of activity for these hormones ranges in minutes; thus, if a peptide hormone's response requires maintenance beyond several minutes, the hormone secretion must continue. Most peptide hormones bind to surface membrane receptors and act through a second messenger. Tissues respond rapidly to peptide hormones compared to the response times of other hormones.

Table 12·2	Storage, Synthesis, Release Mechanism, Transport Medium, Receptor Location and Receptor-Ligand Binding, and Target Organ Response of the Peptide, Steroid, and Amine Hormones			
			Amine Hormones	
	Peptide Hormones	**Steroid Hormones**	**Catecholamines**	**Thyroid Hormones**
Examples	Insulin, glucagons, leptin, IGF-1	Androgens, DHEA, cortisol	Epinephrine, norepinephrine	Thyroxine (T_4)
Synthesis and storage	Made in advance; stored in secretory vesicles	Synthesized on demand from precursors	Made in advance; stored in secretory vesicles	Made in advance; precursor stored in secretory vesicles
Release from parent cell	Exocytosis[a]	Simple diffusion	Exocytosis	Simple diffusion
Transport medium	Dissolved in plasma	Bound to carrier proteins	Dissolved in plasma	Bound to carrier proteins
Lifespan (half-life[b])	Short	Long	Short	Long
Receptor location	On cell membrane	Cytoplasm or nucleus; some have membrane receptors	On cell membrane	Nucleus
Response to receptor-ligand binding[c]	Activation of second messenger systems; may activate genes	Activate genes for transcription and translation; may have nongenomic actions	Activation of second messenger systems	Activate genes for transcription and translation
General target response	Modification of existing proteins and induction of new protein synthesis	Induction of new protein synthesis	Modification of existing proteins	Induction of new protein synthesis

[a]Process in which intracellular vesicles fuse with the cell membrane and release their contents into the extracellular fluid.
[b]Amount of time required to reduce hormone concentration by one-half.
[c]A ligand (the molecule that binds to a receptor) binds to a membrane protein, which triggers endocytosis (process by which a cell brings molecules into the cytoplasm in vesicles formed from the cell membrane).

Steroid Hormones   All steroid hormones have a similar chemical structure because of their derivation from cholesterol. But unlike peptide hormones made in diverse tissues, only the adrenal cortex, gonads, and placenta (in pregnancy) construct steroid hormones. These hormones diffuse easily across cell membranes, both out of the parent cell and into their target tissue. Steroid-secreting cells cannot store hormones; instead, they synthesize their hormones as needed. Steroid hormones move out of the secreting cell by simple diffusion. Steroid hormones are minimally soluble in plasma and other body fluids, so they bind to protein carrier molecules in the blood. To produce an effect on a target, the hormone must unbind from the protein.

Amine Hormones   Small molecules created from one or two amino acids comprise the amine hormones. The amine catecholamines (epinephrine and norepinephrine) are neurohormones that bind to cell membrane receptors similar to typical peptide hormones.

How Hormones Function

Most hormones do not directly affect cellular activity, but rather combine with a specific receptor molecule on the cell surface. The cell then discharges a second chemical that initiates a cascade of cellular events. The binding hormone acts as "**first messenger**" to react with the enzyme **adenyl cyclase** in the plasma membrane to form **cyclic 3,5-adenosine monophosphate (cyclic-AMP)**. This compound then acts as "**second messenger**" or mediator to influence cellular function by initiating a predictable series of actions within the target cell.

Hormone action at specific target cells occurs by one of four mechanisms:

1. Changing the synthesis rate of intracellular proteins
2. Altering enzyme activity
3. Modifying cell membrane transport
4. Inducing secretory activity

A target cell's response to a hormone depends largely on the presence of specific protein receptors on its membrane or in its interior.

Three factors determine a hormone's plasma concentration:

1. Sum of synthesis and release by the host gland
2. Rate of receptor tissue uptake
3. Rate of removal from the blood by the liver and kidneys

In most cases, hormone removal rate, which is usually measured in the urine, equals rate of release.

Hormone Effects on Enzymes   Alteration of enzymatic activity and enzyme-mediated membrane transport constitute the major mechanisms of hormone action. Hormones affect enzyme activity in one of three ways:

1. Stimulate enzyme synthesis
2. Combine with the enzyme to change its shape through allosteric modulation, which increases or decreases the enzyme's ability to interact with a substrate
3. Activate many inactive enzyme forms to increase total enzyme activity

In addition to altering enzyme activity, hormones either facilitate or inhibit transport of substances into cells. Insulin, for example, promotes glucose uptake through the plasma membrane. In contrast, the hormone epinephrine inhibits a cell's glucose uptake.

Control of Hormone Secretion

Endocrine glands are stimulated in three ways: hormonal, humoral, or neural. Each of these stimulation methods function as a reflex pathway, singly or in com-

Questions & Notes

List 3 different chemical structures of hormones.

1.

2.

3.

Give one example of an amine hormone.

FOR YOUR INFORMATION

The Human Pheromone Discovery
Pheromones, like other chemical signaling molecules, communicate information. For example, several sea creatures secrete "alarm pheromones" to warn other fish when danger threatens; ants secrete "trail pheromones" to attract other ants to food. Pheromones secreted by different species (fruit flies, dogs, cats, and cattle) attract members of the opposite sex for mating purposes. By the late 1970s, animal pheromones were so well understood that manufacturers marketed them for pest control; pheromones can lure and divert animals and bugs to traps to prevent crop and flower damage. Research suggests that women and men emit pheromones into the atmosphere. In one double-blind study, 38 heterosexual men, aged 26 to 42 years, who completed a 2-week baseline period and 6-week placebo-controlled, double-blind trial using an aftershave containing a pheromone experienced improved "romance" (see: *http://www.athenainstitute.com/science.html*).

FOR YOUR INFORMATION

Caffeine Stimulates Lipolysis
Caffeine augments cyclic-AMP activity in fat cells; cyclic-AMP activates hormone-sensitive lipases to promote lipolysis and release free fatty acids into the plasma. Increased plasma free-fatty acid levels stimulate fat oxidation, thus conserving liver and muscle glycogen.

bination, to ultimately trigger (and regulate) a specific hormone secretion. All reflex pathways exhibit similar components: stimulus, input signal, integration of the signal, output signal, and response. In endocrine reflexes, the output signal represents a hormone or neurohormone.

Figure 12.2 illustrates a negative feedback system that serves to turn off hormone production. In this example, an increase in blood glucose concentration following a meal initiates insulin secretion; insulin then travels in the blood to its target tissues to increase glucose uptake and metabolism. The resultant decrease in blood glucose concentration provides a negative feedback signal and turns off the reflex, ending further release of insulin. This illustration also shows insulin production triggered by input signals from the nervous system.

Hormonal Stimulation   Hormones often influence other hormones' secretions. For example, hormones from the hypothalamus (trophic releasing and inhibiting hormones, see Table 12.1) induce the discharge of most anterior pituitary hormones. The anterior pituitary hormones, in turn, stimulate other "target gland" endocrine organs to release their hormones into the circulation. Increased blood levels of these hormones provide feedback to inhibit release of anterior pituitary hormones; this ultimately inhibits target gland secretion.

Humoral Stimulation   Fluctuating blood levels of ions, nutrients, and bile stimulate hormone release. The term **humoral** denotes these stimuli to distinguish them from "fluid-borne" hormonal stimuli. An increase in the humoral agent blood glucose stimulates insulin release from the pancreas. Because insulin promotes glucose entry into cells, blood sugar levels decline, ending the humoral initiative for insulin release.

Neural Stimulation   Nerve fibers affect hormone release. For example, during stress, sympathetic nervous system activation of the adrenal medulla initiates release of epinephrine and norepinephrine. In this case, the nervous system augments normal endocrine control to maintain homeostasis.

Neurohormones serve as chemical signals released into the blood by a neuron. The nervous system produces three major groups of neurohormones:

1. Catecholamines synthesized by modified neurons in the adrenal medulla
2. Hypothalamic neurohormones secreted from the posterior pituitary
3. Hypothalamic neurohormones that control hormone release from the anterior pituitary

Hormone–Hormone Interactions

Multiple hormones present at the same time control many cells and tissues. Three types of interactions of diverse hormones exist:

1. **Synergism:** Different hormones act together to augment the effect on specific tissues. For example, the pancreatic hormone glucagon including cortisol and epinephrine act synergistically to elevate blood glucose levels. When two or more hormones interact, the combined effect on the target often exceeds the additive effect of each hormone separately.
2. **Permissiveness:** One hormone cannot exert its full effect without the presence of a second hormone, or a greater quantity of the first hormone.
3. **Antagonism:** One hormone opposes the action of another hormone to diminish the first hormone's effectiveness. Glucagon and growth hormone, for example, both raise blood glucose concentration to counter the glucose-lowering effect of insulin.

PATTERNS OF HORMONE RELEASE

Most hormones respond to peripheral stimuli on an as-needed basis, while others release at regular intervals dur-

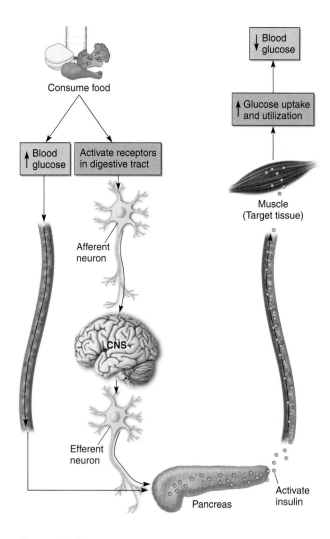

Figure 12.2.   Multiple stimuli for insulin secretion. Insulin is triggered by an increase in blood glucose levels or through nervous stimulation triggered by ingestion of a meal.

ing a 24-hour cycle (referred to as diurnal variation). Some secretory cycles span several weeks, while others follow daily cycles. These cycling patterns are not confined to one category of hormones.

Assessing pulsatile hormone release patterns reveals information not available from a single blood sample. Patterns of release and/or amplitude and frequency of discharge provide more meaningful information about hormone dynamics than a hormone's concentration examined at a single time period.

RESTING AND EXERCISE-INDUCED ENDOCRINE SECRETIONS

The following sections review important hormones, their functions during rest and exercise, and specific host-gland-hormone responses to exercise training.

ANTERIOR PITUITARY HORMONES

Figure 12.3 shows the **pituitary gland** (**hypophysis**), its secretions and various target glands, and their hormone secretions. The pituitary gland consists of distinct anterior and posterior lobes (each with different hormone secretions). The gland attaches to the hypothalamus by neural elements that innervate the posterior pituitary. This nerve bundle (**hypophyseal stalk**) serves as a conduit for hormone movement from its site of synthesis in the hypothalamus to storage in the pituitary. Located beneath the base of the brain, the **anterior pituitary** secretes at least six different polypeptide hormones and influences the secretion of several others.

The **posterior pituitary**, an extension of hypothalamic neurons, secretes the hormones oxytocin, which acts on breast and uterus to stimulate milk production and induce labor and delivery, and antidiuretic hormone (ADH or vasopressin),

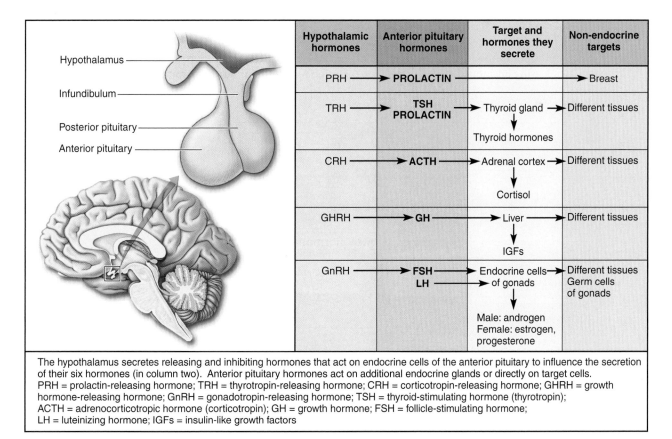

	Hypothalamic hormones	Anterior pituitary hormones	Target and hormones they secrete	Non-endocrine targets
	PRH →	PROLACTIN		→ Breast
	TRH →	TSH PROLACTIN	→ Thyroid gland → Thyroid hormones	Different tissues
	CRH →	ACTH	→ Adrenal cortex → Cortisol	Different tissues
	GHRH →	GH	→ Liver → IGFs	Different tissues
	GnRH →	FSH LH	→ Endocrine cells → of gonads → Male: androgen Female: estrogen, progesterone	Different tissues Germ cells of gonads

Labels: Hypothalamus, Infundibulum, Posterior pituitary, Anterior pituitary

The hypothalamus secretes releasing and inhibiting hormones that act on endocrine cells of the anterior pituitary to influence the secretion of their six hormones (in column two). Anterior pituitary hormones act on additional endocrine glands or directly on target cells.
PRH = prolactin-releasing hormone; TRH = thyrotropin-releasing hormone; CRH = corticotropin-releasing hormone; GHRH = growth hormone-releasing hormone; GnRH = gonadotropin-releasing hormone; TSH = thyroid-stimulating hormone (thyrotropin); ACTH = adrenocorticotropic hormone (corticotropin); GH = growth hormone; FSH = follicle-stimulating hormone; LH = luteinizing hormone; IGFs = insulin-like growth factors

Figure 12.3. The pituitary gland, its secretions and various target glands, and hormone secretions.

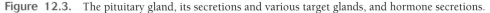

which acts on the kidneys to decrease urine output and control fluid balance.

Growth Hormone

Human growth hormone (**GH** or **somatotropin**) promotes cell division and proliferation throughout the body. This hormone facilitates protein synthesis by:

1. Increasing amino acid transport through plasma membranes
2. Stimulating RNA formation
3. Activating cellular ribosomes that increase protein synthesis

GH release also depresses carbohydrate utilization, while increasing fat use for energy. Insufficient GH secretion early in life blunts skeletal growth (dwarfism), whereas excess production produces extreme growth (gigantism). Excessive GH secretion in post-puberty causes continued soft tissue growth and bone thickening, a condition termed **acromegly**. Many of the growth-promoting effects of GH arise from intermediary chemical messengers on different target tissues rather than a direct action of GH itself. These peptide messengers are termed **somatomedins** or **insulin-like growth factors** (IGFs) because of their structural similarity to insulin. Two IGFs have been identified, IGF-1 and IGF-2, which the liver directly releases under the stimulation.

Hypothalamic secretion of GH-releasing hormone stimulates the anterior pituitary gland's production of GH. Another hormone, hypothalamic **somatostatin**, inhibits GH release. *Each primary pituitary hormone has its own hypothalamic releasing factor.* Anxiety, stress, and physical activity provide neural input to the hypothalamus, causing it to discharge its releasing hormones.

Exercise, GH, and Tissue Synthesis GH secretion increases a few minutes after exercise begins. Increasing exercise intensity increases GH production and its total secretion. Moreover, GH secretion relates more closely to peak exercise intensity than exercise duration or total exercise volume. The exact stimulus for GH release with exercise remains unknown; neural factors most likely provide primary control.

One hypothesis maintains that exercise directly activates GH production, which in turn stimulates anabolic processes. For example, exercise doubles GH pulse frequency and amplitude. Exercise also stimulates endogenous opiate release; these hormones facilitate GH discharge by inhibiting the liver's production of somatostatin, a hormone that blunts GH release.

Figure 12.4 illustrates the overall actions and regulation of GH. Elevated plasma GH stimulates triacylglycerol release from adipose tissue while inhibiting cellular glucose uptake (anti-insulin effect). Inhibiting carbohydrate catabolism while maintaining blood glucose levels sustains prolonged exercise. Concurrently, GH promotes its anabolic, tissue-building effects (mediated via somatomedins) on diverse tissues that include bone and skeletal muscle. Elevated GH and somatomedins trigger the hypothalamus to release more GH-inhibiting hormone. This action depresses the release of growth hormone-releasing hormone, thus inhibiting anterior pituitary release of GH.

Thyrotropin

Thyrotropin (**thyroid-stimulating hormone** or **TSH**) maintains growth and thyroid gland development, including regulation of hormone output from thyroid cells. The

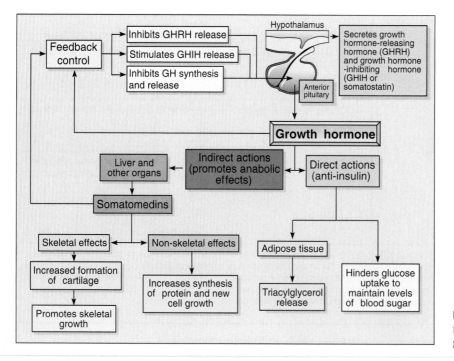

Figure 12.4. Overview for classifying the actions and regulation of human growth hormone (GH).

thyroid gland plays an important role to control cellular metabolism. Physical activity usually increases anterior pituitary TSH output.

Corticotropin

The hypothalamus secretes corticotropin-releasing hormone (CRH) into the hypothalamic-hypophyseal portal system. CRH is then transported to the anterior pituitary where it stimulates the release of **corticotropin (adrenocorticotropic hormone or ACTH)**. ACTH in turn acts on the adrenal cortex to promote synthesis and release of cortisol, much like TSH controls thyroid secretions. ACTH directly enhances triacylglycerol mobilization from adipose tissue, increases the rate of gluconeogenesis, and stimulates protein catabolism. ACTH concentrations increase with exercise duration if intensity exceeds 25% of aerobic capacity.

ACTH synthesizes from a large glycoprotein called proopiomelanocortin or POMC. POMC produces a variety of biologically active peptides in addition to ACTH. In the pituitary, POMC products include beta-endorphin, an endogenous opiate that binds to receptors that block pain perception.

Gonadotropic Hormones

The gonadotropic hormones include **follicle-stimulating hormone (FSH)** and **luteinizing hormone (LH)**. In females, FSH initiates follicle growth in the ovaries and stimulates ovarian secretion of estrogens, one type of female sex hormone. The combination of LH and FSH stimulates estrogen secretion and initiates rupture of the follicle to allow the ovum to pass through the fallopian tube for fertilization. In males, FSH stimulates germinal epithelial growth in the testes to promote sperm development. LH stimulates the testes to secrete the hormone testosterone.

The nature of gonadotropin release confounds interpretation of any exercise-associated alterations in FSH and LH. LH normally releases in a pulsatile manner so it is difficult to separate any specific exercise-related change from the normal secretory pattern. Anxiety affects LH levels via action of the "stress" hormone norepinephrine, thus LH increases in anticipation of exercise and reaches its peak during recovery.

Prolactin

Prolactin (PRL) governs milk secretion from the mammary glands. PRL levels increase with higher exercise intensities and return toward baseline within 45 minutes of recovery. PRL plays an important role in female sexual function, making repeated exercise-induced PRL release inhibit the ovaries and disrupt the normal menstrual cycle, often observed among athletic women. The significance of an increased PRL in men following acute maximal exercise remains unknown.

POSTERIOR PITUITARY HORMONES

Figure 12.3 also depicts the **posterior pituitary gland (neurohypophysis)** formed as an outgrowth of the hypothalamus. This gland stores two hormones, **antidiuretic hormone (ADH or vasopressin)** and **oxytocin**. The posterior pituitary does not synthesize its hormones. Instead, it receives them from the hypothalamus for release to the general circulation via neural stimulation.

ADH primarily limits how much urine the kidneys produce. Oxytocin stimulates uterine muscle activity and milk ejection from the breasts during lactation; thus, oxytocin contributes importantly to birthing and nursing.

Exercise stimulates ADH secretion. This secretion increases water reabsorption by the kidney tubules during and after exercise. ADH release (stimulated by sweating) preserves body fluids, particularly in hot-weather exercise accompanied by dehydration risk. Excessive fluid intake inhibits ADH release, with urine volume increasing proportionately.

Questions & Notes

Give the 4 ways hormones act at specific target cells.

1.

2.

3.

4.

Name the true "master gland."

List the 3 factors that activate target cells by hormone-receptor interaction.

1.

2.

3.

Name the 2 gonadotropic hormones.

1.

2.

FOR YOUR INFORMATION

Obesity, Aldosterone, and Teenage Hypertension
Obese teenagers commonly have high blood pressure associated with increased aldosterone production. This form of hypertension relates to (1) decreased salt sensitivity (and hence increases total body water), (2) increased sodium intake, and (3) decreased sensitivity to insulin's effects (hyperinsulinemia). These interrelationships suggest a direct link between obesity and hypertension.

THYROID HORMONES

The butterfly-shaped thyroid gland weighs approximately 15 to 20 g and is located just below the larynx at the base of the throat (**Figure 12.5**). This larger endocrine gland has two distinct endocrine cell types that secrete calcitonin, a calcium-regulating hormone, and two protein-iodine bound **hormones, thyroxine** (T_4) and **triiodothyronine** (T_3). TSH release by the anterior pituitary gland stimulates the thyroid gland to release its hormones.

Thyroid Hormones Affect Quality of Life

Although thyroid hormones are not directly essential for life, they do affect its quality. In children, full expression of GH requires thyroid activity. Thyroid hormones provide essential stimulation for normal growth and development, especially of nerve tissue.

Hypersecretion of thyroid hormones (**hyperthyroidism**) has the following effects:

1. Increases oxygen uptake and metabolic heat production during rest (heat intolerance a common complaint)
2. Increases protein catabolism and subsequent muscle weakness and weight loss
3. Heightened reflex activity and psychological disturbances that range from irritability and insomnia to psychosis
4. Rapid heart rate (tachycardia)

Hyposecretion of thyroid hormones (**hypothyroidism**) produces the following four effects:

1. Reduces metabolic rate; cold-intolerance from reduced internal heat production
2. Decreases protein synthesis resulting in brittle nails, thinning hair, and dry, thin skin

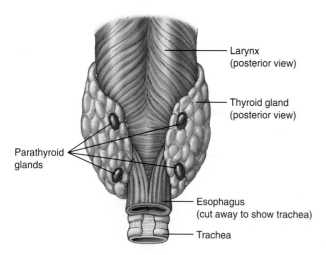

Larynx (posterior view)

Thyroid gland (posterior view)

Parathyroid glands

Esophagus (cut away to show trachea)

Trachea

Figure 12.5. Thyroid gland located on both sides of the neck in the larynx region. Not visible externally under normal conditions.

3. Depresses reflexes activity, slows speech and thought processes, and causes feelings of fatigue; in infancy, causes cretinism (marked by decreased mental capacity)
4. Slows heart rate (bradycardia)

Blood levels of free T_4 (not bound to plasma protein) increase during exercise. This could result from core temperature increases with exercise that alter protein binding of several hormones including T_4. The importance of these transient alterations in hormone levels remains unknown.

PARATHYROID HORMONE

Four small sections of tissue comprise the **parathyroid gland** within thyroid tissue (see Fig. 12.5). This gland secretes the calcium-regulating parathyroid hormone (**PTH** or **parathormone**) to decrease plasma calcium (Ca^{++}) concentration. PTH (a peptide) raises plasma Ca^{++} concentrations in three ways:

1. Mobilizes Ca^{++} from bone
2. Enhances renal Ca^{++} reabsorption
3. Indirectly increases intestinal Ca^{++} absorption by its influence on vitamin D_3

ADRENAL HORMONES

Figure 12.6 shows the flattened, cap-like **adrenal glands** located just above each kidney. The glands form two distinct parts: the **adrenal medulla** (inner portion) and **adrenal cortex** (outer portion). Each portion secretes a different type of hormone.

Adrenal Medulla Hormones

The adrenal medulla forms part of the sympathetic nervous system. It prolongs and augments sympathetic neural effects by secreting two hormones, **epinephrine** and **norepinephrine** (collectively termed **catecholamines**). Neural outflow from the hypothalamus directly influences adrenal medulla secretions (80% as epinephrine), which affect the heart, blood vessels, and glands in the same but slower way as direct sympathetic nervous system stimulation.

Exercise intensity directly governs the quantity of adrenal medulla secretion. For example, norepinephrine levels increase two to six times throughout exercise gradations from light to maximum. Exercise duration also influences catecholamine response, as revealed by the direct relationship between plasma epinephrine and norepinephrine levels and mileage run. Other factors that determine catecholamine response to exercise include age (greater catecholamine secretion in older subjects at the same exercise intensity) and gender (greater epinephrine secretion in males than females at the same relative exercise intensity).

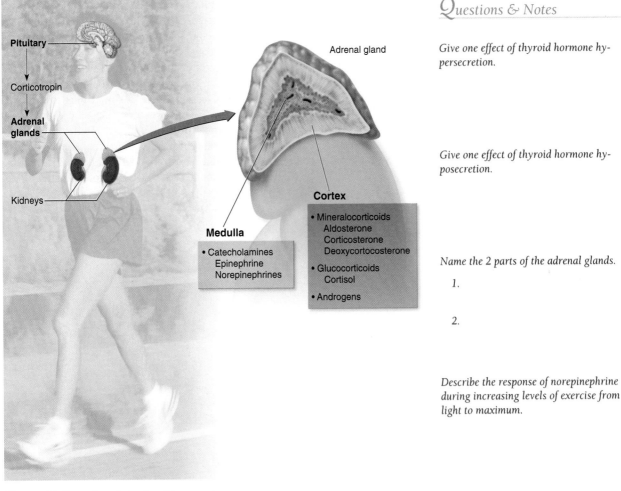

Figure 12.6.   Adrenal gland and its secretions.

Questions & Notes

Give one effect of thyroid hormone hypersecretion.

Give one effect of thyroid hormone hyposecretion.

Name the 2 parts of the adrenal glands.

  1.

  2.

Describe the response of norepinephrine during increasing levels of exercise from light to maximum.

Give the factor that governs the quantity of adrenal medulla secretion.

Adrenal Cortex Hormones

The adrenal cortex secretes **adrenocortical hormones** in response to ACTH stimulation from the pituitary gland. These steroid hormones are categorized by function into one of three groups: **mineralocorticoids**, **glucocorticoids**, and **androgens**; each is produced in a different zone or layer of the adrenal cortex.

Mineralocorticoids   Mineralocorticoids regulate the mineral salts sodium and potassium in the extracellular fluid space. **Aldosterone**, the most physiologically important hormone, comprises almost 95% of all mineralocorticoids.

Aldosterone regulates sodium reabsorption in the kidneys' distal tubules. Increased aldosterone secretion moves sodium ions (which also draw fluid) from the renal filtrate back into the blood, with little sodium passing into the urine. Conservation of fluid via sodium reabsorption increases plasma volume, often with a concomitant increase in cardiac output and arterial blood pressure. In contrast, sodium and fluid literally pour into the urine when aldosterone secretion ceases.

Because the kidneys exchange either a potassium or hydrogen ion for each reabsorbed sodium ion, aldosterone indirectly stabilizes serum potassium and pH. Mineral balance preserves nerve transmission and muscle function; neuromuscular activity would cease without proper regulation of sodium and potassium.

Name the 3 types of steroid hormones secreted by the adrenal cortex.

  1.

  2.

  3.

Chapter 12   Hormones, Exercise, and Training   •   413

Outflow from the sympathetic nervous system during exercise constricts blood vessels to the kidneys. Reduced renal blood flow stimulates the kidneys to release the enzyme **renin** into the blood. Renin in turn stimulates the production of **angiotensin**, a potent vasoconstrictor that also activates aldosterone secretion from the adrenal cortex. Aldosterone secretion increases progressively during exercise, with peak plasma levels as high as six times the resting value. The **renin-angiotensin mechanism** during rest controls aldosterone secretion to changes in blood pressure in the kidneys' afferent arterioles.

Glucocorticoids **Figure 12.7** shows the factors that affect secretion of **cortisol** (**hydrocortisone**), the major steroid glucocorticoid of the adrenal cortex, and its actions on target tissues. Cortisol secretes with a strong diurnal rhythm; secretion normally peaks in the morning and diminishes during the night. Cortisol secretion also increases with stress; thus, it is sometimes called the "stress" hormone. Even though cortisol is considered a catabolic hormone, cortisol's important effect counters hypoglycemia making it essential for life. Animals whose adrenal glands have been removed die if exposed to significant environmental stress. Because cortisol is required

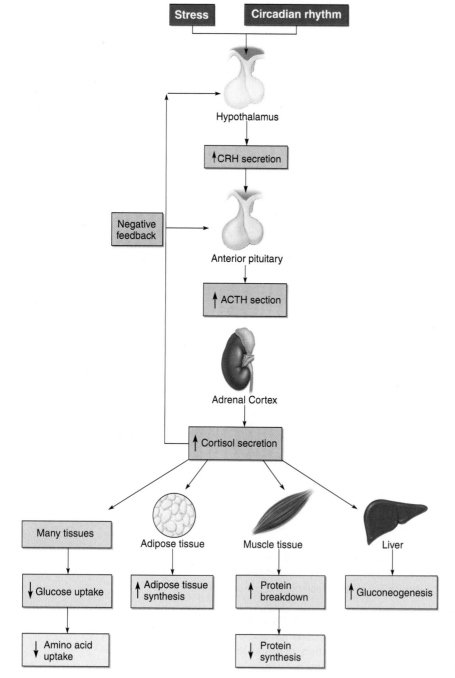

Figure 12.7. Factors that affect cortisol secretion and its actions on target tissues.

for full activity of glucagon and the catecholamines, and has a *permissive effect* on those hormones.

Cortisol's main effects include:

1. Promotes liver gluconeogenesis
2. Breakdown skeletal muscle proteins for gluconeogenic substrate
3. Enhances lipolysis (fat breakdown) during low energy intake and prolonged, moderate physical activity
4. Suppresses the immune system
5. Promotes negative calcium balance
6. Influences brain function, including mood changes and alterations in memory and learning

Physical activity varies cortisol response depending on exercise intensity and duration, fitness level, nutritional status, and even circadian rhythm. Cortisol output increases with exercise intensity. High cortisol levels also occur in prolonged marathon running, long-duration cycling, and hiking. Plasma cortisol increases at relatively low levels of sustained exercise and remains elevated for up to 2 hours in recovery.

Excess cortisol secretion (hypercortisolism) results from hormone-secreting tumors or from exogenous administration of the hormone. This results in **Cushing's syndrome** (Dr. H. Cushing first described the condition in 1932). The condition results from excess gluconeogenesis causing hyperglycemia (mimics diabetes); excessive muscle protein breakdown and lipolysis produce tissue wasting.

Addison's disease (from hyposecretion of all adrenal steroid hormones) is usually caused by autoimmune destruction of the adrenal cortex. Hypoglycemia and poor tolerance to stress characterize this disease. Cortisol hyposecretion also can result from an inherited defect. Hyposecretion of cortisol occurs less commonly than hypersecretion in Cushing's syndrome.

Androgens   The adrenal glands and ovaries (in females) and testes (in males) produce sex steroid hormones collectively termed **androgens**. Specifically, the ovaries provide the primary source of **estradiol (estrogen)** and luteal phase **progesterone**; the adrenal glands in males and females synthesize **dehydroepiandrosterone (DHEA)** and its sulfate, DHEAS. The testes produce **testosterone**, also secreted in small amounts by ovaries; conversely, testosterone converts to estrogen in peripheral tissues.

Plasma testosterone concentration in females, about one-tenth the level in males, increases with exercise (as do estradiol and progesterone). Both resistance exercise and moderate aerobic exercise increase serum and free testosterone levels in untrained males after about 15 to 20 minutes. Testosterone decreases below resting values during longer-duration, higher-intensity aerobic exercise.

PANCREATIC HORMONES

The pancreas is about 14 cm long and weighs 60 g, and lies just below the stomach. **Figure 12.8** illustrates the location of the pancreas and its different endocrine cells. German microscopic anatomist and physician Paul Langerhans (1847–1888) first described the clusters of cells throughout the pancreas in his 1869 dissertation. These clusters, numbering close to 1 million, were named the **islets of Langerhans** to honor him. They contain four distinct cell types, each associated with a different peptide hormone. About three-quarters of the islet cells are **beta cells** that produce **insulin** and a peptide called amylin; another 20% are **alpha cells** that secrete **glucagon**. The remaining cells are **somatostatin**-secreting D cells and PP cells that produce **pancreatic polypeptide**.

Insulin and glucagon act in antagonistic fashion to modulate plasma glucose levels. The blood contains both hormones most of the time; the ratio of the two hormones determines which hormone and its action dominates.

Reduced renal blood flow stimulates the kidneys to release the enzyme _____ into the blood.

Name 3 tissues affected by cortisol's secretion.

1.

2.

3.

Cortisol secretion increases with

_____.

List 3 main effects of cortisol.

1.

2.

3.

Name 3 adrogens.

1.

2.

3.

Name 3 hormones secreted by the pancreas.

1.

2.

3.

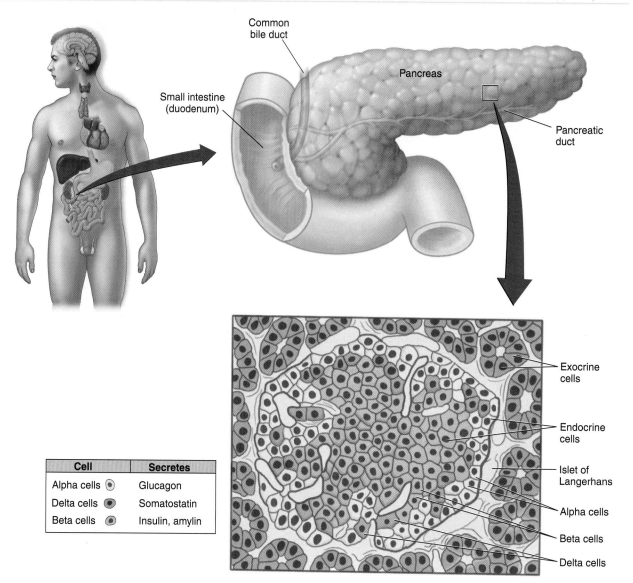

Cell	Secretes
Alpha cells ⊙	Glucagon
Delta cells ⊙	Somatostatin
Beta cells ⊙	Insulin, amylin

Figure 12.8. Location of the pancreas and its different endocrine cells.

In the postabsorptive-fed condition, insulin dominates and the body remains in a state of net anabolism (**Fig. 12.9A**). Ingested glucose provides substrate for energy production; any excess is stored as glycogen or becomes synthesized to fat and protein. In the fasted state, in contrast, glucagon dominates (Fig. 12.9B) to prevent low plasma glucose concentrations (hypoglycemia).

Insulin Secretion

The following five factors influence insulin release following a meal:

1. **Increased glucose concentrations**: Plasma glucose concentrations greater than 100 mg·dL^{-1} represent the main stimulus to insulin secretion. Glucose absorbed from the small intestine travels in the blood-

stream to the pancreas' beta cells where a transporter (GLUT-2) initiates insulin release.

2. **Increased amino acid concentrations**: Increased plasma amino acid concentration, which typically occurs after a meal, triggers insulin release.

3. **Gastrointestinal tract hormones**: Several hormones released from the intestinal tract following a meal travel in the circulation to the beta cells to stimulate insulin release. The two most important of these hormones are glucagon-like peptide-1 (GLP-1) and glucose-dependent insulinotropic peptide (GIP). Both hormones trigger insulin release even before glucose reaches the beta cells.

4. **Parasympathetic nervous system stimulation**: During and following a meal, an increase occurs in parasympathetic stimulation of the intestinal region and pancreas and directly promotes insulin release.

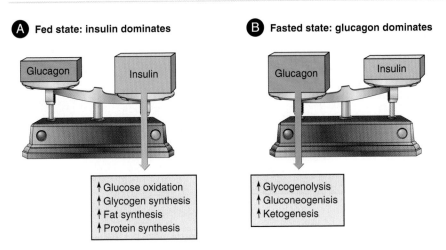

Figure 12.9.   The insulin-to-glucagon ratio regulates blood glucose. In the fed state **(A)**, insulin dominates. In the fasted state **(B)**, glucagon dominates.

FOR YOUR INFORMATION

Insulin Commercialization

Danish Nobel Laureate August Krogh (1920, see Chapter 1) received permission in 1922 from the original patent holders (Board of Governors of the University of Toronto in the names of the those who first discovered insulin, researchers Banting, Collip, and Best) to govern the quality of insulin production in Denmark, Norway, and Sweden. In 1923, Krogh and colleagues founded the Nordisk Insulin Laboratory, which in 1989 became Novo Nordisk Pharmaceutical, Inc., the world's largest producer of insulin and diabetes care systems. (Bodil Schmidt-Nielson, daughter of August and Marie Krogh, provides intimate details about the initial discovery of insulin, including many conflicts and controversies, in her insightful and highly recommended book, *August & Marie Krogh. Lives in Science*. New York: American Physiological Society, 1995.)

5. **Sympathetic nervous system stimulation**: Increased sympathetic activity inhibits insulin secretion. During stress, sympathetic input to the pancreas increases to inhibit insulin secretion and stimulate gluconeogenesis; this provides extra glucose fuel for the nervous system and skeletal musculature.

Insulin's Functions

Primary target tissues for insulin include the liver, adipose tissue, and skeletal muscle.

Insulin's major function regulates glucose metabolism by facilitating cellular glucose uptake in all tissues except the brain. Insulin exerts its action on glucose in the following four ways:

1. *Increases glucose transport into most, but not all, insulin-sensitive cells.* Adipose tissue and resting skeletal muscle do require insulin for glucose uptake during rest. Exercising skeletal muscle does *not* depend on insulin for its glucose uptake. When muscles act, GLUT-4 transporters activate without insulin stimulation to increase glucose uptake. The intracellular signal for this appears to be Ca^{++} and inorganic phosphate (P_i).
2. *Enhances cellular utilization and storage of glucose.* Insulin activates enzymes for glucose utilization (glycolysis) and glycogen and fat synthesis (glycogenesis and lipogenesis). Insulin simultaneously inhibits enzymes for glycogen breakdown (glycogenolysis), glucose synthesis (gluconeogenesis), and fat breakdown (lipolysis) to ensure that metabolism moves towards anabolism. If more glucose is ingested than needed (for energy metabolism), the excess converts to glycogen or fatty acids.
3. *Enhances utilization of amino acids.* Insulin activates enzymes for protein synthesis and inhibits enzymes that promote protein breakdown (beta-oxidation).
4. *Promotes fat synthesis.* Insulin inhibits beta-oxidation of fatty acids to promote conversion of excess glucose or amino acids into triacylglycerols (lipogenesis).

Figure 12.10 illustrates that the anabolic functions of insulin promote glycogen, protein, and fat synthesis. With insulin deficiency, the action of glucagon predominates and cells engage in catabolic activity.

Glucagon Secretion

The alpha cells of the islets of Langerhans secrete glucagon, the "insulin antagonist" hormone. In contrast to insulin, glucagon increases blood glucose levels and

FOR YOUR INFORMATION

Diabetes and Amylin

Amylin, a peptide hormone similar to insulin and co-secreted from the pancreatic beta cells, was discovered in 1987. Like insulin, this hormone helps regulate glucose transport following a meal. It slows gastric emptying and gastric acid secretion, thus delaying sugar digestion and absorption. The combined actions of amylin and two other peptides (gastric inhibitory peptide, *GIP*; and glucagons-like peptide-1, *GLP-1*) initiate a self-regulating cycle. Intestinal glucose stimulates GIP and GLP-1 release, which initiates insulin and amylin secretion. Amylin then returns to the GI tract to slow the rate that food enters the intestine. In the future, an amylin-agonist drug may effectively treat diabetes and/or obesity.

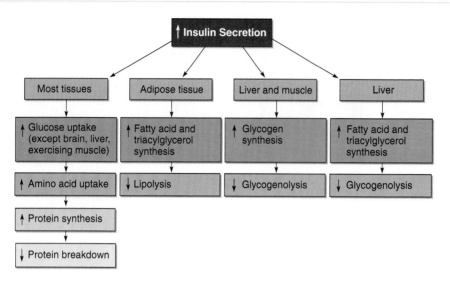

Figure 12.10. Increased insulin promotes glycogen, protein, and fat synthesis.

stimulates liver glycogenolysis and gluconeogenesis and lipid catabolism.

Similar to insulin, blood glucose level regulates the pancreas' glucagon release. A decline in plasma glucose concentration below 100 mg·dL^{-1} stimulates the alpha cells' release of glucagon, resulting in an instantaneous glucose release from the liver. Glucagon contributes to blood glucose regulation during long-duration exercise and starvation; both conditions markedly decrease blood glucose and glycogen reserves.

Interestingly, glucagon release is also stimulated by plasma amino acids. This pathway prevents hypoglycemia after ingesting a pure protein meal. If a meal contains protein without carbohydrate, amino acids in the food trigger insulin secretion. Even though no glucose has been absorbed, insulin-stimulated glucose uptake increases and plasma glucose concentration falls. Co-secretion of glucagon in this situation prevents hypoglycemia by stimulating hepatic glucose output. Because amino acids were ingested, both glucose and amino acids become available to peripheral tissues.

Glucagon's Functions

Figure 12.11 shows that, when the action of glucagon predominates, cells engage in catabolic activity. The liver is glucagon's primary target tissue, stimulating glycogenolysis and gluconeogenesis to increase glucose output. During an overnight fast, 75% of the glucose produced by the liver comes from its glycogen stores, with the remaining 25% produced from gluconeogenic reactions. Glucagon also has a catabolic effect on adipose tissue throughout the body (Fig. 12.11).

DIABETES MELLITUS

As early as the 1st or 2nd century A. D., Greek physicians described the symptoms of diabetes mellitus (*mellitus* is Latin for sweetened with honey). A translation of an early Greek description of diabetes attributed to Areteus the Cappadocian reveals a general misunderstanding of the nature of the disease and the unfortunate outcome:

"Diabetes is a wonderful affliction, not very frequent among men, being a melting down of the flesh and limbs into urine. The patients never stop making water. The flow is incessant, as in the opening of aqueducts. Life is short, disgusting and painful; thirst unquenchable; excessive drinking, which, however, is disproportionate to the large quantity of urine, for more urine is passed; and one cannot stop them from drinking or making water; and at no distant term they expire."

The Chinese physician Chen Chuan, in the 7th century A. D., recorded that the urine of those afflicted with diabetes tasted sweet. Diabetes during the Middle Ages was known as "the pissing evil." Eleven centuries later, physicians in concert with anatomists discovered a link between the pancreas (Langerhans islet cells) and diabetes.

Twenty-one years after Langerhan's discovery, researchers surgically removed the pancreas from a dog and discovered that the animal exhibited the full symptoms of diabetes—*tremendous thirst, increased urine flow, elevated blood glucose, glucose in the urine, and generalized wasting of body mass.* In 1921, the Canadian physician Sir Frederick Banting (1891–1941) of the University of Toronto first described how administration of insulin to dogs whose pancreas was surgically removed "cured" the dogs of diabetes. Banting with co-recipient John Richard Macleod (1876–1935) were awarded the 1923 Nobel Prize in physiology or medicine for this pioneering and life-saving discovery.

Diabetes mellitus consists of four subgroups of disorders that exhibit different pathophysiologies:

1. **Type 1 diabetes** results from the body's failure to produce insulin. Between 5% and 10% of Americans diagnosed with diabetes have the type 1 subgroup.
2. **Type 2 diabetes** is a relative insulin deficiency that results in hyperglycemia. Insulin resistance is a com-

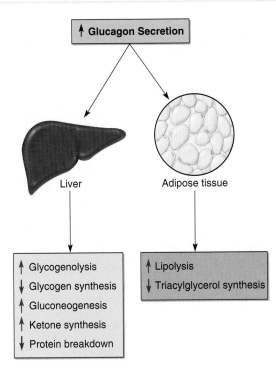

Figure 12.11. Glucagon secretion and its actions on target tissues.

Questions & Notes

Name 4 factors that influence insulin release following a meal.

1.

2.

3.

4.

Describe 3 functions of insulin.

1.

2.

3.

Name the "insulin antagonist" hormone.

Give the major function of glucagon.

Briefly describe the 2 types of diabetic disorders and give one fact about each.

mon symptom. Approximately 90% to 95% (17 million) of Americans diagnosed with diabetes exhibit insulin resistance.

3. **Gestational diabetes** afflicts about 4% of all pregnant women or about 135,000 cases in the United States each year.

4. **Pre-diabetes** is a condition where a person's blood glucose reaches higher than normal levels but not high enough for a diagnosis of type 2 diabetes. More than 20.1 million Americans classify as pre-diabetic in addition to the 18.2 million with either type 1 or type 2 diabetes.

Clinicians have discontinued the former use of the terms **insulin-dependent diabetes mellitus** (IDDM; type 1) and **noninsulin-dependent diabetes mellitus** (NIDDM; type 2) because these diseases often require treatments that overlap and vary, rather than reflect the underlying pathogenesis. For example, many people with type 2 diabetes require exogenous insulin to compensate for their relative insulin deficiency.

Diabetes Symptoms

Diabetes often progresses undiagnosed because many of its symptoms seem harmless. Importantly, early detection of diabetes symptoms and subsequent treatment decrease the chance of developing the more serious complications of diabetes.
Diabetes symptoms include:

- Elevated blood glucose (hyperglycemia)
- Frequent urination (polyuria)
- Excessive thirst (polydipsia)
- Extreme hunger (polyphagia)
- High levels of blood ketones from reliance on excessive fat catabolism
- Unexplained weight loss
- Increased fatigue
- Irritability
- Blurry vision
- Numbness or tingling in the extremities (hands, feet)

Box 12–1 • CLOSE UP

HOW TO DETECT DIABETES MELLITUS

Complications from diabetes mellitus can cause blindness, kidney failure, need for amputation, and birth defects. It also contributes to atherosclerosis and hypertension.

About one-half of the people each year who learn they have diabetes go untreated.

Differences Between the Two Major Forms of Diabetes Mellitus

CONDITION	TYPE 1	TYPE 2
Other names	Type 1-IDDM	Type II-NIDDM
	Juvenile-onset	Adult-onset
	Ketosis-prone	Ketosis-resistant
	Brittle	Stable
Age of onset	<20 y (mean = 12 y)	>40 y; increasingly
	<40 y in some cases	prevalent in youth
Other condition	Viral infection	Obesity
Insulin required	Yes	Sometimes
Insulin receptors	Normal	Low or normal
Symptoms	Relatively severe	Relatively moderate
Prevalence in diabetic population	5 to 10 %	90 to 95 %

Key Blood Tests for Detecting Diabetes Mellitus

SUBSTANCE	NORMAL VALUES	DECISION LEVEL
Fasting plasma glucose (FPG); following 8-h fast	<110 mg $\cdot$ dL^{-1}	≤ 45 mg $\cdot$ dL^{-1}–indicates **hypoglycemia** and a prediabetic condition 110–125 mg $\cdot$ dL^{-1}–indicates **impaired range** >126 mg $\cdot$ dL^{-1}–indicates **suspected diabetes**
Total cholesterol	<200 mg $\cdot$ dL^{-1}	>240 mg $\cdot$ dL^{-1}–patients with diabetes often have elevated plasma cholesterol
Triacylglycerol	40–160 mg $\cdot$ dL^{-1}, males 35–135 mg $\cdot$ dL^{-1}, females	>250 mg $\cdot$ dL^{-1}–patients with diabetes often have elevated plasma triacylglycerols
Oral Glucose-Tolerance Test[a]	**Upper Limit of Normal**	**Diabetic Values**
Time = 0	115 mg $\cdot$ dL^{-1}	>140 mg $\cdot$ dL^{-1}
Time = 60 min	200 mg $\cdot$ dL^{-1}	>200 mg $\cdot$ dL^{-1}
Time = 120 min	140 mg $\cdot$ dL^{-1}	>200 mg $\cdot$ dL^{-1}

[a]Previously preferred but an expensive, time consuming, and unpleasant test. Blood drawn following ingestion of a standard glucose load. Ordinarily, blood glucose rises initially and then returns to normal. In diabetes mellitus blood glucose remains elevated during the recovery period. Many variations exist in the timing of blood sampling and quantity of glucose ingested. A fasting plasma glucose (FPG) test is recommended.

- Slow-healing wounds or sores
- Abnormally high frequency of infection

Go to the following Internet site to calculate your diabetes risk: *http://www.dia-betes.org/risk-test.jsp.*

The Genetics of Diabetes

A simple pattern of inherited characteristics does not fully explain the risk of contracting diabetes. Two factors predispose a person to diabetes: (1) individuals inherit a predisposition to the disease; and (2) something in the environment triggers its activation (onset).

Type 1 Diabetes Most type 1 diabetics inherit risk factors from both parents, with inherited traits more common in whites than blacks or Asians. The most prominent "environmental triggers" for type 1 diabetes include cold weather exposure (develops more often in winter than summer and more frequently in places with cold climates), viral infection, and early diet (less common in those who were breastfed and in those who first ate solid foods at a later age). The development of type 1 diabetes seems to take many years.

For a man with type 1 diabetes, the odds of his child contracting the disease is 1 in 17. For a woman with type 1 diabetes who gave birth before age 25, the child's risk is 1 in 25; the risk decreases to 1 in 100 if the mother gave birth after age 25. A child's risk doubles if the mother developed diabetes before age 11. If both parents are type 1 diabetics, the child's risk ranges between 1 in 10 and 1 in 4. An exception exists to these risks in that about 1 in every 7 type 1 diabetics has a condition called **type 2 polyglandular autoimmune syndrome**. In addition to having diabetes, these individuals also have thyroid disease, a dysfunctional adrenal gland, and often other immune system disorders. The child's risk of contracting this autoimmune syndrome, including type 1 diabetes, rises to 1 in 2.

Type 2 Diabetes Type 2 diabetes has a stronger genetic basis than type 1, yet its occurrence also depends more on environmental factors. Family history of type 2 diabetes provides one of the strongest risk factors for the disease but *only* for people living a typical Western lifestyle (high-fat diet, low intake of complex carbohydrates and fiber, and too little exercise). Overfatness (obesity) provides a considerable risk factor for type 2 diabetes. The ethnic groups in the United States with the highest risk for developing type 2 diabetes are African-Americans, Mexican-Americans, and Pima Indians.

The tendency for type 2 diabetes to run in families relates to children growing up with poor diets and little physical activity. In addition to these environmental influences, a strong genetic basis also exists. In general, if one parent has type 2 diabetes diagnosed before age 50, the risk of the child getting diabetes is 1 in 7; the risk decreases to 1 in 13 if the diagnosis of one parent occurs after age 50. If both parents have type 2 diabetes, the child's risk averages about 1 in 2.

Diabetes Statistics

For many years, physicians viewed type 2 diabetes as an adult-only disease. The last 20 years reveal an alarming increase in type 2 diabetes among children. *Statistics from 2002 (http://www.diabetes.org) indicate that one-third of all new diabetic cases occur in children under age 16 years. This has led many to declare type 2 diabetes a pediatric disease.*

Alarming data also exist for the prevalence of all forms of diabetes among people 20 years or older in the United States. For the year 2002, 18.2 million (8.7%) of all men and women had been diagnosed with diabetes. **Figure 12.12** illustrates the prevalence of all forms of diabetes by race/ethnicity among people aged 20 years or older. A greater incidence of diabetes exists for minorities: 8.4% of all

Give the upper limit of fasting blood glucose that indicates type 1 diabetes.

Give 2 risk factors that predispose a person to type 1 diabetes.

1.

2.

Give 2 risk factors that predispose a person to type 2 diabetes.

1.

2.

FOR YOUR INFORMATION

Diabetes Oral Medications
Many oral medications treat (*http://www.diabetes.org/type-2diabetes/oral-medications.jsp*) type 2 diabetes. Each type helps to lower blood glucose in a different way.

1. Sulfonylureas (SUL-fah-nil-YOO-ree-ahs) stimulate the pancreas to synthesize more insulin.
2. Biguanides (by-GWAN-ides) decrease the amount of glucose synthesized by the liver.
3. Alpha-glucosidase inhibitors (AL-fa gloo-KOS-ih-dayss in-HIB-it-ers) slow the absorption of ingested starches.
4. Thiazolidinediones (THIGH-ah-ZO-li-deen-DYE-owns) increase sensitivity to insulin.
5. Meglitinides (meh-GLIT-in-ides) stimulate the pancreas and synthesis of insulin.
6. D-phenylalanine (dee-fen-nel-AL-ah-neen) derivatives stimulate the rapid synthesis of insulin by the pancreas.

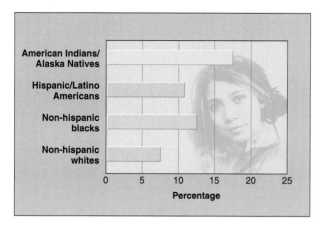

Figure 12.12. Age-adjusted prevalence of all forms of diabetes in people aged 20 years or older by race/ethnicity in the United States in 2002.

non-Hispanic whites, 11.4% of all non-Hispanic blacks, and more than 17% of American Indians and Alaska Natives.

Hispanic/Latino Americans experience 1.5 times more diabetes than non-Hispanic whites of similar age. Mexican-Americans, the largest Hispanic/Latino subgroup, are more than twice as likely to have diabetes than non-Hispanic white counterparts. Similarly, residents of Puerto Rico contract diabetes at 1.8 times the rate of U.S. non-Hispanic whites.

Tests for Diabetes

Several tests diagnose diabetes. The American Diabetes Association (*http://www.diabetes.org/home.jsp*) recommends the **fasting plasma glucose test** (**FPG**) rather than the popular oral glucose tolerance test. The latter evaluates blood sugar levels over a 2-hour interval after drinking a glucose-containing solution (see *How to Detect Diabetes Mellitus*, page 420). The FPG test measures plasma glucose after an 8-hour fast.

The current value for suspected diabetes (FPG >126 mg·dL^{-1}) is lower than the previous standard of 140 mg·dL^{-1} and acknowledges that patients can be asymptomatic with microvascular complications (small blood vessel damage) with FPG values in the low to mid 120 mg·dL^{-1} range. The impaired range represents a transition between normal and diabetes where the body no longer responds properly to insulin or fails to secrete adequate amounts. These individuals require close monitoring because they run a high risk for developing full-blown diabetes.

METABOLIC SYNDROME X

Metabolic syndrome X (or simply **metabolic syndrome**), first described in 1988 by Dr. Gerald Raven at Stanford University, represents a multifaceted grouping of coronary artery disease risks. This "disease of modern civilization"

afflicts millions of adults (more common in men than women) in Western industrialized countries. Disease occurrence relates to genetic, hormonal, and lifestyle factors that include obesity, physical inactivity, and nutrient excesses, including high intakes of saturated and *trans* fatty acids. The clustering of insulin resistance and hyperinsulinemia characterizes the syndrome; it also coincides with dyslipidemia (atherogenic plasma lipid profile), essential hypertension, abdominal (visceral) obesity, and glucose intolerance. Because these individuals are at higher risk for coronary artery disease, they should receive special attention in terms of diagnosis and treatment.

Psychosocial stress, socioeconomic disadvantage, and abnormal psychiatric traits have also been linked to the syndrome's pathogenesis. Such factors likely relate to a central neuroendocrine origin as enhanced activation of the hypothalamic–pituitary–adrenal axis. The endpoints of hyperinsulinemia, obesity, coronary artery disease, type 2 diabetes, stroke, and increased colorectal cancer risk.

DIABETES AND EXERCISE

Hypoglycemia during exercise represents the most common disturbance of glucose homeostasis in type 1 diabetes. During prolonged moderate exercise, hepatic glucose release does not keep pace with active muscle's increased glucose utilization. Reduced plasma glucose becomes severe in those patients who require intensive insulin therapy throughout the day to normalize glucose levels. Sedentary lifestyle and excessive body fat reduce exercise tolerance of type 1 and type 2 diabetics, independent of blood glucose regulation.

Exercise Training in Diabetes

The clinical use of exercise training to control glucose in type 1 diabetics remains unclear, despite the clear association between regular exercise and improved insulin sensitivity by peripheral tissues. These individuals must exercise with caution because of increased insulin sensitivity and because fast delivery of injected insulin via the rapid circulation with exercise accelerates glucose removal from plasma, possibly inducing serious hypoglycemia and diabetic shock.

As a consequence of obesity (and possibly poor diet), many overweight men and women experience reduced glucose tolerance due to generalized insulin resistance; this triggers excessive insulin output from the pancreas (hyperinsulinemia). For individuals who eventually develop type 2 diabetes, exercise training often reduces fasting plasma insulin levels and lowers insulin output (thus indicating improved insulin sensitivity).

Exercise Benefits for Diabetics

Without doubt, exercise training provides important non-pharmacologic therapy for type 2 diabetics. Regular physical activity for the type 2 diabetic improves glycemic control, cardiovascular function, body composition, psychological profile, and reduces a broad array of heart disease risks. Some patients with type 1 diabetes improve their control of blood glucose (with lower daily insulin requirements) with regular exercise, but the results are less consistent than for type 2 patients. Despite this limitation, type 1 and type 2 diabetic patients most likely profit equally from the exercise-related benefits that improve physical fitness, blood pressure, weight control, and blood lipid profile and lower overall heart disease risk.

Glycemic Control   An acute exercise bout abruptly decreases plasma glucose levels in type 2 diabetics. Improved glucose regulation with acute exercise may persist for hours to days, due to the muscles' increased insulin sensitivity. Insulin sensitivity is also increased with acute exercise. Improved longer term glycemic control in the physically active diabetic may occur from the cumulative effects of each acute exercise session, rather than from changes in physical fitness per se. The hyperinsulinemic patient shows the greatest benefit from regular exercise, a response consistent with the notion that exercise reverses insulin resistance (i.e., increases insulin sensitivity).

Cardiovascular Effects   Increased morbidity (disease state) and mortality (ratio of deaths in an area to the population of that area; expressed per 1,000 per year) in type 2 diabetes occur from coronary heart disease, stroke, and peripheral vascular and nerve disease due, in part, to accelerated atherosclerosis and elevated blood glucose. Regular physical activity favorably modifies plasma lipoproteins, hyperinsulinemia, hyperglycemia, some blood coagulation parameters, local vascularization, and blood pressure.

Weight Loss   Exercise without diet therapy only moderately reduces body weight among type 2 diabetics. A moderate effect should not be underestimated because small changes in body weight with exercise may not reflect the more favorable changes in overall body composition. For both the diabetic and non-diabetic individual, body fat loss occurs most effectively by combining diet *plus* exercise.

Psychological Benefits   Regular, moderate-intensity exercise for diabetics and non-diabetics decreases anxiety, improves mood and self-esteem, increases sense of well-being, and enhances overall quality of life.

Exercise Risks for Diabetics

The potential complications of exercise for diabetics must be minimized through proper patient screening before they begin an exercise program and careful monitoring during exercise. **Figure 12.13** lists some potential adverse effects of exercise for the diabetic.

ENDURANCE TRAINING AND ENDOCRINE FUNCTION

Few studies have studied changes in hormonal response to systematic alterations in frequency, intensity, and duration of exercise. Most of what we know about changes in hormonal dynamics with exercise training comes from studies where hormone assessment occurred secondarily to other variables. Nevertheless, a picture has emerged of the integrated response of different hormones to training, particularly with respect to fluid balance, energy modulation, glycemic control, cardiovascular changes, and growth and development. **Table 12.3** lists endocrine hormones and their general responses to regular exercise. Because of complex interactions between endocrine secretions and central nervous system function, limited research exists concerning multiple hormone secretions and chronic exercise adaptations.

Endurance training generally decreases the magnitude of hormonal response to a standard exercise level. Exercise at the same absolute intensity produces a

Briefly describe metabolic syndrome X and its associated health risks.

FOR YOUR INFORMATION

Exercise Guidelines for Type 1 Diabetics

1. Ingest 15 to 30 g of carbohydrate for each 30 minutes of intense exercise.
2. Consume a carbohydrate snack following exercise.
3. Decrease insulin dose:
   a. Intermediate-acting insulin — decrease dose by 30 to 35% on the day of exercise.
   b. Intermediate-acting and short-acting insulin — omit dose if it precedes exercise.
   c. Multiple doses of short-acting insulin — reduce dose before exercise by 30% and supplement carbohydrate intake.
   d. Continuous subcutaneous insulin infusion — eliminate mealtime bolus or insulin increment that precedes or follows exercise.
4. Avoid exercising for 1 hour those muscles receiving a short-acting insulin injection.
5. Avoid exercising in the late evening.

Potential problems with exercise in type 2 diabetes	
System	**Potential Problem**
Systemic	• Retinal hemorrhage • Increased proteinuria • Acceleration of microvascular lesions
Cardiovascular	• Cardiac arrhythmias • Ischemic heart disease (often silent) • Excessive rise in blood pressure • Post-exercise orthostatic hypotension
Metabolic	• Increased hyperglycemia • Increased ketosis
Musculoskeletal	• Foot ulcers (in presence of neuropathy) • Orthopedic injury related to neuropathy • Accelerated degenerative joint disease • Eye injuries and retinal hemorrhage

Figure 12.13. Potential physical and physiologic problems for individuals with type 2 diabetes who begin an exercise program.

lower hormonal response of trained subjects compared with untrained counterparts. Adjusting exercise intensity to a percentage of each person's maximum capacity (i.e., same relative intensity) eliminates the training-related difference in hormonal response. With maximal exercise, trained subjects have an identical or slightly higher catecholamine and pituitary hormonal response than untrained subjects.

Anterior Pituitary Hormones

Growth Hormone and Long-Term Exercise Training

Most research of GH involves responses to a single exercise session. Less information exists on GH levels during prolonged exercise training. Research on the dynamics of GH secretions with chronic exercise takes on significance because of the causal relationship between GH availability and the maintenance of fat-free body mass (FFM) with aging and weight loss.

Figure 12.14 shows the effects of a run training program on 24-hour integrated serum GH concentrations in 21 healthy, eumenorrheic women. The study involved two training groups; one group ran at speeds corresponding to the lactate threshold (@LT), while the other group ran at speeds above lactate threshold (>LT). Nontraining subjects served as controls (C).

Both training groups completed similar weekly mileage. The distance covered during the first week equaled 5 miles; weekly mileage gradually increased to 24 miles by week 20 and continued at this distance un-

Table 12·3   Hormonal Response to Exercise Training

HORMONE	TRAINING RESPONSE
Hypothalamus-Pituitary Hormones	
GH	Resting values increased: trained tend to have less dramatic rise during exercise
TSH	No known training effect
ACTH	Trained have increased exercise values
PRL	Some evidence that training lowers resting values
FSH, LH, and Testosterone	Trained females have depressed values; testosterone levels may increase in males with long-term strength training
Posterior Pituitary Hormones	
Vasopressin (ADH)	Some evidence that training slightly reduces ADH at a given workload
Oxytocin	No research available
Thyroid Hormones	
Thyroxine (T_4)	Reduced concentration of total T_3 and increased free thyroxine at rest
Triiodothyronine (T_3)	Increased turnover of T_3 and T_4 during exercise
Adrenal Hormones	
Aldosterone	No significant training adaptation
Cortisol	Trained exhibit slight elevations during exercise
Epinephrine	Decrease in secretion at rest and same absolute exercise
Norepinephrine	intensity after training
Pancreatic Hormones	
Insulin	Training increases sensitivity to insulin; normal decrease in insulin during exercise is greatly reduced in response to training
Glucagon	Smaller increase in glucose levels during exercise at both absolute and relative workloads
Kidney Hormones	
Renin (enzyme)	No apparent training effect
Angiotensin	

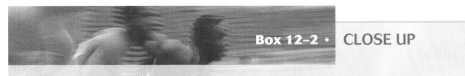

Box 12–2 • CLOSE UP

ALTERNATIVE TREATMENTS FOR DIABETES

A number of alternative treatments exist for diabetes. However, these therapies are not widely accepted, mainly due to lack of scientific consensus. Such treatments include:

- **Acupuncture**: Eastern medical treatment that inserts needles at various centers in the body to release natural painkillers; this may help to manage painful nerve damage in diabetes.
- **Biofeedback**: psychological technique using meditation, relaxation, and stress-reduction methods to manage and relieve pain in diabetics.

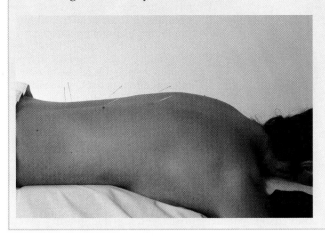

- **Chromium**: supplemental chromium may stimulate production of a glucose-tolerance factor that improves insulin action. The scientific information on chromium supplementation for diabetes is not clear.
- **Magnesium**: diabetics tend to be deficient in magnesium, which can worsen the complications of diabetes, especially type 2 diabetes. The exact nature of the relationship between magnesium and diabetes remains unresolved.
- **Vanadium**: vanadium may normalize blood glucose in type 1 and 2 diabetic animals, but insufficient information exists for humans. This area is currently under research.
- **Pancreatic islet transplantation**: represents a promising development for the future and perhaps permanent treatment for type 1 diabetes. This technique removes islets from the pancreas of a deceased donor and injects them into the liver of a diabetic patient. The islet cells eventually attach to new blood vessels and begin releasing insulin. Rejection of the donor's tissue remains a major problem, but hopefully will be resolved by future research.

For more information on alternative treatments, see the NIDDK bulletin at: *http://diabetes.niddk.nih.gov/dm/pubs/alternativetherapies/index.htm*.

---

til week 40. Thereafter, weekly mileage increased by 1.25 miles each additional 3 weeks. Subjects ran between 35 and 40 miles per week by the end of the study.

The year-long training program increased $\dot{V}O_{2max}$ by 9.9% for the @LT group and 11.8% for the >LT group. In addition, the @LT group increased exercise $\dot{V}O_2$ at lactate threshold ($\dot{V}O_2$–LT) by 21.5%, while the >LT group's $\dot{V}O_2$–LT increased by 28%. The control group did not change. No differences in body mass, percentage body fat, or body fat mass emerged among groups. FFM increased for both training groups.

For GH, the >LT group showed a marked 50% increase in integrated 24-hour resting GH concentration after training. GH concentrations remained unaffected by exercise training for the @LT and control groups. The researchers hypothesized that relatively strenuous exercise above the lactate threshold increased GH pulsatile secretion through the stimulating effect of endogenous opiates and catecholamines, while at the same time, such exercise inhibited somatostatin release. Research must determine whether training at intensities above LT counters GH decrease in aging and how this affects body weight loss and associated deleterious effects on body composition.

Questions & Notes

List 3 potential problems for type 2 diabetics who regularly exercise.

1.

2.

3.

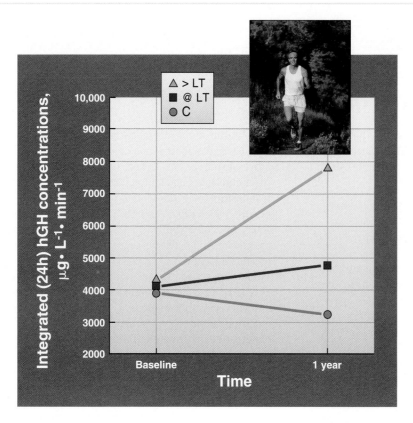

Figure 12.14. Integrated 24-hour hGH concentrations for subjects training at the lactate threshold (@LT), training above the lactate threshold (>LT), and non-training controls (C). Note the large (50%) increase in hGH concentrations for the >LT group compared with the @LT and C groups. (Data from Weltman, A., et al.: Endurance training amplifies the pulsatile release of growth hormone: effects of training intensity. *J. Appl. Physiol.*, 72:2188, 1992.)

Corticotropin (ACTH)   Corticotropin stimulates the adrenal cortex and thus increases fat mobilization for energy. Exercise training raises ACTH levels during physical activity. Enhanced fatty acid oxidation also spares glycogen to benefit prolonged exercise performance.

Prolactin (PRL)   It remains unclear whether long-term training alters PRL, other than the training-induced changes mediated by sympathetic activity or other multiple hormone interactions.

Follicle-Stimulating Hormone (FSH), Luteinizing Hormone (LH), and Testosterone   Women with a history of exercise participation have altered FSH and LH levels at different phases of the menstrual cycle. Alterations in these hormones often cause menstrual dysfunction. FSH levels decrease in trained women throughout an abbreviated anovulatory menstrual cycle, whereas LH and progesterone concentrations rise in the cycle's follicular phase. Factors other than acute and long-term exercise can alter reproductive function in women athletes; these include weight loss, dietary changes, changes in lean-to-fat ratio, emotional stress of training and competition, and altered clearance rates of gonadal steroid hormones.

Endurance training in men affects pituitary-gonadal function, including testosterone and PRL concentrations. **Figure 12.15** compares testosterone, LH, and FSH levels among 46 male runners (64 km average weekly distance) and 18 non-runners matched for age, stature, and body mass. The runners had depressed testosterone levels without significant difference in LH and FSH compared with non-runners.

Reduced testosterone concentration (both increased clearance and decreased production) in endurance-trained men parallels the sex steroid reductions in women who undergo endurance training and associated lower body fat levels. Because LH and FSH do not differ between trained and untrained persons, impaired gonadotropin release from the anterior pituitary does not explain reduced testosterone levels in the trained state. Resistance training presents a different picture because elite male athletes have elevated serum testosterone, LH, and FSH.

In a well-controlled training study on the effects of a supraphysiologic dose of exogenous testosterone, 43 normal men were randomly assigned to one of four groups: placebo with no exercise; testosterone with no exercise; placebo plus exercise; and testosterone plus exercise. The men received injections of 600 mg of testosterone or placebo weekly for 10 weeks. The exercise groups performed standardized weight-lifting for the arms and legs three times weekly. Before and after the treatment period, FFM was determined by underwater weighing, muscle size was determined by magnetic resonance imaging, and the strength of the arms and legs was determined with bench-press and squatting exercises, respectively. For the no-exercise groups, men given testosterone experienced a 14% increase in arm muscle size compared to the placebo group and a 9% increase in arm strength. Similar results occurred for the lower body. Those men assigned to testosterone and exercise showed significantly greater increases in FFM

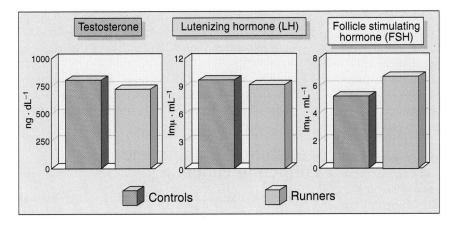

Figure 12.15. Comparison of testosterone, LH, and FSH levels among runners and untrained controls. Runners demonstrate significantly lower testosterone levels with no difference in LH and FSH compared with controls. (Data from Wheeler, G.D, et al.: Reduced serum testosterone and prolactin levels in male distance runners. *JAMA*, 252:514, 1984.)

and muscle size of the arms and legs compared to the testosterone with no exercise group. Neither mood nor behavior changed in any of the groups during training. These data support the conclusion that a supraphysiologic dose of testosterone, especially when combined with resistance training, increases FFM and muscle size and strength in healthy men.

Posterior Pituitary Hormones

Vasopressin (ADH)   Maximal exhaustive exercise or prolonged submaximal exercise at the same relative intensity produces no difference in ADH response between trained and untrained individuals. ADH concentration decreases with training in response to submaximal exercise at the same absolute intensity.

Oxytocin   As of August 2005, we are unaware of research on humans involving training-induced changes for this hormone.

Thyroid Hormones

Exercise training coordinates a pituitary-thyroid response that increases turnover of thyroid hormones, which is a response usually associated with excessive hormonal action that leads to hyperthyroidism. No evidence indicates that hyperthyroidism develops in highly trained individuals. BMR and resting core temperature remain normal with training. The increased T_4 turnover that accompanies chronic exercise occurs through a mechanism that differs from this hormone's normal dynamics.

Research on women who train for a marathon reveals interesting responses for thyroid turnover. From a baseline of relatively sedentary living to training 48 km a week mildly depressed thyroid function as reflected by *decreased* T_3 and T_4 levels. In contrast, extending training distance to 80 km a week *increased* the levels of these hormones. Changes in body composition that accompany a high training volume may contribute to discrepancies in an exercise-induced change in thyroid function in females.

Adrenal Hormones

Aldosterone   The response of the renin-angiotensin-aldosterone system during exercise contributes to homeostatic control of fluid and electrolytes. This represents a transient response because exercise training does not affect resting levels of these compounds or their normal response to exercise.

Questions & Notes

List 3 benefits of exercise for type 2 diabetics.

1.

2.

3.

List 3 potential complications of exercise for type 1 diabetics.

1.

2.

3.

Briefly describe the hormonal response to exercise training for the following hormones.

GH –

ADH –

Insulin –

Glucagon –

Thyroxine –

Cortisol –

Epinephrine –

Name the 2 primary hormones in resistance training adaptations.

1.

2.

Name the hormone thought to produce an "exercise high" response in some individuals.

Cortisol Plasma cortisol levels increase less in trained compared with sedentary subjects during the same moderate exercise levels. Greater cortisol output among untrained individuals may partly result from heightened psychological stress experienced during exercise testing. Elevated cortisol levels promote fatty acid and protein catabolism to provide fuel for energy and substrates for tissue repair following exercise.

Epinephrine and Norepinephrine An important aspect of the catecholamine response to exercise and training involves the **sympathoadrenal response**, rather than the typical adrenal gland response. **Figure 12.16** shows a large initial decrease in epinephrine and norepinephrine concentrations to a standard bout of intense exercise during the first 2 weeks of training. Bradycardia and a smaller increase in blood pressure during submaximal exercise represent the most familiar sympathoadrenal adaptive responses to exercise training. Both responses favorably lower myocardial oxygen demands to exercise and other stressors. Reduced catecholamine output may reflect the benefits of regular physical activity in diminishing the body's response to stressful situations.

Pancreatic Hormones

Insulin and Glucagon Endurance training maintains plasma insulin and glucagon levels in exercise similar to resting values. This seemingly depressed hormonal response with training occurs through two mechanisms:

1. Increased muscle and fat tissue sensitivity to insulin. Exercise training reduces the insulin requirement to regulate blood glucose. Improved insulin sensitivity most likely occurs from improved insulin binding capacity to receptor sites on individual muscle fibers and adipocytes. Liver cells also increase their insulin sensitivity.

2. Increased percentage contribution of fat catabolism for fuel during submaximal exercise; decreased carbohydrate metabolism lowers the insulin requirement.

Resistance Training and Endocrine Function

The large variation among individuals in muscular strength and hypertrophy with similar programs of resistance training suggests considerable individual differences in endocrine dynamics with chronic muscle overload. Muscle remodeling with resistance training reflects a complex process that involves cell receptor interaction with specific hormones, which stimulates DNA synthesis of contractile proteins. The magnitude of the change links to the configuration of the exercise stimulus (e.g., frequency, intensity, volume, and mode of training) and more than likely the hormonal response.

Testosterone and growth hormone represent the two primary hormones in resistance training adaptations. Testosterone augments GH release and interacts with nervous system dynamics. The importance of these functions may exceed any direct anabolic effect of testosterone on muscle structure and function. Not all research demonstrates a direct GH increase with resistance training. In this regard, GH's stimulatory response requires a threshold of exercise training intensity or training duration. *In general, resistance training increases the frequency and amplitude of testosterone and GH secretion, thereby contributing to hypertrophic (growth) effects on muscle.*

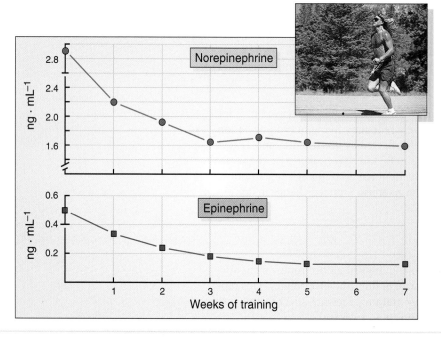

Figure 12.16. Week-by-week changes in plasma catecholamines during a 5-minute exercise bout at 243 watts for six male subjects. Training consisted of running and stationary cycling 6 days a week. Catecholamine levels decreased progressively during training, with the most rapid decline in the early training phase. (Data from Winder, W.W., et al.: Time course of sympathoadrenal adaptations to endurance exercise training in man. *J. Appl. Physiol.*, 45:370, 1968.)

Opioid Peptides and Exercise

Researchers in the 1970s isolated and purified two opioid pentapeptides, methionine and leucine enkephalin (enkephalin, Greek meaning "in the head"). These breakthrough discoveries provided the first direct evidence that endogenous substances behaved like opiates. By the early 1980s, researchers discovered groups of endogenous opioid compounds now generically termed "endorphins" that bind to families of receptors. By definition, the term endorphin characterizes a group of endogenous peptides whose pharmacological action mimics opium and its analogs. Opioid substances include beta-lipotrophin, beta-endorphin, and dynorphin, the most potent opioid peptide. Endorphins regulate menstruation and modulate the response of GH, ACTH, PRL, catecholamines, and cortisol.

Beta-endorphin and **beta-lipotrophin** opioids generally increase with acute exercise. Plasma beta-endorphin in exercising men and women increase five times over resting levels, with higher values probably occurring within the brain. The most notable postulated exercise-related endorphin effect has been its role in triggering a state of euphoria and exhilaration ("**exercise high**") as duration of moderate to intense exercise increases. The endorphin effect may also increase pain tolerance, improve appetite control, and reduce anxiety, tension, anger, and confusion; all of these changes are proposed benefits of regular exercise.

The effect of chronic exercise on endorphin response remains controversial. One could hypothesize that physical training increases an individual's sensitivity to opioid effects so it takes less of the hormone to induce a specific effect. In this sense, regular exercise could be viewed as a "positive addiction." Opiates produced in the body during exercise may degrade more slowly in the blood of trained compared with untrained individuals. A slower disposal rate would facilitate a given opiate response; it might even augment one's tolerance for extended exercise.

Questions & Notes

List 3 opioid substances.

1.

2.

3.

Does resistance training increase or decrease growth hormone secretions?

SUMMARY

1. The endocrine system consists of a host organ, a hormone, and a target or receptor organ. Hormones exist as either steroids or amino acid (polypeptide) derivatives.

2. Hormones alter rates of cellular reactions by acting at specific receptor sites to enhance or inhibit enzyme function.

3. Blood hormone concentration depends on the amount of hormone synthesized, the amount released, the amount taken up by the target organ, and its rate of removal from the blood.

4. The anterior pituitary secretes at least six hormones: PRL, the gonadotropic hormones FSH and LH, corticotropin, thyrotropin, and GH. The anterior pituitary also releases endorphins.

5. GH promotes cell division and cellular proliferation; TSH controls the amount of hormone secreted by the thyroid gland; ACTH regulates the output of the hormones of the adrenal cortex; PRL affects reproduction and development of female secondary sex characteristics; FSH and LH stimulate the ovaries to secrete estrogen and progesterone in women and testosterone in men.

6. The posterior pituitary secretes antidiuretic hormone to control kidney water excretion. It also secretes oxytocin, important in birthing and milk secretion.

7. Thyroxine elevates metabolic rate in all cells and increases carbohydrate and fat breakdown in energy metabolism.

8. The inner (medulla) and outer (cortex) components of the adrenal gland secrete two different types of hormones. The medulla secretes the catecholamines epinephrine and norepinephrine. The adrenal cortex secretes mineralocorticoids (regulate extracellular sodium and potassium), glucocorticoids (stimulate gluconeogenesis and serve as an insulin antagonist), and androgens (control secondary sex characteristics).

9. Insulin secreted by the pancreas' beta cells increases glucose transport into cells to control the body's rate of carbohydrate metabolism. The alpha cells of the pancreas secrete glucagon, an insulin antagonist that raises blood sugar.

10. Type 1 and type 2 diabetes represent the most prevalent diabetes subgroups. Type 1 diabetes causes insulin deficiency by destroying the pancreas' insulin-

producing beta cells. Type 2 diabetes generally occurs in overweight, sedentary, middle-aged individuals with a family history of the disease. It arises mainly from insulin resistance (body tissues require greater than normal insulin for glucose regulation). Eventually, even a large insulin output fails to regulate blood sugar.

11. The increase in diabetes in children and adults has reached epidemic proportions worldwide. More than one-third of all new cases occur in children under age 16.

12. Diabetes risk in minorities also has increased; 8.4% of all non-Hispanic whites, 11.4% of all non-Hispanic blacks, and more than 17% of American Indians and Alaskan Natives.

13. Exercise training exerts differential effects on resting and exercise-induced hormone production and release. Training elevates hormone response during exercise for ACTH and cortisol, and depresses GH, PRL, FSH, LH, testosterone, ADH, T_4, and insulin; no known training response occurs for aldosterone and angiotensin.

14. Exercise, stress, and illness represent interactive factors, each affecting the body's immune system and disease resistance.

15. Exercise-induced elevation of beta-endorphins coincides with euphoria, increased pain tolerance, the "exercise high," and menstrual dysfunction.

THOUGHT QUESTIONS

1. Visit a local health food store and list the supplements that claim to enhance exercise performance. Identify the ingredients and their alleged effects. Which supplements purport to simulate hormonal release? Based on your knowledge of hormonal regulation and function, can any of these products deliver on their claims?

2. Discuss how hormones act as silent messengers to integrate the body as a unit.

3. Hormones play crucial roles in normal growth and development and physiologic function. Give specific examples of why *more* is not necessarily *better* regarding these chemicals.

SELECTED REFERENCES

ADA/ACSM: Diabetes Mellitus and Exercise: Joint Position Paper. *Med. Sci. Sports Exerc.*, 29:1, 1997.

Ahtiainen, J.P., et al.: Acute hormonal and neuromuscular responses and recovery to forced vs maximum repetitions multiple resistance exercises. *Int. J. Sports Med.*, 24:410, 2003.

Ahtiainen, J.P., et al.: Acute hormonal responses to heavy resistance exercise in strength athletes versus nonathletes. *Can. J. Appl. Physiol.*, 29:527, 2004.

American College of Sports Medicine: Position Stand. The recommended quantity and quality of exercise for developing and maintaining cardiorespiratory and muscular fitness, and flexibility in healthy adults. *Med. Sci. Sports Exerc.*, 30:975, 1998.

Baylor, L.S., and Hackney, A.C.: Resting thyroid and leptin hormone changes in women following intense, prolonged exercise training. *Eur. J. Appl. Physiol.*, 88:480, 2003.

Berggren, J.R., et al.: Weight loss and exercise: Implications for muscle lipid metabolism and insulin action. *Med. Sci. Sports Exerc.*, 36:1191, 2004.

Bertoli, A., et al.: Lipid profile, BMI, body fat distribution, and aerobic fitness in men with metabolic syndrome. *Acta. Diabetol.*, 40(Suppl 1):S130, 2003.

Björntorp, P., et al.: Hypertension and the metabolic syndrome: closely related central origin? *Blood Press*, 9:71, 2000.

Borer, K.: *Exercise Endocrinology*. Champaign, IL: Human Kinetics Press, 2003.

Bruce, C.R., Hawley, J.A.: Improvements in insulin resistance with aerobic exercise training: a lipocentric approach. *Med. Sci. Sports Exerc.*, 36:1196, 2004.

Chwalbinska-Moneta, J., et al.: Early effects of short-term endurance training on hormonal responses to graded exercise. *J. Physiol. Pharmacol.*, 56:87, 2005.

Daly, W., et al.: Relationship between stress hormones and testosterone with prolonged endurance exercise. *Eur. J. Appl. Physiol.*, 93:375, 2005.

Di Luigi, L., et al.: Heredity and pituitary response to exercise-related stress in trained men. *Int. J. Sports Med.*, 24:551, 2003.

Doucet, E., et al.: Greater than predicted decrease in energy expenditure during exercise after body weight loss in obese men. *Clin. Sci. (Lond).*, 105:89, 2003.

Ford, E.S., et al.: Prevalence of the metabolic syndrome among US adults: findings from the third National Health and Nutrition Examination Survey. *JAMA*, 287:356, 2002.

Gleeson, M., Bishop, N.C.: Elite athlete immunology: importance of nutrition. *Int. J. Sports Nutr.*, 21 Supplement 1:S44, 2000.

Gomez-Merino, D., et al.: Immune and hormonal changes following intense military training. *Mil. Med.* 168:1034, 2003.

Goto, K., et al.: The impact of metabolic stress on hormonal responses and muscular adaptations. *Med. Sci. Sports Exerc.*, 37:955, 2005.

Healy, M.L., et al.: High dose growth hormone exerts an anabolic effect at rest and during exercise in endurance-trained athletes. *J. Clin. Endocrinol. Metab.*, 88:5221, 2003.

Huang, W.S., et al.: Effect of treadmill exercise on circulating thyroid hormone measurements. *Med. Princ. Pract.*, 13:15, 2004.

Iemitsu, M., et al.: Exercise training improves cardiac function-related gene levels through thyroid hormone receptor signaling in aged rats. *Am. J. Physiol. Heart Circ. Physiol.*, 286:H1696, 2004.

Ivy, J.L.: Muscle insulin resistance amended with exercise training: role of GLUT4 expression. *Med. Sci. Sports Exerc.*, 36:1207, 2004.

Izquierdo, M., et al.: Maximal strength and power, muscle mass, endurance and serum hormones in weightlifters and road cyclists. *J. Sports Sci.*, 22:465, 2004.

Kasa-Vubu, J.Z., et al.: Differences in endocrine function with varying fitness capacity in postpubertal females across the weight spectrum. *Arch. Pediatr. Adolesc. Med.*, 158:333, 2004.

Kraemer, W.J., et al.: Cortitrol supplementation reduces serum cortisol responses to physical stress. *Metabolism*, 54:657, 2005.

Kraemer, W.J., et al.: Influence of muscle strength and total work on exercise-induced plasma growth hormone isoforms in women. *J. Sci. Med. Sport*, 6:295, 2003.

Kraemer, W.J., Ratamess, N.A.: Hormonal responses and adaptations to resistance exercise and training. *Sports Med.*, 35:339, 2005.

Kraemer, W.J., et al.: Changes in exercise performance and hormonal concentrations over a big ten soccer season in starters and nonstarters. *J. Strength Cond. Res.*, 18:121, 2004.

Kroll, M.H.: Parathyroid hormone temporal effects on bone formation and resorption. *Bull. Math. Biol.*, 62: 163, 2000.

Malecki, M.T.: Genetics of type 2 diabetes mellitus. *Diabetes Res. Clin. Pract.*, 68 Suppl 1:S10, 2005.

Marliss, E.B., et al.: Gender differences in glucoregulatory responses to intense exercise. *J. Appl. Physiol.*, 88:457, 2000.

McMurray, R.G., Hackney, A.C.: Interactions of metabolic hormones, adipose tissue and exercise. *Sports Med.*, 35:393, 2005.

Mora-Rodriguez, R., Coyle, E.F.: Effects of plasma epinephrine on fat metabolism during exercise: interactions with exercise intensity. *Am. J. Physiol.*, 278:E669, 2000.

Nieman, D.C., Pedersen, B.K.: *Nutrition and Exercise Immunology.* Boca Raton, FL: CRC Press, 2000.

Nindl B.C., et al.: Growth hormone molecular heterogeneity and exercise. *Exerc. Sport Sci. Rev.*, 31:161, 2003.

Panciera, D.L., et al.: Plasma thyroid hormone concentrations in dogs competing in a long-distance sled dog race. *J. Vet. Intern. Med.*, 17:593, 2003.

Peres, S.B., et al.: Endurance exercise training increases insulin responsiveness in isolated adipocytes through IRS/PI3-kinase/Akt pathway. *J. Appl. Physiol.*, 98:1037, 2005.

Permutt, M.A., et al.: Genetic epidemiology of diabetes. *J. Clin. Invest.*, 115:1431, 2005.

Ratamess, N.A., et al.: Androgen receptor content following heavy resistance exercise in men. *J. Steroid Biochem. Mol. Biol.*, 93:35, 2005.

Rubin, M.R., et al.: High-affinity growth hormone binding protein and acute heavy resistance exercise. *Med. Sci. Sports Exerc.*, 37:395, 2005.

Sinha-Hikim, I., et al.: Testosterone-induced muscle hypertrophy is associated with an increase in satellite cell number in healthy, young men. *Am. J. Physiol. Endocrinol. Metab.*, 285:E197, 2003.

Stich, V., et al.: Adipose tissue lipolysis is increased during a repeated bout of aerobic exercise. *J. Appl. Physiol.*, 88:1277. 2000.

Storer, T.W. et al.: Testosterone dose-dependently increases maximal voluntary strength and leg power, but does not affect fatigability or specific tension. *J. Clin. Endocrinol. Metab.*, 88:1478, 2003.

Teran-Garcia, M., et al.: Endurance training-induced changes in insulin sensitivity and gene expression. *Am. J. Physiol. Endocrinol. Metab.*, 288:E1168, 2005.

Tremblay, M.S., et al.: Effect of training status and exercise mode on endogenous steroid hormones in men. *J. Appl. Physiol.*, 96:531, 2004.

Vaananen, I., et al.: Hormonal responses to 100 km cross-country skiing during 2 days. *J. Sports Med. Phys. Fitness*, 44:309, 2004.

Volek, J.S.: Influence of nutrition on responses to resistance training. *Med. Sci. Sports. Exerc.*, 36:689, 2004.

Warren, M.P., Goodman, L.R.: Exercise-induced endocrine pathologies. *J. Endocrinol. Invest.*, 26:873, 2003.

Weiss, E.P., et al.: Endurance training-induced changes in the insulin response to oral glucose are associated with the peroxisome proliferator-activated receptor-gamma2 Pro12Ala genotype in men but not in women. *Metabolism*, 54:97, 2005.

Wesche, M.F., and Wiersinga, W.M.: Relation between lean body mass and thyroid volume in competition rowers before and during intensive physical training. *Horm. Metab. Res.*, 33:423, 2001.

Section V

Exercise Training and Adaptations

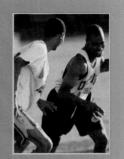

Exercise training for sports often entails more art than science. Individual achievements or win-loss records rather than scientific inquiry and discovery frequently gauge the success of diverse conditioning programs. For example, basketball and soccer coaches frequently place considerable importance on developing aerobic capacity yet may not devote enough time to vigorous anaerobic training. These sports require a relatively steady release of aerobic energy yet crucial game situations frequently demand maximal effort. A poorly trained anaerobic energy transfer system can prevent a player from performing at full potential.

Training the anaerobic capacity of endurance athletes, on the other hand, proves wasteful because of the minimal contribution of anaerobic energy transfer to successful performance. Instead, endurance activities demand a highly conditioned heart and vascular system capable of delivering large quantities of blood (oxygen) to muscles with high capacity to generate ATP aerobically. At the other extreme, one's aerobic metabolic capacity contributes little to overall success in sprint activities and sports like football. In these sports, performance largely depends on muscular strength and power, which require energy generated in reactions without oxygen.

Developing a training program to achieve optimum exercise and sports performance requires a clear understanding of energy transfer and how specific training affects energy delivery and utilization systems.

Chapters 13 and 14 focus on training for aerobic and anaerobic power and muscular strength, the physiologic consequences of such training, and important factors that affect training success. Chapter 15 examines how different environmental conditions and special aids affect physiologic function and exercise performance.

> The test of a first-rate intelligence is the ability to hold two opposed ideas in mind at the same time and still retain the ability to function.
>
> —F. Scott Fitzgerald

CHAPTER OBJECTIVES

- Define each of the following four principles of exercise training: (1) overload, (2) specificity, (3) individual differences, and (4) reversibility.

- Discuss the overload principle for training the intramuscular high-energy phosphates and glycolytic systems. Outline the specific adaptations in each system with exercise training.

- Describe how the following factors affect an aerobic training program: (1) initial fitness level, (2) genetics, (3) training frequency, (4) training duration, and (5) training intensity.

- List five cardiovascular and pulmonary adaptations to aerobic training.

- Explain how exercise heart rate can establish the appropriate exercise intensity for aerobic training.

- Define the training-sensitive zone.

- Explain the need to adjust the training-sensitive zone for swimming and other modes of upper-body exercise.

- Explain the influence of age on maximum heart rate and training-sensitive zone.

- Contrast continuous versus intermittent aerobic exercise training, including advantages and disadvantages of each.

- Outline five potential benefits and risks of exercising during pregnancy.

CHAPTER OUTLINE

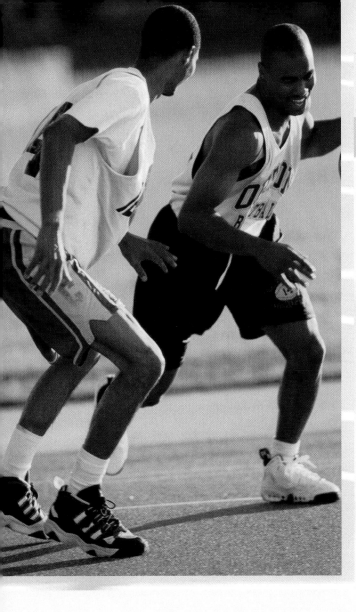

13

Training the Anaerobic and Aerobic Energy Systems

TRAINING MUST FOCUS ON ENERGY REQUIREMENTS

Many forms of physical activity require rapid bursts of power where energy requirements far exceed the body's oxygen delivery capacity. Even with available oxygen, cellular energy transfer from aerobic reactions progresses too slowly to match energy demands. This means that rapid anaerobic (not aerobic) energy transfer capacity determines how fast a running back plows through the line in American football, a volleyball player spikes the ball over the net, and a softball player beats out an infield hit. Even longer-duration basketball, tennis, field hockey, lacrosse, and soccer involve sprinting, dashing, darting, and stop-and-go where capacity to generate short bursts of anaerobic power play an important role.

At the other extreme, success in endurance activities necessitates a highly trained aerobic energy system. This requires a cardiovascular system capable of delivering large quantities of blood to active tissues for an extended time and a musculature with high capacity to process oxygen for the aerobic resynthesis of ATP.

ENERGY FOR EXERCISE: KNOWING WHAT TO TRAIN FOR

Training for a particular sport or performance goal requires careful evaluation of the activity's energy components. This forms the basis to effectively partition one's time for specific training of the appropriate energy transfer system.

Keep in mind that the three energy systems (ATP-PCr system, lactic acid [glycolytic] system, and aerobic system) often operate concurrently. Their contributions to the total energy requirement can differ markedly depending on exercise duration and intensity.

A maximum burst of effort for a tennis serve, golf swing, front-flip in gymnastics, and even a 60- or 100-m sprint requires immediate energy transfer. This occurs anaerobically, almost exclusively from the intramuscular high-energy phosphates ATP and PCr. In performances lasting up to 90 seconds in duration (100-m swim or 440-m run), anaerobic energy transfer reactions still predominate. In this case, the initial glycolytic phase of carbohydrate breakdown with subsequent lactate formation provides the primary energy source. One's capacity and tolerance for lactate accumulation determine the magnitude of energy generated from anaerobic sources. Training for anaerobic-type activities must reach sufficient intensity and duration to overload the glycolytic energy transfer system

Wrestling, boxing, ice hockey, a 200-m swim, 1500-m run, or a full-court press in basketball all require rapid anaerobic energy transfer, including the important contribution of aerobic energy metabolism. As exercise intensity diminishes somewhat, and duration extends between 2 to 4 minutes, reliance on energy from anaerobic metabolism decreases, whereas energy release from oxygen-consuming reactions predominates. Beyond 4 minutes, exercise becomes progressively more dependent on aerobic metabolism; energy from aerobic reactions almost exclusively powers a marathon run, long-distance swim, or 25-mile continuous bicycle ride.

GENERAL TRAINING PRINCIPLES

Effective physiologic conditioning requires adherence to carefully planned and executed physical activity. Attention focuses on frequency and length of workouts, type of training, speed, intensity, duration, and repetition of the activity, and appropriate competition. These factors vary depending on the performance goal. Several general principles of physiologic conditioning underlie the performance classifications based on intensity and duration of activity shown in **Figure 13.1**.

Overload Principle

The regular application of a specific exercise overload enhances physiologic function to produce a training response. Exercising at intensities greater than normal induces a variety of highly specific adaptations that enable the body to function more efficiently. Achieving the appropriate overload requires manipulating combinations of training frequency, intensity, and duration, with focus on exercise mode. These factors are discussed later in this chapter.

The concept of overload applies to athletes, sedentary persons, disabled persons, and even cardiac patients. An increasing number of people in this latter group have applied appropriate exercise rehabilitation to walk, jog, and eventually participate in marathons and ultraendurance events.

Specificity Principle

Exercise training specificity refers to adaptations in metabolic and physiologic systems that depend on the type of overload imposed. In a broad sense, an exercise stress, like strength-power training develops specific strength-power adaptations; likewise, regular aerobic (cardiovascular) exercise elicits specific endurance-training adaptations with essentially no transfer effects between strength training and aerobic training. The specificity principle also encompasses activities with *identical* metabolic components. For example, aerobic fitness for swimming, bicycling, running, or rowing improves most effectively when the exerciser trains the specific muscles required for the specific activity. In essence, specific exercise elicits specific adaptations, creating specific training effects (referred to as the **SAID principle—Specific Adaptations to Imposed Demands**).

Individual Differences Principle

Many factors contribute to variations in training responses among individuals. One important factor is rela-

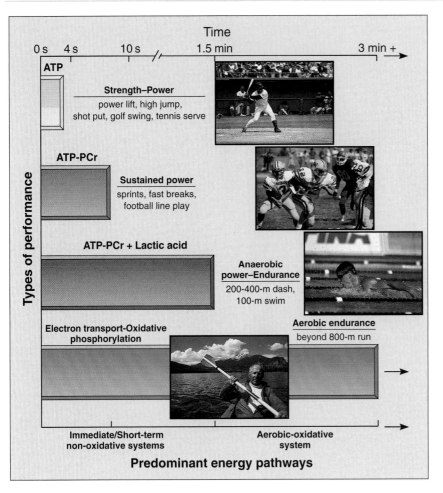

Figure 13.1   Performance classifications based on the duration of all-out exercise and corresponding predominant intracellular energy pathways.

tive fitness level at the start of training. People vary in their initial fitness and state of training at the start of a conditioning program and thus may respond differently to the same training stimulus. Insisting that all performers on a team (or even those in the same event) train the same way and at the same relative or absolute exercise intensity does not optimize training by recognizing individual differences in training responsiveness. Training programs must meet individual needs and capacities. Coaches and trainers should recognize how athletes and trainees respond to a given exercise stimulus and adjust the exercise prescription based on that response.

Reversibility Principle

Detraining occurs relatively rapidly when a person quits their exercise training regimen. After only a week or two of detraining, measurable reductions occur in physiologic function and exercise capacity, with a total loss of training improvements occurring within several months. **Figure 13.2** shows the average percentage of decreases reported from several studies for the changes in physiologic and metabolic variables with detraining (including bed rest).

In one experiment, $\dot{V}O_{2max}$ decreased 25% in five subjects confined to bed for 20 consecutive days; a similar decrease in maximal stroke volume and cardiac output accompanied the loss of aerobic capacity (roughly 1% per day). Capillary number within trained muscle also decreased 14% to 25% over the detraining period.

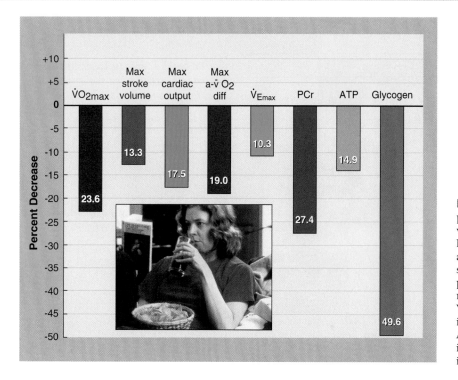

Figure 13.2 Average changes in physiologic and metabolic variables with different durations of detraining. Based on data from six studies. Values are as follows: $\dot{V}O_{2max}$ in $L \cdot min^{-1}$; stroke volume in $mL \cdot b^{-1}$; cardiac output in $L \cdot min^{-1}$; a-$\bar{v}O_2$ diff = arteriovenous oxygen differences in $mL \cdot dL^{-1}$; $\dot{V}_{Emax}$ = maximum minute ventilation in $L \cdot min^{-1}$; PCr in $mmol \cdot g$ wet muscle; ATP in $mmol \cdot g$ wet muscle^{-1}; glycogen in $mmol \cdot g$ wet muscle^{-1}; max heart rate in $b \cdot min^{-1}$.

The above results clearly highlight the transient and reversible nature of exercise training improvements, even among high performance athletes. For this reason, athletes begin a reconditioning program several months before the start of the competitive season, or maintain some moderate level of off-season, sport-specific exercise to slow down the rate of deconditioning.

ADAPTATIONS TO EXERCISE TRAINING

Not all people respond similarly to the same training regimen. Individual differences in improvement generally represent the rule rather than the exception, particularly among children and older adults. Among individuals in the same exercise-training program, one person might show ten times more improvement than another. For example, improvement in $\dot{V}O_{2max}$ for subjects who trained similarly for 9 to 12 months ranged between 0 and 43%. Such variation in results is not uncommon; simply stated—some individuals respond more readily than do others to an identical training stimulus.

The concept of **responders** and **nonresponders** emerged from training data collected on identical twins. Ten pairs of identical twins, separated at birth and reared in different environments completed the same 20-week endurance-training program. The results showed a strong genetic component for improvements in cardiovascular and metabolic variables. Both members of the twin pair showed nearly the same training response; a large improvement in one twin mirrored similar improvement in the other and vice versa. In the mid-1960s, the renowned Swedish physiologist Dr. Per-Olof Åstrand prophetically

commented concerning the yet to be quantified role of genetics in exercise performance: *"To be an Olympic-caliber performer, you must choose your parents wisely."* Future research in molecular genetics may someday uncover a practical means to identify responders and nonresponders and individualize conditioning programs to optimize overall improvements for each.

Exercise Adherence   Less than 13% of U.S. adults exercise regularly at sufficient intensity and duration to attain a minimum fitness level. More than 60% of those who initiate or renew a personal exercise program do not maintain it at the appropriate level. Adherence rates to regular exercise range between 9% and 90% for worksite, commercial, and community-based programs. Remarkably, the dropout rate for exercise programs duplicates that for other behavior-oriented smoking, alcohol, drug cessation, weight loss, and psychotherapy programs.

Figure 13.3 presents factors related to high and low adherence success to regular exercise. *Proper leadership exerts the greatest positive influence on exercise compliance.*

Anaerobic System Changes

Figure 13.4 presents a generalized summary of the metabolic adaptations in anaerobic function that accompany strenuous physical training that requires considerable overload of the anaerobic systems of energy transfer. Changes in anaerobic power and capacity occur without concomitant increases in aerobic functions. Adaptations with sprint-power training include:

1. *Increased levels of anaerobic substrates.* Muscle biopsies taken before and after resistance training reveal in-

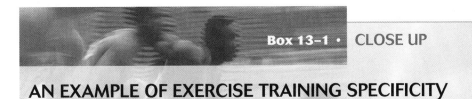

Box 13–1 • CLOSE UP

AN EXAMPLE OF EXERCISE TRAINING SPECIFICITY

In an experiment in one of our laboratories on aerobic training specificity, 15 men swam 1 hour a day, 3 days a week, for 10 weeks at heart rates between 85% and 95% of maximum (HR_{max}). $\dot{V}O_{2max}$ was measured during treadmill running and tethered swimming before and after training. Because vigorous swim training overloads the central circulation (as reflected by high exercise heart rates), we anticipated at least some transfer in aerobic power improvements from swim training to running. This did not occur; an almost total specificity accompanied the $\dot{V}O_{2max}$ improvement with swim training.

The accompanying figure illustrates that swim training improved $\dot{V}O_{2max}$ by 11% when measured during swimming, but only by 1.5% when measured during running. If only treadmill

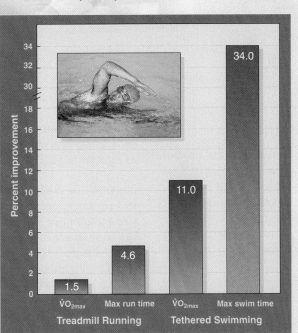

running had been used to evaluate swim training effects, we would mistakenly have concluded that there was *no training effect*. For maximum performance during testing, subjects improved 34% in swim time to exhaustion but only 4.6% in run time on the treadmill test.

These findings and other research studies strongly indicate that training for specific aerobic activities must provide an appropriate general level of cardiovascular stress *and* over-load the *specific muscles* required by the activity. Little improvement results when a dissimilar exercise measures aerobic capacity or exercise performance. In contrast, considerable improvements emerge when the exercise training mode evaluates aerobic adaptations.

creases in the trained muscle's resting levels of ATP, PCr, free creatine, and glycogen, accompanied by a significant improvement in muscular strength. Other studies show higher levels of ATP and total creatine content in the trained muscles of sprint runners and track speed cyclists compared with distance runners and road racers.

2. *Increased quantity and activity of key enzymes that control the anaerobic phase of glucose catabolism.* The most dramatic increases in anaerobic enzyme function and fiber size occur in fast-twitch muscle fibers. These changes do not reach the magnitude observed for oxidative enzymes with aerobic training.

3. *Increased capacity to generate high levels of blood lactate during all-out exercise.* Enhanced lactate-producing capacity probably results from (1) increased levels of glycogen and glycolytic enzymes and (2) improved motivation and "pain" tolerance to fatiguing exercise.

Improved Buffering Capacity?   Individuals who engage in anaerobic training tolerate higher blood lactate levels (and lower pH values) than untrained counterparts. This raises speculation that anaerobic training improves the body's capacity for acid-base regulation, perhaps by enhancing chemical buffers or alkaline reserve. No research has demonstrated that exercise training augments buffering capacity. Motivational factors probably improve training-induced tolerance to elevated plasma acidity.

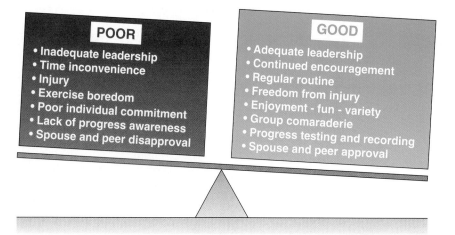

Figure 13.3 Variables related to good and poor adherence to regular exercise. (From Franklin, B.A.: Program factors that influence exercise adherence. In: *Exercise Adherence: Its Impact on Public Health*. Dishman, R.K. (ed.) Champaign, IL: Human Kinetics, 1988.)

Aerobic System Changes

Table 13.1 summarizes important metabolic and physiologic differences when comparing typical values of healthy untrained individuals and endurance athletes. Aerobic adaptations to training generally occur independent of gender and age. They also take place in medically cleared individuals with cancer, coronary heart disease, diabetes, hypertension, and obstructive pulmonary disease (see Chapter 17).

Metabolic Adaptations Aerobic exercise training induces intracellular changes that enhance a muscle fiber's capacity to aerobically generate ATP.

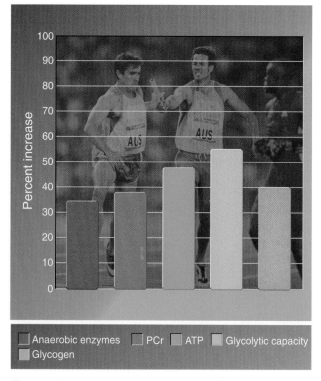

Figure 13.4 Generalized potential for increases in anaerobic energy metabolism of skeletal muscle with intense training.

Metabolic Machinery An increase in mitochondrial size and number in aerobically trained skeletal muscle improves its capacity to generate ATP by oxidative phosphorylation.

Enzymes A twofold increase in the level of aerobic system enzymes compliments the increase in mitochondrial size and number. These adaptations likely allow the athlete to sustain a high percentage of aerobic capacity during prolonged exercise without accumulating blood lactate (i.e., higher blood lactate threshold). An increase in enzyme activity per unit of mitochondrial protein does not enhance enzymatic metabolism, but rather increases in *total* mitochondrial substrate.

Fat Catabolism *Regular aerobic exercise profoundly improves ability to oxidize fatty acids, particularly triacylglycerols stored within active muscle during steady-rate exercise* (**Fig. 13.5**). Lipolysis increases from greater blood flow within trained muscle and a higher quantity of fat-mobilizing (from adipocytes) and fat-metabolizing (within muscle fibers) enzymes. This allows the endurance athlete to exercise at a higher absolute level of submaximal exercise before experiencing the fatiguing effects of glycogen depletion compared with an untrained person.

Carbohydrate Catabolism *Aerobically trained muscle exhibits an enhanced capacity to oxidize carbohydrate.* Consequently, a considerable quantity of pyruvate moves through the aerobic energy pathways during intense endurance exercise. A trained muscle's greater mitochondrial oxidative capacity and increased glycogen storage contributes to the enhanced capacity for carbohydrate breakdown. Increased carbohydrate catabolism during intense aerobic exercise serves two important functions:

1. Provides for a considerably faster aerobic energy transfer than from fat breakdown
2. Liberates about 6% more energy than fat per quantity of oxygen consumed

Muscle Fiber Type and Size Endurance training produces aerobic metabolic adaptations in *both* muscle fiber

| Table 13·1 | Typical Metabolic and Physiologic Values for Healthy Endurance-Trained and Untrained Men[a] | | | |

VARIABLE	UNTRAINED	TRAINED	PERCENTAGE DIFFERENCE[b]
Glycogen, mmol·g wet muscle^{-1}	85.0	120	41
Number of mitochondria, mmol^3	0.59	1.20	103
Mitochondrial volume, % muscle cell	2.15	8.00	272
Resting ATP, mmol·g wet muscle^{-1}	3.0	6.0	100
Resting PCr, mmol·g wet muscle^{-1}	11.0	18.0	64
Resting creatine, mmol·g wet muscle^{-1}	10.7	14.5	35
Glycolytic enzymes			
Phosphofructokinase, mmol·g wet muscle^{-1}	50.0	50.0	0
Phosphorylase, mmol·g wet muscle^{-1}	4–6	6–9	60
Aerobic enzymes			
Succinate dehydrogenase, mmol·kg wet muscle^{-1}	5–10	15–20	133
Max lactate, mmol·kg wet muscle^{-1}	110	150	36
Muscle fibers			
Fast twitch, %	50	20–30	−50
Slow twitch, %	50	60	20
Max stroke volume, mL·b^{-1}	120	180	50
Max cardiac output, L·min^{-1}	20	30–40	75
Resting heart rate, b·min^{-1}	70	40	−43
HR$_{max}$, b·min^{-1}	190	180	−5
Max a-$\bar{v}$O$_2$ diff, mL·100 mL^{-1}	14.5	16.0	10
$\dot{V}$O$_{2max}$, mL·kg^{-1}·min^{-1}	30–40	65–80	107
Heart volume, L	7.5	9.5	27
Blood volume, L	4.7	6.0	28
$\dot{V}$E$_{max}$, L·min^{-1}	110	190	73
Percent body fat	15	11	−27

[a] In some cases, we list approximate values. In all cases, the trained values represent data from endurance athletes. We advise caution in assuming that the percentage differences between trained and untrained men necessarily result from training because genetic differences between individuals probably exert a strong influence on many of these factors.
[b] Computed as the percentage that the value for the trained differs from the corresponding value for the untrained.

types. This enhances each fiber's existing aerobic capacity and lactate threshold level without modifying muscle fiber type. Selective hypertrophy also occurs in the different muscle fiber types in specific overload training. Highly trained endurance athletes have larger slow-twitch fibers than fast-twitch fibers in the same muscle. Conversely, for athletes trained in anaerobic-power activities, fast-twitch fibers occupy more of the muscle's cross-sectional area. As might be expected, slow-twitch muscle fibers with high capacity to generate ATP aerobically contain relatively large quantities of myoglobin. Among animals, a muscle's myoglobin content relates to their level of physical activity. The leg muscles of hunting dogs, for example, contain more myoglobin than the muscles of sedentary house pets; similar findings exist for grazing cattle compared with penned animals. Whether regular exercise exerts any effect on myoglobin levels in humans remains unclear.

Cardiovascular Adaptations   Figure 13.6 summarizes important adaptations in cardiovascular function with aerobic exercise training. Endurance training produces significant dimensional and functional cardiovascular adaptations because of the intimate linkage of the cardiovascular system to aerobic processes.

Heart Size   Aerobic training normally enlarges the heart by increasing left ventricular cavity size and by inducing a slight thickening of its walls. Cardiac enlargement of this type, termed **eccentric hypertrophy**, improves stroke volume. With reduced training intensity, myocardial structure returns to control levels. Myocardial overload stimulates greater cellular protein synthesis, with concomitant reductions in protein breakdown. Accelerated protein synthesis occurs largely from an increase in the trained myocardium's RNA content. Individual

FOR YOUR INFORMATION

Generality for Cardiac Training
A high degree of specificity in training exists for aerobic fitness, yet more general effects occur in cardiac function (e.g., ventricular contractility). This indicates that the heart muscle per se becomes conditioned through a variety of big-muscle exercise modes that increase demand for blood flow.

FOR YOUR INFORMATION

Prolonged Recovery
Recovery time can be considerable with intense exercise that elevates core temperature, disrupts internal equilibrium, and elevates blood lactate. For this reason, apply intervals of anaerobic training at the end of a workout. Otherwise, fatigue from training carries over and perhaps hinders ability to perform subsequent aerobic training.

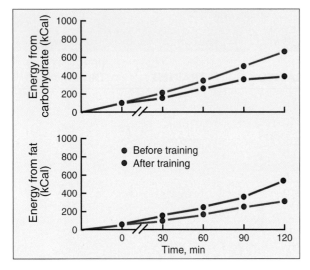

Figure 13.5 Training enhances fat burning during submaximal exercise. This carbohydrate-sparing results from a facilitated release of fatty acids from adipose tissue depots, an increased intramuscular fat content, and enhanced mitochondrial fat oxidation capacity in endurance-trained muscle. (Data from Hurley, B.F., et al.: Muscle triglyceride utilization during exercise: Effect of training. *J. Appl. Physiol.*, 5:62, 1986.)

myofibrils thicken, while the number of these contractile filaments concurrently increases.

Plasma Volume Only four training sessions can increase plasma volume up to 20%. This adaptation en-

hances circulatory and thermoregulatory dynamics and facilitates oxygen delivery to muscle during exercise. The rapid increase in plasma volume with aerobic training also contributes to training-induced eccentric hypertrophy.

Stroke Volume **Figure 13.7** illustrates the stroke volume response for two groups of men during upright exercise of increasing intensity. One group of six endurance athletes had trained for several years; three sedentary college students comprised the other group. Graded exercise on a bicycle ergometer evaluated the students' responses before and after a 55-day training program designed to improve aerobic fitness.

These data reveal important (and representative) findings concerning aerobic training adaptations:

1. The endurance athlete's heart has a considerably larger stroke volume during rest and exercise than an untrained person of similar age.
2. For trained and untrained individuals, the greatest increase in stroke volume in upright exercise occurs in the transition from rest to moderate exercise. Further increases in exercise intensity increase stroke volume only minimally.
3. The heart's stroke volume achieves near-maximum values at 40% to 50% of $\dot{V}O_{2max}$; in young adults, this usually represents a heart rate between 120 and 140 beats per minute.

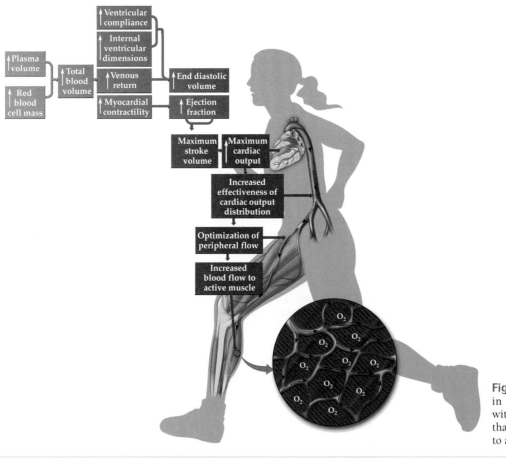

Figure 13.6 Adaptations in cardiovascular function with aerobic exercise training that increase oxygen delivery to active muscles.

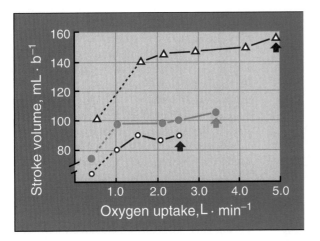

Figure 13.7   Stroke volume in relation to oxygen uptake during upright exercise in endurance athletes (open triangles) and sedentary college students before (open circles) and after (filled circles) 55 days of aerobic training; (arrows = maximal values). (From Saltin, B.: Physiological effects of physical conditioning. *Med. Sci. Sports,* 1:50, 1969.)

4. For untrained individuals, only a small stroke volume increase occurs in the transition from rest to exercise. For them, acceleration in heart rate produces the major increase in cardiac output. For trained endurance athletes, *both* heart rate and stroke volume increases augment cardiac output, with stroke volume increasing 50% to 60% above resting values.

5. For previously sedentary subjects, 8 weeks of aerobic training substantially increases stroke volume, but these values remain well below the average of elite athletes. The precise reason for this difference remains unknown. More than likely, prolonged intense training, genetics, or a combination of both factors contributes to the differences.

Heart Rate   A proportionate reduction in heart rate during submaximal exercise accompanies the large stroke volume of elite endurance athletes and stroke volume increase of sedentary subjects following aerobic training. **Figure 13.8** illustrates this training effect on the relationship between heart rate and oxygen uptake (exercise intensity) for endurance athletes and sedentary students before and after training.

A linear relationship between heart rate and oxygen uptake exists for both groups throughout the major portion of the exercise range. As exercise intensity increases, the heart rates of the athletes accelerate to a lesser extent than untrained students; the slope (or rate of change) in the lines differ considerably. Consequently, the athlete (or trained student) with an efficient cardiovascular response to exercise achieves a higher oxygen uptake before reaching a particular submaximal heart rate than a sedentary student. At an oxygen uptake of 2.0 $L \cdot min^{-1}$, for example, the athletes' heart rate averages 70 $b \cdot min^{-1}$ lower than the heart rate of the sedentary students. After 55 days of training for the student, the difference in submaximal heart rate decreases to 40 $b \cdot min^{-1}$. In each instance, cardiac output remains about the same. This means that larger stroke volumes account for the lower exercise heart rates. If the heart pumps a large quantity of blood with each beat, then adequate blood (oxygen) delivery to the active muscles requires only a small heart rate increase, and vice versa for a heart with a relatively small stroke volume.

Cardiac Output   An increase in maximum cardiac output represents the most significant change in cardiovascular function with aerobic training (**Fig. 13.9**). Maximum heart rate may decrease slightly with training, so the heart's increased outflow capacity results directly from improved stroke volume.

List 5 specific metabolic adaptations to aerobic training.

1.

2.

3.

4.

5.

Endurance-trained muscle contains
_____ and
_____ mitochondria
than untrained muscle fibers.

List 4 factors that explain enhanced fat catabolism with endurance training.

1.

2.

3.

4.

Give 2 reasons why endurance training reduces total carbohydrate catabolism in submaximal exercise.

1.

2.

List 2 important adaptations in cardiovascular function with aerobic exercise training.

1.

2.

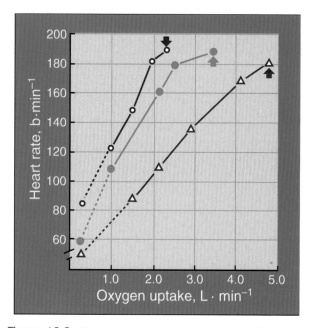

Figure 13.8 Heart rate in relation to oxygen uptake during upright exercise in endurance athletes (open triangles) and sedentary college students before (open circles) and after (filled circles) 55 days of aerobic training (arrows = maximal values). (From Saltin, B.: Physiological effects of physical conditioning. *Med. Sci. Sports*, 1:50, 1969.)

Research in the 1960s showed that training, while improving the maximal cardiac output, reduced the heart's minute volume during moderate exercise. In one study, average cardiac output of young men after 16 weeks of

aerobic training decreased by 1.1 and 1.5 L·min^{-1} at a specific submaximal oxygen consumption. As expected, maximal cardiac output increased 8% from 22.4 to 24.2 L·min^{-1}. With a reduced submaximal cardiac output, a corresponding increase in oxygen extraction in the active muscles matches the exercise oxygen requirement. A training-induced reduction in submaximal cardiac output presumably reflects two factors: (1) more effective distribution of blood flow and (2) trained muscles generate more ATP aerobically at a lower tissue PO_2.

Oxygen Extraction   Aerobic training increases the maximum quantity of oxygen extracted from arterial blood during exercise. A more effective distribution of cardiac output to working muscles and enhanced capacity of muscle fibers to metabolize oxygen produce the increase in a-$\bar{v}O_2$ difference.

Figure 13.10 compares the relationship between oxygen extraction (a-$\bar{v}O_2$ difference) and exercise intensity for trained athletes and untrained students. For the students, the a-$\bar{v}O_2$ difference increases steadily during light and moderate exercise to a maximum of 15 mL of oxygen per deciliter (dL) of blood. Following 55 days of training, the students' maximum oxygen extraction increased 13% to 17 mL of oxygen per dL. This means that during intense exercise, arterial blood released approximately 85% of its oxygen content. Actually, the active muscles extract even more oxygen because the a-$\bar{v}O_2$ difference reflects an average based on sampling of mixed-venous blood. This sample contains blood returning from tissues that use much less oxygen during exercise than active muscle (e.g., skin, kidneys, non-active mus-

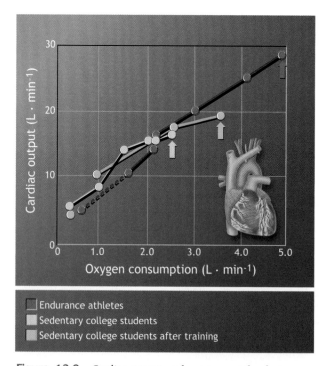

Figure 13.9 Cardiac output and oxygen uptake during upright exercise in endurance athletes (■) and sedentary college students before (■) and after (□) 55 days of aerobic training (↑ = max values). (From Saltin, B.: Physiological effects of physical conditioning. *Med. Sci. Sports*, 1:50, 1969.)

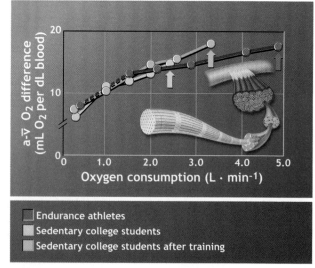

Figure 13.10 The a-$\bar{v}$ O$_2$ difference and oxygen consumption during upright exercise in endurance athletes (■) and sedentary college students before (■) and after (□) 55 days of aerobic training (↑ = max values). (From Saltin, B.: Physiological effects of physical conditioning. *Med. Sci. Sports*, 1:50, 1969.)

culature). The posttraining value for maximal a-v̄O_2 difference for the students equals the value of the endurance athletes. Obviously, the students' lower cardiac output capacity (Fig. 13.9) explains the large difference in $\dot{V}O_{2max}$ that still differentiates athletes and relatively untrained students.

Blood Flow and Distribution   Three factors explain why aerobic training causes large increases in muscle blood flow during maximal exercise:

1. Improvements in maximum cardiac output
2. Redistribution (shunting) of blood from non-active areas that temporarily compromise blood flow in all-out exercise effort
3. Increased capillarization within the trained muscle tissues

Blood Pressure   Aerobic exercise training decreases systolic and diastolic blood pressures during rest and submaximal exercise. The most apparent effect occurs for systolic pressure, particularly for hypertensive subjects. **Table 13.2** shows that the average resting systolic pressure of seven middle-aged male patients decreased from 139 to 133 mm Hg after 4 to 6 weeks of interval training. Systolic pressure in submaximal exercise declined from 173 to 155 mm Hg, while diastolic pressure decreased from 92 to 79 mm Hg. *Systolic and diastolic blood pressures generally decline approximately 6 to 10 mm Hg with regular aerobic exercise for previously sedentary adult men and women of all ages.*

Training-induced reduction in sympathetic nervous system hormones (catecholamines) causes the lowering effect of exercise on blood pressure. This response decreases peripheral vascular resistance to blood flow, causing blood pressure to decrease. Exercise training also facilitates sodium elimination by the kidneys that subsequently reduces fluid volume and blood pressure. *Regular aerobic exercise represents a prudent first line of defense in most therapeutic programs to manage borderline hypertension.* More severe elevations in blood pressure require combinations of diet, weight loss, exercise, and pharmacologic therapy.

Pulmonary Adaptations   Aerobic training induces alterations in pulmonary dynamics during exercise. Such changes contribute to a more effective ventilatory response to the stress of physical activity.

Maximal Exercise   Improvements in maximal oxygen uptake with training increase maximal exercise minute ventilation. This adaptation makes sense physio-

Questions & Notes

Give the most significant change in cardiovascular function with aerobic training.

Does heart rate max increase or decrease with aerobic training?

Does oxygen extraction increase or decrease in maximal exercise with aerobic training?

Give 2 reasons why aerobic training causes large increases in muscle blood flow during maximal exercise.

1.

2.

Table 13·2	Measures of Blood Pressure During Rest and Submaximal Exercise Before and After 4 to 6 Weeks of Aerobic Training in Seven Middle-Aged Patients with Coronary Heart Disease[a]					
	REST			**SUBMAXIMAL EXERCISE**		
	MEAN VALUE		**DIFFERENCE (%)**	**MEAN VALUE**		**DIFFERENCE (%)**
MEASURE[b]	**BEFORE**	**AFTER**		**BEFORE**	**AFTER**	
Systolic blood pressure (mm Hg)	139	133	−4.3	173	155	−10.4
Diastolic blood pressure (mm Hg)	78	73	−6.4	92	79	−14.1
Mean arterial blood pressure (mm Hg)	97	92	−5.2	127	109	−14.3

[a] Modified from Clausen, J.P., et al.: Physical training in the management of coronary artery disease. *Circulation*, 40:143, 1969.
[b] Blood pressure measured directly by a pressure transducer inserted into the brachial artery.

logically because improved aerobic capacity reflects larger oxygen utilization and need to eliminate greater quantities of carbon dioxide via increased alveolar ventilation.

Submaximal Exercise Exercise training improves ability to sustain high levels of submaximal ventilation. For example, 20 weeks of regular run training increased ventilatory muscle endurance by 16% in healthy adult men and women. Less lactate accumulated during submaximal breathing exercise, probably from the increase in aerobic enzyme levels in the ventilatory musculature. Enhanced ventilatory endurance reduces the feeling of breathlessness and pulmonary discomfort frequently experienced by untrained persons who perform prolonged submaximal exercise.

Only 4 weeks of training considerably reduces the ventilation equivalent for oxygen ($\dot{V}_E/\dot{V}O_2$) in submaximal exercise. Consequently, a particular level of submaximal oxygen uptake requires breathing less air; this reduces the percentage of the total oxygen cost of exercise attributable to breathing. Enhanced ventilatory economy contributes to endurance performance in two ways:

1. Reduces the fatiguing effects of exercise on ventilatory musculature
2. Frees oxygen from the respiratory muscles for use by non-respiratory active muscles

The precise mechanism for reduced ventilatory equivalent during submaximal exercise after training remains unresolved. The change is consistently observed in adolescents and adults. In general, tidal volume increases, breathing frequency decreases, and air remains in the lungs for a longer time interval between breaths. Slower breathing increases the amount of oxygen the alveoli captures (extracts) from the inspired air. For example, the exhaled air of trained individuals contains only 14% to 15% oxygen during submaximal exercise, whereas the untrained person's expired air contains about 17% oxygen at the same exercise intensity. This means the untrained person must ventilate proportionately more air to achieve the same submaximal oxygen uptake.

Blood Lactate Concentration

Figure 13.11 illustrates the generalized effect of endurance training in lowering blood lactate levels and extending the level of exercise intensity before the onset of blood lactate accumulation (OBLA) during exercise of progressively increasing intensity. The explanation underlying this effect centers on three possibilities related to central and peripheral adaptations to training discussed in this chapter: (1) decreased rate of lactate formation during exercise, (2) increased rate of lactate clearance (removal) during exercise, and (3) combined effects of decreased lactate clearance and increased lactate removal. More than likely, the combination of both factors exerts the influence.

Body Composition Changes

For the overfat or borderline overfat person, regular aerobic exercise reduces body mass and body fat. Significant increases in fat-free body mass also accompany resistance training. Exercise only or exercise combined with calorie restriction reduces body fat more than fat lost with only dieting because exercise conserves the body's lean tissue.

Body Heat Transfer

Well-hydrated, aerobically trained individuals exercise more comfortably in hot environments because of a larger plasma volume and more-responsive thermoregulatory mechanisms. Trained men and women dissipate heat faster and more effectively than the untrained. Metabolic heat generated by exercise poses less of a detriment to exercise performance and overall safety.

Endurance Performance Changes

Enhanced endurance accompanies the physiologic adaptations with training. **Figure 13.12** depicts the results of cycling performance following training performed 4 days per week for 40 to 60 minutes for 10 weeks at an intensity of 85% $\dot{V}O_{2max}$. The performance test required subjects to attempt to maintain a constant work rate of 265 watts for 8 minutes. Training produced less drop-off in power output during the prescribed 8-minute exercise test.

Psychological Benefits

Regular exercise (either aerobic or resistance training) produces significant psychological benefits regardless of age. Adaptations often occur to a degree equal to that achieved with other therapeutic interventions including pharmacologic therapy.

FACTORS AFFECTING THE AEROBIC TRAINING RESPONSE

Figure 13.13 illustrates the two major goals of aerobic training:

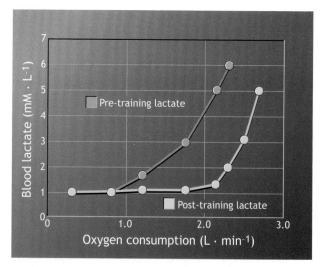

Figure 13.11 Generalized response for pre- and posttraining lactate accumulation during graded exercise. (Plots based on data from the Applied Physiology Laboratory, University of Michigan, Ann Arbor, MI.)

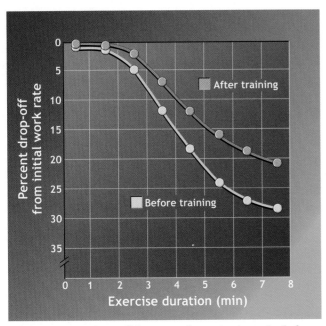

Figure 13.12   Percentage drop-off from initial exercise intensity before and after 10 weeks of endurance cycling training. (From the Applied Physiology Laboratory, University of Michigan, Ann Arbor, MI.)

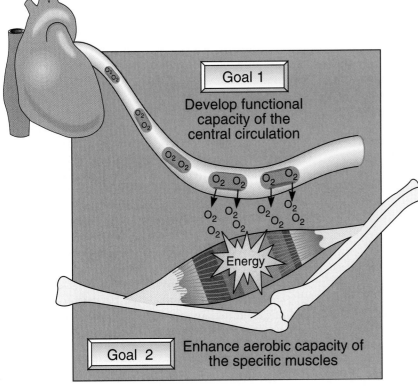

Figure 13.13   Two major goals of aerobic training.

Questions & Notes

Briefly describe the effects of endurance training on the blood pressure response at rest and during submaximal exercise.

Which decreases more in response to aerobic training for a hypertensive individual, systolic or diastolic pressure?

Give the major benefit of improved pulmonary adaptations with exercise training.

Discuss whether maximal pulmonary ventilation increases or decreases as $\dot{V}O_{2max}$ improves with aerobic training.

Endurance training _____ the ventilatory equivalent for oxygen during submaximal exercise.

List 2 factors to explain why endurance training lowers blood lactate levels during exercise of progressively increasing intensity.

1.

2.

Give one change in body composition resulting from aerobic training.

1. Enhance the capacity of the central circulation to deliver oxygen
2. Increase the capacity of active muscles to consume oxygen

Several factors influence the outcome of aerobic training, including initial level of cardiovascular fitness and training frequency, training duration, and training intensity.

Initial Level of Cardiorespiratory Fitness

As a general rule, the initial level of cardiorespiratory fitness affects the magnitude of training improvement. Improvement occurs if one's initial fitness is low; conversely, an exceptionally high level of initial fitness leaves little room for improvement. For example, a 5% improvement in physiologic function for an elite athlete can be more significant than a 25% increase for a sedentary person. As a general guideline, aerobic fitness improvements generally range between 5% and 25% with endurance training. Some of this improvement occurs within the first week of training.

Training Frequency

Exercising at least 3 days a week generally initiates adaptive changes in the aerobic system. Several research studies have reported improvements when training only 1 day a week. Those subjects, however, had been sedentary; for them, any form of overload stimulates improvement. *In general, a training response occurs with exercise performed at least three times weekly for at least six weeks.* Interestingly, several studies show that training four or five times a week generated only *slightly* greater physiologic improvements compared with thrice-weekly exercise. For the average person, the small improvement in physiologic function (as measured by $\dot{V}O_{2max}$) may not warrant the extra 1- or 2-day time investment in training. In contrast, the extra caloric expenditure from daily exercise justifies more frequent exercise for weight control. Current emphasis on the relationship between frequency of exercise and health status indicates that individuals should exercise on most days to derive maximum health benefits. We discuss the health benefits of regular physical activity in Chapter 17.

Training Duration

A common inquiry about exercise participation concerns the duration of daily workouts. For example, does 10 minutes of jogging provide twice the benefits of 5 minutes? Would a 2- or 3-minute run repeated eight to ten times provide greater training benefits than a continuous 20- to 30-minute run at similar intensity? Precise answers to these questions remain elusive because of an incomplete understanding of the mechanisms underlying aerobic fitness improvements. Both continuous and more intense intermittent exercise overload improve aerobic

capacity. In general, performing less exhaustive, moderate-paced exercise for at least 30 minutes each session sets a realistic exercise recommendation for the average person. In contrast, most competitive endurance athletes devote several hours each training session to activities that enhance the aerobic system's functional capacity.

As for training volume, more does not necessarily produce greater results. In a study of collegiate swimmers, one group trained for 1.5 hours daily, while another group performed two 1.5-hour exercise sessions each day. Despite one group exercising at twice the daily exercise volume, no differences in the improvement in swimming power, endurance, or performance time emerged between groups. About 60 minutes of daily physical activity provides optimal health benefits.

Training Intensity

Exercise intensity represents the most critical factor for successful aerobic training. Intensity reflects the activity's energy requirements per unit time and specific energy systems activated. One can express exercise intensity in several ways:

1. Calories expended per unit time
2. Exercise level or power output
3. Level of exercise below, at, or above the blood lactate threshold
4. Percentage of $\dot{V}O_{2max}$
5. Heart rate or percentage of maximum heart rate
6. Multiples of resting metabolic rate (METs)

By far, exercise heart rate provides the most practical way to assess exercise strenuousness. Researchers frequently use heart rate to structure a training program and evaluate the effectiveness of various training intensities. For college-age men and women, exercise must reach an intensity to raise heart rate to at least 130 to 140 b·min^{-1}. This equals about 50% to 55% of $\dot{V}O_{2max}$ or 70% of HR$_{max}$. As a general rule, this exercise intensity represents the minimal or threshold stimulus for cardiovascular improvement. More intense exercise proves even more effective. Conversely, extending exercise duration induces fitness improvement if intensity of effort does not meet the threshold level.

Overly Strenuous Exercise Not Necessary
An exercise heart rate at 70% HR$_{max}$ (140 b·min^{-1} for most young adults) represents only moderate exercise that can continue for a long duration with little or no physiologic discomfort. The term **conversational exercise** describes this training level (i.e., sufficiently intense to stimulate a training effect yet not so strenuous it limits a person from talking during the workout).

Figure 13.14 shows that heart rate at a given level of submaximal exercise or oxygen uptake gradually decreases as aerobic fitness improves. Consequently, the absolute exercise level (running or swimming speed, power output on a cycle ergometer) must increase accordingly to

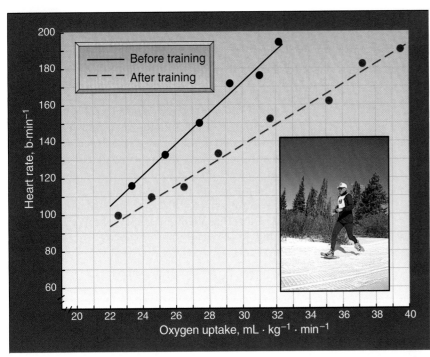

Figure 13.14   Improvements in heart rate response to oxygen uptake with aerobic training. Reduced submaximal exercise heart rate with training usually reflects an enhanced stroke volume of the heart.

Questions & Notes

Name the 2 major goals of aerobic training.

1.

2.

List 4 factors that affect the magnitude of the aerobic training response.

1.

2.

3.

4.

Give the generally expected range for percentage improvement in $\dot{V}O_{2max}$ with training.

List 5 ways to express exercise intensity.

1.

2.

3.

4.

5.

Give the best practical way to estimate the strenuousness of physical activity.

achieve the desired target heart rate. A person who began training by slow walking now walks more briskly; eventually periods of the workout include jogging. Ultimately, exercising at the training heart rate requires continuous running.

A minimal threshold intensity exists, below which a training effect does not occur; a ceiling may also exist where higher intensity exercise produces no further gains. The lower and upper limits of the training zone depend on the participant's age, initial fitness level, and state of training. For people with relatively poor aerobic fitness (including older men and women), the training threshold approaches 60% to 65% HR_{max}, which corresponds to about 45% $\dot{V}O_{2max}$; more fit individuals generally require a higher threshold level. The ceiling for training intensity remains unknown, although 85% $\dot{V}O_{2max}$ (90% HR_{max}) probably represents the upper limit. Above this level, increases in intensity primarily overload the anaerobic system for energy transfer. The Close Up on page 454 discusses heart rate to establish the appropriate exercise level for aerobic training.

How Long Before Improvement Occurs?

Positive adaptations in cardiorespiratory fitness and aerobic capacity with training generally occur within several weeks after beginning an exercise program. **Figure 13.15** shows absolute and percentage improvements in $\dot{V}O_{2max}$ for men who trained 6 days a week for 10 weeks. Training consisted of 30 minutes of bicycling 3 days a week combined with running for up to 40 minutes on alternate days. This produced a continuous week-by-week improvement in aerobic capacity. Adaptive responses to training eventually level off as a person reaches the genetically determined maximum. *Women and men show similar adaptations to aerobic training.*

Trainability and Genes

The limits for developing fitness capacity link closely to natural endowment. For two individuals in the same exercise program, one might show 10 times more improvement than the other. Genetics research indicates a genotype dependency for

FOR YOUR INFORMATION

Ideal Aerobic Workout
The ideal workout to improve cardiorespiratory fitness for the average person consists of a 5-minute warm-up of easy stretching and light aerobic exercise, 30–60 minutes of rhythmic, big-muscle activity at an intensity between 70% and 85% of HR_{max}, and a 5- to 10-minute recovery (cool down) of less intense exercise. The 30- to 60-minute exercise period represents the conditioning phase of the aerobic workout.

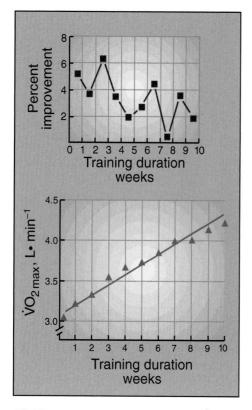

Figure 13.15   Continuous improvements in $\dot{V}O_{2max}$ during 10 weeks of high-intensity, aerobic training. (From Hickson, R.C., et al.: Linear increases in aerobic power induced by a program of endurance exercise. *J. Appl. Physiol.*, 42:373, 1977.)

much of one's sensitivity in responding to maximal aerobic and anaerobic power training, including adaptations of most muscle enzymes. Genetic makeup plays such a predominant role in training responsiveness that it makes it almost impossible to predict a specific individual's response to a given training stimulus.

Maintenance of Aerobic Fitness Gains

An important question concerns the optimal exercise frequency, duration, and intensity to maintain aerobic improvements with training. In one study, healthy young adults increased $\dot{V}O_{2max}$ 25% with 10 weeks of interval training by bicycling and running for 40 minutes, 6 days a week. They then joined one of two groups that continued to exercise for an additional 15 weeks at the same intensity and duration but at a reduced frequency of either 4 or 2 days a week. Both groups maintained their gains in aerobic capacity despite up to two-thirds reduction in training frequency.

Aerobic capacity improvement involves somewhat different training requirements than its maintenance. With intensity held constant, the frequency and duration of exercise required to maintain a certain level of aerobic fitness remain considerably lower than required for its improvement. A small decline in exercise intensity, in contrast, reduces $\dot{V}O_{2max}$. *This indicates that exercise intensity plays a principal role in maintaining the increase in maximal aerobic power achieved through training.*

Fitness components other than $\dot{V}O_{2max}$ more readily suffer adverse effects of reduced exercise training volume. Well-trained endurance athletes who normally trained 6 to 10 hours a week reduced weekly training to one 35-minute session; this did not decrease $\dot{V}O_{2max}$ over a 4-week period. Endurance capacity at 75% $\dot{V}O_{2max}$ significantly decreased, which related to reduced pre-exercise glycogen stores and a diminished level of fat oxidation during exercise. These findings indicate that a single measure, such as $\dot{V}O_{2max}$, cannot adequately evaluate all factors that affect the adaptations to training and detraining.

Tapering for Peak Performance

In most instances, little improvement occurs in the aerobic systems during the competitive season. At best, athletes strive to prevent physiologic and performance deteriorations as the season progresses. Before major competition, athletes often reduce or taper training intensity and/or volume, believing that such adjustments produce peak performance. The taper period and exact alterations in training vary by sport.

No clear answers exist about optimum taper duration or training modification. From a physiologic perspective, 4 to 7 days probably provides sufficient time for maximum muscle and liver glycogen replenishment, optimal nutritional support and restoration, alleviation of residual muscle soreness, and healing of minor injuries.

FORMULATING AN AEROBIC TRAINING PROGRAM

This section presents guidelines for initiating aerobic training and describes a method to gauge and adjust training intensity. We also discuss advantages and possible limitations of aerobic training through intermittent and continuous procedures.

General Guidelines

Regardless of present physiologic fitness, some basic guidelines (based on both research and common sense) provide important structure when initiating an aerobic exercise training program:

- **Start slowly.** Injury can occur when initiating vigorous activity after years of sedentary living. Minor muscle aches and twinges of joint pain normally follow the start of an exercise program, particularly with eccentric muscle actions (see Chapter 14). Severe muscular discomfort and excessive cardiovascular strain offer no additional training benefits; excessive fatigue frequently discourages the beginner from continuing a regular exercise program.

- **Allow a warm-up period.** Mild stretching and aerobic exercise (running in place, jogging on a treadmill, skipping rope, rowing, calisthenics, or stationary cycling) for several minutes provides adequate muscular and cardiovascular warm-up immediately before the aerobic workout phase. Rhythmic, moderate exercise at a heart rate between 50% to 60% of maximum also adjusts coronary blood flow for more favorable myocardial oxygenation.
- **Allow a cool-down period.** After the training phase of exercise, slow down gradually before stopping to allow metabolism to progress to resting levels. More importantly, a gradual cool down prevents blood from pooling in the large veins of the previously exercised muscles. Venous pooling could decrease blood pressure and reduce blood flow to the heart and brain. This produces dizziness, nausea, and even fainting. Reduced blood to the myocardium often precipitates a series of irregular heart beats that could trigger a catastrophic cardiac episode.

Guidelines for Children

Children are not small adults. Their physical activity programs should be general in nature compared with specific formulations used to "train" adults. Guidelines from the National Association for Sport and Physical Education recommend the following:

1. Accumulate more than 60 minutes, and up to several hours per day, of age and developmentally appropriate activities for elementary school children.
2. Some of the child's physical activity each day should be in periods lasting 10 to 15 minutes or more and include moderate to vigorous activity. This activity will be intermittent in nature, involving alternating moderate to vigorous activity with brief rest and recovery periods.
3. Extended periods of inactivity are *not* appropriate for normal, healthy children.
4. Elementary school children should participate in a variety of physical activities of various levels of intensities.

Cardiorespiratory Fitness Standards for Children   Because of the relatively strong association between aerobic capacity and exercise performance (higher $\dot{V}O_{2max}$ relates to better performance), a valid method to evaluate cardiorespiratory fitness in children uses time to complete a 1-mile walk-run. **Table 13.3** presents criterion standards (a minimum $\dot{V}O_{2max}$ consistent with good health), for $\dot{V}O_{2max}$ and 1-mile times for children of different ages.

Questions & Notes

Give the "ceiling" for training intensity for exercise heart rate and %$\dot{V}O_{2max}$.

   Heart rate:

   %$\dot{V}O_{2max}$:

Women and men show _____ adaptations to aerobic training.

Give the principle exercise training variable to maintain a training-induced increase in $\dot{V}O_{2max}$.

Write 2 formulae to predict maximum heart rate from age.

   1.

   2.

Table 13·3	Criterion Standards for 1-Mile Walk–Run Times and $\dot{V}O_{2max}$ for Children Ages 10 to 17 Years	
Age, y	**1-Mile Time min:s**	**$\dot{V}O_{2max}$ mL·kg^{-1}·min^{-1}**
10	12:30	39
11	12:00	38
12	12:00	37
13	11:30	36
14	11:00	35
15	10:30	35
16	10:30	35
17	10:00	35

From Institute for Aerobic Research: *The Prudential FITNESSGRAM Test Administration Manual.* Dallas: Institute for Aerobics Research, 1992.

FOR YOUR INFORMATION

Improvement for the Average Person
As a broad guideline, individuals classified as average for $\dot{V}O_{2max}$ can improve aerobic power between 5% to 25% during a 12-week aerobic training program.

Setting fitness standards for children requires careful attention. Although $\dot{V}O_{2max}$ ($mL \cdot kg^{-1} \cdot min^{-1}$) remains relatively stable or decreases slightly between ages 5 and 19 years, walk-run performance almost doubles from growth and development and improved exercise economy during this period (a 12-year-old runs a mile twice as fast as a 5-year-old). Also, $\dot{V}O_{2max}$ improves only slightly for children who undergo aerobic training, whereas exercise performance increases considerably. This raises the question of whether aerobic capacity or exercise performance represents the "best" expression of cardiorespiratory fitness in children and its improvement with training.

Applying a mathematical equation generated to predict $\dot{V}O_{2max}$ based on a walk-run test in children poses problems because of continually increasing levels of running economy as a child ages. Variations in exercise economy alter the relationship between aerobic fitness and running performance through all stages of growth and development.

ESTABLISHING TRAINING INTENSITY

What represents a considerable aerobic exercise stress for a sedentary person falls below an elite athlete's threshold training intensity. Consequently, exercise intensity must be assessed relative to the stress it places on a person's aerobic system. Within this framework, one could justifiably maintain that three individuals performing their best marathon times of 2.5, 3.0, and 4.0 hours experience equivalent levels of physiologic stress despite large variations in running speed.

Train at Percentage of $\dot{V}O_{2max}$

In this method, an individual trains at a percentage of $\dot{V}O_{2max}$ determined directly or estimated from exercise intensity. For example, if running at 5.5 mph requires an oxygen uptake of 33 $mL \cdot kg^{-1} \cdot min^{-1}$, and $\dot{V}O_{2max}$ equals 60 $mL \cdot kg^{-1} \cdot min^{-1}$, the exercise represents a stress of 55% of aerobic capacity. For another individual with a lower $\dot{V}O_{2max}$ of 40 $mL \cdot kg^{-1} \cdot min^{-1}$, the oxygen cost of running at 5.5 mph still requires 33 $mL \cdot kg^{-1} \cdot min^{-1}$, yet this person must exercise at 83% of maximum. To provide a similar overload (intensity) of 83% of $\dot{V}O_{2max}$ for the first jogger, the pace must increase to a speed requiring 48 $mL\ O_2$ $mL \cdot kg^{-1} \cdot min^{-1}$ or 8.6 mph.

Train at Percentage of Maximum Heart Rate

Assessing exercise intensity accurately by direct measurement of oxygen uptake requires laboratory measurements. A more practical alternative uses heart rate to classify exercise by intensity (strenuousness) and individualizes aerobic training to keep pace as fitness improves.

This approach applies the well-established relationship between percentage $\dot{V}O_{2max}$ and percentage HR_{max}.

The error in estimating percentage $\dot{V}O_{2max}$ from percentage HR_{max}, or vice versa, averages about $\pm 8\%$. From this intrinsic relationship, one need only monitor exercise heart rate to estimate percentage $\dot{V}O_{2max}$. *The relationship between percentage $\dot{V}O_{2max}$ and percentage HR_{max} remains the same for arm or leg exercise among healthy subjects, normal weight and obese groups, cardiac patients, and people with spinal cord injury.* Importantly, a lower HR_{max} occurs in arm compared with leg exercise; one must consider this difference in formulating the exercise prescription for different exercise modes.

To train at a percentage of maximum heart rate requires knowledge of the heart rate in near-maximal exercise. Three or four minutes of all-out running or swimming elicit HR_{max} values. Such intense exercise requires considerable motivation and endangers those predisposed to coronary heart disease. For this reason, predicting HR_{max} has become standard practice. Although the most common formula to predict HR_{max} is 220 − age, more resent research suggests substantial individual differences using this method when applied to all individuals. New formulae predict HR_{max} results with less error. The accompanying *Close Up* presents the formula and shows the most common methods that use heart rate to establish individual training levels.

Effectiveness of Less Intense Exercise   The recommendation to train at 70% of HR_{max} as the threshold for aerobic improvement represents a *general guideline* for a comfortable yet effective exercise intensity. Twenty to 30 minutes of continuous exercise at the 70% level stimulates a training effect; exercise at a lower intensity of 60% to 65% HR_{max} for 45 minutes also proves beneficial. *In general, longer exercise duration offsets lower exercise intensity, particularly for older and less fit individuals.* Regardless of exercise level, more is not necessarily better because excessive exercise increases the chance for sustaining bone, joint, and muscle injuries.

Train at a Perception of Effort

In addition to oxygen consumption, heart rate, and blood lactate as indicators of exercise intensity, one also can use the **rating of perceived exertion** (RPE). With this psychophysiologic approach, the exerciser rates on a numerical scale (called the Borg scale, named after researcher Gunnar Borg who developed this scaling system) perceived feelings relative to exertion level. Monitoring and adjusting RPE during exercise is an effective way to prescribe exercise on the basis of an individual's perception of effort that coincides with objective measures of physiologic/metabolic strain (%HR_{max}, %$\dot{V}O_{2max}$, blood lactate concentration). Exercise levels corresponding to higher levels of energy expenditure and physiologic strain produce higher RPE ratings. For example, an RPE of 13 or 14 (exercise that feels "somewhat hard"; **Fig. 13.16**) coincides with about 70% HR_{max} during cycle ergometer and

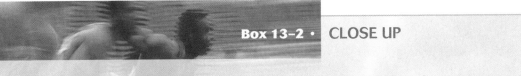

Box 13–2 • CLOSE UP

CARDIOVASCULAR FITNESS CATEGORIES USING $\dot{V}O_{2MAX}$

The $\dot{V}O_{2max}$ test represents the most often cited criterion of cardiorespiratory fitness. Current practice evaluates the $\dot{V}O_{2max}$ score against **criterion-referenced standards** rather than norm-referenced standards. Criterion-referenced standards establish a minimum $\dot{V}O_{2max}$ consistent with good health (similar to blood pressure and cholesterol standards), independent of the score's percentile ranking within a particular normative data set. The accompanying table presents a 5-part classification scheme for $\dot{V}O_{2max}$ for men and women of different ages. The poor category for each age group represents the lower limit of cardiorespiratory fitness below which probably places the individual at increased risk for cardiovascular disease.

The highest $\dot{V}O_{2max}$ values are generally achieved by individuals who compete in distance running, swimming, bicycling, and cross-country skiing. These athletes have almost double the $\dot{V}O_{2max}$ of sedentary individuals.

Cardiovascular Fitness Classifications Based on $\dot{V}O_{2max}$ ($mL \cdot kg^{-1} \cdot min^{-1}$)

GENDER	AGE	POOR	FAIR	AVERAGE	GOOD	EXCELLENT
Men	≤29	≤24.9	25–33.9	34–43.9	44–52.9	≥53
	30–39	≤22.9	23–30.9	31–41.9	42–49.9	≥50
	40–49	≤19.9	20–26.9	27–38.9	39–44.9	≥45
	50–59	≤17.9	18–24.9	25–37.9	38–42.9	≥43
	60–69	≤15.9	16–22.9	23–35.9	36–40.9	≥41
Women	≤29	≤23.9	24–30.9	31–38.9	39–48.9	≥49
	30–39	≤19.9	20–27.9	28–36.9	37–44.9	≥45
	40–49	≤16.9	17–24.9	25–34.9	35–41.9	≥42
	50–59	≤14.9	15–21.9	22–33.9	34–39.9	≥40
	50–69	≤12.9	13–20.9	21–32.9	33–36.9	≥37

treadmill exercise; an RPE between 11 and 12 corresponds to exercise at the lactate threshold for trained and untrained individuals. Individuals learn quickly to exercise at a specific RPE. In this sense, the axiom "listen to your body" becomes apropos.

Train at the Lactate Threshold

Exercising at or slightly above the lactate threshold provides effective aerobic training, with the higher exercise levels producing the greatest benefits, particularly for fit individuals. Many coaches use the 4-mM blood lactate level as the optimal aerobic training intensity, yet no convincing evidence exists to justify this particular blood lactate level as "ideal." Regardless of the specific blood lactate level chosen for endurance training, the blood lactate–exercise intensity relationship should be evaluated periodically, with exercise intensity adjusted to meet aerobic fitness improvements. If regular blood lactate measurement proves impractical, the exercise heart rate at the initial lactate determination remains a convenient and relatively stable marker for setting the appropriate predetermined exercise intensity. This is because no systematic training-induced change occurs in the heart rate–blood lactate relationship during incremental exercise.

METHODS OF TRAINING

Each year, performance improvements occur in almost all athletic competitions. These advances generally relate to increased opportunities for participation; indi-

FOR YOUR INFORMATION

A Regular Dose of Aerobic Exercise Combats Obesity

Sixty minutes of moderate daily exercise (low-impact walking or aerobic dancing, swimming, stationary cycling) reduces excess body fat. Exercise can be divided into 10-, 20-, or 30-minute sessions, as long as the daily total equals 60 minutes or more. For an individual who weighs 216 pounds, the caloric expenditure during slow walking equals 7.8 kCal each minute (470 kCal per hour). Over 1 month, total exercise calories would accumulate to 14,100 kCal (470 kCal × 30 days), the equivalent of 4.0 pounds of body fat—14,100 kCal ÷ 3500 kCal per pound of adipose tissue. In 1 year, as long as caloric intake remains constant, fat loss (without dieting) would amount to nearly 50 pounds.

Box 13-3 · CLOSE UP

PREDICTING MAXIMUM HEART-RATE AND THE TRAINING SENSITIVE ZONE

Percentage of maximum HR predicts exercise intensity (an activity's relative energy requirements).

HR_{max} in beats per min (bpm) can be predicted by age, independent of gender and physical activity status. For *nonfat* men and women, HR_{max} predicts as:

$$HR_{max} = 208 - 0.7 \times (Age, y)$$

Example

Calculate the HR_{max} for a 20-year-old male.

$$HR_{max} = 208 - 0.7 \times (Age, y)$$
$$= 194 \text{ bpm}$$

PREDICTING HR_{MAX} FOR MEN AND WOMEN WITH ≥ 30% BODY FAT

For overfat men and women with percentage body fat levels ≥ 30%, HR_{max} predicts as:

$$HR_{max} = 200 - 0.5 \times (Age, y)$$

Example

Calculate the HR_{max} for a 25-year-old female with a percentage body fat of 32%.

$$HR_{max} = 200 - 0.5 \times (Age, y)$$
$$= 188 \text{ bpm}$$

COMPUTING LOWER- AND UPPER-LIMIT TRAINING HEART RATES

For men and women below the age of 60, the minimal or **lower-limit target (threshold) heart rate (LL_{THR})** stimulus for cardiovascular improvement ranges between 60% and 70% of HR_{max}, representing about 50% to 60% of $\dot{V}O_{2max}$. The **upper-limit target heart rate (UL_{THR})** equals about 90% of HR_{max}, representing about 85%–90% of $\dot{V}O_{2max}$. In individuals above the age of 60, LL_{THR} equals 60% and UL_{THR} equals 75% of HR_{max}.

Method 1: Percentage Method

This method calculates the lower-limit and upper-limit target heart rate as a simple percentage of the age-predicted HR_{max}.

1. Calculate LL_{THR} as:

$$LL_{THR} = \text{Predicted } HR_{max}$$
$$\times \text{ lower-limit percentage for age}$$

where the lower-limit percentage = 70% for men and women ≤ 60 years and 60% for men and women > 60 years.

2. Calculate UL_{THR} as:

$$UL_{THR} = \text{Predicted } HR_{max}$$
$$\times \text{ upper-limit percentage for age}$$

where the upper-limit percentage = 90% for men and women ≤ 60 years and 80% for men and women > 60 years.

Example

Data: Male, age 55 years.

1. Calculate predicted HR_{max}

$$HR_{max} = 208 - 0.7 \times (Age, y)$$
$$= 170 \text{ bpm}$$

$$LL_{THR} = 170$$
$$\times \text{ lower-limit percentage for age}$$
$$= 170 \times 0.70$$
$$= 119 \text{ bpm}$$

2. Calculate UL_{THR}

$$UL_{THR} = HR_{max}$$
$$\times \text{ upper-limit percentage for age}$$
$$= 170 \times 0.90$$
$$= 153 \text{ bpm}$$

Box 13-3 •   CLOSE UP *(Continued)*

Method 2: Karvonen Method (Heart Rate Reserve)

An alternate, equally effective method calculates the lower- and upper-threshold HR levels at a percentage of the difference between resting and maximum HR, termed **heart rate reserve** (**HRR**; also referred to as the **Karvonen method** named after the Finnish physiologist who introduced this method). Karvonen's method produces somewhat higher values compared to heart rate computed as percentage of HR_{max}. The Karvonen method uses about 50% of HRR the as the LL_{THR} and 85% of HRR as UL_{THR}.

1. Calculate predicted HR_{max}:

$$HR_{max} = 208 - 0.7 \times Age, y$$

2. Calculate LL_{THR}:

$$LL_{THR} = [(HR_{max} - HR_{rest}) \times 0.50] + HR_{rest}$$

3. Calculate UL_{THR}:

$$UL_{THR} = [(HR_{max} - HR_{rest}) \times 0.85] + HR_{rest}$$

Example

Data: Male, age 55 years, $HR_{rest} = 60$ b·min^{-1}.

1. Calculate predicted HR_{max}:

$$HR_{max} = 208 - 0.7 \times Age, y$$
$$= 170 \ bpm$$

2. Calculate LL_{THR}:

$$LL_{THR} = [(HR_{max} - HR_{rest}) \times 0.50] + HR_{rest}$$
$$= [(170 - 60) \times 0.50] + 60$$
$$= 115 \ bpm$$

3. Calculate UL_{THR}:

$$UL_{THR} = [(HR_{max} - HR_{rest}) \times 0.85] + HR_{rest}$$
$$= [(170 - 60) \times 0.85] + 60$$
$$= 154 \ bpm$$

Adjust for Swimming and Other Upper-Body Exercises

In trained and untrained subjects, swimming HR_{max} averages about 13 bpm lower than in running. The smaller arm muscle mass activated during swimming probably causes this difference. Consequently, HR_{max} must be adjusted downward for swimming or other upper-body exercise. Subtract 13 bpm from the age-predicted HR_{max} values to calculate training HR during swimming. For example, a 25-year-old person wanting to swim at 80% of HR_{max} should select a swimming speed that produces an exercise heart rate (percentage method) of about 142 bpm ($0.80 \times [191 - 13]$).

REFERENCES

1. Davis, J.A., and Convertino, V.A.: A comparison of heart rate methods for predicting endurance training intensity. *Med. Sci. Sports Exerc.*, 7:295, 1975.
2. Karvonen, M., et al.: The effects of training on heart rate. A longitudinal study. *Ann. Med. Exp. Biol. Fenn.*, 35:307, 1957.
3. Miller, W.C., et al.: Predicting max HR and the HR-VO$_2$ relationship for exercise prescription in obesity. *Med. Sci. Sports Exerc.*, 25:1077, 1993.
4. Tanaka, H., et al.: Age-predicted maximal heart rate revisited. *J. Am. Coll. Cardiol.*, 37:153, 2001.

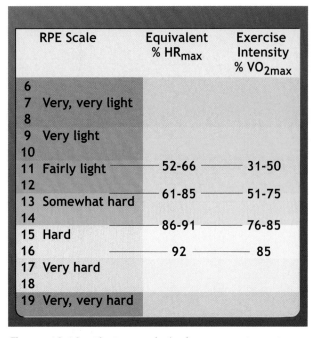

	RPE Scale	Equivalent % HR$_{max}$	Exercise Intensity % VO$_{2max}$
6			
7	Very, very light		
8			
9	Very light		
10			
11	Fairly light	52–66	31–50
12			
13	Somewhat hard	61–85	51–75
14			
15	Hard	86–91	76–85
16		92	85
17	Very hard		
18			
19	Very, very hard		

Figure 13.16 The Borg scale (and accompanying estimates of relative exercise intensity) for obtaining the RPE during exercise. (Modified from Borg, G.A.: Psychological basis of physical exertion. *Med. Sci. Sports Exerc.*, 14:377, 1982.)

viduals with "natural endowment" more likely become exposed to particular sports. Also, improved nutrition and health care, better equipment, and more systematic and scientific approaches to athletic training contribute to superior performance. The following sections present general guidelines for anaerobic and aerobic training.

Anaerobic Training

The capacity to perform all-out exercise for up to 60 seconds largely depends on ATP generated by the immediate and short-term anaerobic systems for energy transfer (see Fig. 13.1).

The Intramuscular High-Energy Phosphates

Football, weightlifting, and other brief, sprint-power sport activities rely almost exclusively on energy derived from ATP and PCr, the muscles' high-energy phosphates. Engaging specific muscles in repeated 5- to 10-second maximum bursts of effort overloads the phosphagen pool. The intramuscular high-energy phosphates supply energy for brief, intense exercise, so little lactate accumulates and recovery progresses rapidly. Thus, exercise can begin again after about a 30-second rest. The use of brief, all-out exercise interspersed with recovery represents a specific application of interval training for anaerobic conditioning.

The activities selected to enhance ATP–PCr energy transfer capacity must engage the specific muscles at the movement speed and power output for which the athlete

desires improved anaerobic power (specificity principle). Not only does this enhance the metabolic capacity of the specifically trained muscle fibers, but it also facilitates recruitment and modulation of firing sequence of the appropriate motor units activated in the movement.

Lactate-Generating Capacity As duration of all-out effort extends beyond 10 seconds, dependence on anaerobic energy from the intramuscular high-energy phosphates decreases, with a proportionate increase in anaerobic energy transfer from anaerobic glycolysis. To improve energy transfer capacity by the short-term lactic acid energy system, training must overload this aspect of energy metabolism.

Anaerobic training requires extreme physiologic and psychological demands and considerable motivation. Repeated bouts of up to 1-minute maximum exercise stopped 30 seconds before subjective feelings of exhaustion cause blood lactate to increase to near-maximum levels. The individual repeats each exercise bout after 3 to 5 minutes of recovery. Repetition of exercise causes "lactate stacking," which results in a higher blood lactate level than with just one bout of all-out exhaustive effort. As with all training, one must exercise the specific muscle groups that require enhanced lactate-producing capacity. A backstroke swimmer trains by swimming the backstroke, a cyclist should bicycle, and basketball, hockey, or soccer players should perform movements and direction changes similar to those required by the sport.

Aerobic Training: Continuous Versus Intermittent Methods

Two types of aerobic training include continuous and intermittent methods.

Continuous Training Continuous (**long slow distance, LSD**) training requires sustained, steady-rate aerobic exercise. Because of its submaximal nature, exercise continues for considerable time in relative comfort. This makes LSD training ideal for people beginning an exercise program or wanting to reduce excess body fat. *The greatest health-related benefits of exercise emerge when a person moves from a sedentary lifestyle to one that incorporates only a moderate level of continuous aerobic exercise.* LSD training generally progresses at the relatively comfortable threshold intensity of 70% HR$_{max}$, although it can be effective at the 85% or 90% level.

Endurance athletes overload the cardiovascular and energy transfer systems using continuous exercise training at nearly the same intensity as competition. This specifically activates slow-twitch muscle fibers in sustained exercise. A champion middle-distance runner may run 5 miles continuously in 25 minutes during workouts at a heart rate of 180 b·min^{-1}; this pace does not exhaust the athlete but still nearly duplicates race conditions. By finishing each exercise session with several all-out sprints stopped 30 to 40 seconds before exhaustion, the athlete also trains the short-term anaerobic system (glycolysis) that contributes to race performance, particularly at the finish. A marathon runner trains at a slightly slower pace than a middle-distance athlete to simulate the intensity and distance of actual competition.

Interval Training   Periods of intense activity interspersed with moderate to low energy expenditure characterize many sport and life activities. **Interval exercise training** simulates this variation in energy transfer intensity through specific spacing of exercise and rest periods. With this approach, a person trains at an inordinately high exercise intensity with minimal fatigue that would normally prove exhausting if done continuously. Rest-to-exercise intervals vary from a few seconds to several minutes depending on the energy system(s) overloaded. Four factors help to formulate the interval training prescription:

1. Intensity of exercise interval
2. Duration of exercise interval
3. Duration of recovery interval
4. Repetitions of exercise-recovery interval

Running continuously at a 4-minute mile pace exhausts most people within a minute due to rapid lactate accumulation. However, running at this speed for only 15 seconds followed by a 30-second rest period enables a person to accomplish 4 minutes of running at this near-record pace. Of course, this does not equate to a 4-minute mile, but during 4 minutes of running, the person covers a one-mile distance even though the combined exercise and rest intervals require 11 minutes 30 seconds.

Rationale for Interval Training   A sound rationale forms the basis for interval training. In the example of a continuous run by an average person at a 4-minute mile pace, the predominant energy for exercise comes from the short-term anaerobic energy pathway with rapid lactate accumulation. The individual becomes exhausted within 60 to 90 seconds. In contrast, running at this speed for 15-second intervals or less places significant demands on the immediate energy system (intramuscular ATP and PCr) with little lactate accumulation. Recovery becomes predominantly "alactic" in nature and occurs rapidly. The subsequent exercise interval can begin after only a brief rest period. Repetitively linking specific exercise and rest intervals (interval training) eventually places considerable demand on aerobic energy metabolism.

In interval training, as with other forms of physiologic conditioning, exercise intensity must overload the specific energy system(s) the person desires to improve. **Table 13.4** outlines a practical method for determining exer-cise intensity for interval training in running and swimming.

Available evidence does *not* support superiority for either continuous or interval training to improve aerobic fitness. Both methods probably can be applied interchangeably. Importantly, continuous LSD training gives the endurance athlete a more "task-specific" cardiovascular and metabolic overload that more closely mimics the duration and intensity of race conditions. Likewise, sprint and middle-distance athletes benefit from the intense metabolic demands and specific neuromuscular and fiber-type activation that interval training provides.

Formulating the Exercise:Relief Interval

Exercise Interval

- Add 1.5 to 5 s to the exerciser's "best time" for training distances between 60 and 220 yd for running and 15 and 55 yd for swimming. If a person covers 60 yd from a running start in 8 s, the exercise duration for each repeat equals 8 + 1.5 or 9.5 s. Add 3 s to the best running time for interval training distances of 110 yd and 5 s to a distance of 220 yd. This particular application of

Table 13·4	Guidelines for Determining Interval-Training Exercise Intensities for Running and Swimming Different Distances[a]

INTERVAL TRAINING DISTANCES (YARDS)		WORK RATE FOR EACH EXERCISE INTERVAL OR REPEAT
Run	**Swim**	
55	15	1.5 ⎫ seconds *slower* than best
110	25	3.0 ⎬ times from a running (or (swimming) start for each
220	55	5.0 ⎭ for each distance
440	110	1 to 4 seconds *faster* than the average run or 110-yd swim time recorded during a 1-mile run or 440-yd swim
660–1320	165–320	3 to 4 seconds *slower* than the average 440-yd run or 100-yard swim time recorded during a 1-mile run or 440-yd swim

[a]From Fox, E. L., and Matthews, D.K.: *Interval Training,* Philadelphia: W. B. Saunders, 1974.

interval training most effectively trains the intramuscular high-energy phosphate component of the anaerobic energy system.

- For training distances of 440 yd running or 110 yd swimming, determine the exercise rate by subtracting 1 to 4 s from the average 440-yd portion of a mile run or 110-yd portion of a 440-yd swim. If a person runs a 7:00-minute mile (averaging 105 s per 440 yd), the interval time for each 440-yd repeat ranges between 104 s (105 − 1) and 101 s (105 − 4).

- For run training intervals beyond 440 yd (and swim intervals beyond 110 yd) add 3 to 4 s to the average 440-yard portion of a mile run or 110-yard portion of a 440-yard swim. In running an 880-yard interval, the 7:00-minute miler runs each interval in about 216 s ([105 + 3] × 2 = 216).

Relief Interval

- The relief (recovery) interval occurs either passively (rest:relief) or actively (exercise:relief). Recovery duration represents a multiple of the exercise interval. A 1:3 ratio overloads the immediate energy system. For a sprinter who runs 10-s intervals, the relief interval equals 30 s. For training the short-term glycolytic energy system, the relief interval doubles (ratio of 1:2). Thus, a 2-min recovery follows a 1-min run or swim. These specified ratios of exercise to relief for training provide for sufficient restoration of high-energy phosphates and lactate removal so subsequent exercise proceeds without undue fatigue.

- For training the long-term aerobic energy system, the exercise:relief interval usually equals 1:1 or 1:1.5. During a 60- to 90-s exercise interval, for example,

oxygen uptake increases rapidly to a high level. Although some lactate accumulates during this relatively intense exercise, duration remains brief enough to prevent exhaustion. A 1- to 2-min recovery permits exercise to begin again before oxygen uptake returns to its pre-exercise level. Consecutive repeat exercise:relief intervals ensures that cardiovascular response and aerobic metabolism eventually maintain near-maximal levels throughout exercise and recovery. Performing continuously at this exercise intensity would exhaust the person within several minutes and training would cease.

Fartlek Training   Fartlek, a Swedish word that means "speed play," represents a training method introduced to the United States in the 1940s. This relatively unscientific blending of interval and continuous training has particular application to exercise out-of-doors over natural terrain. The system uses alternate running at fast and slow speeds over both level and hilly terrain.

In contrast to the precise exercise-interval training prescription, fartlek training does not require systematic manipulation of exercise and relief intervals. Instead, the performer determines the training schema based on "how it feels" at the time, in a way similar to gauging exercise intensity based on one's rating of perceived exertion. If used properly, this method will overload one or all of the energy systems. Fartlek training provides an ideal means of general conditioning and off-season training, but it lacks the systematic quantified approaches of interval and continuous training. It also adds freedom and variety in workouts.

Insufficient evidence prevents proclaiming superiority of any specific training method for improving aerobic capacity.

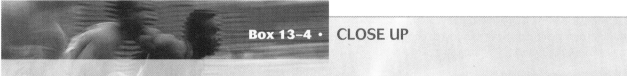

Box 13-4 · CLOSE UP

DETERMINE 10,000-M RUNNING PACE FROM LACTATE THRESHOLD

Physiologic measurements during exercise help to (1) pinpoint strengths and weaknesses about an individual's performance capacity and potential and (2) optimize training intensity for the most effective outcome. For example, research indicates that athletes run 10,000 m at a pace approximately 5 m·min^{-1} faster than the running speed associated with their lactate threshold (LT). Knowledge of the exercise intensity associated with LT should provide the athlete and coach with a realistic performance expectation based on an individualized assessment of the aerobic metabolic response to exercise. This information puts into a biologic perspective (for both coach and athlete) an answer to the questions: "How fast can I perform this event?" and "What training pace is best for me?"

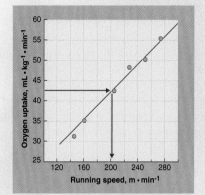
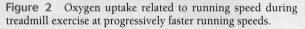

Figure 2   Oxygen uptake related to running speed during treadmill exercise at progressively faster running speeds.

TESTING

Step 1. Determine the LT (see Chapter 9; if you cannot directly measure blood lactate, use the ventilatory threshold method). Figure 1 shows the relationship between blood lactate and oxygen uptake ($\dot{V}O_2$) during graded treadmill exercise, with LT indicated by the arrow. In this example, LT occurred at a $\dot{V}O_2$ of 43.5 mL·kg^{-1}·min^{-1}.

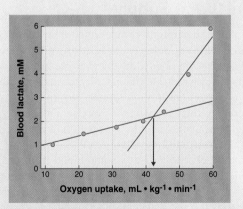

Figure 1   Determination of LT from measures of blood lactate and $\dot{V}O_2$ during graded treadmill exercise.

Step 2. Determine the relationship between $\dot{V}O_2$ (mL·kg^{-1}·min^{-1}; either actual or estimated) and running speed (m·min^{-1}). The subject runs on a treadmill for 5 minutes at each of six different submaximal speeds. Construct a graph relating $\dot{V}O_2$ versus running speed (Fig. 2). Draw a best-fit line through the plotted points.

Step 3. Convert the $\dot{V}O_2$ at LT (43.5 mL·kg^{-1}·min^{-1}; Fig. 1) to a running speed using the best-fit line presented in Figure 2. Draw a horizontal line from the oxygen uptake value on the Y-axis until it intersects the line of best fit; from this intersection, draw a perpendicular line to the X-axis that indicates running speed. The arrow shows the corresponding speed (m·min^{-1}) as 204 m·min^{-1}.

COMPUTING EXPECTED PERFORMANCE

Assume an athlete exceeds by 5 m·min^{-1} his or her running speed at LT during training (and competition) for 10,000 m (and other endurance events); the projected average running speed for this person equals 209 m·min^{-1} (204 m·min^{-1} + 5 m·min^{-1}).

DETERMINE THE PROJECTED RACE TIME FOR THE 10,000-M RUN

Use the data from Figures 1 and 2 to estimate the time for a 10,000-m race.

$$\text{Estimated time} = \text{Distance} \div \text{Speed}$$
$$= 10,000 \text{ m} \div 209 \text{ m·min}^{-1}$$
$$= 47.85 \text{ min } (47 \text{ min:}51 \text{ s})$$

This analysis based on LT measurements indicates that the athlete should complete the 10,000-m run in 47 minutes and 51 seconds. It also represents a realistic estimate of an appropriate training intensity to achieve the performance goal.

Each form of training produces success. One can probably use the various methods interchangeably, particularly to modify training and achieve a more psychologically pleasing exercise regimen.

THE OVERTRAINING SYNDROME

Ten to 20 percent of athletes experience the syndrome of **overtraining**, or "staleness." As a result of complex interactions among biologic and psychological influences, an athlete can fail to endure and adapt to training, so that normal exercise performance deteriorates and the individual encounters increasing difficulty fully recovering from a workout. This takes on crucial importance for elite athletes for whom performance decrements of 1% to 3% might cause a gold medalist to fail to qualify for competition.

Two clinical forms of overtraining have been described:

1. The less common **sympathetic form** is characterized by increased sympathetic activity during rest and is generally typified by hyperexcitability, restlessness, and impaired exercise performance. This form of overtraining may reflect excessive psychological/emotional stress that accompanies the interaction among training, competition, and responsibilities of normal living.
2. The more common **parasympathetic form** is characterized by predominance of vagal activity during rest and exercise. More properly termed **overreaching** in the early stages (within as few as 10 days), the syndrome is qualitatively similar in symptoms to the full-blown parasympathetic overtraining syndrome but of shorter duration. Overreaching generally results from excessive and protracted exercise overload with inadequate recovery and rest. Initially, maintenance of exercise performance requires greater effort, which eventually leads to performance deterioration in training and competition. Short-term rest intervention of a few days up to several weeks usually restores full function. Untreated overreaching eventually progresses to the overtraining syndrome.

Symptoms of Overtraining and Staleness

The eight most common overtraining characteristics include:

1. Unexplained and persistently poor performance and high fatigue ratings
2. Prolonged recovery from typical training sessions or competitive events
3. Disturbed mood states characterized by general fatigue, apathy, depression, irritability, and loss of competitive drive
4. Persistent feelings of muscle soreness and stiffness in muscles and joints
5. Elevated resting pulse, and increased susceptibility to

upper respiratory tract infections (altered immune function) and gastrointestinal disturbances
6. Insomnia
7. Loss of appetite, weight loss, and inability to maintain proper body weight for competition
8. Overuse injuries

No simple, reliable method can diagnose overtraining in its earliest stages. Deterioration in physical performance and alterations in mood rather than immune function changes provide the best indications.

EXERCISE TRAINING DURING PREGNANCY

Walking, swimming, and aerobics are the most popular physical activities during pregnancy. Older mothers, women who delivered more than one child or had previous children, and women with unfavorable reproductive histories are less likely to exercise during pregnancy.

Energy Cost and Physiologic Demands of Exercise

Cardiovascular responses during exercise in pregnancy follow normal patterns. An uncomplicated pregnancy offers no greater physiologic strain to the mother during moderate exercise other than provided by the additional weight gain and possible encumbrance of fetal tissue. Increases in maternal body mass add significantly to exercise effort in weight-bearing activities like walking, jogging, and stair climbing.

Fetal Blood Supply

Any factor that might compromise fetal blood supply raises concern regarding exercise during pregnancy. Studies of uterine blood flow during exercise in various mammalian species indicate that healthy animals maintain adequate oxygen supply to the developing fetus during moderate to intense maternal exercise. Fetal oxygen supply decreases considerably with maternal exercise in animals with restricted placental circulation.

Exercise probably diverts some blood from the uterus and visceral organs for preferential distribution to active muscles; thus, intense exercise could pose a hazard to a fetus with restricted placental blood flow. In addition, elevated maternal core temperature hinders heat dissipation from the fetus through the placenta. Maternal hyperthermia negatively affects fetal development (e.g., increased risk for neural tube defect) early in pregnancy. During warm weather, pregnant women should exercise in the cool part of the day and for shorter intervals while maintaining regular fluid intake.

Current medical opinion maintains that 30 or 40 minutes of moderate aerobic exercise by a previously active, healthy, low-risk woman during an uncomplicated pregnancy does not compromise fetal oxygen supply, acid-base status, or produce other adverse effects to mother or fetus. Performed regularly, moderate exercise maintains cardiovascular fitness and also produces a training effect.

Pregnancy Course and Outcome

Until recently, no overall consensus existed on whether regular exercise enhanced the course of pregnancy, including labor, delivery, and outcome. We believe current data support a recommendation for regular, moderate physical activity during pregnancy, even after the first trimester. In many ways, maternal physiologic responses and adaptations to exercise beneficially interact with physiologic changes in pregnancy.

Research indicates that regular aerobic exercise throughout pregnancy reduces birth weight, birth weight percentile, and the offspring's calculated percentage body fat and fat mass. Follow-up studies of children whose mothers regularly exercised during the second and third trimesters of pregnancy indicated that these children maintained similar height and head girth, but weighed less and had significantly lower sum of five skinfolds and lower upper-arm fat than children of sedentary women during pregnancy. Surprisingly, the offspring of active mothers performed significantly better on intelligence tests and had superior oral language skills. Some stimulus associated with regular exercise during pregnancy (e.g., intermittent stress, vibration, sound, motion, accelerated heartbeat) most likely benefits fetal neurological development and increased mental capacity. *The offspring of exercising women did not show evidence of a comparative deficit in any area examined.* These findings should reassure active women who chose to continue exercising during an uncomplicated pregnancy.

Questions & Notes

Give a "comfortable" exercise training threshold intensity level for most individuals.

List 2 factors used to formulate an interval training prescription.

1.

2.

Briefly explain fartlek training.

True or False:

Interval training is the single best form of exercise training to improve aerobic capacity.

Give the 2 clinical forms of overtraining.

1.

2.

List 3 common symptoms of the overtraining syndrome.

1.

2.

3.

List 3 contraindications for exercising during pregnancy.

1.

2.

3.

Box 13–5 • CLOSE UP

HOW TO PRESCRIBE EXERCISE DURING PREGNANCY

Pregnancy places extraordinary demands on a women's physiology, necessitating some modification in exercise prescription. Pregnant women should consult a physician prior to initiating an exercise program (or before modifying an existing program) to rule out possible complications. This pertains particularly to women of low fitness status and little exercise experience prior to pregnancy. The table lists 14 common contraindications to exercising during pregnancy.

Exercise during pregnancy should heighten awareness about heat dissipation, adequate calorie and nutrient intake, and knowing when to reduce exercise intensity. For a normal, uncomplicated pregnancy, light to moderate exercise does not negatively affect fetal development; the benefits of properly prescribed regular exercise during pregnancy generally outweigh potential risks.

EXERCISE GUIDELINES

Exercise Mode

Avoid exercise in the supine position, particularly after the first trimester. Supine exercise can impair venous return (mass of the fetus compresses the inferior vena cava), which could ultimately reduce cardiac output and uterine blood flow. Non-weight-bearing exercise (e.g., cycling, swimming) minimizes gravity's effects and the effects of added mass associated with fetal development. Weight-bearing exercise in moderation should not pose a risk.

Exercise Frequency

Exercise frequency can be 3 days a week emphasizing continuous, steady-rate effort. With more frequent exercise, reduce the intensity.

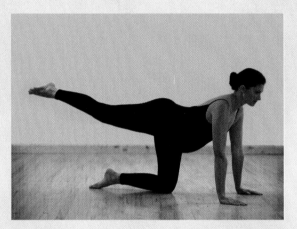

Contraindications for Exercising During Pregnancy

- Pregnancy-induced hypertension
- Pre-term labor during the prior or current pregnancy
- Persistent second to third trimester bleeding
- Type 1 diabetes
- Multiple pregnancy
- Excessive alcohol intake
- Anemia

- Pre-term rupture of membranes
- Incompetent cervix
- Intrauterine growth retardation
- History of two or more spontaneous abortions
- Smoking
- History of premature labor
- Excessive obesity

Box 13–5 • CLOSE UP (Continued)

Exercise Duration

Durations of 30 to 40 minutes are appropriate, depending on how the woman feels.

Exercise Intensity

Pregnancy alters the relationship between heart rate and oxygen uptake, making it difficult to establish exercise guidelines from heart rate. An effective alternative establishes exercise intensity based on rating of perceived exertion (RPE), which should range between 11 ("fairly light") to 13 ("somewhat hard").

Rate of Progression

Perform exercise on a regular basis; moderate aerobic exercise maintains cardiovascular fitness and typically produces a small training effect. For most women, exercise progression to induce training effects should not be a goal. Rather, goals should include maintenance of cardiorespiratory fitness, muscle mass, and physician-recommended weight gain. The combined effects of pregnancy per se and regular exercise often produce improved fitness after delivery.

Other Issues

Hyperthermia can negatively affect fetal development (increased risk for neural tube defect) chiefly during the first trimester of pregnancy. Thus, exercise during hot weather should occur in the cool part of the day (for shorter intervals) while maintaining adequate fluid intake. Periodic rest intervals minimize excessive fatigue and thermal stress. *Using a sauna or hot tub immersion increases fetal hyperthermia risk and impaired development.*

When to Stop Exercise and Seek Medical Advice

Immediately discontinue exercise under the following conditions:

- Any signs of vaginal bleeding
- Any gush of fluid from the vagina (premature rupture of membranes)
- Sudden swelling of ankles, hands, or face
- Persistent, severe headaches and/or disturbances in vision; unexplained lightheadedness or dizziness
- Elevated pulse rate or blood pressure that does not rapidly return to normal following exercise
- Excessive fatigue, palpitations, or chest pain
- Persistent uterine contractions (more than 6 to 8 per h)
- Unexplained or unusual abdominal pain
- Insufficient weight gain (less than 1.0 kg per month during the last two trimesters)

SUMMARY

1. Activation of a specific energy transfer system in exercise provides a means to classify diverse physical activities. Effective training allocates appropriate time to overload the energy system(s) involved in the activity.

2. Exercise intensity and duration largely determine the degree of anaerobic and aerobic energy transfer during physical activity. During sprint-power activities, primary energy transfer involves the immediate and short-term energy systems. The long-term aerobic system becomes progressively more important in activities longer than 2 minutes in duration.

3. Proper exercise training recognizes four principles for producing and maintaining optimum improvements: overload, specificity, individual differences, and reversibility.

4. Anaerobic training increases resting intramuscular anaerobic substrates and key glycolytic enzymes that typically increase all-out, sprint-power exercise performance.

5. Aerobic training must overload both circulatory function and metabolic capacity of specific muscles. Peripheral adaptations in active tissues exert a substantial benefit to exercise performance.

6. The major factors that affect aerobic training improvement include initial fitness level, frequency of training, duration of exercise, and exercise intensity. Of these four factors, exercise intensity exerts the most profound influence.

7. Aerobic training adaptations include increases in mitochondrial size and number, improved activity of

aerobic enzymes, greater capillarization of trained muscle, and enhanced oxidation of fats during submaximal exercise. Each factor increases a muscle's potential to generate ATP aerobically.

8. Aerobic training induces functional and dimensional changes in the cardiovascular system. These include a decrease in resting and submaximal exercise heart rate, enlarged left ventricular cavity, enhanced stroke volume and cardiac output, and an expanded $a\text{-}\bar{v}O_2$ difference.

9. Two ways establish training intensity: (1) on an absolute basis (standard exercise load or oxygen uptake), or (2) on a relative basis geared to an individual's physiologic response ($\%\dot{V}O_{2max}$ or $\%HR_{max}$).

10. The most effective methods to prescribe exercise are based on (1) percentage of HR_{max} (at least 65% to 70% age-predicted HR_{max}), or (2) rating of perceived exertion.

11. Three days minimum per week represents an effective frequency for aerobic training. Optimal frequency levels have not been established.

12. When intensity, duration, and frequency remain constant, similar training improvements emerge regardless of training mode provided the evaluation test utilizes the training exercise.

13. If exercise intensity remains at the training level, exercise frequency and duration can decrease by two-thirds without compromising gains in $\dot{V}O_{2max}$.

14. Prolonged and intense training can lead to the syndrome of overtraining or staleness with associated alterations in neuroendocrine and immune functions. The syndrome includes chronic fatigue, poor exercise performance, frequent infections, and general loss of interest in training.

15. Moderate aerobic exercise by a previously active, healthy, low-risk woman during an uncomplicated pregnancy does not compromise fetal well-being or produce adverse maternal effects.

THOUGHT QUESTIONS

1. Discuss whether regular physical activity benefits a person, even if exercise remains insufficient to stimulate a training effect.

2. Your personal training client insists that a single mode of cross-training exercise improves aerobic fitness for all physical activities requiring a high level of aerobic fitness. Give your opinion regarding the effectiveness of single-mode cross-training exercise.

3. Respond to the question: "How long must I exercise to get in shape?"

4. What information do you need to develop a program to effectively improve and evaluate aerobic capacity for the specific physical job performance requirements for (1) firefighters, (2) police officers, and (3) oilfield workers?

SELECTED REFERENCES

Albertus, Y., et al.: Effect of distance feedback on pacing strategy and perceived exertion during cycling. *Med. Sci. Sports Exerc.*, 37:461, 2005.

American College of Sports Medicine: *Guidelines for Exercise Testing and Prescription.* 7th Ed. Baltimore: Lippincott, Williams & Wilkins, 2006.

American College of Sports Medicine: Position stand on the recommended quantity and quality of exercise for developing and maintaining cardiorespiratory and muscular fitness, and flexibility in healthy adults. *Med. Sci. Sports Exerc.*, 30:975, 1998.

Atlaoui, D., et al.: The 24-h urinary cortisol/cortisone ratio for monitoring training in elite swimmers. *Med. Sci. Sports Exerc.*, 36:218, 2004.

Barak, Y., et al.: Transferability of strength gains from limited to full range of motion. *Med. Sci. Sports Exerc.*, 36:1413, 2004.

Bautmans, I., et al.: Biochemical changes in response to intensive resistance exercise training in the elderly. *Gerontology*, 51:253, 2005.

Borg, G.A.: Psychological basis of physical exertion. *Med. Sci. Sports Exerc.*, 14:377, 1982.

Borg-Stein, J., et al.: Musculoskeletal aspects of pregnancy. *Am. J. Phys. Med. Rehabil.*, 84:180, 2005.

Boule, N.G., et al.: HERITAGE Family Study. Effects of exercise training on glucose homeostasis: the HERITAGE Family Study. *Diabetes Care*, 28:108, 2005.

Boule, N.G., et al.: Physical fitness and the metabolic syndrome in adults from the Quebec Family Study. *Can. J. Appl. Physiol.*, 30:140, 2005.

Bourdin, M., et al.: Laboratory blood lactate profile is suited to on water training monitoring in highly trained rowers. *J. Sports Med. Phys. Fitness*, 44:337, 2004.

Cam, F.S., et al.: Association between the ACE I/D gene polymorphism and physical performance in a homogeneous non-elite cohort. *Can. J. Appl. Physiol.*, 30:74, 2005.

Caputo, F., Denadai, B.S.: Effects of aerobic endurance training status and specificity on oxygen uptake kinetics during maximal exercise. *Eur. J. Appl. Physiol.*, 93:87, 2004.

Clapp, J.F. III, et al.: Beginning regular exercise in early pregnancy: effect on fetoplacental growth. *Am. J. Obstet. Gynecol.*, 183:1484, 2000.

Coyle, E.F.: Improved muscular efficiency displayed as Tour de France champion matures. *J. Appl. Physiol.*, 98:2191, 2005.

Coyle, E.F.: Very intense exercise-training is extremely potent and time efficient: a reminder. *J. Appl. Physiol.*, 98:1983, 2005.

Dawes, H.N., et al.: Borg's rating of perceived exertion scales: do the verbal anchors mean the same for different clinical groups? *Arch. Phys. Med. Rehabil.*, 86(5):912, 2005.

de Vos, N.J., et al.: Optimal load for increasing muscle power during explosive resistance training in older adults. *J. Gerontol. A. Biol. Sci. Med. Sci.*, 60:638, 2005.

Delmonico, M.J., et al.: Blood pressure response to strength training may be influenced by angiotensinogen A-20C and angiotensin II type I receptor A1166C genotypes in older men and women. *J. Am. Geriatr. Soc.*, 53:204, 2005.

Denadai, B.S., Higino, W.P.: Effect of the passive recovery period on the lactate minimum speed in sprinters and endurance runners. *J. Sci. Med. Sport*, 7:488, 2004.

Diffee, G.M.: Adaptation of cardiac myocyte contractile properties to exercise training. *Exerc. Sport Sci. Rev.*, 32:112, 2004.

Duffield, R., et al.: Energy system contribution to 400-metre and 800-metre track running. *J. Sports Sci.*, 23:299, 2005.

Eston, R.G., et al.: The validity of predicting maximal oxygen uptake from a perceptually-regulated graded exercise test. *Eur. J. Appl. Physiol.*, 94:221, 2005.

Fischer, C.P., et al.: Endurance training reduces the contraction-induced interleukin-6 mRNA expression in human skeletal muscle. *Am. J. Physiol. Endocrinol. Metab.*, 287:E1189, 2004.

Flerreira, I., et al.: Longitudinal changes in $\dot{V}O_{2max}$: associations with carotid IMT and arterial stiffness. *Med. Sci. Sports Exerc.*, 35:1670, 2003.

Friedmann, B., et al.: Exercise with the intensity of the individual anaerobic threshold in acute hypoxia. *Med. Sci. Sports Exerc.*, 36:1737, 2004.

Glowacki, S.P., et al.: Effects of resistance, endurance, and concurrent exercise on training outcomes in men. *Med. Sci. Sports Exerc.*, 36:2119, 2004.

Goodman, J.M., et al.: Left ventricular adaptations following short-term endurance training. *J. Appl. Physiol.*, 98 454, 2005.

Green, J.M., et al.: RPE-lactate dissociation during extended cycling. *Eur. J. Appl. Physiol.*, 94:145, 2005.

Hagberg, J.M., et al.: Specific genetic markers of endurance performance and $\dot{V}O_{2max}$. *Exer. Sport Sci. Rev.*, 29:15, 2001.

Hartmann, U., Mester, J.: Training and overtraining markers in selected sport events. *Med. Sci. Sports Exerc.*, 32:209, 2000.

Holloszy, J.O., Coyle, E.F.: Adaptations of skeletal muscle to endurance exercise and their metabolic consequences. *J. Appl. Physiol.*, 56:831, 1984.

Holloszy, J.O.: Metabolic consequences of endurance training. In:

Exercise, Nutrition, and Energy Metabolism. Horton ES. and Terjung R L. (eds.). New York: Macmillan, 1988.

Horowitz, J.F.: Regulation of lipid mobilization and oxidation during exercise in obesity. *Exer. Sport Sci. Rev.*, 29:42, 2001.

Kang, J., et al.: Metabolic and perceptual responses during spinning cycle exercise. *Med. Sci. Sports Exerc.*, 37:853, 2005.

Kardel, K.R.: Effects of intense training during and after pregnancy in top-level athletes. *Scand. J. Med. Sci. Sports*, 15:79, 2005.

Kemi, O.J., et al.: Moderate vs. high exercise intensity: differential effects on aerobic fitness, cardiomyocyte contractility, and endothelial function. *Cardiovasc. Res.*, 67:161, 2005.

Keytel, L.R., et al.: Prediction of energy expenditure from heart rate monitoring during submaximal exercise. *J. Sports Sci.*, 23:289, 2005.

Koch, L.G., et al.: Test of the principle of initial value in rat genetic models of exercise capacity. *Am. J. Physiol. Regul. Integr. Comp. Physiol.*, 288:R466, 2005.

Kraemer, W.J., et al.: Effects of concurrent resistance and aerobic training on load-bearing performance and the Army physical fitness test. *Mil. Med.*, 169:994, 2004.

Larsson, L., Lindqvist, P.G.: Low-impact exercise during pregnancy—a study of safety. *Acta. Obstet. Gynecol. Scand.*, 84:34, 2005.

Lawton, T., et al.: The effect of continuous repetition training and intra-set rest training on bench press strength and power. *J. Sports Med. Phys. Fitness*, 44:361, 2004.

Lee, C.M., et al.: Influence of short-term endurance exercise training on heart rate variability. *Med. Sci. Sports Exerc.*, 35:961, 2003.

Lee, I-M., et al.: Physical activity and coronary heart disease in women: is "no pain no gain" passé? *JAMA*, 285:1447, 2001.

Mador, M.J., et al.: Endurance and strength training in patients with COPD. *Chest*, 125:2036, 2004.

Magel, J.R., et al.: Metabolic and cardiovascular adjustment to arm training. *J. Appl. Physiol.*, 45:75, 1978.

Matsakas, A., et al.: Short-term endurance training results in a muscle-specific decrease of myostatin mRNA content in the rat. *Acta. Physiol. Scand.*, 183:299, 2005.

Mayo, M.J., et al.: Exercise-induced weight loss preferentially reduces abdominal fat. *Med. Sci. Sports Exerc.* 35:207, 2003.

McArdle, W.D., et al.: Specificity of run training on $\dot{V}O_{2max}$ and heart rate changes during running and swimming. *Med. Sci. Sports*, 10:16, 1978.

McConnell, A.K., Sharpe, G.R.: The effect of inspiratory muscle training upon maximum lactate steady-state and blood lactate concentration. *Eur. J. Appl. Physiol.*, 94:277, 2005.

McMillan, K., et al.: Lactate threshold responses to a season of professional British youth soccer. *Br. J. Sports Med.*, 39:432, 2005.

Messonnier, L., et al.: Are the effects of training on fat metabolism involved in the improvement of performance during high-intensity exercise? *Eur. J. Appl. Physiol.*, 94:434, 2005.

Meyer, T., et al.: A conceptual framework for performance diagnosis and training prescription from submaximal gas exchange parameters—theory and application. *Int. J. Sports Med.*, 26 Suppl 1:S38, 2005.

Mizunoya, W., et al.: Dietary conjugated linoleic acid increases endurance capacity and fat oxidation in mice during exercise. *Lipids*, 40:265, 2005.

Morris, S.N., Johnson, N.R.: Exercise during pregnancy: a critical appraisal of the literature. *J. Reprod. Med.*, 50:181, 2005.

Murtagh, E.M., et al.: The effects of 60 minutes of brisk walking per week, accumulated in two different patterns, on cardiovascular risk. *Prev. Med.*, 41:92, 2005.

Neary, J.P., et al.: Effects of taper on endurance cycling capacity and single muscle fiber properties. *Med. Sci. Sports Exerc.*, 35:1875, 2003.

Newcomer, B.R., et al.: Exercise over-stress and maximal muscle oxidative metabolism: a 31P magnetic resonance spectroscopy case report. *Br. J. Sports Med.*, 39:302, 2005.

Ogonovszky, H., et al.: The effects of moderate, strenuous, and overtraining on oxidative stress markers and DNA repair in rat liver. *Can. J. Appl. Physiol.*, 30:186, 2005.

Parise, G., et al.: Antioxidant enzyme activity is up-regulated after unilateral resistance exercise training in older adults. *Free Radic. Biol. Med.*, 39:289, 2005.

Pechar, G.S., et al.: Specificity of cardiorespiratory adaptation to bicycle and treadmill training. *J. Appl. Physiol.*, 36:753, 1974.

Perseghin, G.: Muscle lipid metabolism in the metabolic syndrome. *Curr. Opin. Lipidol.*, 16:416, 2005.

Persinger, R.C., et al.: Consistency of the talk test for exercise prescription. *Med. Sci. Sports Exerc.*, 36:1632, 2004.

Plumm, B.M., et al.: The athlete's heart: a meta-analysis of cardiac structure. *Circulation*, 101:336, 2000.

Rankinen, T., et al.: The human gene map for performance and health-related fitness phenotypes: the 2003 update. *Med. Sci. Sports Exerc.*, 36:1451, 2004.

Rhea, M.R., Alderman, B.L.: A meta-analysis of periodized versus nonperiodized strength and power training programs. *Res. Q. Exerc. Sport*, 75:413, 2004.

Ricardo, D.R., et al.: Initial and final exercise heart rate transients: influence of gender, aerobic fitness, and clinical status. *Chest*, 127:318, 2005.

Robergs, R.A., et al.: Biochemistry of exercise-induced metabolic acidosis. *Am. J. Physiol. Regul. Integr. Comp. Physiol.*, 287:R502, 2004.

Scharhag, J., et al.: Does prolonged cycling of moderate

intensity affect immune cell function? *Br. J. Sports Med.*, 39:171, 2005.

Skew, C.D., et al.: Skeletal muscle phenotype is associated with exercise tolerance in patients with peripheral arterial disease. *J. Vasc. Surg.*, 41:802, 2005.

Stanton, R., et al.: The effect of short-term Swiss ball training on core stability and running economy. *J. Strength Cond. Res.*, 18:522, 2004.

Stewart, K.J.: Exercise training and the cardiovascular consequences of type 2 diabetes and hypertension: plausible mechanisms for improving cardiovascular health. *JAMA*, 288:1622, 2002.

Taivassalo, T., Haller, R.G.: Implications of exercise training in mtDNA defects—use it or lose it? *Biochim. Biophys. Acta.*, 1659:221, 2004.

Tanasescu, M., et al.: Exercise type and intensity in relation to coronary heart disease in men. *JAMA*, 288:1994, 2002.

Teran-Garcia, M., et al.: Hepatic lipase gene variant -514C>T is associated with lipoprotein and insulin sensitivity response to regular exercise: The HERITAGE Family Study. *Diabetes*, 2005; 54:2251, 2005.

Timmons, J.A., et al.: Human muscle gene expression responses to endurance training provide a novel perspective on Duchenne muscular dystrophy. *FASEB J.*, 19:750, 2005.

Weissgerber, T.L., et al.: The role of regular physical activity in preeclampsia prevention. *Med. Sci. Sports Exerc.*, 36:2024, 2004.

Weltman, A., et al.: Exercise training at and above lactate threshold in previously untrained women. *Int. J. Sports Med.*, 13:257, 1992.

Weltman, A., et al.: Repeated bouts of exercise alter the blood lactate-RPE relation. *Med. Sci. Sports Exerc.*, 30:1113, 1998.

Willardson, J.M., Bressel, E.: Predicting a 10 repetition maximum for the free weight parallel squat using the 45 degrees angled leg press. *J. Strength Cond. Res.*, 18:567, 2004.

Wolfarth, B., et al.: The human gene map for performance and health-related fitness phenotypes: the 2004 update. *Med. Sci. Sports Exerc.*, 37:881, 2005.

Zaryski, C., Smith, D.J.: Training principles and issues for ultra-endurance athletes. *Curr. Sports Med. Rep.*, 4:165, 2005.

CHAPTER OUTLINE

CHAPTER OBJECTIVES

- Describe the following four methods to assess muscular strength: (1) cable tensiometry, (2) dynamometry, (3) one-repetition maximum (1-RM), and (4) computer-assisted isokinetic dynamometry.

- Outline the procedure to assess 1-RM for the bench press and leg press.

- Explain how to ensure test standardization and fairness when evaluating muscular strength.

- Compare absolute and relative upper- and lower-body muscular strength in men and women.

- Define concentric, eccentric, and isometric muscle actions, including examples of each.

- Recommend appropriate frequency, overload, and sets and repetitions for dynamic exercise resistance training.

- Explain the specificity of training response for muscular strength related to enhanced performance in sports and occupational tasks.

- Compare isokinetic resistance training to conventional dynamic and static resistance training.

- Describe the rationale for plyometric training to improve muscular strength and power, and give examples of exercises used for this purpose.

- Indicate how psychological and muscular factors influence maximum strength capacity.

- Outline the major physiologic adaptations to resistance training.

- Develop a circuit resistance training program to improve muscular strength and aerobic fitness simultaneously.

- Describe tests to assess muscular endurance of the abdominals and chest-shoulder areas.

- Describe delayed-onset muscle soreness (DOMS) related to (1) type of exercise most frequently associated with DOMS, (2) best way to minimize DOMS effects when beginning a training program, and (3) cellular factors related to DOMS.

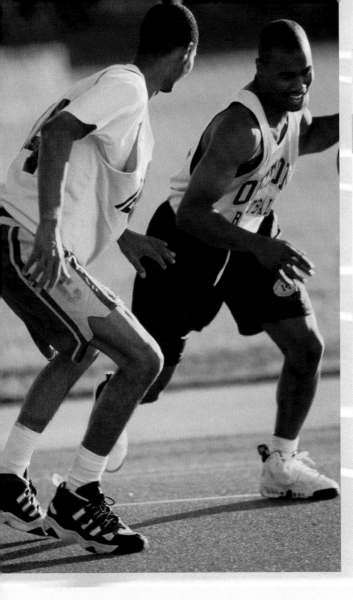

Training Muscles to Become Stronger

PART 1 •
Muscular Strength: Measurement and Improvement

Weightlifting began as a spectator sport in America in the early 1840s practiced by "strong-men" showcasing their prowess in traveling carnivals and sideshows. By the mid-1880s, measuring muscular strength became a popular way to evaluate an individual's physical fitness, particularly in schools and colleges. In 1897 at a meeting of College Gymnasium Directors, strength contests were established to determine overall body strength based on back, leg, arm, and chest strength. The first six colleges to participate included Amherst College, Columbia University, Harvard University, The University of Minnesota, Dickinson College, and Wesleyan College. The overall winner of the competition was Harvard followed closely by Columbia. By the mid-1900s, physical culture specialists, body builders, competitive weight lifters, field-event athletes, and some wrestlers used weightlifting exercises. Research in the late 1950s and early 1960s showed that muscle-strengthening exercises did not reduce movement speed or flexibility as previously believed.

In the following sections, we explore the underlying rationale for strength (resistance) training, including acute and chronic physiologic adjustments as muscles become stronger with training.

FOUNDATIONS FOR STUDYING MUSCULAR STRENGTH

The inclusion of strength development programs as part of athletic training regimens is not new; it prepared men for warfare in ancient China, Greece, and Rome. When the ancient Olympic games first began in 776 B.C., athletes trained nearly year-round and incorporated muscle-strengthening exercises into their training routines.

The scientific foundations for strength training for athletes began with the Chinese in 3600 B.C. In the Chou dynasty (1122–249 B.C.), conscripts had to pass weight-lifting tests before they became soldiers. Weight training also took place in ancient Egypt and India; sculptures and illustrations depict athletes training with heavy stone weights. Women also practiced weight training; wall mosaics recovered from Roman villas showed young girls exercising with hand-held weights. During the "Age of Strength" in the 6th century, weight lifting competitions often took place between soldiers and athletes. Galen, the famous early Greek physician (see Chapter 1), refers to exercising with weights (halters) in his insightful treatise, *The Preservation of Health*.

The quest to develop muscular strength led to different systems of resistance training. The first modern text detailing a strength training system appears to be the 1561 text by Sir Thomas Elyot entitled *The Boke Named The Gouenour*. Elyot's treatise details a curriculum of study, including intellectual and artistic pursuits and physical education, about the role of gymnastics and strength development standards to which a "governor" (landed gentry) should aspire. In the 1860s, Archibald MacLaren, a Scotsman, compiled the first system of physical training with dumbbells and barbells for use by the British army.

OBJECTIVES OF RESISTANCE TRAINING

Resistance training and strength development, besides having a theoretical basis, apply to six main areas:

1. Weight lifting and power lifting competition (who is strongest?)
2. Body building (maximize muscular development for aesthetic goals)
3. General strength training (fitness and health enhancement)
4. Physical therapy (rehabilitation from injury or disease)
5. Sport-specific resistance training (maximize sport performance)
6. Muscle physiology (understanding muscle function and structure)

RESISTANCE TRAINING VOCABULARY

Terms and jargon abound in the area of resistance training, yet certain terms consistently appear in the research literature and popular writings about resistance training methods and outcomes. **Table 14.1** defines common resistance training terms.

TYPES OF MUSCLE ACTION

Three types of muscle action include:

1. **Concentric action** (also called miometric) represents the most common form of muscle action; it occurs in dynamic activities where muscles shorten and produce tension through the range of motion (ROM). **Figure 14.1A** illustrates a concentric muscle action by raising a dumbbell from the extended to flexed elbow position. Because a concentric muscle action shortens the muscle, the word *"contraction"* frequently describes this process.
2. **Eccentric action** (also called lengthening, stretching, or plyometric) occurs when external resistance exceeds muscle force, and muscle lengthens as tension develops. Figure 14.1B shows a weight slowly lowered against the force of gravity. The muscles of the upper arm increase in length as they brake to prevent the weight from crashing to the floor.
3. **Isometric action** (also called static or stationary) occurs when a muscle attempts to shorten but cannot overcome the external resistance. Considerable force

Table 14·1	Definition of Selected Terms Apppearing in the Resistance Training Literature

1. **Cheating.** Breaking from strict form when performing an exercise (e.g., rather than maintaining an erect upper body when performing a standing arm curl, a slight body swing at the start the movement allows the person to lift a heavier weight or the same weight more times). Cheating increases injury risk if performed improperly.
2. **Circuit Resistance Training (CRT).** Series of resistance training exercises performed in sequence with minimal rest between exercises. More frequent repetitions with less resistance (usually 40% to 50% of 1-RM) stimulate the cardiovascular system to produce an aerobic training effect.
3. **Concentric Action.** Muscle shortening during force application.
4. **Dynamic Constant External Resistance (DCER) Training.** Resistance training where external resistance or weight does not change; joint flexion and extension occurs with each repetition. Formerly (but incorrectly) referred to as "isotonic" exercise.
5. **Eccentric Action.** Muscle lengthening occurs during force application.
6. **Exercise Intensity.** Muscle force expressed as a percentage of muscle's maximum force-generating capacity or some level of maximum.
7. **Isokinetic Action.** Muscle action performed at constant angular limb velocity.
8. **Isometric Action.** Muscle action without noticeable change in muscle length.
9. **Maximal Voluntary Muscle Action (MVMA).** Maximal force generated in one repetition (1-RM), or performing a series of submaximal actions to momentary failure.
10. **Muscular Endurance.** Sustaining maximum (or submaximum) force; often determined by assessing maximum number of exercise repetitions at a percentage of maximum strength.
11. **Overload.** A muscle acting against a resistance normally not encountered (unaccustomed stress).
12. **Periodization.** Variation in training volume and intensity over a specified time period; goal to prevent staleness while peaking physiologically for competition.
13. **Plyometrics.** Resistance training involving eccentric-to-concentric actions performed quickly so a muscle stretches slightly prior to the concentric action; utilizes stretch reflex to augment the muscle's force-generating capacity.
14. **Power.** Rate of performing work (Force × Distance ÷ Time, or Force × Velocity). Power applied to weightlifting relates to the mass lifted times the vertical distance it moves, divided by the time to complete the movement. If 100 pounds moves vertically 3 feet in 1 second, then the power generated = 100 lb × 3 ft ÷ 1 s or 300 ft-lb·s^{-1}.
15. **Progressive Overload.** Incrementally increasing the stress placed on a muscle to produce greater force or greater endurance.
16. **Range of Motion (ROM).** Maximum range of movement through an arc of a joint.
17. **Repetition.** One complete exercise movement, usually consisting of concentric and eccentric muscle actions or one complete isometric muscle action.
18. **Repetition Maximum (RM).** Greatest force generated for one repetition of a movement (1-RM), or predetermined number of repetitions (e.g., 5-RM or 10-RM).
19. **Set.** Pre-established number of repetitions performed.
20. **Sticking Point.** Region in an exercise movement (against a set resistance) that provides the greatest difficulty to complete the movement.
21. **Strength.** Maximum force-generating capacity of a muscle or group of muscles.
22. **Torque.** Force that produces a turning, twisting, or rotary movement in any plane about an axis (i.e., movement of bones about a joint); commonly expressed in newton-meters (Nm).
23. **Training Volume.** Total work performed in a single training session.
24. **Variable Resistance Training.** Training with equipment that uses a lever arm, cam, hydraulic system, or pulley to alter the resistance to match the increases and decreases in a muscle's capacity throughout a joint's ROM.

generates during an isometric action without noticeable muscle lengthening or shortening or joint movement. Figure 14.1C illustrates an isometric muscular action against an immovable bar.

The term **isotonic** commonly describes concentric and eccentric muscle actions because movement occurs in both cases. This term comes from the Greek

Questions & Notes

List 2 objectives of resistance training.

1.

2.

List the 3 types of muscle action.

1.

2.

3.

Define the following terms:

Eccentric:

Concentric:

Muscular endurance:

Torque:

FOR YOUR INFORMATION

Objectives of Resistance Training for Overall Fitness and Sports Performance
- Increase maximal strength
- Increase explosive power (achieve maximum force rapidly)
- Improve repetitive rate of maximal power output
- Improve repetitive rate of submaximal power output (muscular endurance)
- Hypertrophy muscle fibers and connective tissue harness

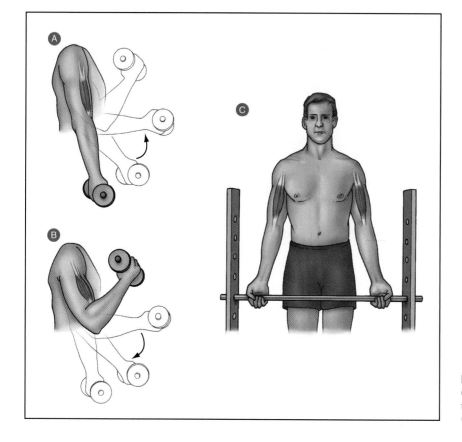

Figure 14.1 Muscular force during **(A)** concentric (shortening), **(B)** eccentric (lengthening), and **(C)** isometric (static) actions.

isotonos (*iso*, meaning the same or equal; *tonos*, meaning tension or strain). This term should not be applied to most dynamic muscle actions that involve movement because the muscle's force-generating capacity varies as the joint angle changes; thus, force output does not remain constant at the same percentage of maximum through the ROM.

Dynamic constant external resistance (DCER) refers to resistance training where external resistance or weight does not change, but lifting (concentric) and lowering (eccentric) phases occur during each repetition. *DCER implies that the external weight or resistance remains constant throughout the movement.*

MEASUREMENT OF MUSCULAR STRENGTH

Four methods commonly assess **muscular strength** (defined as the maximum force, tension, or torque generated by a muscle or muscle groups): cable tensiometry, dynamometry, one-repetition maximum, and computer-assisted electromechanical and isokinetic determinations.

Cable Tensiometry

Figure 14.2A shows how a **cable tensiometer** assesses static muscular force during knee extension. Increased force on the cable depresses a riser over which the cable

passes; this deflects the pointer and indicates the amount of force applied. The application of the tensiometer for strength measurements differs considerably from its original use for measuring tension on steel cables linking various parts of an airplane.

Cable tensiometry isolates a muscle at a specific joint angle to determine strength before and after training and rehabilitation. This strength assessment provides a unique advantage. One can measure force capacity at different points of the movement phase, so the strength (or weakness) of particular muscles can be determined at diverse joint angles throughout the ROM. This cannot be accomplished with standard weight-lifting equipment.

Dynamometry

Figures 14.2B and C display hand-grip and back-lift **dynamometers** to assess static strength. Both devices operate on the principle of compression. Application of external force to the dynamometer compresses a steel spring and moves a pointer. By knowing how much force must move the pointer a given distance, one can determine how much external "static" force has been applied to the dynamometer.

One-Repetition Maximum

The **one-repetition maximum (1-RM)** technique refers to a dynamic method to assess muscular strength. To test **1-**

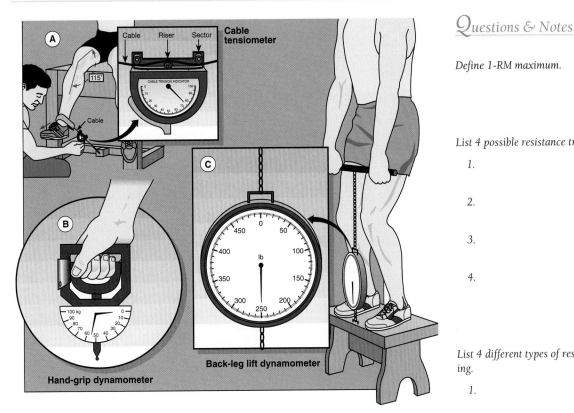

Figure 14.2 Measurement of static strength by **(A)** cable tensiometer, **(B)** hand-grip dynamometer, and **(C)** back-leg lift dynamometer.

RM for single or multiple muscle groups, choose the initial weight close to, but below maximum lifting capacity (see Close Up *How to Assess and Evaluate One-Repetition Maximum for Bench Press and Leg Press* on page 474). Depending on the muscle group, the weight increment usually ranges from 1 to 5 kg. The 1-RM maneuver requires concentric and eccentric muscle actions, but only the concentric phase of the action evaluates 1-RM.

In addition to the 1-RM (maximum) method, **Figure 14.3** illustrates two submaximal methods (and the percentage of maximum each represents) to evaluate a muscle's force- and power-generating capacity. In these tests, the greatest amount of weight lifted 5 or 10 times becomes the repetition maximum to assess strength. The measurement procedure in these cases assesses 5-RM (generally 90% of maximum) or 10-RM (about 78% of maximum). The 5-RM and 10-RM methods provide appropriate markers of muscular strength, particularly when testing children and older adults where maximal lifting may be contraindicated.

Estimating 1-RM Strength Using Submaximum Repetitions-to-Fatigue Test Scores

A strong inverse relationship exits between muscular endurance (number of repetitions-to-fatigue using a submaximum resistance) and the percentage of 1-RM lifted; that is, the heavier the load, the fewer number of repetitions performed. In situations where 1-RM testing is unwarranted or ill-advised (child/youth, older individuals, individuals with physical limitations, the poorly conditioned), 1-RM strength can be predicted using repetitions-to-fatigue with a submaximum weight.

Testing Protocol   Determine the maximum number of repetitions-to-fatigue a person can achieve at a given weight lifted. Use this number to predict the

(text continues on page 476)

Questions & Notes

Define 1-RM maximum.

List 4 possible resistance training goals.

1.

2.

3.

4.

List 4 different types of resistance training.

1.

2.

3.

4.

List 3 different types of muscle action.

1.

2.

3.

What is the most popular method for measuring strength?

Box 14–1 • CLOSE UP

HOW TO ASSESS AND EVALUATE ONE-REPETITION MAXIMUM FOR BENCH PRESS AND LEG

Muscle strength refers to a muscle's maximum force-generating capacity. The maximum weight (resistance) lifted with proper form for one repetition (1-RM) for a particular muscle action measures dynamic muscular strength. A trial-and-error approach determines the 1-RM strength value. After each successful single lift, the weight increases by 5 to 10 pounds until achieving the maximum. The individual rests 2 to 3 minutes between attempts.

The 1-RM bench press (illustrated on page 475) assesses maximum muscular strength of major muscle groups of the upper body; the leg press assesses maximum strength of major portions of the lower-body musculature. Dividing the 1-RM score by body weight (1-RM, lb ÷ body weight, lb) assesses relative muscular strength and provides a frame of reference to evaluate different body weight comparisons (see table below).

Reference Values for 1-RM Bench Press and Leg Press Expressed Relative to Body Weight[a]

	AGE, y			
Rating	**20–29**	**30–39**	**40–49**	**50–59**
Men				
Excellent				
Bench Press	>1.26	>1.08	>0.97	>0.86
Leg Press	>2.08	>1.88	>1.76	>1.66
Good				
Bench Press	1.17–1.25	1.01–1.07	0.91–0.96	0.81–0.85
Leg Press	2.00–2.07	1.80–1.87	1.70–1.75	1.60–1.65
Average				
Bench Press	0.97–1.16	0.86–1.00	0.78–0.90	0.70–0.80
Leg Press	1.83–1.99	1.63–1.79	1.56–1.69	1.46–1.59
Fair				
Bench Press	0.88–0.96	0.79–0.85	0.72–0.77	0.65–0.69
Leg Press	1.65–1.82	1.55–1.62	1.50–1.55	1.40–1.45
Poor				
Bench Press	<0.87	<0.78	<0.71	<0.60
Leg Press	<1.64	<1.54	<1.49	<1.39
Women				
Excellent				
Bench Press	>0.78	>0.66	>0.61	>0.54
Leg Press	>1.63	>1.42	>1.32	>1.26
Good				
Bench Press	0.72–0.77	0.62–0.65	0.57–0.60	0.51–0.53
Leg Press	1.54–1.62	1.35–1.41	1.26–1.31	1.13–1.25
Average				
Bench Press	0.59–0.71	0.53–0.61	0.48–0.56	0.43–0.50
Leg Press	1.35–1.53	1.20–1.34	1.12–1.25	0.99–1.12
Fair				
Bench Press	0.53–0.58	0.49–0.52	0.44–0.47	0.40–0.42
Leg Press	1.25–1.34	1.13–1.19	1.06–1.11	0.86–0.98
Poor				
Bench Press	<0.52	<0.48	<0.43	<0.39
Leg Press	<1.25	<1.12	<1.05	<0.85

Adapted from: Cooper Institute for Aerobics Research, 1997.
[a]Score = 1-RM, lb ÷ Body weight, lb.

Box 14–1 • **CLOSE UP** *(Continued)*

PROCEDURES FOR BENCH PRESS TEST

Muscle Groups

Shoulder flexors and adductors; elbow extensors.

Equipment

Barbell or bench press station on a single- or multi-station resistance machine.

Starting Position

1. Overhand (pronated) grip, slightly wider than shoulder-width apart.
2. Lay supine on a bench, feet on the floor straddling the bench.
3. Signal a spotter to position the bar at arms length above the chest with arms extended.

Movement

1. Downward movement: lower the bar until it touches the chest.
2. Upward movement: push the bar up to full elbow extension while maintaining body position without arching the back. The spotter maintains grip on the bar throughout the movement without offering assistance; also helps to place the bar on the supports.

PROCEDURES FOR LEG PRESS TEST

Muscle Groups

Knee extensors and hip extensors.

Equipment

Leg press on a single- or multi-station resistance machine.

Starting Position

1. Sit with the legs parallel and the feet on the machine's foot rests.
2. Grasp the seat's handle.

Movement

1. Forward movement: push the foot rests steadily forward; do not forcefully lock out the knees during extension.
2. Backward movement: move the footrests slowly back to the starting position.

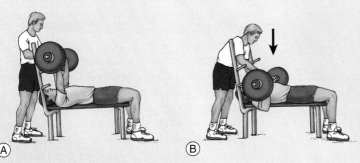

Beginning (**A**), downward (**B**), and upward (**C**) positions for the bench press.

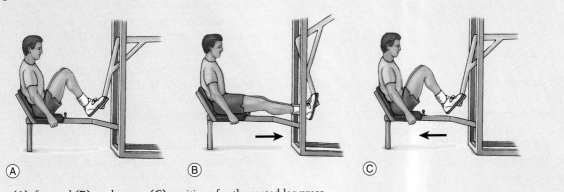

Beginning (**A**), forward (**B**), and return (**C**) positions for the seated leg press.

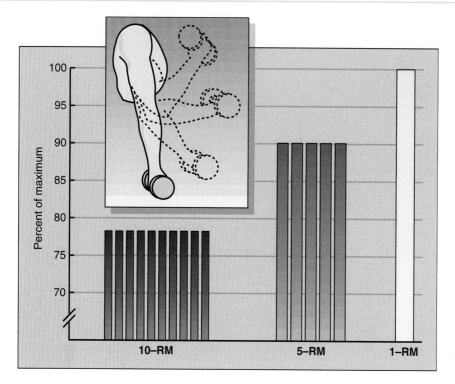

Figure 14.3 Three methods to assess force-generating capacity in a dynamic movement.

1-RM. [Refer to the Close Up, *How To Assign Load (Resistance) and Repetition Number to Achieve Different Training Goals* for procedures to determine the maximum number of repetitions on page 478.] Use the data in **Table 14.2** derived from several sources to determine 1-RM as follows:

1. Read across the Max Reps (RM) row and find the number of repetitions completed.
2. Read down the column to the load lifted (weight completed, in lb).
3. Read across the row to the far left to find the estimated 1-RM.

An example follows for an individual who performs a 5-RM test and lifts 174 pounds.

1. Read across the Max Reps (RM) row and find the number 5 (number of repetitions-to-fatigue).
2. Read down the column to the number 174 (the load lifted in lb).
3. Read across the row to the far left, and find the estimated 1-RM (in this example, 200 lb).

The data in Table 14.2 can also estimate the load (weight in lb) at a given percentage of 1-RM. For example, find the 1-RM load in column 1 (e.g., 120 lb); go across to the desired percentage in row 2 (%1-RM; 80%) and find the weight (in lb) corresponding to that percentage in the intersecting cell (in this example, 96 lb).

Computer-Assisted Electromechanical and Isokinetic Determinations

Microprocessor technology integrated with exercise equipment quantifies muscular force and power during a variety of movements. Modern instrumentation measures force, acceleration, and velocity of body segments in various movement patterns. Force platforms measure the external application of muscular force by limbs during jumping. Other electromechanical devices measure forces generated during all movement phases of cycling, rowing, supine bench press, seated and upright leg press, and exercises for other trunk, arm, and leg movements.

An **isokinetic dynamometer**, an electromechanical instrument with a speed-controlling mechanism, accelerates to a preset, constant speed with applied force regardless of the force exerted on the movement arm. *Maximum force (or any percentage of maximum effort) can be applied during all phases of movement at a constant velocity.* A load cell within the dynamometer continuously records the applied force to calculate average force, power output, and total work throughout the ROM.

The interface of computer technology with mechanical devices provides valuable data for evaluating muscle function and prescribing exercise. Many devotees who still consider a maximum lift (1-RM) as the best criterion to assess overall muscular strength reject technologic advances that assess strength by computer. The argument to

Table 14·2 — Estimating 1-RM from Submaximum Load (Weight) and Number of Repetitions

To use the table, do the following: (1) read across the Max Reps (RM) row and find the number of repetitions completed; (2) read down the column to the load (weight completed, lb) lifted; (3) read across the row to the far left to find the estimated 1-RM.

Max Reps (RM)	1	2	3	4	5	6	7	8	9	10	12	15
%1-RM	100	95	93	90	87	85	83	80	77	75	67	65
Load lifted (weight completed, lb)												
10	10	10	9	9	9	9	8	8	8	8	7	7
20	20	9	19	18	17	17	17	16	15	15	13	13
30	30	9	28	27	26	26	25	24	23	23	20	20
40	40	38	37	36	35	34	33	32	31	30	27	26
50	50	48	47	45	44	43	42	40	39	38	34	33
60	60	57	56	54	52	51	50	48	46	45	40	39
70	70	67	65	63	61	60	58	56	54	53	47	46
80	80	76	74	72	70	68	66	64	62	60	54	52
90	90	86	84	81	78	77	75	72	69	68	60	59
100	100	95	93	90	87	85	83	80	77	75	67	65
110	110	105	102	99	96	94	91	88	85	83	74	72
120	120	114	112	108	104	102	100	96	92	90	80	78
130	130	124	121	117	113	111	108	104	100	98	87	85
140	140	133	130	126	122	119	116	112	108	105	94	91
150	150	143	140	135	131	128	125	120	116	113	101	98
160	160	152	149	144	139	136	133	128	123	120	107	104
170	170	162	158	153	148	145	141	136	131	128	114	111
180	180	171	167	162	157	153	149	144	139	135	121	117
190	190	181	177	171	165	162	158	152	146	143	127	124
200	200	190	186	180	174	170	166	160	154	150	134	130
210	210	200	195	189	183	179	174	168	162	158	141	137
220	220	209	205	198	191	187	183	176	169	165	147	143
230	230	219	214	207	200	196	191	184	177	173	154	150
240	240	228	223	216	209	204	199	192	185	180	161	156
250	250	238	233	225	218	213	208	200	193	188	168	163
260	260	247	242	234	226	221	206	208	200	195	174	169
270	270	257	251	243	235	230	224	216	208	203	181	176
280	280	266	260	252	244	238	232	224	216	210	188	182
290	290	276	270	261	252	247	241	232	223	218	194	189
300	300	285	279	270	261	255	249	240	231	225	201	195
310	310	295	288	279	270	264	257	248	239	233	208	202
320	320	304	298	288	278	272	266	256	246	240	214	208
330	330	314	307	297	287	281	274	264	254	248	221	215
340	340	323	316	306	296	289	282	272	262	255	228	221
350	350	333	326	315	305	298	291	280	270	263	235	228
360	360	342	335	324	313	306	299	288	277	270	241	234
370	370	352	344	333	322	315	307	296	285	278	248	241
380	380	361	353	342	331	323	315	304	293	285	255	247
390	390	371	363	351	339	332	324	312	300	293	261	254
400	400	380	372	360	348	340	332	320	308	300	268	260

From Baechle, T.R., et al.: Resistance Training. In: *Essentials of Strength Training and Conditioning.* 2nd Ed. Champaign, IL: Human Kinetics Press, 2000.

support isokinetic methodology maintains that muscle strength dynamics involve considerably more than a final outcome from a 1-RM, 5-RM, or 10-RM lift. Even if two people achieve the same 1-RM, the force-time curves could considerably differ. Differences in force dynamics (e.g., time to peak tension or rate of force development) reflect differences in how neuromuscular factors interact. The newer cyber-technologies assess many components of muscle dynamics, not *just* the maximum weight an individual can bench press or squat.

Box 14-2 • CLOSE UP

HOW TO ASSIGN LOAD (RESISTANCE) AND REPETITION NUMBER TO ACHIEVE DIFFERENT TRAINING GOALS

Assigning combinations of load (resistance) and repetition number (reps) constitutes the most important aspects of establishing a resistance training program. Research and practical experience indicate that resistances producing a maximum of 6 or less reps elicit the greatest increase in strength and maximal power output. Resistances that produce 10 to 15 or even 20 and above reps greatly impact muscular endurance development. This knowledge makes it possible to specifically train for a desired type of muscular performance.

IDENTIFYING TRAINING GOALS

Age, physical maturity, training history, and psychological and physical tolerance should formulate training goals or program design. Training goals center around four major objectives:

1. **Strength development** of specific muscle groups (i.e. upper and/or lower body, abdomen, back) for purposes relating to sports or job performance

2. **Power development** for specific sports performance (i.e., running back in football, basketball rebounder, high jumper, shot putter)
3. **Hypertrophic development** for appearance or to alter body size (i.e., weight gain) and to improve overall muscular strength
4. **Muscle endurance development** related to enhanced job or sports performance

Specific program characteristics apply to each of the above resistance training objectives (**Table 1**).

ASSIGNING LOAD AND REPETITION

Table 2 recommends specific repetition maximums (RM) and load, expressed as a percentage of 1-RM (%1-RM).

The following 5-step sequence to determine loads and repetition number for individualized training makes use of data from Table 2:

Table 1	Program Characteristics for Different Types of Training		
Strength Training	**Power Training**	**Hypertrophy Training**	**Endurance Training**
• Choice of exercise and movement patterns need to be stressed • Usually emphasized early in training or during off-season • Applies heavy loads with few repetitions (usually ≤6-RM) • Longer rest periods between sets required • Usually includes 1–4 sets	• Choice of exercise and movement patterns need to be stressed • Usually emphasized early in training or during off-season • High-intensity (usually <10-RM) resistance is varied over time • Applies more repetitions than strength training, but rarely more than 10-RM • Moderate amount of rest between sets • Usually includes moderate to high number of sets (4–10)	• Uses a variety of exercise choices • Includes many isolation exercises • Moderate to high resistance/repetitions used (6- to 12-RM) • Often uses back-to-back sets of same muscles • Large number of sets used (>3)	• Choice of exercise and movement patterns need to be stressed • Low load, high repetitions used (12- to 20-RM) • Short rest periods between sets • Two to three sets

Box 14–2 •   CLOSE UP *(Continued)*

1. Determine the 1-RM in kg or lb as follows:
   a. Warm-up (complete 5–7 reps) using a light resistance
   b. Rest for 1–2 minutes; perform slow stretching
   c. Increase load by 10–20 lb (4–9 kg) or 8%–10% for upper-body exercise and by 30–40 lb (14–18 kg) or 10%–20% for lower-body exercise; Complete 3–10 reps; stop at 10 reps
   d. Rest for 1–2 minutes; perform slow stretching
   e. Increase load above previous level (step c above), attempting to approach "near" maximum; increase 10–20 lb (4–9 kg) or 8%–10% for upper-body exercise and 30–40 lb (14–18 kg) or 10%–20% for lower-body exercise; complete as many reps as possible (at this load, maximum reps will probably range between 2–6)
   f. Rest 2–3 minutes; perform slow stretching
   g. Increase load above previous level (step e above), attempting to approach "near" maximum; increase 10–20 lb (4–9 kg) or 8%–10% for upper-body exercise and 30–40 lb (14–18 kg) or 10%–20% for lower-body exercise. Complete as many reps as possible (at this load repetitions will probably range between 1–4)
   h. Rest 2–3 minutes; perform slow stretching
   i. If previous load produced ≥1-RM, rest 2–3 minutes (perform slow stretching). Increase load 5–10 lb (2–4 kg) or 1%–5% and attempt again. If previous load could not be completed one time, rest 2–3 minutes (perform slow stretching) and decrease load by 5–10 lb (2–4 kg) or 1%–5% for upper-body exercise and by 10–20 lb (4–9 kg) for lower-body exercise; attempt lift again trying to achieve the 1-RM.
2. Determine training goal(s) [e.g., strength, power, hypertrophy, endurance]
3. Determine appropriate *repetition number* for the specific training goal
   a. (see Table 2)
4. Determine specific *%1-RM* based on repetition number
   a. (see Table 2)

Table 2	Load:Repetition Continuum for Specific Training Goals	
Training Goal	**Load (%1-RM)**	**Goal Repetitions**
Strength	≥85	≤6
High Power	80–90	1–2
Low Power	75–85	3–5
Hypertrophy	67–85	6–12
Endurance	≤67	≥12

From Baechle, T.R., et al.: Resistance Training. Chapter 18. In: Baechle, T.R., and Earle, R.W. (eds.). *Essentials of Strength Training and Conditioning.* 2nd Ed. Champaign, IL: Human Kinetics Press, 2000.

5. Determine training load (weight)
   a. Multiple 1-RM load by the %1-RM (expressed as a decimal) selected for training

EXAMPLES

A person's training goal is to achieve muscle hypertrophy, and 1-RM was determined at 200 pounds.

Follow the 5-step procedure outlined previously to determine load and repetition number:

---

1. **Determine 1-RM**
   1-RM = 200 lb
2. **Determine training goal**
   Muscle hypertrophy
3. **Determine appropriate repetition number** for the specific training goal (see Table 2)
   Repetition number is 6–12; use 8
4. **Determine specific %1-RM** based on repetition number (see Table 2)
   For goal repetitions 6–12, the %1-RM is 67%–85%; use 75%
5. **Determine training load** (weight); multiply 1-RM load by the %1-RM (expressed as a decimal) selected for training
   Training load = 200 × 0.75 = 150 lbs

This person would train using 8 reps with a weight of 150 pounds. Retest the 1-RM as improvement progresses (every 2 weeks or so) to adjust the training load.

REFERENCES

Baechle, T.R., and Earle, R.W. (eds.): *Essentials of Strength Training and Conditioning.* 2nd Ed. Champaign, IL: Human Kinetics Press, 2000.

Fleck, S.J., and Kraemer, W.J.: *Designing Resistance Training*

Programs. 2nd Ed. Champaign, IL: Human Kinetics Press, 1997.

Kraemer, W.J., and Koziris, L.P.: Muscle strength training: Techniques and considerations. *Phys. Ther. Pract.,* 2:54, 1992.

STRENGTH TESTING CONSIDERATIONS

The following factors need to be considered when strength testing, regardless of methodology:

1. Give standardized instructions.
2. Allow a warm-up of uniform duration (e.g., 3 to 5 min) and intensity (e.g., 50% of previously established 1-RM).
3. Provide adequate practice several days before testing to minimize "learning" that could compromise initial results or inflate evaluation of true training effects.
4. Ensure constancy of limb position and/or measurement angle.
5. Provide several trials (repetitions) to establish a strength criterion score.
6. Administer strength tests with established high reliability (reproducibility) of scores (r > 0.85).
7. Consider individual differences in body size and composition when comparing strength scores among individuals and groups.

Physical Testing in the Occupational Setting

No *one* best measure of muscular strength exists. Each individual possesses an array of muscular strengths and powers. Often, these expressions of physiologic function and performance do not correlate highly to each other. Likewise, a person has diverse capabilities for aerobic capacity, depending on the muscle mass activated in exercise. A 12-minute run to infer aerobic capacity for fire fighting or lumbering (both requiring considerable upper-body aerobic metabolism) or a static grip or leg strength measure to evaluate the diverse dynamic strengths and powers required in such occupations is physiologically unwise in light of current knowledge about physical performance specificity. *Measurement in the occupational setting must mimic specific job tasks and measure the physiologic demands of intensity, duration, and pace.* For example, it would be inappropriate to assess the ability to carry 20 kg of firehose by measuring leg press or squat strength. Instead, a functional test that assessed the ability to carry the 20-kg hose a distance of 30 m and then ascend 20 stairs more accurately reflects the requirements of performance specificity in the occupational setting.

TRAINING MUSCLES TO BECOME STRONGER

Strengthening muscles requires adherence to exercise training principles and specific guidelines.

Overload and Intensity

Resistance training applies the **overload principle** with weights (dumbbells or barbells), immovable bars, straps, pulleys, or springs, and oil, air, and water hydraulic devices. *In each case, the muscle responds to the intensity of the overload rather than the* form *of overload.*

The amount of overload reflects a percentage of the maximum strength (1-RM) of a nonfatigued muscle or muscle group. Performing a **voluntary maximal muscle action** means the muscle must exert as much force as its *present* capacity allows. A partially fatigued muscle cannot generate the same force as a nonfatigued muscle. The last repetition to momentary failure in a set denotes a voluntary maximal muscle action. Muscular overload in resistance training usually requires such voluntary maximal muscle actions.

Three approaches (either singularly or in combination) apply muscular overload in resistance training:

1. Increase load or resistance
2. Increase number of repetitions
3. Increase speed of muscle action

The degree of muscular overload, often called training intensity, represents the most important factor in strength development; it requires training above a minimum threshold level to induce a training response. *Minimal intensity for muscular overload occurs between 60% and 70% of 1-RM.* This means that performing a large number of repetitions with light resistance (low percentage of 1-RM) produces only minimal strength improvements.

Force–Velocity Relationship

Different physical activities require different amounts of strength (force) and power. Absolute or peak force generated in a movement depends on the speed of muscle lengthening and shortening. **Figure 14.4** shows the **force–velocity relationship** for concentric and eccentric muscle actions. Muscles shorten (and lengthen) at different maximum velocities (horizontal axis of graph) depending on the load placed on them. *As the load increases, maximum shortening velocity decreases. Conversely, a muscle's force-generating capacity (vertical axis of graph) rapidly declines with increased shortening velocity.* This explains the difficulty attempting to move a heavy weight rapidly.

A shortening (concentric) action becomes a lengthening (eccentric) action when the external load exceeds a muscle's maximum isometric force capacity (noted as point 0 on the horizontal axis). In contrast to a concentric muscle action, rapid eccentric actions generate the greatest force. This may explain the relatively greater muscle damage and delayed muscle soreness accompanying a bout of eccentric exercise. Force at zero velocity of shortening (isometric action) exceeds all forces generated with concentric actions. Muscle fiber type also influences the force–velocity relationships; fast-twitch muscle fibers produce greater muscle force at fast movement speeds than slow-twitch fibers because they possess higher ATPase activity, which accelerates the breakdown of ATP. Athletes who possess a high percentage of fast-twitch fibers have a distinct performance advantage in power-type physical activities.

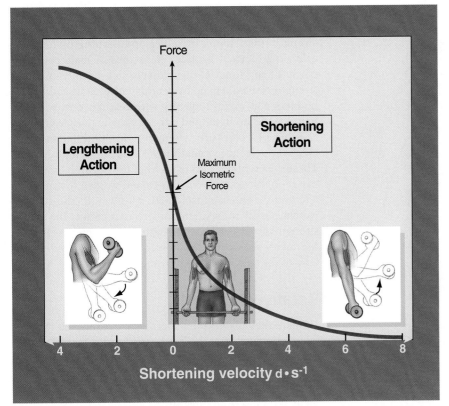

Figure 14.4 Maximum force–velocity relationship for shortening and lengthening muscle actions. Rapid shortening velocities (degrees per second, $d \cdot s^{-1}$) generate the least maximum force. Shortening velocity becomes zero (maximum isometric force) when the curve crosses the Y-axis. Force-generating capacity increases to its highest as the muscle lengthens at rapid velocities.

Power–Velocity Relationship

Figure 14.5 shows an inverted U relationship between a muscle's maximal power output and speed of limb movement during concentric muscle action. Peak power rapidly increases with increasing velocity to a **peak velocity region**. Thereafter, maximal power output decreases because of reduced maximum force at faster movement speeds (Fig. 14.4). *Each muscle group has an optimum movement speed to produce maximum power.* Similar to the force–velocity relationship, greater peak power occurs in fast-twitch fibers than in slow-twitch fibers at any velocity of movement.

Load–Repetition Relationship

The total work accomplished by muscle action depends on the load (resistance) placed on the muscle. One can perform high repetitions with light loads but few repetitions with near-maximal loads. **Figure 14.6A** shows this relationship for the full range of percentages of 1-RM. The area from 60% to 100% 1-RM represents the **strength training zone**, the training stimulus that optimizes strength improvement.

MALE AND FEMALE DIFFERENCES IN MUSCULAR STRENGTH

Two strength-testing approaches determine whether true gender differences exist in muscular strength.

Questions & Notes

List 4 factors to consider when strength testing.

 1.

 2.

 3.

 4.

Give the most important aspect of strength testing in the occupational setting.

Muscle responds to the _____ of the overload rather than the form of overload.

List 3 approaches to apply muscular overload in resistance training.

 1.

 2.

 3.

Give the minimum intensity for muscular overload to induce a training response.

As load increases, maximum shortening velocity _____.

A muscle's force-generating capacity rapidly declines with increased _____ _____.

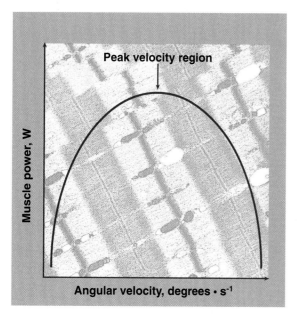

Figure 14.5 Power–velocity relationship. Power (work per unit time) increases as a function of movement velocity up to a peak velocity region. Thereafter, power decreases with further increases in angular velocity.

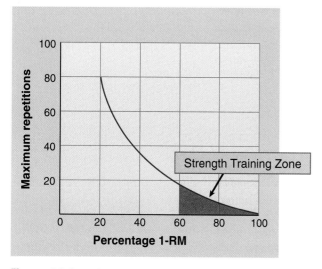

Figure 14.6 Relationship between maximum number of repetitions to failure and load at 20% to 100% 1-RM. From Siff, M.C., and Verkhoshansky, Y.V.: *Supertraining: Special Strength Training for Sporting Excellence*. Perry, OH: Strength Coach, Inc., 1997.)

1. Assess absolute strength (total force exerted)
2. Assess relative strength (force exerted related to body mass, fat-free body mass [FFM], or muscle cross-sectional area)

Absolute Strength

When comparing **absolute strength** (total force in lb or kg), men score considerably higher than women in all muscle groups regardless of test mode. Gender differences in absolute strength clearly emerge for upper-body strength evaluations; women exhibit about 50% less strength than men. In lower-body strength, females achieve 20% to 30% below the scores of male counterparts. Exceptions to these disparities usually include strength-trained female track and field athletes and bodybuilders who train diligently with resistance exercise to increase the strength (and size) of specific muscle groups.

Table 14.3 shows the strength ratios for different muscle groups (female strength score ÷ male strength score). These data represent averages from the research literature based on strength scores of men and women for concentric and eccentric muscle actions. Overall, the typical woman's total body strength represents 64% of the man's strength; for upper-body strength, women average 56% of the men's score, whereas lower-body strength averages 72% of the values achieved by men.

Relative Strength

Human skeletal muscle fibers *in vitro* (outside of the body) generate 16 to 30 Newtons (N) maximal force per square centimeter of **muscle cross-sectional area (MCSA)** regardless of gender. In the body (*in vivo*), force-output capacity varies depending on the bony lever's arrangement and muscle architecture.

Figure 14.7 compares arm flexor strength of men and women related to MCSA. The strong linear relationship (r = 0.95) suggests that individuals with the largest MCSA generate the greatest muscular force. The inset graph shows equality in strength between men and women when arm flexor strength is expressed per unit MCSA. See the accompanying Close Up on page 484 for determining MCSA.

Relative strength is computed using body mass (strength score in lb or kg ÷ body mass in lb or kg), segmental or total fat-free mass (strength score in lb or kg ÷ fat-free

	Ratio of Female Strength to Male Strength for Different Muscle Groups[a]	
Table 14·3		
MUSCLE GROUP		**STRENGTH RATIO (FEMALE ÷ MALE)**
Elbow flexors		0.55
Elbow extensors		0.48
Knee flexors		0.69
Knee extensors		0.68
Shoulder flexors		0.55
Trunk extensor and flexors		0.60
Hip extensors and flexors		0.80
Finger flexors		0.60

[a] Data represent an average of values in the literature that reported female–male data. The ratios were obtained by dividing the female mean strength for a given muscle(s) by the mean male strength score. These data can be used to (1) evaluate performance of women relative to men, (2) select first approximations of suitable loads for females based on male data, or (3) approximate male data if only female data are available.

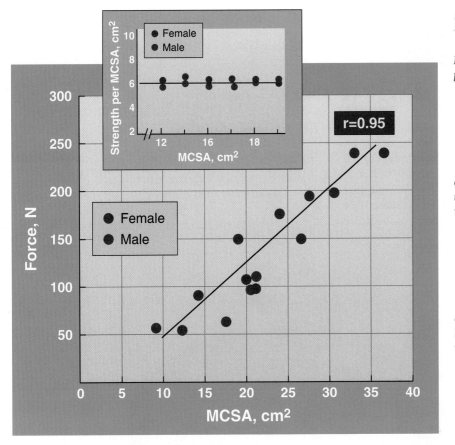

Figure 14.7 Plot of force (Newtons, N) versus muscle cross-sectional area (MCSA, cm²). Data represent elbow flexion. The inset figure shows the strength per unit MCSA. (Data from Miller, J.D., et al.: Gender differences in strength and muscle fiber characteristics. *Eur. J. Appl. Physiol.*, 66:254, 1992; and Ikai, M., and Fukunaga, R.: Calculation of muscle strength per unit cross-sectional area of human muscle by means of ultrasonic measurements. *Arbeitsphysiologie*, 26:26, 1968.)

Questions & Notes

Describe the shape of the curve of the power–velocity relationship.

Give the average percentage increase in upper-body strength for men compared to women.

Give the average percentage increase in lower-body strength for men compared to women.

Give the range of forces (N) that human muscle can generate per square centimeter of muscle cross-sectional area.

mass in lb or kg), or MCSA (strength score in lb or kg ÷ MCSA). These relative ratio scores to express strength look strange because most people more readily relate to a 225-pound bench press than a ratio expression of this weight-lifting performance. A relative score increases the "fairness" when comparing two individuals' strength performances (or the same person assessed before, during, and after a training regimen or weight-loss program).

Resistance Training for Children

Resistance training for children has gained popularity, yet its benefits and possible risks remain fertile ground for further research. Incomplete skeletal development in young children and adolescents, raises concern about the potential for bone and joint injury with heavy muscular overload. One might question whether resistance training improves strength at a relatively young age because the hormonal profile continues to develop, particularly for the tissue-building hormone testosterone. *Limited evidence indicates that closely supervised resistance training programs using concentric-only muscle actions with high repetitions and low resistance significantly improve children's muscular strength without adverse effect on bone or muscle.* **Table 14.4** provides basic guidelines for resistance exercise progressions for children at different ages.

For Your Information

All About Power

Power [(force × distance) ÷ time)] represents the product of strength and speed of movement expressed in watts (W; 1 W = 0.73756 ft-lb·s⁻¹, 6.12 kg-m·min⁻¹, or 0.01433 kCal·min⁻¹).

For Your Information

Muscular Strength and Puberty

Until puberty, boys maintain about 10% greater muscle strength than girls. After age 12, boys continue to increase in strength while strength plateaus in girls. Gender-related changes in body composition account for much of the strength difference.

Box 14–3 • CLOSE UP

DETERMINING UPPER-ARM MUSCLE AND FAT AREAS

Girth measurements include bone surrounded by a mass of muscle tissue ringed by a layer of subcutaneous fat (Fig. A). Muscle represents the largest component of the girth (except in the obese and elderly), so girth indicates one's relative muscularity. Estimating limb muscle area assumes similarity between a limb and a cylinder, with subcutaneous fat evenly distributed around the cylinder (Fig. A).

MEASUREMENTS

Determine the following:

1. Upper-arm girth (relaxed triceps; G_{arm}): Measure with arm extended relaxed at the side (or parallel to the ground in an abducted position). Measure girth (cm) midway between the acromial and olecranon process (Fig. B).

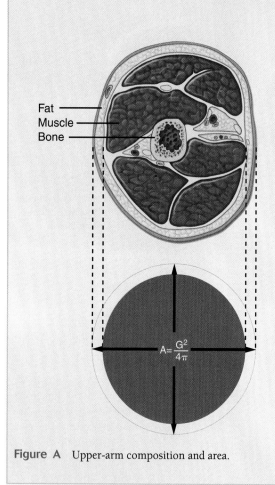

Fat
Muscle
Bone

$$A = \frac{G^2}{4\pi}$$

Figure A Upper-arm composition and area.

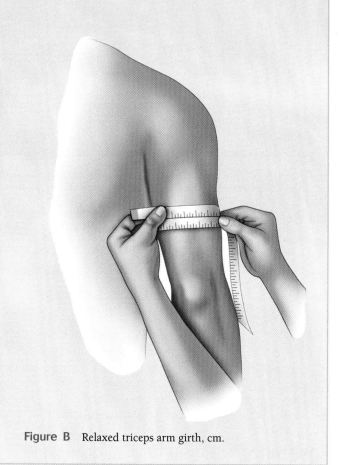

Figure B Relaxed triceps arm girth, cm.

SYSTEMS OF RESISTANCE TRAINING

Five different but interrelated systems of training develop muscular strength:

1. Isometric training
2. Dynamic constant external resistance training
3. Variable resistance training
4. Isokinetic training
5. Plyometric training

Isometric Training (Static Exercise)

Isometric strength training gained popularity between 1955 and 1965. Research in Germany during this time showed a 5% per week increase in isometric strength from

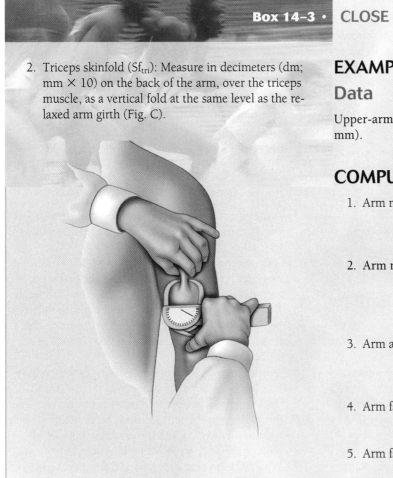

Box 14–3 • CLOSE UP *(Continued)*

2. Triceps skinfold (Sf_{tri}): Measure in decimeters (dm; mm $\times$ 10) on the back of the arm, over the triceps muscle, as a vertical fold at the same level as the relaxed arm girth (Fig. C).

Figure C Triceps skinfold, mm.

EXAMPLE

Data

Upper-arm girth (G_{arm}) in cm, 30.0; Sf_{tri} 2.5 dm (25 mm).

COMPUTATIONS

1. Arm muscle girth, cm $= G_{arm} - (\pi Sf_{tri})$
$= 30.0 \text{ cm} - (\pi 2.5 \text{ dm})$
$= 30.0 - 7.854$
$= 22.1 \text{ cm}$

2. Arm muscle area, cm^2 $= [G_{arm} - (\pi Sf_{tri})] \div 4\pi$
$= (30.0 \text{ cm}) - (\pi 2.5 \text{ dm})^2$
$\div 4\pi$
$= 488.4 \div 12.566$
$= 38.9 \text{ cm}^2$

3. Arm area (A), cm^2 $= (G_{arm})^2 \div 4\pi$
$= (30.0 \text{ cm})^2 \div 4\pi$
$= 900 \div 12.566$
$= 71.6 \text{ cm}^2$

4. Arm fat area, cm^2 $=$ arm area $-$ arm muscle area
$= 71.6 \text{ cm}^2 - 38.9 \text{ cm}^2$
$= 32.7 \text{ cm}^2$

5. Arm fat index, % fat area $=$ (arm fat area
$\div$ arm area) $\times$ 100
$= (32.7 \text{ cm}^2 \div 71.6 \text{ cm}^2) \times 100$
$= 45.7\%$

Table 14•4	Guidelines for Resistance Exercise for Children[a]
AGE, y	**GUIDELINES**
5–7	Introduce child to basic exercises with little or no weight; develop the concept of a training session; teach exercise techniques; progress from body weight calisthenics, partner exercises, and lightly resisted exercises; keep volume low
8–10	Gradually increase exercise number; practice exercise techniques for all lifts; start gradual progressive loading of exercises; keep exercises simple; increase volume slowly; carefully monitor tolerance to exercise stress
11–13	Teach all basic exercise techniques; continue progressive loading of each exercise; emphasize exercise technique; introduce more advanced exercises with little or no resistance
14–15	Progress to more advanced resistance exercise programs; add sport-specific components; emphasize exercise techniques; increase volume
16+	Entry level into adult programs after the person masters all background experience

[a]Note: If a child at a particular age level has no previous experience, progression must start at previous levels and move to more advanced levels as exercise tolerance, skill, and understanding permit.
From Kraemer, W.J., and Fleck S.J.: *Designing Resistance Training Programs.* Champaign, IL: Human Kinetics, 1997.

only a daily, single, two-thirds maximum isometric action for 6 seconds in duration. Repeating this action 5 to 10 times increased isometric strength. Strength gains from this simple exercise seemed beyond belief, and subsequent research demonstrated that isometric strength gains progressed at a slower rate. Research also showed that gains in strength from isometrics related to repetitions, duration of muscle action, and training frequency.

Research since 1965 has revealed the following information regarding isometric training:

1. Maximal voluntary isometric actions (100% of maximum) produce greater gains in isometric strength than submaximal isometric actions.
2. Duration of muscle activation directly relates to increases in isometric strength.
3. One daily isometric action does not increase isometric strength as effectively as repeated actions.
4. An optimal isometric training program consists of daily repeated isometric actions.
5. Isometric training does not provide a consistent stimulus for muscular hypertrophy.
6. Gains in isometric strength occur predominantly at the joint angle used in training.

Limitations of Isometrics A drawback to isometric training involves difficulty in monitoring exercise intensity and training results. Essentially no movement occurs and it becomes difficult to determine objectively if the person's strength actually improves and whether the person applies an appropriate overload force during training. Isometric force measurement requires specialized equipment (e.g., strain gauge or cable tensiometer) not readily available at most exercise facilities.

Benefits of Isometrics Isometric exercise effectively improves strength of a particular muscle or group of muscles when the applied isometric force covers four or five joint angles through the ROM. Isometric training works well in orthopedic applications that isolate strengthening movements during rehabilitation. Isometric measurement pinpoints an area of muscle weakness, and isometric training strengthens muscles at the appropriate joint angle.

Dynamic Constant External Resistance (DCER) Training

This popular system of resistance training involves lifting (concentric) and lowering (eccentric) phases with each repetition using weight plates (barbells and dumbbells) or exercise machines that feature different applications of muscle overload.

Progressive Resistance Exercise Researchers in rehabilitation medicine after World War II devised a method of resistance training to improve the force-generating capacity of previously injured patients. Their method involved three sets of exercise, each consisting of 10 repetitions done consecutively without rest. The first set involved one-half the maximum weight lifted 10 times or one-half 10-RM; the second set used three-quarters 10-RM; the final set required maximum weight for 10 repetitions or 10-RM. As patients became stronger, the resistance increased periodically to match strength improvements. This technique of **progressive resistance exercise** (**PRE**), a practical application of the overload principle, forms the basis for most resistance training programs.

Variations of PRE Research has varied PRE to determine an optimal number of sets and repetitions and frequency and relative intensity of training to improve strength. The findings can be summarized as follows:

1. Performing between 3-RM and 9-RM yields the most effective number of repetitions to increase muscular strength.
2. PRE training once weekly with only 1-RM for one set increases strength significantly after the first week of training, and each week up to at least the sixth week.
3. No particular sequence of PRE training with different percentages of 10-RM improves strength more effectively, provided each training session consists of one set of 10-RM.
4. Smaller strength increases occur when performing one set of an exercise rather than two or three sets, and three sets produce greater improvement than two sets.
5. For beginners, strength increases occur with only one training day weekly, but the optimum number of training days per week with PRE remains unknown.
6. When PRE training uses several different exercises, training four or five days a week can be less effective for increasing strength than training two or three times weekly. More frequent training prevents sufficient recuperation between exercise sessions; this could minimize neuromuscular adaptations, energy replenishment, and strength development.
7. A fast rate of movement for a given resistance generates greater strength improvement than lifting at a slower rate. Neither free weights (barbells or dumbbells) nor concentric-eccentric-type weight machines produce inherently superior results compared with other strength development methods.

Responses of Men and Women to DCER Training Figure 14.8 shows strength changes for men and women with DCER training. These data represent an average from 12 experiments. Women achieved higher percentage improvement than men, although considerable overlap existed among individuals. These findings indicate a relative equality in trainability between women and men, at least with short-duration resistance training.

Variable Resistance Training

A limitation of typical DCER weight-lifting exercise involves failure of muscles to generate maximum force

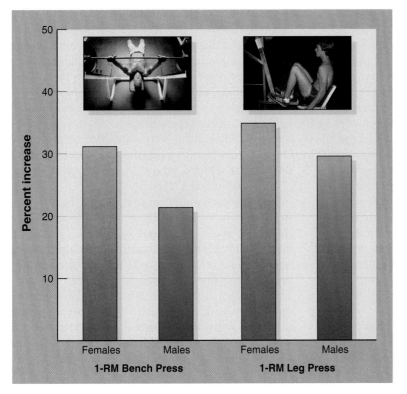

List 5 different systems of resistance training.

1.

2.

3.

4.

5.

Give one limitation of isometric strength training.

Figure 14.8 Percentage increase in 1-RM bench press and leg press of females and males in response to resistance training. Values represent average of 12 studies using dynamic constant external resistance (DCER) training for a minimum of 9 weeks duration, 3 days per week, and two or more sets per session.

Define RPE and give its physiologic significance.

through all movement phases. **Variable resistance training equipment** alters external resistance to movement by use of a lever arm, irregularly shaped metal cam, hydraulics, or a pulley so as to match increases and decreases in force capacity related to joint angle (lever characteristics) throughout a ROM. This adjustment, based on average physical dimensions of a population, theoretically should facilitate strength gains because it allows near-maximal force production throughout the full ROM.

Biomechanical research shows that a single cam device cannot possibly compensate fully for individual differences in mechanics and force applications at all phases of a particular movement. Variations in limb length, point of attachment of muscle tendons to bone, body size, and strength at different joint angles all affect maximum force generated throughout a ROM. In most cases, cams produce too much resistance during the first half and too little resistance during the second half of flexion and extension exercises. Despite these limitations, variable resistance devices improve strength comparable to other weight-lifting (resistance) equipment.

List 2 factors responsible for low back syndrome.

1.

2.

Special Consideration: The Lower Back

Approximately 60% of manual workers in the United States suffer back problems at some time in their careers, and back problems represent the primary cause for job-related disability claims. Such disability translates into millions of lost hours, chronic physical discomfort, and billions of dollars spent on visits to health-care professionals. The causes for this malady are not always apparent, and a cure remains elusive. Prime factors in **low back syndrome** include muscular weakness (particularly the abdominal region) and poor lower back and leg flexibility. Strengthening and flexibility exercises help alleviate and rehabilitate chronic low-back strain. Even continuing normal daily activities (within limits dictated by pain tolerance) leads to a more rapid recovery from an episode of acute back pain than does bed rest.

Resistance-training exercise poses a dilemma for those with low back syndrome. If done properly, resistance training strengthens the abdominal muscles and lumbar extensor muscles of the lower back that support and protect the spine. Unfortunately, the novice exerciser frequently performs exercises incorrectly while attempting to create excessive force. Incorrect movements recruit additional muscle groups, improperly align the spinal column (especially with the back arching, a form of weight-lifting cheating), and trigger lower back strain. A seemingly simple sit-up exercise, if done improperly with legs stiff, back arched, and head thrown back, places unnecessary strain on the lower spine (sit-ups should always be done with the knees flexed and chin tucked to chest). Pressing and curling exercises with weights performed with excessive hyperextension or back arch (another form of "cheating") creates shearing forces that produce undesirable muscle strain or spinal pressure.

Wearing a weightlifting belt during heavy lifts (squats, dead lifts, clean-and-jerk maneuvers) reduces intra-abdominal pressure compared to lifting without a belt. A belt reduces the potentially injurious compressive forces on spinal discs during heavy lifting as in most Olympic and power-lifting events. A person who trains with a belt should generally refrain from lifting without one. Further recommendations include performing at least some submaximal resistance training without a belt to strengthen the deep abdominal muscles and to develop the proper pattern of muscle recruitment to generate high intra-abdominal pressures without a belt.

General Back Exercises   Figure 14.9 illustrates 12 exercises for general strengthening of the abdomen and lower back, and improving hamstring and lower back flexibility for individuals with no apparent lower back and spinal injuries. Those with low back syndrome may require other more specific exercises.

Isokinetic Training

Isokinetic resistance training differs markedly from isometric, DCER, and variable resistance methods. Isokinetic training employs a muscle action performed at constant angular limb velocity. Unlike dynamic resistance exercise, isokinetic exercise does not require a specified initial resistance; rather, the isokinetic device controls movement velocity. The muscles exert maximal forces throughout the ROM while shortening (concentric action) at a specific velocity. Advocates of isokinetic training argue that exerting maximal force throughout the full ROM optimizes strength development. Also, concentric-only actions minimize potential for muscle and joint injury and pain.

Experiments With Isokinetic Exercise and Training   Experiments using isokinetic exercise ex-

plored the force-velocity relationship in various exercises and related this to the muscle's fiber-type composition. **Figure 14.10** displays the progressive decline in concentric peak torque output with increasing angular velocity of the knee extensor muscles in two groups that differed in sports training and muscle fiber composition. For movement at $180°·s^{-1}$, power athletes, (elite Swedish track and field sprinters and jumpers) achieved significantly higher torque per kilogram of body mass than competition walkers and cross-country runners (endurance athletes). At this angular velocity, maximal torque equaled about 55% of maximal isometric force ($0°·s^{-1}$).

The athletes' muscle fiber composition distinguishes the two curves in Figure 14.10. At zero velocity shortening (isometric action), the same peak force (per unit body mass) occurred for athletes with relatively high (power athletes) or low (endurance athletes) percentages of fast-twitch muscle fibers; this indicated that maximal isometric knee extension activated both fast- and slow-twitch motor units. Increasing movement velocity produced greater torque by individuals with a higher percentage of fast-twitch fibers. More than likely, fast-twitch muscle fibers favor performance in power activities where high torque generation at rapid movement velocities often dictates success.

Plyometric Training

Athletes who require specific, powerful movements (e.g., football, volleyball, sprinting, and basketball) often perform exercise training termed **plyometrics**. Plyometric training movements make use of the inherent stretch-recoil characteristics of skeletal muscle and neurological modulation via the stretch or myotatic reflex (see Chapter 11). Consider walking. When the foot first hits the ground, the quadriceps initially act eccentrically (stretch), then briefly isometrically, before the shortening phase of muscle action begins. The term **stretch-shortening cycle** describes the sequence of linked, eccentric-isometric-concentric muscle actions. When stretching occurs rapidly, stored elastic energy in muscle fibers and initiation of the myotatic reflex combine to produce a powerful concentric action. Faster recruitment of muscle fibers and recruitment of more muscle fibers with prior stretching may also augment a muscle's responsiveness.

Vertical jumping provides an example of the stretch-shortening cycle to enhance performance. During a normal vertical jump, the jumper bends at the knees and hips (eccentric action), pauses briefly (isometric action), and rapidly reverses direction (concentric action) to explode upward as fast (and high) as possible. If this same movement stops for several seconds following the knee bend (just before reversing movement direction), the subsequent jump (concentric action) produces a lower jump height compared with a performance that uses the rapid and complete stretch-shortening cycle.

Practical Applications   A plyometric training drill incorporates body mass and gravity to provide the all-

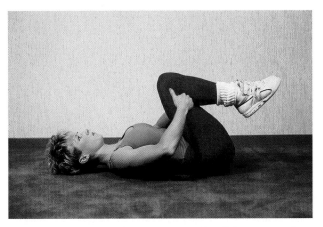

(A) *Knees-to-chest stretch*: Lie supine and pull knees into chest while keeping lower back flat on the surface.

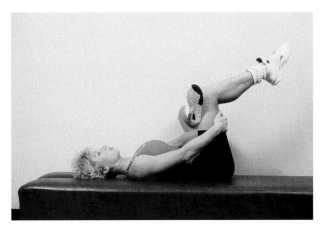

(B) *Cross-leg stretch*: Cross legs like sitting male. Cross legs and pull 90°-flexed knee toward chest.

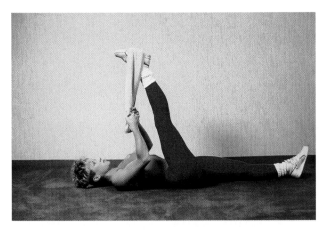

(C) *Hamstring stretch*: Wrap strap over foot, keeping lower back flat; pull leg upward toward head.

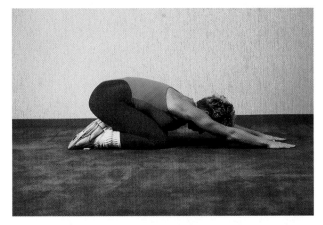

(D) *Allah stretch*: Sit with buttocks on bilateral heels; move hands as far forward along the surface as possible.

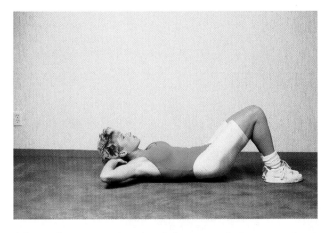

(E) *Bent-knee sit-up*: Keep hands low on neck (or across chest) with head positioned over the shoulders. Roll up slowly, engaging one row of the abdominals at a time. Raise the shoulders 4 to 6 inches off the surface.

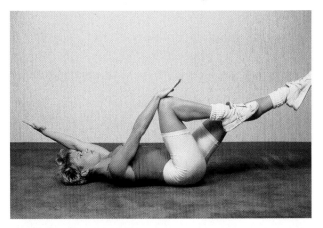

(F) *Dying bug*: Flex the pelvis to flatten the lower back against the surface. Over one side, bring an extended arm and flexed knee together. The opposing side should extend a straight arm overhead and straight leg backward. Maintain pelvic flexion while exchanging opposing arms and legs in this position.

Figure 14.9   Exercises to strengthen the abdomen and lower back and increase hamstring and lower back flexibility. (Photos courtesy of Dr. Bob Swanson, Santa Barbara Back and Neck Care Center. Santa Barbara, CA.)

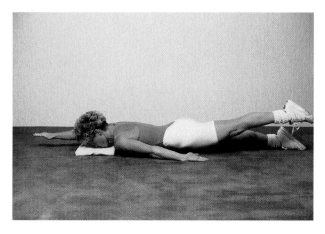

(G) *Dry-land swimming*: Lying prone with pelvic flexion, alternate lifting opposite arm and legs.

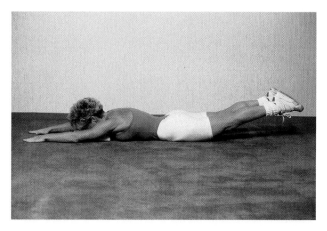

(H) *Both legs up*: Lying prone with pelvic flexion, lift both legs simultaneously while keeping the head on the floor.

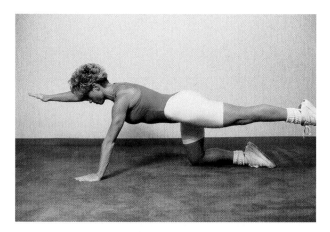

(I) *Pointer (bird dog)*: Start with hands and knees on the floor. Flex pelvis into counter position. Exchange pointing opposite arm and leg while keeping the torso level.

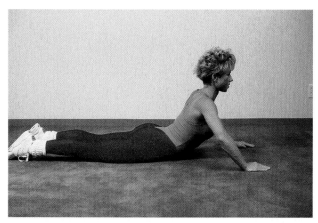

(J) *Upper body up*: Lying prone with pelvic flexion and arms outstretched or behind the back, lift the upper torso while keeping the legs on the floor.

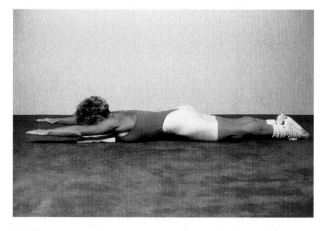

(K) *Prone cobra push-up*: Keep the pelvis on the floor while pressing up with the arms, causing lower back extension.

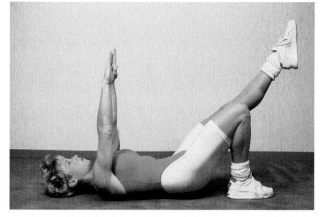

(L) *Leg pointer*: Lie supine on the floor and flex the pelvis with the lower abdominals to flatten the lower back into the surface. Extend one arm upward and one leg outward while keeping the quadriceps level.

Figure 14.9 *(continued)*

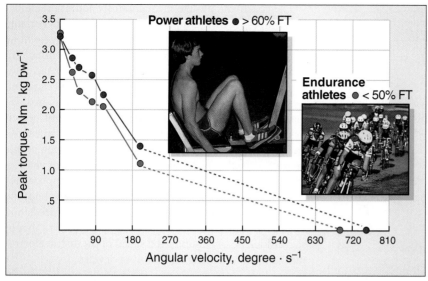

Figure 14.10   Peak torque per unit body mass related to angular velocity in two groups of athletes with different muscle fiber compositions. The torque–velocity curves were extrapolated (dashed line) to an estimated maximal velocity for knee extension. (Data from Throstensson, A.: Muscle strength, fiber types, and enzyme activities in man. *Acta. Physiol. Scand.*, Suppl:443, 1976.)

Questions & Notes

Briefly describe isokinetic training.

Briefly describe plyometric training.

True or false:

Training with plyometric methods produces greater injuries than other training modes.

important rapid prestretch or cocking phase that activates the stretch reflex and the muscle's natural elastic recoil elements. Lower-body plyometric drills include a standing jump, multiple jumps, repetitive jumping in place, depth or drop jumps (from 1- to 4-ft heights), and various modifications of single- and double-leg jumps. Repeating these exercises regularly supposedly provides both neurological and muscular training to enhance power performance of the specific muscles. **Figure 14.11** shows examples of plyometric exercises, including general jumping exercises and depth jumps for strength-power development using resistance and other apparatus.

The _____ principle dictates the best exercise training system based on the particular needs of an individual.

Research with Plyometric Exercises   Testimonials and opinions abound
to promote the beneficial effects of plyometric training, but carefully controlled scientific evaluations remain scarce. No consensus exists about optimal jump number with untrained subjects. Similarly, insufficient evidence makes it difficult to recommend optimal height for performing depth jumps (heights from 19 to 32 inches have produced varying degrees of success).

Performing plyometric exercise while wearing a weighted vest or belt (up to 12% of body mass) augments the training effect. When individuals performed resistance training and plyometric exercises two to three times weekly for 4 to 10 weeks, vertical jump height increased between 1.2 to 4.2 inches. Plyometric training also improves standing long jump and sprint running performances. Concurrent resistance training with plyometrics improves performance to a greater extent than either method alone.

Training with plyometric methods does not produce greater injuries than other training modes, even in untrained individuals. Common sense dictates that plyometric training should be introduced slowly into the total training regimen. Clearly, plyometrics should not serve as the main form of resistance training; instead, plyometrics can serve as an adjunct to a diverse muscle-strengthening program.

Define the term periodization.

COMPARISON OF TRAINING SYSTEMS

Few studies have directly compared different training systems within the same experimental protocol. Some studies compare two different training systems (e.g.,

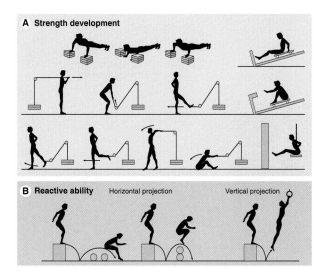

Figure 14.11 Examples of stretch-shortening cycle (plyometric) exercises. **(A)** Strength development; and **(B)** reactive ability.

isometric versus variable resistance; isometric versus isokinetic; and isometric versus eccentric). The results generally support the specificity and individual differences principles. When training and testing incorporate the same system, strength increases regardless of the training system. When testing uses a different system than in training, strength increases occur, and in some experiments, improvements become nonexistent. Difficulties also arise in trying to compare different training systems because of methodologic problems that equate training volume (sets and repetitions), total work, total training time, and most importantly, training intensity. This makes it almost impossible to directly prove that one strength training system fares better than another. Moreover, for unknown reasons, some individuals simply respond more favorably to one system over another. More than likely, *the specificity of training principle dictates the best training system for an individual based on desired outcomes and performance needs.*

Practical Implications of Training Specificity

The complex interaction between the nervous and muscular systems partially explains why leg muscles strengthened using squats or deep knee bends do not show equivalent improvement in another leg movement such as jumping. Strengthening muscles for golf, rowing, swimming, or football requires more than just identifying and overloading the muscles involved in the movement. Newly acquired strength does not simply transfer to other patterns of movement, even movements involving the same muscles. For older men, a 227% increase in leg extension strength occurred through standard weight training when weight lifting assessed strength improvement. In contrast, when an isokinetic dynamometer evaluated peak leg extensor torque, only a 10% to 17% improvement occurred.

The coach and athlete must carefully address the muscle group(s) involved in a particular movement. *Training should develop maximum force-generating capacity for those muscle groups throughout the ROM at a movement pattern and speed that closely mimics actual sports performance.* Isometric training cannot accomplish this goal because no limb movement takes place; isokinetic actions provide maximal overload potential at diverse movement velocities because movement speed with electromechanical dynamometers can approach $400°·s^{-1}$. Even moving at this relatively "fast" speed does not mimic movement velocity during some sports where limb velocity approaches $2000°·s^{-1}$. For example, arm velocity measured about the elbow joint during a baseball pitch routinely exceeds 600 to $700°·s^{-1}$, and leg velocity during a football, rugby, or soccer kick nearly doubles the speed of the fastest electromechanical measuring and training devices.

PERIODIZATION

Periodization refers to organizing resistance training into phases of different types of exercise at varying intensities and volumes for a specific time period. In essence, the training model decreases training volume and increases training intensity as the program progresses. Fractionating the **macrocycle** (usually a 1-year time period) into component parts (**mesocycles**) enables manipulation of training intensity, volume, frequency, sets, repetitions, and rest periods to prevent overtraining, and provides the means to alter the variety of workouts. This apparently reduces any negative effects from overtraining or "staleness" and enables the competitive athlete to achieve peak performance to coincide with competition. **Figure 14.12** depicts the basic design for periodization and a typical macrocycle with four distinct mesocycle phases. As competition approaches, periodization gradually decreases training volume while concurrently increases training intensity.

Periodization produces an inverse relation between training volume and training intensity up through the competition phase and then decreases both aspects during the second transition or recuperation period. Note the increase in the time devoted to technique training as competition approaches, with training volume at the lowest point of the cycle.

Sport-specific training principles apply in periodization as the coach designs training based on the sport's particular strength, power, and endurance requirements. A detailed analysis of metabolic and technical requirements of the sport also frames the training paradigm. The concept of periodization makes intuitive sense, yet few if any studies present conclusive evidence for this training approach. Confounding factors include difficulty controlling for differences in training intensity, training volume, and the participants' fitness capacities. One critical review of periodized strength training concluded that it produced greater improvements in muscular strength, body mass, lean body mass,

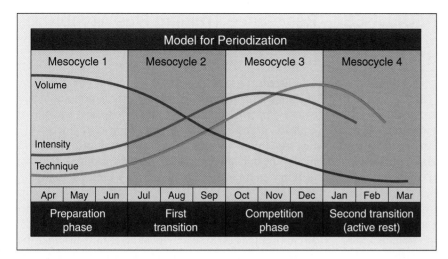

Figure 14.12 Basic periodization scheme comprising four transition phases. The periodization concept subdivides a macrocycle into distinct phases or mesocycles. These, in turn, usually separate into weekly microcycles. (Red line = volume; blue line = intensity; green line = technique.)

and percentage body fat than nonperiodized multi-set and single-set training programs. More research must evaluate periodization, particularly relating to fitness status, age, gender, and specific sports performance. Studies must equate and then manipulate training loads and intensities and evaluate additional factors such as biomechanics and motor control in the sport skill, changes in segmental and whole-body composition, biochemical and ultrastructural tissue adaptations, and transfer of newly acquired fitness to specific performance measures.

PRACTICAL RECOMMENDATIONS FOR INITIATING A RESISTANCE-TRAINING PROGRAM

1. Avoid maximum lifts in the beginning stages of resistance training. Excessive resistance contributes little to strength development and greatly increases risk of muscle or joint injury. A load equal to 60% to 80% of a muscle's force-generating capacity sufficiently stimulates increase in muscular strength. This load generally allows completion of about 10 repetitions of a particular movement.
2. Use lighter resistance to perform more repetitions at the start of training. Novices should initially attempt 12 to 15 repetitions. This regimen does not place excessive strain on the musculoskeletal system during the early phase of the program. Use a heavier load if 12 repetitions feel too easy. The resistance is too heavy if the exerciser cannot complete 12 repetitions. This trial-and-error process may take several exercise sessions to establish the proper starting weight.
3. After several weeks of training, when the muscles adapt and the exerciser learns the correct movements, repetitions can decrease to between 6 and 8.
4. Add more resistance after reaching the target number of repetitions. This regimen represents progressive resistance training; as muscles become stronger, resistance increases with the lifting of a heavier load.
5. The exercise sequence should proceed from larger to smaller muscle groups to avoid premature fatigue of the smaller group.

RESISTANCE TRAINING GUIDELINES FOR SEDENTARY ADULTS, THE ELDERLY, AND CARDIAC PATIENTS

Currently, the American College of Sports Medicine, American Heart Association, Centers for Disease Control and Prevention, American Association of Cardiovascular and Pulmonary Rehabilitation, and the U.S. Surgeon General's Office consider regular resistance exercise an important component of a comprehensive, health-related physical fitness program. Resistance training goals for competitive athletes focus on optimizing muscular strength, power, and muscular hypertrophy "with high-intensity" 1-RM to 6-RM training loads. In contrast, goals for most middle-aged and older adults focus on maintenance (and possible increase) of muscle and bone mass and muscular strength and muscular endurance to enhance the overall health and physical-fitness profile. Adequate muscular strength in midlife maintains a margin of safety above the necessary threshold required to prevent injury in later life.

The resistance-training program recommended for middle-aged and older men and women classifies as "moderate intensity." In contrast to the multiple-set, heavy-resistance approach used by younger athletes, the program uses single sets of diverse exercises performed between 8- and 15-RM a minimum of twice weekly.

Resistance Training Plus Aerobic Training Equals Less Strength Improvement

Concurrent resistance and aerobic training programs produce less muscular strength and power improvement than training for strength only. This partly explains why power athletes and body builders refrain from endurance activities while participating in resistance training. More than likely, the added energy (and perhaps protein) demands of heavy endurance training impose a limit on a muscle's growth and metabolic responsiveness to resistance training. Also, a short-term bout of high-intensity endurance exercise inhibits performance in subsequent muscular strength activities. Research must determine whether this effect on maximal force output limits ability to overload skeletal muscle optimally to a degree that impairs strength development with concurrent strength and endurance training. If it does, then a 20- to 30-minute recovery between aerobic and strength training components might enhance the quality of the subsequent strength workout. These considerations should not deter those desiring a well-rounded conditioning program offering the specific fitness and health benefits available from both exercise training modes.

SUMMARY

1. The four common methods to measure muscular strength include: (1) tensiometry, (2) dynamometry, (3) 1-RM testing with weights, (4) computer-assisted force and work-output determinations including isokinetic measurement.

2. Substantial physiologic and performance specificity in the response to training cast doubt on the appropriateness of general fitness measures (including strength tests) to determine success in specific physical tasks or occupations.

3. Human skeletal muscle theoretically generates a maximum of 16 to 30 N of maximum force per cm^2 of muscle cross-section regardless of gender.

4. On an absolute basis, men outperform women on tests of strength because of the male's larger quantity of muscle mass. These differences are greatest in upper-body muscular strength.

5. Muscles become stronger with overload training that (1) increases the load, (2) increases the speed of muscle action, or (3) combines both factors.

6. Strength gains occur when the overload represents at least 60% to 80% of a muscle's maximum force-generating capacity.

7. Closely supervised resistance training for children, using moderate levels of concentric exercise, improves muscular strength with no adverse effects on bone or muscle.

8. Three major exercise systems develop muscular strength: (1) dynamic constant external resistance training, (2) isometric training, and (3) isokinetic training. Each system produces highly specific strength gains that relate directly to training mode.

9. Resistance training exercises performed incorrectly with excessive hyperextension or back arch create shearing forces that produce undesirable muscle strain or spinal pressure and trigger low back pain.

10. Isokinetic training generates maximum force throughout the full range of motion (ROM) at different limb movement velocities. Thus, this training method offers a unique way to apply resistance training to enhance specific sports performance.

11. Plyometric training uses the inherent stretch-recoil characteristics of the neuromuscular system to develop specific muscular power. Research must determine risks, benefits, and proper applications of plyometric training.

12. Resistance training for specific sports should develop maximum force-generating capacity throughout a muscle's ROM at a speed that closely mimics the actual performance.

THOUGHT QUESTIONS

1. Explain why athletes have spotters apply external force to the bar in the early phase of a bench press to increase difficulty and then provide assistance toward its completion.

2. Based on your knowledge of gender-related differences in muscular strength, devise a physical test that (1) minimizes and (2) maximizes performance differences between men and women.

3. Discuss the statement: "There is no one best system of resistance training."

PART 2 •
Adaptations to Resistance Training

Resistance training produces both acute responses and chronic adaptations. *An acute response refers to immediate changes (in muscle or other cells, tissues, or systems) during or immediately after a single bout of exercise.* For example, energy stores and cardiovascular dynamics change in response to specific muscle actions. Repeated exposure to the stimulus produces a longer lasting change that affects the acute response over time (e.g., less disruption in cellular integrity [muscle damage] with a given level of exercise). *Adaptation refers to how the body adjusts to a repeated (chronic) stimulus.*

Knowing the acute and chronic responses to resistance training facilitates exercise prescription and program design. Adaptations to repeated muscular overload ultimately determine a training program's effectiveness. The time-course of adaptations varies among individuals and depends on the nature and magnitude of prior adaptations. Also, a resistance-training program must consider the expression of individual differences in adaptation (training responsiveness).

Adaptations to resistance training occur from the cellular to systemic levels. **Figure 14.13** displays six factors that impact muscle mass development and maintenance. More than likely, genetic factors strongly influence the effect of each factor on the ultimate training outcome. Resistance training contributes little to tissue growth without appropriate nutrition. Similarly, training outcome depends on specific hormones and patterns of nervous system activation. Without muscular overload, however, each of the other factors cannot effectively increase muscle mass and muscle strength.

NEURAL ADAPTATIONS

Well-documented changes from overload training occur in the gross structural and microscopic architecture within muscle tissue. **Figure 14.14** shows the adaptation of variables, broadly classified as neural and muscular, with regular resistance training.

A classic series of experiments clearly illustrated the importance of neural factors in expressing muscular strength. In one protocol, researchers measured upper-arm strength while they fired intermittent gunshots behind the subjects just before they performed a maximal voluntary contraction. At another time, subjects shouted or screamed loudly at the moment they exerted force. In addition to the "shoot and shout" series, the experimenters measured subjects' strength under the influence of two disinhibitory drugs, alcohol and amphetamines ("pep

FOR YOUR INFORMATION

Hold That Stretch!
Stretching with fast, bouncing, jerky movements that use the body's momentum can strain or tear muscles, and create a reflex action that resists the muscle stretch.

FOR YOUR INFORMATION

Neural Adaptations Important
Three factors enhance neural adaptations with resistance training:
1. Increased central nervous system activation
2. Improved motor unit synchronization
3. Lowered neural inhibitory reflexes

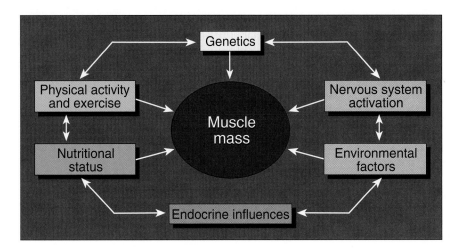

Figure 14.13 Six factors that impact muscle mass.

pills"). They also measured strength during hypnosis; subjects were told their strength would exceed their prior strength and they should not fear injury. Arm strength increased in almost all of the psychological conditions. The greatest strength increases occurred under hypnosis, the most "mental" of the treatments.

To explain these observations, the researchers suggested that *physical factors (size and type of muscle fibers and anatomic lever arrangement of bone and muscle) ultimately determine a person's muscular strength capacity.* They claimed that psychological or mental factors within the central nervous system prevent most people from fully fulfilling strength capacity. Neural inhibitions might result from social conditioning, unpleasant past experiences with physical activity, or an overprotective home environment. When performing under intense emotional conditions like athletic competition, emergency situations, or posthypnotic suggestion, however, the inhibitory neural

mechanisms decrease considerably, and the person achieves a super performance that more closely matches the physiologically determined capacity. Such observations help to explain the apparent beneficial effects of "psyching" or almost self-induced hypnosis that athletes achieve immediately prior to competitive performance.

Excellent examples of disinhibition occur in weightlifters and powerlifters, high-jumpers and other track and field competitors, and self-defense experts who perform nontraditional skills like smashing cement bricks with their hands, feet, or head. Great feats of strength during emergency situations also fit into this explanation. In addition, rapid improvements in muscular strength during the first few weeks of strength training largely result from a learning phenomenon, or lessening of fear and psychological inhibition, as the novice becomes familiar with the specific strength activity (e.g., proper form in bench press or squat exercise).

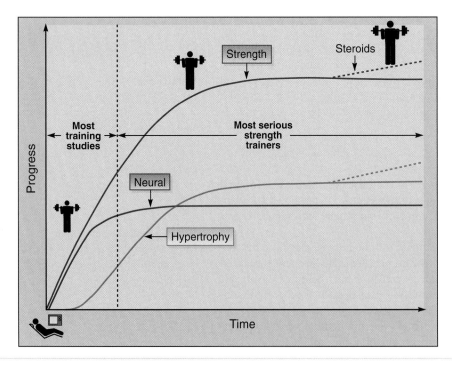

Figure 14.14 Relative roles of neural and muscular adaptations during strength training. Note that neural adaptation predominates in the early phase of training. This phase also encompasses most training studies. In intermediate and advanced training, progress becomes limited by the extent of muscular adaptation, notably hypertrophy; this increases the temptation to try anabolic steroids when hypertrophy by training alone becomes difficult. (Data from Sale, D.G.: Neural adaptation to resistance training. *Med. Sci. Sports Exerc.*, 20:135, 1988.)

Motor Unit Activation: Size Principle   Recruitment of motor units occurs in sequence from low to high thresholds and thus, from low to high muscle force output. An increased rate of motor unit firing also increases a muscle's force output. These two factors, recruitment of motor units and increase in their firing rate, produce a continuum of voluntary force output from muscle.

Type II motor units have a high twitch force; they become activated in activities requiring significant force. In contrast, type I motor units activate under lower force requirements that generate less force. Individuals unaccustomed to high physical demands probably cannot voluntarily recruit all higher threshold type II motor units; thus, they cannot maximally tap their muscle's true strength potential. An adaptation to resistance training develops how well an untrained person recruits more motor units to achieve a maximal muscle action. Increased synchronization of motor unit firing provides another neural adjustment to increase force production with training. Greater synchronization causes more motor units to fire simultaneously.

In advanced weight lifters, neural components also contribute to strength improvement. In one study, minimal changes took place in muscle fiber size, yet 2 years of training increased absolute strength and power. EMG analysis revealed enhanced voluntary activation of muscle over the training period. This suggests that the neural component contributes significantly to strength improvements.

MUSCLE ADAPTATIONS

Psychological inhibitions and learning factors greatly modify muscular strength, but anatomic and physiologic factors within the muscle determine the ultimate limit of strength development. Gross and ultrastructural changes in muscle with chronic resistance training generally produce adaptations in the contractile apparatus accompanied by substantial gains in muscular strength and power. Increase in muscle external size represents the most visible adaptation to resistance training. **Muscle fiber hypertrophy** (increased size of individual fibers) usually explains increases in gross muscle size, although increased fiber number (**fiber hyperplasia**) provides a controversial complimentary hypothesis.

Muscle Fiber Hypertrophy

Muscle hypertrophy with resistance training represents a fundamental biologic adaptation. The extraordinarily large muscle size and definition of weight lifters and body builders results from enlargement of individual muscle cells, mainly the fast-twitch fibers. Growth takes place from one or more of the following adaptations:

1. Increased amounts of contractile proteins (actin and myosin)
2. Increased number and size of myofibrils per muscle fiber
3. Increased amounts of connective, tendinous, and ligamentous tissues
4. Increased quantity of enzymes and stored nutrients

Not all muscle fibers undergo the same degree of enlargement with resistance training. *Muscle growth depends on the muscle fiber type activated and the recruitment pattern.* With initiation of resistance training, alterations in various muscle proteins begin within several workouts. As training continues, contractile proteins increase in conjunction with enlargement of muscle fiber cross-sectional area. **Table 14.5** lists important cellular adaptations in muscle to resistance training.

Significant Metabolic Adaptations Occur   Success at elite levels of sport performance undoubtedly requires a particular muscle fiber distribution. The relatively fixed nature of muscle fiber type suggests an obvious genetic predisposition for exceptional performance. However, considerable plasticity exists for metabolic potential, as specific training enhances the anaerobic and aerobic energy transfer capacity of both fiber types. The heightened oxidative capacity of fast-twitch fibers

Briefly describe the difference between an acute and chronic response to exercise.

List 4 factors that impact development and maintenance of muscle mass.

1.

2.

3.

4.

List 2 factors that determine a person's muscular strength capacity.

1.

2.

Give one example of neural disinhibition in athletics.

Briefly describe the size principle of motor unit recruitment.

List 3 adaptations in muscle that influence muscle growth.

1.

2.

3.

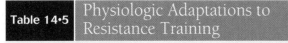

Table 14•5	Physiologic Adaptations to Resistance Training	
SYSTEM/VARIABLE		**RESPONSE**
Muscle Fibers		
Number		Equivocal
Size		Increase
Type		Unknown
Capillary Density		
In bodybuilders		No change
In powerlifters		Decrease
Mitochondria		
Volume		Decrease
Density		Decrease
Twitch Contraction Time		Decrease
Enzymes		
Creatine phosphokinase		Increase
Myokinase		Increase
Enzymes of Glycolysis		
Phosphofructokinase		Increase
Lactate dehydrogenase		No change
Aerobic Metabolism Enzymes		
Carbohydrate		Increase
Triacylglycerol		Not known
Intramuscular Fuel Stores		
Adenosine triphosphate		Increase
Phosphocreatine		Increase
Glycogen		Increase
Triacylglycerols		Not known
$\dot{V}O_{2max}$		
Circuit resistance training		Increase
Heavy resistance training		No change
Connective Tissue		
Ligament strength		Increase
Tendon strength		Increase
Collagen content of muscle		No change
Bone		
Mineral content		Increase
Cross-sectional area		No change
Resistance to fracture		Increase

Modified from Fleck, S.J., and Kramer, W.J.: Resistance training: Physiological responses and adaptations (Part 2 of 4). *Phys. Sports Med.*, 16:108, 1988.

with endurance training brings them to a level nearly equal to the aerobic capacity of the slow-twitch fibers of untrained counterparts. Age presents no barrier to training adaptations of muscle fibers. With an adequate training stimulus, skeletal muscles of older men and women (fiber size, capillarization, and glycolytic and respiratory enzymes) adapt to both endurance and resistance training similar to younger persons.

Endurance training induces some conversion of type IIb fibers to the more aerobic type IIa fibers. The well-documented increase in mitochondrial size and number and corresponding increase in total quantity of citric acid cycle and electron transport enzymes accompany these fiber subdivision changes. Only specifically trained muscle fibers adapt to regular exercise; this explains why well-trained athletes who change to a sport requiring different muscle groups (or different portions of the same muscle) often feel untrained for the new activity. Within this frame-

work, swimmers or canoeists (with well-trained upper-body musculature) do not necessarily transfer their upper body fitness to a running sport that relies predominantly on a highly conditioned lower-body musculature.

Muscle Remodeling: Can Fiber Type Be Changed?

Skeletal muscle represents dynamic tissue whose cells do not remain as fixed populations throughout life. Rather, muscle fibers undergo regeneration and remodeling in response to diverse functional demands (e.g., resistance or endurance training) to alter their phenotypic profile. Activation of muscle via specific types and intensities of long-term use stimulates otherwise dormant myogenic stem cells (**satellite cells**) beneath a muscle fiber's basement membrane to proliferate and differentiate to form new fibers. Fusion of satellite cell nuclei and their incorporation into existing muscle fibers probably enables the fiber to synthesize more proteins to form additional myofibrils. This most likely contributes directly to muscular hypertrophy with chronic overload and may stimulate transformation of existing fibers from one type to another. A variety of extracellular signal molecules, primarily peptide growth factors (e.g., insulin-like growth factor [IGF], fibroblast growth factors, transforming growth factors, and hepatocyte growth factor) govern satellite cell activity and possibly exercise-induced muscle fiber proliferation and differentiation.

Studies with humans and animals support the concept that skeletal muscle adapts to altered functional demands. For example, *arduous training can induce transformation in fiber type.* In one study, four athletes trained anaerobically for 11 weeks followed by 18 weeks of aerobic training. Anaerobic training increased the percentage of type IIc fibers and decreased the percentage of type I fibers; the opposite occurred during the aerobic training phase. Similarly, 4 to 6 weeks of sprint training significantly increased the percentage of fast-twitch fibers with a commensurate decrease in slow-twitch fiber percentage. Increasing daily training duration also increases the fast- to slow-twitch shift in myosin heavy-chain phenotype in rat hindlimb muscles. Such findings suggest that specific training (and perhaps inactivity) may convert type I to type II fibers or vice versa. Available evidence does not permit definitive statements concerning the fixed nature of a muscle's fiber composition. More than likely, the genetic code exerts the greatest influence on fiber-type distribution. The major direction of a muscle's fiber composition probably becomes fixed before birth or during the first few years of life. The possibility does exist that some fiber-type transformation occurs with specific exercise training.

The Middle Aged and Elderly Respond Women and men experience considerable physiologic and performance adaptations with resistance training, independent of aging effects. A study of five older healthy men (average age 68 years) clearly demonstrates the remarkable plasticity of human skeletal muscle among the middle aged. The men

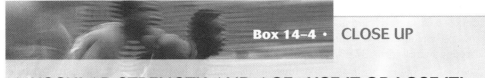

Box 14–4 • CLOSE UP

MUSCULAR STRENGTH AND AGE—USE IT OR LOSE IT!

The well-documented decline in muscular strength with age remains poorly understood. Contributing factors certainly include biologic aging per se, the cumulative effects of disease, a sedentary lifestyle, and nutritional inadequacies. If the strength decline in the elderly results largely from a "disuse syndrome," an appropriate resistance training program should reverse or at least slow down loss of muscle function.

Resistance training by the elderly is rare, mainly because of safety considerations, but also because of the belief that "old" muscle does not respond to overload training. Fortunately, recent research has seriously challenged such tenets. In one study, 10 subjects who averaged 90.2 years of age participated in an 8-week resistance training program. Concentric and eccentric muscle actions during a seated leg extension/flexion movement trained the quadriceps and hamstring muscles. Training, conducted 3 days a week, consisted of three sets of eight repetitions (6 to 9 s per rep) with a 1- to 2-minute rest between sets. During the first week of training, resistance equaled 50% 1-RM (measured every 2 weeks); by the second week, the load increased to 80% 1-RM and remained the same for an additional 8 weeks.

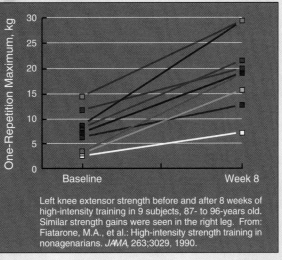

Left knee extensor strength before and after 8 weeks of high-intensity training in 9 subjects, 87- to 96-years old. Similar strength gains were seen in the right leg. From: Fiatarone, M.A., et al.: High-intensity strength training in nonagenarians. *JAMA,* 263;3029, 1990.

The figure shows changes in 1-RM strength for the left leg from the pretraining baseline to after 8 weeks of training for each of the nine subjects. The changes averaged an impressive 174% (167% for the right leg.) The absolute weight lifted increased from 8.0 kg to 20.6 kg for the right leg and from 7.6 kg to 19.3 kg for the left leg. Strength increases progressed throughout the 8 weeks and did not plateau with continued training. Also, no differences in strength improvement occurred between women and men. Interestingly, each subject increased functional mobility, including rising out of a chair and increased walking speed, and two subjects no longer needed a cane to walk. After the resistance training program, subjects returned to their sedentary lifestyle. Within only 4 weeks of detraining, strength decreased 32%.

The old adage "use it or lose it" seems all too apropos. The study's remarkable results demonstrate the desirability of conventional resistance training for older-age adults; training profoundly reversed the effects of aging on muscular strength.

REFERENCES

ACSM Position Stand on Exercise and Physical Activity for Older Adults. *Med. Sci. Sports Exerc.,* 30:992, 1998.

Evans, W.J.: Exercise training guidelines for the elderly. *Med. Sci. Sports Exerc.,* 31:12, 1999.

Hurley, B.F., and Hagberg, J.M.: Optimizing health in older persons: Aerobic or strength training? *Exerc. Sport Sci. Rev.,* 26:61, 1998.

Wescott, W.L., and Baechle, T.R.: *Strength Training Past 50.* Champaign, IL: Human Kinetics, 1998.

trained for 12 weeks using heavy-resistance, isokinetic, and free-weight exercises. Training increased muscle volume and cross-sectional area of the biceps brachii (13.9%) and brachialis (26.0%), while hypertrophy increased by 37.2% in the type II muscle fibers. Increases of 46.0% in peak torque and 28.6% in total work output accompanied these cellular adaptations.

Equally impressive training responses occur for elderly persons. One hundred nursing home residents (average age, 87.1 years) trained for 10 weeks with high-intensity resistance training. For the 63 women and 37 men who participated, muscle strength increased an average of 113%. Strength increases also paralleled improved function, reflected by an 11.8% increase in normal gait velocity and 28.4% increase in stair-climbing speed; thigh muscle cross-sectional area increased by 2.7%.

Changes in Muscle Fiber-Type Composition With Resistance Training   Research has evaluated the effects of 8 weeks of resistance exercise on muscle fiber size and fiber composition for the leg extensor muscles of 14 men who performed three sets of 6-RM leg squats three times weekly. Biopsy specimens from the vastus lateralis muscle before and after training showed no change in percentage distribution of fast- and slow-twitch muscle fibers with resistance training (as indicated by the activity level of myofibrillar ATPase). It remains unclear whether specific resistance training early in life or for the prolonged periods engaged in by Olympic-caliber athletes alters a muscle fiber's inherent twitch (speed of shortening) characteristics.

Metabolic characteristics of specific fibers and fiber subdivisions undergo modification within 4 to 8 weeks of resistance training. This occurs despite the lack of dramatic changes in inherent muscle fiber type with chronic exercise. A decrease in the percentage of type IIb and a corresponding increase in type IIa fibers denotes one of the more prominent and rapid resistance training adaptations.

Muscle Fiber Hypertrophy and Testosterone Levels   Popular belief maintains that the chief male sex hormone testosterone facilitates muscle hypertrophy with resistance training. Testosterone binds with special receptor sites on muscle and other tissues to contribute to male secondary sex characteristics. These characteristics include gender differences in muscle mass and strength that develop at puberty's onset. Variation in testosterone levels would then explain individual differences in muscular enlargement with resistance training and the smaller hypertrophic response of women to muscular overload. Research to date does not support such notions about female's response to overload training and testosterone. *Essentially no correlation exists between plasma testosterone levels and body composition and muscular strength in men and women.* Individuals with high muscle strength and/or FFM often have either high or low testosterone levels. While acute increases in sex hormone release follow a single bout of maximal resistance training (or any maximal effort exercise), the effect remains transient and probably of little consequence to training responsiveness.

Muscle Fiber Hypertrophy: Male Versus Female
Computed tomography scans to evaluate muscle cross-sectional area show that men and women experience *similar* hypertrophic responses to resistance training. Men achieve a greater absolute increase in muscle size because of a larger initial total muscle mass, but without a difference in muscle enlargement on a percentage basis compared with women of similar training status.

Other comparisons between elite male and female bodybuilders verify these observations. *Limited data from short-term studies indicate that women can use conventional resistance training and gain strength and size on a similar percentage basis as men without developing overly large muscles (i.e., a large absolute increase in muscle girth).*

Muscle Fiber Hyperplasia

A common question concerns whether resistance training increases the number of muscle cells (hyperplasia). If this does occur, to what extent does it contribute to muscle enlargement? Chronic overload of skeletal muscle in various animal species develops new muscle fibers from satellite cells between the basement layer and plasma membrane or by longitudinal splitting. Under conditions of stress, neuromuscular disease, and muscle injury, the normally dormant satellite cells develop into new muscle fibers. With longitudinal splitting, a relatively large muscle fiber splits into two or more smaller individual daughter cells through lateral budding. These fibers function more efficiently than the large single fiber from where they originated.

Generalizing findings from research on animals to humans poses a problem. The massive cellular hypertrophy in humans with resistance training does not occur in many animal species. In cats, for example, muscle fiber proliferation (hyperplasia) reflects the primary compensatory adjustment to muscular overload. *Some evidence supporting hyperplasia in humans does exist.* Autopsy data from young, healthy men who died accidentally show that muscle fiber counts of the larger and stronger leg (the leg opposite the dominant hand) contained 10% more muscle fibers than the smaller leg. Cross-sectional studies of body builders with large limb circumferences and muscle mass failed to show they possessed above-normal-size individual muscle fibers. The possibility does exist that some of the body builders inherited an initially large number of small muscle fibers that then "hypertrophy" to normal size with resistance training, yet the findings suggest the likelihood of hyperplasia with certain forms of resistance training. Muscle fibers may adapt differently to high-volume, high-intensity training used by body builders than to the typical low-repetition, heavy-load system favored by strength and power athletes. *Even if other human studies replicate a training-induced hyperplasia (and even if the response reflects a positive adjustment), enlargement of existing individual muscle fibers (hypertrophy) represents the most important contribution to increased muscle size from overload training.*

CONNECTIVE TISSUE AND BONE ADAPTATIONS

Supporting ligaments, tendons, and bone strengthen as muscle strength and size increase. Ligament and tendon strength increases generally parallel the rate of muscle fiber adaptation, while bone changes improve more slowly, perhaps over a 6- to 12-month period. Connective tissue proliferates around individual muscle fibers; this thickens and strengthens the muscle's connective tissue harness. Such adaptations from resistance training protect joints and muscles from injury and justify resistance exercise for preventive and rehabilitative purposes. Resistance training also positively affects bone dynamics in young individuals. For example, elite 14- to 17-year-old junior Olympic weight lifters have higher bone densities in the hip and femur regions than age-matched controls or adults.

CARDIOVASCULAR ADAPTATIONS

Training volume and intensity influence the effect of resistance training on cardiovascular system adaptations (**Table 14.6**).

Subtle yet important differences exist between myocardial enlargement from resistance training (**physiologic hypertrophy**) and enlargement from chronic hypertension (**pathologic hypertrophy**). In pathologic conditions, ventricular wall thickness increases beyond normal limits independent of assessment method and evaluative criteria. Dilation and weakening of the left ventricle, a frequent response to chronic hypertension (and subsequent congestive heart failure), do not accompany the compensatory increase in myocardial wall thickness that occurs with resistance training. The hearts of resistance-trained athletes usually exceed the size of untrained counterparts, but heart size generally falls within the upper-range of normal limits related to body size or cardiac function variables.

Resistance exercise more acutely increases blood pressure than lower-intensity dynamic movements but does *not* produce any long-term increase in resting

Table 14•6	Cardiovascular Adaptations to Resistance Training	
VARIABLE	**ADAPTATION**	
Rest		
Heart rate	No change	
Blood pressure		
Diastolic	Decrease or no change	
Systolic	Decrease or no change	
Rate-pressure product (HR × SBP)	Decrease or no change	
Stroke volume	Increase or no change	
Cardiac function	Increase or no change	
Left ventricular wall thickness	Increase	
Right ventricular wall thickness	No change	
Left ventricular chamber volume	No change	
Right ventricular chamber volume	No change	
Left ventricular mass	Increase	
Lipid profile		
Total cholesterol	Decrease	
HDL-C	Increase or no change	
LDL-C	Decrease or no change	
During exercise		
Heart rate	No change	
Blood pressure		
Diastolic	Decrease	
Systolic	Decrease	
Rate-pressure product	Decrease	
Stroke volume	Increase or no change	
Cardiac output	Increase or no change	
$\dot{V}O_{2peak}$	Increase or no change	

Questions & Notes

Indicate (with an up or down arrow) the specific physiologic adaptations to resistance training that occur for the following variables:

Muscle fiber size:

Mitochondria volume:

Mitochondria density:

Twitch contraction time:

Connective tissue ligament strength:

Bone mineral content:

True or False:

There is no possibility for fiber-type transformation with specific exercise training.

Briefly describe the possible role of testosterone in the hypertrophic response to resistance training.

List 3 cardiovascular adaptations that result from resistance training.

1.

2.

3.

blood pressure. Weight lifters and body builders with hypertension probably have existing essential hypertension, experience chronic overtraining syndrome, use steroids, or possess an undesirable level of body fat or other hypertension risks established for the general population.

Metabolic Stress of Resistance Training

Metabolic and cardiovascular evaluations indicate that traditional resistance training methods offer little benefit for aerobic fitness or weight control or for significantly modifying risk factors related to cardiovascular disease. Oxygen uptake for both isometric and typical weight-lifting exercises would classify as "light to moderate" for energy expenditure, even though subjects reported considerable muscular stress. A person can perform 15 or 20 different resistance exercises during a 1-hour training session, yet the total time devoted to exercise usually lasts no longer than 6 or 7 minutes. This relatively brief activity period (with only moderate energy expenditure) reinforces that traditional resistance training programs would not improve endurance capacity for running, cycling, or swimming. Resistance training exercises also serve only limited value as the primary activities in a weight-loss program because of the typically low total energy expenditure during a training session.

Circuit Resistance Training: Increased Energy Expenditure
Modifying standard resistance training by de-emphasizing heavy overload increases exercise caloric expenditure and workout volume, thus improving more than one aspect of physical fitness. Research has focused on the energy cost and cardiorespiratory demands of **circuit resistance training** (CRT). In CRT, a pre-established exercise-rest sequence usually consists of eight to 15 different exercise stations, with 15 to 20 repetitions performed for each exercise. *Exercise resistance requires between 40% and 50% of 1-RM.* After a 15- to 30-second rest interval, participants move to succeeding exercise stations to complete the circuit. **Figure 14.15** outlines the sequence of progression through a multi-level, 5- to 12-station circuit.

In one experiment, 20 men and 20 women performed three exercise circuits (10 stations per circuit using weight machines) with a 15-second rest between exercises (22.5 min to perform the three circuits). Net energy expended (excluding resting metabolism) equaled 129 kCal for men and 95 kCal for women over the total exercise period. Heart rate averaged 142 b·min^{-1} (72% HR$_{max}$; 40% $\dot{V}O_{2max}$) for men and 158 b·min^{-1} (82% HR$_{max}$; 45% $\dot{V}O_{2max}$) for women.

CRT provides an alternative for fitness enthusiasts who desire a general conditioning program that improves both muscular strength and aerobic capacity. It can also supplement an off-season fitness program for sports requiring a high level of strength, power, and muscular endurance.

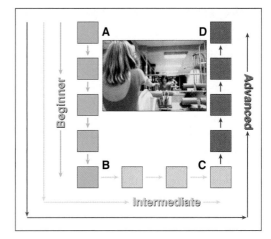

Figure 14.15 A basic multi-level exercise circuit. Beginners can work twice through the circuit from A to B; after several weeks, they progress three times through this portion of the circuit; finally, they increase the number of circuit revolutions up to six, depending on the number of stations. At the intermediate level, add several stations; participants proceed three to six times through circuit A to C. Build progression into each circuit by increasing the number of stations (A to D) and/or exercise load, repetitions, and duration.

Table 14.7 presents energy expenditure data for different types of resistance-type exercises compared to walking on the level. Isokinetic CRT procedures produced the highest energy expenditures.

BODY COMPOSITION ADAPTATIONS

Table 14.8 shows changes in body composition with DCER training from different experiments. For the most part, small decreases occur in body fat, with minimal increases in total body mass and FFM. The largest FFM increases amount to about 3 kg (6.6 lb) over 10 weeks, or about 0.3 kg weekly, with results about the same for men and women. Body composition data for other dynamic strength training systems show similar results. No one resistance training system proves superior for changing body composition.

MUSCLE SORENESS AND STIFFNESS

Most people experience soreness and stiffness in the exercised joints and muscles following an extended layoff from exercise. Temporary soreness may persist for several hours immediately after unaccustomed exercise, whereas a residual **delayed-onset muscle soreness (DOMS)** appears later and can last for 3 or 4 days. The following seven factors can produce DOMS:

1. Minute tears in muscle tissue or damage to its contractile components with accompanying release of creatine kinase, myoglobin, and troponin I, the muscle-specific marker of muscle fiber damage

Table 14·7	Energy Expenditure for Different Modes of Resistance Exercise Compared to Walking[a]			
MODE	**SEX**	**KJ·MIN^{-1}**	**KCAL·MIN^{-1}**
Nautilus, circuit	M	29.7	7.1
	F	24.3	5.8
Nautilus, circuit	M	22.6	5.4
Universal, circuit	M	33.1	7.9
	F	28.5	6.8
Isokinetic, slow	M	40.2	9.6
Isokinetic, fast	M	41.4	9.9
Isometric and free-weight	M	25.1	6.0
Hydra-Fitness, circuit	M	37.7	9.0
Walking on level	M	22.6	5.4

[a] Based on a body weight of 68 kg.
Data from Katch, F.I., et al.: Evaluation of acute cardiorespiratory responses to hydraulic resistance exercise. *Med. Sci. Sports Exerc.,* 17:168, 1985.

2. Osmotic pressure changes that cause fluid retention in the surrounding tissues
3. Muscle spasms
4. Overstretching and perhaps tearing of portions of the muscle's connective tissue harness
5. Acute inflammation
6. Alteration in the cell's mechanism for calcium regulation
7. Combination of the above factors

Eccentric Actions Produce Muscle Soreness

The precise cause of muscle soreness remains unknown. The degree of discomfort and muscle disturbance depends largely on the intensity and duration of effort and type of exercise performed. The magnitude of active strain imposed on a muscle fiber (rather than absolute force) precipitates muscle damage and soreness. Eccentric and, to some extent, isometric muscle actions generally trigger the greatest postexercise discomfort, magnified among older individuals. Existing muscle damage or soreness from previous exercise does not exacerbate subsequent muscle damage or impair the regenerative process.

In one study, subjects rated muscle soreness immediately after exercise and 24, 48, and 72 hours later. Greater soreness resulted from exercise involving repeated intense strain during active lengthening in eccentric actions than from concentric and isometric actions. Soreness did not relate to lactate buildup because high-intensity,

(text continues on page 507)

(text continues on page 507)

Questions & Notes

True or False:

Supporting ligaments, tendons, and bone strengthen as muscle strength and size increase.

List 3 cardiovascular adaptations resulting from resistance training.

1.

2.

3.

FOR YOUR INFORMATION

Low Energy Expenditure
Standard resistance training with weights and barbells "burns" a relatively small number of calories during a workout. The total energy expended equals about the same number of calories walking on level ground at 4 mph, gardening, or swimming slowly for the equivalent time period.

Table 14·8	Body Composition Changes with Resistance Training[a]				
			BODY COMPOSITION CHANGES		
GENDER	**TRAINING DURATION, WK**	**# OF EXERCISES**	**BODY MASS, KG**	**FFM, KG**	**% BODY FAT**
F	10	10	0.1	1.3	−1.8
M	20	10	0.7	1.7	−1.5
M	9	5	0.5	1.4	−1.0
F	24	4	−0.04	1.0	−2.1
F	9	11	0.4	1.5	−1.3
M	8	10	1.0	3.1	−2.9
M	10	11	1.7	2.4	−9.1
F	10	8	−0.1	1.1	−1.9
M	10	8	0.3	1.2	−1.3
M	20	10	0.5	1.8	−1.7

[a] Data from different studies in the literature. F = female; M = male; FFM = fat-free mass.

Box 14–5 • CLOSE UP

HOW TO ASSESS MUSCULAR ENDURANCE

Muscular endurance represents how well a muscle (or muscle group) exerts submaximum force repeatedly within a given time period, or the duration a given muscle action can sustain a percentage of its 1-RM either dynamically or isometrically. The number of total repetitions of a muscle action in a given time (e.g., number of curl-ups, sit-ups, or push-ups within 1 minute or while maintaining a given cadence) provides a common yardstick for expressing muscular endurance. Muscular endurance depends somewhat on a muscle's maximum strength but little on cardiorespiratory fitness because components of aerobic fitness represent separate physiological (and fitness) entities. To test muscular endurance using weights, the weight lifted should coincide with either a percentage of body weight (**Table 1**) or a percentage of 1-RM, so total repetition number averages between 15 and 20.

Two of the more popular muscular endurance tests do not require weights to assess endurance of the abdominal (curl-up) and upper-body (push-up) musculatures.

CURL-UP MUSCULAR ENDURANCE TEST

Initial Position

The individual lies supine with knees flexed and feet about one foot from the buttocks. The arms extend forward with fingers palm-down on the thighs pointing towards the knees (**Fig. 1A**). The tester kneels behind the person with hands cupped (about 2 inches off the floor) under the individual's head.

Movement

The person curls up slowly, sliding the fingers up the legs until the fingertips touch the patellae (knee caps; **Fig. 1B**), followed by slowly returning to the starting position with the back of the head touching the tester's hands. To reduce lower back strain, minimize rectus femoris involvement and emphasize abdominal muscle action; no assistance should anchor or support the feet.

Table 1	Recommended Percentage of Body Weight Lifted in Different Resistance Exercise Movements to Assess Muscular Endurance		
		PERCENTAGE OF BODY WEIGHT	
EXERCISE		**MEN**	**WOMEN**
Arm curl		0.33	0.25
Bench press		0.66	0.50
Lateral pull down		0.66	0.50
Triceps extension		0.33	0.33
Leg extension		0.50	0.50
Leg curl		0.33	0.33

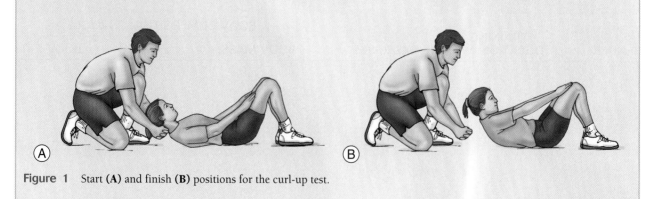

Ⓐ Ⓑ

Figure 1 Start (**A**) and finish (**B**) positions for the curl-up test.

Box 14–5 • CLOSE UP *(Continued)*

The Test and Standards

Required curl-up rate equals 20 repetitions per minute (3 s per curl-up; metronome set at 40 b·min^{-1}, or 2 beats per curl-up and recovery). Individuals perform as many curl-ups as possible at a cadence (which must be maintained) to a maximum of 75. **Table 2** presents standards for evaluating scores on the curl-up test.

PUSH-UP MUSCULAR ENDURANCE TEST

The push-up muscular endurance test can be performed in one of two ways: (1) full-body push-up, and (2) modified push-up that reduces the body mass above the arms, chest, and shoulders. The modified push-up serves as an alternative to assess individual differences in up-

per-body strength for females because they possess considerably less relative strength in upper-body musculature compared with males.

Initial Position

Full-Body Push-Up: The person assumes a relatively stiff prone position from head to ankles, keeping the hands shoulder-width apart and arms fully extended (Fig. 2A).

   Modified Push-Up: The person assumes the bent-knee position with hips and buttocks pressing downward in line with the neck and shoulders (Fig. 2B).

Movement

Full-Body Push-Up and Modified Push-Up: The body lowers until the elbows reach 90° of flexion; the return

Table 2	Test Standards to Assess Curl-Up Performance		
	NUMBER OF CURL-UPS COMPLETED		
	AGE, y		
RATING	**<35**	**35–44**	**>45**
Excellent			
Men	60	50	40
Women	50	40	30
Good			
Men	45	40	25
Women	40	25	15
Fair			
Men	30	25	15
Women	25	15	10
Poor			
Men	15	10	5
Women	10	6	4

From Faulkner, R.A., et al.: A partial curl-up protocol for adults based on an analysis of two procedures. *Can. J. Sport Sci.*, 14:135, 1989; Sparling, P.B., et al.: Development of a cadence curl-up for college students. *Res. Q. Exerc. Sport.*, 68:309, 1997.

Box 14–5 • CLOSE UP *(Continued)*

action requires pushing up until the arms fully extend. The push-up action should proceed in a continuous motion without rest pauses between flexion-extension movements.

Standards

Table 3 presents standards for scoring the full body push-up (men) and modified push-up (women) tests.

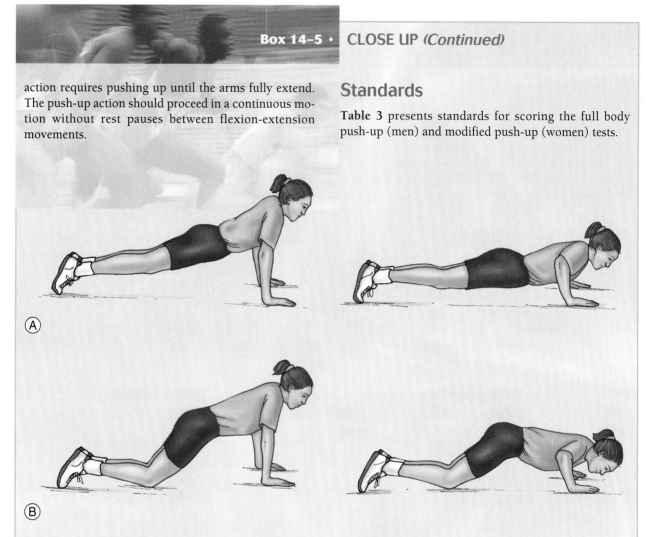

Figure 2   Start and finish positions for **(A)** full-body push-up and **(B)** modified push-up.

| Table 3 | Test Standards to Assess Push-Up Performance of Men (Full-Body Push-Up) and Women (Modified Push-Up) |

| | NUMBER OF PUSH-UPS COMPLETED | | | | |
| | AGE, y | | | | |
RATING	20–29	30–39	40–49	50–59	60+
Full-body push-up					
Excellent	>54	>44	>39	>34	>29
Good	45–54	35–44	30–39	25–34	20–29
Average	35–44	25–34	20–29	15–24	10–19
Fair	20–34	15–24	12–19	8–14	5–9
Poor	<20	<15	<12	<8	<5
Modified push-up					
Excellent	>48	>39	>34	>29	>19
Good	34–48	25–39	20–34	15–29	5–19
Average	17–33	12–24	8–19	6–14	3–4
Fair	6–16	4–11	3–7	2–5	1–2
Poor	<6	<4	<3	<2	<1

From Pollock, M.L., et al.: *Health and Fitness Through Physical Activity.* New York: John Wiley & Sons, 1984.

level running (concentric actions) produced no residual soreness despite considerable elevations in blood lactate. In contrast, downhill running (eccentric actions) caused moderate-to-severe DOMS without lactate elevation during exercise.

Cell Damage

DOMS develops 42 hours following downhill running. Corresponding increases occur for serum levels of the muscle-specific enzyme creatine kinase (CK) and myoglobin (Mb), both common markers of muscle damage. Subjects were retested on the same exercise after 3, 6, and 9 weeks. **Figure 14.16** shows the perceived soreness rating for the leg muscles in relation to time postexercise for the three study durations. For the 3- and 6-week comparisons, differences between exercise bouts reached statistical significance, with diminished DOM noted in the second trial (open squares).

Similar patterns emerged for CK and Mb related to perception of muscle soreness. Interestingly, peak soreness ratings achieved at 48 hours did not relate to absolute or relative changes in CK or Mb. Individuals reporting the greatest muscle soreness did not necessarily have the highest CK and Mb values.

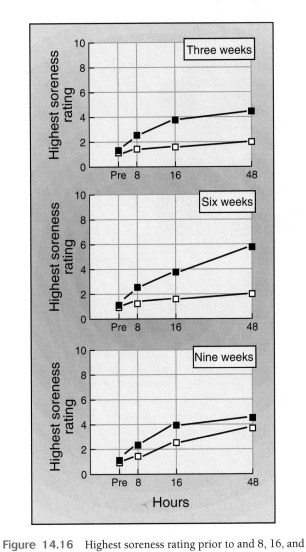

Figure 14.16   Highest soreness rating prior to and 8, 16, and 48 hours following bout 1 (closed square) and bout 2 (open square) performed 3, 6, and 9 weeks later. Similar results were obtained for creatine kinase and myoglobin. (Data from Byrnes, W.C., et al.: Delayed onset muscle soreness following repeated bouts of downhill running. *J. Appl. Physiol.*, 59:710, 1985.)

Give the most important body composition alteration that results from resistance training.

Define DOMS.

List 4 factors that can produce DOMS.

1.

2.

3

4.

Name the type of muscle overload that produces the greatest level of DOMS.

Describe 2 tests to assess muscular endurance.

1.

2.

When does DOMS usually develop following exercise?

Describe one procedure to reduce the soreness from DOMS.

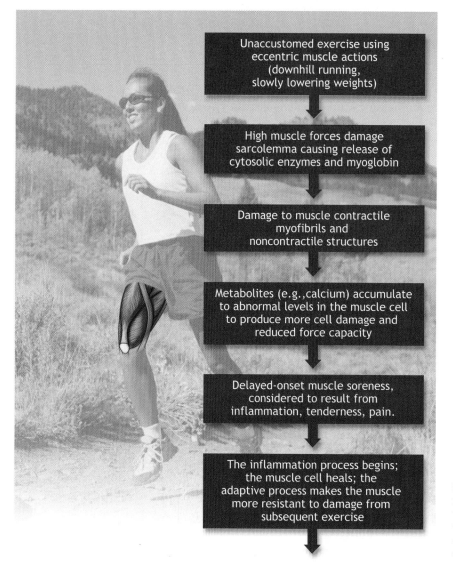

Unaccustomed exercise using eccentric muscle actions (downhill running, slowly lowering weights)

High muscle forces damage sarcolemma causing release of cytosolic enzymes and myoglobin

Damage to muscle contractile myofibrils and noncontractile structures

Metabolites (e.g.,calcium) accumulate to abnormal levels in the muscle cell to produce more cell damage and reduced force capacity

Delayed-onset muscle soreness, considered to result from inflammation, tenderness, pain.

The inflammation process begins; the muscle cell heals; the adaptive process makes the muscle more resistant to damage from subsequent exercise

Figure 14.17 Proposed sequence for delayed-onset muscle soreness after unaccustomed exercise. Cellular adaptations to short-term exercise provide enhanced resistance to subsequent damage and pain.

The first bout of repetitive, unaccustomed physical activity disrupts the integrity of the cells' internal environment. This can produce microlesions and temporary ultrastructural damage in a pool of stress-susceptible or degenerating muscle fibers. Damage becomes more extensive several days after exercise than in the immediate postexercise period. A single bout of moderate concentric exercise provides a prophylactic effect on muscle soreness from subsequent high-force eccentric exercise, with the beneficial effect lasting up to 6 weeks. *Such results support the wisdom of initiating a training program with repetitive, moderate concentric exercise to protect against the muscle soreness that occurs following exercise with an eccentric component.*

Altered Sarcoplasmic Reticulum

Changes in pH, intramuscular high-energy phosphates, ionic balance, or temperature with unaccustomed exercise produce major alterations in sarcoplasmic reticulum structure and function. These effects depress rates of Ca^{++} uptake and release and increase free Ca^{++} concentration as the mineral rapidly moves into the cytosol of the damaged fibers. An overload of intracellular Ca^{++} may contribute to the autolytic process within damaged muscle fibers that degrades both contractile and noncontractile structures, leading to reduced force capacity and eventual muscle soreness. Vitamin E supplementation protects against cellular membrane disruption and enzyme loss following muscle damage from heavy resistance exercise.

Current DOMS Model

Figure 14.17 diagrams the probable steps in the development of DOMS and subsequent recuperation. An area of current controversy concerns whether the liberal use of nonsteroidal anti-inflammatory agents to treat soft-tissue injury or acute pain from DOMS provides any benefit (or harm) to short- and long-term recuperation.

SUMMARY

1. Genetic, exercise, nutritional, hormonal, environmental, and neural factors interact to regulate skeletal muscle mass and corresponding strength development.

2. Physiologic factors (e.g., size and type of muscle fibers and anatomic-lever arrangement of bone and muscle) ultimately determine an individual's muscular strength. Neural influences from the central nervous system that activate prime movers in a specific movement greatly affect one's ability to express this strength.

3. Muscular strength increases with resistance training from (1) improved capacity for neuromuscular activation, and (2) significant alterations in a muscle fiber's contractile elements.

4. As overloaded muscles become stronger, individual fibers normally grow larger (hypertrophy). Total muscle enlargement involves (1) increased protein synthesis within the fiber's contractile elements, and (2) proliferation of cells that thicken and strengthen the muscle's connective tissue harness.

5. Muscle fiber hypertrophy involves (1) structural changes within the contractile mechanism of individual fibers (particularly fast-twitch fibers), and (2) increases in intramuscular anaerobic energy stores. If new muscle fibers develop, their contribution to muscular enlargement remains unknown.

6. Intense resistance training does not induce cellular component adaptations to enhance aerobic energy transfer.

7. Women and men improve strength and muscle size to about the same relative extent (percentage) with resistance training.

8. Conventional resistance-training exercises contribute little to cardiovascular-aerobic fitness. Most resistance training programs would not reduce body fat significantly because of the relatively low caloric cost.

9. Circuit resistance training using lower resistance and higher repetitions combines the muscle-training benefits of resistance exercise with cardiovascular, calorie-burning benefits of continuous exercise.

10. Eccentric muscle actions produce significantly more delayed-onset muscle soreness (DOMS) compared with concentric only and isometric exercise.

11. Muscle tears and connective tissue damage cause DOMS.

THOUGHT QUESTIONS

1. How would you apply the principle of specificity to (1) evaluate current muscular strength and power, and (2) improve muscular performance for a football lineman?

2. Outline steps in designing a resistance-training program for sedentary, middle-age men and women.

3. Outline tests to evaluate muscular performance to best reflect the force-power requirements for firefighters.

4. Respond to a friend who comments: "I run and work out with free weights regularly, yet every spring my muscles are sore a day or two after a few hours of yard work."

SELECTED REFERENCES

Alkner, B.A., Tesch, P.A.: Knee extensor and plantar flexor muscle size and function following 90 days of bed rest with or without resistance exercise. *Eur. J. Appl. Physiol.*, 93:294, 2004.

Andersen, L.L., et al.: Neuromuscular adaptations to detraining following resistance training in previously untrained subjects. *Eur. J. Appl. Physiol.*, 93:511, 2005.

Andersen, L.L., et al.: The effect of resistance training combined with timed ingestion of protein on muscle fiber size and muscle strength. *Metabolism*, 54:151, 2005.

Baker, D., Newton, R.U.: Acute effect on power output of alternating an agonist and antagonist muscle exercise during complex training. *J. Strength Cond. Res.*, 19:202, 2005.

Bazzucchi, I., et al.: Differences between young and older women in maximal force, force fluctuations, and surface EMG during isometric knee extension and elbow flexion. *Muscle Nerve*, 30:626, 2004.

Brandenburg, J.P.: The acute effects of prior dynamic resistance exercise using different loads on subsequent upper-body explosive performance in resistance-trained men. *J. Strength Cond. Res.*, 19:427, 2005.

Brocherie, F., et al.: Electrostimulation training effects on the physical performance of ice hockey players. *Med. Sci. Sports Exerc.*, 37:455, 2005.

Brock Symons, T., et al.: Effects of deep heat as a preventative mechanism on delayed onset muscle soreness. *J. Strength Cond. Res.*, 18:155, 2004.

Burgomaster, K.A., et al.: Resistance training with vascular occlusion: metabolic adaptations in human muscle. *Med. Sci. Sports Exerc.*, 35:1203, 2003.

Cronin, J., Crewther, B.: Training volume and strength and power development. *J. Sci. Med. Sport*, 7:144, 2004.

Cronin, J.B., Hansen, K.T.: Strength and power predictors of sports speed. *J. Strength Cond. Res.*, 19:349, 2005.

Dannecker, E.A., et al.: Sex differences in delayed onset muscle pain. *Clin. J. Pain*, 21:120, 2005.

de Vos, N.J., et al.: Optimal load for increasing muscle power during explosive resistance training in older adults. *J. Gerontol. A. Biol. Sci. Med. Sci.*, 60:638, 2005.

DeLorme, T.L., Watkins, A.L.: *Progressive Resistance Exercise*. New York: Appleton-Century-Crofts, 1951.

Goto, K., et al.: The impact of metabolic stress on hormonal responses and muscular adaptations. *Med. Sci. Sports Exerc.*, 37:955, 2005.

Gotshalk, L.A., et al.: Cardiovascular responses to a high-volume continuous circuit resistance training protocol. *J. Strength Cond. Res.*, 18:760, 2004.

Graves, J.E., et al.: Specificity of limited range of motion variable resistance training. *Med. Sci. Sports Exerc.*, 21:84, 1989.

Gruber, M., Gollhofer, A.: Impact of sensorimotor training on the rate of force development and neural activation. *Eur. J. Appl. Physiol.*, 92:98, 2004.

Hakkinen, A., et al.: Effects of home strength training and stretching versus stretching alone after lumbar disk surgery: a randomized study with a 1-year follow-up. *Arch. Phys. Med. Rehabil.*, 86:865, 2005.

Hamnegard, C.H., et al.: Quadriceps strength assessed by magnetic stimulation of the femoral nerve in normal subjects. *Clin. Physiol. Funct. Imaging*, 24:276, 2004.

Harber, M.P., et al.: Single muscle fiber contractile properties during a competitive season in male runners. *Am. J. Physiol. Regul. Integr. Comp. Physiol.*, 287:R1124, 2004.

Harmon, E.: Resistive torque analysis of 5 Nautilus exercise machines. *Med. Sci. Sports Exerc.*, 5:113, 1983.

Henwood, T.R., Taaffe, D.R.: Improved physical performance in older adults undertaking a short-term programme of high-velocity resistance training. *Gerontology*, 51:108, 2005.

Herman, S., et al.: Upper and lower limb muscle power relationships in mobility-limited older adults. *J. Gerontol. A. Biol. Sci. Med. Sci.*, 60:476, 2005.

Ikai, M., Steinhaus, A.H.: Some factors modifying the expression of human strength. *J. Appl. Physiol.*, 16:157, 1961.

Kasikcioglu, E., et al.: Angiotensin-converting enzyme gene polymorphism, left ventricular remodeling, and exercise capacity in strength-trained athletes. *Heart Vessels*, 19:287, 2004.

Katch, F.I., et al.: Evaluation of acute cardiorespiratory responses to hydraulic resistance exercise. *Med. Sci. Sports Exerc.*, 17:168, 1985.

Kawamori, N., Haff, G.G.: The optimal training load for the development of muscular power. *J. Strength Cond. Res.*, 18:675, 2004.

Kemmler, W.K., et al.: Effects of single- vs. multiple-set resistance training on maximum strength and body composition in trained postmenopausal women. *J. Strength Cond. Res.*, 18:689, 2004.

Leonard, C.T., et al.: Comparison of surface electromyography and myotonometric measurements during voluntary isometric contractions. *J. Electromyogr. Kinesiol.*, 14:709, 2004.

Lieber, R.L.: *Skeletal Muscle Structure, Function, and Plasticity: The Physiological Basis of Rehabilitation*. Baltimore: Lippincott, Williams & Wilkins, 2002.

Lund, H., et al.: Learning effect of isokinetic measurements in healthy subjects, and reliability and comparability of Biodex and Lido dynamometers. *Clin. Physiol. Funct. Imaging*, 25:75, 2005.

Massey, C.D., et al.: An analysis of full range of motion vs. partial range of motion training in the development of strength in untrained men. *J. Strength Cond. Res.*, 18:518, 2004.

McCurdy, K.W., et al.: The effects of short-term unilateral and bilateral lower-body resistance training on measures of strength and power. *J. Strength Cond. Res.*, 19:9, 2005.

Mjolsnes, R., et al.: A 10-week randomized trial comparing eccentric vs. concentric hamstring strength training in well-trained soccer players. *Scand. J. Med. Sci. Sports*, 14:311, 2004.

Nosaka, K., et al.: Partial protection against muscle damage by eccentric actions at short muscle lengths. *Med. Sci. Sports Exerc.*, 37:746, 2005.

Petrella, J.K., et al.: Age differences in knee extension power, contractile velocity, and fatigability. *J. Appl. Physiol.*, 98:211, 2005.

Raue, U., et al.: Effects of short-term concentric vs. eccentric resistance training on single muscle fiber MHC distribution in humans. *Int. J. Sports Med.*, 26:339, 2005.

Reeves, N.D., et al.: Plasticity of dynamic muscle performance with strength training in elderly humans. *Muscle Nerve*, 31:355, 2005.

Sale, D.G.: Influence of exercise and training on motor unit activation. In: *Exercise and Sport Sciences Reviews*. Vol. 15. Pandolf KB. (ed.) New York: Macmillan, 1987.

Seger, J.Y., et al.: Specific effects of eccentric and concentric training on muscle strength and morphology in humans. *Eur. J. Appl. Physiol.*, 79:49, 1998.

Seger, J.Y., Thorstensson, A.: Effects of eccentric versus concentric training on thigh muscle strength and EMG. *Int. J. Sports Med.*, 26:45, 2005.

Shepstone, T.N., et al.: Short-term high- vs low-velocity isokinetic lengthening training results in greater hypertrophy of the elbow flexors in young men. *Scand. J. Med. Sci. Sports*, 15:135, 2005.

Signorile, J.F., et al.: Early plateaus of power and torque gains during high- and low-speed resistance training of older women. *J. Appl. Physiol.*, 98:1213, 2005.

Symons, T.B., et al.: Effects of maximal isometric and isokinetic resistance training on strength and functional mobility in older adults. *J. Gerontol. A. Biol. Sci. Med. Sci.*, 60:777, 2005.

Symons, T.B., et al.: Reliability of a single-session isokinetic and isometric strength measurement protocol in older men. *J. Gerontol. A. Biol. Sci. Med. Sci.*, 60:114, 2005.

Symons, T.B., et al.: Reliability of isokinetic and isometric knee-extensor force in older women. *J. Aging Phys. Act.*, 12:525, 2004.

Toji, H., Kaneko, M.: Effect of multiple-load training on the force-velocity relationship. *J. Strength Cond. Res.*, 18:792, 2004.

Trappe, S., et al.: Human single muscle fibre function with 84 day bed-rest and resistance exercise. *J. Physiol.*, 557:501, 2004.

Tsang, W.W., Hui-Chan, C.W.: Comparison of muscle torque, balance, and confidence in older tai chi and healthy adults. *Med. Sci. Sports Exerc.,* 37:280, 2005.

Weiss, L.W., et al.: Strength/power augmentation subsequent to short-term training abstinence. *J. Strength Cond. Res.*, 18:765, 2004.

Weltman, A.W., et al.: The effects of hydraulic resistance strength training in pre-pubertal males. *Med. Sci. Sports Exerc.*, 18: 629, 1986.

Wood, L.E., et al.: Elbow flexion and extension strength relative to body or muscle size in children. *Med. Sci. Sports Exerc.*, 36:1977, 2004.

CHAPTER OBJECTIVES

- Explain the statement: The hypothalamus plays the most important role in regulating thermal balance.
- Name four physical factors that contribute to heat exchange during rest and exercise.
- Describe how the circulatory system serves as a "workhorse" for thermoregulation.
- List desirable clothing characteristics for exercising in cold and warm weather.
- Describe how cardiac output, heart rate, and stroke volume respond during submaximal and maximal exercise during environmental heat stress.
- Describe circulatory adjustments that maintain blood pressure during exercise in the heat.
- Quantify fluid loss during hot-weather exercise.
- Identify the physiologic consequences of dehydration.
- Explain how acclimatization, training, age, gender, and body fat modify heat tolerance during exercise.
- Identify factors that comprise the Heat Stress Index.
- Explain the purpose of the Wind Chill Index.
- Describe the physiologic adjustments to cold stress.
- Outline the effects of increasingly higher altitudes on (1) partial pressure of oxygen in ambient air, (2) saturation of hemoglobin with oxygen in the pulmonary capillaries, and (3) $\dot{V}O_{2max}$.
- Describe the immediate and long-term physiologic adjustments to altitude exposure.
- Outline three approaches for creating an altitude environment at sea level so an athlete can spend sufficient time to stimulate an acclimatization response.
- Describe the typical time course for red blood cell reinfusion and mechanism for its ergogenic effect on endurance performance and aerobic capacity.
- Discuss the medical use of erythropoietin and its potential dangers for healthy athletes.
- Contrast "general warm-up" and "specific warm-up."
- Identify potential cardiovascular benefits of moderate warm-up immediately prior to extreme physical effort.
- Provide a rationale for breathing a hyperoxic gas mixture to enhance exercise performance, and quantify its potential to increase tissue oxygen availability.

CHAPTER OUTLINE

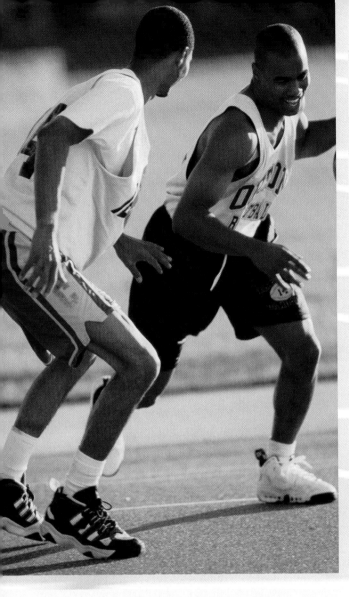

chapter

15

Factors Affecting Physiologic Function: The Environment and Special Aids to Performance

The environment can influence the body's physiology in a way that augments the stress of exercise and reduces performance. Altitude impairs the normal sea level oxygenation of blood flowing through the lungs during sport competiton. Above a certain elevation, the capacity to generate energy aerobically becomes severely compromised. Exercise in a hot humid environment or extreme cold often imposes a severe thermal stress that dramatically affects not only exercise performance but also the participant's health and safety. How an environmental stressor deviates from neutral conditions and duration of exposure determines its total effect. Several environmental stressors operating at the same time (e.g., extreme cold exposure at high altitude) may exceed and override the simple additive effects of each stressor acting singularly.

Coaches and athletes continually search for additional ways to gain the competitive "edge" and improve athletic performance. It should occasion little surprise that athletes routinely use a variety of substances and procedures at almost all competitive levels, often without regard for potential health dangers or lack of scientific evidence to support their effectiveness.

This chapter discusses the specific problems encountered during exercise in hot and cold environments and at high altitude. We present this information within the framework of the immediate physiologic adjustments and longer-term adaptations as the body strives to maintain internal consistency despite an environmental challenge. We also explore three common ergogenic interventions (blood doping, warm-up, and hyperoxic gas) to improve physiologic function, exercise capacity, and athletic performance.

PART 1 •
Mechanisms of Thermoregulation

THERMOREGULATION

Normal body temperature fluctuates several degrees during the day in response to physical activity, emotions, and ambient temperature variations, with oral temperature averaging about 1.0°F (0.56°C) less than rectal temperature. Body temperature also exhibits diurnal fluctuations; lowest temperatures occur during sleep, and slightly higher temperatures persist when awake, even when the person remains relaxed in bed.

Thermoregulation plays such an important role in the body's homeostatic balance that the price of failure is death. A person can tolerate a drop in core temperature of 18°F (10°C) but only an increase of 5°C (9°F). More than 100 times over the past 20 years, football players have died from excessive heat stress during practice or competition, as have collegiate wrestlers. Heat injury also commonly

occurs during military operations and longer-duration athletic events, as it often does in industry (mining) and farming operations (migrant pickers).

Understanding thermoregulation and the most effective ways to support temperature control mechanisms can dramatically reduce heat-related tragedies. Coaches, athletes, and race and event organizers must reduce factors that promote heat gain and dehydration. Concern should also focus on the most effective behavioral approaches (e.g., prudent scheduling of events, acclimatization, proper clothing, and fluid and electrolyte replacement before, during, and after exercise) to blunt the potential for negative effects on performance and safety.

THERMAL BALANCE

Figure 15.1 lists factors that contribute to heat gain and heat loss as the body attempts to maintain thermal neutrality. This balance results from integrative mechanisms that:

1. Alter heat transfer to the periphery (**shell**)
2. Regulate evaporative cooling
3. Vary the rate of heat production

The temperature of the deeper tissues (**core**) rises quickly when heat gain exceeds heat loss during vigorous exercise in a warm environment. In the cold, in contrast, heat loss often exceeds heat production that reduces core temperature.

Body Temperature Measurement

A thermal gradient exists within the body, with core body temperature (T_{core}) the highest and shell temperature ($\overline{T}_{skin}$) the lowest. Mean body temperature ($\overline{T}_{body}$) represents an average of skin and internal temperatures. Common sites to estimate average core temperature ($\overline{T}_{core}$) include the rectum, eardrum (tympanic temperature), and esophagus (esophageal temperature). The values in these regions do estimate the temperature in the brain's hypothalamus, the area that controls thermoregulation. Temperature sensors (thermistors) placed at various skin locations estimate T_{skin}. Mean skin temperature ($\overline{T}_{skin}$) denotes the weighted average of different skin temperatures that reflect the portion of the body's surface each site represents (e.g., arm, trunk, leg, head). $\overline{T}_{body}$ computes as follows:

$$\overline{T}_{body} = (0.6 \times \overline{T}_{core}) + (0.4 \times \overline{T}_{skin})$$

The relative proportion of the body's average temperature represented by the core equals 0.6 (60%) and 0.4 (40%) for the skin.

HYPOTHALAMIC REGULATION OF TEMPERATURE

The hypothalamus contains the central coordinating center for temperature regulation. This group of specialized neu-

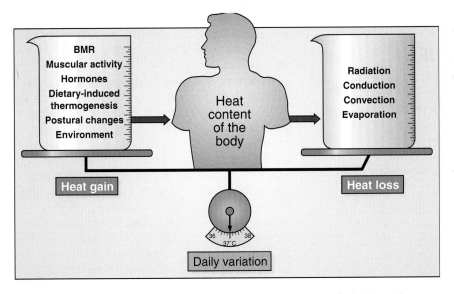

Figure 15.1. Factors that contribute to heat gain and heat loss as the body regulates core temperature at approximately 98.6°F (37°C).

*Q*uestions & Notes

Give the average difference between oral and rectal temperature.

List 3 factors that result in body heat gain.

1.

2.

3.

List 3 factors that result in body heat loss.

1.

2.

3.

Name the central coordinating center for temperature regulation.

Name the 2 ways the body's temperature-regulating mechanisms become activated.

1.

2.

rons at the floor of the brain serves as a thermostat to carefully regulate temperature within a narrow range of 37°C ± 1°C (98.6°F ± 1.8°F). Unlike a home thermostat, however, the hypothalamus cannot turn off the heat; it only initiates responses to protect the body when core temperature changes from its "norm" due to heat gain or heat loss. Temperature-regulating mechanisms become activated in two ways:

1. Thermal receptors in the skin provide peripheral input to the hypothalamic central control center.
2. Temperature changes in blood that perfuses the hypothalamus directly stimulate the hypothalamic central control center.

The central hypothalamic regulatory center plays the most important role in maintaining thermal balance. Cells in the anterior hypothalamus directly detect changes in blood temperature in addition to receiving peripheral input. The cells then activate either the posterior hypothalamus to initiate coordinated responses for heat conservation or the anterior hypothalamus for heat loss. Peripheral receptors primarily detect cold; the hypothalamus monitors body warmth by the temperature of the blood that perfuses this area. **Table 15.1** summarizes the mechanisms that regulate body temperature; each responds in a graded manner, increasing or decreasing as required.

Table 15•1	Mechanisms for Temperature Regulation	
Stimulated by cold		
• Decreases heat loss	• Vasoconstriction of skin vessels; postural reduction of surface area (curling up)	
• Increases heat producton	• Shivering and increased voluntary activity; increased thyroxine and epinephrine secretion	
Stimulated by heat		
• Increases heat loss	• Vasodilation of subcutaneous skin vessels; sweating	
• Decreases heat production	• Decreased muscle tone and voluntary activity; decreased thyroxine and epinephrine secretion	

FOR YOUR INFORMATION

Inaccuracy of Oral Temperature
Oral temperature does not accurately measure deep body (core) temperature after strenuous exercise. For example, large and consistent differences occurred between oral and rectal temperatures after a 14-mile race in a tropical climate; the rectal temperature averaged 103.5°F (39.7°C), whereas oral temperature remained a normal 98.6°F (37°C). This discrepancy partly results from evaporative cooling of the mouth and airways from relatively high ventilatory volumes during and immediately after intense exercise.

REGULATING BODY TEMPERATURE DURING COLD AND HEAT EXPOSURE

Cold Stress

In extreme cold, excessive heat loss occurs at rest. This increases the body's heat production and slows heat loss as physiologic adjustments combat the predictable decrease in core temperature.

Three integrated factors regulate body temperature during cold exposure:

1. **Vascular Adjustments.** Circulatory adjustments "fine tune" temperature regulation. Stimulation of cutaneous cold receptors constricts peripheral blood vessels. Vasoconstriction immediately reduces the flow of warm blood to the body's cooler surface and redirects it to the warmer core (cranial, thoracic, and abdominal cavities and portions of the muscle mass). Consequently, skin temperature decreases toward ambient temperature to optimize the insulatory benefits of skin and subcutaneous fat.

2. **Muscular Activity.** The greatest contribution of muscle in defending against cold occurs during physical activity, although shivering also generates considerable metabolic heat (maximum of 3 to 5 times resting metabolism). Exercise energy metabolism can sustain a constant core temperature when air temperatures dip to −30°C (−22°F) without the need for heavy clothing.

3. **Hormonal Output.** Increased epinephrine and norepinephrine partially account for increased basal heat production during cold exposure. Prolonged cold stress also increases the release of thyroxine to elevate resting metabolism.

Heat Stress

Thermoregulatory mechanisms primarily protect against overheating. Thwarting excessive body heat buildup becomes important during sustained intense exercise where metabolic rate often increases 20 to 25 times the resting level—heat production that could increase core temperature by 1.8°F (1°C) every 5 minutes. Here, rivalry exists between mechanisms that maintain a large muscle blood flow and mechanisms that regulate body temperature. **Figure 15.2** illustrates four potential avenues for heat exchange when exercising. Body heat loss occurs in four ways:

1. **Radiation:** Objects continually emit electromagnetic heat waves. Because the body is usually warmer than the environment, the net exchange of radiant heat energy occurs from the body through the air to solid, cooler objects in the environment. Despite subfreezing temperatures, a person can remain warm by absorbing sufficient radiant heat energy from direct sunlight or reflected from the snow, sand, or water.

The body absorbs radiant heat energy when the temperature of objects in the environment exceeds skin temperature, making evaporative cooling the only avenue for heat loss.

2. **Conduction:** Heat loss by conduction directly transfers heat through a liquid, solid, or gas from one molecule to another. Circulation transports most of the body heat to the shell, but a small amount continually moves by conduction directly through the warmer deep tissues to the cooler surface. Conductive heat loss then warms air molecules and cooler surfaces that contact the skin. The rate of conductive heat loss depends on the temperature gradient between the skin and surrounding surfaces and their thermal qualities. For example, when hiking outdoors in the heat, some relief (cooling) can come from lying on a cool rock shielded from the sun. Conductance between the rock's colder surface and the hiker's warmer surface facilitates body heat loss until the rock warms to body temperature.

3. **Convection:** The effectiveness of heat loss by conduction depends on how rapidly air near the body exchanges once it becomes warmed. With little or no air movement (convection), air next to the skin warms and acts as a zone of insulation, minimizing further conductive heat loss. Conversely, if cooler air continuously replaces warmer air surrounding the body (as it does on a breezy day, in a room with a fan, or during running), heat loss increases because convective currents carry the heat away. For example, air currents at 4 mph cool twice as effectively as air moving at 1 mph.

4. **Evaporation:** Evaporation provides the major physiologic defense against overheating. Water vaporization from the respiratory passages and skin surface continually transfers heat to the environment (see Close Up on page 518). In response to heat stress, the body's 2 to 4 million sweat (eccrine) glands secrete large quantities of hypotonic saline solution (0.2% to 0.4% NaCl). Cooling occurs when sweat reaches the skin and fluid evaporates. The cooled skin then cools the blood shunted from the interior to the surface. Along with heat loss through sweating, approximately 350 mL of water seeps through the skin (insensible perspiration) each day and evaporates to the environment. Also, 300 mL of water vaporizes daily from respiratory passages' moist mucous membranes. In cold weather, respiratory tract evaporation appears as "foggy breath."

Evaporative Heat Loss at High Ambient Temperatures

Increased ambient temperature reduces the effectiveness of heat loss by conduction, convection, and radiation. When ambient temperature exceeds body temperature, these three mechanisms of thermal transfer actually contribute to heat gain. When this occurs (or when conduction, convection, and radiation cannot adequately dissipate a large metabolic heat load), sweat evaporation

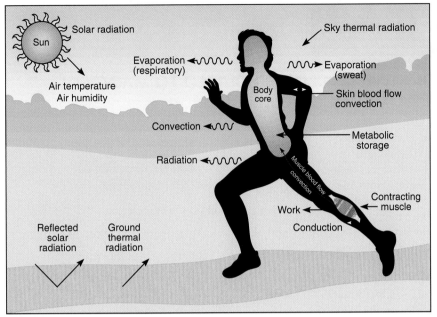

Figure 15.2. Heat production within active muscle and its subsequent transfer to the core and skin. Excess body heat dissipates to the environment and core temperature regulates within a narrow range.

Questions & Notes

List 3 factors that regulate body temperature during cold exposure.

1.

2.

3.

List 4 ways the body loses heat.

1.

2.

3.

4.

For each liter of water evaporated from the skin's surface, _____ kCal of heat energy transfers to the environment.

and water vaporization from the respiratory tract provide the *only* avenue for dissipating heat. For someone relaxing in a hot, humid environment, the normal 2-L daily fluid requirement doubles or even triples from evaporative fluid loss.

Heat Loss in High Humidity   Sweat evaporation from the skin depends on three factors:

1. Surface exposed to the environment
2. Temperature and relative humidity of ambient air
3. Convective air currents around the body

By far, **relative humidity** *exerts the greatest impact on the effectiveness of evaporative heat loss.*

With high humidity, ambient air's vapor pressure approaches that of moist skin (approximately 40 mm Hg). When this happens, evaporation decreases even though large quantities of sweat bead on the skin and eventually roll off. This response represents a useless water loss that can precipitate dehydration and overheating. Continually drying the skin with a towel before sweat evaporates also hinders evaporative cooling. *Sweat does not cool the skin; rather, skin cooling occurs when sweat evaporates.* Individuals can tolerate relatively high environmental temperatures when humidity remains low. For this reason, hot, dry desert climates are more thermally "comforting" than cooler but more humid tropical climates.

INTEGRATION OF HEAT-DISSIPATING MECHANISMS

Heat dissipation involves the integration of three physiologic mechanisms: circulation, evaporation, and hormonal adjustments.

Circulation   *The circulatory system serves as the "workhorse" for thermal balance.* At rest in hot weather, heart rate and cardiac output increase, while superficial arte-

List 3 factors that influence sweat evaporation from the skin.

1.

2.

3.

Give the main environmental factor that affects the magnitude of evaporative heat loss.

FOR YOUR INFORMATION

Air Contains Water
Relative humidity describes the ratio of water in ambient air to its total capacity for moisture at a particular ambient temperature, expressed as a percentage. For example, 40% relative humidity means that ambient air contains only 40% of the air's moisture-carrying capacity at a specific temperature.

Box 15–1 • CLOSE UP

ESTIMATING THE EVAPORATIVE COOLING REQUIRED TO MAINTAIN CONSTANT CORE TEMPERATURE DURING EXERCISE

Evaporation describes the conversion of a substance from liquid form into a gaseous state. The process requires heat energy to overcome the cohesive forces that hold molecules together to form the vapor. Heat loss from water evaporation accounts for nearly 25% of all heat lost at rest and at least 75% during exercise. Heat transfers from the body to water on the skin and pulmonary surfaces. Evaporation results from a vapor pressure gradient (the pressure exerted by water molecules as they convert to a gas or water vapor) between the skin and ambient air (see figure on next page). A large vapor pressure gradient between water molecules on the skin and in ambient air facilitates evaporation and subsequent body cooling. An increase in ambient air's relative humidity increases its vapor pressure, thwarting evaporative skin cooling because of a diminished vapor pressure gradient between the skin and air. This explains the difficulty in dissipating body heat via evaporative cooling during vigorous exercise in a humid environment.

Each 1 liter of water evaporated from the skin and pulmonary airways transfers 580 kCal of heat energy (0.58 kCal per mL) to the environment. If evaporative cooling provided the *only* mechanism for heat dissipation, one can estimate the magnitude of evaporation required to maintain a constant core temperature during exercise.

PROBLEM

An individual walks at 3.5 mph for 60 minutes on the level at an oxygen uptake of 0.8 L·min^{-1}. Estimate the following:

1. Heat production during exercise
2. Magnitude of evaporative cooling required to prevent a rise in core temperature

SOLUTION

A. Determine Exercise Total Energy Expenditure (TEE)

1. Compute total $\dot{V}O_2$ during exercise.

$$\text{Total } \dot{V}O_2 = \dot{V}O_2, \text{L·min}^{-1} \times \text{exercise, min}$$
$$= 0.8 \text{ L·min}^{-1} \times 60 \text{ min}$$
$$= 48.0 \text{ L}$$

2. Convert total $\dot{V}O_2$ to energy expenditure (assume 1 L O_2 = 5.05 kCal).

$$\text{TEE} = 48.0 \text{ L} \times 5.05 \text{ kCal}$$
$$= 242.4 \text{ kCal}$$

B. Determine Total Heat Produced During Exercise

Computation of total heat production must consider mechanical efficiency for exercise (i.e., % total energy converted to mechanical work versus % total energy dissipated as heat); assume 22% mechanical efficiency for walking. Consequently, of the total energy required for exercise, 78% appears as heat (100% − 22%).

$$\begin{aligned}\text{Total heat} \\ \text{produced, kCal} &= \text{TEE, kCal} \\ &\quad \times \text{ percent lost as heat} \\ &= 242.4 \text{ kCal} \times 0.78 \\ &= 189.1 \text{ kCal}\end{aligned}$$

C. Calculate Total Evaporation Required to Prevent Core Temperature Increase

$$\begin{aligned}\text{Total evaporation} &= \text{total heat produced, kCal} \\ &\quad \div \text{ kCal heat loss per L} \\ &\quad \text{ evaporation} \\ &= 189.1 \text{ kCal} \div 580 \text{ kCal·L}^{-1} \\ &= 0.326 \text{ L (326 mL or 11 oz)}\end{aligned}$$

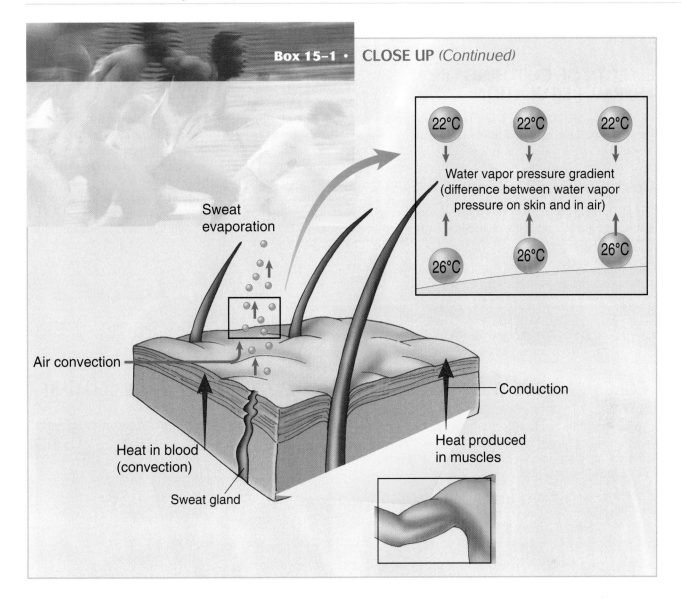

Box 15–1 • CLOSE UP *(Continued)*

rial and venous blood vessels dilate to divert warm blood to the body's cooler shell. Peripheral vasodilation causes a flushed or reddened face on a hot day or during vigorous exercise. With extreme heat stress, 15% to 25% of the cardiac output passes through the skin, greatly increasing thermal conductance of peripheral tissues. This favors radiative heat loss to the environment, mostly from the hands, forehead, forearms, ears, and tibial region.

Evaporation Sweating begins several seconds after initiation of vigorous exercise. After about 30 minutes, it reaches equilibrium that directly relates to exercise load. A large cutaneous blood flow coupled with evaporative cooling usually produces an effective thermal defense. The cooled peripheral blood then returns to deeper tissues to acquire additional heat on its return to the heart.

Hormonal Adjustments Heat stress initiates hormonal adjustments to conserve salts and fluid lost in sweat. The pituitary gland releases **vasopressin (antidiuretic hormone** or **ADH)** in response to a thermal challenge. *ADH stimulates water reabsorption from kidney tubules, forming more concentrated urine during heat stress.* Concurrently, with even a single bout of exercise or repeated days of exercise in hot weather, the adrenal cortex releases the sodium-conserving hormone **aldosterone** to increase the renal tubules' reabsorption of sodium. Aldosterone

Questions & Notes

Explain why superficial arterial and venous blood vessels dilate during exposure to external heat.

also acts on sweat glands to reduce sweat's osmolality to further conserve electrolytes.

EFFECTS OF CLOTHING ON THERMOREGULATION

Clothing insulates the body from its surroundings. It reduces radiant heat gain in a hot environment or retards conductive and convective heat loss in the cold.

Cold-Weather Clothing

The mesh of the clothing's fibers traps air and warms it to insulate from the cold. This establishes a barrier to heat loss because cloth and air both conduct heat poorly. A thicker zone of trapped air next to the skin provides more effective insulation. Several layers of light clothing, or garments lined with animal fur, feathers, or synthetic fabrics (with numerous layers of trapped air), insulate better than a single bulky layer of winter clothing.

The clothing layer against the skin must transport moisture away from the body's surface to the next clothing layer (the insulating layer) for subsequent evaporation. Wool or synthetics (e.g., polypropylene) that insulate well and dry quickly serve this purpose. When clothing becomes wet, either through external moisture or condensation from sweating, it loses nearly 90% of its insulating properties. Wet clothing facilitates heat trans-

---

Box 15–2 • CLOSE UP

COMPUTING THE THERMAL INSULATION OF CLOTHES USING THE CLO UNIT

To remain comfortable, the human body must maintain a skin temperature of about 33°C (91°F) and remain in thermal equilibrium with the environment. Three factors control thermal comfort:

1. Heat production
2. Insulation value of clothing
3. Environmental temperature

Clothing Insulation (Clo Units)

The **Clo unit** represents an index of thermal resistance, reflecting the insulatory capacity provided by any layer of air trapped between the skin and clothing, including clothing's insulation value. Assuming an external environment with no wind and no body movement to disturb the insulatory layer of air about the body, one Clo unit maintains a sedentary person at 1 MET (approximately 3.5 mL $O_2 \cdot kg^{-1} \cdot min^{-1}$; 1.5 kCal·min^{-1}) indefinitely in an environment of 21°C (68.8°F) and 50% relative humidity.

Table 1 shows Clo values for different items of clothes. To determine the total insulatory value of what a person wears, add the individual Clo values for the different garments.

Without wind penetration or air movement around the clothing, the Clo value for a given weight of clothes equals 0.15 times clothing weight in pounds. For example, wearing 10 pounds of clothes produces a Clo value of 1.5 (0.15 × 10 lb = 1.5 Clo).

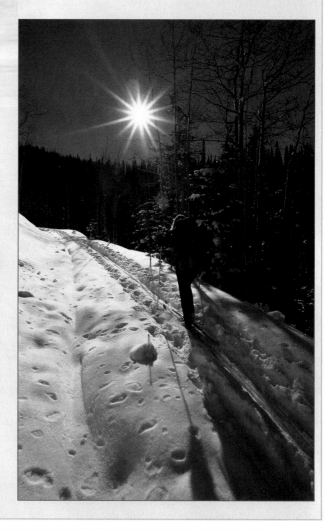

Box 15-2 • CLOSE UP *(Continued)*

Effects of Metabolic Rate and Environmental Temperature on CLO Requirement

An individual's metabolic rate at a given environmental temperature affects the Clo requirement to maintain core temperature. For example, Table 2 considers six different conditions of metabolic intensity from sleeping to intense exercise (expressed in MET units) at three environmental temperatures (0°C, −20°C, −50°C). Note

that, for each condition, the Clo unit requirement to maintain a person equivalent to resting (1.0 MET) at 21°C (68.8°F) and 50% relative humidity, with negligible air movement (thermal equilibrium with the environment), increases almost proportionally from sleeping to intense physical effort at the three extreme temperatures. In other words, at any given temperature, the less physical activity there is, the more clothing required. Conversely, less clothing is required at higher levels of physical activity.

Table 1	Clo Values for Different Garments [Higher Clo units indicate greater insulatory capacity]		

GARMENT	CLO UNIT	GARMENT	CLO UNIT
Underwear, pants		**Jackets**	
Pantyhose	0.02	Vest	0.13
Women's underwear	0.03	Light summer jacket	0.25
Men's briefs	0.04	Normal jacket	0.35
Pants, long leg	0.1		
Underwear, shirts		**Coats, jackets**	
Bra	0.1	Normal coat	0.6
Shirt, sleeveless	0.06	Down jacket	0.55
T-shirt	0.09	Parka	0.7
Shirt, long sleeve	0.12		
Half-slip, nylon	0.14		
Shirts		**Accessories**	
Tube top	0.06	Socks	0.02
Short sleeve	0.09	Thick, ankle socks	0.05
Light-weight blouse, short sleeves	0.15	Thick, long socks	0.1
		Slippers, quilted	0.03
Light-weight blouse, long sleeves	0.2	Shoes, thin soled	0.02
		Shoes, thick soled	0.04
Normal, long sleeves	0.25	Boots, gloves	0.05
Flannel, long sleeves	0.3		
Trousers		**Skirts, dresses**	
Shorts	0.06	Light skirt, 15 cm above knee	0.10
Walking shorts	0.11	Light skirt, 15 cm below knee	0.18
Light-weight	0.2	Heavy skirt, knee-length	0.25
Normal weight	0.25	Light dress, sleeveless	0.25
Flannel	0.28	Winter dress, long sleeves	0.4
Overalls	0.28		
Sweaters		**Sleepwear**	
Sleeveless vest	0.12	Long-sleeve gown	0.3
Thin sweater	0.2	Thin-strap, short gown	0.15
Turtleneck, thin	0.26	Hopital gown	0.31
Turtleneck, thick	0.37	Long-sleeve, long pajamas	0.5
Normal sweater	0.28		
Thick sweater	0.35		
Robes		**Coverall**	
Long-sleeve, wrap, long	0.53	Daily wear, belted, work	0.49
		Highly insulating, multicomponent, filling	1.03
Long-sleeve, wrap, short	0.41	Fiber-pelt	1.13

Box 15-2 • CLOSE UP *(Continued)*

Table 2	Clo Units Required to Maintain Core Temperature Related to Activity Level and Ambient Temperature		

	TEMPERATURE IN DEGREES CELSIUS		
ACTIVITY LEVEL METS	0°C	−20°C	−50°C
	CLO UNITS REQUIRED		
Heavy work, 6.0	1.0	1.6	2.2
Moderate work, 3.0	1.6	2.8	4.2
Light work, 2.0	2.6	4.0	6.2
Very light work, 1.5	3.4	5.6	8.2
Resting, 1.0	5.4	8.3	12.4
Sleeping, 0.8	6.7	10.6	15.5

Six factors affect clothing insulation (Clo) value:

1. *Wind speed:* increased speed disrupts the zone of insulation about the body.
2. *Body movements:* pumping actions of arms and legs disturb the zone of insulation.
3. *Chimney effect:* loosely hanging clothing ventilates the trapped air layers to reduce the zone of insulation.
4. *Bellows effect:* vigorous body movements increase ventilation of air layers to reduce the zone of insulation.
5. *Water vapor transfer:* clothing resists the passage of water vapor and thus decreases body heat loss by evaporative cooling.
6. *Permeation efficiency factor:* how well clothing absorbs liquid (sweat) by capillary action (wicking). Wicking of sweat away from body surface reduces evaporation's cooling effect, thus improving clothing's insulatory effectiveness.

Effects of Physical Activity

Physical activity markedly affects the amount of insulation required to maintain thermal comfort (Table 2). This factor must be considered when choosing a garment for a particular activity. For example, cross-country skiers produce heat at a rate of about 290 kCal·h^{-1} while active and thus remain comfortable at −25°F with 2.0 Clo of insulation. On the other hand, a soldier standing (heat production 105 kCal·h^{-1}) in an Arctic environment at −4°F, requires 4.3 Clo of insulation to remain comfortable.

A value for average physical activity estimates the amount of clothes required to remain warm. Downhill skiers spend considerable time inactive on a chair lift where their needs for insulation become considerable, but during periods of extended activity, they may need to vent excess heat away by adjustable cuffs, zippers, and drawstrings. These factors help extend the overall comfort range of well-engineered clothing.

fer from the body because water conducts heat faster than air.

When working or exercising in cold air, adequacy of insulation does not usually present a problem; rather, the key factor involves dissipation of metabolic heat (and sweat) through a thick air-clothing barrier. Cross-country skiers alleviate this dilemma by removing layers of clothing as the body warms. This maintains core temperature without reliance on evaporative cooling.

Warm-Weather Clothing

Dry clothing, no matter how lightweight, *retards* heat exchange more than the same clothing soaking wet. The common practice of switching to a dry tennis, basketball, or football uniform in hot weather makes little sense for temperature regulation because evaporative heat loss occurs only when clothing becomes wet throughout. A dry uniform simply prolongs the time between sweating and cooling.

Different materials absorb water at different rates. Cottons and linens, for example, readily absorb moisture. In contrast, heavy sweatshirts and rubber or plastic garments produce high relative humidity close to the skin, thus retarding sweat evaporation and cooling. Individuals should wear loose-fitting clothing to permit free convection of air between the skin and environment to promote evaporation from the skin. Moisture-wicking fabrics (e.g., polypropylene, coolmax, drylite) adhere closely to the skin to optimally transfer heat and moisture from the skin to the environment, particularly during high-intensity exercise in hot weather. These fabrics wick moisture away from the skin. They also offer benefits during exercise in cold environments because dry clothing (in contrast to sweat-drenched clothing) greatly reduces hypothermia risk. Color also plays an important role; dark colors absorb light rays and add to radiant heat gain, whereas lighter color clothing reflects heat rays.

Football Uniforms   Of all athletic uniforms and equipment, football gear presents the most significant barrier to heat dissipation. The 6 or 7 kg of equipment, carried over a relatively hot artificial playing surface, also adds considerably to the total metabolic load.

Wearing football gear while exercising produced significantly higher rectal and skin temperatures during exercise and recovery than the other exercise conditions. Skin temperature directly beneath the padding averaged only 1°C less than rectal temperature. This indicates that subcutaneous blood in these areas cooled only about one-fifth as much as blood near the skin surface directly exposed to the environment. Rectal temperature remained elevated in recovery with uniforms, making a rest period of limited value in normalizing thermal status unless the athlete removes the uniform.

SUMMARY

1. Humans tolerate only relatively small variations in internal (core) temperature. Exposure to heat or cold stress initiates thermoregulatory responses that either generate or conserve heat at low ambient temperatures and dissipate heat at high temperatures.

2. Oral temperature does not accurately measure core temperature following strenuous exercise. This discrepancy partly results from evaporative cooling of the mouth and airways at high rates of pulmonary ventilation.

3. The hypothalamus serves as the "thermostat" for temperature regulation. This coordination center initiates regulatory adjustments from peripheral thermal receptors in skin and changes in hypothalamic blood temperature.

4. Heat conservation in cold stress occurs by vascular adjustments that shunt blood from the cooler periphery to the warmer deep tissues of the body's core. If this proves ineffective, shivering increases metabolic heat. Thermogenic hormones initiate an additional small but prolonged increase in resting metabolism.

5. Heat stress causes warm blood to divert from the body's core to the shell. Heat loss occurs by radiation, conduction, convection, and evaporation. Evaporation provides the major physiologic defense against overheating at high ambient temperatures and during exercise.

6. Humid environments dramatically decrease the effectiveness of evaporative heat loss. This makes a physically active person particularly vulnerable to a dangerous state of dehydration and spiraling core temperature.

7. Ideal warm-weather clothing includes lightweight, loose-fitting, and light-color clothes. Even when wearing ideal clothing, heat loss slows until evaporative cooling achieves optimal levels.

8. Several layers of light clothing provide a thick zone of trapped air near the skin for more effective insulation than a single thick layer of clothing. Wet clothing decreases insulation, and heat flows readily from the body.

1. What mechanism might explain how improved aerobic fitness increases exercise tolerance in a warm, humid environment?

2. From the standpoint of survival, discuss why the body's physiology is more geared to regulate temperature in heat stress than in cold stress.

3 Describe the ideal personal physical and physiologic characteristics that minimize heat injury risk in exercise during environmental heat stress.

4 How should a person dress who wants to play 90 minutes of outdoor paddle tennis at 20°F (26.7°C)?

PART 2 •
Exercise, the Environment, and Thermoregulation

EXERCISE IN THE HEAT

Cardiovascular adjustments and evaporative cooling facilitate metabolic heat dissipation during exercise, particularly in hot weather. A trade-off occurs because fluid loss in thermoregulation (sweating) often creates a relative state of dehydration. Excessive sweating leads to more serious fluid loss that reduces plasma volume. The extreme end result involves circulatory failure and core temperature increases to lethal levels.

Circulatory Adjustments

Two competitive cardiovascular demands exist when exercising in hot weather:

1. Oxygen delivery to active muscles must increase to sustain exercise energy metabolism.
2. Peripheral blood flow to the skin must increase to transport metabolic heat from exercise for dissipation at the body's surface; this blood no longer remains available to active muscles.

Cardiac output remains the same during submaximal exercise in hot and cold environments, but the heart's stroke volume becomes smaller when exercising in the heat. In fact, stroke volume decreases in proportion to the fluid deficit created during exercise, producing *higher* heart rates at all submaximal exercise levels. Maximal cardiac output and aerobic capacity decrease during exercise in the heat because the compensatory increase in heart rate does not offset the decrease in stroke volume.

Vascular Constriction and Dilation   Adequate skin and muscle blood flow during heat stress occurs at the expense of other tissues that temporarily compromise their blood supply. For example, compensatory constriction of the splanchnic vascular bed and renal tissues rapidly counters vasodilation of the subcutaneous vessels. A prolonged reduction in blood flow to visceral tissues probably contributes to liver and renal complications sometimes noted with exertional heat stress.

Maintaining Blood Pressure   Arterial blood pressure remains stable during exercise in the heat because visceral vasoconstriction increases total vascular resistance, as blood redirects to areas in need. During near maximal exercise with accompanying dehydration, relatively less blood diverts to peripheral areas for heat dissipation. This reflects the body's attempt to maintain cardiac output despite sweat-induced decreases in plasma volume. *Circulatory regulation and maintenance of muscle blood flow take precedence over temperature regulation, often at the expense of a spiraling core temperature and accompanying health risk.*

Core Temperature During Exercise

Heat generated by active muscles can increase core temperature to fever levels that would incapacitate a person if caused by external heat stress alone. Champion distance runners show no ill effects from rectal temperatures as high as 105.8°F (41°C) recorded at the end of a 3-mile race.

Within limits, increased core temperature with exercise does not reflect heat-dissipation failure. To the contrary, this well-regulated response occurs even during cold-weather exercise. **Figure 15.3** illustrates the relationship between esophageal (core) temperature and oxygen uptake (expressed as a percentage of $\dot{V}O_{2max}$) during exercise of increasing severity for five men and two women of varying fitness levels. Core temperature increases in proportion to exercise intensity. *More than likely, a modest core temperature increase reflects favorable internal adjustments that create an optimal thermal environment for physiologic and metabolic function.*

Water Loss in the Heat

Dehydration induced by a few hours of intense exercise in the heat can reach levels that impede heat dissipation and severely compromise cardiovascular function and exercise capacity. **Figure 15.4** shows average water loss per hour

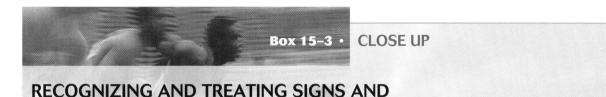

Box 15–3 • CLOSE UP

RECOGNIZING AND TREATING SIGNS AND SYMPTOMS OF HEAT-RELATED DISORDERS

Human heat dissipation occurs by:

1. Redistribution of blood from deeper tissues to the periphery
2. Activation of the cooling mechanism provided by evaporation of sweat from the skin's surface and respiratory passages

What Happens During Heat Stress?

During heat stress at rest, cardiac output increases, vasoconstriction and vasodilation move central blood volume towards the skin, and thousands of previously dormant capillaries threading through the upper skin layer open to accommodate blood flow. Conduction of heat away from warm blood at the skin's cooled surface is accomplished without undue strain on the body's heat-dissipating functions. In contrast, heat production during physical activity often strains heat-dissipating mech-anisms, especially in high ambient temperature and high humidity.

Signs and Symptoms of Heat-Related Disorders

The signs and symptoms, collectively termed **heat ill-ness**, range in severity from mild to life threatening. In order of increased severity, **heat cramps**, **heat syncope**, **heat exhaustion**, and **heat stroke** represent the major categories of heat illness. No clear-cut demarcation exists among these maladies because symptoms often overlap. When symptoms of serious heat illness occur, immediate action must include reducing heat stress and rehydrating the person until medical help arrives. **Table 1** lists the causes, signs, and symptoms and preventive methods for the four categories of heat illness.

Table 1	Heat Illness: Causes, Signs and Symptoms, and Prevention		
CONDITION	**CAUSES**	**SIGNS AND SYMPTOMS**	**PREVENTION**
Heat Cramps	Intense, prolonged exercise in the heat	Tightening, cramps, involuntary spasms of active muscles; low serum Na^+	Cease exercise; rehydrate
Heat Syncope	Peripheal vasodilatation and pooling of venous blood; hypotension; hypohydration	Lightheadedness; syncope, mostly in upright position during rest or exercise; pallor; high rectal temperature	Ensure acclimatization and fluid replenishment; reduce exertion on hot days; avoid standing
Heat Exhaustion	Cumulative negative water balance	Exhaustion; hypohydration, flushed skin; reduced sweating in extreme dehydration syncope, high rectal temperature	Proper hydration before exercise and adequate replenishment during exercise; ensure acclimatization
Heat Stroke	Extreme hyperthermia leads to thermoregulatory failure; aggravated by dehydration	Acute medical emergency; includes hyperpyrexia (rectal temperature >41°C, 105.8°F); lack of sweating and neurologic deficit (disorientation, twitching, seizures, coma)	Ensure acclimatization; identify and exclude individuals at risk; adapt activities to climatic constraints

from sweating at various air temperatures for a typical adult during rest and light and moderate activity.

Magnitude of Exercise Fluid Loss For an acclimatized person, sweat loss peaks at about 3 $L \cdot h^{-1}$ during intense exercise in the heat and averages nearly 12

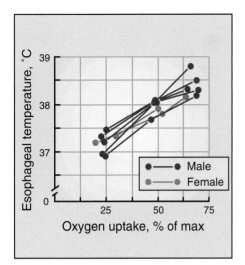

Figure 15.3. Relationship between esophageal temperature and oxygen uptake expressed as a percentage of $\dot{V}O_{2max}$. (Data from Saltin, B., and Hermansen, L.: Esophageal, rectal, and muscle temperature during exercise. *J. Appl. Physiol.*, 21:1757, 1966.)

L (26 lb) on a daily basis. Intense sweating for several hours can induce sweat-gland fatigue that impairs core temperature regulation. Elite marathon runners frequently sweat in excess of 5 L of fluid during competition; this represents 6% to 10% of body mass. For slower-paced marathons or ultramarathons, average fluid loss rarely exceeds 500 $mL \cdot h^{-1}$. For more intense exercise, even in a temperate climate, soccer players averaged 2 L of sweat loss during a 90-minute game played at about 50°F (10°C).

Hot, humid environments impede the effectiveness of evaporative cooling (because of the high vapor pressure of ambient air) and promote large fluid losses. **Figure 15.5** illustrates a linear relationship between sweat rate during rest and exercise and the air's moisture content (expressed as wet bulb temperature; see pages 533–534). Ironically, excessive sweat output in high humidity contributes little to cooling because minimal evaporation takes place. In this regard, clothing that retards rapid evaporation of sweat creates an extremely humid microclimate at the skin's surface that promotes dehydration and overheating.

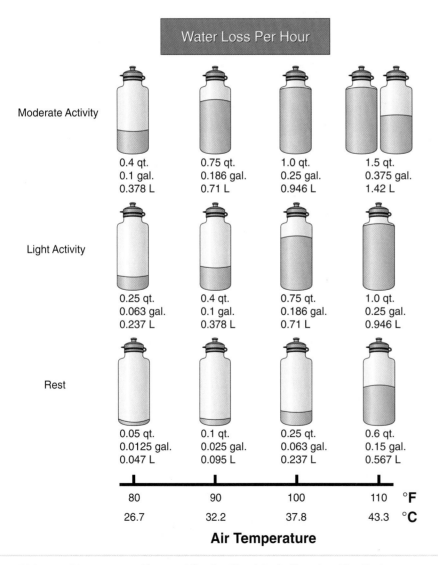

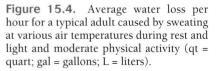

Figure 15.4. Average water loss per hour for a typical adult caused by sweating at various air temperatures during rest and light and moderate physical activity (qt = quart; gal = gallons; L = liters).

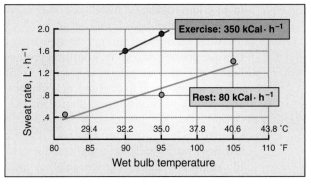

Figure 15.5. Effects of humidity (wet-bulb temperature) on sweat rate during rest and exercise in the heat. Ambient temperature (dry-bulb) equaled 43.3°C (110°F). (Data from Iampietro, P.F.: Exercise in hot environments. In: *Frontiers of Fitness*. Shephard, R.J. (ed.). Springfield, IL: Charles C. Thomas, 1971.)

Consequences of Dehydration

Just about any degree of dehydration impairs physiologic function and thermoregulation. When plasma volume decreases as dehydration progresses, peripheral blood flow and sweating rate also decrease to make thermoregulation progressively more difficult. Compared with normal hydration, premature fatigue occurs from reduced plasma volume that increases heart rate, perception of effort, and core temperature. A fluid loss equivalent to only 1% of body mass increases rectal temperature compared with the same exercise performed fully hydrated. Dehydration equivalent to 5% of body mass increases rectal temperature and heart rate while decreasing sweating rate, $\dot{V}O_{2max}$, and exercise capacity compared with the normally hydrated condition.

Blood plasma supplies most of the water lost through sweating; thus, maintaining cardiac output becomes problematic as sweat loss progresses. Loss of plasma volume (1) initiates increases in systemic vascular resistance to maintain blood pressure, and (2) reduces skin blood flow. Reduced cutaneous blood flow thwarts a major avenue for heat dissipation. *Dehydration reduces circulatory and temperature-regulating capacity to meet the metabolic and thermal demands of exercise.*

Seven factors affect sweat-loss dehydration: exercise intensity, exercise duration, environmental temperature, solar load, wind speed, relative humidity, and clothing. **Table 15.2** shows theoretical water requirements at different ambient temperatures and relative humidities with and without a solar load. A 100°F

Questions & Notes

Give the degree of dehydration that can impair physiologic function and thermoregulation.

Name 3 body functions negatively affected by dehydration.

   1.

   2.

   3.

Give 2 physiologic consequences of loss of plasma volume due to dehydration.

   1.

   2.

Give the most effective defense against heat stress.

True or False:

The thirst mechanism can precisely gauge a persons water needs.

Name the component of the triacylglycerol molecule that can increase the body's fluid volume.

AIR TEMP (°F) AND RH*	INDOORS (NO SOLAR LOAD)				OUTDOORS (CLEAR SKY)			
	REST	LIGHT	MEDIUM	HEAVY	REST	LIGHT	MEDIUM	HEAVY
85° @ 50%	0.2	0.5	1.0	1.5	0.5	0.9	1.3	1.8
96° @ 30%	0.3	0.9	1.3	1.9	0.8	1.2	1.7	2.0
105° @ 30%	0.6	1.0	1.5	2.0	0.9	1.3	1.9	2.0
115° @ 20%	0.8	1.2	1.7	2.0	1.1	1.5	2.0	2.0
120° @ 20%	0.9	1.3	1.9	2.0	1.3	1.7	2.0	2.0

Table 15•2 Water Requirements ($L \cdot h^{-1}$) for Rest and Varying Intensities of Work in the Heat: Indoors and Outdoors at Diverse Temperatures and Relative Humidity

*RH = relative himidity

From Askew, E.C.: Nutrition and performance in hot, cold, and high altitude environments. In: *Nutrition in Exercise and Sport.* 3rd Ed., Wolinsky, I., (ed.). Boca Raton, FL: CRC Press, 1997.

In addition, cold stress increases urine production, which also adds to total body fluid loss. Ironically, many people overdress for outdoor winter activities. Sweating begins as exercise progresses because body heat production exceeds heat loss. This discrepancy can magnify if individuals consider it unimportant to consume fluids before, during, and after strenuous exercise in cold weather.

Diuretic Use   Athletes who take diuretics to rapidly lose body water (and body weight) reduce plasma volume; this negatively affects thermoregulation and cardiovascular function. Diuretic drugs can also impair neuromuscular function not noted when comparable fluid loss occurs by exercise. Athletes who vomit and take laxatives to lose weight not only become dehydrated but also lose minerals. These practices weaken muscles and impair motor function.

Water Replacement and Rehydration

Adequate fluid replacement sustains evaporative cooling of acclimatized humans. Properly scheduling fluid replacement maintains plasma volume so that circulation and sweating progress optimally. This, however, may be "easier said than done" because some coaches and athletes cling to the misguided notion that water consumption hinders performance. When left on their own, most athletes voluntarily replace only about one-half of water lost during exercise (< 500 mL·h^{-1}).

Chronic dehydration to lose weight becomes a "way of life" for many athletes, from ballet dancers who strive to maintain a thin appearance to power athletes who try to make weight to compete in a lighter-weight category. The enlightened coach and exercise specialist must remain vigilant about an athlete's hydration status and its impact on exercise performance and safety. *All participants in sports and recreation activities from novice to champion must replenish fluids regularly!*

Cold treatments (e.g., periodic application of cold towels to the forehead and abdomen during exercise, or taking a cold shower before exercising in a hot environment) at best provide only minimal benefits to facilitate heat transfer at the body's surface compared with the same exercise without skin wetting. Adequate hydration provides the most effective defense against heat stress by balancing water loss with water intake, not by pouring water over the head or body. *A well-hydrated athlete always functions at a higher physiologic and performance level than a dehydrated one.*

Determining Rate and Quantity of Rehydration

Table 15.3 shows sample computations for determining the quantity and rate of fluid loss in exercise. The data listed under headings A to H show the calculations of sweat rate (column H) for a person who exercises for 90 minutes (column G), with a urine volume (in mL; column

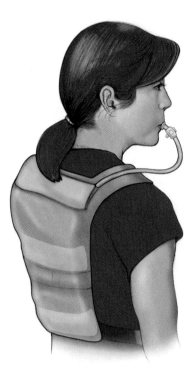

Figure 15.6. Back-mounted pack provides for readily-available fluid during prolonged outdoor exercise.

(37.8°C) ambient air temperature increases the resting water requirement by 50% to 60%. Adding physical activity and radiant heat increases the requirement even more. Eight hours of heavy outdoor work at temperatures of 96°F or higher (relative humidity 20% or greater) could increase total water intake requirements to 15 L. Replacing this much fluid requires drinking water at regular intervals throughout the day. First initiated during the 1990–1991 Desert War in Iraq and Kuwait, and continued in the 2003 war in Iraq, the U.S. military imposed forced water intake through a planned drinking program before, during, and after job tasks. They also outfitted each soldier with a personal fluid-replacement pack. **Figure 15.6** shows an example of the Army's water-pack system. The Army attributed the relatively low incidence of heat casualties to the discipline of planned hydration and use of water packs.

Fluid Loss in Winter Environments   Dehydration can become a serious risk during vigorous cold-weather exercise. For example, colder air contains less moisture than air at a warmer temperature, particularly at higher altitudes. Fluid volume loss increases from the respiratory passages as incoming cold, dry air fully humidifies and warms to body temperature (1 L of fluid can be lost daily).

Table 15·3	Computing the Magnitude of Sweat Loss and Rate of Sweating in Exercise						
A	**B**	**C**	**D**	**E**	**F**	**G**	**H**
BM Before Exercise	*BM After Exercise*	*DBM (A-B)*	*Drink Volume*	*Urine Volume Output*	*Sweat Loss (C + D − E)*	*Exercise Time*	*Sweat Rate (F ÷ G)*
61.7 kg	60.3 kg	1400 g	420 mL	90 mL[a]	1730 mL	90 min (1.5 h)	19.2 mL · min^{-1}[b] (1152 mL · h^{-1})

[a] Weight of urine should be subtracted if urine was excreted prior to postexercise body weight measurement.
[b] 1152 mL·h^{-1}; in this example, a person should drink about 1000 mL (32 oz) of fluid during each hour of activity (250 mL [8.5 oz] every 15 min) to remain well hydrated.
Calculations of sweat rate (column H) for a person who exercises for 90 min (column G) and who consumes 420 mL of fluid (column D); BM = body mass; DBM = difference in body mass before and after exercise (column C); urine volume (in mL; column E) measured prior to postexercise body mass measurement.
(Modified from: Gatorade Sports Science Institute, Vol. 9, No. 4 [suppl 63], 1996.)

E) measured prior to post-exercise body mass measurements (columns A, B, and C). With a sweat rate of 1152 mL·h^{-1}, the person would need to consume about 1000 mL (32 oz) during each hour to match total fluid loss during activity at a rate of 250 mL (8.5 oz) at 15-minute intervals.

Partitioning rehydration periods into 10- to 15-minute intervals allows for the maintenance of optimal stomach volume and properly matches fluid loss with fluid intake. Provide for unrestricted access to water during practice and competition. *Athletes must rehydrate on a regular schedule because the thirst mechanism imprecisely gauges water needs.*

Exogenous Glycerol Use Glycerol is (1) a component of the triacylglycerol molecule, (2) a gluconeogenic substrate, (3) an important constituent of the cells' phospholipid plasma membrane, and (4) an osmotically active natural metabolite. Ingesting a concentrated mixture of glycerol (banned by the United States Olympic Committee [USOC]) plus water increases the body's fluid volume.

The typically recommended pre-exercise glycerol dosage of 1.0 g of glycerol per kg of body mass in 1 to 2 L of water lasts up to 6 hours. This glycerol solution facilitates water absorption from the intestine and causes extracellular fluid retention, mainly in the plasma fluid compartment. Advocates maintain that the hyperhydration effect of glycerol supplementation reduces overall heat stress during exercise as reflected by increased sweating rate; this lowers heart rate and body temperature during exercise and enhances endurance performance under heat stress. Reducing heat stress with hyperhydration using glycerol plus water supplementation prior to exercise increases safety for the exercise participant.

Questions & Notes

Name the 3 physiologic mechanisms that facilitate heat loss from the body.

1.

2.

3.

Name the hormone released from the pituitary gland in response to a thermal challenge.

Box 15–4 • CLOSE UP

HOW TO OPTIMALLY REHYDRATE FOR EXERCISE

Pre-Exercise Hyperhydration

Ingesting "extra" water (**hyperhydration**) prior to exercise in the heat offers some protection because it delays hypohydration, increases sweating during exercise, and brings about a smaller rise in core temperature.

Acute hyperhydration results from consuming (1) at least 500 mL of water before sleeping the night before exercising in the heat, (2) another 500 mL upon awakening, and (3) 400 to 600 mL (13 to 20 oz) of cold water about 20 minutes before exercising in the heat. This final pre-exercise intake provides fluid and increases stomach volume to optimize gastric emptying. An extended regimen of pre-exercise hyperhydration (4.5 L fluid per day, starting a few days before heat exposure) increases body water reserves and improves temperature regulation.

During intense exercise in the heat, matching fluid loss with fluid intake becomes virtually impossible because only 800 to 1000 mL of fluid empty from the stomach each hour. This rate of stomach emptying does not match a water loss that may average nearly 2000 mL per hour. Under these conditions, pre-exercise hyperhydration would prove beneficial.

Adequacy of Rehydration

Changes in body weight indicate water loss and the adequacy of rehydration. Voiding small volumes of dark yellow urine with a strong odor also provides a qualitative indication of inadequate hydration. Well-hydrated individuals typically produce urine in large volumes that does not give off a strong smell.

Table 1 presents recommendations for fluid intake with acute weight (fluid) loss during exercise.

Each 1 pound of weight lost represents 450 mL (15 fluid oz) of dehydration.

Periodic water breaks listed in the table during activity can deter fluid depletion. Alcohol-containing beverages generally impede restoration of fluid balance, particularly if the rehydration fluid contains 4% or more alcohol content.

Electrolyte Replacement

The volume of ingested fluid following exercise must exceed by 25% to 50% of the exercise sweat loss to restore fluid balance because the kidneys continually form urine regardless of hydration status. Unless the beverage contains sufficiently high sodium content, excess fluid intake merely increases urine output without benefit to rehydration. Maintaining a relatively high plasma concentration of sodium (by adding sodium to ingested fluid) sustains the thirst drive, promotes retention of ingested fluids (less urine output), and more rapidly restores lost plasma volume.

With prolonged exercise in the heat, sweat loss can deplete the body of 13 to 17 g of salt (2.3 to 3.4 g per L of sweat) daily, about 8 g more than typically consumed. Thus, to replace lost sodium by adding about one-third teaspoon of table salt to 1 liter of water. With heavy sweating, increasing the intake of potassium-rich foods (citrus fruits and bananas) replaces potassium losses. A glass of orange juice or tomato juice replaces almost all the potassium, calcium, and magnesium excreted in 3 L of sweat.

Table 1	Recommended Fluid Intake with Weight Loss in the Heat[a]			
WEIGHT LOSS		**MINUTES BETWEEN WATER BREAKS**	**FLUID PER BREAK**	
lb	**kg**		**oz**	**mL**
8	3.6	Discontinue activity;		
7.5	3.4	immediate fluid required		
7	3.2	10	8-10	266
6.5	3.0	10	8-9	251
6	2.7	10	8-9	251
5.5	2.5	15	10-12	325
5	2.3	15	10-11	311
4.5	2.1	15	9-10	281
4	1.8	15	8-9	251
3.5	1.6	20	10-11	311
3	1.4	20	9-10	281
2.5	1.1	20	7-8	222
2	0.9	30	8	237
1.5	0.7	30	6	177
1	0.5	45	6	177
0.5	0.2	60	6	177

[a]Based on an 80% replacement of weight loss.

Not all research demonstrates meaningful thermoregulatory or exercise performance benefits of glycerol hyperhydration over pre-exercise hyperhydration with plain water. Side effects of exogenous glycerol ingestion include nausea, dizziness, bloating, and light-headedness. Proponents of glycerol supplementation argue that failure to reverse the USOC's glycerol ban only increases the elite athletes' risk of heat injury, including potentially fatal heat stroke. Clearly, this area requires further research.

FACTORS AFFECTING HEAT TOLERANCE

Factors that affect heat tolerance include: acclimatization, exercise training, age, gender, and body composition.

Acclimatization

Relatively light exercise performed easily in cool weather becomes taxing if attempted on the first hot day of spring. The early stages of spring training often prove hazardous for heat injury because thermoregulatory mechanisms have not adjusted to the dual challenge of exercise and environmental heat. *Repeated exposure to hot environments, when combined with exercise, improves capacity for exercise with less discomfort during heat stress.*

Heat acclimatization refers to the physiologic adaptive changes that improve heat tolerance. **Figure 15.7** shows that 2 to 4 hours daily of heat exposure produce essentially complete acclimatization after 10 days. In practical terms, the first several exercise sessions in a hot environment should be light in intensity and last about 15 to 20 minutes. Thereafter, exercise sessions can increase systematically to reach normal training duration and intensity.

Table 15.4 summarizes the main physiologic adjustments during heat acclimatization. Optimal acclimatization necessitates adequate hydration. As acclimatization progresses, proportionately larger quantities of blood transfer to cutaneous vessels, which facilitates heat exchange from the core to the shell. More effective

Questions & Notes

Name 4 heat-related illnesses.

1.

2.

3.

4.

Each 1 pound of weight loss represents _____ mL of dehydration.

Give 2 reasons to add a small amount of electrolyte to a rehydration fluid.

1.

2.

Name 5 factors that affect heat tolerance.

1.

2.

3.

4.

5.

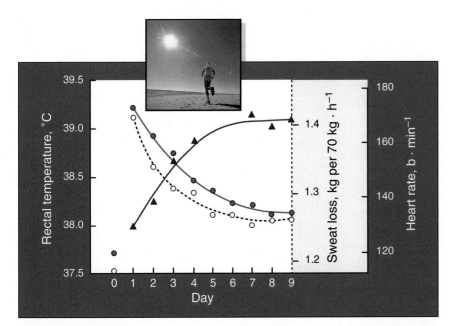

Figure 15.7. Average rectal temperature (○), heart rate (●), and sweat loss (▲) during 100 minutes of daily heat-exercise exposure for 9 consecutive days. On day 0, the men walked on a treadmill at an exercise intensity of 300 kCal·h⁻¹ in a cool climate. Thereafter, they performed the same daily exercise in the heat at 48.9°C (26.7°C wet-bulb). (Data from Lind, A.R., and Bass, D.E.: Optimal exposure time for development of acclimatization to heat. *Fed. Proc.*, 22:704, 1963.)

Table 15•4	Physiologic Adjustments During Heat Acclimatization
ACCLIMATIZATION RESPONSE	**EFFECT**
• Improved cutaneous blood flow	• Transports metabolic heat from deep tissues to the body's shell
• Effective distribution of cardiac output	• Appropriate circulation to skin and muscles to meet demands of metabolism and thermoregulation; greater stability in blood pressure during exercise
• Lowered threshold for start of sweating	• Evaporative cooling begins early in exercise
• More effective distribution of sweat over skin surface	• Optimum use of effective surface for evaporative cooling
• Increased sweat output	• Maximizes evaporative cooling
• Lowered sweat's salt concentration	• Dilute sweat preserves electrolytes in extracellular fluid

cardiac output distribution maintains blood pressure during exercise; a lowered threshold (earlier onset) for sweating complements this circulatory acclimatization. These responses initiate cooling before internal temperature increases substantially. After 10 days of heat exposure, sweating capacity nearly doubles, and sweat dilutes (less salt lost) and more evenly distributes on the skin surface to facilitate greater cooling. For an acclimatized individual, increased sweat loss increases the need to rehydrate during and following exercise. A heat-acclimatized person exercises with a lower skin and core temperature and heart rate than an unacclimatized individual because of adjustments in circulatory function and evaporative cooling. Unfortunately, the major benefits of acclimatization to hot environments dissipate within 2 to 3 weeks after return to more temperate conditions.

Exercise Training

The normal exercise-induced "internal" heat stress from strenuous physical activity in a cool environment adjusts peripheral circulation and evaporative cooling in a manner qualitatively similar to hot ambient temperature acclimatization. This enables well-conditioned men and women to respond more effectively to severe heat stress than sedentary counterparts.

Exercise training increases sweating response sensitivity and capacity so sweating begins at a lower core temperature. It also produces larger volumes of more dilute sweat. These beneficial responses relate to the increase in plasma volume that occurs early in endurance training. Increased plasma volume supports sweat gland function during heat stress and maintains adequate plasma volume to support skin and muscle blood flow demands of exercise. A

trained person stores less heat early during exercise and reaches a thermal steady state sooner and at a lower core temperature than an untrained person. The training advantage for thermoregulation occurs *only* if the individual fully hydrates during exercise.

As might be expected, exercise "heat conditioning" in cool weather proves less effective than acclimatization from similar exercise training in the heat. *Full heat acclimatization does not occur without exposure to environmental heat stress.* Athletes who train and compete in hot weather have a distinct thermoregulatory advantage over those who train in cooler climates but periodically compete in hot weather.

Age

Studies that consider body size and composition, aerobic fitness level, hydration level, and degree of acclimatization show little age-related effects on thermoregulatory capacity or acclimatization to heat stress. For example, in comparing young and middle-aged competitive runners, no age-related decrements emerged in thermoregulatory ability during marathon running. Likewise, temperature regulation was not impaired in physically trained 50-year-old men compared with younger men.

Children Prepubescent children show a lower sweating rate and higher core temperature during heat stress than adolescents and adults, despite their larger number of heat-activated sweat glands per unit of skin area. Thermoregulatory differences probably last through puberty without limiting exercise capacity except during extreme environmental heat stress. Sweat composition also differs between children and adults; children show higher concentrations of sodium and chlorine but lower lactate, H^+, and potassium concentrations. Children also take longer to acclimatize to heat compared with adolescents and young adults. *From a practical and health standpoint, children exposed to environmental heat stress should exercise at a reduced intensity and receive additional time to acclimatize than more mature competitors.*

Gender

Women and men equally tolerate the physiologic and thermal stress of exercise when matched for fitness and acclimatization levels; both genders acclimatize to a similar degree. However, gender differences occur for the following four thermoregulatory mechanisms:

1. **Sweating:** Women possess more heat-activated sweat glands per unit of skin area than men. Women begin sweating at higher skin and core temperatures; they also produce less sweat for a similar heat-exercise load, even when acclimatized comparably to men.
2. **Evaporative Versus Circulatory Cooling:** Despite a lower sweat output, women show heat tolerance similar to men of equal aerobic fitness at the same exer-

cise level. Women probably rely more on circulatory mechanisms for heat dissipation, whereas men exhibit greater evaporative cooling. Women who sweat less to maintain thermal balance have less chance of suffering dehydration during exercise at high ambient temperatures.

3. **Body Surface Area-to-Mass Ratio:** Women possess a larger body surface area-to-mass ratio, a favorable dimensional characteristic to dissipate heat. Thus, under identical conditions of heat exposure, women cool at a rate faster than men through a smaller body mass across a relatively large surface area. In this regard, children also possess a "geometric" advantage during heat stress because boys and girls have larger surface areas per unit of body mass compared with adults.

4. **Menstruation:** Initiation of sweating requires a higher core temperature threshold during the luteal phase of menstruation. This change in thermoregulatory sensitivity during the menstrual cycle does not affect ability to exercise or perform strenuous physical work in a hot environment.

Excess Body Fat

Excess body fat negatively impacts exercise performance in hot environments. Fat's specific heat exceeds that of muscle tissue and subsequently insulates the body's shell to retard heat conduction to the periphery. The large, overfat person also possesses a small body surface area-to-mass ratio for sweat evaporation compared with a leaner, smaller person. Excess body fat directly adds to the metabolic cost of weight-bearing activities, and retards effective heat exchange. When these effects are compounded by the evaporation-retarding characteristics and weight of equipment (e.g., football and lacrosse gear), intense competition, and a hot, humid environment, the overfat athlete experiences considerable difficulty regulating body temperature. Fatal heat stroke occurs 3.5 times more frequently in obese young adults than nonobese counterparts.

EVALUATING ENVIRONMENTAL HEAT STRESS

Nine factors other than air temperature determine the physiologic strain imposed by heat.

1. Individual variations in body size and fatness
2. State of training
3. Degree of acclimatization
4. Level of hydration
5. Convective air currents
6. Radiant heat gain
7. Intensity of exercise
8. Amount, type, and color of clothing
9. Relative humidity (several football deaths from heat injury occurred when air temperature dipped below 75°F [23.9°C] but relative humidity exceeded 95%)

Prevention remains the most effective way to manage heat-stress injuries. Acclimatization minimizes the chances for heat injury. Another defense involves evaluating the environment for its potential for heat stress with the **wet bulb–globe temperature (WB–GT)** guide. This index of environmental thermal challenge developed by the United States military relies on ambient temperature, relative humidity, and radiant heat to calculate WB–GT. Wet-bulb (WB) temperature records by an ordinary mercury thermometer and a thermometer with a wet wick that surrounds the mercury bulb (wet bulb) exposed to rapid air movement in direct sunlight (most industrial supply companies sell inexpensive wet-bulb thermometers). On a dry day (low relative humidity), significant evaporation occurs from the wetted bulb. This creates a cooling effect that maximizes the difference between the two thermometer readings. A small difference between readings indicates high rela-

Questions & Notes

Define a "Clo" unit and describe its use.

Explain why stroke volume decreases during exercise in the heat.

What happens to arterial blood pressure during exercise in the heat?

Describe the association between oxygen uptake (expressed as a percentage of maximum) and core temperature during exercise of increasing intensity.

Give an average peak sweat loss per hour during intense exercise in the heat.

FOR YOUR INFORMATION

American College of Sports Medicine Ambient Temperature Recommendations for Participation in Continuous Activities Like Endurance Running and Cycling

TEMPERATURE	CATEGORY	RECOMMENDATION
Above 28°C (82°F)	Very high risk	Postpone competitive activity
23 to 28°C (73–82°F)	High risk	Heat-sensitive individuals (e.g., obese, low physical fitness, unacclimatized, dehydrated, previous history of heat injury) should not compete
18 to 23°C (65–73°F)	Moderate risk	
Below 18°C (65°F)	Low risk	

tive humidity whereas a large difference indicates little air moisture and a high rate of evaporation. A standard thermometer with a black metal sphere around the bulb records the globe temperature (GT). The black globe absorbs radiant energy from the surroundings to provide a measure of this important source of heat gain.

Figure 15.8 presents WB–GT guidelines for purposes of reducing the chance of heat injury during athletic activities. These standards apply to lightly clothed humans; they do not consider the specific heat load imposed by football uniforms or other types of equipment. For football, the lower end of each temperature range serves as a more prudent guide. Figure 15.8 (bottom) also presents heat stress recommendations based only on the WBT.

By use of relative humidity (obtained from local meteorological stations or media reports), the **Heat Stress Index** can evaluate relative degree of environmental heat stress (Fig. 15.9). To eliminate potential error from using meteorological data some distance from the event site, determine the index close to the actual competition site. Data collected on the 24-hour trend for ambient temperature and relative humidity can establish starting times for different sporting events when heat overload becomes of concern.

EXERCISE IN THE COLD

The physiologic strain imposed by the cold depends largely on three factors:

1. Environmental temperature
2. Level of energy metabolism
3. Resistance to heat flow provided by body fat

Water represents an excellent medium to study physiologic adjustment to cold; the body loses heat about two to four times faster in cool water compared with air at the same temperature. Metabolic heat generated by muscular activity contributes to thermoregulation during cold stress. Shivering frequently results if people remain inactive in a pool or ocean environment because of a large conductive heat loss. Swimming at a submaximal pace in 18°C (64°F) water requires about 500 mL more oxygen each minute than similar swimming in 26°C (79°F) water. The extra oxygen directly relates to the added energy cost of shivering as the body attempts to combat heat loss. Often, the additional metabolic heat from shivering and exercise cannot counter the large thermal drain, so core temperature declines.

Individual differences in body fat content exert a considerable effect on physiologic function in a cold environment during rest and exercise. Successful distance swimmers have more subcutaneous fat than other endurance athletes. The additional fat greatly increases effective insulation because blood in the periphery moves centrally to the body's core in cold water. These athletes often swim in ocean waters with almost no decrease in core temperature compared to leaner swimmers who cannot counter the heat drain to the water.

Acclimatization to Cold

Humans adapt more successfully to chronic heat exposure than regular cold exposure. Avoiding the cold or minimizing its effects represents the basic response of Eskimos and Laplanders. The clothing of these cold-weather inhabitants provides a near-tropical microclimate, and the temperature inside an igloo averages about 70°F (21°C).

Some indication of cold adaptation comes from studies of the Ama, the women divers of Korea and southern Japan. They tolerate daily prolonged exposure to diving for food in water as cold as 50°F (10°C). In addition to an apparent psychological toughness, a 25% increase in resting metabolism probably contributes to their cold tolerance. Interestingly, the Ama divers possess similar body fat levels as nondiving females.

WB–GT Range		Recommendations
°F	°C	
80–84	26.5–28.8	• Use discretion, especially if unconditioned or unacclimatized
85–87	29.5–30.5	• Avoid strenuous activity in the sun
>88	>31.2	• Avoid exercise training

WBT Range		Recommendations
°F	°C	
60	15.5	• No prevention necessary
61–65	16.2–18.4	• Alert all participants to problems of heat stress and importance of adequate hydration
66–70	18.8–21.1	• Insist that appropriate quantity of fluid be ingested
71–75	21.6–23.8	• Rest periods and water breaks every 20 to 30 minutes; limits placed on intense activity
76–79	24.5–26.1	• Practice curtailed and modified considerably
>80	>26.5	• Practice cancelled

Figure 15.8. Wet bulb–globe temperature (WB–GT) and wet-bulb temperature (WBT) guide for outdoor activity. (Data from Iampietro, P.F.: Exercise in hot environments. In: *Frontiers of Fitness.* Shephard, R.J. (ed.). Springfield, IL: Charles C. Thomas, 1971.)

Heat Stress Index

Air temperature (°F) / Heat sensation

Relative humidity	70°	75°	80°	85°	90°	95°	100°	105°	110°	115°	120°
0%	64°	69°	73°	78°	83°	87°	91°	95°	99°	103°	107°
10%	65°	70°	75°	80°	85°	90°	95°	100°	105°	111°	116°
20%	66°	72°	77°	82°	87°	93°	99°	105°	112°	120°	130°
30%	67°	73°	78°	84°	90°	96°	104°	113°	123°	135°	148°
40%	68°	74°	79°	86°	93°	101°	110°	123°	137°	151°	
50%	69°	75°	81°	88°	96°	107°	120°	135°	150°		
60%	70°	76°	82°	90°	100°	114°	132°	149°			
70%	70°	77°	85°	93°	106°	124°	144°				
80%	71°	78°	86°	97°	113°	136°					
90%	71°	79°	88°	102°	122°						
100%	72°	80°	91°	108°							

Heat sensation	Risk of heat injury
90°–105°	Possibility of heat cramps
105°–130°	Heat cramps or heat exhaustion likely Heat stroke possible
130°+	Heat stroke a definite risk

Figure 15.9. Heat Stress Index. Stress on the body relates directly to air temperature and relative humidity.

A type of general cold adaptation occurs following prolonged cold-air exposure. Increased heat production does not accompany body heat loss, and individuals regulate at a lower core temperature in the cold. Some peripheral adaptations also reflect a form of acclimation with severe localized cold stress. Repeated cold exposure of the hands or feet brings about blood flow increases through these areas during cold stress as occurs in fishermen who handle nets and fish in the cold. Although such local adaptations actually facilitate regional heat loss, they provide a form of self-defense because vigorous circulation in exposed areas defends against tissue damage from localized hypothermia (frostbite).

EVALUATING ENVIRONMENTAL COLD STRESS

Heightened participation in outdoor winter activities increases cold injuries from overexposure. Pronounced peripheral vasoconstriction during severe cold exposure causes skin temperature in the extremities to decline to dangerous levels. *Early warning signs of cold injury include a tingling and numbness in the fingers and toes or a burning sensation in the nose and ears.* Disregarding these signs of overexposure leads to frostbite; when irreversible damage occurs, the tissue must be removed surgically.

Wind Chill Index

The **Wind Chill Index** (Fig. 15.10) illustrates the cooling effects of increased wind velocity on bare skin for different air temperatures. For example, 30°F (−1°C) with wind speed at 25 mph produces the same chilling effect as 0°F (−17.8°C) in calm air; a 25-mph wind at 10°F (−12.2°C) causes the same effect as calm air at −29°F (−34°C). When a person runs, skis, or skates into the wind, the effective cooling from the wind increases directly with the exerciser's veloc-

Questions & Notes

Give the most effective way to manage heat injury.

Define wet bulb–globe temperature.

Give the 3 factors that increase physiologic strain during cold exposure.

1.

2.

3.

Physiologic adaptation occurs more readily to chronic ________ exposure than to chronic ________ exposure.

Give 3 early warning signs of cold injury.

1.

2.

3.

Define the wind chill index.

Ambient temperature, °F*													
40	35	30	25	20	15	10	5	0	−5	−10	−15	−20	−25	−30

Equivalent temperature, °F

Calm	40	35	30	25	20	15	10	5	0	−5	−10	−15	−20	−25	−30	Calm
5	37	33	27	21	16	12	6	1	−5	−11	−15	−20	−26	−31	−35	5
10	28	21	16	9	4	−2	−9	−15	−21	−27	−33	−38	−46	−52	−58	10
15	22	16	11	1	−5	−11	−18	−25	−36	−40	−45	−51	−58	−65	−70	15
20	18	12	3	−4	−10	−17	−25	−32	−39	−46	−53	−60	−67	−76	−81	20
25	16	7	0	−7	−15	−22	−29	−37	−44	−52	−59	−67	−74	−83	−89	25
30	13	5	−2	−11	−18	−26	−33	−41	−48	−56	−63	−70	−79	−87	−94	30
35	11	3	−4	−13	−20	−27	−35	−43	−49	−60	−67	−72	−82	−90	−98	35
**40	10	1	−6	−15	−21	−29	−37	−45	−53	−62	−69	−76	−85	−94	−101	40**

■ Little danger   ■ Danger   ▨ Great danger

* °C= 0.556 (°F −32)
** Convective heat loss at wind speeds above 40 mph has little additional effect on body cooling

Figure 15.10.   Wind Chill Index.

ity. Thus, running at 8 mph into a 12-mph headwind produces the effect of a 20-mph headwind. Conversely, running at 8 mph with a 12-mph tailwind creates a relative wind speed of only 4 mph. The yellow-shaded zone on the left of Figure 15.10 indicates relatively little danger from cold exposure for a person properly clothed. In contrast, in the orange-shaded zone (which generally begins at an ambient air temperature of about 18°F [−7.8°C]), increasing danger exists to exposed flesh, particularly ears, nose, and fingers. In the red zone on the right, the equivalent temperatures pose serious danger of exposed flesh freezing within minutes.

Perhaps an Exaggeration   Assessments by several groups of researchers indicate that the wind-chill index, based on Antarctic expeditions in the 1940s that measured the time that cans of water froze at different temperatures and wind speeds, significantly *overestimates* cold air's effects on human skin. The National Weather Service reassessed its computer model to calculate the wind-chill index as a public health tool to reduce hypothermia, frostbite, and related cold injuries. Critics maintain that the index does not consider the difference between body heat loss in the sun and shade or rates of freezing for different areas of the human body. The following table is an example of a modification of the wind chill index for an air temperature of 10°F relative to current assessments displayed in Figure 15.10.

PROPOSED MODIFICATION OF WIND CHILL INDEX FOR AIR TEMPERATURE OF 10°F

Wind Speed (mph)	Current Wind Chill[a]	Proposed Wind Chill[a]
5	6	10
10	−9	0
15	−18	−8
20	−25	−14
25	−29	−19
30	−33	−23
35	−35	−26
40	−37	−29

[a]Equivalent air temperature, °F.

Respiratory Tract During Cold-Weather Exercise

Cold ambient air does not damage respiratory passages. Even in extreme cold, incoming air warms to between 80°F (27°C) and 90°F (32°C) as it reaches the bronchi. Warming an incoming breath of cold air greatly increases its capacity to hold moisture. Thus, humidification of inspired cold air produces water and heat loss from the respiratory tract, especially with large ventilatory volumes during demanding exercise. This contributes to dryness of mouth, a burning sensation in the throat, irritation of the respiratory passages, and general dehydration. Wearing a scarf or mask-type "baklava" that covers the nose and mouth and traps the water in exhaled air (and warms and moistens the next incoming breath) reduces uncomfortable respiratory symptoms.

SUMMARY

1. Cutaneous and muscle blood flow increase during exercise in the heat, whereas other tissues temporally compromise their blood supply.

2. Core temperature normally increases during exercise; the relative stress of exercise determines the magnitude of the increase.

3. Excessive sweating strains fluid reserves, creating a relative state of dehydration. Sweating without fluid replacement decreases plasma volume and causes a precipitous, dangerous rise in core temperature.

4. Exercise in a hot, humid environment poses a thermoregulatory challenge because the large sweat loss in high humidity contributes little to evaporative cooling.

5. A relatively small degree of dehydration impedes heat dissipation, compromises cardiovascular function, and diminishes exercise capacity.

6. Adequate fluid replacement preserves plasma volume to maintain circulation and sweating at optimal levels. The ideal fluid replacement schedule during exercise matches fluid intake to fluid loss, a process effectively monitored by changes in body weight.

7. A small amount of electrolytes added to the rehydration beverage replenishes fluid more effectively than drinking plain water.

8. Repeated heat stress initiates thermoregulatory adjustments that improve exercise capacity and reduce discomfort on subsequent heat exposure. Heat acclimatization favorably redistributes cardiac output while increasing sweating capacity. Full acclimatization generally requires about 10 days of heat exposure.

9. Studies that consider body size and composition, aerobic fitness, level of hydration, and degree of acclimatization show little age-related decrement in thermoregulatory capacity during moderate heat-exercise stress or ability to acclimatize to heat stress.

10. When equated for level of fitness and acclimatization, women and men show equivalent efficiency in thermoregulation during exercise, but women sweat less than men at the same core temperature.

11. The Heat Stress Index uses ambient temperature and relative humidity to evaluate the environment's potential heat challenge to an exercising person.

12. Water conducts heat about 25 times greater than air; thus, immersion in water of only 28 to 30°C provides considerable cold stress. This initiates rapid thermoregulatory adjustments to conserve body heat.

13. Subcutaneous fat provides excellent insulation against cold stress. It enhances the effectiveness of vasomotor adjustments to maintain a large percentage of metabolic heat.

14. Enhanced insulation from body fat becomes apparent in cold water, where fatter individuals exhibit less thermal and cardiovascular strain and greater exercise tolerance than leaner counterparts.

15. Appropriate clothing enables humans to tolerate the coldest climates on earth.

16. Ambient temperature and wind speed determine the environment's "coldness." The wind chill index determines the interacting effects of ambient temperature and wind speed on exposed flesh.

17. Inspired ambient air temperature does not pose a danger to the respiratory tract. Considerable water evaporation from the respiratory passages during cold-weather exercise magnifies fluid loss.

THOUGHT QUESTIONS

1. What information contributes to predicting an individual's survival time during extreme cold exposure?

2. In deciding on the starting time for an upcoming summer marathon in Florida, indicate what past meteorological information would be most valuable and why.

3. Explain whether marathoners should splash water over their body as they run.

4 Suppose you had to jog across a desert for 8 hours (sea level, 115°F [46.1°C], 20% relative humidity) while carrying only a backpack. What items would you take? Why?

PART 3 •
Exercise at Altitude

High-altitude natives live in permanent settlements in the Andes and Himalayan mountains as high as 5486 m (18,000 ft). Prolonged exposure of an unacclimatized person to this high altitude can cause death from ambient air's subnormal oxygen pressure (**hypoxia**), even if the person remains inactive. The physiologic challenge of even medium altitude becomes apparent during physical activity for unacclimatized newcomers to oxygen's decreased partial pressure.

STRESS OF ALTITUDE

Figure 15.11 illustrates the barometric pressure, pressures of the respired gases, and percentage saturation of hemoglobin at various terrestrial elevations. The density of air decreases progressively with ascents above sea level. For example, the barometric pressure at sea level averages 760 mm Hg, whereas at 3048 m, the barometer reads 510 mm Hg; at an elevation of 5486 m, the pressure of a column of air at the earth's surface represents about one-half of its pressure at sea level. Dry ambient air, whether at sea level or altitude, contains 20.9% oxygen. The P_{O_2} (density of oxygen molecules) decreases proportionately to the decrease in barometric pressure upon ascending to higher elevations ($P_{O_2} = 0.209 \times$ barometric pressure). Ambient P_{O_2} at sea level averages 150 mm Hg but averages only 107 mm Hg at 3048 m. *Reduced P_{O_2} and accompanying arterial hypoxia precipitates the immediate physiologic adjustments to altitude and longer-term acclimatization.*

Oxygen Loading at Altitude

The inherent nature of the oxyhemoglobin dissociation curve (Chapter 9) dictates that only a small change in hemoglobin's percentage saturation occurs with decreasing P_{O_2} until about 3048 m. At 1981 m (6500 ft), for example, alveolar P_{O_2} lowers from its sea level value of 100 mm Hg to 78 mm Hg, yet hemoglobin still remains 90% saturated with oxygen. This relatively small decrease in oxy-

gen carried by blood has little effect on a resting or mildly active individual but exerts a major effect on more intense endurance performance.

In the transition from moderate to higher elevations, values for alveolar (arterial) oxygen partial pressure exist on the steep part of the oxyhemoglobin dissociation curve. This reduces hemoglobin oxygenation and negatively impacts even moderate aerobic activities. An acute exposure to 4300 m, for example, reduces aerobic capacity 32% compared with the sea level value. Above 5182 m (17,000 ft) permanent living becomes nearly impossible, and mountain climbing usually progresses with the aid of oxygen equipment. However, acclimatized mountaineers have lived for weeks at 6706 m (22,002 ft) breathing only ambient air. Members of two Swiss expeditions to Mt. Everest remained at the summit for 2 hours without using oxygen equipment (an impressive feat considering arterial P_{O_2} equals 28 mm Hg with a corresponding 58% oxygen saturation of arterial blood). An unacclimatized person under these conditions becomes unconscious within 30 seconds. Although such performances clearly represent an exception, they demonstrate the enormous adaptive capability of humans to work and survive without external support at extreme terrestrial elevations.

ACCLIMATIZATION

Altitude acclimatization broadly describes the adaptive responses in physiology and metabolism that improve tolerance to altitude hypoxia. Acclimatization adjustments occur progressively to each higher elevation, and full acclimatization requires time. As a broad guideline, it takes about 2 weeks to adapt to 2300 m. Thereafter, each 610-m altitude increase requires an additional week for full adaptation up to 4572 m. As summarized in **Table 15.5**, compensatory responses to altitude occur almost immediately, whereas others take weeks or even months.

Immediate Adjustments

At elevations above 2300 m, rapid physiologic adjustments compensate for the thinner air and reduced alveolar oxygen pressure. The most important of these responses include:

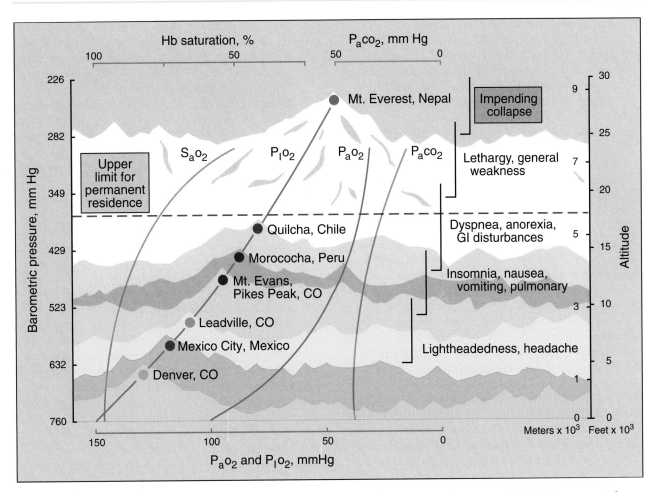

Figure 15.11. Changes in environmental and physiological variables with progressive elevations in altitude (P_aO_2 = partial pressure of arterial oxygen; P_aCO_2 = partial pressure of arterial carbon dioxide; P_IO_2 = partial pressure of oxygen in inspired air; S_aO_2 = oxygen saturation of hemoglobin).

Table 15•5	Immediate and Longer-term Adjustments to Altitude Hypoxia	
SYSTEM	**IMMEDIATE**	**LONGER-TERM**
Pulmonary Acid-Base	Hyperventilation Body fluids become more alkaline due to reduced CO_2 (H_2CO_3) with hyperventilation	Hyperventilation Excretion of base (HCO_3^-) via the kidneys with reduced alkaline reserve
Cardiovascular	Increased submaximal heart rate Increased submaximal cardiac output Stroke volume remains the same or lowers slightly Maximum cardiac output remains the same or lowers slightly	Submaximal heart rate remains elevated Submaximal cardiac output falls to or below sea-level values Stroke volume lowers Maximum cardiac output lowers
Hematologic		Decreased plasma volume Increased hematocrit Increased hemoglobin concentration Increased total number of red blood cells Possible increased capillarization of skeletal muscle
Local		Increased red-blood-cell 2,3-DPG Increased mitochondria Increased aerobic enzymes

1. **Hyperventilation triggered by increased respiratory drive.** *Hyperventilation represents the immediate first line of defense to altitude exposure.* Chemoreceptors located in the aortic arch and branching of the carotid arteries in the neck detect reductions in arterial P_{O_2}. Chemoreceptor stimulation increases ventilation, raising alveolar oxygen concentration toward the level in ambient air. Any increase in alveolar P_{O_2} with hyperventilation facilitates oxygen loading in the lungs.

2. **Increased blood flow (cardiac output) during rest and submaximal exercise.** Submaximal heart rate and cardiac output can increase 50% above sea level values in the early stages of altitude acclimatization, whereas the heart's stroke volume remains essentially unchanged. Sea level and altitude exercise oxygen uptake remain similar, but increased submaximal exercise blood flow at altitude compensates for the reduced arterial oxygen content. In contrast, the circulatory adjustments to acute altitude exposure with maximal exercise cannot compensate for the lower oxygen content of arterial blood dramatically decreasing $\dot{V}O_{2max}$ and exercise capacity.

Fluid Loss A decreased thirst sensation at altitude negatively affects the body's fluid balance. The cool and dry air in mountainous regions also causes considerable body water to evaporate as air warms and moistens in the respiratory passages. Respiratory fluid loss often leads to moderate dehydration and accompanying symptoms of dryness of the lips, mouth, and throat, particularly for active people with relatively large daily pulmonary ventilations (and exercise-related sweat loss). For these active people, body weight should be checked frequently (to ensure against dehydration), augmented with unlimited fluid availability.

Longer-Term Adjustments

Hyperventilation and increased submaximal cardiac output provide a rapid, effective counter to the acute altitude challenge. Other *slower acting* physiologic adjustments commence during a prolonged altitude stay. The three most important adjustments include:

1. **Acid-base adjustment.** Hyperventilation at altitude favorably increases alveolar oxygen concentration, while carbon dioxide concentration decreases. The ambient air contains essentially no carbon dioxide, so increased alveolar ventilation at altitude washes out (dilutes) carbon dioxide in the alveoli. This creates a larger than normal gradient for carbon dioxide diffusion from blood into the lungs, reducing arterial carbon dioxide considerably. During prolonged high-altitude exposure, alveolar carbon dioxide pressure can decrease to 10 mm Hg compared with the sea level value of 40 mm Hg. Carbon dioxide loss from body fluids causes pH to increase as the blood becomes more alkaline.

(Recall from Chapter 10 that carbonic acid transports the largest amount of the body's carbon dioxide.) Control of respiratory alkalosis produced by hyperventilation occurs through the kidneys, which slowly excrete base (HCO_3^-) through the renal tubules. The establishment of acid-base equilibrium with acclimatization occurs with a loss of alkaline reserve. Altitude does not affect the anaerobic metabolic pathways per se, but the blood's buffering capacity for acids gradually decreases, reducing the critical level for accumulation of acid metabolites like lactate.

2. **Hematological changes.** An increase in the blood's oxygen-carrying capacity provides the most important long-term adaptation to altitude. A rapid decrease in plasma volume increases red blood cell (RBC) concentration during the first few days at altitude. This response causes arterial blood's oxygen content to increase significantly above values observed on immediate ascent to altitude. The reduced arterial P_{O_2} stimulates a concurrent increase in RBC mass, a response termed **polycythemia** that directly increases the blood's capacity to transport oxygen. The kidneys release the erythrocyte-stimulating hormone **erythropoietin** within 15 hours after altitude ascent. In the weeks that follow, RBC production in the marrow of the long bones increases considerably and remains elevated. For example, oxygen-carrying capacity of blood for high-altitude residents of Peru averages 28% above sea level values. For well-acclimatized mountaineers, oxygen transport capacity for each dL (100 mL) of blood (at sea level P_{O_2}) ranges between 25 and 31 mL compared to about 20 mL for lowland residents. Even with hemoglobin's reduced oxygen saturation at altitude, the actual *quantity* of oxygen in arterial blood of elite mountaineers at altitude nearly equals sea level values. **Figure 15.12** illustrates the general trend for increased hemoglobin and hematocrit during altitude acclimatization for eight young women at the University of Missouri (altitude 213 m) who lived and worked for 10 weeks at the 4267-m summit of Pikes Peak. Upon reaching Pikes Peak, red blood cell concentration increased rapidly because of a reduced plasma volume during the first 24 hours. Over the following month, hemoglobin concentration and hematocrit continued to rise and then stabilized for the remainder of the stay. Two weeks after the women returned to Missouri, hemoglobin and hematocrit returned to pre-altitude values.

3. **Cellular adaptations.** Long-term acclimatization initiates peripheral changes that facilitate aerobic metabolism. These changes (1) increase capillary concentration in skeletal muscle, reducing the distance for oxygen diffusion between blood and tissues; (2) add mitochondria number and aerobic enzyme concentration; and expand (3) oxygen storage within specific muscle fibers that facilitates intracellular oxygen delivery and utilization, particularly at low tissue P_{O_2}.

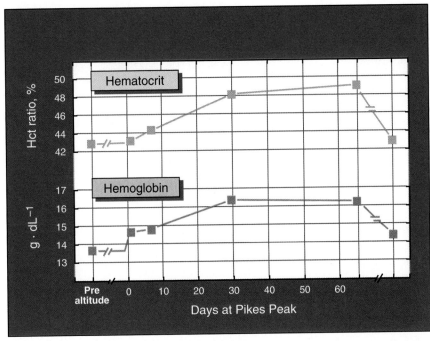

Figure 15.12. Effects of altitude on hemoglobin and hematocrit levels of eight young women before, during, and 2 weeks after exposure to 4267 m (From Hannon, J.P., et al.: Effects of altitude acclimatization on blood composition of women. *J. Appl. Physiol*, 26:540, 1968.)

ALTITUDE-RELATED MEDICAL PROBLEMS

Natives who live and work at high altitudes and newcomers to altitude encounter medical problems associated with reduced ambient PO_2. Some mild problems dissipate within hours or several days, depending on the rapidity of ascent and degree of exposure; other medical complications become severe and compromise overall health and safety. Three medical conditions discussed in the Close Up on page 544 pose potential problems: (1) acute mountain sickness, (2) high-altitude pulmonary edema, and (3) high-altitude cerebral edema.

EXERCISE CAPACITY AT ALTITUDE

The stress of high altitude imposes meaningful limitations on exercise capacity and physiologic function. Even at lower altitudes, the body's adjustments do not fully compensate for reduced oxygen pressure and diminishing exercise performance.

Aerobic Capacity

Aerobic capacity progressively and somewhat linearly decreases from arterial oxygen desaturation as altitude increases. Trained and untrained individuals can generally expect a 1.5% to 3.5% reduction in $\dot{V}O_{2max}$ for every 305-m (1000 ft) increase above 1524 m (5000 ft), with a slightly greater rate of decrease for elite athletes. The aerobic capacity of a relatively fit man on top Mt. Everest equals only about 1000 mL of oxygen per minute (14 to 18 mL·kg^{-1}·min^{-1}).

Circulatory Factors

Aerobic capacity remains below sea level values even after several months of acclimatization. Reduced circulatory efficiency in moderate and strenuous exercise offsets the benefits of acclimatization. During submaximal exercise, the immediate altitude response increases submaximal exercise blood flow; cardiac output decreases in the days that follow and does not improve with longer altitude exposure. A decrease in stroke volume as the altitude stay progresses accounts for diminished cardiac output. At maximal exercise, a decrease in maximum cardiac output occurs after about a week above 3048 m and persists throughout the altitude stay. *Reduced maximum exercise blood flow results from the combined effect of decreased maximum heart rate and maximum stroke volume.*

Fit subjects experience a 2% to 13% decrement in 1- and 3-mile running performance at medium altitude (2300 m). The effects become more pronounced at higher elevations. Even after 4 weeks of acclimatization, endurance performance at altitude remains below sea level values. The small improvements in endurance at altitude during acclimatization probably relate to increases in (1) minute ventilation (ventilatory acclimatization), and (2) arterial oxygen saturation.

ALTITUDE TRAINING AND SEA LEVEL PERFORMANCE

Unquestionably, altitude acclimatization improves one's capacity to exercise at altitude. However, the effect of altitude exposure and altitude training on $\dot{V}O_{2max}$ and endurance performance immediately on return to sea level remains equivocal. Altitude adaptations in local circulation and cellular function and compensatory increases in the blood's oxygen-carrying capacity should enhance sea-level exercise performance. Unfortunately, much of the altitude research has not adequately evaluated this possibility. Often, poor control exists over the subjects' physical activity level, making it difficult to determine whether any improved sea-level $\dot{V}O_{2max}$ or performance score on return from altitude represents a training effect, an altitude effect, or synergism between altitude and training.

$\dot{V}O_{2max}$ on Return to Sea Level

Sea level performance does not significantly improve after living at altitude when aerobic capacity serves as the criterion. Compared to pre-altitude measures, no change in $\dot{V}O_{2max}$ occurred for young runners on return to sea level after 18 days at 3100 m. Training in chambers designed to simulate altitude provided no additional benefit to sea level performance compared to similar training at sea level. As expected, the altitude-trained group showed superior physical performance in the altitude experiments compared to their sea level counterparts.

Some physiologic changes produced during prolonged altitude exposure actually *negate* adaptations that could improve exercise performance upon return to sea level. The residual effects of muscle mass loss and reduced maximum heart rate and stroke volume observed with pro-

longed altitude exposure would not enhance immediate performance on return to sea level. Any reduction in maximum cardiac output during a stay at altitude offsets benefits derived from the blood's greater oxygen-carrying capacity.

Can Sea Level Training Be Maintained at Altitude?

Exposure to 2300 m and higher makes it nearly impossible for athletes to train at the same intensity as at sea level. At 4000 m, for example, runners can only train at 40% of their sea level $\dot{V}O_{2max}$ compared with 80% of this value at sea level. This altitude-related reduction in absolute training intensity makes it difficult for athletes to maintain peak condition for sea-level competition.

Altitude Training Versus Sea Level Training

To evaluate the effectiveness of exercise training at altitude, middle-distance runners trained at sea level for 3 weeks at 75% of sea level $\dot{V}O_{2max}$. Another group of six runners trained an equivalent distance at the same percentage $\dot{V}O_{2max}$ measured at 2300 m. The groups then exchanged training sites and continued 3 weeks of similar training. Initially, 2-mile run times decreased by 7.2% at altitude compared to sea level. The times improved about 2.0% for both groups after altitude training, but post-altitude performance on return to sea level remained unchanged compared to pre-altitude sea level runs. The $\dot{V}O_{2max}$ for both groups at altitude decreased initially by about 17% and improved only slightly after 20 days of altitude training. When the runners returned to sea level, aerobic capacity averaged 2.8% below pre-altitude sea level values! Clearly, for these well-conditioned runners, no synergistic effect occurred with hard aerobic training at medium altitude compared with equally severe training at sea level.

"Live High–Train Low"   *Failure to maintain the muscular power outputs of sea level training at altitude may initiate a detraining effect.* For these reasons, elite endurance athletes have resorted to the banned (and dangerous) practices of blood doping or erythropoietin injections to increase hematocrit and hemoglobin concentration without the bother and negative effects of an altitude stay.

Athletes who lived at 2500 m but returned regularly to 1250 m to train (i.e., "live high–train low") showed greater performance increases in the 5000-m run than athletes who lived and trained at 2500 m or athletes who lived and trained at sea level. Altitude acclimatization and maintaining sea level training intensity provide important additive benefits to endurance at sea level.

At-Home Acclimatization

At-Home Acclimatization   The method of at-home acclimatization makes use of the observation that altitude's beneficial effects on erythropoiesis and aerobic capacity require relatively short-term exposures to hypoxia. For example, daily intermittent exposures of 3 to 5 hours for 9 days to simulated altitudes of 4000 to 5500 m in a hypobaric chamber increased endurance performance, RBC count, and hemoglobin concentration in elite mountain climbers. Intermittent hypoxic training under normobaric conditions provides an added bonus with clinical and cardioprotective implications because such exercise augments training's effect on selected metabolic and cardiovascular risk factors.

In the absence of a hypobaric chamber, three approaches create an "altitude" environment where an athlete, mountaineer, or hot-air balloonist living at sea level spends a large enough portion of the day to stimulate an altitude acclimatization response.

1. **Gamow Hypobaric Chamber** (named after its inventor, Rustem Igor Gamow [University of Colorado], son of the famed physicist George Gamow, co-author of the Big Bang Theory). A person rests and sleeps in a small chamber; reducing the chamber's total air pressure simulates the barometric pressure of a given altitude. Reductions in barometric pressure bring about proportionate reductions in inspired air's P_{O_2}.

2. **Increasing air's nitrogen concentration.** To eliminate the necessity of constructing an enclosure to withstand differentials between ambient sea level air and reduced pressure within the hypobaric chamber, altitude has been simulated at sea level by increasing the nitrogen percentage of the air within an enclosure. Increased nitrogen percentage reduces the air's oxygen percentage, thus decreasing the P_{O_2} of inspired air. Nordic skiers have applied this technique by living for 3 to 4 weeks in a specially constructed house that provides air with only 15.3% oxygen compared with the normal concentration of 20.9%. This system does require nitrogen gas and careful monitoring of the breathing mixture.

3. **Wallace Altitude Tent.** A suitcase-sized unit (**Fig. 15.13**), developed by British Olympic cyclist Shaun Wallace, continuously supplies air with an oxygen content that eventually equilibrates at 15% to simulate an altitude of 2500 m (8200 ft). The 70-pound unit consists of a portable tent that fits over a normal bed; a hypoxic generator (housed in an airline suitcase) continually feeds altitude-simulating hypoxic air into the tent. The porosity of the tent's material limits the diffusion rate of outside oxygen into the tent to maintain the 15% value for oxygen within the tent. Equilibration of the tent's environment at the 15% oxygen level requires about 90 minutes.

Questions & Notes

Define hypoxia.

List the 2 factors that precipitate the immediate physiologic adjustments to altitude.

1.

2.

Give the altitude level (in meters) where P_{O_2} starts to change abruptly.

Give the formula for calculating P_{O_2}.

At an altitude of 4300m, aerobic capacity is reduced by about _____% compared with the value at sea level.

FOR YOUR INFORMATION

The Lactate Paradox

On ascent to high altitude, lactate production at a given submaximal exercise intensity increases compared with sea level exercise, presumably from altitude hypoxia and added reliance on anaerobic glycolysis. Surprisingly, the lactate response to exercise after acclimatization results in *lower* lactate production, despite failure of either $\dot{V}O_{2max}$ or regional blood flow to increase. Thus, the following question arises concerning this apparent physiologic contradiction, called the **lactate paradox:** How can reduced lactate accumulation occur without a concomitant increase in tissue oxygenation? Research points to a reduced output of the glucose-mobilizing hormone epinephrine during chronic altitude exposure. Glucose and glycogen provide the only macronutrient sources for anaerobic energy (and lactate formation). This reduced glucose mobilization blunts capacity for lactate formation. Reductions in intracellular ADP during chronic altitude exposure may also inhibit glycolytic pathway activation. Reduced lactate levels during maximal exercise have been partly attributed to reduced central nervous system drive that diminishes capacity for all-out effort.

Box 15–5 • CLOSE UP

RECOGNIZING AND TREATING SIGNS AND SYMPTOMS OF HIGH-ALTITUDE MEDICAL PROBLEMS

Newcomers and sometimes high-altitude natives risk a variety of medical problems associated with reduced P_{O_2} at higher elevations. Some of these problems remain mild and dissipate within several days depending on the rapidity of ascent and degree of exposure. Three primary medical conditions threaten those who ascend to high altitude:

1. **Acute mountain sickness (AMS)**, the most common malady
2. **High-altitude pulmonary edema (HAPE)**, which reverses if the person returns quickly to a lower altitude

3. **High-altitude cerebral edema (HACE)**, a potentially fatal condition if not diagnosed and treated immediately
4. **High-altitude retinal hemorrhage (HARH)**, a condition that results in bleeding in the macula of the eye to produce irreversible visual defects.

Table 1 summarizes the causes, symptoms, and associated treatments for these conditions.

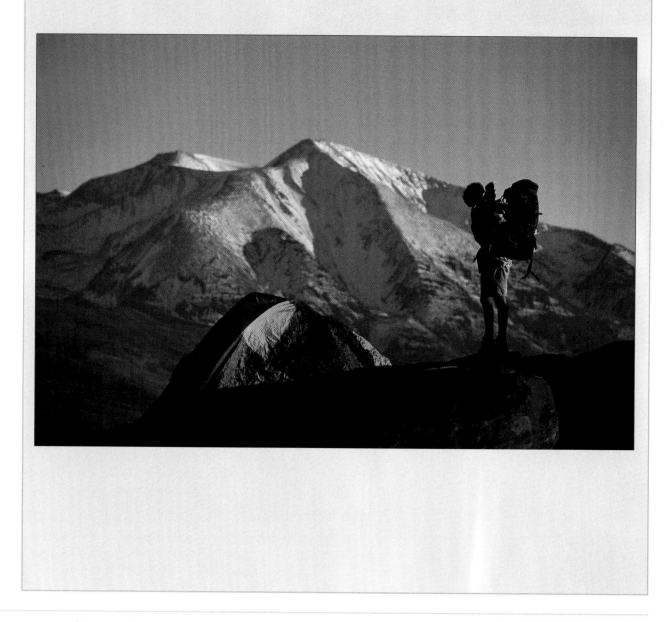

Box 15-5 • CLOSE UP *(Continued)*

Table 1 High-Altitude Medical Problems

CONDITION	CAUSES	SYMPTOMS	TREATMENT
Acute Mountain Sickness (AMS)—Relatively benign condition that becomes exacerbated by exercise in the first few hours of exposure.	Occurs most often in people who ascend rapidly to high altitude (>3000 m, 10,000 ft) without benefiting from gradual and progressive acclimatization to lower altitudes.	Symptoms begin within 4-12 h after exposure, and dissipate within one week. Some people have symptoms at altitudes as low as 2500 m (8000 ft), but most symptoms become prevalent above 3000 m (10,000 ft). Rapid ascent to 4200 m (14,000 ft) guarantees symptoms. Decreased thirst and severe appetite suppression occurs during the early stages, often resulting in a 40% reduction in energy intake and consequent body mass loss. Even moderate exercise becomes intolerable with AMS symptoms. <u>Common Symptoms</u> • Headache (result of increased cerebral hemodynamics from acute hyperventilation) • Dizziness • Nausea • Constipation • Vomiting • Depressed urine output (even with adequate hydration) • Dimness of vision • Insomnia • Generalized weakness	Rest and gradual acclimatization is preferred treatment. Symptoms subside with acclimatization and often disappear shortly thereafter. Acclimatizing slowly to moderate altitudes below 3048 m followed by a slow progression to higher elevations usually prevents AMS.
High-Altitude Pulmonary Edema (HAPE)—Fluid accumulates in the brain and lungs in this life-threatening condition.	Predisposing factors include altitude, rate of ascent, and individual susceptibility.	Symptoms usually manifest within 23 to 96 h following rapid ascent. <u>Common symptoms</u> • General fatigue • Dyspnea upon exertion • Persistent dry, irritating cough without phlegm and without pre-existing pumonary infection • Pain or pressure in the substernal area • Headache and nausea • Chest examination reveals wheezy and raspy sounds known as rales. Well-acclimatized individuals can develop symptoms with severe exertion at elevations above 5486 m (18,000 ft) (the result of increased pulmonary artery pressure).	To prevent severe disability or death requires immediate descent to lower altitude on a stretcher (or flown to safety). Any physical activity potentiates complications. Supplemental oxygen, 2-4 L·min⁻¹ is common if medical facilities are available. If descent or oxygen are not available administer 20 mg nifedipine slow-release formulation every 6 hrs until descent, or use of a hyperbaric chamber. With treatment, symptoms decrease within hours and complete clinical recovery within several days. HAPE poses no problem at altitudes below 1676 m (5500 ft).
High-Altitude Cerebral Edema (HACE)—A potentially fatal neurologic syndrome that develops within hours or days in individuals with AMS. HACE occurs in about 1% of people exposed to altitudes >2700 m (9000 ft). Involves increased intracranial pressure causing coma and death if untreated.	Cerebral edema results from cerebral vasodilation and elevations in capillary hydrostatic pressures causing movement of fluid and protein from the vascular compartment across the blood-brain barrier. An enlarged cerebral fluid volume eventually distorts brain structures, particularly the brain's white matter, which exacerbates symptoms and increases sympathetic nervous system activity.	Early symptoms, similar to AMS and HAPE, progressively worsen as the altitude stay progresses. <u>Common Symptoms</u> • Debilitating headache and severe fatigue • Altered mental status and neurologic deterioration including disruption of vision and bladder and bowel dysfunction • Loss of coordination of trunk muscles • Paralysis on one side of the body, and generally poor reflexes	Because of the difficulty diagnosing HACE at high altitude, immediate descent to a lower elevation becomes mandatory treatment. Use of supplemental oxygen, drugs and/or a hyperbaric chamber are effective.
High Altitude Retinal Hemorrhage (HARH)—Hemorrhage in the macula of the eye (the oval "yellow spot" region in the back of the eyeball close to the optic disc) produces irreversible visual defects.	Retinal bleeding probably results from surges in blood pressure with exercise that causes blood vessels in the eye to dilate and rupture from increased cerebral blood flow.		Immediate descent to a lower elevation becomes mandatory treatment. Use of supplemental oxygen, drugs, and/or a hyperbaric chamber are effective.

Reference: Armstrong L.E.: *Performing in Extreme Environments*. Champaign, IL: Human Kinetics Press, 2000.

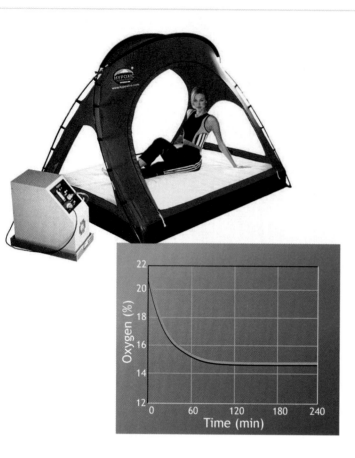

Figure 15.13. The Wallace Altitude Tent fits over a double or queen-size bed or can be constructed for in-home use as a semipermanent cubicle. Patches of "breathable" nylon permit diffusion of ambient oxygen (at higher P_{O_2}) into the tent (at lower P_{O_2}) to maintain the percentage of oxygen within the tent at about 15%. A hypoxic generator (*outside of tent*) continuously supplies air with oxygen content that equilibrates within the tent at near 15%. The *inset* shows the time course for equilibration of air within the tent to reach the 15% oxygen level. (Photo courtesy of Shaun Wallace, Hypoxico Inc., Cardiff, CA.)

SUMMARY

1. Inadequate oxygenation of hemoglobin occurs from the reduction in ambient P_{O_2} upon altitude ascent. This produces noticeable performance decrements in aerobic physical activities at 2000 m and higher.

2. Reduced arterial P_{O_2} and accompanying tissue hypoxia at altitude stimulate physiologic responses that improve altitude tolerance during rest and exercise. The primary immediate responses include hyperventilation and increased submaximal cardiac output via an elevated heart rate.

3. Longer-term acclimatization involves physiologic adjustments that greatly improve tolerance to altitude hypoxia. The main adjustments involve (1) re-establishing acid-base balance of body fluids, (2) increased hemoglobin and red blood cell synthesis, and (3) enhanced local circulation and cellular metabolic functions. Adjustments (2) and (3) facilitate oxygen transport, delivery, and utilization.

4. Altitude level dictates the rate and magnitude of acclimatization. Noticeable improvements occur within several days, but major adjustments require about 2 weeks. Near-full acclimatization to high altitude takes 4 to 6 weeks.

5. For individuals at a simulated altitude that approaches the summit of Mt. Everest, alveolar P_{O_2} equals 25 mm Hg. This reduces $\dot{V}O_{2max}$ by 70%. Unacclimatized individuals at this altitude become unconscious within 30 seconds.

6. Acclimatization does not fully compensate for altitude stress. Even after acclimatization, $\dot{V}O_{2max}$ decreases about 2% for every 300 m above 1500 m. Impaired endurance performance generally parallels the reduced aerobic capacity.

7. Altitude-related decrements in maximum heart rate and stroke volume offset the beneficial effects of acclimatization. This partially explains the inability to achieve sea level $\dot{V}O_{2max}$ values at altitude.

8. Sea level $\dot{V}O_{2max}$ and endurance performance do not improve following altitude acclimatization. More than likely, reduced circulatory efficiency in exercise (and possibly detraining and a decreased muscle mass) offsets acclimatization benefits.

9. Altitude training provides no additional benefit to sea level exercise performance compared with equivalent training only at sea level.

THOUGHT QUESTIONS

1. To climb Mt. Everest, elite mountaineers take 3 months to establish base camps at 16,600 ft (4216 m), 19,500 ft (4953 m), 21,300 ft (5410 m), 24,000 ft (6096 m), and 26,000 ft (6604 m) before the final ascent. Explain the physiologic rational for this "stage ascent" approach to mountaineering.

2. If altitude acclimatization improves endurance exercise performance at altitude, why doesn't it improve similar performance immediately upon return to sea level?

3. Explain whether periodic breath holding while exercising at sea level brings about similar physiologic adaptations as training at altitude.

4. Advise an athlete who plans to train for an endurance race at high altitude in two months.

PART 4 •
Use of Physiologic Agents to Enhance Exercise Performance

Red blood cell (RBC) reinfusion, exogenous use of the hormone erythropoietin, pre-exercise warm-up, and breathing hyperoxic gas mixtures represent four common non-nutritional, non-pharmacologic procedures to enhance physiologic response to exercise and increase performance.

RED BLOOD CELL REINFUSION

RBC reinfusion, often called induced erythrocythemia, blood boosting, or blood doping, came into public prominence as a possible ergogenic technique during the 1972 Munich Olympics. Gold-medal winner endurance athlete Lasse Viren allegedly used this technique to prepare for his endurance runs in the 5000- and 10,000-m events.

How It Works

RBC reinfusion requires withdrawal of between one and four units (1 unit = 450 mL) of a person's blood. Plasma is removed and immediately reinfused, and the packed RBCs are frozen for storage. To prevent significant reductions in blood cell concentration, removal of each unit of blood occurs over 3 to 8 weeks because it takes this duration to re-establish normal RBC levels. Reinfusion of stored RBCs (referred to as autologous transfusion) occurs up to 7 days before endurance competition. (Homologous transfusion infuses type-matched donor's blood.) This increases hematocrit and hemoglobin levels by 8% to 20% and increases average hemoglobin concentration for men from a normal of 15 g per dL of blood to 19 g per dL (hematocrit increases from a normal value of 40% up to 60%). Theoretically, the added blood volume increases maximal cardiac output while the increased hematocrit augments the blood's oxygen-carrying capacity to increase the oxygen available to working muscles. This effect benefits the endurance athlete, especially long-distance runners, for whom oxygen transport often limits exercise capacity.

Infusing 900 to 1800 mL of freeze-preserved autologous blood usually provides ergogenic benefits. Each 500-mL infusion of whole blood, or its equivalent of 275 mL of packed red cells, adds about 100 mL of oxygen to the blood's total oxygen-carrying capacity. This occurs because each dL of whole blood normally carries about 20 mL of oxygen. An endurance athlete's total blood volume circulates five times each minute in high-intensity exercise. The potential "extra" oxygen avail-

Questions & Notes

Give another name for red blood cell re-infusion.

Briefly explain why blood boosting works.

Give 2 possible negative effects of blood doping.

1.

2.

Give the average increase in $\dot{V}O_{2max}$ generally achieved with blood doping.

able to the tissues from each unit of reinfused blood (or its packed red cell component) equals 0.5 L (5 × 100 mL extra O₂).

Blood doping also creates opposite effects to those intended. A large infusion of packed RBCs (and resulting inordinately large increase in cellular concentration) could increase blood viscosity and decrease cardiac output; this effect would reduce aerobic capacity. Certainly, any large increase in blood viscosity or thickness compromises blood flow through atherosclerotic vessels of individuals with coronary artery disease.

Does It Work?

Research generally confirms physiologic and performance improvements with RBC reinfusion. Differences among various research studies originate largely from blood storage methods. Frozen RBCs store in excess of 6 weeks without loss of cells compared to conventional storage at 4°C (used in earlier studies); substantial hemolysis (destruction) occurs at 4°C after only 3 weeks. This is important because it usually takes a person about 6 weeks to replenish blood cells after withdrawal of two units of whole blood (**Fig. 15.14**).

RBC reinfusion elevates hematologic characteristics in men and women. This effect translates to a 5% to 13% increase in aerobic capacity, reduced submaximal heart rate and blood lactate for a standard exercise task, and improved endurance at sea level and altitude. **Table 15.6** illustrates hematologic, physiologic, and performance responses for five adult men during submaximal and maximal exercise before and 24 hours after a compara-

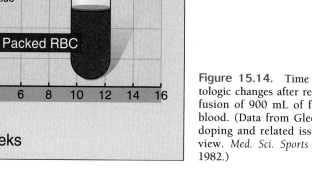

Figure 15.14. Time course of hematologic changes after removal and reinfusion of 900 mL of freeze-preserved blood. (Data from Gledhill, N.: Blood doping and related issues: A brief review. *Med. Sci. Sports Exerc.*, 14:183, 1982.)

Table 15·6	Physiologic, Performance, and Hematologic Characteristics Prior to and 24 Hours After the Reinfusion of 750 mL of Packed Red Blood Cells			
VARIABLE	**PRE-INFUSION**	**POST-INFUSION**	**DIFFERENCE**	**DIFFERENCE, %**
Hemoglobin, g · 100 mL blood⁻¹	13.8	17.6	3.8[b]	+27.5[b]
Hematocrit, %[a]	43.3	54.8	11.5[b]	+26.5[b]
Submaximal $\dot{V}O_2$, L · min⁻¹	1.6	1.5	−0.01	−0.6
Submaximal HR, b · min⁻¹	127.4	109.2	18.2	−14.3[b]
$\dot{V}O_{2max}$, L · min⁻¹	3.3	3.7	0.4[b]	+12.8[b]
HR$_{max}$, b · min⁻¹	181.6	180.0	−1.6	−0.9
Treadmill run time, s	793	918	125[b]	+15.8

[a]Hematocrit presented as the percent (%) of 100 mL of whole blood occupied by red blood cells.
[b]Statistically significant difference.
From Robertson, R.J., et al.: Effect of induced erythrocytemia on hypoxia tolerance during exercise. *J. Appl. Physiol.*, 53:490, 1982.

tively large 750-mL infusion of packed RBC. These response patterns generally reflect the results of the more recent research in this area.

A New Twist: Hormonal Blood Boosting

To eliminate the somewhat cumbersome and lengthy process of blood doping, endurance athletes have used **erythropoietin**, a hormone normally produced by the kidneys. This hormone stimulates bone marrow to increase production of RBCs. From a medical standpoint, erythropoietin combats anemia in patients with severe kidney disease. Normally, with low hematocrit or when arterial oxygen pressure decreases (as in severe lung disease or ascent to high altitude), erythropoietin release stimulates RBC production. Unfortunately, if administered exogenously in an unregulated and unmonitored fashion (simply injecting the hormone requires much less sophistication than blood doping procedures), hematocrit can dangerously exceed levels in excess of 60%. Excessive hemoconcentration increases blood viscosity and greatly augments the exercise-induced increase in systolic blood pressure. This potentiates the likelihood for stroke, heart attack, heart failure, pulmonary embolism, and even death.

WARM-UP

Coaches, trainers, and athletes at all levels of competition believe in the benefit of some type of mild physical activity or **warm-up** before vigorous exercise. They accept that preliminary exercise enables the performer to (1) prepare either physiologically or psychologically for an event, and (2) reduce likelihood of joint and muscle injury. For animals, it requires greater forces and increases in muscle length to injure a "warmed-up" muscle compared with a muscle in a "cold" condition. The explanation maintains that warming up stretches the muscle-tendon unit to allow for greater length and less tension at any given load.

Two categories classify warm-up, although considerable overlap exists:

1. **General warm-up** involves calisthenics, stretching, and general body movements or "loosening-up" exercises usually *unrelated* to the specific neuromuscular actions of the anticipated performance.
2. **Specific warm-up** provides *skill rehearsal* for the actual activity. Swinging a golf club, throwing a baseball or football, practicing tennis or basketball, and preliminary lead-up in the high jump or pole vault are examples.

Psychological Considerations

Competitors at all levels believe that some prior activity prepares them mentally for their event so they can concentrate on the upcoming performance. *Evidence supports that a specific warm-up related to the activity improves required skill and coordination patterns.* Sports requiring accuracy, timing, and precise movements benefit from specific or formal preliminary practice.

Competitors also believe that prior exercise, particularly before strenuous effort, gradually prepares them to go "all out" with less fear of injury. The ritual warm-up of baseball pitchers provides a case in point. A starting or relief pitcher would never enter a game throwing at competitive speeds without previously warming up. Would any elite athlete begin competition without first engaging in a particular form, intensity, or duration of warm-up? Because topflight athletes believe in warming up, it becomes nearly impossible to design an experiment with these individuals to resolve whether or not warm-up actually improves subsequent performance and reduces injury potential.

In certain situations, peak performance occurs when play begins, without time for warming up. When a reserve player enters a game in the last few minutes, no time exists for preliminary stretching, vigorous calisthenics, or taking practice shots. The player must go all out with no warm-up except for that done before the

Describe erythropoientin's effect as an ergogenic substance.

Give a possible negative effect of erythropoientin infusion.

Name 2 sports that generally benefit from specific warm-up.

1.

2.

Describe 3 physiologic mechanisms that may improve exercise performance.

1.

2.

3.

game or at intermission. Do more injuries occur in such cases? Does poorer basketball defense or rebounding or football line play take place during the first few minutes of an "unwarmed" condition than after a performance preceded by a warm-up or performance later in the game?

Effects on Exercise Performance

Little evidence exists that warm-up per se directly improves subsequent exercise performance. Lack of scientific justification does not mean that warm-up should be disregarded. Because of the strong psychological component and "possible" physical benefits of warming up, whether passive (massage, heat applications, and diathermy), general (calisthenics and jogging), or specific (practice of the actual movements), we recommend that such procedures continue. Until substantial evidence justifies elimination, a brief warm-up provides a comfortable way to lead into more vigorous exercise. A gradual warm-up should increase muscle and core temperature without inducing fatigue or reducing immediate energy stores. This consideration makes the warm-up highly individualized because, for example, the duration and intensity of an Olympic swimmer's warm-up would exhaust a recreational swimmer. The competitive event or activity should begin within several minutes from the end of the warm-up. Engage specific muscles in a way that mimics the anticipated activity and brings about a full range of joint motion.

Warm-Up and Sudden Strenuous Exercise

Several studies have evaluated the effects of preliminary exercise on cardiovascular responses to sudden, strenuous exercise. The findings provide a different physiologic framework for justifying warm-up for individuals in adult fitness and cardiac rehabilitation programs and occupations and sports requiring a sudden burst of high-intensity exercise.

In one study, 44 men free from overt symptoms of coronary heart disease performed high-intensity treadmill exercise for 10 to 15 seconds without prior warm-up. Evaluation of post-exercise electrocardiograms (ECG) revealed that 70% of subjects displayed abnormal ECG changes attributed to inadequate myocardial oxygen supply. These changes did not relate to age or fitness level. To evaluate warm-up, 22 of the men jogged in place at moderate intensity with a heart rate of 145 b·min^{-1} for 2 minutes before the treadmill run. With warm-up, 10 men with previously abnormal ECG responses to the treadmill run showed normal tracings and 10 men improved their ECGs; only two subjects showed ischemic changes (poor oxygen supply) after the warm-up. Warm-up also improved the blood pressure response. For seven subjects with no warm-up, systolic blood pressure averaged 168 mm Hg immediately after the treadmill run. This decreased to 140 mm Hg with the 2-minute warm-up.

Coronary blood flow adaptation to sudden, intense exercise does not occur instantaneously, and transient myocardial ischemia can occur in apparently healthy and fit individuals. The positive effect of prior warm-up (at least 2 min of easy jogging) on the ECG and blood pressure indicates a more favorable relationship between myocardial oxygen supply and demand.

Warm-up preceding strenuous exercise probably benefits all people, yet the greatest effect occurs for those with compromised myocardial oxygen supply. A brief pre-exercise warm-up optimizes blood pressure and hormonal adjustments at the onset of subsequent strenuous exercise. Warm-up serves two purposes: (1) it reduces myocardial workload and thus myocardial oxygen requirement, and (2) it enhances coronary blood flow to augment myocardial oxygen supply.

BREATHING HYPEROXIC GAS

Athletes often breathe oxygen-enriched or **hyperoxic gas mixtures** during time out, at half-time, or after strenuous exercise. They believe this procedure enhances the blood's oxygen-carrying capacity, thus facilitating recovery from prior exercise. When healthy people breathe ambient air at sea level, hemoglobin in arterial blood leaving the lungs contains 95% to 98% of its full oxygen complement. In physiologic terms:

1. Breathing higher than normal concentrations of oxygen (hyperoxic mixtures) at sea level increases hemoglobin's oxygen transport by only 10 mL of extra oxygen for every 1000 mL of blood.
2. Oxygen dissolved in plasma when breathing a hyperoxic mixture increases only slightly from its normal quantity of 3 mL to about 7 mL per 1000 mL of blood.

This means that breathing hyperoxic gas at sea level increases the oxygen-carrying capacity by 14 mL of oxygen for every 1000 mL of blood; 10 mL extra is attached to hemoglobin, and 4 mL extra is dissolved in plasma.

Before Exercise

The blood volume of a 70-kg person equals approximately 5000 mL. Therefore, a hyperoxic breathing mixture potentially adds about 70 mL of oxygen in the total blood volume (5000 mL blood $\times$ 14.0 mL extra O_2 per 1000 mL blood = 70 mL O_2). Despite any potential psychological benefit to the athlete who believes that pre-exercise oxygen breathing helps performance, only a slight performance advantage exists from the small amount of extra oxygen (70 mL). Any advantage occurs only if subsequent exercise took place *immediately* after hyperoxic breathing. This means the athlete cannot breathe ambient air in the interval between hyperoxic breathing and exercise. Breathing ambient air (considerably lower P_{O_2} than the previously inspired hyperoxic mixture) facilitates oxygen's movement from the body back into the environment. The halfback who breathes oxygen on the sideline before returning to the game, or the swimmer who takes a few breaths of oxygen before moving to the blocks for starting instructions (while breathing ambient air) gains no competitive edge because of physiologic benefits. This is particularly ironic in American football because the energy to power each play is generated almost completely from metabolic reactions that do *not* require oxygen!

During Exercise

Breathing hyperoxic gas during submaximal and maximal aerobic exercise enhances endurance performance. Oxygen breathing during submaximal aerobic exercise reduces blood lactate, heart rate, and ventilation volume and increases maximal oxygen uptake.

In one study, subjects performed a 6.5-minute endurance ride on a bicycle ergometer at an exercise level equivalent to 115% of $\dot{V}O_{2max}$ while breathing either room air or 100% oxygen. Subjects breathed both air and oxygen from identical tanks of compressed gas to mask knowledge of the breathing mixture.

Figure 15.15 gives the details of the endurance ride showing superiority in endurance (with less drop-off in pedal revolutions) during the hyperoxic trials. Figure 15.15B shows oxygen uptake curves during the endurance ride while breathing either oxygen or room air. A higher oxygen uptake occurred when breathing 100% oxygen, with a correspondingly faster increase in oxygen uptake early in exercise. The small increase in hemoglobin saturation with hyperoxic breathing and the additional oxygen dissolved in plasma increase oxygen availability during maximal exercise where total blood volume circulates up to seven times each minute in an elite endurance athlete. Quantitatively, the 70 mL of extra oxygen in the total blood volume with hyperoxic breathing (circulated seven times each minute) provides an additional 490 mL of oxygen each minute during intense aerobic exercise. Also, increased partial pressure of oxygen in solution while breathing hyperoxic gas facilitates oxygen diffusion across the tissue-capillary membrane to mitochondria. This accounts for a more rapid oxygen utilization early in exercise. Although it provides physiologic benefit during some forms of exercise, the sports application of breathing hyperoxic mixtures seems limited. The added weight of an appropriate breathing system would negate any ergogenic benefit. The legality of the system's use during competition seems unlikely.

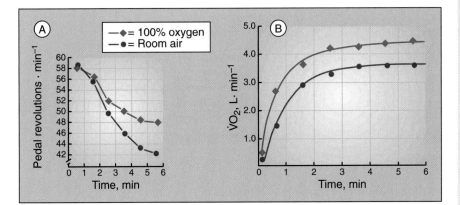

Figure 15.15. **(A)** Superiority of endurance (measured by pedal revolutions each minute) breathing pure oxygen versus breathing ambient air at sea level. **(B)** Oxygen uptake curves during the endurance rides show enhanced oxygen uptake while breathing pure oxygen. (Data from Weltman, A., et al.: Effects of increasing oxygen availability on bicycle ergometer endurance performance. *Ergonomics*, 21:427, 1978.)

In Recovery

Figure 15.16 illustrates the effects of breathing hyperoxic gas during recovery from strenuous exercise on subsequent exercise performance. After 1 minute of all-out bicycle ergometer exercise, subjects recovered passively (quiet sitting) or actively (light pedaling) while breathing room air or 100% oxygen for either 10 or 20 minutes. They then repeated the all-out bicycle ride. No differences emerged in the 6-second revolutions and cumulative revolutions (top graph) for the 1-minute ride after breathing either room air or pure oxygen in recovery. No difference resulted between trials breathing either room air or oxygen when comparing blood lactate levels at 10 and 20 minutes of recovery. This indicated that oxygen inhalation did not preferentially alter lactate removal. These findings do not support the use of hyperoxic breathing mixtures to facilitate recovery or as an adjuvant to performance after different durations of recovery from prior exercise.

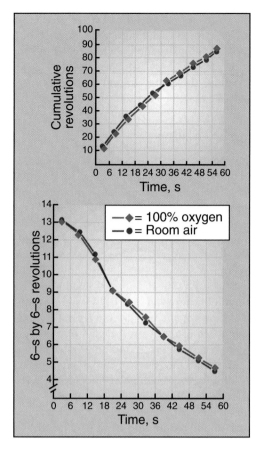

Figure 15.16. Cumulative **(top)** and absolute **(bottom)** pedal revolutions on a bicycle ergometer during 1 minute of maximal exercise subsequent to breathing either oxygen or ambient air during recovery from a previous maximal exercise bout. (Data from Weltman, A., et al.: Exercise recovery, lactate removal, and subsequent high intensity exercise performance. *Res. Q.*, 48:786, 1977.)

SUMMARY

1. RBC reinfusion (blood doping) involves drawing, storing, and reinfusing concentrated RBCs for use several weeks later. The added blood volume and RBC concentration theoretically create a larger maximum cardiac output and increase the blood's oxygen-carrying capacity; both factors increase $\dot{V}O_{2max}$.

2. Research supports the ergogenic benefits of RBC reinfusion for aerobic exercise performance and thermoregulation.

3. Diverse physiologic rationales justify warm-up for ergogenic purposes and injury prevention. These include potential benefits for muscular contraction speed and efficiency, tissue compliance, enhanced oxygen delivery and utilization, and facilitated nerve impulse transmission. Limited research supports the performance benefits of warm-up other than its potential positive effect on psychological factors.

4. A moderate cardiovascular warm-up before sudden strenuous exercise reduces cardiac workload and enhances coronary blood flow by depressing transient myocardial ischemia at the onset of intense physical activity.

5. Breathing 100% oxygen during exercise extends endurance by increasing oxygen uptake, reducing blood lactate, and lowering pulmonary ventilation. Breathing hyperoxic mixtures before or after exercise provides no ergogenic benefit.

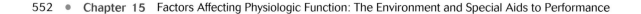

THOUGHT QUESTIONS

1. As a basketball coach, what warm-up procedures would you recommend prior to a game?

2. Explain the rationale for oxygen inhalation at the sidelines during a football game played at the moderately high altitude of Denver, Colorado.

SELECTED REFERENCES

American College of Sports Medicine: American College of Sports Medicine position stand on heat and cold illnesses during distance running. *Med. Sci. Sports Exerc.*, 28:1, 1996.

Armstrong, L.E., and Maresh, C.M.: Effects of training, environment, and host factors on the sweating response to exercise. *Int. J. Sports Med.*, 19(Suppl 2):s103, 1998.

Ashenden, M.J., et al.: "Live high, train low" does not change the total haemoglobin mass of male endurance athletes sleeping at a simulated altitude of 3000 m for 23 nights. *Eur. J. Appl. Physiol.*, 80:479, 1999.

Bailey, D.M., et al.: Implications of moderate altitude training for sea-level endurance in elite distance runners. *Eur. J. Appl. Physiol.*, 78:360, 1998.

Barnard, R.J., et al.: Ischemic response to sudden strenuous exercise in healthy men. *Circulation*, 48:936, 1973.

Bärtsh, P.: High altitude pulmonary edema. *Med. Sci. Sports Exerc.*, 31(Suppl):S23, 1999.

Beidleman, B.A., et al.: Exercise responses after altitude acclimatization are retained during reintroduction to altitude. *Med. Sci. Sports Exerc.*, 29:1588, 1997.

Brandenburg, J.P.: The acute effects of prior dynamic resistance exercise using different loads on subsequent upper-body explosive performance in resistance-trained men. *J. Strength Cond. Res.*, 19:427, 2005.

Brien, A.J., and Simon, T.L.: The effects of red blood cell infusion on 10-km race time. *JAMA*, 257:2761, 1987.

Burnley, M., et al.: Effects of prior warm-up regime on severe-intensity cycling performance. *Med. Sci. Sports Exerc.*, 37:838, 2005.

Chapman, R.F., et al.: Individual variation in responses to altitude training. *J. Appl. Physiol.*, 85:1448, 1998.

Clark, S.A., et al.: Effects of live high, train low hypoxic exposure on lactate metabolism in trained humans. *J. Appl. Physiol.*, 96:517, 2004.

Cymerman, A., et al.: Operation Everest II: Maximal oxygen uptake at extreme altitude. *J. Appl. Physiol.*, 66:2446, 1989.

Dematte, J.E., et al.: Near-fatal heat stroke during the 1995 heat wave in Chicago. *Arch. Intern. Med.*, 129:173, 1998.

Drust, B., et al.: Elevations in core and muscle temperature impairs repeated sprint performance. *Acta. Physiol. Scand.*, 183:181, 2005.

Edwards, R.J., et al.: The effect of an angiotensin-converting enzyme inhibitor and a K+(ATP) channel opener on warm up angina. *Eur. Heart J.*, 26:598, 2005.

Eiken, O., et al.: Human skeletal muscle function and metabolism during intense exercise at high O2 and N2 pressures. *J. Appl. Physiol.*, 63:571, 1987.

Emonson, D.L., et al.: Training-induced increases in sea level $\dot{V}O_{2max}$ and endurance training are not enhanced by acute hypobaric exposure. *Eur. J. Appl. Physiol.*, 76:8, 1997.

Faigenbaum, A.D., et al.: Acute effects of different warm-up protocols on fitness performance in children. *J. Strength Cond. Res.*, 19:376, 2005.

Falk, B.: Exercise in the pediatric population: Effects of thermal stress. In: *Environmental and Exercise Physiology*. Doubt, T. (ed.). Champaign, IL: Human Kinetics, 1997.

Franke, W.W., and Berendonk, B.: Hormonal doping and androgenization of athletes: A secret program of the German Democratic Republic government. *Clin. Chem.*, 43:1262, 1997.

Godek, S.F., et al.: Sweat rate and fluid turnover in American football players compared with runners in a hot and humid environment. *Br. J. Sports Med.*, 39:205, 2005.

Gonzalez-Alonso, J.R., et al.: Influence of body temperature on the development of fatigue during prolonged exercise in the heat. *J. Appl. Physiol.*, 86:1032, 1999.

Hales, J.R.S.: Hyperthermia and heat illness: Pathological implications for avoidance and treatment. *Ann. N.Y. Acad. Sci.*, 813:534, 1997.

Hasegawa, H., et al.: Wearing a cooling jacket during exercise reduces thermal strain and improves endurance exercise performance in a warm environment. *J. Strength Cond. Res.*, 19:122, 2005.

Hornery, D.J., et al.: Physiological and performance benefits of halftime cooling. *J. Sci. Med. Sport*, 8:15, 2005.

Hsu, A.R., et al.: Effects of heat removal through the hand on metabolism and performance during cycling exercise in the heat. *Can. J. Appl. Physiol.*, 30:87, 2005.

Inoue, Y., et al.: Mechanisms underlying the age-related decrement in the human sweating response. *Eur. J. Appl. Physiol.*, 79:121, 1999.

Jacobs, I., et al.: Thermoregulatory thermogenesis in humans during cold stress. *Exerc. Sport Sci. Rev.*, 22:221, 1994.

Jansen, G.F., et al.: Cerebral vasomotor reactivity at high altitude in humans. *J. Appl. Physiol.*, 86:681, 1999.

Jung, A.P., et al.: Influence of hydration and electrolyte supplementation on incidence and time to onset of exercise-associated muscle cramps. *J. Athl. Train.*, 40:71, 2005.

Kenney, W.L.: Thermoregulation at rest and during exercise in healthy older adults. *Exerc. Sport Sci. Rev.*, 25:41, 1997.

Kuwahara, T., et al.: Effects of menstrual cycle and physical training on heat loss responses during dynamic exercise at moderate intensity in a temperate environment. *Am. J. Physiol. Regul. Integr. Comp. Physiol.*, 288:R1347, 2005.

Leiper, J.B., et al.: The effect of intermittent high-intensity running on gastric emptying of fluids in man. *Med. Sci. Sports Exerc.*, 37:240, 2005.

Levine, B.D., and Stray-Gunderson, J.: "Living high-training low": Effect of moderate-altitude acclimatization with low-altitude training on performance. *J. Appl. Physiol.*, 83:102, 1997.

Liu, Y., et al.: Effect of "living high-training low" on the cardiac functions at sea level. *Int. J. Sports Med.*, 19:380, 1998.

Magnani, M., et al.: Monitoring erythropoietin abuse in athletes. *Br. J. Haematol.*, 106:260, 1999.

Maughan, R.J., et al.: Fluid and electrolyte balance in elite male football (soccer) players training in a cool environment. *J. Sports Sci.*, 23:73, 2005.

Maxwell, N.S., et al.: Intermittent running: Muscle metabolism in the heat and effect of hypohydration. *Med. Sci. Sports Exerc.*, 31:675, 1999.

McAnulty, S.R., et al.: Hyperthermia increases exercise-induced oxidative stress. *Int. J. Sports Med.*, 26:188, 2005.

McArdle, W.D., et al.: Thermal adjustment to cold-water exposure in exercising men and women. *J. Appl. Physiol.*, 56:1572, 1984.

McArdle, W.D., et al.: Thermal responses of men and women during cold-water immersion: Influences of exercise intensity. *Eur. J. Appl. Physiol.*, 65:265, 1992.

McCullough, E.A., Kenney, W.L.: Thermal insulation and evaporative resistance of football uniforms. *Med. Sci. Sports Exerc.*, 35:832, 2003.

Mendel, R.W., et al.: Effects of creatine on thermoregulatory responses while exercising in the heat. *Nutrition*, 21:301, 2005.

Morgan, R.M., et al.: Acute effects of dehydration on sweat composition in men during prolonged exercise in the heat. *Acta. Physiol. Scand.*, 182:37, 2004.

Nielsen, B.: Heat acclimatization—Mechanisms of adaptation to exercise in the heat. *Int. J. Sports Med.*, 19(Suppl 2):s1534, 1998.

Pandolf, K.B., et al.: Does erythrocyte infusion improve 3.2-km run performance at high altitude? *Eur. J. Appl. Physiol.*, 79:1, 1998.

Paraskevaidis, I.A., et al.: Repeated exercise stress testing identifies early and late preconditioning. *Int. J. Cardiol.*, 98:221, 2005.

Pilmanis, A.A., et al.: Exercise-induced altitude decompression sickness. *Aviat. Space Environ. Med.*, 70:22, 1999.

Pugh, L.C.G.E.: Athletes at altitude. *J. Physiol. (London)*, 192:619, 1967.

Pugh, L.C.G.E.: Muscular exercise on Mount Everest. *J. Physiol. (London)*, 141:233, 1958.

Pugh, L.C.G.E.: Physiological and medical aspects of the Himalayan Scientific and Mountaineering Expedition, 1960–61. *Br. Med. J.*, 2:621, 1962.

Purvis, A.J., Tunstall, H.: Effects of sock type on foot skin temperature and thermal demand during exercise. *Ergonomics*, 47:1657, 2004.

Rav-Acha, M., et al.: Cold injuries among Israeli soldiers operating and training in a semiarid zone: a 10-year review. *Mil. Med.*, 169:702, 2004.

Reisman, S., et al.: Warm-up stretches reduce sensations of stiffness and soreness after eccentric exercise. *Med. Sci. Sports Exerc.*, 37:929, 2005.

Roels, B., et al.: Effects of hypoxic interval training on cycling performance. *Med. Sci. Sports Exerc.*, 37:138, 2005.

Safran, M.R., et al.: The role of warm up in muscular injury prevention. *Am. J. Sports Med.*, 16:123, 1988.

Saltin, B.: Exercise and the environment: Focus on altitude. *Res. Q. Exerc. Sport*, 67:1, 1996.

Sarvazyan, A., et al.: Ultrasonic assessment of tissue hydration status. *Ultrasonics*, 43:661, 2005.

Saunders, A.G., et al.: The effects of different air velocities on heat storage and body temperature in humans cycling in a hot, humid environment. *Acta. Physiol. Scand.*, 183:241, 2005.

Sawka, M.N., and Coyle, E.F.: Influence of body water and blood volume on thermoregulation and exercise performance in the heat. *Exerc. Sport Sci. Rev.*, 27:167, 1999.

Sharwood, K.A., et al.: Weight changes, medical complications, and performance during an Ironman triathlon. *Br. J. Sports Med.*, 38:718, 2004.

Shirreffs, S.M., et al.: Fluid and electrolyte needs for preparation and recovery from training and competition. *J. Sports Sci.*, 22:57, 2004.

Shirreffs, S.M., et al.: The sweating response of elite professional soccer players to training in the heat. *Int. J. Sports Med.*, 26:90, 2005.

Strachan, A.T., et al.: Serotonin2C receptor blockade and thermoregulation during exercise in the heat. *Med. Sci. Sports Exerc.*, 37:389, 2005.

Townsend, N.E., et al.: Hypoxic ventilatory response is correlated with increased submaximal exercise ventilation after live high, train low. *Eur. J. Appl. Physiol.*, 94:207, 2005.

van Nieuwenhoven, M.A., et al.: The effect of two sports drinks and water on GI complaints and performance during an 18-km run. *Int. J. Sports Med.*, 26:281, 2005.

Watson, P., et al.: Blood–brain barrier integrity may be threatened by exercise in a warm environment. *Am. J. Physiol. Regul. Integr. Comp. Physiol.*, 288:R1689, 2005.

West, J.B.: *High Life: A History of High Altitude Physiology and Medicine*. Oxford, England: Oxford University Press, 1998.

Williams, M.H.: *The Ergogenics Edge: Pushing the Limits of Sports Performance*. Champaign, IL: Human Kinetics, 1998.

Young, A.J., et al.: Exertional fatigue, sleep loss, and negative energy balance increase susceptibility to hypothermia. *J. Appl. Physiol.*, 85:1210, 1998.

Section VI

Optimizing Body Composition, Successful Aging, and Health-Related Exercise Benefits

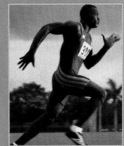

Estimates indicate that one-third of all deaths globally occur from aliments linked to lifestyle characteristics of excess body weight, diminished physical activity, and smoking, and this trend knows no economic borders.

Coupled with expanding girth is the graying of the population. Thirty years ago, age 65 represented the onset of old age. Now gerontologists mark 85 as a demarcation of "oldest-old" and age 75 as "young old." Demographers estimate that nearly one-half of the children born in 1996 will survive to age 95 or 100 years. Within this framework, the "new gerontology" addresses areas beyond age-related diseases and recognizes that *successful aging* requires enhanced physiologic function and improved physical fitness.

The physiologic and exercise capacities of older people generally rate below those of younger counterparts, yet one can question whether such differences reflect true biologic aging or simply the effect of disuse (brought on by alterations in lifestyle as people age). A meaningful upswing has occurred in participation of "senior citizens" in a broad range of physical activities. An active lifestyle retains a relatively high level of functional capacity, thus enabling older men and women to safely engage in more vigorous sports and physical activities. In addition, maintaining this lifestyle offers considerable protection against obesity and other diseases related to skeletal and cardiovascular health.

Clinical exercise physiologists have become part of a team approach to health care. The exercise physiologist primarily focuses on restoring the patient's mobility and functional capacity while working closely with the physical therapist, occupational therapist, and physician. To this end, exercise physiologists assume an increasingly more important clinical role in sports medicine to evaluate and recondition individuals with diverse diseases and physical disabilities.

In this section, Chapter 16 focuses on body composition: its components and assessment, differences between men and women and trained and untrained individuals, and topics relevant to obesity, including the role of diet and increased physical activity for effective weight loss and weight maintenance. In Chapters 17 and 18, we explore aspects of the aging process and the role played by the exercise physiologist as a healthcare professional in the clinical setting.

"From the glaciers of the Arctic to the palm-fringed beaches of the South Pacific, there are now more fat people in the world than hungry people! Obesity has become one of the world's leading causes of morbidity and mortality.

—ANONYMOUS

CHAPTER OBJECTIVES

- Outline body composition characteristics of the "reference man" and "reference woman."

- Define (1) lean body mass, (2) fat-free body mass, and (3) minimal weight.

- Describe Archimedes' principle applied to human body volume measurement.

- List assumptions for computing percentage body fat from body density.

- Explain how population-specific skinfold and girth equations predict body fat.

- Give strengths and weaknesses of the body mass index for assessing excess weight, excess fat, and disease risk.

- Describe the current status of overweight and obesity among American adults and children.

- List the significant health risks of obesity.

- Describe the criterion for obesity.

- Define fat cell hypertrophy and fat cell hyperplasia, and explain how each contributes to obesity and how each is modified with changes in body weight.

- Outline how "unbalancing" the energy balance equation affects body weight.

- Explain the rationale for including regular physical activity in a prudent weight loss program.

- Explain how a moderate increase in physical activity for a previously sedentary, overweight person affects: (1) daily food intake and (2) overall energy expenditure.

- Explain the rationale for and effectiveness of specific exercise for localized fat loss.

- Give diet and exercise advice to a person who wants to gain weight to enhance sports performance.

CHAPTER OUTLINE

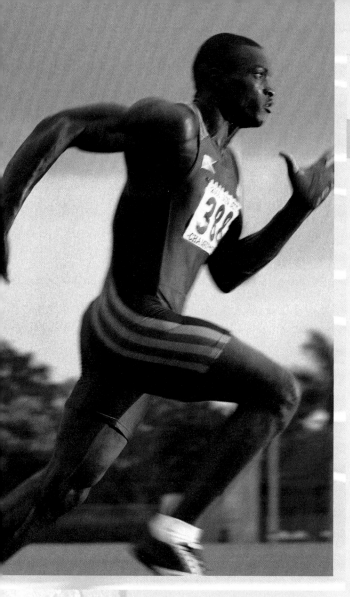

Body Composition, Obesity, and Weight Control

This chapter describes the gross composition of the human body and presents the rationale of direct and indirect methods to partition the body into two basic compartments: body fat mass and fat-free body mass. It also presents simple, noninvasive methods to analyze an individual's body composition and explores the role of exercise and diet, individually and in combination, to achieve optimal body composition.

PART 1 •
Gross Composition
of the Human Body

Over the past 70 years, numerous studies have focused on body composition and how best to measure its various components. Most methodologies partition the body into two distinct compartments: (1) fat-free body mass, and (2) body fat mass. The density of homogenized samples of fat-free body tissues in small mammals equals 1.100 g·cm^{-3} at 37°C. Fat stored in adipose tissue has a density of 0.900 g·cm^{-3} at 37°C. Subsequent body composition studies expanded the two-component model to account for biologic variability in three (water, protein, fat) or four (water, protein, bone mineral, fat) distinct components. Women and men differ in relative quantities of specific body composition components. Consequently, gender-specific reference standards provide a framework for evaluating "normal" body composition.

MULTICOMPONENT MODEL OF BODY COMPOSITION

Figure 16.1 shows a proposed five-level model for examining the human body. Each level of the model becomes more elaborate (atoms, molecules, cells, tissue systems, and whole body) as the body's complexity of biologic organization increases in accord with advances in physics and chemistry assessment techniques. Note that subdivisions exist within each of the five levels. The model primarily attempts to identify and then quantify each level's various components. An essential feature provides separate and distinct levels, each with directly or indirectly measurable characteristics.

Body composition analysis often focuses on the tissue and whole-body levels, primarily because of methodological and practical limitations. Gender differences in several of the body's compositional components provide a convenient framework for understanding body composition using the concept of a reference man and reference woman developed in the 1960s by Dr. Albert Behnke (1898–1993; ACSM Honor Award; Navy physician and research scientist).

BEHNKE'S REFERENCE MAN AND WOMAN MODEL

Figure 16.2 presents the body composition of the reference man and women first proposed by Behnke. The schema partitions body mass into lean body mass, muscle, and bone, with total body fat subdivided into storage and essential fat components. This model integrates the average physical dimensions from thousands of individuals measured in large-scale civilian and military anthropometric surveys with data from laboratory studies of tissue composition and structure.

The reference man is taller and heavier, his skeleton weighs more, and he possesses a larger muscle mass and lower body fat content than the reference woman. These differences exist even when one expresses fat, muscle, and bone as a percentage of body mass. Just how much of the gender difference in body fat relates to biologic and behavioral factors (perhaps from lifestyle differences) remains unclear. More than likely, hormonal differences play an important role. The reference model proves useful for statistical comparisons and interpretations of data from individuals and groups.

Essential and Storage Fat

In the reference model, total body fat exists in two storage sites or depots: **essential fat** and **storage fat**. Essential fat consists of the fat in the heart, lungs, liver, spleen, kidneys, intestines, muscles, and lipid-rich tissues of the central nervous system and bone marrow. Normal physiologic functioning requires this fat. In the heart, for example, dissectible fat from cadavers represents approximately 18.4 g or 5.3% of an average heart weighing 349 g in males and 22.7 g or 8.6% of a heart weighing 256 g in females. In the female, essential fat also includes additional **sex-specific fat**.

The storage fat depot includes fat (triacylglycerol) primarily in adipose tissue. The adipose tissue energy reserve contains approximately 83% pure fat, 2% protein, and 15% water within its supporting structures. Storage fat includes the visceral fatty tissues that protect the various internal organs within the thoracic and abdominal cavities from trauma and the larger adipose tissue volume deposited beneath the skin's surface. A similar proportional distribution of storage fat exists in men and women (12% of body mass in men and 15% in women), but total percentage of essential fat in women, which includes the sex-specific fat, averages four times that in men. More than likely, the additional essential fat in women serves biologically important functions for child bearing and other hormone-related functions. Considering the reference body's total quantity of approximately 8.5 kg of storage fat, this depot theoretically represents 63,500 kCal of available energy, or the energy equivalent of running nonstop at a 9-minute-per-mile pace for 114 hours!

Figure 16.3 partitions the distribution of body fat for the reference woman. As part of the 5% to 9% sex-specific

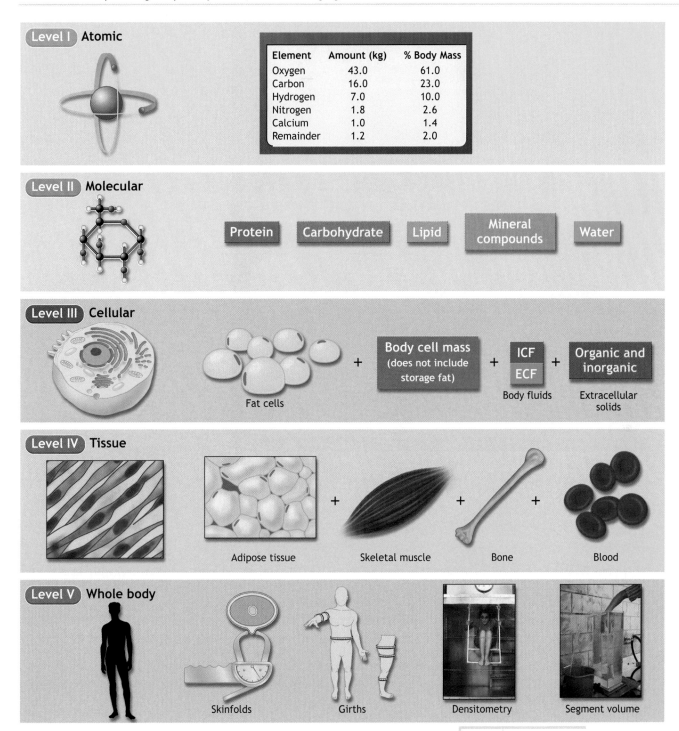

Level I   **Atomic**

Element	Amount (kg)	% Body Mass
Oxygen	43.0	61.0
Carbon	16.0	23.0
Hydrogen	7.0	10.0
Nitrogen	1.8	2.6
Calcium	1.0	1.4
Remainder	1.2	2.0

Level II   **Molecular**

Protein   Carbohydrate   Lipid   Mineral compounds   Water

Level III   **Cellular**

Fat cells   +   Body cell mass (does not include storage fat)   +   ICF / ECF   +   Organic and inorganic

Body fluids   Extracellular solids

Level IV   **Tissue**

Adipose tissue   +   Skeletal muscle   +   Bone   +   Blood

Level V   **Whole body**

Skinfolds   Girths   Densitometry   Segment volume

Figure 16.1.   Theoretical model for body fat distribution for the reference woman with body mass of 56.7 kg, stature, 163.8 cm, and 27% body fat. ICF = intracellular fluid; ECF = extracellular fluid. (From Katch, V.L., et al.: Contribution of breast volume and weight to body fat distribution in females. *Am. J. Phys. Anthropol.*, 53:93, 1980.)

fat reserves, breast fat probably contributes no more than 4% of body mass for women whose total fat content ranges between 14% and 35%. We interpret this to mean that other substantial sex-specific fat depots exist (e.g., pelvic, buttock, and thigh regions) that contribute to the female's body fat stores. **Table 16.1** presents data for percentage body fat for selected groups of male and female athletes. Striking differences exist among these groups.

FOR YOUR INFORMATION

Frame Size and Body Fat

Do individuals with a large frame size possess more body fat than persons with a small or medium bony frame? Many people justify their large body mass (and extra fat) on the basis of a large skeletal structure. Limited research indicates that when properly classified by frame size and body composition, bony structure and body fatness do not relate.

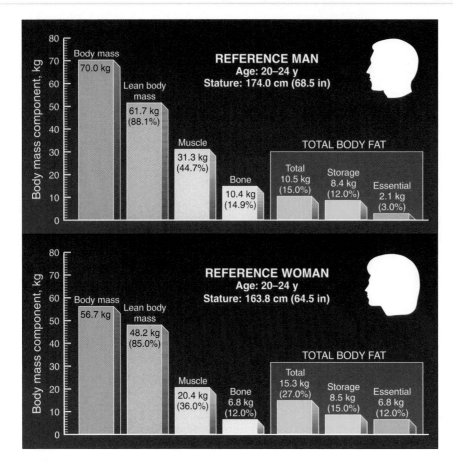

Figure 16.2. Body composition of the reference man and reference woman.

Fat-Free Body Mass and Lean Body Mass

The terms fat-free body mass (FFM) and lean body mass (LBM) refer to specific entities. Many researchers use these terms interchangeably; technically, the differences are subtle but real. LBM (a theoretical entity) contains the small percentage of non–sex-specific essential fat equivalent to approximately 3% of body mass (located chiefly within the central nervous system, bone marrow, and internal organs). In contrast, FFM represents the body mass devoid of all extractable fat (FFM = body mass − fat mass). Behnke points out that FFM refers to an **in vitro** entity (*"in an artificial environment outside the living organism"*) appropriate to carcass analysis. Behnke considered the LBM an **in vivo** (*"within a living organism"*) entity relatively constant in water, organic matter, and mineral content throughout the active adult's life span. In normally hydrated, healthy adults, the FFM and LBM differ only in the essential fat component (approximately 3% of total body mass).

Figure 16.2 shows that the lean body mass in men and **minimal body mass** in women consist chiefly of essential fat (plus sex-specific fat for females), muscle, water, and bone. The whole-body density of the reference man

with 12% storage fat and 3% essential fat is 1.070 g·cm⁻³; the density of his FFM equals 1.094 g·cm⁻³. If the reference man's total body fat percentage equals 15.0% (storage fat plus essential fat), the density of a hypothetical fat-free body attains the upper limit of 1.100 g·cm⁻³.

In the reference woman, the average whole-body density of 1.040 g·cm⁻³ represents a body fat percentage of 27%; of this, approximately 12% consists of essential body fat. A density of 1.072 g·cm⁻³ represents the minimal body mass of 48.5 kg. In actual practice, density values exceeding 1.068 for women (14.8% body fat) and 1.088 g·cm⁻³ for men (5% body fat) rarely occur except in young, lean athletes.

Minimal Leanness Standards

A biologic lower limit probably exists beyond which a person's body mass cannot decrease without lowering the fat-free mass to a degree that impairs health status or alters normal physiologic functions.

Men   To estimate the lower body fat limit in men (i.e., lean body mass), subtract storage fat from body mass. For

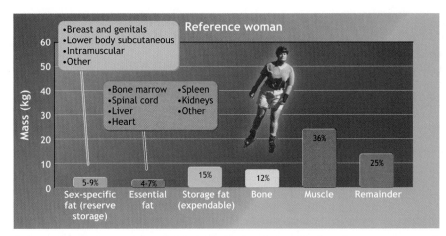

Figure 16.3. Theoretical model for body fat distribution for the reference woman with body mass of 56.7 kg, stature, 163.8 cm, and 27% body fat. (From Katch V.L., et al. Contribution of breast volume and weight to body fat distribution in females. *Am J Phys Anthropol* 1980;53:93.)

the reference man, the lean body mass (61.7 kg) includes approximately 3% (2.1 kg) essential body fat. Encroachment into this reserve may impair optimal health and capacity for exercise.

Low body fat values exist for male world-class endurance athletes and some conscientious objectors to military service who voluntarily reduced body fat stores during a prolonged experiment with semistarvation. The low fat levels of marathon runners, ranging from 1% to 8% of body mass, probably reflect an adaptation to severe training for distance running and a low caloric intake. Relatively low body fat level reduces the energy cost of weight-bearing exercise; it also provides a more effective gradient to dissipate metabolic heat generated during prolonged, high-intensity exercise.

Women   In contrast to the lower limit of body mass for the reference man (with 3% essential fat), the lower limit for the reference woman is approximately 12% essential fat. This theoretical limit, termed **minimal body mass**, represents 48.5 kg for the reference woman. Generally, the leanest women in the population do not fall below 10% to 12% body fat, which is a narrow range probably at the lower limit for most women in good health. Behnke's theoretical concept of minimal body mass in women, incorporating approximately 12% essential fat, corresponds to the lean body mass in men that includes 3% essential fat.

Underweight and Thin

The terms *underweight* and *thin* describe considerably different physical conditions. Measurements in our laboratories have focused on the structural characteristics of "apparently" thin females. We initially screened subjects subjectively as thin or "skinny." Twenty-six women were measured for skinfolds, circumferences, and bone diameters, and percentage body fat and FFM by hydrodensitometry (see page 567).

Unexpectedly, the women's percentage of body fat averaged 18.2%, which is only 7 to 9 percentage points below the values of 25% to 27% body fat typically reported for young adult women. Another striking finding included equivalence in four trunk and four extremity bone diameter measurements for the thin-appearing women compared with 174 women who averaged 25.6% fat and 31 women who averaged 31.4% body fat. Thus, appearing thin or skinny did not nec-

Table 16·1	Percentage Body Fat of Male and Female Athletes		
	PERCENTAGE BODY FAT		
SPORT	**MALE**		**FEMALE**
Ballet dancing	8–14		13–20
Baseball/softball	12–15		12–18
Basketball	6–12		20–27
Body building	5–8		10–15
Canoe/Kayak	6–12		10–16
Cycling	5–15		15–20
Football			
Backs	9–12		
Linebackers	13–14		
Lineman	15–19		
Quarterbacks	12–14		
Gymnastics	5–12		10–16
Horse racing	8–12		10–16
Ice/Field hockey	8–15		12–18
Orienteering	5–12		12–24
Racquetball	8–13		15–22
Rock climbing	5–10		13–18
Rowing	6–14		12–18
Rugby			10–17
Skiing			
Alpine	7–14		18–24
Cross-country	7–12		16–22
Jumping	10–15		12–18
Speed skating	10–14		15–24
Synchronized swimming			12–24
Swimming	9–12		14–24
Tennis	12–16		16–24
Track and field			
Discus throwers	14–18		22–27
Jumpers	7–12		10–18
Long distance	6–13		12–20
Shot putters	16–20		20–28
Sprinters	8–10		12–20
Decathletes	8–10		
Triathlon	5–12		10–15
Volleyball	11–14		16–25
Weightlifters	9–16		
Wrestling	5–16		

Data compiled from the research literature.

essarily correspond to a diminutive frame size or critically low body fat percentage proposed in the Behnke model for the lower limits of minimal body mass and essential body fat.

We recommend three criteria to designate an underweight adult female:

1. Body mass lower than minimal body mass calculated from skeletal measurements
2. Body mass lower than the 20th percentile by stature
3. Percentage body fat lower than 17% assessed by a criterion method

LEANNESS, REGULAR EXERCISE, AND MENSTRUAL IRREGULARITY

Physically active women, particularly participants in the "low weight" or "appearance" sports (e.g., distance running, body building, figure skating, diving, ballet, and gymnastics), increase their likelihood for one of three maladies:

1. Delayed onset of menstruation
2. Irregular menstrual cycle (**oligomenorrhea**)
3. Complete cessation of menses (**amenorrhea**)

Menstrual and ovarian dysfunction results largely from changes in the pituitary gland's normal pulsatile secretion of luteinizing hormone, regulated by gonadotropin-releasing hormone from the hypothalamus.

Amenorrhea occurs in 2% to 5% of women of reproductive age in the general population, but it reaches 40% in some athletic groups. As a group, ballet dancers remain lean and exhibit a greater incidence of menstrual dysfunction and eating disorders and a higher mean age at menarche than age-matched, nondance counterparts. One-third to one-half of female endurance athletes exhibit some menstrual irregularity. In premenopausal women, irregularity or absence of menses accelerates bone loss and increases the risk of musculoskeletal injury during exercise and, thus, increases interruption of training.

A high level of chronic physical stress may disrupt the hypothalamic-pituitary-adrenal axis and modify the output of gonadotropin-releasing hormone to cause irregular menstruation (*exercise stress hypothesis*). A concurrent hypothesis maintains that an energy reserve inadequate to sustain pregnancy induces cessation of ovulation (*energy availability hypothesis*). Proponents of this "energy deficit" explanation maintain that exercise per se exerts no deleterious effect on the reproductive system other than the potential impact of its additional energy cost on creating a negative energy balance.

Some researchers argue that 17% body fat represents a critical level for onset of menstruation, with 22% fat needed to sustain a normal cycle. They reason that body fat below these levels triggers hormonal and metabolic disturbances that affect the menses. Research with animals has identified **leptin**, a hormone intimately linked to body fat levels and appetite control, as a principal chemical that initiates puberty. Thus, a link may exist between hormonal regulation of sexual maturity onset (and perhaps continued optimal sexual function) and the level of stored energy reflected by accumulated body fat.

The lean body mass-to-body fat ratio may play a key role in normal menstrual function. This could occur through peripheral fat's role in converting androgens to estrogens or through leptin production in adipose tissue. Other factors may also be operative. Many physically active females who are below the supposedly critical 17% body fat level have normal menstrual cycles with a high level of physiologic and exercise capacity. Conversely, some amenorrheic athletes maintain body fat levels considered average for the population. Potential causes of menstrual dysfunction include the complex interplay of physical, nutritional, genetic, hormonal, regional fat distribution, psychological, and environmental factors. An intense exercise bout triggers release of an array of hormones, some of which can disrupt normal reproductive function. Intense and/or prolonged exercise that releases cortisol and other stress-related hormones may alter ovarian function via the hypothalamic-pituitary-adrenal axis.

In all likelihood, 13% to 17% body fat probably represents the minimum associated with regular menstrual function. The effects and risks of sustained amenorrhea on the reproductive system remain unknown. A gynecologist/endocrinologist should evaluate failure to menstruate or cessation of the normal cycle because it may signal a significant medical condition (such as pituitary or thyroid gland malfunction or premature menopause).

FOR YOUR INFORMATION

When a Model Is Not Ideal
In 1967, only an 8% difference existed in body weight between professional fashion models and the average American woman. Today, a model's body weight averages 23% lower than the national average. Twenty years ago, gymnasts weighed about 20 pounds more than their present day counterparts. Thus, it should come as little surprise that disordered eating patterns and unrealistic weight goals (and general dissatisfaction with one's body) remain so common among females of all ages.

SUMMARY

1. Total body fat consists of essential fat and storage fat. Essential fat contains fat in bone marrow, nerve tissue, and organs; it does not represent an energy reserve but is an important component for normal biologic function. Storage fat, the energy reserve, accumulates mainly as adipose tissue beneath the skin and in the deeper visceral depots.

2. Storage fat averages 12% of body mass for young adult men and 15% of body mass for women.

3. True sex differences exist for essential fat. It averages 3% body mass for men and 12% body mass for women. The greater percentage of essential fat for females probably relates to child bearing and hormonal functions (i.e., sex-specific essential fat).

4. A person probably cannot reduce body fat below the essential fat level and still maintain good health and optimal exercise capacity.

5. Menstrual dysfunction occurs among female athletes who train hard, incur an energy deficit, and maintain low levels of body fat. The precise interaction among menstrual dysfunction and the physiologic and psychological stress of regular training and competition, hormonal balance, energy and nutrient intake, and body fat requires further study.

THOUGHT QUESTION

What arguments counter the position that no true sex difference exists in body fat, but only a difference caused by gender-related patterns of regular physical activity and caloric intake?

PART 2 •
Methods to Assess Body Size and Composition

Two general approaches determine the fat and fat-free components of the human body:

1. Direct measurement by chemical analysis or dissection
2. Indirect estimation by hydrostatic weighing, anthropometric measurements, and other simple procedures including body stature and mass

DIRECT ASSESSMENT

Two methods directly assess body composition. In one technique, a chemical solution literally dissolves the body into its fat and nonfat (fat-free) components. **Figure 16.4** presents the chemical analyses data from five disease-free human cadavers. Water content equaled 60%, and ranged between 50% and 70%. Nearly identical averages emerged for protein (17%) and fat (18%), but twice the range in individual values existed for body fat. Ash (total major and trace mineral content) represented 5% of body mass. These data exhibit variation in total body fatness, yet the composition of skeletal mass and fat-free tissues remain relatively stable. Compositional consistency of various tis-

sues provides a theoretical basis to formulate mathematical equations to estimate body fat percentage from noninvasive, indirect measures.

The other direct assessment approach involves physical dissection of fat, fat-free adipose tissue, muscle, and bone. Such analyses require extensive time, meticulous attention to detail, and specialized laboratory equipment and pose ethical questions and legal problems in obtaining cadavers for research purposes. The most complete physical dissection study was published in 1984. **Figure 16.5** pre-

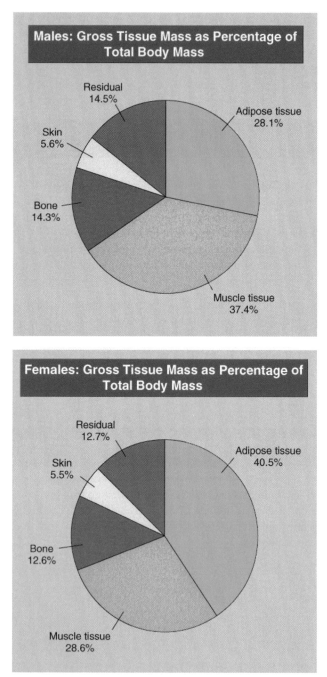

Figure 16.5. Various tissues in the adult male and female body expressed as a percentage of total body mass (in kg). (From Clarys, J.P., et al.: Gross tissue weights in the human body by cadaver dissection. *Hum. Biol.*, 56:459, 1984.)

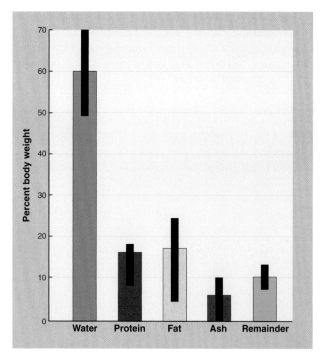

Figure 16.4. Body composition of five cadavers determined by direct chemical analysis. The height of the individual bars indicates the arithmetic mean for the five cadavers, and the black vertical bars represent the range. [Data from Widdowson, E.M.: In: *Human Body Composition: Approaches and Applications.* Brožek, J. (ed.). London: Pergamon Press, 1965.]

sents results from 25 cadavers ranging in age from 55 to 94 years. The sample included 12 embalmed (six males and six females) and 13 nonembalmed (six males and seven females) whites. Analyses for each cadaver included removing skeletal muscle and other major organs (brain, heart, lungs, liver, kidneys, and spleen). Bones were then separated at their articulations and scraped to leave surfaces free of muscle and adipose tissue. Muscle included the ligaments, and bone retained the cartilage of any articular surface. Airtight plastic buckets stored all dissected tissues, including scrapings. The tissues were weighed to within 0.1 g, and their densities were determined (ratio of mass to volume: mass ÷ volume). Complete dissection took approximately 15 hours and required a team of 10 to 12 anatomists and kinesiologists. Figure 16.5 shows an average adipose tissue mass equivalent to 40.5% of total body mass in females and 28.1% in males. The researchers introduced the concept of adipose tissue-free weight (ATFW)—the whole-body mass minus the mass of all dissectible adipose tissue that contains about 83% pure fat. Muscle accounted for 52% of the ATFW in males and 48.1% in females, whereas bone constituted 19.9% of ATFW in males and 21.3% in females. Combining the data for males and females, the average proportion of the ATFW included 8.5% skin, 50.0% muscle, and 20.6% bone.

INDIRECT ASSESSMENT

Many indirect procedures assess body composition, including Archimedes' principle applied to **hydrostatic weighing** (also known as **underwater weighing** and **hydrodensitometry**). This method computes percentage body fat from **body density**. Other procedures to predict body fat use skinfold thickness and girth measurements, x-ray, total-body electrical conductivity or impedance, near-infrared interactance, ultrasound, computed tomography, air plethysmography, magnetic resonance imaging, and dual-energy x-ray absorptiometry.

Hydrostatic Weighing (Archimedes' Principle)

The Greek mathematician and inventor Archimedes (287–212 BC) discovered a fundamental principle still applied to evaluate human body composition. An itinerant scholar of that time described the interesting circumstances surrounding the event:

> "King Hieron of Syracuse suspected that his pure gold crown had been altered by substitution of silver for gold. The King directed Archimedes to devise a method for testing the crown for its gold content without dismantling it. Archimedes pondered over this problem for many weeks without succeeding, until one day, he stepped into a bath filled to the top with water and observed the overflow. He thought about this for a moment, and then, wild with joy, jumped from the bath and ran naked through the streets of Syracuse shouting, 'Eureka! Eureka!' I have discovered a way to solve the mystery of the King's crown."

Archimedes reasoned that gold must have a volume in proportion to its mass, and to measure the volume of an irregularly shaped object required submersion in water with collection of the overflow. Archimedes took lumps of gold and silver, each having the same mass as the crown, and submerged each in a container full of water. To his delight, he discovered the crown displaced more water than the lump of gold and less than the lump of silver. This could only mean the crown consisted of *both* silver and gold as the King suspected.

Essentially, Archimedes evaluated the **specific gravity** of the crown (i.e., the ratio of the crown's mass to the mass of an equal volume of water) compared with the specific gravities for gold and silver. Archimedes also reasoned that an object submerged or floating in water becomes buoyed up by a counterforce that equaled the weight of the volume of water it displaces. This buoyant force supports an immersed object against the downward pull of gravity. Thus, an object "loses weight in water." *Because the object's loss of weight in water equals the weight of the volume*

Describe the differences between essential and storage fat.

What is the difference between "fat-free mass" and "lean body mass"?

Which tissue component accounts for the greatest part of the fat-free mass?

List 3 criteria for determining underweightness.

1.

2.

3.

Give another name for underwater weighing.

of water it displaces, the specific gravity refers to the ratio of the weight of an object in air divided by its loss of weight in water. The loss of weight in water equals the weight in air minus the weight in water.

$$\text{Specific gravity} = \text{Weight in air} \div \text{Loss of weight in water}$$

In practical terms, suppose a crown weighed 2.27 kg in air and 0.13 kg less (2.14 kg) when weighed underwater (**Fig. 16.6**). Dividing the weight of the crown (2.27 kg) by its loss of weight in water (0.13 kg) results in a specific gravity of 17.5. Because this ratio differs considerably from the specific gravity of gold (19.3), we too can conclude: *"Eureka, the crown must be fraudulent!"*

Archimedes' principle allows the application of hydrodensitometry to determine the body's volume and, from this, body density and an estimate of percentage body fat.

Determining Body Density For illustrative purposes, suppose a 50-kg woman weighs 2 kg when submerged in water. According to Archimedes' principle, a 48-kg *loss* of weight in water equals the weight of the displaced water. The volume of water displaced can be computed easily because chemists have determined the density of water at any temperature. In this example, 48 kg of

water equals 48 L, or 48,000 cm³ (1 g of water = 1 cm³ by volume at 39.2°F). If the woman were measured at the cold-water temperature of 39.2°F, no density correction for water would be necessary. In practice, researchers use warmer water and apply the density value for water at the particular weighing temperature. The whole-body density of this person, computed as mass ÷ volume, equals 50,000 g (50 kg) ÷ 48,000 cm³, or 1.0417 g·cm⁻³.

Computing Percentage Body Fat, Fat Mass, and Fat-Free Body Mass The equation that incorporates whole-body density to estimate the body's fat percentage is derived from the following three premises:

1. Densities of fat mass (all extractable lipid from adipose and other body tissues) and FFM (remaining lipid-free tissues and chemicals, including water) remain relatively constant (fat tissue = 0.90 g·cm⁻³; fat-free tissue = 1.10 g·cm⁻³), even with variations in total body fat and the FFM components of bone and muscle.
2. Densities for the components of the FFM at a body temperature of 37°C remain constant within and among individuals: water, 0.9937 g·cm⁻³ (73.8% of FFM); mineral, 3.038 g·cm⁻³ (6.8% of FFM); protein, 1.340 g·cm⁻³ (19.4% of FFM).
3. The person measured differs from the reference body only in fat content (reference body assumed to possess 73.8% water, 19.4% protein, and 6.8% mineral).

The following equation, derived by Berkeley physicist Dr. William Siri, computes percentage body fat from whole-body density:

Siri Equation

$$\text{Percentage body fat} = 495 \div \text{Body density} - 450$$

Based on the previous three assumptions, the following example incorporates the body density value of 1.0417 g·cm⁻³ (determined for the woman in the previous example) in the **Siri equation** to estimate percentage body fat:

$$\begin{aligned}
\text{Percentage body fat} &= 495 \div \text{Body density} - 450 \\
&= 495 \div 1.0417 - 450 \\
&= 25.2\%
\end{aligned}$$

The mass of body fat can be calculated by multiplying body mass by percentage fat:

$$\begin{aligned}
\text{Fat mass (kg)} &= \text{Body mass (kg)} \times (\text{Percentage fat} \div 100) \\
&= 50 \text{ kg} \times 0.252 \\
&= 12.6 \text{ kg}
\end{aligned}$$

Subtracting mass of fat from body mass yields FFM:

$$\begin{aligned}
\text{FFM (kg)} &= \text{Body mass (kg)} - \text{Fat mass (kg)} \\
&= 50 \text{ kg} - 12.6 \text{ kg} \\
&= 37.4 \text{ kg}
\end{aligned}$$

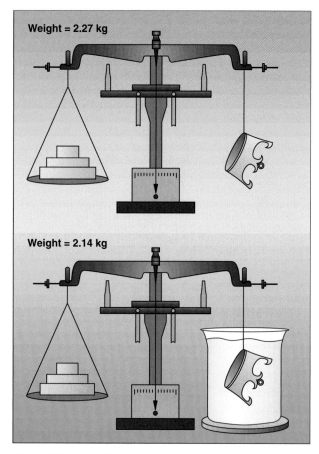

Weight = 2.27 kg

Weight = 2.14 kg

Figure 16.6. Archimedes' principle for determining the volume and specific gravity of the king's crown.

In this example, 25.2% or 12.6 kg of the 50-kg body mass consists of fat, with the remaining 37.4 kg representing the FFM component.

Limitations and Errors in Hydrostatic Weighing   The generalized density values for fat-free tissue (1.10 g·cm^{-3}) and fat tissue (0.90 g·cm^{-3}) represent average values for young and middle-aged adults. These constants vary among individuals and groups, particularly the density and chemical composition of the FFM. This variation impacts the accuracy of predicting percentage body fat from whole-body density. For example, African Americans and Hispanics have larger FFM densities than Whites (1.113 g·cm^{-3} for African Americans, 1.105 g·cm^{-3} for Hispanics, and 1.100 g·cm^{-3} for Whites). Consequently, using the existing density-to-fat equations (based on assumptions for Whites) to calculate body composition for African Americans or Hispanics *overestimates* FFM and *underestimates* percentage body fat. The following modification of the Siri equation computes percentage body fat from body density for African Americans:

Modification for African Americans

Percentage body fat = 437.4 ÷ Body density − 392.8

Applying constant density values for the various tissues for children (who are growing) or for aging adults also introduces errors in determining body composition from whole-body density values. For example, the water and mineral contents of the FFM continually change during the growth period, and demineralization from osteoporosis occurs with aging. Lower bone density makes density of the fat-free tissues of young children and the elderly lower than the assumed constant of 1.10 g·cm^{-3}, thus overestimating percentage body fat. For this reason, many researchers do not convert body density to percentage body fat in children and aging adults. Others apply a multicompartment model to adjust for such factors in computing percentage body fat from body density in prepubertal children. **Table 16.2** presents equations adjusted to maturation level to determine body fat percentage from whole-body density of boys and girls ages 7 to 17 years.

Table 16.3 presents density estimates of FFM for different adult male and female population subgroups and equations to predict percentage body fat from whole-body density based on assumptions regarding the densities and proportions of the body's protein, mineral, and water content. Obviously, different equations to convert body density to percentage body fat yield different values, depending on their underlying assumptions. This variation does not reflect an inherent error in the underwater weighing method; rather, careful use of hydrostatic weighing to assess body volume generates a technical error for this variable of less than 1%.

Body Volume Measurement   **Figure 16.7** illustrates three examples of body volume measurements by hydrostatic weighing. First the subject's body mass in air is assessed, usually to the nearest ±50 g. A diver's belt secured around the waist prevents less dense (more fat) subjects from floating to the surface during submersion. Seated with the head out of water, the subject then makes a forced maximal exhalation while lowering the head beneath the water. The breath is held for several seconds while the underwater weight is recorded. The subject repeats this procedure 8 to 12 times to obtain a dependable or "true" underwater weight score. Even when achieving a full exhalation, a small volume of air, the **residual lung volume (RLV)**, remains in the lungs. The calculation of body volume requires subtraction of the buoyant effect of the residual lung volume, measured immediately before, during, or after the underwater weighing.

Questions & Notes

Write the Siri equation for estimating percentage body fat.

What is the difference between density and specific gravity?

Compute the percentage body fat for a person with a body density of 1.0399 g·mL^{-1}.

Calculate the pounds of fat in a person who weighs 150 lbs with 15% body fat.

FOR YOUR INFORMATION

Residual Lung Volume Affects Computed Body Density
Not accounting for residual lung volume causes the computed body density value to decrease because the lungs' air volume contributes to buoyancy (lighter underwater weight) without affecting body mass. A lower body density makes a person "fatter" when converting body density to percentage body fat.

Table 16·2	Percentage Body Fat Estimated From Body Density (Db) Using Age- and Gender-Specific Conversion Constants to Account for Changes in the Density of the Fat-Free Body Mass as a Child Matures	
AGE (YEARS)	**BOYS**	**GIRLS**
7–9	%Fat = (5.38/Db − 4.97) × 100	%Fat = (5.43/Db − 5.03) × 100
9–11	%Fat = (5.30/Db − 4.86) × 100	%Fat = (5.35/Db − 4.95) × 100
11–13	%Fat = (5.23/Db − 4.81) × 100	%Fat = (5.25/Db − 4.84) × 100
13–15	%Fat = (5.08/Db − 4.64) × 100	%Fat = (5.12/Db − 4.69) × 100
15–17	%Fat = (5.03/Db − 4.59) × 100	%Fat = (5.07/Db − 4.64) × 100

From: Lohman T. Applicability of body composition techniques and constants for children and youth. *Exer Sports Sci Rev* 1986; 14:325.

Table 16·3	Equations to Predict Percentage Body Fat From Body Density (Db) Based on Different Estimates of the Fat-Free Body Density (FFDb)	
AGE, y	**EQUATION**	**FFDb[a]**
Male		
White		
7–12	%fat = 5.08/Db − 4.89	1.084
13–16	%fat = 5.07/Db − 4.64	1.094
17–19	%fat = 4.99/Db − 4.55	1.098
20–80	%fat = 4.95/Db − 4.50	1.100
African American		
18–22	%fat = 4.37/Db − 3.93	1.113
Japanese		
18–48	%fat = 4.97/Db − 4.52	1.099
61–78	%fat = 4.87/Db − 4.41	1.105
Female		
White		
7–12	%fat = 5.35/Db − 4.95	1.082
13–16	%fat = 5.10/Db − 4.66	1.093
17–19	%fat = 5.05/Db − 4.62	1.095
20–80	%fat = 5.01/Db − 4.57	1.097
Native American		
18–60	%fat = 4.81/Db − 4.34	1.108
African American		
24–79	%fat = 4.85/Db − 4.39	1.106
Hispanic		
20–40	%fat = 4.87/Db − 4.41	1.105
Japanese		
18–48	%fat = 4.76/Db − 4.28	1.111
61–78	%fat = 4.95/Db − 4.50	1.100
Anorexic		
15–30	%fat = 5.26/Db − 4.83	1.087
Obese		
17–62	%fat = 5.00/Db − 4.56	1.098

Equations from the research literature.
[a] Each estimate of the fat-free body density (FFDb) uses slightly different values for the proportions of the body's protein, mineral, and water content.

A Word About Residual Volume   The greatest source of error in calculating body volume by hydrostatic weighing results from errors in measuring RLV. Its measurement requires specialized equipment and trained personnel. In situations that do not demand research-level accuracy (general screening, teaching laboratories), RLV predictions based on age, stature, body mass, or vital capacity provide an appropriate estimate (see Close Up on page 572).

Body Volume Measurement by Air Displacement Techniques other than hydrodensitometry can measure body volume. **Figure 16.8** illustrates the **BOD POD**, a plethysmographic device to assess body volume. Essentially, body volume equals the chamber's reduced air volume when the subject enters the chamber. The subject sits in a structure comprised of two chambers, each of known volume. A molded fiberglass seat forms a common wall separating the front (test) and rear (reference) chambers. A volume-perturbing element (a moving diaphragm) connects the two chambers. Changes in pressure between the two chambers oscillate the diaphragm, which directly reflects any change in chamber volume. The subject makes several breaths into an air circuit to assess thoracic gas volume (which when subtracted from measured body volume yields true body volume). Body density computes as body mass (measured in air) ÷ body volume (measured by BOD POD). The Siri equation converts body density to percentage body fat.

Skinfold Measurements

Simple anthropometric procedures successfully predict body fatness. The most common of these procedures uses **skinfolds**. The rationale for using skinfolds to estimate the body's fat composition results from the close relationships among three factors: (1) fat in adipose tissue deposits directly beneath the skin (**subcutaneous fat**), (2) the body's internal fat stores, and (3) body density of the intact human body.

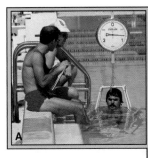

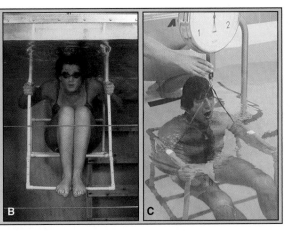

Figure 16.7. Measuring body volume by underwater weighing. (A) In a swimming pool. (B) In a stainless steel pool with plexiglas front in the laboratory. (C) Seated in a therapy pool.

Figure 16.8. **Top**, BOD POD for measuring total body volume by air displacement. **Bottom**, Diagrammatic representation of the major system components of the air displacement chamber. Photo courtesy of Life Sciences Instruments, Concord, CA.

Questions & Notes

Compute the percentage fat for a Hispanic female with a body density of 1.0417 g·mL^{-1}.

Compute the percentage fat for an African American male with a body density of 1.0611 g·mL^{-1}.

Compute the percentage fat for a 15-year-old boy with a body density of 1.0444 g·mL^{-1}.

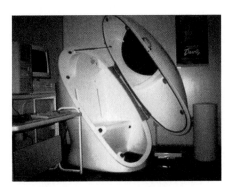

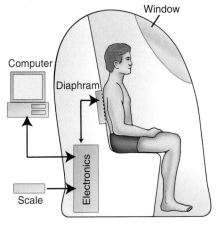

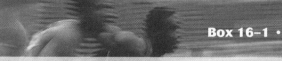

Box 16–1 • CLOSE UP

PREDICTING RESIDUAL LUNG VOLUME

Hydrostatic weighing represents a valid and reliable laboratory technique to assess body composition. The procedure accurately assesses body volume in the course of determining whole-body density (body mass ÷ body volume). Body volume equals the difference between body mass measured in air minus body weight measured underwater (subtracting residual lung volume [RLV] and air in the GI tract) and corrected for water density at the weighing temperature. The small volume of air trapped in the GI tract (<100 mL) can be disregarded. In contrast, RLV represents a large and variable gas volume that must be subtracted to accurately determine body volume.

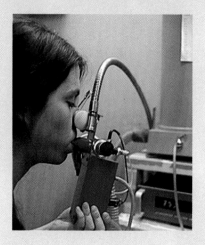

Laboratory techniques of helium dilution, nitrogen washout, or oxygen dilution routinely measure RLV. Each procedure requires complicated and expensive laboratory equipment. An alternate, although less valid, approach estimates RLV with gender-specific prediction equations based on age, stature, and body mass. The standard error of estimate to predict RLV ranges between ±325 to 500 mL; this can correspond to errors in predicting percentage body fat of up to ±2.5% or more body fat units.

RLV PREDICTION EQUATIONS

Variables: age, y; stature (St), cm; body mass (BM), kg
Normal-weight males:

$$\text{RLV, L} = (0.022 \times \text{Age}) + (0.0198 \times \text{St}) - (0.015 \times \text{BM}) - 1.54$$

Normal-weight females (uses only age and stature):

$$\text{RLV, L} = (0.007 \times \text{Age}) + (0.0268 \times \text{St}) - 3.42$$

Overfat males (%fat ≥ 25) and females (%fat ≥ 30):

$$\text{RLV, L} = (0.0167 \times \text{Age}) + (0.0130 \times \text{BM}) + (0.0185 \times \text{St}) - 3.3413$$

EXAMPLES

1. Male: age, 21 y; body mass; 80 kg (176.4 lb); stature, 182.9 cm (72 in)

$$\begin{aligned}\text{RLV (L)} &= (0.022 \times 21) + (0.0198 \times 182.9) \\ &\quad - (0.015 \times 80) - 1.54 \\ &= 0.462 + 3.621 - 1.2 - 1.54 \\ &= 1.34 \text{ L}\end{aligned}$$

2. Female: age, 19 y; stature, 160.0 cm (63 in)

$$\begin{aligned}\text{RLV (L)} &= (0.007 \times 19) + (0.0268 \times 160.0) \\ &\quad - 3.42 \\ &= 0.133 + 4.288 - 3.42 \\ &= 1.00 \text{ L}\end{aligned}$$

3. Overfat male: age, 35 y; body mass, 104 kg (229.3 lb); stature, 179.5 cm (70.7 in)

$$\begin{aligned}\text{RLV (L)} &= (0.0167 \times 35) + (0.0130 \times 104) \\ &\quad + (0.0185 \times 179.5) - 3.3413 \\ &= 0.5845 + 1.352 + 3.321 - 3.3413 \\ &= 1.39 \text{ L}\end{aligned}$$

REFERENCES

Grimby, G., and Söderholm, B.: Spirometric studies in normal subjects. III: Static lung volumes and maximum ventilatory ventilation in adults with a note on physical fitness. *Acta. Med. Scand.,* 2:199, 1963.

Miller, W.C.T., et al.: Derivation of prediction equations for RV in overweight men and women. *Med. Sci. Sports Exerc.,* 30:322, 1998.

The Caliper   By 1930, a special pincer-type caliper accurately measured subcutaneous fat at selected body sites. The **skinfold caliper (Fig. 16.9)** works on the same principle as a micrometer to measure the distance between two points. The pincer jaws exert a constant tension of 10 g·mm^{-2} at the point of contact with the double layer of skin plus subcutaneous tissue. The caliper dial indicates skinfold thickness in millimeters.

Figure 16.9 shows three different types of skinfold calipers. Compared with the most costly calipers (Harpenden and Lange), the less expensive models are less precise, exert nonconstant jaw tension throughout the range of measurement, usually have a smaller measurement scale (<60 mm), and produce less consistent scores at the same skinfold site when used by inexperienced testers.

Measuring skinfold thickness requires grasping a fold of skin and subcutaneous fat firmly with the thumb and forefingers and pulling it away from the underlying muscle tissue following the skinfold's natural contour. The skinfold is recorded within 2 seconds after applying the full force of the caliper. This time limitation avoids skinfold compression (see Close Up, *When Should Skinfold Readings Be Taken?*, page 574). For research purposes, the investigator should have considerable experience in taking measurements and demonstrate consistency in duplicating skinfold values at multiple sites for the same subject made on the same day, consecutive days, or even weeks apart. A good rule of thumb to achieve consistency requires taking duplicate or triplicate practice measurements at all skinfold sites on approximately 50 individuals who range in body fat from "thin" to "obese." Careful attention to details usually ensures greater measurement reproducibility.

Questions & Notes

Compute the residual lung volume for a 22-year-old male with a body mass of 79 kg and a stature of 73 inches.

Compute the residual lung volume for a 22-year-old female with a stature of 62 inches.

List one advantage of using the BOD POD compared to skinfolds.

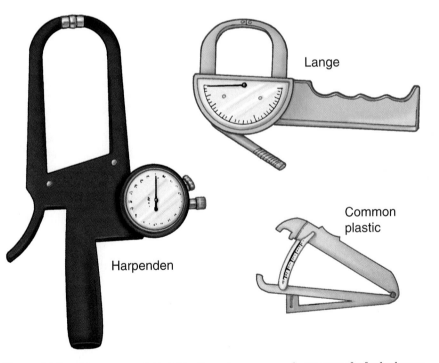

Lange

Common plastic

Harpenden

Figure 16.9.   Three types of skinfold calipers to measure subcutaneous fat for body composition assessment.

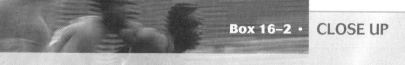

Box 16-2 • CLOSE UP

WHEN SHOULD SKINFOLD READINGS BE TAKEN?

A frequently asked question about taking skinfold measurements concerns when to read the caliper value. Should you leave the caliper on the site for 1, 3, or 5 seconds, or until the pointer stops moving?

Research-quality skinfold calipers exert an average compression force of 10 g per mm^2 at all jaw openings. This means that the caliper always exerts the same pressure regardless of skin-plus-fat thickness. Once applied to the skinfold site, the caliper continues to displace subcutaneous interstitial water, connective tissue, and fat throughout the measurement period until the skinfold's rebound force counteracts the caliper pressure.

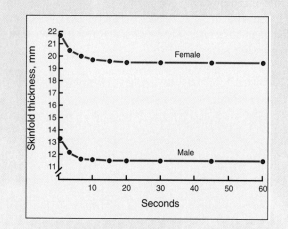

The inset shows the compression data for triceps skinfold for 18 males and 18 females. Modification of the caliper provided for an instantaneous record of skinfold thickness throughout the measurement period. More than 70% of the total compression of skin and underlying fat takes place within the first 4 seconds after applying the caliper. Thus, to record the uncompressed skin-plus-fat measurement, the reading should be made when applying the caliper to the skin (as it exerts its full pressure) and certainly within 1 or 2 seconds. Any prolonged delay in reading the caliper *underestimates* the actual skinfold value.

The absolute change in skinfold thickness among subjects over 60 seconds ranged between 0.3 mm and 4.5 mm. Although not a dramatic absolute change, this error can affect the accuracy of percentage body fat when using skinfold prediction equations. For example, using the initial uncompressed versus the final compressed skinfold value (after 60 s) produced differences in predicted percentage body fat that ranged between 2 and 8 fat percentage units (a 10% to 50% error). This large error cannot be ignored. Almost all of the research studies using skinfolds have not specified when they recorded their readings. One can only surmise that it occurred immediately after placing the calipers on the skin to obtain an uncompressed value.

REFERENCE

Becque, D.M., et al.: Time course of skin-plus-fat compression in males and females. *Hum. Biol.*, 58:33, 1986.

Skinfold Sites The most common skinfold sites include the triceps, subscapular, suprailiac, abdominal, and upper thigh. An average of two or three measurements at each site on the right side of the body with the subject standing represents the skinfold score. **Figure 16.10** shows the anatomic location for five of the most frequently measured skinfold sites:

1. **Triceps:** Vertical fold at the posterior midline of the upper arm, halfway between the tip of the shoulder and tip of the elbow; elbow remains in an extended, relaxed position.
2. **Subscapular:** Oblique fold just below the bottom tip of the scapula.

3. **Suprailiac (iliac crest):** Slightly oblique fold just above the hip bone (crest of ileum); the fold follows the natural diagonal line.
4. **Abdomen:** Vertical fold 1 inch to the right of the umbilicus.
5. **Thigh:** Vertical fold at the midline of the thigh, two-thirds of the distance from the middle of the patella (knee cap) to the hip.

Other sites include:

6. **Chest (males):** Diagonal fold (with its long axis directed towards the nipple) on the anterior axillary fold as high as possible.
7. **Biceps:** Vertical fold at the posterior midline of the upper arm.

Using Skinfold Data   Skinfolds can provide meaningful information about body fat and its distribution. There are two ways to use skinfolds:

1. Sum the individual skinfold values (Σskf). This "sum of skinfolds" indicates relative fatness among individuals; it also reflects absolute or percentage changes in fatness before and after physical conditioning or diet regimen.
2. Apply mathematical equations to predict body density or percentage body fat from the individual skinfold values or the Σskf. These equations apply to specific populations because they predict fatness fairly accurately for subjects similar in age, gender, training state, fatness, and race to those used to derive the equations.

In young adults, approximately one-half of the body's total fat consists of subcutaneous fat, with the remainder visceral and organ fat. With advancing age, a proportionately greater quantity of fat deposits internally compared with subcu-

How long after taking a skinfold should you wait before you read the caliper dial?

List the 7 most common skinfold sites.

  1.

  2.

  3.

  4.

  5

  6.

  7.

List one way to apply skinfold scores (besides using an equation) to assess body composition.

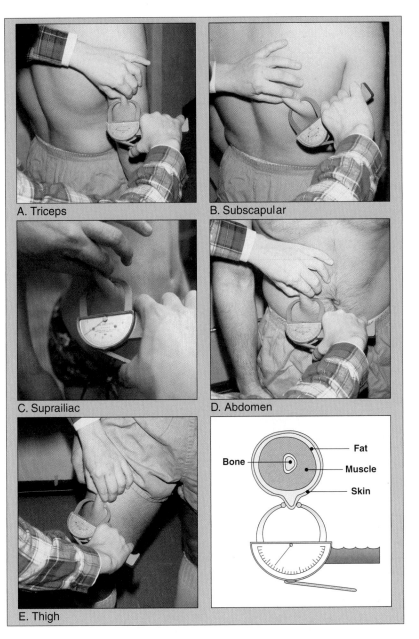

A. Triceps
B. Subscapular
C. Suprailiac
D. Abdomen
E. Thigh

Bone — Fat
Muscle
Skin

Figure 16.10.   Anatomic location of five common skinfold sites: (**A**) Triceps. (**B**) Subscapular. (**C**) Suprailiac. (**D**) Abdomen. (**E**) Thigh. Except for the subscapular and suprailiac sites, which are measured diagonally, measurements are taken in the vertical plane. The lower right schematic shows a skinfold caliper and the compression of a double layer of skin and underlying tissue during the measurement.

Box 16–3 • CLOSE UP

CHOOSING APPROPRIATE SKINFOLD EQUATIONS TO PREDICT BODY FAT IN DIVERSE POPULATIONS

More than 100 different equations exist to predict body density and percentage body fat from skinfolds. The equations, often formulated from homogeneous groups, incorporate between two and seven measurement sites to predict body density, which then converts to percentage body fat using an appropriate equation for the specific population. The different equations yield predicted values that (at best) usually fall within ±3% to 5% body fat units assessed by hydrostatic weighing.

DIFFERENT EQUATIONS

The table presents examples of skinfold equations for different populations. The following abbreviations apply (all skinfolds in mm): Skf = skinfolds; Σ = sum; tri = tricep; calf = calf; scap = subscapular; midax = midaxillary; iliac = suprailiac; abdo = abdomen; thigh = thigh; Db = body density, $g \cdot cm^{-3}$; BF = body fat; age in years (y).

Equations to Predict Percentage Body Fat From Skinfolds

POPULATION	AGE, y	VARIABLES	EQUATION	COMMENTS
Children				
Boys	6–10	tri + calf	%BF = 0.735 (Σ2Skf) + 1.0	
		tri + scap	%BF = 0.783 (Σ2Skf) + 1.6	Use when ΣSkf > 35 mm
Girls	6–10	tri + calf	%BF = 0.610 (Σ2Skf) + 5.1	
		tri + scap	%BF = 0.546 (Σ2Skf) + 9.7	Use when ΣSkf > 35 mm
Native Americans				
Women	18–60	tri + midax + iliac	Db = 1.061 − 0.000385 (Σ3Skf) − 0.000204 (age)	%BF = [(4.81 ÷ Db) − 4.34]100
African Americans				
Women	18–55	chest + abdo + thigh + tri + scap + iliac + midax	Db = 1.0970 − 0.00046971 (Σ7Skf) + 0.00000056(Σ7Skf)² − 0.00012828 (age)	%BF = [(4.85 ÷ Db) − 4.39]100
Men	8–61	chest + abdo + thigh + tri + scap + iliac + midax	Db = 1.1120 − 0.00043499 (Σ7Skf) + 0.00000055(Σ7Skf)² − 0.00028826 (age)	%BF = [(4.37 ÷ Db) − 3.93]100
Hispanics				
Women	20–40	chest + abdo + thigh + tri + scap + iliac + midax	Db = 1.10970 − 0.00046971 (Σ7Skf) + 0.00000056(Σ7Skf)² − 0.00012828 (age)	%BF = [(4.87 ÷ Db) − 4.41]100
Native Japanese				
Women	18–23	tri + scap	Db = 1.0897 − 0.00133 (Σ2Skf)	%BF = [(4.76 ÷ Db) − 4.28]100
Men	18–27	tri + scap	Db = 1.0913 − 0.00116 (Σ2Skf)	%BF = [(4.97 ÷ Db) − 4.52]100
White Americans				
Women	18–55	tri + iliac + thigh	Db = 1.0994921 − 0.0009929 (Σ3Skf) + 0.0000023 (Σ3Skf)² − 0.0001392 (age)	%BF = [(5.01 ÷ Db) − 4.57]100
Men	18–55	chest + abdo + thigh	Db = 1.109380 − 0.0008267 (Σ3Skf) + 0.0000016 (Σ3Skf)² − 0.0002574 (age)	%BF = [(4.95 ÷ Db) − 4.50]100
Athletes (all sports)				
Men	18–29	tri + iliac + abdo + thigh	Db = 1.112 − 0.00043499 (Σ7Skf) + 0.00000055 (Σ7Skf)² − 0.00028826 (age)	%BF = [(5.01 ÷ Db) − 4.57]100
Women	18–29	chest + midax + tri + scap + abdo + iliac + thigh	Db = 1.096095 − 0.0006952 (Σ4Skf) + 0.0000011 (Σ4Skf)² − 0.0000714 (age)	%BF = [(4.95 ÷ Db) − 4.50]100

taneous fat. Thus, the same skinfold score reflects a *greater* percentage body fat as a person grows older. *For this reason, use age-adjusted, generalized equations to predict body fat from skinfolds that apply to a broad age range of adult men and women* (see Close Up, *Choosing Appropriate Skinfold Equations to Predict Body Fat in Diverse Populations* on page 576). We recommend both options (sum of skinfolds and specific equations) as a best alternative to more accurately estimate the body's amount and distribution of fat.

A person can become a skilled skinfold technician by adhering to the following guidelines:

1. Take great care in locating (and marking) anatomical landmarks for each site prior to measurement.
2. Read the caliper dial to the nearest one-half marking (e.g., 0.5 mm).
3. Take a minimum of two measurements at each site, and use the average in subsequent calculations.
4. Take duplicate (or triplicate) measurements in rotational order rather than consecutive readings at each site to avoid a compression effect.
5. Do not take measurements immediately after exercise; the shift in body fluid to the skin spuriously increases the reading.
6. Practice on at least 50 subjects making multiple measurements at the different skinfold sites to gain experience.
7. Obtain training from skilled technicians in how to take skinfolds; this will allow you to compare your results with an "expert."
8. Take measurements on dry, lotion-free skin.
9. If possible, enroll in a course that deals with body composition assessment; some continuing education providers offer such a course that awards a certification of completion in body composition assessment procedures (*http://www.sportsnutritionsociety.org/site/bccissn.php*).

Girth Measurements

Figure 16.11 shows the six most common sites for girth measurements. Girths offer an easily administered and valid alternative to skinfolds. Apply a linen or plastic measuring tape lightly to the skin surface so the tape remains taut but not tight. This avoids skin compression. Take duplicate measurements at each site and average the scores. The six most common girth sites with their specific anatomic landmarks are listed below:

A. **Right upper arm (biceps):** Palm up, arm straight, and extended in front of the body; taken at the midpoint between shoulder and elbow
B. **Right forearm:** Maximum girth with arm extended in front of the body with palm up
C. **Abdomen:** 1 inch above the umbilicus
D. **Hips (buttocks):** Maximum protrusion with heels together
E. **Right thigh:** Upper thigh just below the buttocks
F. **Right calf:** Widest girth midway between ankle and knee

Usefulness of Girth Measurements The equations and constants presented in Appendix F for young and older men and women predict an individual's percentage body fat within $\pm 2.5\%$ to $\pm 4.0\%$ body fat units of the actual value, provided the individual's physical characteristics resemble the original validation group. Relatively small prediction errors make population-specific girth equations useful to those without access to laboratory facilities. These equations should not be used to predict fatness in individuals who appear excessively thin or fat or who participate regularly in strenuous sports or resistance training that can increase girth without altering subcutaneous fat. Girths also can analyze patterns of body fat distribution (**fat patterning**), including changes in fat distribution during weight loss and gain.

Questions & Notes

List the 3 most important guidelines that one should follow to become a skilled skinfold technician.

1.

2.

3.

List the 6 most common girth measurement sites.

1.

2.

3.

4.

5.

6.

Predict percentage body fat for a 10-year-old female with a tricep skinfold of 20 mm and a subscapular skinfold of 18 mm.

Compute percentage body fat for an athletic female with a body density of 1.04225 g·mL⁻¹.

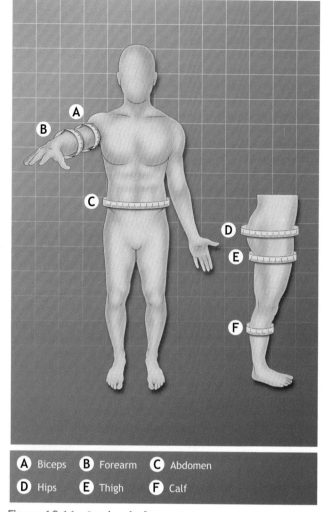

| **A** Biceps | **B** Forearm | **C** Abdomen |
| **D** Hips | **E** Thigh | **F** Calf |

Figure 16.11   Landmarks for measuring various girths at six common anatomical sites (see text for description).

Step 3. Compute percent body fat by substituting the appropriate constants in the formula for young men shown at the bottom of Chart 1 in Appendix F as:

$$\textbf{Percentage fat} = \textbf{Constant A} + \textbf{Constant B} - \textbf{Constant C} - 10.2$$

$$= 42.56 + 40.68 - 58.37 - 10.2$$

$$= 83.24 - 58.37 - 10.2$$

$$= 24.87 - 10.2$$

$$= 14.7\%$$

Step 4. Calculate the mass of body fat as:

$$\textbf{Fat mass} = \textbf{Body mass} \times (\% \textbf{ fat} \div 100)$$

$$= 79.1 \text{ kg} \times (14.7 \div 100)$$

$$= 79.1 \text{ kg} \times 0.147$$

$$= 11.6 \text{ kg}$$

Step 5. Determine FFM as:

$$\textbf{FFM} = \textbf{Body mass} - \textbf{Fat mass}$$

$$= 79.1 \text{ kg} - 11.63 \text{ kg}$$

$$= 67.5 \text{ kg}$$

Bioelectrical Impedance Analysis

A small, alternating current flowing between two electrodes passes more rapidly through hydrated fat-free body tissues and extracellular water compared with fat or bone tissue because of the greater electrolyte content (lower electrical resistance) of the fat-free component. Consequently, impedance to electric current flow relates to the quantity of total body water, which in turn relates to FFM, body density, and percentage body fat.

Bioelectrical Impedance Analysis (BIA) requires measurement by trained personnel under strictly standardized conditions, particularly for electrode placement and subject's body position, hydration status, previous food and beverage intake, skin temperature, and recent physical activity. The person lies on a flat, nonconducting surface. Injector (source) electrodes attach on the dorsal surfaces of the foot and wrist, and detector (sink) electrodes attach between the radius and ulna (styloid process) and at the ankle between the medial and lateral malleoli (**Fig. 16.12**).

The person receives a painless, localized electrical current with impedance (resistance) to current flow be-

Predicting Body Fat from Girths   From the appropriate tables in Appendix F, substitute the corresponding constants A, B, and C in the formula shown at the bottom of each table. This requires one addition and two subtraction steps. The following five-step example shows how to compute percentage fat, fat mass, and FFM for a 21-year-old man who weighs 79.1 kg:

Step 1. Measure the upper arm, abdomen, and right forearm girths with a cloth tape to the nearest 0.25 in (0.6 cm): upper arm = 11.5 in (29.21 cm); abdomen = 31.0 in (78.74 cm); right forearm = 10.75 in (27.30 cm).

Step 2. Determine the three constants A, B, and C corresponding to the three girths from Appendix F: Constant A corresponding to 11.5 in = 42.56; Constant B corresponding to 31.0 in = 40.68; and Constant C corresponding to 10.75 in = 58.37.

tween the source and detector electrodes determined. Conversion of the impedance value to body density—adding body mass and stature, gender, age, and
sometimes race, level of fatness, and several girths to the equation—computes
percentage body fat from the Siri equation or other similar density conversion
equation.

Hydration level affects BIA accuracy. Either hypohydration or hyperhydration
alters the body's normal electrolyte concentrations; this modifies current flow independent of a real change in body composition. For example, impedance decreases from body water loss through sweating in prior exercise or voluntary fluid
restriction. This produces a lower percentage body fat estimate, whereas hyperhydration produces the opposite effect (higher fat estimate).

Skin temperature (influenced by ambient conditions) also affects whole-body
resistance and, thus, the BIA prediction of body fat. A lower predicted body fat occurs in a warm environment (less impedance to electrical flow) compared with a
cold environment.

Even under normal hydration and environmental temperature, body fat predictions may be questionable compared with hydrostatic weighing. BIA tends to
overpredict body fat in lean and athletic subjects and underpredict fat in the
obese. BIA may be no more accurate than anthropometric methods that use girths
and skinfolds to predict body fat. Also, conflicting evidence exists whether BIA
can detect small changes in body composition during weight loss.

Questions & Notes

*Does the electrical current used in the
BIA technique put the subject at risk?*

List 2 factors that can affect BIA results.

1.

2.

*Of the 3 prediction methods—girths,
skinfold, and BIA—which one appears
most accurate and easiest to use?*

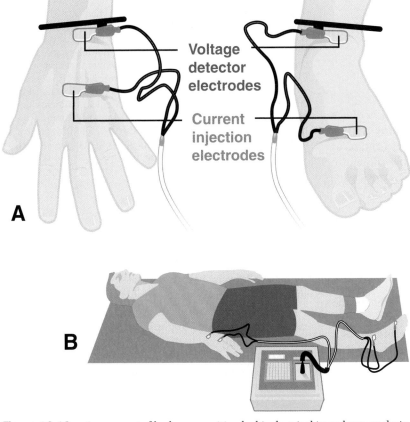

Figure 16.12.   Assessment of body composition by bioelectrical impedance analysis. (**A**)
Standard placement of electrodes. (**B**) Proper body position.

Dual-Energy X-Ray Absorptiometry

Dual-energy x-ray absorptiometry (DXA), a high-technology procedure routinely used to assess bone mineral density in osteoporosis screening, permits quantification of fat and muscle around bony areas of the body, including regions without bone present. When used for body composition assessment, DXA does not require assumptions about the biologic constancy of the fat and fat-free components, as does hydrostatic weighing.

Two distinct x-ray energies (short exposure with low-radiation dosage) penetrate into bone and soft tissue areas to a depth of about 30 cm. Specialized computer software reconstructs an image of the underlying tissues. The computer-generated report quantifies bone mineral content, total fat mass, and FFM. Selected body regions also can be targeted for more in-depth analysis (**Fig. 16.13**).

Body Mass Index

Clinicians and researchers frequently use the **body mass index (BMI)**, derived from body mass related to stature, to assess the "normalcy" of one's body weight.

$$BMI = Body\ mass,\ kg \div Stature,\ m^2$$

Example:
Male: Stature = 175.3 cm, 1.753 m (69 in); body mass = 97.1 kg (214.1 lb)

$$BMI = 97.1\ kg \div (1.753\ m \times 1.753\ m)$$
$$= 97.1 \div 3.073$$
$$= 31.6$$

The importance of this easy-to-obtain index is its curvilinear relationship to all-cause mortality; as BMI becomes larger, risk increases for cardiovascular complications (including hypertension), diabetes, certain cancers and renal disease (**Fig. 16.14**). The level of disease risk along the bottom of Figure 16.4 represents the degree of risk with each 5-unit change in BMI. The lowest health risk category occurs for BMIs in the range of 20 to 25, with the highest risk for BMIs exceeding 40. For women, 21.3 to 22.1 represents the desirable BMI range; the corresponding range for men equals 21.9 to 22.4. An increased disease incidence occurs when BMI exceeds 27.8 for men and 27.3 for women.

Based on classifications established in June, 1998 by the 24-member expert panel convened by the National Heart, Lung and Blood Institute, "**overweight**" is classified as a BMI of 25 to 29.9, and "**obesity**" is classified as a BMI ≥ 30 (see Part 3).

Limitations of BMI for Athletes

As with height-weight tables, BMI does not consider the body's proportional composition. Specifically, factors other than excess body fat (bone and muscle mass, and even the increased plasma volume induced by exercise training) affect the

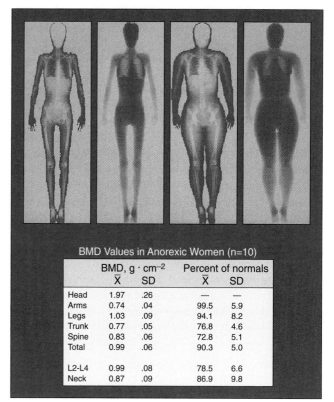

BMD Values in Anorexic Women (n=10)

	BMD, g · cm⁻²		Percent of normals	
	X̄	SD	X̄	SD
Head	1.97	.26	—	—
Arms	0.74	.04	99.5	5.9
Legs	1.03	.09	94.1	8.2
Trunk	0.77	.05	76.8	4.6
Spine	0.83	.06	72.8	5.1
Total	0.99	.06	90.3	5.0
L2-L4	0.99	.08	78.5	6.6
Neck	0.87	.09	86.9	9.8

Figure 16.13. Dual-energy X-ray absorptiometry (DXA). Example of an anorexic female (two left images) and a typical female (two right images) whose body fat percentage averages 25% of her total body mass of 56.7 kg (125 lb). The average anorexic subject weighed 44.4 kg (97.9 lb) with DXA-estimated 7.5% body fat from the fat percentages at the arms, legs, and trunk regions. The values in the right column of the inset table present the average percentage values for bone mineral density (BMD) for different regional body areas in the anorexic group compared with a group of 287 normal females aged 20 to 40 years. (Photo courtesy of R.B. Mazess, Department of Medical Physics, University of Wisconsin, Madison, WI, and the Lunar Radiation Corporation, Madison, WI. Data from Mazess, R.B., et al.: Skeletal and body composition effects of anorexia nervosa. Paper presented at the international Symposium on In Vivo Body Composition Studies, June 20–23, Toronto, Ontario, Canada, 1989.)

numerator of the BMI equation. A high BMI could lead to an incorrect interpretation of overweightness in lean individuals with excessive muscle mass, when in fact, genetic makeup or exercise training could cause elevated BMI.

The possibility of misclassifying someone as overweight using BMI standards applies particularly to large-size, field-event athletes, bodybuilders, weightlifters, upper-weight class wrestlers, and professional football players. For example, the BMI for seven defensive linemen from a former NFL Super Bowl team averaged 31.9 (team BMI averaged 28.7), clearly signaling these professional athletes as overweight and placing them in the moderate category for mortality risk. However, their body fat content, 18.0% for lineman and 12.1% for the team, misclassified them for fatness using BMI as the overweight standard.

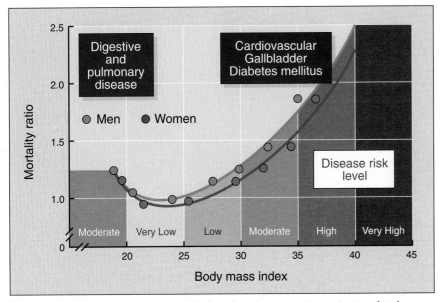

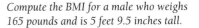

Compute your BMI.

Compute the BMI for a male who weighs 165 pounds and is 5 feet 9.5 inches tall.

Figure 16.14. Curvilinear relationship based on American Cancer Society data between all-cause mortality and body mass index (BMI). At extremely low BMIs, the risk for digestive and pulmonary diseases increases, while cardiovascular, gallbladder, and type 2 diabetes risk increases with higher BMIs. (Modified from Bray, G.A.: Pathophysiology of obesity. *Am. J. Clin. Nutr.*, 55:488S, 1992).

Classify the body weight of a person with a BMI of 32.

In contrast to the professional football players, the average player in the National Basketball Association for the 1993–1994 season had a BMI of only 24.5. This relatively low BMI places them at low risk and keeps them out of the overweight category, although they would be classified as overweight by height-weight standards.

At what BMI does mortality risk due to cardiovascular disease begin to rise?

OTHER INDIRECT PROCEDURES TO ESTIMATE BODY COMPOSITION

Near-Infrared Interactance

Near-infrared interactance (NIR) applies technology developed by the U.S. Department of Agriculture to assess body composition of livestock and the lipid content of various grains. The commercial versions to assess body composition in humans use a safe, portable, lightweight monitor, require minimal training, and necessitate little physical contact with the subject during measurement. These test administration aspects make NIR popular for body composition assessment in health clubs, hospitals, and weight-loss centers. Unfortunately, research with humans has not confirmed NIR's validity compared to hydrostatic weighing and skinfold measurements. NIR does not accurately predict body fat across a broad range of body fat levels; NIR provides less accuracy than skinfolds. It overestimates body fat in lean men and women and underestimates it in fatter subjects.

In terms of body composition analysis, what does ultrasound measure?

Predict percentage fat for a 29-year-old white female who is 5 feet 4 inches tall and has a BMI of 30.

Ultrasound

Ultrasound technology can (1) assess the thickness of different tissues (fat and muscle), and (2) obtain an image of the deeper tissues such as a muscle's cross-sectional area. The method converts electrical energy through a probe into high-frequency (pulsed) sound waves that penetrate the skin surface into the underlying tissues. The sound waves pass through adipose tissue and penetrate the muscle layer. They then reflect from the fat–muscle interface (after reflection from a bony surface) to produce an echo, which returns to a receiver within the

Box 16–4 • CLOSE UP

PREDICTING PERCENTAGE BODY FAT FROM BODY MASS INDEX

Many clinicians now view a BMI in excess of 25 to represent overweight and a BMI in excess of 30 to represent the obese state. A lower healthy BMI limit of 18.5 has also been recognized. The basic assumption underlying BMI guidelines lies in its supposed close association with body fatness and consequent morbidity and mortality. This measure exhibits a somewhat higher yet still moderate association with body fat and disease risk than estimates based simply on stature and body mass. Several formulae predict percentage body fat (%BF) from BMI and provide a better indication of health risk than BMI alone.

INDEPENDENT VARIABLES

The following independent variables predict %BF:

1. BMI
2. Age – years
3. Sex – male, female
4. Race – White, African American, Asian

Calculate BMI

Use the following formula to calculate body mass index (BMI) using metric or nonmetric data.

Metric data

$$\text{BMI (kg·m}^{-2}) = \text{body mass (kg)} \div \text{stature (m)} \times \text{stature (m)}$$

Nonmetric data

$$\text{BMI (lb·in}^{-2}) = \text{body weight (lb)} \times 703 \div \text{height (in)} \times \text{height (in)}$$

EQUATION TO PREDICT PERCENTAGE BODY FAT

$$\%BF = 63.7 - 864 \times (1 \div BMI) - 12.1 \times sex + 0.12 \times age + 129 \times Asian \times (1 \div BMI) - 0.091 \times Asian \times age - 0.030 \times African\ American \times age$$

where sex = 1 for male and 0 for female; Asian = 1 and 0 for other races; African American = 1 and 0 for other races; age in years; BMI = body weight in kg ÷ stature^2 in m^2.

EXAMPLES

Example #1: African American Male; Age = 30 y; BMI = 25

$$\%BF = 63.7 - [864 \times (1 \div BMI)]$$
$$- (12.1 \times sex) + (0.12 \times age)$$
$$+ [129 \times Asian \times (1 \div BMI)]$$
$$- (0.091 \times Asian \times age)$$
$$- (0.030 \times African\ American \times age)$$
$$= 63.7 - (864 \times 0.04) - (12.1 \times 1)$$
$$+ (0.12 \times 30) + (129 \times 0 \times 0.04)$$
$$- (0.091 \times 0 \times 30)$$
$$- (0.030 \times 1 \times 30)$$
$$= 63.7 - (34.56) - (12.1) + (3.6)$$
$$+ (0) - (0) - (0.9)$$
$$= 19.7\%$$

Example #2: Asian Female; Age = 50 y; BMI = 30

$$\%BF = 63.7 - [864 \times (1 \div BMI)]$$
$$- (12.1 \times sex) + (0.12 \times age)$$
$$+ [129 \times Asian \times (1 \div BMI)]$$
$$- (0.091 \times Asian \times age)$$
$$- (0.030 \times African\ American \times age)$$
$$= 63.7 - (864 \times 0.0333) - (12.1 \times 0)$$
$$+ (0.12 \times 50) + (129 \times 1 \times 0.0333)$$
$$- (0.091 \times 1 \times 50)$$
$$- (0.030 \times 0 \times 50)$$
$$= 63.7 - (28.80) - (0) + (6.0)$$
$$+ (4.295) - (4.55) - (0)$$
$$= 40.7\%$$

Example #3: Asian Male; Age = 70 y; BMI = 28

$$\%BF = 63.7 - [864 \times (1 \div BMI)]$$
$$- (12.1 \times sex) + (0.12 \times age)$$
$$+ [129 \times Asian \times (1 \div BMI)]$$
$$- (0.091 \times Asian \times age)$$
$$- (0.030 \times African\ American \times age)$$

Box 16–4 • CLOSE UP *(Continued)*

$$= 63.7 - (864 \times 0.03571) - (12.1 \times 1)$$
$$+ (0.12 \times 70) + (129 \times 1 \times 0.03571)$$
$$- (0.091 \times 1 \times 70)$$
$$- (0.030 \times 0 \times 70)$$
$$= 63.7 - (30.853) - (12.1) + (8.4)$$
$$+ (4.61) - (6.37) - (0)$$
$$= 25.4\%$$

Example #4: White Male; Age = 55 y; BMI = 24.5

$$\%BF = 63.7 - [864 \times (1 \div BMI)]$$
$$- (12.1 \times sex) + (0.12 \times age)$$
$$+ [129 \times Asian \times (1 \div BMI)]$$
$$- (0.091 \times Asian \times age)$$
$$- (0.030 \times African\ American \times age)$$
$$= 63.7 - (864 \times 0.0408) - (12.1 \times 1)$$
$$+ (0.12 \times 55) + (129 \times 0 \times 0.0408)$$
$$- (0.091 \times 0 \times 55)$$
$$- (0.030 \times 0 \times 55)$$

$$= 63.7 - (35.25) - (12.1) + (6.6)$$
$$+ (0) - (0) - (0)$$
$$= 22.9\%$$

ACCURACY

The correlation between predicted %BF (using the above formulae) and measured %BF (using a 4-compartment model to estimate body fat) is r = 0.89 with a standard error for estimating an individual's %BF equal to ±3.9% body fat units. This compares favorably with other prediction methods that use skinfolds and girths.

PREDICTED PERCENTAGE FAT AT GIVEN CRITICAL BMI VALUES

The table presents predicted %BF values for different threshold BMI values for males and females of different ethnicity. These data provide a research-based approach for developing healthy percentage body fat ranges from guidelines based on BMI.

Table 1 Predicted Percentage Body Fat by Sex and Ethnicity Related to BMI Healthy Weight Guidelines

	FEMALES			MALES		
AGE AND BMI	AFRICAN AMERICANS	ASIANS	WHITE	AFRICAN AMERICANS	ASIANS	WHITE
20-39 y						
BMI <18.5	20%	25%	21%	8%	13%	8%
BMI ≥25	32%	35%	33%	20%	23%	21%
BMI ≥30	38%	40%	39%	26%	28%	26%
40-59 y						
BMI <18.5	21%	25%	23%	23%	13%	11%
BMI ≥25	34%	36%	35%	35%	24%	23%
BMI ≥30	39%	41%	42%	41%	29%	29%
60-79 y						
BMI <18.5	23%	26%	25%	11%	14%	13%
BMI ≥25	35%	36%	38%	23%	24%	25%
BMI ≥30	41%	41%	43%	29%	29%	31%

REFERENCE

Gallagher, D., et al.: Healthy percentage body fat ranges: An approach for developing guidelines based on body mass index. *Am. J. Clin. Nutr.*, 72:694, 2000.

probe. The time required for sound wave transmission through the tissues and back to the transducer converts to a distance score to indicate fat or muscle thickness. Ultrasound exhibits high reliability for repeat measurements of subcutaneous fat thickness at multiple sites in the lying and standing positions on the same day and different days. The technique has application for determining total and segmental subcutaneous adipose tissue volume. Ultrasound to map muscle and fat thickness at different body regions can quantify changes in the topographic fat pattern and serve as a valuable adjunct to whole-body composition assessment. In hospitalized patients, ultrasonic fat and muscle thickness determinations aid in nutritional assessment during weight loss and gain.

Computed Tomography and Magnetic Resonance Imaging

Computed Tomography   Computed tomography (CT) generates detailed cross-sectional, two-dimensional radiographic images of different body segments when an x-ray beam (ionizing radiation) passes through tissues of different densities. The CT scan produces pictorial and quantitative information about total tissue area, total fat and muscle area, and thickness and volume of tissues within an organ.

Figure 16.15, A and B, shows CT scans of the upper legs and a cross section at the midthigh of a professional walker who walked 11,200 miles through the 50 United States in 50 weeks. Total cross section and muscle cross section increased and subcutaneous fat decreased correspondingly in the midthigh region in the "after" scans (not shown). CT scans have established the relationship between simple anthropometric measures (skinfolds and girths) at the abdomen and total adipose tissue volume measured from single or multiple pictorial "slices" through this region. The single cut through the L4–L5 region minimizes radiation dose and provides the best view of visceral and subcutaneous fat.

Magnetic Resonance Imaging   Magnetic resonance imaging (MRI) offers a valuable, noninvasive assessment of the body's tissue compartments. Figure 16.16 shows a color-enhanced MRI transaxial image of the midthigh of a 30-year-old male middle-distance runner. Computer software subtracts fat and bony tissues (lighter-colored areas) to compute thigh muscle cross-sectional area (red area). With MRI, electromagnetic radiation (not ionizing radiation as in CT scans) in a strong magnetic field excites the hydrogen nuclei of the body's water and lipid molecules. The nuclei then project a detectable signal that rearranges under computer control to visually represent the various body tissues. MRI effectively quantifies total and subcutaneous adipose tissue in individuals with varying degrees of body fatness.

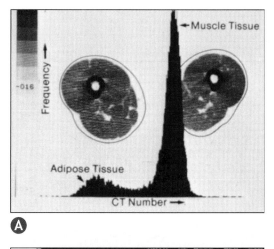

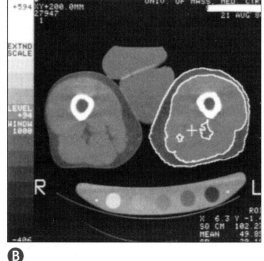

Figure 16.15.   CT scans. (A) Plot of pixel elements illustrating the extent of adipose and muscle tissue in a cross section of the thigh. (B) A cross section of the midthigh (CT scans courtesy of Dr. Steven Heymsfeld, Obesity Research Center, St. Luke's-Roosevelt Hospital, Columbia University, College of Physicians and Surgeons, New York, NY.)

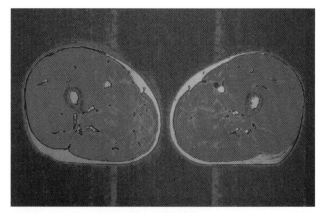

Figure 16.16.   MRI scans of the midthigh of a 30-year-old male middle-distance runner. (MRI scans courtesy of J. Staab, Department of the Army, USARIEM, Natick, MA.)

AVERAGE VALUES FOR BODY COMPOSITION

Table 16.4 presents average values for percentage body fat in men and women from different areas of the United States. The column headed "68% Variation Limits" indicates the range for percentage body fat that includes ±1 standard deviation, or about 68 of every 100 persons measured. As an example, the average percentage body fat of 15.0% for young men from the New York sample includes the ±68% variation limits from 8.9% to 21.1% body fat. Interpreting this statistically, for 68 of every 100 young men measured, percentage fat ranges between 8.9% and 21.1%. Of the remaining 32 young men, 16 would possess more than 21.1% body fat, whereas the 16 other men would have a body fat percentage of less than 8.9%. *Percentage body fat for young adult men averages between 12% and 15%; the average fat value for women falls between 25% and 28%.*

DETERMINING GOAL BODY WEIGHT

No one really knows the optimum body fat or body weight for a particular individual. Inherited genetic factors greatly influence body fat distribution and play an important role in programming of body size as the individual ages. Values for percentage body fat for young adults average approximately 15% for men and 25% for women. Women and men who exercise regularly or train for athletic

FOR YOUR INFORMATION

A Desirable Range for Goal Body Weight

For practical purposes, recommend a "desirable body weight range" rather than a single goal weight. This range should lie within 2 pounds of the computed "goal body weight." For example, if goal body weight equals 135 pounds, the person should strive for a weight between 133 and 137 pounds.

Table 16·4	Average Percentage Body Fat for Younger and Older Women and Men From Selected Studies				
STUDY	AGE RANGE, y	STATURE, cm	BODY MASS, kg	% FAT	68% VARIATION LIMITS
Younger Women					
North Carolina, 1962	17–25	165.0	55.5	22.9	17.5–28.5
New York, 1962	16–30	167.5	59.0	28.7	24.6–32.9
California, 1968	19–23	165.9	58.4	21.9	17.0–26.9
California, 1970	17–29	164.9	58.6	25.5	21.0–30.1
Air Force, 1972	17–22	164.1	55.8	28.7	22.3–35.3
New York, 1973	17–26	160.4	59.0	26.2	23.4–33.3
North Carolina, 1975		166.1	57.5	24.6	—
Army recruits, 1986	17–25	162.0	58.6	28.4	23.9–32.9
Massachusetts, 1994	17–30	165.3	57.7	21.8	16.7–27.8
Older Women					
Minnesota, 1953	31–45	163.3	60.7	28.9	25.1–32.8
	43–68	160.0	60.9	34.2	28.0–40.5
New York, 1963	30–40	164.9	59.6	28.6	22.1–35.3
	40–50	163.1	56.4	34.4	29.5–39.5
North Carolina, 1975	33–50	—	—	29.7	23.1–36.5
Massachusetts, 1993	31–50	165.2	58.9	25.2	19.2–31.2
Younger Men					
Minnesota, 1951	17–26	177.8	69.1	11.8	5.9–11.8
Colorado, 1956	17–25	172.4	68.3	13.5	8.2–18.8
Indiana, 1966	18–23	180.1	75.5	12.6	8.7–16.5
California, 1968	16–31	175.7	74.1	15.2	6.3–24.2
New York, 1973	17–26	176.4	71.4	15.0	8.9–21.1
Texas, 1977	18–24	179.9	74.6	13.4	7.4–19.4
Army recruits, 1986	17–25	174.7	70.5	15.6	10.0–21.2
Massachusetts, 1994	17–30	178.2	76.3	12.9	7.8–18.9
Older Men					
Indiana, 1966	24–38	179.0	76.6	17.8	11.3–24.3
	40–48	177.0	80.5	22.3	16.3–28.3
North Carolina, 1976	27–50	—	—	23.7	17.9–30.1
Texas, 1977	27–59	180.0	85.3	27.1	23.7–30.5
Massachusetts, 1993	31–50	177.1	77.5	19.9	13.2–26.5

competition typically have lower body fat levels than age-matched sedentary counterparts. In contact sports and activities requiring muscular power, successful performance usually requires a large body mass with average to low body fat. In contrast, weight-bearing endurance activities require a lighter body mass and a minimal level of body fat.

Proper assessment of body composition, not body weight, should determine an individual's ideal body weight. Compute a "goal" body weight target that uses a desired (and prudent) percentage of body fat as follows:

Goal body weight = Fat-free body mass
$$\div (1.00 - \% \text{ fat desired})$$

Suppose a 23-year-old, 120-kg (265 lb) male power athlete, currently with 24% body fat, wants to know how much fat weight to lose to attain a body fat composition of 15% (average value for young males). The following computations provide this information:

Fat mass = Body mass, kg × Decimal % body fat
$$= 120 \text{ kg} \times 0.24$$
$$= 28.8 \text{ kg}$$

Fat-free body mass = Body mass, kg − Fat mass, kg
$$= 120 \text{ kg} - 28.8 \text{ kg}$$
$$= 91.2 \text{ kg}$$

Goal body weight = Fat-free body mass, kg $\div$ (1.00 − Decimal % fat desired)
$$= 91.2 \text{ kg} \div (1.00 - 0.15)$$
$$= 91.2 \text{ kg} \div 0.85$$
$$= 107.3 \text{ kg (236.6 lb)}$$

Desirable fat loss = Present body weight, kg − Goal body weight, kg
$$= 120 \text{ kg} - 107.3 \text{ k}$$
$$= 12.7 \text{ kg (28.0 lb)}$$

If this person lost 12.7 kg of body fat, his new body mass of 91.2 kg would have a fat content equal to 15% of body mass. These calculations assume no change in FFM during weight loss. Moderate caloric restriction plus increased daily energy expenditure reduces body fat (and conserves lean tissue). Part 4 of this chapter discusses prudent yet effective approaches to reducing body fat.

SUMMARY

1. Two approaches directly assess body composition. In one technique, a chemical solution literally dissolves the body into its fat and nonfat (fat-free) components. The other approach involves physical dissection of fat, fat-free adipose tissue, muscle, and bone.

2. Hydrostatic weighing determines body volume (body density) with subsequent estimation of percentage body fat. The computation assumes a constant density for the body's components of fat and fat-free tissues. Subtracting fat mass from body mass yields fat-free body mass (FFM).

3. Part of the error inherent in predicting body fat from whole-body density lies in the assumptions concerning the densities of the body's fat and fat-free components. These densities, principally FFM, differ from assumed constants because of race, age, and athletic experience.

4. An air displacement method (BOD POD) offers an alternative means to quantify body composition because of ease of administration and high reproducibility of body volume scores and generally high validity compared with hydrostatic weighing.

5. Common field methods to assess body composition use prediction equations from relationships among selected skinfolds and girths and body density and percentage body fat. These equations show population specificity because they predict most accurately with subjects similar to those who participated in the equations' original derivation.

6. Body mass index (BMI) relates more closely to body fat and health risk than simply body mass and stature. As with height-weight tables, BMI does not consider the body's proportional composition.

7. The concept of bioelectrical impedance analysis states that hydrated, fat-free body tissues and extracellular water facilitate electrical flow better compared with fat tissue because of the greater electrolyte content of the

fat-free component. Impedance to electric current flow relates directly to the body's fat content.

8. Near-infrared interactance should be used with caution when assessing body composition; this methodology currently lacks verification of adequate validity.

9. Ultrasound, CT, MRI, and DXA indirectly assess body composition. Each has a unique application and special limitations for expanding knowledge of the compositional components of the live human body.

10. Based on data from healthy young adults, the average male has 15% body fat and the average female possesses 25%. These values can serve as a yardstick to evaluate deviations from "average" for the body fat of individual athletes and specific athletic groups.

11. Goal body weight computes as fat-free body mass ÷ 1.00 − desired %fat.

12. Topflight male and female endurance runners represent the lower end of the fat-to-lean continuum.

THOUGHT QUESTIONS

1. How would you use anthropometric data to estimate optimal body composition?

2. Discuss whether the established differences in body composition between men and women justify using gender-specific normative standards for evaluating diverse components of physical fitness and motor performance.

3. A friend complains that three fitness centers determined her percentage body fat from skinfolds as 21%, 25%, and 31%. How can you reconcile these discrepancies?

PART 3 •
Overfatness and Obesity

Questions & Notes

Compute the desired body weight for a 24-year-old female who weighs 75 kg with a body fat percentage of 32.

In our modern scientific era, in which molecular geneticists routinely unravel intimate secrets of subcellular function, researchers cannot yet provide an answer to a seemingly simple question: "Why have so many people become so fat, and what can be done to ameliorate the problem?" A random-digit telephone survey of nearly 110,000 adults in the United States found that nearly 70% struggle to lose weight or just maintain body weight. Fifty-eight percent of Americans would like to lose weight, 36% are following a particular diet plan, yet less than 19% of those following such plans closely track their intake of fats, carbohydrates, proteins, and calories. Only one-fifth of the 45 to 50 million Americans trying to lose weight use the recommended combination of eating fewer calories and engaging in at least 150 minutes of weekly leisure-time physical activity. Those attempting to lose weight spend nearly $40 billion annually on weight-reduction products and services, often using potentially harmful dietary practices and drugs while ignoring sensible weight-loss programs. Approximately 2 million Americans pay more than $125 million on appetite-suppressing, over-the-counter diet pills that line drugstore, health food, fitness center, and supermarket shelves, not to mention TV and radio direct marketing and mail order and Internet sales. Despite the upswing in attempts to lose weight, Americans are considerably more overweight than a generation ago, and the trend is for further increases in all regions of the United States.

Compute the desirable fat loss in pounds for a 22-year-old female who weighs 155 pounds with 29% body fat.

According to the latest 2004 data from the Centers for Disease Control Behavioral Risk Factor Surveillance Survey (*www.cdc.gov/nccdphp/dnpa/obesity/ trend/maps/*), Mississippi has the highest prevalence of obesity (29.5%; followed by Alabama, 28.9%; West Virginia, 27.6%; Tennessee, 27.2%) than any other state! Only six states were lower than 20% (Colorado, 16.8%; Massachusetts, 18.4%; Vermont, 18.7%; Rhode Island, 19.0%; Connecticut and Montana, 19.7%). Interestingly, two of the states with the highest adult obesity rates also have the highest adult prevalence of diabetes (West Virginia, 10.9%; Mississippi, 9.6%). The full 2005 report, "How Obesity Policies are Failing in America," from the Trust for Americans Health (*http://healthyamericans.org/reports/obesity2005/ Obesity2005Report.pdf*) provides illuminating data and trends about current State policies and strategies (including school nutrition and physical activity policies) concerned with the consequences of the United States obesity epidemic.

OVERWEIGHT, OVERFATNESS, AND OBESITY

Considerable confusion surrounds the precise meaning of the terms overweight, overfat, and obesity as applied to body composition. Each term often takes on a different meaning depending on the situation and context of use. The medical literature indicates that the term *overweight* refers to an overfat condition, despite the absence of accompanying body fat measures. Within this context, *obesity* refers to individuals at the extreme of the overfat continuum. This frame of reference delineates the body fat range by body mass index.

Research and contemporary discussion among diverse disciplines emphasizes the need to distinguish between overweight, overfat, and obesity to ensure consistency in use and interpretation. In general, weight-for-height at a given age has provided the most convenient (and easily obtained) index to infer body fat and accompanying health risks. In proper context, the *overweight* condition refers to a body weight that exceeds some average for stature, and perhaps age, usually by some standard deviation unit or percentage. The overweight condition frequently accompanies an increase in body fat, but not always (e.g., male power athletes), and may or may not coincide with the comorbidities of glucose intolerance, insulin resistance, dyslipidemia, and hypertension (e.g., physically fit overfat men and women).

When body fat measures are available, it becomes possible to more accurately place an individual's body fat level on a continuum from low to high, independent of body weight. *Overfatness* then would refer to a condition where body fat exceeds an age- and/or gender-appropriate average by a predetermined amount. In most situations, "overfatness" represents the correct term to assess individual and group body fat levels.

The term *obesity* refers to the overfat condition that accompanies a constellation of comorbidities that include one or all of the following components of the "**obese syndrome**": glucose intolerance, insulin resistance, dyslipidemia, type 2 diabetes, hypertension, elevated plasma leptin concentrations, increased visceral adipose tissue, and

increased risk of coronary heart disease and some cancers. Limited research suggests that excess body fat, not excess body weight per se, explains the relationship between above average body weight and disease risk. Such findings emphasize the importance of distinguishing the composition of excess body weight to determine an overweight person's disease risk.

Men and women may be overweight or overfat and yet do not exhibit components of the "obese syndrome." We urge caution in using the term obesity in all cases of excessive body weight. We acknowledge that the terms overweight, overfat, and obese are often used interchangeably to refer to the same condition.

OBESITY: A GLOBAL EPIDEMIC

According to the World Health Organization (WHO; July, 2004), obesity represents a complex condition with serious social and psychological dimensions that significantly impacts all age and socioeconomic groups and threatens to overwhelm both developed and developing countries. In 1995, an estimated 200 million obese adults worldwide and another 18 million children under the age of 5 years classified as overweight. In 2000, the number of clinically obese adults increased by 100 million to over 310 million. The WHO points out that the obesity epidemic does not just affect industrialized societies; in developing countries, over 115 million people suffer from obesity-related problems. The WHO posits that increased consumption of more energy-dense, nutrient-poor foods with high levels of sugar and saturated fats, combined with reduced physical activity, have led to obesity rates that have risen threefold or more since 1980 in some areas of North America, the United Kingdom, Eastern Europe, the Middle East, the Pacific Islands, Australia, and China. This makes every fourth person on the planet overfat! Viewed from this perspective, more than 1.7 billion people need to reduce excess body weight and fat.

Table 16•5	BMI Classifications of Obesity and Associated Risk of Illness	
CLASSIFICATION	**BMI**	**RISK OF ASSOCIATED IILLNESS**
Underweight	<18.5	Low
Normal range	18.5-24.9	Average
Overweight	≥25.0	
Pre-Obese	25-29.9	Increased
Obese Class I	30.0-34.9	Moderate
Obese Class II	35.0-39.9	Severe
Obese Class III	≥40.0	Very Severe

From: National Task Force on the Prevention and Treatment of Obesity. Overweight, Obesity and Health Risk. *Arch Intern Med*, 160:898, 2000.

Table 16.5 presents BMI classifications of obesity and associated illness risk. Obesity in adults is defined as a BMI ≥ 30. According to this definition, the prevalence of overweightness and obesity in adults numbers about 130 million Americans (65% of adults age 20 years or older, including 35% of college students). As of February 2006, more than 31% of the adult population classifies as obese compared with only 14.5% in 1980. Five percent of the adult population and 15% of African American women have Class III obesity (defined as BMI ≥ 40).

Researchers maintain that if this worldwide trend continues, particularly in the United States (and there is little reason to think otherwise), then 70% to 75% of the United States adult population may reach overweight or obesity status by the year 2010, with essentially the entire population becoming overweight within one to two generations.

Obesity in developing countries is now accelerating at a faster rate than in the United States, prompted mainly by changes in appetite, feeding patterns, and the global food supply. Consider the following:

- Some of the highest levels of adult obesity in the world occur in the Pacific Islands. Obesity rates range from around 2% of the adult population in highland Papua New Guinea to nearly 80% in Nauru (a small oval-shaped island in the western Pacific Ocean, 26 miles south of the equator; population, 10,000). In most Pacific Islands, obesity is well above 20% for adults and twice that for adolescents.
- China soon will become the world's biggest country in more ways than sheer population. Pursuing a new doctrine of a "well-off society," Chinese cities represent the world's largest growth market for restaurants. A new KFC, Pizza Hut, McDonald's, or Taco Bell opens almost every day, and the rates of obesity have followed: nearly one in four Chinese children are now overfat for their age.
- The majority of the Greek population, birthplace of the Olympic Games, no longer adheres to the traditional Mediterranean diet. Instead, consumption of a typical "western diet" prevails, as have the rates of obesity among the younger portion of the population. One in five children under age 5 is now considered obese; this represents 20% of this age population. But Greece is not alone; Bulgaria, Norway, the United Kingdom, Croatia, Spain, Malta, and Italy report similar percentages of obese children. The rest of Europe is not far behind, with the majority of countries reporting at least 10% or more childhood obesity.

Childhood Obesity in America

Particularly disturbing are trends of increased obesity and obesity-related diseases among young American children and adolescents. Overweight in these groups is defined as a BMI equal to or greater than (≥) the 95th percentile of the Center for Disease Control growth charts for children of the same age and gender. A BMI ≥ the 95th percentile in a young adult corresponds to an obese classification, yet the term "overweight" describes children and adolescents with a BMI ≥ the 95th percentile. Approximately 15% to 20% of American children and 12% of adolescents (up from 7.6% in 1976–1980) meet this criterion.

Excessive fatness in one's youth represents even more of an adult health risk than adult acquired overfatness. Regardless of their final body weight as adults, overweight children and adolescents exhibit a greater risk for a broad range of illnesses as adults compared with adults who were normal weight during their youth.

CAUSES OF OBESITY

Obesity frequently begins in childhood. For these children, the chances of becoming obese adults increase threefold compared with children of normal body weight. Simply stated, a child usually does not grow out of obesity. Tracking body weight through generations indicates that obese parents likely give birth to children who become overweight and whose offspring also often become overweight. This pattern continues from generation to generation.

Excessive fatness also develops slowly through adulthood, with most of the weight gain occurring between ages 25 to 44 years. In one longitudinal study, the fat content of 27 adult men increased an average of 6.5 kg over a 12-year period from age 32 to 44 years. Women gained the most weight; about 14% gained 13.6 kg (30 lb) between ages 25 and 34. The typical American man (beginning at age 30) and woman (beginning at age 27) gains between 0.2 to 0.8 kg (0.5 to 1.8 lb) of body weight each year until age 60, despite a progressive decrease in total food intake. The degree to which this creeping obesity during adulthood reflects a normal biologic pattern of aging remains unclear.

Overeating and Other Causative Factors

Human obesity results from a complex interaction of factors, including genetic, environmental, metabolic, physiologic, behavioral, social, and perhaps racial influences. Individual differences in specific factors that predispose humans to excessive weight gain include eating patterns and eating environment; food packaging, body image, and variations related to resting metabolic rate; diet-induced thermogenesis; level of spontaneous activity or "fidgeting"; basal body temperature; susceptibility to specific viral infections; levels of cellular adenosine triphosphatase, lipoprotein lipase, and other enzymes; and levels of metabolically active brown adipose tissue.

Regardless of the specific causes of obesity and their interactions, common treatment procedures—such as diets, surgery, drugs, psychological methods, and exercise, either alone or in combination—have failed miserably on a long-term basis. Nonetheless, researchers continue to devise strategies to prevent and treat this health catastrophe.

Effect of Global Changing of Dietary Patterns

Changes in diet and reduced energy expenditure via patterns of work and leisure, often referred to as the "**nutrition transition**," contribute greatly to the increase in obesity worldwide. Moreover, the pace of these changes is accelerating, especially in the low-income and middle-income countries of the world. Dietary changes that characterize the nutrition transition include quantitative and qualitative changes. The adverse changes include shifts in dietary structure towards higher energy density with greater fat and added sugars, greater saturated fat (mostly from animal sources), reduced complex carbohydrates and dietary fiber, and reduced fruit and vegetable intakes. These trends in food consumption suggest a causal link to rising obesity rates.

Food consumption, expressed in kCal per capita per day, provides a key variable for measuring and evaluating energy storage. Analysis of worldwide data show steadily increasing daily kCal per capita from the mid-1960s to the late 1990s, increasing globally by approximately 450 kCal and by over 600 kCal in developing countries (**Table 16.6**). These data, coupled with decreased energy expenditure for all populations of the world, help to explain the worldwide creeping obesity epidemic.

Fast Food and Obesity Link in Adolescents An estimated 75% of all U.S. adolescents (aged 12 to 18 years) eat fast food one or more times per week. This increase in fast-food consumption parallels the escalating obesity epidemic, raising the possibility of a causal relationship. Characteristics of fast food linked to excess energy intake and subsequent adiposity include enormous portion size, high-energy density, palatability, excessive amounts of refined starch and added sugars, high fat content, and low levels of dietary fiber. Research demonstrates that fast-food consumption directly relates to total energy intake and inversely relates to diet quality; moreover, a direct and positive association exits between fast food and body weight in adolescents (primarily overweight and obese).

Table 16·6	Global and Regional Per Capita Food Consumption (kCal per capita per day)					
REGION	**1964-1966**	**1974-1976**	**1984-1986**	**1997-1999**	**2015**	**2030**
World	2358	2435	2655	2803	2940	3050
Developing Countries	2054	2152	2450	2681	2850	2980
Near East and North Africa	2290	2591	2953	3006	3090	3170
Sub-Saharan Africa (excluding South Africa)	2058	2079	2057	2195	2360	2540
Latin America + Caribbean	2393	2546	2689	2824	2980	3140
East Asia	1957	2105	2559	2992	3060	3190
South Asia	2017	1986	2205	2403	2700	2900
Industrialized Countries	2947	3065	3206	3380	3440	3500

From: Diet, Nutrition and The Prevention of Chronic Diseases. WHO Technical Report Series #916. Report of a Joint WHO/FAO Expert Consultation. Geneva, Switzerland: World Health Organization; 2003.

A recent study sheds light on the fast food–obesity relationship. Twenty-eight lean (BMI ≤ 85th percentile for age and sex) and 26 overweight (BMI = 85-88th percentile for age and sex) adolescents were served "extra large" fast-food fare during a lunch hour at a local restaurant. Subjects were instructed to eat as much as desired, and extra portions (refills) were available on request. In a follow-up, the subjects were required to recall all food consumed and their energy expenditure on the fast-food day and one other similar but non-fast food day during the week.

When instructed to eat as much or little fast food as desired, the overweight participants consumed more than lean participants whether energy intake was expressed in absolute terms or relative to estimated needs (overweight participants consumed 1860 kCal [66.5% of their estimated total energy expenditure], whereas lean participants consumed 1458 kCal [57.0 % of their estimated total energy expenditure]). The overweight participants consumed more total energy on fast food days versus days without fast food, the lean participants consumed virtually the same total on both days. These observations suggest that overweight individuals do not compensate energy intake for the massive portion sizes characteristic of fast food, whereas lean participants adjust portion size to maintain balanced caloric intake.

Genetics Play a Role

Genetic makeup does not necessarily cause obesity, but it does lower the threshold for its development; it contributes to differences in weight gain for individuals fed identical daily caloric excess. **Figure 16.17** summarizes findings from a large number of individuals representing nine different types of backgrounds. Genetic factors determined about 25% of the transmissible variation among people

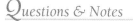
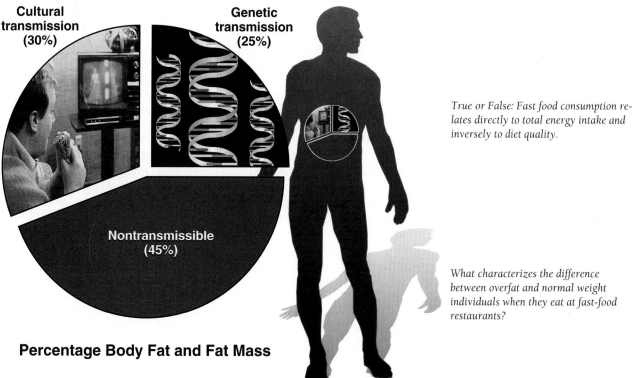

Cultural transmission (30%)

Genetic transmission (25%)

Nontransmissible (45%)

Percentage Body Fat and Fat Mass

Figure 16.17.   Total transmissible variance for body fat. Total body fat and percentage body fat determined by hydrostatic weighing. (Data from Bouchard, C., et al.: Inheritance of the amount and distribution of human body fat. *Int. J. Obes.*, 12:205, 1988.)

in percentage body fat and total fat mass, whereas the largest transmissible variation related to a cultural effect. *In an obesity-producing environment (sedentary and stressful with easy access to calorie-dense food), the genetically susceptible individual gains weight.*

A Mutant Gene? Studies of twins, adopted children, and specific segments of the population show a link between genetic factors that explain up to 80% of the risk of becoming obese. Little risk exists for an overweight toddler to grow into an obese adult if both parents are of normal weight. For a child under age 10, regardless of current body weight, with one or both obese parents (BMI ≥ 30), the child's risk of becoming an obese adult doubles compared to the general population; the risk further increases with the severity of obesity in the biologic family members. If a first-degree relative's BMI exceeds 35, the child's obesity risk increases to three times normal; a BMI of 40 corresponds to five times the risk.

Researchers now link some forms of human obesity to a mutant gene. Studies at the University of Cambridge in England identified a specific defect in two genes that control body weight. Two cousins from a Pakistani family in England inherited a defect in the gene that makes **leptin** (derived from the Greek root *leptos*, meaning thin), an important hormone in body weight regulation. Congenital absence of leptin produced continual hunger and marked obesity in these children. The second genetic defect, observed in an English patient, affected the body's response to the "signal" leptin provided. The signal largely determines how much one eats, how much energy one expends, and, ultimately, one's adult body weight.

Leptin Studies with animals provide fundamental information about the genetic link to obesity and associated diseases. For example, a strain of hybrid mice that balloon up to five times the girth of normal mice supports research in humans that some individuals appear genetically "predestined" to become overfat. The mutation of a gene called "obese," or simply "*ob*," may disrupt hormonal signals that regulate metabolism, fat storage, and appetite and may fundamentally change the brain's circuitry in areas that control appetite. These factors would tip the sensitive energy balance equation toward body fat accumulation.

The model in **Figure 16.18** proposes that the *ob* gene normally becomes activated in adipose tissue (and perhaps muscle tissue). In these tissues, it encodes and stimulates production of a body fat–signaling, hormone-like protein (ob–protein, or leptin) that enters the bloodstream. This satiety signal molecule travels to the ventromedial nucleus, the hypothalamic area that controls appetite and metabolism and develops soon after birth. Normally, leptin blunts the urge to eat when caloric intake maintains ideal fat stores. Leptin may affect certain neurons in the hypothalamus in a way to (1) stimulate production of chemicals that suppress appetite, and/or (2) reduce the levels of brain chemicals that stimulate appetite. These mechanisms would explain how body fat could remain intimately "connected" via a physiologic pathway to the brain for energy balance regulation. In a way, the adipocyte serves an endocrine-like function. With a gene defective for either adipocyte leptin production and/or hypothalamic leptin sensitivity (as probably exists in humans), the brain cannot adequately assess the body's adipose tissue status. Thus, the urge to eat remains constant. Based on studies with animals, it also appears that leptin acts during a critical period early in life to shape the brain's neural circuitry, strengthening circuits that inhibit eating and weakening ones that stimulate appetite. In essence, leptin availability, or lack thereof, not only affects the neurochemistry of appetite, but also the dynamic "wiring" of the brain to possibly affect appetite and obesity in adulthood.

The hormone–hypothalamic biologic control mechanism may explain the extreme difficulty the overfat have in sustaining fat loss. In children and adults, plasma leptin circulates in direct proportion to adipose tissue mass when energy balance remains in steady state. Four times more leptin occurs in overfat subjects than in lean subjects. Consequently, human obesity resembles a relative state of **leptin resistance**, which is similar to obesity-related insulin resistance. In fact, high blood leptin concentrations are strongly associated with the combination of upper-body obesity, glucose intolerance, hypertriglyceridemia, and hypertension. These core metabolic disturbances occur in the insulin-resistant or metabolic syndrome.

The linkage of genetic and molecular abnormalities to obesity allows researchers to view overfatness as a disease instead of a psychological flaw. Early identification of one's genetic predisposition toward obesity makes it possible to begin diet and exercise intervention before obesity sets in and fat loss becomes exceedingly difficult. Pharmaceutical companies may eventually synthesize compounds that produce satiety or affect the resting rate of fat catabolism. These chemicals would produce weight control with a smaller caloric intake and fewer feelings of hunger and deprivation that often accompany conventional diet plans.

Physical Inactivity: An Important Component in Fat Accumulation Maintaining a physically active lifestyle blunts the "normal" tendency to gain fat during adulthood. For young and middle-aged men who exercised regularly, time spent in physical activity related inversely to body fat level (the more exercise performed, the less body fat). Surprisingly, no relationship emerged between body fat and caloric intake. This suggests that less demanding activity, not greater food intake, produced the greater body fat levels observed among the active middle-aged men compared with younger, more active counterparts.

From age 3 months to 1 year, the total energy expenditure of infants who later became overweight averaged 21% less than infants with normal weight gain. Native Americans with low daily energy expenditure were at a four times greater risk of gaining more than 7.5 kg over a 2-year period than tribal members with higher energy expenditure.

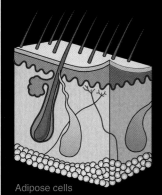

Step 1
The gene inside of the fat cell creates a hormone responsible for satiety

Adipose cells

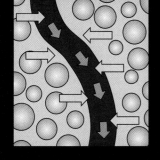

Step 2
The satiety hormone moves from the fat cells and enters the bloodstream

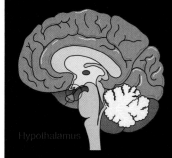

Step 3
The satiety hormone signals the hypothalamus to reduce or stop the drive to eat after the "set point" is reached for the body's total quantity of fat.

Hypothalamus

Figure 16.18. Genetic model for obesity. A malfunction of the satiety gene affects production of the satiety hormone leptin. Underproduction of leptin disrupts proper function of the hypothalamus (Step #3), the center that regulates the body's fat level. (Model based on research conducted at Rockefeller University, New York, NY).

Questions & Notes

How important are genetic factors in determining percentage body fat and total fat mass?

What is the risk for a child with one or both obese parents of becoming obese?

Describe the effect of too little leptin production.

Describe the 2 ways leptin can affect body fat levels.
  1.

  2.

True or False: Human obesity resembles a state of leptin resistance.

HEALTH RISKS OF OBESITY

In 1998, obesity joined cigarette smoking, hypertension, elevated serum cholesterol, and physical inactivity in the American Heart Association's list of primary coronary heart disease risk factors. Clear associations exist among obesity and hypertension, type 2 diabetes, and various lipid abnormalities (dyslipidemia), including increased risk of cerebrovascular disease, alterations in fatty acid metabolism, and atherosclerosis. The 10 major health consequences of obesity include:

1. Cardiovascular disease
2. Type 2 diabetes
3. Hypertension
4. Dyslipidemia
5. Ischemic stroke
6. Sleep apnea
7. Degenerative joint disease

FOR YOUR INFORMATION

Potent Heart Disease Risk
An 8-year study of nearly 116,000 female nurses concluded that all but the thinnest women showed increased risk for heart attack and chest pains. Women of average body weight had 30% more heart attacks than women of low body weight, while the risk for moderately overweight nurses averaged 80% higher than for the lightest women. Women who gained just 9 kg (20 lb) from their late teens to middle age doubled their heart attack risk.

8. Some types of cancer
9. Gallstones
10. Fertility problems

Staggering economic expenses arise from obesity-related medical complications; the costs associated with adult obesity are estimated at over $100 billion per year, or approximately 10% to 12% of the U.S. national healthcare budget. The combined effects of poor diet and physical inactivity caused about 400,000 deaths in the year 2000, or 16.6% of the total death rate. If the size of Americans continues to increase at the current rate, by 2020 one in five healthcare dollars spent on middle-aged Americans will result from obesity. Hospitalization rates among children and adolescents for common problems associated with obesity increased rapidly between 1979 and 1999, while the costs of hospitalization for obesity-related diagnoses increased threefold.

CRITERIA FOR EXCESSIVE BODY FAT: HOW FAT IS TOO FAT?

Three criteria can directly evaluate a person's body fat status:

1. Percentage body fat
2. Fat patterning
3. Fat cell size and number

Percentage Body Fat

The demarcation often becomes arbitrary between normal body fat levels and obesity. In Part 1 of this chapter, we identified the normal range of body fat in adult men and women as plus or minus one unit of variation (standard deviation) from the average population value. That variation unit equals 5% body fat for men and women between ages 17 and 50 years. Within this statistical boundary, overfatness corresponds to any percentage body fat value above the average value for age and gender, plus 5 percentage points. For young men, whose fat mass averages 15% of body mass, borderline obesity equals 20% body fat. For older men, average percentage fat approximates 25%. Consequently, a body fat content in excess of 30% represents overfatness for this group. For young women, obesity corresponds to a body fat content above 30%, whereas for older women, borderline obesity begins at 37% body fat.

Age-specific demarcations for obesity assumes that men and women normally become fatter with age. However, this does not necessarily occur for physically active older men and women. If lifestyle accounts for the greatest portion of body fat increase during adulthood, then the criterion for overfatness could justifiably represent the standard for younger men and women:

Men: >20% body fat

Women: >30% body fat

Gradations of obesity progress from the upper limit of normal to as high as 50% to 70% of body mass as fat. Common terms for gradations in obesity include pleasantly plump for those just above the cut-off and the more clinical demarcations of moderately obese, massively obese, and morbidly obese. The last category includes people who weigh in the range of 170 to 275 kg (385 to 600 lb) and whose fat content exceeds 55%. In such cases, body fat can exceed FFM.

Fat Patterning

Fat cells (adipocytes) display remarkable diversity depending on their anatomic location. Some cells efficiently "capture" excess nutrient calories from the bloodstream and synthesize them into triacylglycerols for storage. Others accumulate triacylglycerols but also readily release this stored energy to other tissues. This explains why certain fat deposits resist shrinkage while others expand readily to the body's changing energy balance. Patterning of adipose tissue distribution, independent of total body fat and body mass, alters the health risk from obesity.

Studies using MRI and CT scanning to precisely discriminate subcutaneous from visceral (intra-abdominal) adipose tissue (**VAT**) show that VAT accumulation relates to an altered metabolic profile that includes these five conditions:

1. Hyperinsulinemia
2. Insulin resistance and glucose intolerance
3. Hypertriglyceridemia
4. Reduced high-density lipoprotein (HDL) cholesterol concentrations
5. Increased apolipoprotein B, the regulatory protein constituent of the harmful low-density lipoprotein (LDL) cholesterol

The excessive insulin production and depressed insulin sensitivity that characterize VAT obesity not only increase risk for type 2 diabetes, but also increase risk for ischemic heart disease. Thus, visceral obesity constitutes an additional component of the insulin-resistant, dyslipidemic syndrome, the most prevalent cause of coronary artery disease in industrialized countries.

The importance of body fat distribution in the clinical assessment of obese patients first emerged in 1947 and has been confirmed in subsequent epidemiological studies. A preferential abdominal fat accumulation, originally described as **android obesity** (male-pattern or central obesity), exists largely among overweight patients with hypertension, type 2 diabetes, and coronary heart disease. This contrasts to the lower health risks of gynoid obesity (female-pattern or peripheral obesity), where the majority of excess fat deposits in the body's gluteal and femoral regions.

The waist-to-hip girth ratio (WHR) has provided the initial clinical assessment of VAT. In general, ratios that exceed 0.80 for women and 0.95 for men indicate excessive visceral fat accumulation. A higher ratio predicts increased risk of death from coronary artery disease and other illnesses with greater accuracy than the BMI. The accompanying Close Up, *Calculating and Interpreting the Waist-to-Hip Girth Ratio* (page 596), describes measurement procedures and health implications of this important measure.

A limitation of the waist-to-hip ratio is that it poorly captures the specific effects of each girth measure. Waist and hip circumferences reflect different aspects of body composition and fat distribution. Each has an independent and often opposite effect on cardiovascular disease risk. **Waist girth**, the so-called malignant form of obesity that reflects central fat deposition, provides a reasonable indication of the accumulation of intra-abdominal (visceral) adipose tissue. Waist girth independently complements BMI. Over a broad range of BMI values, men and women with large waist circumference values possess greater relative risk for cardiovascular disease, type 2 diabetes, cancer, and cataracts (the leading cause of blindness worldwide), than individuals with similar BMIs but with low waist circumference or with peripheral obesity. For this reason, we recommend that either WHR or waist girth be used as the "**second dimension of obesity**" (percentage body fat being the first dimension) in comprehensive assessment of body composition and health-risk profile.

Fat Cell Size and Number

The size and number of fat cells provide a view of the structure, form, and dimensions of normal and abnormal levels of body fatness. Increases in adipose tissue mass occurs in two ways:

1. Enlarging (filling) of existing fat cells with more fat: **fat cell hypertrophy**
2. Increasing the total number of fat cells: **fat cell hyperplasia**

The technique for assessing adipocyte size and number involves sucking small fragments of subcutaneous tissue, usually from the upper back, buttocks, abdomen, and back of the upper arm, into a syringe through a needle inserted directly into the fat depot (**Fig. 16.19**). Chemical treatment of the biopsy sample enables the researcher to separate and count the fat cells. Dividing the amount of fat in the sample by the total number of cells it contains determines the average quantity of fat per cell. The quantity of total body fat divided by the average fat content per cell reasonably estimates total fat cell number.

Fat Cell Size and Number in Normal and Obese Adults
The data in the left side of **Figure 16.20** illustrates the strong association between total fat mass in obese individuals and their number of fat cells. The person with the lowest body fat content had the fewest number of fat cells, while the fattest subject had considerably more adipocytes. In contrast, the data displayed in the right panel of the figure show little relationship between total body fat and average fat cell size in the obese. This suggests that a biologic upper limit exists for fat cell size. After reaching this size, cell number probably becomes the key factor that determines the extent of extreme obesity. Even doubling the size of normal fat cells would not account for the tremendous difference in the fat content between obese and nonobese people. It seems reasonable to conclude, therefore, that the excessive adipose tissue mass in severe obesity occurs by fat cell hyperplasia. As a frame of reference, an average person has about 25 to 30 billion fat cells. For the moderately obese, this number ranges between 60 and 100 billion, whereas the fat cell number for the massively obese may increase to 360 billion or more.

$\mathcal{Q}$*uestions & Notes*

List 5 major health risks of obesity.

1.

2.

3.

4.

5.

List 3 criteria to evaluate a person's body fat status.

1.

2.

3.

Give the cut-off percentage fat values for adult males and females for defining overfatness.

Males:

Females:

FOR YOUR INFORMATION

Waist Girth: The Second Dimension of Obesity
The following box represents gender-neutral guidelines for abdominal girth that corresponds to visceral adipose tissue equal to and exceeding the "risky" quantity of 130 cm.

Age	Waist Girth
< 40 years	≥ 100 cm (39.4 in)
40–60 years	≥ 90 cm (35.4 in)

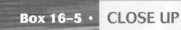

Box 16-5 • CLOSE UP

CALCULATING AND INTERPRETING THE WAIST-TO-HIP GIRTH RATIO

Waist-to-hip girth ratio (WHR) indicates relative fat distribution in adults and risk of disease (see table). A higher ratio reflects a greater proportion of abdominal fat with greater risk for hyperinsulinemia, insulin resistance, type 2 diabetes, endometrial cancer, hypercholesterolemia, hypertension, and atherosclerosis.

WHR computes as abdominal girth (cm or in) ÷ hip girth (cm or in); waist girth represents the smallest girth around the abdomen (the natural waist), and hip girth reflects the largest girth measured around the buttocks (see figure).

Waist-Hip Ratio and Disease Risk

	AGE, y	LOW	MODERATE	RISK LEVEL HIGH	VERY HIGH
Men	20–29	<0.83	0.83–0.88	0.89–0.94	>0.94
	30–39	<0.84	0.84–0.91	0.92–0.96	>0.96
	40–49	<0.88	0.88–0.95	0.96–1.00	>1.00
	50–59	<0.90	0.90–0.96	0.97–1.02	>1.02
	60–69	<0.91	0.91–0.98	0.99–1.03	>1.03
Women	20–29	<0.71	0.71–0.77	0.78–0.82	>0.82
	30–39	<0.72	0.72–0.78	0.79–0.84	>0.84
	40–49	<0.73	0.73–0.79	0.80–0.87	>0.87
	50–59	<0.74	0.74–0.81	0.82–0.88	>0.88
	60–69	<0.76	0.76–0.83	0.84–0.90	>0.90

CALCULATING WHR

Example #1

Male: age, 21 y; abdominal girth, 101.6 cm; hip girth, 93.5 cm.

WHR = abdominal girth (cm) ÷ hip girth (cm)

= 101.6 ÷ 93.5

= 1.08 (very high disease risk)

Example #2

Female: age 41 y; abdominal girth, 83.2 cm; hip girth, 101 cm.

WHR = abdomen girth (cm) ÷ hip girth (cm)

= 83.2 ÷ 101

= 0.82 (high disease risk)

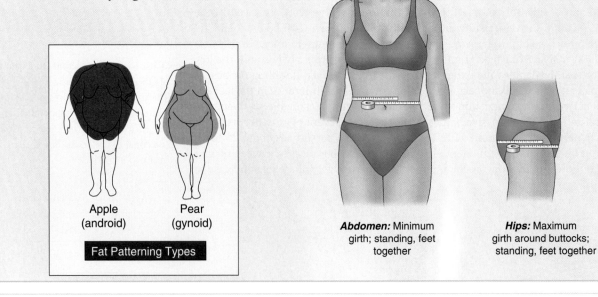

Apple (android)   Pear (gynoid)

Fat Patterning Types

Abdomen: Minimum girth; standing, feet together

Hips: Maximum girth around buttocks; standing, feet together

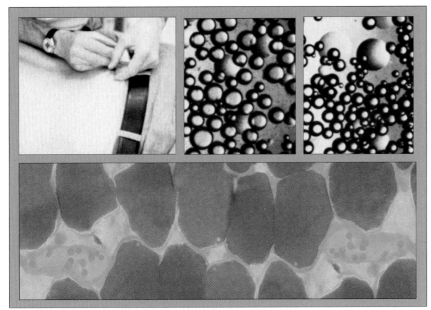

Figure 16.19.   Upper panel: Needle biopsy procedure to extract fat cells of the upper buttocks region. The area is sterilized, anesthetized, and the biopsy needle placed beneath the skin surface. The syringe sucks small tissue fragments from the site. The two photomicrographs indicate fat cells biopsied from the buttocks of a physically active professor prior to (center) and after (right) 6 months of marathon training. The average fat cell diameter averaged 8.6% smaller after training. The volume of fat in each cell decreased by 18.2%. The large spherical structures in the background represent intracellular lipid droplets. (Photomicrographs courtesy of P.M. Clarkson, Muscle Biochemistry Laboratory, University of Massachusetts, Amherst, MA.) **Lower panel:** Cross section of human fat cells magnified ×440. (From Geneser, F.: *Color Atlas of Histology*. Philadelphia: Lea & Febiger, 1985.)

List the waist:hip ratio (WHR) cut-off values that indicate excessive visceral fat accumulation for males and females.

Males:

Females:

List the waist girth cut-off values that indicate excessive visceral fat accumulation for males and females.

Males:

Females:

List the 2 ways that adipose tissue increases.

1.

2.

What evidence indicates that there may be an upper limit for fat cell size?

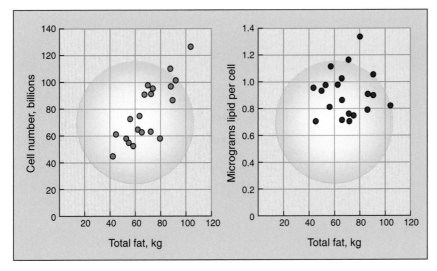

Figure 16.20.   Adipose cell number (**left**) and size (**right**) related to the body's total fat mass.

SUMMARY

1. Overfatness, defined as an excessive quantity of body fat, represents a complex disorder involving interrelated factors that tip energy balance in favor of weight gain.

2. Over the past 25 years, the average body weight of adult Americans has increased considerably. Currently, 30% of adults (59 million) classify as obese (BMI ≥ 30), and nearly 65% (130 million adults) are either overweight or obese (BMI ≥ 25).

3. Genetic factors probably account for 25% to 30% of excessive body fat accumulation. Genetic predisposition does not necessarily cause obesity, but given the right environment, the genetically susceptible individual gains body fat.

4. Fifteen to 20% of American children and 12% of adolescents (up from 7.6% in 1976–1980) classify as overweight. Excessive body fatness, childhood's most common chronic disorder, is particularly prevalent among poor and minority children.

5. Obesity represents a medical condition that includes overfatness and other conditions such as dyslipidemia, hypertension, insulin resistance, and glucose intolerance.

6. Probably no biologic reason fully accounts for the typical body fat increases observed for American men and women with aging. Therefore, body fat standards for borderline overfatness in adult men and women could justifiably be the values for younger adults: 20% body fat for men and 30% for women.

7. Adipose tissue patterning on the body provides important health-related information. Fat distributed in the abdominal-visceral region (android-type obesity) poses a greater health risk compared to fat deposited at the thigh, hips, and buttocks (gynoid-type obesity).

8. Waist girth provides a second dimension of obesity when assessing the health-risk profile. Men and women with large waist circumference possess greater relative risk for cardiovascular disease, type 2 diabetes, cancer, and cataracts than individuals with small waist circumferences.

9. Size and number of adipocytes provides another obesity classification. Before adulthood, body fat increases by (1) enlargement of individual fat cells (fat cell hypertrophy), and (2) increases in total number of fat cells (fat cell hyperplasia). Because cell size probably reaches some biologic upper limit, cell number plays the key role in determining the ultimate extent of obesity.

THOUGHT QUESTIONS

1. Discuss the possibility that body fat accumulation in children and adults does not necessarily result from excessive food intake.

2. What possible explanation(s) accounts for the rapid increase in body fat worldwide?

3. In your opinion, what are the leading causes of childhood obesity?

4. Explain if and why different body fat standards should apply to people of different ages.

PART 4 •
Achieving Optimal Body Composition Through Diet and Exercise

Describe the prognosis for successful weight loss for most people.

The following statement by University of Pennsylvania obesity specialist Dr. Albert Stunkard presents a realistic view about the possibility of long-term weight loss for the obese:

> *"Most obese persons will not stay in treatment. Of those who stay in treatment, most will not lose weight, and of those who do lose weight, most will regain it."*

This bleak outlook delivered more than three decades ago buttresses the majority of subsequent research showing that initial modifications in body weight have little relation to long-term success. Participants who remain in supervised weight-loss programs reduce about 10% of their original body weight. Unfortunately, individuals typically regain one- to two-thirds of the lost weight within 1 year and almost all of it within 5 years. **Figure 16.21** illustrates that over a 7.3-year follow-up of 121 patients, the tendency to regain lost weight occurred independent of length of fasting (up to 2 months), extent of weight loss (up to 41.4 kg), or age at overfatness onset. One-half of the subjects returned to their original weight within 3 years, and only seven patients remained at their reduced body weight. Such discouraging statistics indicate the difficulty in sustaining long-term weight loss, particularly in the relaxed atmosphere of one's own home, which often provides ready access to food and little emotional support. Although prognosis for long-term success remains poor, some individuals achieve success. These men and women frequently reduce one-third of their original weight and keep it off for a lifetime (see page 616).

Describe the relationship between fat cell number and total body fat.

THE ENERGY BALANCE EQUATION: THE KEY TO WEIGHT CONTROL

The rationale underlying the energy balance equation forms the basis for a weight-loss program. **Figure 16.22** (top) shows the ideal situation where energy input (calories in food) balances energy output (calories expended in daily physical activities) to maintain a desirable body weight. The middle part of the figure depicts what happens all too frequently when energy input exceeds energy out-

Describe the energy balance equation.

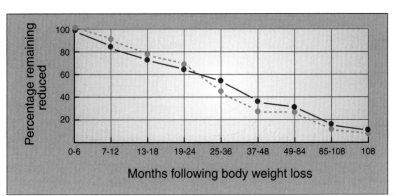

Figure 16.21. Percentage of patients remaining at reduced body weights at various time intervals following accomplished weight loss. The red line represents 60 subjects with obesity onset before age 21; green line indicates 42 subjects with obesity onset after age 21. (Data from Johnson, D., and Drenick, E.J.: Therapeutic fasting in morbid obesity. *Arch. Intern. Med.*, 137:1381, 1977.)

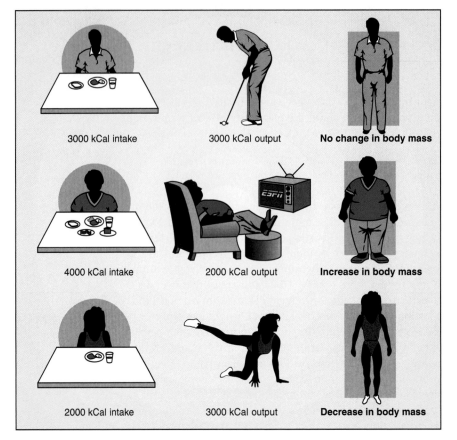

Figure 16.22.   The energy balance equation.

put. Under such conditions, calories store as fat in adipose tissue. *Approximately 3500 "extra" kCal through either increased energy intake or decreased energy output equals the energy equivalent of 1 pound (0.45 kg) of stored body fat (adipose tissue).* The bottom of the figure illustrates what occurs when energy intake falls below energy output. In this case, the body obtains required calories from its energy stores with a reduction in body weight and body fat.

There are three ways to "unbalance" the energy balance equation to cause weight loss:

1. Maintain caloric output and decrease caloric intake below daily energy requirements
2. Maintain caloric intake and increase caloric output above daily requirements through additional physical activity
3. Combine methods 1 and 2 by decreasing daily food intake and increasing daily energy expenditure

To appreciate the sensitivity of the energy balance equation for weight control, consider what happens when daily calorie intake exceeds output by only 100 kCal. This could occur by eating one extra banana daily. Annually, the "extra" number of ingested calories equals 36,500 kCal (365 days × 100 kCal). Because 0.45 kg (1 lb) of body fat contains about 3500 kCal, the small daily in-

crease in caloric intake would cause a yearly gain of 4.7 kg (10.4 lb) of body fat. If this energy imbalance continued, then theoretically fat mass would increase by 23.6 kg (52 lb) over 5 years. Reducing daily food intake by only 100 kCal and increasing energy expenditure a similar amount by walking 1 additional mile each day would reduce total body fat by 9.5 kg (21 lb) in a year!

Personal Assessment

An objective assessment of food intake and energy expenditure provides the frame of reference for unbalancing the energy balance equation to favorably modify body mass and body composition.

Energy Intake   Estimates of caloric intake from daily food intake records usually fall within ±10% of the number of calories consumed. For example, suppose the actual energy value of a person's daily food intake averaged 2130 kCal. Based on a careful 3-day dietary history to estimate caloric intake, the daily value would fall between 1920 and 2350 kCal.

Careful record keeping of food intake also provides the dieter with an objective list of foods consumed (rather than a "*guesstimate*") and triggers an important behavioral aspect of the weight control process—awareness of current food habits and preferences.

Energy Output   In addition to caloric restriction through dieting, a physically active lifestyle becomes crucial to long-term success at weight loss. This does not mean playing a token game of tennis twice a year, going for a swim on weekends during the summer, or walking to the store when the car needs repair. Modifying personal exercise habits entails a serious commitment to changing daily routines to include regular periods of moderate to vigorous physical activity. The accompanying Close Up on page 602 illustrates how to compute daily energy (kCal) requirement (including exercise) for weight maintenance and/or weight loss.

DIETING TO TIP THE ENERGY BALANCE EQUATION

Many people believe that only calories from dietary lipids increase body fat. Individuals reduce fat intake to achieve body fat loss (generally a good idea) but often disproportionately increase carbohydrate and protein intakes so total caloric intake remains unchanged or even increases. The prudent dietary approach to weight loss unbalances the energy balance equation by reducing daily energy intake 500 to 1000 kCal *below* the daily energy expenditure while consuming well-balanced meals. Compared with more severe energy restriction, which augments lean tissue loss, a moderate reduction in food intake produces a greater fat loss relative to energy deficit. *Total energy intake, not the mixture of macronutrients, determines the effectiveness of weight loss with low-energy diets.* Most people do not tolerate prolonged daily caloric restriction of more than 1000 kCal; more extreme semi-starvation also increases the likelihood for malnourishment, depletion of glycogen reserves, and loss of lean tissue.

Practical Illustration

Suppose a physically active college male who consumes 3800 kCal daily and maintains body mass at 80 kg (176 lb) wants to reduce 5 kg (11 lb). He decides to maintain his activity level but decrease food intake to create a daily caloric deficit of 1000 kCal. Thus, instead of consuming 3800 kCal, he takes in only 2800 kCal daily. In 7 days, the accumulated deficit equals 7000 kCal (1000 kCal·d^{-1} × 7 d), or the energy equivalent of 0.9 kg (2 lb) of body fat. Actually, during the first week of caloric restriction, considerably more than 0.9 kg would be lost because the body's energy deficit initially comes mainly from glycogen stores. This stored nutrient contains fewer calories per gram and more water than stored fat. For this reason, short periods of caloric restriction often encourage the dieter but result in large percentages of water and carbohydrate loss per unit weight loss with only a small decrease in body fat. As weight loss continues, the energy deficit created by food restriction requires a larger proportion of body fat breakdown. By adhering to the 2800 kCal diet, the person reduces body fat at the rate of 0.45 kg of fat every 3.5 days, provided daily energy output remains unchanged.

Results Not Always Predictable

The mathematics of weight loss through caloric restriction seems straightforward, but results do not always follow. First, one assumes that daily energy expenditure remains relatively unchanged throughout the dieting period. Some people experience lethargy (because caloric restriction depletes the body's glycogen stores), which actually decreases daily energy expenditure. Second, the energy cost of physical activity decreases in proportion to the weight lost. This also shrinks the energy output side of the energy balance equation. If weight loss indeed progressed in proportion to caloric restriction, a progressive decrease in body

Questions & Notes

One pound of stored body fat contains how many kCal of energy?

List the 3 ways to unbalance the energy balance equation.

   1.

   2.

   3.

How accurate are 3-day daily food intake records to estimate total caloric intake?

Which determines the effectiveness of weight loss with low-energy diets, total energy intake or the mixture of macronutrients consumed?

During the first week of weight loss, does the body lose more water or fat per unit of weight lost?

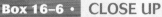

Box 16-6 • CLOSE UP

COMPUTING DAILY ENERGY (CALORIC) REQUIREMENT (INCLUDING EXERCISE) FOR WEIGHT MAINTENANCE AND/OR WEIGHT LOSS

Successful weight loss requires a negative energy balance, where total calorie (kCal) expenditure exceeds total kCal intake. Foods consumed in the diet provide the energy the body requires to carry out its metabolic functions. Total daily energy expenditure (TDEE), often referred to as the body's "energy requirement," includes:

1. Normal daily energy expenditure (includes sleeping and "normal" daily living conditions), excluding energy expenditure during physical activity.
2. Energy expenditure during physical activity (includes energy expenditure above "normal" daily living activities).

Weight maintenance occurs when kCal intake equals TDEE. Determining TDEE allows one to compute the change in food consumption necessary for weight maintenance *or* weight loss.

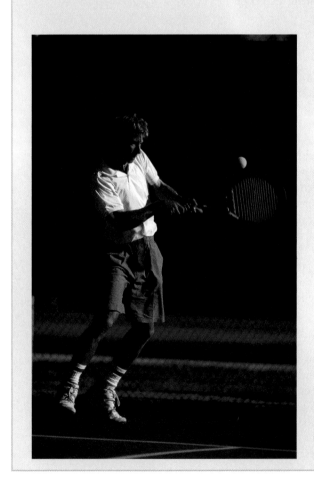

COMPUTING TOTAL DAILY ENERGY EXPENDITURE TO MAINTAIN BODY WEIGHT

Table 1 presents the computational steps to determine TDEE, including kCal expenditure of physical activity and target number of calories to achieve a given weight loss.

Example Computations

The following example illustrates the computations for a 24-year-old male who weighs 72.6 kg (160 lbs) and who participates in moderate daily physical activity. (Refer to Table 1.)

1. Record body weight (BW) . . . . .160 lb
2. Record caloric requirement per pound BW *(See Table 2)* 15.0
3. Compute daily caloric requirement without physical activity to maintain current BW *(Multiply Step #1 × Step #2)* .2400 kCal
4. Select physical activity *See Table 3 (if more than one physical activity is selected, estimate the average daily calories burned as a result of each additional activity [Steps #4 through #11] and add all of these totals to Step #12)* . . . .**jogging**
5. Record the number of exercise sessions completed weekly 4
6. Record the duration of each exercise session in minutes . . . . .60 min
7. Compute the total *weekly* exercise time in minutes *(Multiply Step #5 by Step #6)* . . . .240 min
8. Compute the average *daily* exercise time in minutes *(Divide Step #7 by 7 [round to nearest whole min])* . . . . .34 min
9. Record the caloric expenditure per pound per minute $(kCal \cdot lb^{-1} \cdot min^{-1})$ for your physical activity *(See Table 3)* 0.090
10. Compute total calories burned per minute $(kCal \cdot min^{-1})$ during physical activity *(Multiply Step #1 by Step #9)* . . . .$14.4 \ kCal \cdot min^{-1}$
11. Compute average daily calorie expenditure (kCal) during physical activity *(Multiply Step #8 by Step #10 [round to nearest whole number])* . . . . .490 kCal
12. Compute daily caloric requirement, including exercise kCal, to maintain current BW (TDEE) *(Add Step #3 plus Step #11)* . . . . .2890 kCal

Box 16–6 • CLOSE UP *(Continued)*

COMPUTATIONS OF TARGET ENERGY INTAKE REQUIRED TO REDUCE BODY WEIGHT

In the above example, the TDEE to maintain body weight equals 2890 kCal. Therefore, total kCal intake must decrease below this value to induce a negative caloric balance for weight loss. The energy deficit should never cause total daily caloric intake to fall below 1200 kCal for women and 1500 kCal for men. This level of energy intake represents a safe level to ensure adequate intake of protein, vitamins, and minerals. Prudent recommendations include subtracting 500 kCal per day if the TDEE is below 3000 kCal and 1000 kCal for daily TDEE above 3000 kCal.

To compute target number of calories for weight loss:

1. Compute number of calories to subtract from requirement to achieve a negative calorie balance *(Subtract 500 kCal if the total daily kCal expenditure [Step #12] is below 3000 kCal, 1000 kCal for daily expenditures above 3000 kCal)* . . . . **500 kCal**
2. Compute target total caloric intake to reduce weight *(Subtract Step #13 from Step #12)* . . . . **2390 kCal**

Table 1	Computation of Daily Total Caloric Requiement and Target Caloric Intake to Lose Weight

1. Record body weight (BW) . . . . ___
2. Record caloric requirement per pound BW *(See Table 2)* . . . . ___
3. Compute daily caloric requirement without physical activity to maintain current BW *(Multiply Step #1 × Step #2)* . . . . ___
4. Select physical activity *See Table 3 (if more than one physical activity is selected, estimate the average daily calories burned as a result of each additional activity [Steps #4 through #11] and add all of these totals to Step #12)* . . . . ___
5. Record the number of exercise sessions you do per week . . . . ___
6. Record the duration of each exercise session in minutes . . . . ___
7. Compute the total weekly exercise time in minutes *(Multiply Step #5 by Step #6)* . . . . ___
8. Compute the average daily exercise time in minutes *(Divide Step #7 by 7 [round to nearest whole min])* . . . . ___

9. Record the caloric expenditure per pound per minute $(kCal \cdot lb^{-1} \cdot min^{-1})$ for your physical activity *(See Table 3)* . . . . ___
10. Compute total calories burned per minute $(kCal \cdot min^{-1})$ during physical activity *(Multiply Step #1 by Step #9)* . . . . ___
11. Compute average daily calorie expenditure (kCal) during physical activity *(Add Step #3 plus Step #11)* . ___
12. Compute daily caloric requirement, including exercise kCal, to maintain current BW (TDEE) . . . . ___
13. Compute number of calories to subtract from requirement to achieve a negative calorie balance *(Subtract 500 kCal if the total daily kCal expenditure [Step #12] is below 3000 kCal, 1000 kCal for daily expenditures above 3000 kCal)* . . . . ___
14. Compute target caloric intake required to lose weight *(Subtract Step #13 from Step #12)* . . . . ___

Table 2	Average 24-h Energy Expenditure Estimated From Body Weight (lb) Based on Different Physical Activity Levels for Men and Women*

	kCal PER POUND**	
ACTIVITY LEVEL	**MALES**	**FEMALES**
Sedentary (limited) physical activity [No regular physical activity outside of work]	13.0	12.0
Moderate physical activity [Planned, systematic light to moderate physical activity 2-3 days per week, outside of work]	15.0	13.5
Strenuous physical activity [Planned, systematic heavy physical activity 4-6 days per week, outside of work]	17.0	15.0

*Pregnant or lactating women add 3.0 kCal per lb.
** For example, the 24-h energy expenditure for a sedentary male weighing 160 lbs equals 2080 kCal (13 kCal per pound × 160 lbs = 2080).

Box 16–6 • CLOSE UP (Continued)

Table 3 Sample Caloric Expenditures in kCal Per Pound of Body Weight Per Minute (kCal·lb^{-1}·min^{-1})

Activity	kCal·lb^{-1}·min^{-1}	Activity	kCal·lb^{-1}·min^{-1}	Activity	kCal·lb^{-1}·min^{-1}
Basketball	0.062	Jumping rope		Volleyball	0.023
Circuit weight training		70 jumps/min	0.075	Walking	
Nautilus	0.042	80 jumps/min	0.080	4.5 mph	0.045
Climbing hills	0.055	Racquetball	0.080	grass track	0.037
Cycling		Running		shallow pool	0.090
5.5 mph	0.032	11 min: 30 s/mile	0.062	Swimming	
10 mph	0.050	9 min/mile	0.087	crawl, slow	0.058
13 mph	0.070	8 min/mile	0.097	crawl, fast	0.071
Aerobic dance		7 min/mile	0.1085	back stroke	0.077
medium	0.047	6 min/mile	0.1231	breast stroke	0.074
intense	0.061	Skiing, soft snow, leisure	0.044	side stroke	0.056
Golf	0.038	Skiing, hard snow,		Canoeing	
Gymnastics	0.030	moderate speed	0054	leisure	0.019
				racing	0.047

REFERENCE

American College of Sports Medicine: Position statement on proper and improper weight loss programs. *Med. Sci. Sports Exerc.*, 15:9, 1993.

weight would depend solely on the extent of caloric deprivation. Metabolic changes also take place during caloric restriction, further blunting the weight loss effort.

Resting Metabolism Lowered A reduction in resting metabolism often occurs when dieting produces weight loss. The decrease in resting metabolism exceeds the decrease attributable to loss of either body mass or FFM; severe caloric restriction can depress resting metabolic rate by 45%! A blunted metabolism characterizes individuals attempting to lose weight, regardless if they dieted previously or were fat or lean. Reduced metabolism conserves energy, causing the diet to become progressively less effective despite a low caloric intake. Weight loss plateaus and further weight loss slows relative to that predicted from the mathematics of the restricted energy intake.

Figure 16.23 displays the results for body weight and resting oxygen uptake (minimal energy requirement) during 31 days of carefully monitored caloric intakes for six obese men. During the pre-diet period, body weight and resting oxygen uptake stabilized on an average daily food intake of 3500 kCal. When subjects switched to a 450 kCal low-calorie diet, body weight and resting metabolism decreased, but the percentage decline in metabolism exceeded the decrease in body weight. The dashed line represents the expected weight loss from the 450-kCal diet. The decline in resting metabolism conserved energy and caused a progressively less effective diet. More than one-half of the total weight loss occurred over the first 8 days of dieting, with the remaining weight loss during the final 16 days. The dieter often becomes frustrated and discouraged when a plateau occurs in the anticipated weight-loss curve.

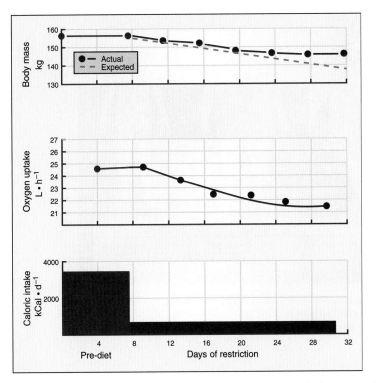

Figure 16.23.   Effects of two levels of caloric intake on changes in body mass and resting oxygen uptake. Often the failure of the actual weight loss to keep pace with predictions based on food restriction leaves the dieter frustrated and discouraged. (Adapted from Bray, G.: Effect of caloric restriction on energy expenditure in obese subjects. *Lancet*, 2:397, 1969.)

Setpoint Theory: A Case Against Dieting

One can lose large amounts of weight in a relatively short time by simply not eating, but success remains short-lived; eventually, the urge to eat wins out, and the lost weight returns. The reason for this failure may be the existence of a "*setpoint*" that differs from that desired by the dieter. The proponents of a **setpoint theory** argue that all people, fat or thin, have a well-regulated internal control mechanism or setpoint. This controller, probably located deep within the brain's lateral hypothalamus (or possibly within fat cells themselves), drives the body to preserve a particular level of body weight and/or body fat. In a practical sense, this would be the body weight one achieves if not counting calories or worrying about weight. Each time the level of body fat decreases below one's natural setpoint, internal adjustments occur (like reducing metabolic rate) to resist this change and conserve or replenish body fat. Even when a person overeats to gain weight above their normal level, resting metabolism increases to resist this change.

Fat Cell Size and Number After Weight Loss

Figure 16.24 shows the results of a classic study of weight loss effects on adipose tissue characteristics of obese adults during two stages of weight loss. Nineteen obese subjects who initially weighed 149 kg reduced body mass by 45.8 kg, weighing 103 kg at the end of the first part of the experiment. Prior to weight reduction, the number of fat cells averaged 75 billion. This number remained essentially unchanged with weight reduction. The average size of the fat cells, on the other hand, decreased by 33% from 0.9 μg to a normal value of 0.6 μg of fat

Questions & Notes

List one factor that may explain why weight loss results are not always predictable.

List the 2 factors that contribute to the total daily energy expenditure (TDEE).

1.

2.

Give the calorie expenditure per min for a 160 lb person for each of the following activities:

Intense aerobic dance –

Golf –

Running (7 min per mile pace) –

Swimming (slow crawl stroke) –

Does resting metabolism increase or decrease with dieting?

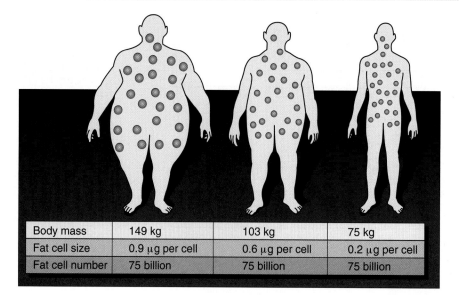

Body mass	149 kg	103 kg	75 kg
Fat cell size	0.9 µg per cell	0.6 µg per cell	0.2 µg per cell
Fat cell number	75 billion	75 billion	75 billion

Figure 16.24. Changes in adipose cellularity with weight reduction in obese subjects (Data from Hirsch, J.: Adipose cellularity in relation to human obesity. In: *Advances in Internal Medicine*, Vol. 17. Stollerman, G.H. (ed.). Chicago: Year Book, 1971.)

per cell. Subjects attained a normal body mass when they lost an additional 28 kg. Cell number again remained unchanged, while cell size continued to shrink to about one-third the size of the fat cells in normal, nonobese subjects. Other experiments have confirmed these findings in young children and adults.

The formerly obese person who reduces body mass and body fat to near average values still does not become "cured" of obesity, at least for adipocyte number. The large number of relatively small fat cells in the reduced obese may somehow relate to appetite control, and the person craves food, overeats, and regains lost weight (fat). This certainly makes sense within the framework of the body fat hormone (leptin)–satiety interaction discussed previously.

Fat cell number significantly increases during three general time periods:

1. Last trimester of pregnancy
2. First year of life
3. Adolescent growth spurt

The total number of fat cells probably cannot be altered to any significant degree during adulthood. Removing large amounts of fat by liposuction (surgically excising fat deposits at selected body sites), which has become the most popular cosmetic procedure performed over 500,000 times in 2005, does not change the person's metabolic profile (i.e., concentration of the hormone leptin, blood cholesterol, triacylglycerols, and blood pressure and insulin levels). Even removing 20 pounds of fat from the abdomen in severely obese females did not improve important risk factors for heart disease. Future research needs to determine if removal of deep visceral or storage fat gives more promising health results than liposuction, which primarily removes "pinchable" subcutaneous fat.

New Fat Cells Can Develop

In adult-onset, severe obesity, new adipocytes develop in addition to the hypertrophy of existing cells as the person becomes even fatter. This probably occurs because fat cells have an upper-size limit of about 1.0 µg of lipid per cell. In the massively obese (60% body fat; 170% of normal weight), almost all adipocytes achieve a hypertrophic limit; for the person to add fat, new cells must proliferate from a preadipocyte cell pool.

How to Select a Diet Plan

The most difficult aspect of dieting involves deciding exactly what foods to include in the daily menu. One can choose from literally hundreds of diet plans: water diets, drinker's diets, zone diets, fruit or vegetable diets, fast-food diets, eat to win diets, and diets named for cities (e.g., South Beach or Beverly Hills diets), including the potentially dangerous varieties of high-fat, low-carbohydrate, and liquid-protein diets. Some authors have even stated that total caloric intake should *not* be considered, but rather the order of eating foods. For individuals desperate to shed excess weight, such misinformation reinforces negative eating behaviors, causing another repeat cycle of failure.

Low Carbohydrate-Ketogenic Diets Ketogenic diets emphasize carbohydrate restriction while generally ignoring total calories and the diet's cholesterol and saturated fat content. Billed as a "diet revolution" and championed by the late Dr. Robert C. Atkins, the diet was first promoted in the late 1800s and has appeared in various forms since then. Long disparaged by the medical establishment, advocates maintain that restricting daily carbohydrate intake to 20 g or less for the initial 2 weeks, with some liberalization afterwards causes the body to mobilize considerable fat for energy. This generates excess plasma ketone bodies—byproducts of incomplete fat breakdown from inadequate carbohydrate catabolism—that supposedly suppress appetite. Theoretically, the ketones lost in the urine represent unused energy that should further facilitate weight loss. Some advocates claim that urinary energy loss becomes so great that dieters can eat all they want as long as they restrict carbohydrates.

The singular focus of the low-carbohydrate diet may eventually reduce caloric intake, despite claims that dieters need not consider calorie intake as long as lipid represents the excess. Initial weight loss may also result largely from dehydration caused by an extra solute load on the kidneys that increases water excretion. Water loss does not reduce body fat. Low-carbohydrate intake also sets the stage for a loss of lean tissue as the body recruits amino acids from muscle to maintain blood glucose via gluconeogenesis—an undesirable side effect for a diet designed to induce body fat loss. It remains unclear whether the ketogenic diet facilitates fat loss compared to a well-balanced, low-calorie diet rich in unrefined, fiber-rich complex carbohydrates. In general, weight loss relates principally to a diet's low caloric content and diet duration rather than reduced carbohydrate content.

Three recent controlled clinical trials compared the Atkins-type, low-carbohydrate diet with traditional low-fat diets for weight loss. The low-carbohydrate diet was more effective in achieving a modest *weight* loss for severely overweight people. Some measures of heart health also improved as reflected by a more favorable lipid profile and glycemic control in those who followed the low-carbohydrate diets for up to 1 year. Such findings add a measure of credibility to low-carbohydrate diets and challenge conventional wisdom concerning the potential dangers from consuming a high-fat diet plan. Recent research suggests that low-carbohydrate dieters lost weight faster than low-fat dieters, at least for the first months; by the end of 12 months, however, the gap in weight loss between low carbohydrate and low fat was small and not statistically significant.

Importantly, Atkins-type, high-fat, low-carbohydrate diets require systematic long-term evaluation (up to 5 years) for safety and effectiveness, particularly to the blood lipid profile. The diet, which places no limit on the amount of meat, fat, eggs, and cheese a person eats, may pose potential hazards. For example, low-carbohydrate, high-protein diets raise serum uric acid levels, potentiate the development of kidney stones, alter electrolyte concentrations to initiate cardiac arrhythmias, cause acidosis, aggravate existing kidney problems from the extra solute burden in the renal filtrate, deplete glycogen reserves to contribute to a fatigued state, decrease calcium balance and increase risk for bone loss, and cause dehydration. This diet is definitely contraindicated during pregnancy because it retards fetal development from inadequate carbohydrate intake. For high-performance endurance athletes who train mainly above 65% of maximum effort, switching to a high-fat diet is ill advised because of the body's need to maintain glucose in the bloodstream and glycogen packed in the active muscles and liver storage depots. Fatigue during high-intensity exercise that lasts for more than 60 minutes occurs more rapidly when athletes have consumed a high-fat diet compared to carbohydrate-rich meals.

In summarizing the low-carbohydrate craze, the noted M.I.T. brain/nutrition researcher Judith Wurtman stated, "It may take a long time, but 10 years from now, people are going to look back on this and say, *'Boy, were we really stupid.'*" (*NY Times*; p. 53, May 3, 2004.)

High-Protein Diets

A modification of a low-carbohydrate ketogenic diet emphasizes a large protein consumption. These diets are promoted to the obese as "last-chance diets." Earlier versions consisted of protein in liquid form adver-

Questions & Notes

Describe the setpoint theory of weight loss.

List the 3 time periods generally associated with fat cell hyperplasia.

1.

2.

3.

Describe the essence of ketogenic diets.

FOR YOUR INFORMATION

Site of Fat Removal May Affect Health Profile
In animal models, surgical removal of fat packed around internal organs (heart, kidneys, pancreas) improved insulin resistance, while fat removal from abdominal subcutaneous sites failed to improve insulin control. Despite various liposuction procedures in extreme adult obesity, fat cell proliferation still occurs. Removal of deep visceral fat may prove helpful in combating future adipose cell proliferation.

tised as "miracle liquid." Unknown to the consumer, the liquid protein mixture often contained a blend of ground-up animal hooves and horns, with pigskin mixed in a broth with enzymes and tenderizers to "predigest" it. Collagen-based blends produced from gelatin hydrolysis (supplemented with small amounts of essential amino acids) often did not contain the highest quality amino acid mixture and lacked required vitamins and minerals (particularly copper). A negative copper balance often coincides with electrocardiographic abnormalities and rapid heart rate. The diet's safety improves if it contains high-quality protein with ample carbohydrate, essential fatty acids, and micronutrients.

Some argue that extremely high protein intake suppresses appetite through reliance on fat mobilization and subsequent ketone formation. The elevated thermic effect of dietary protein, with its relatively low coefficient of digestibility (particularly for plant protein), ultimately reduces the net calories available from ingested protein compared with a well-balanced meal of equivalent caloric value. This point has some validity, but one must consider other factors when formulating a sound weight-loss program, particularly for the physically active individual. Four important considerations include a high-protein diet's potential for (1) strain on liver and kidney function and accompanying dehydration, (2) electrolyte imbalance, (3) glycogen depletion, and (4) lean-tissue loss.

Semi-Starvation Diets

A therapeutic fast, or **very low-calorie diet (VLCD)**, may benefit the obese whose body fat exceeds 40% to 50% of body mass. The diet provides between 400 and 800 kCal daily as high-quality protein foods or liquid meal replacements. Dietary prescriptions usually last for up to 3 months but only as a "last resort" before undertaking more extreme medical approaches for morbid obesity (>100 lb above ideal weight) that include various surgical treatments (collectively called **bariatric surgery**). In laparoscopic surgery, a slender, tubular instrument inserted into the abdominal cavity bands the stomach to reduce its proximal volume. Concurrently, the small intestine is often rearranged to minimize the surface for food absorption. In 2005, the number of morbidly obese patients who had the stomach-reducing surgery increased more than threefold since 2000. These procedures carry a serious risk of complications, including death.

Dieting with VLCD requires close supervision, usually in a hospital setting. Proponents maintain that severe food restriction breaks established dietary habits, which in turn, improves the long-term prospects for success. These diets also may depress appetite to aid compliance. Daily medications that accompany a VLCD include calcium carbonate for nausea, bicarbonate of soda and potassium chloride to maintain consistency of body fluids, mouthwash and sugar-free chewing gum for bad breath (from a high level of ketones from fatty acid catabolism), and bath oils for dry skin. Semi-starvation does not compose an "ul-

timate diet" or the proper approach to weight control. Because a VLCD provides inadequate carbohydrate, the glycogen-storage depots in the liver and muscles deplete rapidly. This impairs physical tasks requiring either high-intensity aerobic effort or shorter duration anaerobic power output. The continuous nitrogen loss with fasting and weight loss reflects an exacerbated lean tissue loss. This may occur disproportionately from critical organs like the heart. Finally, prolonged fasting has a poor success rate.

Table 16.7 summarizes the principles and the main advantages and disadvantages of some popular dietary approaches to weight loss.

The Well-Balanced Dietary Approach

Calories do count! Weight loss occurs on any calorie-restricted diet regardless of its composition. The "secret" of successful dieters who keep pounds off is that they skip gimmicks and focus on healthful eating and lifestyle habits they can sustain throughout life.

What comprises a healthful diet that can be maintained throughout life? Diets rich in fiber and complex carbohydrates found in fruits, vegetables, beans, and whole grains are associated with longevity, lasting weight control, reduced risk of cardiovascular disease, diabetes, gastrointestinal disorders, possibly cancer, and overall health promotion. If one maintains a caloric deficit, diet composition should not effect on the magnitude of weight loss.

EXERCISING TO TIP THE ENERGY BALANCE EQUATION

Despite debate about the precise contributions of physical inactivity and excessive caloric intake to body fat accretion, a sedentary lifestyle consistently emerges as an important factor in weight gain by children, adolescents, and adults.

Excess weight gain often parallels reduced physical activity rather than increased caloric intake. Physically active individuals who eat the most often weigh the least and maintain the highest fitness levels. Obese infants do not characteristically ingest more calories than recommended dietary standards. For overweight children ages 4 to 6 years, daily energy expenditure averaged 25% below the current recommendation for energy intake at this age. A low level of daily physical activity primarily caused the depressed energy output. More specifically, 50% of boys and 75% of girls in the United States fail to engage in even moderate physical activity three or more times weekly. Time-in-motion photography to document activity patterns of elementary-school children showed that overweight children remained considerably less active than normal-weight peers; excess body weight did not relate to food intake. Excessive fatness relates directly to the number of hours spent watching television (a consistent marker of inactivity) among children, adolescents, and adults (See Close Up on page 614.) Television watching, playing video games, and otherwise remaining physically inactive characterizes minority teens. Minimizing time devoted to such behaviors can help to combat childhood obesity.

Overfat children often eat the same or even less than peers of average body weight, which also pertains to less physically active adults as they progressively gain weight. Overweight individuals do not eat more on average than persons of normal weight. Consequently, it remains neither prudent nor justifiable to emphasize dieting alone to effectively induce long-term weight loss.

Increasing Energy Output

Physically active men and women maintain a desirable body composition. An increased level of regular physical activity combined with dietary restraint maintains weight loss more effectively than long-term caloric restriction alone. A negative energy balance induced by increased caloric expenditure, through either lifestyle activities or formal exercise programs, unbalances the energy balance equation for weight loss, improves physical fitness, and favorably alters body composition and body fat distribution. Regular exercise possibly produces less accumulation of central adipose tissue associated with aging. Additional spin-off from regular exercise includes reduced risk of adult-onset obesity, improved obesity-related comorbidities, decreased mortality, and beneficial effects on existing chronic diseases.

Misconceptions About Exercise and Weight Loss   Two main arguments attempt to counter the exercise approach to weight loss.

1. **Exercise increases appetite so a proportionate increase in food intake negates the caloric deficit exercise produces.** In considering the effects of exercise on appetite and food intake, one must distinguish exercise type and duration and the participant's body fat status. Lumberjacks, farm laborers, and endurance athletes consume about twice as many daily calories as sedentary individuals. More specifically, marathon runners, cross-country skiers, and endurance cyclists consume about 4000 to 6000 kCal daily, yet they are the leanest people in the population. Obviously, their large caloric intake meets the energy requirements of training while maintaining a relatively lean body composition. For the overweight person, the extra energy required for exercise more than offsets any small compensatory appetite-stimulating effect of moderate physical activity. To some extent, the large energy reserve of the overfat person makes it easier to tolerate weight loss and exercise without an obligatory increase in caloric intake so common for leaner counterparts. *A weak coupling exists between the short-term energy deficit induced by exercise and energy intake. Increased physical activity by overweight, sedentary individuals does not necessarily alter physiologic needs and automatically produce compensatory increases in food intake to balance any additional energy expenditure.*
2. **The relatively small calorie-burning effect of a normal exercise workout does not "dent" the body's fat reserves compared with food restriction.** A common misconception concerns the contribution to weight loss of the calories expended in typical exercise. Some argue correctly that it requires an inordinate amount of short-term exercise to reduce just 1 pound of body fat: for example, chopping wood for 10 hours, playing golf for 20 hours, performing mild calisthenics for 22 hours, or playing ping-pong for 28 hours or volleyball for 32 hours. Consequently, a 2- or 3-month exercise regimen produces only a small fat loss in an overfat person. From a different perspective, however, if one played golf (no cart) for 2 hours daily (350 kCal) 2 days per week (700 kCal), it would take about 5 weeks to lose 1 pound of body fat. Assuming the person plays year-round, golfing 2 days a week produces about a 10-pound yearly fat loss, provided food intake remains constant. Even an activity as innocuous as chewing gum burns an extra 11 kCal each hour, a 20% increase compared to normal resting metabolism. Simply stated, the

Questions & Notes

Is a low carbohydrate-ketogenic diet recommended for athletes? Why? Why not?

Describe conditions under which you would prescribe a VLCD eating plan.

Name the major factor that consistently emerges as an important factor in weight gain by children, adolescents, and adults.

List one disadvantage for each of the following weight-loss methods:

Surgery:

Fasting:

Low-CHO, high-fat diet:

High-CHO, low-fat diet:

Table 16•7	Principles and Main Advantages and Disadvantages of Some Popular Weight Loss Methods			
METHOD	**PRINCIPLE**	**ADVANTAGES**	**DISADVANTAGES**	**COMMENTS**
Surgical procedures	Alteration of the gastrointestinal tract changes capacity or amount of absorptive surface	Caloric restriciton is less necessary	Risks of surgery and postsurgical complications can include death	Radical procedures include stapling of the stomach and removal of a section of the small intestine (intestinal jejunoileal bypass)
Fasting	Decreased energy input assures negative energy balance	Weight loss is rapid	Ketogenic A large portion of weight lost is from lean body mass Nutrients are lacking	Medical supervision mandatory and hospitalization recommended
Protein-sparing modified fast	Same as fasting except protein or protein with carbohydrate intake may preserve lean body mass	Weight loss is rapid	Ketogenic Nutrients are lasking Some unconfirmed deaths have been reported, possibly from electrolyte depletion	Medical supervision mandatory Popular presentation in Linn's *The Last Chance Diet*
One-food-centered diets	Low-caloric intake favors negative energy balance	Being easy to follow has initial psychological appeal	Being too restrictive means that nutrients are probably lacking Repetitious nature may cause boredom	No food or food combination can "burn off" fat Examples include the grapefruit diet and the egg diet
Low-carbohydrate/ high-fat diets	Increased ketone excretion removes energy-containing substances from the body Fat intake is often voluntarily decreased; results in a low caloric intake	Inclusion of rich foods may have pschological appeal Initial rapid loss of water may be an incentive	Ketogenic High-fat intake contraindicated for heart and diabetes patients Nutrients are lacking	Popular versions have been offered by Taller and Atkins; some have been called the "Mayo", "Drinking Man's", "South Beach" and "Air Force" diets
Low-carbohydrate/ high-protein diets	Low caloric intake favors negative energy balance	Initial rapid loss of water weight may be an incentive Increased thermic effect of protein	Expensive and repetitious; difficult to sustain	If meat emphasized, the diet becomes high in fat
High-carbohydrate/ low-fat diets	Low caloric intake favors negative energy balance	Wise food selections can make the diet nutritionally sound	Initial water retention (from glycogen storage) may be discouraging	The Pennington diet The Pritikin diet

Modified and reprinted by permission from Reed, P.B.: *Nutrition: An Applied Science.* Copyright © 1980 by West Publishing Co. All Rights Reserved.

calorie-expending effects of exercise add up. A caloric deficit of 3500 kCal equals a 1-pound body fat loss, whether the deficit occurs rapidly or systematically over time.

Effectiveness of Regular Exercise

The effectiveness of regular exercise for weight loss relates closely to the degree of excess body fat. Overfat persons lose weight and fat more readily with exercise than normal-weight persons. Aerobic exercise and resistance training, even without dietary restriction, provide considerable positive spin-off to the weight loss effort. These exercises favorably alter body composition (reduced body fat with a small increase in FFM) for the healthy overweight person, postmenopausal woman, cardiac patient, and physically challenged individual. For example, overfat children who exercised 40 minutes a day, 5 days a week for 4 months without dietary restriction accumulated less visceral adipose tissue than nonexercising controls. The active children also gained more FFM and lost more total fat mass and percentage body fat. Even when an exercise program produces no loss in body weight, substantial reductions still can occur in both abdominal subcutaneous and visceral fat. This response certainly blunts a tendency toward insulin resistance and predisposition to type 2 diabetes.

Adding exercise to a weight-loss program favorably modifies the composition of the weight lost in the direction of greater fat loss. In a pioneering study, each of three groups of adult women maintained a daily energy deficit of 500 kCal for 16 weeks. The diet group reduced daily food intake by 500 kCal, while the exercise group increased energy output by 500 kCal with a supervised walking and exercise program 5 days weekly. The women using diet plus exercise created a daily 500 kCal deficit by reducing food intake by 250 kCal and increasing energy output by 250 kCal through exercise. No significant difference emerged among the three groups for weight loss; each group lost approximately 5 kg. This finding shows that a caloric deficit produces body weight loss regardless of the method to create the energy imbalance. For body fat reduction, combining diet and exercise proved most effective. FFM increased by 0.9 kg (exercise group) and 0.5 kg (combination group) with exercise, while dieters lost 1.1 kg of lean tissue.

Table 16.8 shows the effects of regular exercise for weight loss by six sedentary, obese young men who exercised 5 days a week for 16 weeks by walking 90 minutes each session. The men lost nearly 6 kg of body fat (a decrease in percentage body fat from 23.5% to 18.6%). Exercise capacity also improved, as did HDL cholesterol (15.6%) and the HDL:LDL cholesterol ratio (25.9%).

Figure 16.25 shows body composition changes for 40 obese women placed into one of four groups: (1) control, no exercise and no diet; (2) diet only, no exercise (DO); (3) diet plus resistance exercise (D+E), and (4) resistance exercise only, no diet (EO). The women trained 3 days a week for 8 weeks. They performed 10 repetitions each of three sets of eight strength exercises. Body mass decreased for the DO (−4.5 kg) and D+E groups (−3.9 kg), compared with the EO group (+0.5 kg) and controls (−0.4 kg). Importantly, FFM increased in the EO group (+1 kg), whereas the DO group lost 0.9 kg of FFM. The authors concluded that augmenting a calorie-restriction program with resistance exercise training preserved FFM, compared with dietary restriction alone.

Most of the health-related metabolic improvements in the obese with regular exercise relate to total exercise volume and quantity of fat loss rather than to improved cardiorespiratory fitness. Ideal exercise for weight loss consists of continuous, large-muscle activities with moderate-to-high caloric cost, such as walking, running, rope skipping, stair stepping, cycling, and swimming. Many recreational sports and games also are effective in weight control, but precise quantification and regulation of energy expenditure becomes difficult. Aerobic exercise stimulates fat catabolism, establishes favorable blood pressure responses, and generally promotes cardiovascular health. No selective effect exists for running, walking, or bicycling; each promotes fat loss with equal effectiveness. Expending an extra 300 kCal daily (e.g., jogging for 30 minutes) should produce a 1-pound fat loss in about 12 days. This represents a yearly caloric deficit equivalent to the energy in 30 pounds of body fat.

Dose-Response Relationship   The total energy expended in physical activity relates in a dose-response manner to the effectiveness of exercise for weight loss. A reasonable goal progressively increases moderate exercise to between 60 and 90 minutes daily or a level that burns up to 2500 kCal on a weekly basis. To combat the obesity epidemic, the public health perspective must promote the population's need to increase total daily energy expenditure substantially and regularly rather than increase exercise intensity to induce a training response. An overly fat person who starts out with light exercise, such as slow walking, can achieve considerable caloric expenditure simply by extending exercise duration. The focus on exercise duration offsets the inadvisability of having the previously sedentary, obese individual begin with more strenuous exercise. Also, the energy cost of weight-bearing exercise relates directly to body mass; thus, the overweight person expends considerably more calories in such exercise than someone of average body weight. In general, greater levels of exercise associate with a greater magnitude of weight loss.

Questions & Notes

What effect does regular physical activity have on a child's body composition and the tendency to accumulate body fat?

Does regular exercise necessarily increase one's appetite?

Which component of body composition, fat mass or the fat-free mass is most affected by regular physical activity?

List 2 examples of the cumulative effects of regular physical activity in a program designed for weight loss.

1.

2.

FOR YOUR INFORMATION

No One "Best" Aerobic Exercise
No selective effect on weight loss occurs for diverse big muscle activities like running, walking, swimming, or bicycling; each produces similar effects in altering body composition, provided equivalence exists for exercise duration, frequency, and intensity.

Box 16–7 • CLOSE UP

RECOGNIZING THE WARNING SIGNS OF DISORDERED EATING

Disordered eating refers to a broad spectrum of complex behaviors, core attitudes, coping strategies, and conditions that share the commonalty of an emotionally based, inordinate, and (often) pathological focus on body size, shape, and weight. **Anorexia nervosa** and **bulimia nervosa** represent the two most common eating disorders. A third category, **binge-eating disorder**, does not include purging behavior.

ANOREXIA NERVOSA

Anorexia nervosa represents a medically unhealthy physical and mental state characterized by a crippling obsession with body size. A "nervous loss of appetite" reflects a compulsive preoccupation with dieting and thinness and refusal to consume enough food to maintain a normal body weight. The relentless pursuit of thinness (present in about 1% to 2 % of the general population) includes an intense fear of weight gain and almost any degree of fatness (despite a low body weight) and failure to menstruate regularly (amenorrhea). Anorectics have a distorted body image; they truly perceive themselves as overly fat despite their emaciation.

Anorexia nervosa usually begins with a normal attempt to lose weight through dieting. With continued dieting, the individual continues to eat less until very little food is consumed on a daily basis. Eventually, food restriction becomes such an obsession that the anorectic achieves no sense of satisfaction despite further weight loss. As weight loss continues, the anorectic person exhibits denial of the accompanying extreme emaciation. In some cases, the intense hunger accompanying near-total food deprivation cannot be continually ignored. This causes episodes of binging and subsequent purging.

WARNING SIGNS OF ANOREXIA NERVOSA

- Preoccupation with being overly fat despite maintenance of normal body weight
- Cessation of menses (amenorrhea)
- Frequently commenting about body weight or shape
- Dramatic loss of body weight
- Weight too low for successful athletic performance
- Ritualistic concern and unusual preoccupation with dieting, counting calories, cooking, and eating meals
- Excessive concern about body weight, size, and shape, even following substantial weight loss
- Feeling of helplessness in the presence of food

- Severe mood shifts
- Guilt about eating
- Compulsive need for continuous, vigorous physical activity that exceeds training requirements for most sports
- Maintenance of a skinny look (body weight less than 85% of expected weight)
- Preferring to eat in isolation
- Refusal to eat to gain weight
- Wearing baggy clothes to disguise thin-looking appearance
- Episodes of binging and purging

BULIMIA NERVOSA

The term *bulimia*, literally meaning "ox hunger," refers to "gorging" or "insatiable appetite." Unlike continual semi-starvation with anorexia nervosa, binge eating characterizes bulimia nervosa. The binger consumes calorically dense food, often at night and usually between 1000 to 10,000 kCal within several hours, followed by fasting, self-induced vomiting, taking laxatives or diuretics (water pills), or compulsive exercising solely to avoid gaining weight after the binge.

WARNING SIGNS OF BULIMIA NERVOSA

- Excessive concern about body weight, body size, and body composition
- Frequent gains and losses in body weight
- Visits to the bathroom following meals
- Fear of not being able to stop eating
- Eating when depressed
- Compulsive dieting after binge-eating episodes
- Severe shifts in mood (depression, loneliness)
- Secretive binge eating but never overeating in front of others
- More frequent criticism of one's body size and shape
- Experiencing personal or family problems with alcohol or drugs
- Irregular menstrual cycle (oligomenorrhea)

BINGE-EATING DISORDER

Episodes of binging without subsequent purging characterize binge-eating disorder, a recently defined eating disorder. Individuals eat more rapidly than normal until they no longer can consume additional food. Food intake ex-

Box 16–7 • CLOSE UP *(Continued)*

ceeds that determined by the internal physiologic drive of hunger. Binge eating, done in private, occurs with feelings of guilt, depression, or self-disgust. The diagnosis of binge-eating disorder requires that the individual experiences a lack of control over eating and a marked psychological distress when it occurs. Individuals must binge at least an average of 2 days a week for 6 months. Binge eating differs from obesity; the same level of self-anger, shame, lack of control, and frustration about binge eating does not usually accompany obesity. Little factual information exists about the prevalence of binge-eating disorder.

ANOREXIA ATHLETICA

The term *anorexia athletica* describes the continuum of subclinical eating behaviors of a large number of athletes who fail to meet the criteria for a true eating disorder, but who exhibit at least one unhealthy method of weight control. These include fasting, vomiting (termed "instrumental vomiting" when used to make weight), and use of diet pills, laxatives, or diuretics (water pills). Patterns of disordered eating behaviors coincide with a specific sport season and terminate when the competitive season ends.

Table 16·8	The Effects of a 16-Week Walking Program on Changes in Body Composition and Blood Lipids in Six Obese Young Adult Men		
VARIABLE	**PRE-TRAINING[a]**	**POST-TRAINING[a]**	**DIFFERENCE**
Body mass, kg	99.1	93.4	−5.7[b]
Body density, g·mL^{-1}	1.044	1.056	+0.012[b]
Body fat, %	23.5	18.6	−4.9[b]
Fat mass, kg	23.3	17.4	−5.9[b]
Fat-free body mass, kg	75.8	76.0	+0.2
Sum of skinfolds, mm	12.9	104.8	−38.1[b]
HDL cholesterol, mg·100 mL^{-1}	32	37	−5.0[b]
HDL/LDL cholesterol	0.27	0.34	+0.07[b]

[a] Values are means
[b] Statistically significant differences
From Leon, A.S., et al.: Effects of a vigorous walking program on body composition, and carbohydrate and lipid metabolism of obese young men. *Am. J. Clin. Nutr.*, 33:1776, 1979.

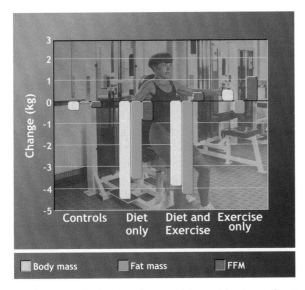

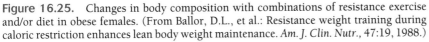

Figure 16.25. Changes in body composition with combinations of resistance exercise and/or diet in obese females. (From Ballor, D.L., et al.: Resistance weight training during caloric restriction enhances lean body weight maintenance. *Am. J. Clin. Nutr.*, 47:19, 1988.)

Questions & Notes

List 3 warning signs of anorexia nervosa.

1.

2.

3.

List 3 warning signs of bulimia nervosa.

1.

2.

3.

FOR YOUR INFORMATION

Exercise Compliance

Cigarette smoking, a previously sedentary lifestyle, lack of family support, and disruptive events, such as illness, all negatively influence an individual's compliance to an exercise program for weight loss. Compliance greatly improves when the person enrolls in a supervised exercise program.

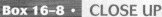

Box 16–8 • CLOSE UP

TELEVISION AND CHILDHOOD OBESITY

The prevalence and persistence of childhood obesity represents a health calamity. An interesting line of research has focused on obesity's relationship to television watching. Children in the United States spend as much time in front of the TV each year as they do attending school. Estimates indicate that children ages 6 to 11 years watch TV an average of 26 hours weekly, whereas adolescents spend about 22 hours each week in front of the television.

Television viewing is also linked to obesity; each hourly increment of weekly TV watching by adolescents reflects a 2% increase in obesity prevalence. A similar pattern emerges for adults; men who view more than 3 hours of daily TV increase their likelihood for obesity to twice that of men who view TV less than 1 hour daily. The question remains: Does the sedentary nature of TV watching causally contribute to obesity, or does the TV-obesity association merely reflect the fact that the obese condition causes one to become sedentary, and watching TV provides a pleasant sedentary pastime.

To answer this question, researchers assessed energy metabolism in 15 obese and 16 normal-weight girls (average age, 10.2 years) for 25 minutes during rest and during rest when viewing TV. The inset figure illustrates that watching television depressed the resting metabolism by 15% in obese girls and 17% in nonobese girls. Obese children watch more daily TV than normal-weight peers; thus, the cumulative effect of a depressed metabolic rate while viewing TV exerts *greater impact* for

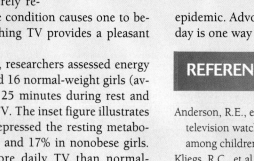

weight gain on the obese. Also, children who watch excessive television further increase their risk for obesity in that resting energy expenditure drops below the value obtained if they simply did nothing at all!

The acute decrease in energy expenditure during TV viewing supports a causal relationship between time spent watching television and excessive weight gain. A vicious cycle develops because children also tend to snack with high-calorie foods while watching TV. These findings become worrisome when coupled with the fact that 30% of American children average less than 30 minutes of daily physical activity.

We believe that parents, teachers, and school administrators should encourage children to exercise 1 hour per day during the elementary school day. Eliminating required physical education in the elementary school curriculum contributes to the national obesity epidemic. Advocating regular exercise during the school day is one way to help.

REFERENCES

Anderson, R.E., et al.: Relationship of physical activity and television watching with body weight and level of fatness among children. *JAMA*, 279:938, 1998.

Kliegs, R.C., et al.: Effects of television on metabolic rate: Potential implications for childhood obesity. *Pediatrics*, 91:281, 1993.

Exercise Frequency   To determine the optimal exercise frequency for weight loss, subjects exercised for 30 to 47 minutes for 20 weeks by either running or walking, with exercise intensity maintained between 80% and 95% of maximum heart rate. Training twice weekly produced no changes in body weight, skinfolds, or percentage body fat, but training 3 and 4 days weekly did. Furthermore, subjects who trained 4 days a week reduced body mass and skinfolds more than subjects who trained 3 days a week. Percentage body fat decreased similarly in both groups. These findings support a recommendation to exercise a minimum of 3 days per week to favorably alter body composition; the additional caloric expenditure with

more frequent exercise produces greater results. The threshold exercise energy expenditure for weight loss probably remains highly individualized. The calorie-burning effect of each exercise session should eventually reach a minimum of 300 kCal whenever possible. This generally occurs with 30 minutes of moderate-to-vigorous running, swimming, bicycling, or circuit-resistance training or 60 minutes of brisk walking.

Self-Selected Energy Expenditures: Mode of Exercise   No selective effect exists among diverse modes of big-muscle aerobic exercise to favorably reduce body weight, body fat, skinfold thickness, and girths, yet other differences may emerge. For individuals without physical activity limitations, running usually provides the most suitable exercise mode for maximizing energy expenditure during self-selected intensities of continuous exercise.

DIET PLUS EXERCISE: THE IDEAL COMBINATION

Combining exercise with diet offers considerably more flexibility for achieving a negative caloric balance than either exercise alone or diet alone. Including regular exercise in a weight control program facilitates longer term maintenance of fat loss than total reliance on food restriction. Most nutrition experts agree that body fat losses up to 2 pounds (0.9 kg) each week fall within acceptable limits, although a steady 0.5- to 1.0-pound a week loss may be even more desirable.

Setting a Target Time   Suppose 20 weeks represents the target time to achieve a 9-kg (20 lb) fat loss. Based on this goal, the weekly deficit would have to average 3500 kCal, or a daily average of 500 kCal (3500 ÷ 7). To achieve this deficit by dieting, daily caloric intake must decrease by 500 kCal for 20 weeks for the desired 9-kg fat loss. However, if the dieter performed an additional 45 minutes of moderate exercise equivalent to 350 extra kCal 3 days a week, then the weekly caloric deficit would increase by 1050 kCal (3 days per week × 350 kCal per exercise session). Consequently, to achieve the weekly desired 0.45-kg fat loss, the weekly caloric intake needs to decrease by only 2400 kCal (about 350 kCal a day) instead of 3500 kCal. If the number of exercise days increases from three to five, daily food intake need only decrease by 250 kCal. If duration of the 5-day per week extra exercise lengthens from 45 minutes to 90 minutes, then the desired weight loss occurs without reducing food intake because the required deficit of 3500 kCal comes entirely from additional physical activity.

If the intensity of the 90-minute exercise performed 5 days a week increased by only 10% (cycling at 22 instead of 20 mph; running one mile in 9 min instead of 10 min; swimming each 50 yd in 54 s instead of 60 s), the number of calories burned each week through exercise increases by 350 kCal (3500 kCal·wk^{-1} × 10%). This new weekly deficit of 3850 kCal (550 kCal·d^{-1}) then permits the dieter to *increase* daily food intake by 50 kCal yet still lose a pound of fat each week.

The effective use of physical activity combined with mild dietary restriction readily unbalances the energy balance equation in the direction of weight loss. This dual approach reduces feelings of intense hunger and psychological stress compared to weight loss exclusively by caloric restriction. In addition, prolonged dieting increases the chances of developing a variety of nutritional deficiencies, which would hinder exercise training and competitive performance.

Adding aerobic exercise and resistance exercise to a weight loss effort protects against the loss of FFM usually observed when relying solely on diet to achieve weight loss. This occurs partly because exercise training enhances fat mobilization from the body's adipose depots and fat catabolism by the active muscles. In addition, exercise protects against protein loss in skeletal muscle (maintains nitrogen balance). The protein-sparing effects of regular exercise helps to explains why weight loss occurs more readily from the fat reserves in a weight-reduction program that employs regular exercise.

MAINTENANCE OF GOAL BODY WEIGHT

The popular and scientific literature is replete with success stories of individuals who have lost considerable amounts of weight using different interventions that include (singularly or in combination) nutritional, exercise, and behavioral approaches. As already detailed in Figure 16.21, the maintenance of goal weight, even if achieved, still remains elusive.

Questions & Notes

What effect does regular exercise have on insulin resistance, independent of weight loss?

Describe the effects of regular exercise on HDL levels.

Is it possible to gain muscle and lose fat during weight loss? Explain.

Do most of the health-related benefits that obese people experience with regular exercise relate to the volume of exercise performed or to whether intensity is sufficient to improve cardiorespiratory fitness?

Weight Cycling: Going No Place Fast

Most weight loss occurs during the first 6 months of a weight loss program. Between 55% and 85% of those starting a weight loss program drop-out, regardless of treatment length, and eventually regain the lost weight.

Controversy exists about whether the failure to keep off weight raises heart disease risk. Initial reports indicated repeated bouts of weight loss and regain, so-called "yo-yo dieting," increased the likelihood of death from heart attack. The risk averaged nearly 70% higher for regainers than for those who maintained body weight. In contrast, data from 6500 originally healthy Japanese American men showed no ill effects from a repeated cycle of weight loss and regain. From a public health perspective, the risks from overweight and obesity far exceed those for weight cycling. The obese should not use concern for the potential hazards of yo-yo dieting as an excuse to abandon efforts to reduce excess body fat. This, in particular, includes efforts to increase "extra" physical activities of daily living and sports and recreational activities.

A delicate balance exists among successful retention strategies, successful weight loss, and strategies for maintaining weight loss. Most overfat individuals try numerous and diverse weight loss programs, each with short-term success but disappointing long-term results. **Figure 16.26** presents data on the body weights of two women who recorded their weight weekly, one for 120 months and the other for 200 months. These data typically depict the plight of most overfat individuals who strive to achieve and then maintain an optimal body weight throughout their life, but with little long-term success. Subject 1 gained about 30 pounds over a 16-year period, while subject 2 gained 22 pounds over 10 years.

Subject 1 participated in six weight loss programs during her recording period. Each of the three formal programs lasted about 5 months, while the three self-directed efforts lasted 2 months. Weight loss for all programs averaged 9.2 pounds; the woman regained an average of 12 pounds within 1 year after each weight loss attempt.

Subject 2 attempted weight loss eight times during the 10 years of recording her body weight. Attempts lasted between 2 to 16 months, with weight loss averaging 8 pounds for all attempts. Similar to subject 1, she regained all lost weight (average gain of 9.9 lb over 9 months).

For both women, gains in body weight occurred over time, despite interruptions from dieting; these gains could not be attributed to menopause, alterations in exercise patterns, pregnancy, changes in smoking status, or seasonal variation. Following each period of weight loss, body weight increased to the original pre-diet level or higher. The trend of steady weight gain for both women when not dieting counters the idea of a fixed setpoint and, instead, supports the hypothesis that physiologic changes occur that facilitate weight gain (and perhaps reset the setpoint) with aging.

Long-Term Success Possible

The outlook for long-term weight loss maintenance remains poor, yet success stories are well documented. Among lifetime members of a commercial weight-loss organization that promotes prudent caloric restriction, behavior modification, group support, and moderate physical activity, more than one-half maintained their original weight loss goal after 2 years, and more than one-third had done so after 5 years. Another project recruited 784 individuals (629 women; 155 men) in the **National Weight Control Registry (NWCR)**, the largest database assembled of individuals who successfully achieved prolonged weight loss. Criteria for NWCR membership included: (1) 18 years of age or older, and (2) weight loss of at least 30 pounds (13.6 kg) maintained for 1 year or longer. Participants had lost, on average, 66 pounds (30 kg), and 14% had lost more than 100 pounds (45.4 kg). Members maintained the required minimum 30-pound weight loss for a 5.5-year average, while 16% of the group maintained this loss for 10 years or longer! Most participants had been overweight since childhood; nearly one-half had one overweight parent, and more than 25% had two overweight parents. Although genetic background may have predisposed these men and women to obesity, their impressive ability to take weight off and keep it off proves that heredity alone need not destine a person to a lifetime of obesity.

About 55% of the NWCR members used either a formal program or professional assistance to lose weight; the rest achieved success on their own. In response to questions about weight loss methods, 89% modified both food intake and physical activity to achieve their goal weight. Only 10% relied singularly on diet, and 1% used exercise exclusively. The diet strategy practiced by nearly 90% of participants restricted intake of certain types and/or amounts of foods (43% counted calories, 33% limited lipid intake, and 25% restricted actual grams of lipid). More than 44% ate the same foods they normally ate, but in reduced amounts (**Table 16.9**).

The registry members' belief in the importance of physical activity for weight maintenance represents a significant finding—nearly all of the men and women used exercise in their weight-control strategy. Ninety-two percent exercised at home, and about one-third exercised regularly with friends. Women primarily walked and did aerobic dancing, while men chose competitive sports and resistance training.

The data in **Table 16.10** show that weight loss had far-reaching, positive effects on the lives of these successful weight losers. At least 85% of the group improved quality of life, level of energy, physical mobility, general mood, self-confidence, and physical health. Only 13 people (1.6%) worsened in any of these areas.

One of the most interesting findings of the NWCR is the large percentage of participants who reported a triggering event or incident (medical, emotional, lifestyle, body weight incident, inspirational) that preceded their suc-

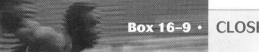

Box 16–9 • CLOSE UP

APPLICATION OF SURFACE ANTHROPOMETRY: THE BODY IMAGE

A matrix of 11 girths illustrated in the top of **Figure 1** constructs a muscular and nonmuscular body image for college versus professional baseball players to provide a quantitative assessment of body shape. If the anthropometric proportions of the individual conform to group symmetry, all of the deviation values on the body image

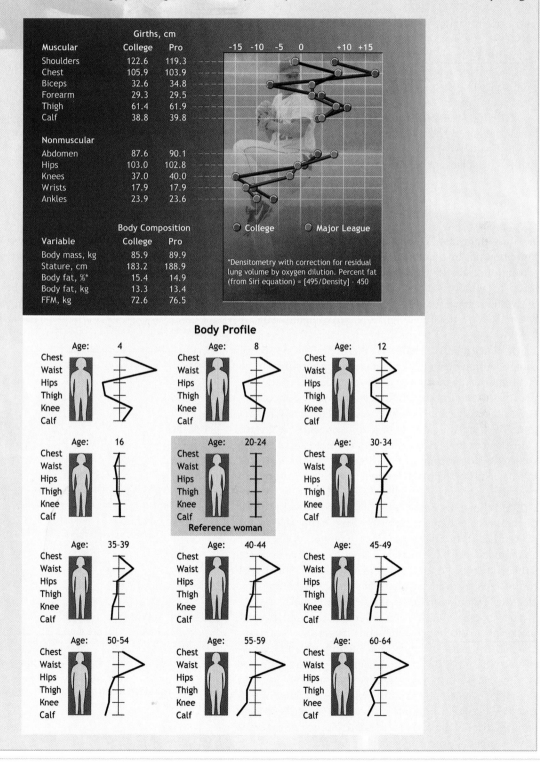

Box 16–9 • CLOSE UP *(Continued)*

would fall within ±2% units of the vertical (zero deviation) reference line.

Practical application of the body image analysis allows quantification of the relative proportions of the body's girth dimensions and charts any changes in physical dimensions due to chronic exercise training, dietary intervention, or aging (*http://www.bodyimagekit.com*). The body profile method also can quantify differences (or similarities) in physique status among athletes in diverse sports (e.g., gymnasts vs. distance swimmers) or within the same sport (e.g., football defensive lineman vs. quarterbacks; soccer goalies vs. forwards; small vs. large bodybuilders; basketball centers vs. guards). The lower part of Figure 1 shows age trends in girth patterns for females aged 4 to 64 years. Note that the waist (designated a nonmuscular region) increases progressively from age

30 to age 64 years. If all of the girths remained in relative proportion with aging, no positive (or negative) deviations would occur in the body profile; all measurements would plot as a vertical line as they do for the reference woman at ages 20 to 24 years.

REFERENCES

Katch, F.I., and Katch, V.L.: The body composition profile: Techniques of measurement and application. *Clin. Sport Med.,* 3:31, 1984.

Katch, F.I., and Katch, V.L.: Computer technology to evaluate body composition, nutrition and exercise. *Prev. Med.,* 12:619, 1983.

---

cessful weight loss. This finding supports why intervention programs by themselves are not effective; instead, intervention strategies must be coupled with "readiness criteria" to achieve success. Despite the success of these individuals, small weight regains were common; very few were able to re-lose the weight after any weight regain.

Spot Reduction: Does It Work? The notion of spot reduction maintains that exercising a specific muscle facilitates relatively greater fat mobilization from the adipose tissue in close proximity to the muscle. Therefore, exercising a specific body area should selectively reduce more fat from that area than if different muscle groups performed exercise of the same caloric value. Advocates of spot reduction recommend performing excessive sit-ups or side bends to reduce abdominal fat, while push-ups and bench presses would be advocated to selectively remove fat from the upper trunk region. The promise of spot reduction conveys not only aesthetic benefits but also an improved health profile (e.g., selective reduction of "risky" abdominal fat). Unfortunately, research evidence does not support localized exercise for spot reduction or the use of topical creams, heat, massage, wraps, magnet therapy, and electrical stimulation for localized fat reduction.

To examine claims for spot reduction, researchers compared the girths and subcutaneous fat stores of the right and left forearms of high-caliber tennis players. As expected, the girth of the dominant, or playing, arm exceeded that of the nondominant arm because of a modest muscular hypertrophy from the exercise overload of tennis. Measurements of skinfold thickness, however, clearly showed that regular and prolonged tennis exercise did not reduce subcutaneous fat deposits in the playing arm.

Another study evaluated fat biopsy specimens from abdominal, subscapular, and buttock sites before and after 27 days of sit-up exercise training. The number of sit-ups increased from 140 at the end of the first week to 336 on day 27. Despite the significant amount of localized exer-

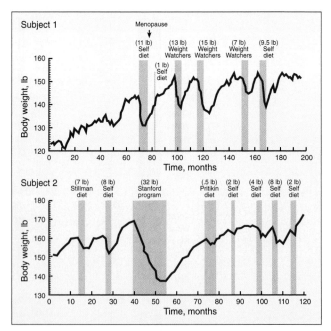

Figure 16.26. Tracking of weekly body weights of two overweight women over a prolonged time. Subject 1 gained 30 pounds over a 16-year period; subject 2 gained 22 pounds over 10 years. (Data from Black, D.R. et al.: A time series analysis of longitudinal weight changes in two adult women. *Int. J. Obes.,* 15:623, 1991.)

cise, adipocytes in the abdominal region were no smaller than those in unexercised buttocks or subscapular control regions.

No one doubts that a negative caloric balance created through regular exercise can reduce total body fat. However, exercise mobilizes fatty acids through hormones that target fat depots throughout the body. Areas of greatest body fat concentration and/or lipid-mobilizing enzyme activity supply the major portion of this energy. No evidence exists for a preferential release of fatty acids from the fat pads directly over the active muscle.

Consumer Beware   The Federal Trade Commission (FTC) (*http://www.ftc.gov/opa/2005/04/abenergizer.htm*) has successfully thwarted the efforts of false claims in a heavily promoted TV infomercial for the *Ab Energizer Exercise System*, a multi-electronic exercise belt that relied on electrical pulses (what the marketers claimed was electrical muscle stimulation or EMS) to cause the abdominal muscles to contract 700 times in minutes to create "six-pack" abs with "no pain, no work, and no situps." In trying to make the case for spot reduction, the Ab Energizer promised to stimulate, tighten, and tone the abdominal muscles to produce a slimmer appearance, and "even cause your friends to think you have lost weight. This is particularly true in stomach areas (men and women), and women's inner and outer thigh muscles." Basically, the Ab Energizer promised spot reduction and toning in the abdominal and upper thigh and buttocks regions without firm scientific verification. In its ruling, the FTC permanently banned the defendants from claiming that the Ab Energizer or any similar device: causes weight loss, inch loss, fat loss, muscle growth, or well-defined abs; is equivalent or superior to abdominal exercise; makes a material contribution to any system or program that produces such results; or is safe for all users. In a follow-up case in May 2005, the San Diego City Attorney's Office and district attorneys in Napa, Solano, and Sonoma Counties in Northern California forced the sports orthopedic medical surgeon who endorsed the Ab Energizer to pay $175,000 in restitution for his product endorsement that he claimed toned muscles and reduced excess fat via repeated electrical stimulation. Target, Walgreens, and Wal-Mart stores also paid more than $1 million dollars in restitution for selling the unapproved "medical device." Notwithstanding the FTC and California judgments, consumers, despite scientific evidence to the contrary, continue to purchase weight loss/muscle toning "miracle" products based on both advertising hype and reliance that a physician's endorsement constitutes "proof" that such devices work.

Questions & Notes

What is the recommended frequency of exercise to favorably alter body composition?

Is one type of aerobic exercise better for weight loss than another?

Explain why it is desirable to add resistance exercises to aerobic training to enhance body composition changes during weight loss.

Discuss the effectiveness of specific exercises to achieve a spot-reducing effect.

When gaining weight, what type of exercises are most beneficial?

Table 16•9	Dietary Strategies to Achieve Weight Loss		
	PERCENTAGE		
STRATEGY	**WOMEN**	**MEN**	**TOTAL**
Restricted intake of certain types or classes of foods	87.8	86.7	87.6
Ate all foods but limited quantity	47.2	32.0	44.2
Counted calories	44.8	39.3	43.7
Limited % of lipid intake	31.1	36.7	33.1
Counted lipid grams	25.7	21.3	25.2
Followed exchange diet	25.2	11.3	22.5
Used liquid formula	19.1	26.0	20.4
Ate only 1 or 2 foods types	5.1	6.7	5.5

From Klem M.L. eta l.: A descriptive study of individuals successful at long-term maintenance of substantial weight loss. *Am. J. Clin. Nutr.*, 66:239, 1997.

FOR YOUR INFORMATION

Excess Calories Accumulate Fat
Each 0.45 kg (1 lb) of adipose tissue contains about 87% pure lipid or 3500 kCal (395 g $\times$ 9 kCal·g^{-1}). An excess intake of 3500 kCal accumulates 0.45 kg of extra fat. Magic potions, trick diets, or special formula foods cannot undo this strategic ratio.

Table 16•10	Effect of Weight Loss on Various Dimensions of Life		
AREA OF LIFE	IMPROVED	NO DIFFERENCE	WORSENED
Quality of life	95.3	4.3	0.4
Level of energy	92.4	6.7	0.9
Mobility	92.3	7.1	0.6
General mood	91.4	6.9	1.6
Self-confidence	90.9	9.0	0.1
Physical health	85.8	12.9	1.3
Interactions with:			
Opposite sex	65.2	32.9	0.9
Same sex	5.0	46.8	0.4
Strangers	69.5	30.4	0.1
Job performance	54.5	45.0	0.6
Hobbies	49.1	36.7	0.4
Spouse interactions	56.3	37.3	5.9

From Klem M.L. eta l.: A descriptive study of individuals successful at long-term maintenance of substantial weight loss. *Am. J. Clin. Nutr.*, 66:239, 1997.

GAINING WEIGHT

For most people, weight loss to reduce body fat and improve overall health and aesthetic appearance becomes the primary focus of any attempt to alter body composition. Many individuals desire to gain weight to improve the body composition profile and/or performance in sport or exercise that requires muscular strength and power. This goal poses a unique dilemma not easily resolved. Gaining weight per se occurs all too easily by tilting the body's energy balance to favor greater caloric intake. In a sedentary person, an accumulated excess intake of 3500 kCal produces a body fat gain of 1 pound because adipocytes store the excess calories. Weight gain for athletes should ideally occur in the form of lean tissue, specifically muscle mass and accompanying connective tissue. Generally, this form of weight gain takes place if an increased caloric intake (adequate carbohydrate for energy and protein sparing, and enough protein for tissue synthesis) accompanies the proper exercise regimen.

Increase Lean, Not Fat

Muscular overload (resistance training) supported by adequate energy and protein intake, with sufficient recovery, increases muscle mass and strength. Adequate energy intake assures that protein available for muscle growth does not catabolize for any energy deficit created by training. Consequently, intense aerobic training should not coincide with resistance training when trying to achieve maximal increases in muscle mass. More than likely, the added energy (and perhaps protein) demands of concurrent resistance and aerobic exercise training impose a limit on

muscle growth and responsiveness to resistance training. A safe recommendation would increase daily protein intake to about 1.5 g per kg of body mass during the resistance-training period. The individual should obtain diverse sources of plant and animal proteins; relying totally on animal sources for increased dietary protein (high in saturated fatty acids and cholesterol) potentially increases risk for heart disease.

If all the calories consumed in excess of energy requirements during resistance training go towards muscle growth, then 2000 to 2500 extra kCal from a well-balanced diet would support each 0.5 kg (1.1 lb) increase in lean tissue. In practical terms, 700 to 1000 kCal added to the daily diet supports a weekly 0.5- to 1.0-kg (1.1- to 2.2-lb) gain in lean tissue and additional energy for training. This ideal situation presupposes that all extra calories synthesize lean tissue.

How Much Gain to Expect

Experience indicates that a 1-year, intense resistance training regimen for young, athletic-type men produces about a 20% increase in body mass, the major portion consisting of lean tissue mass. The rate of lean tissue gain then rapidly plateaus as training progresses beyond the first year. For athletic women, first year gains in lean tissue mass average 50% to 75% of absolute values for men, probably due to women's smaller initial lean body mass. Individual differences in the amount of nitrogen incorporated into body protein (and protein incorporated into muscle) each day may explain variations in lean tissue gains with resistance training. Regularly monitoring body mass and body fat by hydrostatic weighing or other validated indirect techniques verifies whether the combination of training and additional food intake increases lean tissue and not body fat.

SUMMARY

1. There are three ways to unbalance the energy balance equation to bring about weight loss: (1) reduce energy intake below daily energy expenditure, (2) maintain normal energy intake and increase energy output, and (3) combine both methods and decrease food intake and increase energy expenditure.

2. Long-term maintenance of weight loss through dietary restriction has a success rate of less than 20%. Typically, one- to two-thirds of the lost weight returns within a year, and almost all of it returns within 5 years.

3. A caloric deficit of 3500 kCal created through either diet or exercise equals the calories in one pound (0.45 kg) of body fat (adipose tissue).

4. Disadvantages of extreme semi-starvation include loss of lean body tissue, lethargy, possible malnutrition and metabolic disorders, and decrease in the basal energy expenditure. These factors conserve energy and reduce the diet's effectiveness.

5. Adipocyte number stabilizes sometime before adulthood; any weight gain or loss thereafter usually relates to a change in fat cell size. In extreme obesity, cell number can increase once adipocytes reach their hypertrophic limit.

6. Increases in adipocyte number involve three general time periods: last trimester of pregnancy, first year of life, and adolescent growth spurt prior to adulthood.

7. The calories expended in exercise accumulate; a modest amount of extra exercise performed routinely creates a dramatic calorie-burning effect over time.

8. For previously sedentary, overfat men and women, moderate increases in physical activity do not necessarily increase food intake proportionately. Most individuals consume adequate calories to counterbalance caloric expenditure.

9. Combining exercise and caloric restriction offers a flexible yet effective means to weight control. Exercise enhances fat mobilization and utilization for energy, improves insulin sensitivity, and retards lean tissue loss.

10. Rapid weight loss during the first few days of caloric deficit comes mainly from body water loss and glycogen depletion. Continued weight reduction occurs at the expense of greater fat loss per unit weight loss.

11. Successful weight losers generally rely on both food intake and physical activity to achieve their goal weight. Increased physical activity for weight maintenance represents a significant component for these individuals.

12. A triggering event or incident (medical, emotional, lifestyle, weight incident, inspirational) usually precedes successful weight loss. For weight loss success, intervention strategies must couple with "readiness criteria."

13. From a public health perspective, the risks from obesity far exceed those from weight cycling.

14. Selective fat reduction at specific body areas by spot exercise does not work. Exercise stimulates fatty acid mobilization through hormones and enzyme action that target fat depots throughout the body. The areas of greatest body fat concentration and/or lipid-mobilizing enzyme activity supply the greatest amount of energy.

15. Athletes should gain weight as lean body tissue (chiefly muscle mass). This occurs most readily with a modest increase in caloric intake plus systematic resistance training.

THOUGHT QUESTIONS

1. What strategy, advice, and words of encouragement can you offer to a person who has attempted several diets yet never achieved long-term weight loss?

2. Respond to this comment: "The only way to lose weight is to stop eating. It's that simple!"

3. Outline a prudent, yet effective plan for losing weight for a middle-age woman whose physician advises her to shed 20 pounds of excess weight. Provide the rationale for each of your recommendations.

SELECTED REFERENCES

Aleman-Mateo, H., et al.: Determination of body composition using air displacement plethysmography, anthropometry and bio-electrical impedance in rural elderly Mexican men and women. *J. Nutr. Health Aging*, 8:344, 2004.

Anderson, J.W., et al.: Long-term weight-loss maintenance: a meta-analysis of US studies. *Am. J. Clin. Nutr.*, 74:579, 2001.

Anderson, R.E.: Effects of lifestyle activity vs structured aerobic exercise in obese women. *JAMA*, 281:335, 1999.

Anderson, R.E., et al.: Relationship of physical activity and television watching with body weight and level of fatness among children. *JAMA*, 279:938, 1998.

Ball, S.D., Altena, T.S.: Comparison of the Bod Pod and dual energy x-ray absorptiometry in men. *Physiol. Meas.*, 25:671, 2004.

Ball, S.D., et al.: Comparison of anthropometry to DXA: a new prediction equation for men. *Eur. J. Clin. Nutr.*, 58:1525, 2004.

Ballard, T.P., et al.: Comparison of Bod Pod and DXA in female collegiate athletes. *Med. Sci. Sports Exerc.*, 36:731, 2004.

Ballor, D.L., and Keesey, R.E.: A meta-analysis of the factors affecting changes in body mass, fat mass and fat-free mass in males and females. *Int. J. Obes.*, 15:717, 1991.

Becque, M.D., et al.: Time course of skin-plus-fat compression in males and females. *Hum. Biol.* 58:33, 1984.

Behnke, A.R., et al.: The specific gravity of healthy men. *JAMA*, 118:495, 1942.

Behnke, A.R., and Wilmore, J.H.: *Evaluation and Regulation of Body Build and Composition.* Englewood Cliffs, NJ: Prentice Hall, 1974.

Booth, F.W., et al.: Waging war on modern chronic diseases: Primary prevention through exercise biology. *J. Appl. Physiol.*, 88:774, 2000.

Bouchard, C.: Human variation in body mass: Evidence for a role of the genes. *Nutr. Rev.*, 55:S21, 1997.

Bowman, B.A., et al.: Effects of fast food consumption on energy intake and diet quality among children in a national household survey. *Pediatrics*, 113:112, 2004.

Brandon, L.J.: Comparison of existing skinfold equations for estimating body fat in African American and white women. *Am. J. Clin. Nutr.*, 67:1115, 1998.

Bray, G.A., and Popkin, B.M.: Dietary fat intake does affect obesity! *Am. J. Clin. Nutr.*, 68:1157, 1998.

Broeder, C.E., et al.: Assessing body composition before and after resistance or endurance training. *Med. Sci. Sports Exerc.*, 29:705, 1997.

Brožek, J., et al.: Densitometric analysis of body composition: Revision of some quantitative assumptions. *Ann. N.Y. Acad. Sci.*, 110:113, 1963.

Buemann, B., et al.: The N363S polymorphism of the glucocorticoid receptor and metabolic syndrome factors in men. *Obes. Res.*, 13:862, 2005.

Cameron, N., et al.: Regression equations to estimate percentage body fat in African prepubertal children aged 9 y. *Am. J. Clin. Nutr.*, 80:70, 2004.

Chakravarthy, M.V., Booth, F.W.: Eating, exercise, and ìthriftyī genotypes: connecting the dots toward an evolutionary understanding of modern chronic diseases. *J. Appl. Physiol.*, 96:10, 2004.

Chan, J.L., Mantzoros, C.S.: Role of leptin in energy-deprivation states: normal human physiology and clinical implications for hypothalamic amenorrhoea and anorexia nervosa. *Lancet.*, 366:74, 2005.

Chanoine, J.P., et al.: Effect of orlistat on weight and body composition in obese adolescents: a randomized controlled trial. *JAMA*, 293:2873, 2005.

Clark, R.R., et al.: Minimum weight prediction methods cross-validated by the four-component model. *Med. Sci. Sports Exerc.*, 36:639, 2004.

Clarys, J.P., et al.: Gross tissue weights in the human body by cadaver dissection. *Hum. Biol.*, 56:459, 1984.

Collins, A.L., et al.: Within- and between-laboratory precision in the measurement of body volume using air displacement plethysmography and its effect on body composition assessment. *Int. J. Obes. Relat. Metab. Disord.*, 28:80, 2004.

Conway, J.M., et al.: A new approach for the estimation of body composition: Infrared interactance. *Am. J. Clin. Nutr.*, 40:1123, 1984.

Coppini, L.Z., et al.: Limitations and validation of bioelectrical impedance analysis in morbidly obese patients. *Curr. Opin. Clin. Nutr. Metab. Care*, 8:329, 2005.

Déspres, J.-P., et al.: Estimation of deep abdominal adipose-tissue accumulation from simple anthropometric measurements in men. *Am. J. Clin. Nutr.*, 54:471, 1991.

Després, J.-P.: Visceral obesity, insulin resistance, and dyslipidemia: Contribution of endurance exercise training to the treatment of the plurimetabolic syndrome. *Exerc. Sport Sci. Rev.*, 25:271, 1997.

Dietz, W.H.: Health consequences of obesity in youth: Childhood predictors of adult disease. *Pediatrics*, 101:518, 1998.

Diliberti, N., et al.: Increased portion size leads to increased energy intake in a restaurant meal. *Obes. Res.*, 12:562, 2004.

Donnelly, J.E., et al.: Effects of 16 mo of verified, supervised aerobic exercise on macronutrient intake in overweight men and women: the Midwest Exercise Trial. *Am. J. Clin. Nutr.*, 78:950, 2003.

Dorsey, K.B., et al.: Diagnosis, evaluation, and treatment of childhood obesity in pediatric practice. *Arch. Pediatr. Adolesc. Med.*, 159:632, 2005.

Eaton, D.K., et al.: Associations of body mass index and perceived weight with suicide ideation and suicide attempts among US high school students. *Arch. Pediatr. Adolesc. Med.*, 159:513, 2005.

Ebbeling, C.B., et al.: Compensation for energy intake from fast food among overweight and lean adolescents. *JAMA*, 291:2828, 2004.

Eisenmann, J.C., et al.: Assessing body composition among 3- to 8-year-old children: anthropometry, BIA, and DXA. *Obes. Res.,* 12:1633, 2004.

Eisenstein, J., et al.: High-protein weight loss diets: Are they safe and do they work? A review of the experimental and epidemiological data. *Nutr. Revs.,* 60:189, 2002.

Epstein, L.H., et al.: Exercise in treating obesity in children and adolescents. *Med. Sci. Sports Exerc.,* 28:428, 1996.

Eston, R.G., et al.: Prediction of DXA-determined whole body fat from skinfolds: importance of including skinfolds from the thigh and calf in young, healthy men and women. *Eur. J. Clin. Nutr.,* 59:695, 2005.

Fernández, J.R., et al.: Is percentage body fat differentially related to body mass index in Hispanic Americans, African Americans, and European Americans? *Am. J. Clin. Nutr.,* 77:71, 2003.

Fields, D.A., et al.: Assessment of body composition by air-displacement plethysmography: influence of body temperature and moisture. *Dyn. Med.,* 3:3, 2004.

Fields, D.A., Hunter, G.R.: Monitoring body fat in the elderly: application of air-displacement plethysmography. *Curr. Opin. Clin. Nutr. Metab. Care,* 7:11, 2004.

Flegal, K.M., et al.: Excess deaths associated with underweight, overweight, and obesity. *JAMA,* 293:1861, 2005.

Foster, G.D., et al.: A randomized trial of a low-carbohydrate diet for obesity. *N. Engl. J. Med.,* 348:2082, 2003.

Frank, L.L., et al.: Effects of exercise on metabolic risk variables in overweight postmenopausal women: a randomized clinical trial. *Obes. Res.,* 13:615, 2005.

Freedman, C.S., et al.: Trends and correlates of class 3 obesity in the United States from 1990 through 2000. JAMA, 288:1758, 2002.

Freedson, P.A., et al.: Physique, body composition, and psychological characteristics of competitive female body builders. *Phys. Sports Med.,* 11:85, 1983.

Frisch, R.E., et al.: Delayed menarche and amenorrhea in ballet dancers. *N. Engl. J. Med.,* 303:17, 1980.

Frisch, R.E., et al.: Lower lifetime occurrence of breast cancer and cancers of the reproductive system among former college athletes. *Am. J. Clin. Nutr.,* 45:328, 1987.

Garcia, A.L., et al.: Improved prediction of body fat by measuring skinfold thickness, circumferences, and bone breadths. *Obes. Res.,* 13:626, 2005.

Gause-Nilsson, I., Dey, D.K.: Percent body fat estimation from skin fold thickness in the elderly. Development of a population-based prediction equation and comparison with published equations in 75-year-olds. *J. Nutr. Health Aging,* 9:19, 2005.

Giannopoulou, I., et al.: Effects of diet and/or exercise on the adipocytokine and inflammatory cytokine levels of postmenopausal women with type 2 diabetes. *Metabolism,* 54:866, 2005.

Giannopoulou, I., et al.: Exercise is required for visceral fat loss in postmenopausal women with type 2 diabetes. *J. Clin. Endocrinol. Metab.,* 90:1511, 2005.

Gortmaker, S.L., et al.: Television viewing as a cause of increasing obesity among children in the United States: 1986–1990. *Arch. Pediatr. Adolesc. Med.,* 150:136, 1996.

Gregg, E.W., et al.: Secular trends in cardiovascular disease risk factors according to body mass index in US adults. *JAMA,* 293:1868, 2005.

Gutin, B., et al.: Plasma leptin concentrations in obese children: Changes during 4-month periods with and without physical training. *Am. J. Clin. Nutr.,* 69:388, 1999.

Harber, V.J.: Menstrual dysfunction in athletes: an energetic challenge. *Exerc. Sport Sci. Rev.,* 1:19, 2000.

Haroun, D., et al.: Composition of the fat-free mass in obese and nonobese children: matched case-control analyses. *Int. J. Obes. Relat. Metab. Disord.,* 29:29, 2005.

Hedley, A., et al.: Prevalence of overweight and obesity among US children, adolescents, and adults, 1999–2002. *JAMA,* 291:2847, 2004.

Heshka, S., et al.: Weight loss with self-help compared with a structured commercial program: a randomized trial. *JAMA,* 289:1792, 2003.

Hill, J.O., et al.: Racial differences in amounts of visceral adipose tissue in young adults: The CARDIA (Coronary Artery Risk Development in Young Adults) Study. *Am. J. Clin. Nutr.,* 69:381, 1999.

Hirsch, J., and Batchelor, B.R.: Adipose tissue cellularity in human obesity. *Clin. Endocrinol. Metab.,* 5:299, 1976.

Hirsch, J., et al.: Diet composition and energy balance in humans. *Am. J. Clin. Nutr.,* 67(Suppl):551S, 1998.

Hirsch, J., and Knittle, J.: Cellularity of obese and non-obese human adipose tissue. *Fed. Proc.,* 29:1518, 1970.

Hirsch, J., et al.: Diet composition and energy balance in humans. *Am. J. Clin. Nutr.,* 67(Suppl):551S, 1998.

Horowitz, J.F.: Regulation of lipid mobilization and oxidation during exercise in obesity. *Exer. Sport Sci. Rev.,* 29:42, 2001.

Hortobagyi, T., et al.: Comparison of four methods to assess body composition in black and white athletes. *Int. J. Sports Nutr.,* 2:60, 1992.

Ibanez, J., et al.: Twice-weekly progressive resistance training decreases abdominal fat and improves insulin sensitivity in older men with type 2 diabetes. *Diabetes Care,* 28:662, 2005.

Jackson, A.S., and Pollock, M.L.: Generalized equations for predicting body density of men. *Br. J. Nutr.,* 40:497, 1978.

Jakicic, J.M., et al.: Effects of intermittent exercise and use of home exercise equipment on adherence, weight loss, and fitness in overweight women. A randomized trial. *JAMA,* 282:1554, 1999.

Jakicic, J.M., Gallagher, K.I.: Exercise considerations for the sedentary, overweight adult. *Exerc. Sport Sci. Rev.,* 31:91, 2003.

Janssen, I., et al.: Body mass index and waist circumference independently contribute to prediction of nonabdominal, abdominal subcutaneous, and visceral fat. *Am. J. Clin. Nutr.,* 75:683, 2002.

Jeffery, R.W., et al.: Physical activity and weight loss: does prescribing higher physical activity goals improve outcome? *Am. J. Clin. Nutr.,* 78:684, 2003.

Jeffrey, R.W., et al.: Epidemic obesity in the United States: Are fast food and television viewing contributing? *Am. J. Public Health,* 88:277, 1998.

Jurimae, J., et al.: Adiponectin is altered after maximal exercise in highly trained male rowers. *Eur. J. Appl. Physiol.,* 93:502, 2005.

Kah-Banerjee, P., et al.: Prospective study of the association of changes in dietary intake, physical activity, alcohol consumption, and smoking with 9-y gain in waist circumference among 16587 US men. *Am. J. Clin. Nutr.*, 78:719, 2003.

Kahn, H.S., Valdez, R.: Metabolic risks identified by the combination of enlarged waist and elevated triacylglycerol concentration. *Am. J. Clin. Nutr.*, 78:928, 2003.†

Katch, F.I., et al.: Effects of situp exercise training on adipose cell size and adiposity. *Res. Q. Exerc. Sport*, 55:242, 1984.

Katch, F.I., et al.: Estimation of body volume by underwater weighing: Description of a simple method. *J. Appl. Physiol.*, 23:811, 1967.

Katch, F.I., et al.: *The Fidget Factor*. Kansas City: McMeel Publishing, 2000.

Katch, F.I., et al.: Validity of bioelectrical impedance to estimate body composition in cardiac and pulmonary patients. *Am. J. Clin. Nutr.*, 43:972, 1986.

Katch, F.I., and McArdle, W.D.: Prediction of body density from simple anthropometric measurements in college-age men and women. *Hum. Biol.*, 45:445, 1973.

Katch, F.I., and McArdle, W.D.: Validity of body composition prediction equations for college men and women. *Am. J. Clin. Nutr.*, 28:105, 1975.

Katch, F.I., and Michael, E.D.: Prediction of body density from skinfold and girth measurements of college females. *J. Appl. Physiol.*, 25:92, 1968.

Katch, F.I.: Practice curves and errors of measurement in estimating underwater weight by hydrostatic weighing. *Med. Sci. Sports*, 1:212, 1969.

Katch, F.I., and Katch, V.L.: Measurement and prediction errors in body composition assessment and the search for the perfect prediction equation. *Res. Q. Exerc. Sport*, 51:249, 1980.

Katch, F.I., and McArdle, W.D.: Validity of body composition prediction equations for college men and women. *Am. J. Clin. Nutr.*, 28:105, 1975.

Katch, V.L., et al.: The underweight female. *Phys. Sports Med.*, 8:55, 1980.

Katch, V.L., et al.: Contribution of breast volume and weight to body fat distribution in females. *Am. J. Phys. Anthropol.*, 53:93, 1980.

Katzmarzyk, P.T., et al.: The economic costs associated with physical inactivity and obesity in Canada: An update. *CJAP*, 29:90, 2004.

Keys, A., and Brožek, J.: Body fat in adult men. *Physiol. Rev.*, 33:245, 1960.

Kim, J., et al.: Intramuscular adipose tissue-free skeletal muscle mass: estimation by dual-energy X-ray absorptiometry in adults. *J. Appl. Physiol.*, 97:655, 2004.

King, N.A., et al.: Effects of exercise on appetite control: Implications for energy balance. *Med. Sci. Sports Exerc.*, 29:1070, 1997.

King, M.A., and Katch, F.I.: Changes in body density, fatfolds, and girths at 2.3 kg increments of weight loss. *Hum. Biol.*, 58:709, 1986.

Kirk, S., et al.: The relationship of health outcomes to improvement in BMI in children and adolescents. *Obes. Res.*, 13:876, 2005.

Kohrt, W.M.: Preliminary evidence that DEXA provides an accurate assessment of body composition. *J. Appl. Physiol.*, 84:372, 1998.

Kondo, M., et al.: Upper limit of fat-free mass in humans: A study of Japanese sumo wrestlers. *Am. J. Hum. Biol.*, 6:613, 1994.

Lafortuna, C.L., et al.: Gender variations of body composition, muscle strength and power output in morbid obesity. *Int. J. Obes. Relat. Metab. Disord.*, 29:833, 2005.

Lafortuna, C.L., et al.: The relationship between body composition and muscle power output in men and women with obesity. *J. Endocrinol. Invest.*, 27:854, 2004.

Lahti-Koski, M., et al.: Associations of body mass index and obesity with physical activity, food choices, alcohol intake, and smoking in the 1982-1997 Finrisk Studies. *Am. J. Clin. Nutr.*, 75:809, 2002.

Larew, K., et al.: Muscle metabolic function, exercise performance, and weight gain. *Med. Sci. Sports Exerc.*, 35:230, 2003.

Lazzer, S., et al.: Assessment of energy expenditure associated with physical activities in free-living obese and nonobese adolescents. *Am. J. Clin. Nutr.*, 78:471, 2003.

Lee, I-M., et al.: Physical activity and coronary heart disease in women: is ìno pain no gainî passÈ? *JAMA*, 285:1447, 2001.

Lohman, T.G., et al.: Assessing body composition and changes in body composition. Another look at dual-energy X-ray absorptiometry. *Ann. N. Y. Acad. Sci.*, 904:45, 2000.

Lohman, T.G., et al.: Body fat measurement goes high-tech: Not all are created equal. *ACSM Health Fitness J.*, 1:30, 1997.

Lohman, T.G., and Going, S.B.: Multicomponent models in body composition research: Opportunities and pitfalls. *Basic Life Sci.*, 60:53, 1993.

Loucks, A.B.: Energy availability, not body fatness, regulates reproductive function in women. *Exerc. Sport Sci. Rev.*, 31:144, 2003.

Lukaski, H.C.: Methods for the assessment of human body composition: Traditional and new. *Am. J. Clin. Nutr.*, 46:537, 1987.

Maddalozzo, G.F., et al.: Concurrent validity of the BOD POD and dual energy x-ray absorptiometry techniques for assessing body composition in young women. *J. Am. Diet Assoc.*, 102:1677, 2002.

Mayer, L., et al.: Body fat redistribution after weight gain in women with anorexia nervosa. *Am. J. Clin. Nutr.*, 81:1286, 2005.

Mayer, J., et al.: Relation between calorie intake, body weight and physical work: Studies in an industrial male population in West Bengal. *Am. J. Clin. Nutr.*, 4:169, 1956.

Maynard, L.M., et al.: Childhood body composition in relation to body mass index. *Pediatrics*, 107:344, 2001.

Mayo, M.J., et al.: Exercise-induced weight loss preferentially reduces abdominal fat. *Med. Sci. Sports Exerc.*, 35:207, 2003.

Mazes, R.A.B., et al.: Total body composition by dual photon (153Gd) absorptiometry. *Am. J. Clin. Nutr.*, 40:834, 1984.

McArdle, W. D., and Toner, M. M.: Application of exercise for weight control: The exercise prescription. In: *Eating Disorders Handbook: Complete Guide to Understanding and Treatment*. Frankle, R., and Yang, M.-U. (eds.). Rockville, MD: Aspen Publishers, 1988.

McMurray, R.G., Hackney, A.C.: Interactions of metabolic hormones, adipose tissue and exercise. *Sports Med.*, 35:393, 2005.

Mei, Z., et al.: Validity of body mass index compared with other body-composition screening indexes for the assessment of body fatness in children and adolescents. *Am. J. Clin. Nutr.*, 75:978, 2002.

Mendez, J., et al.: Density of fat and bone mineral of mammalian body. *Metabolism*, 9:472, 1960.

Mendez, M.A., et al.: Overweight exceeds underweight among women in most developing countries. *Am. J. Clin. Nutr.*, 81:714, 2005.

Meyer, H.E., et al.: Body mass index and mortality: the influence of physical activity and smoking. *Med. Sci. Sports Exerc.*, 34:1065, 2002.

National Task Force on the Prevention and Treatment of Obesity: Long-term pharmacotherapy in the management of obesity. *JAMA*, 276:1907, 1996.

National Task Force on the Prevention and Treatment of Obesity: Obesity, overweight and health risk. *Arch. Intern Med.*, 160:898, 2000.

Ogden, C.L., et al.: Prevalence and trends in overweight among US children and adolescents, 1999-2000. *JAMA*, 288:1728, 2002.

Omar, H.A., Rager, K.: Prevalence of obesity and lack of physical activity among Kentucky adolescents. Int. *J. Adolesc. Med. Health*, 17:79, 2005.

Ozcelik, O., et al.: Exercise training as an adjunct to orlistat therapy reduces oxidative stress in obese subjects. *Tohoku J. Exp. Med.*, 206:313, 2005.

Perseghin, G.: Muscle lipid metabolism in the metabolic syndrome. *Curr. Opin. Lipidol.*, 16:416, 2005.

Pérusse, L., et al.: Familial aggregation of abdominal visceral fat level: Results from the Quebec family. *Metabolism*, 45:378, 1996.

Pérusse, L., et al.: Acute and chronic effects of exercise on leptin levels in humans. *J. Appl. Physiol.*, 83:5, 1997.

Peterson, M.J., et al.: Development and validation of skinfold-thickness prediction equations with a 4-compartment model. *Am. J. Clin. Nutr.*, 77:1186, 2003.

Petroni, M.L., et al.: Feasibility of air plethysmography (BOD POD) in morbid obesity: a pilot study. *Acta. Diabetol.*, 40 Suppl 1:S59, 2003.

Phelan, S., et al.: Recovery from relapse among successful weight maintainers. *Am. J. Clin. Nutr.*, 78:1079, 2003.

Phillips, S.M., et al.: A longitudinal comparison of body composition by total body water and bioelectrical impedance in adolescent girls. *J. Nutr.*, 133:1419, 2003.

Plasqui, G., Westerterp, K.R.: Accelerometry and heart rate as a measure of physical fitness: proof of concept. *Med. Sci. Sports Exerc.*, 37:872, 2005.

Pollock, M.L., et al.: Twenty-year follow-up of aerobic power and body composition of older track athletes. *J. Appl. Physiol.*, 82:1508, 1997.

Racette, S.B., et al.: Modest weight loss improves insulin action in obese African Americans. *Metabolism*, 54:960, 2005.

Rathbun, E.N., and Pace, N.: Studies on body composition. *J. Biol. Chem.*, 158:667, 1945.

Roche, L.F., et al. (eds.). *Human Body Composition*. Champaign, IL: Human Kinetics, 1996.

Ross, R., et al.: Exercise alone is an effective strategy for reducing obesity and related comorbidities. *Exer. Sport Sci. Rev.*, 28:165, 2000.

Salans, L.B., et al.: Experimental obesity in man: Cellular character of the adipose tissue. *J. Clin. Invest.*, 50:1005, 1971.

Samaha, F.F., et al.: A low-carbohydrate as compared with a low-fat diet in severe obesity. *N. Engl. J. Med.*, 348:2074, 2003.

Schoeller, D.A.: Balancing energy expenditure and body weight. *Am. J. Clin. Nutr.*, 68(Suppl):956S, 1998.

Schoeller, D.A., et al.: How much physical activity is need to minimize weight gain in previously obese women. *Am. J. Clin. Nutr.*, 66:551, 1997.

Schutte, J.E., et al.: Density of lean body mass is greater in Blacks than Whites. *J. Appl. Physiol.*, 56:1647, 1984.

Seidell, J.C., et al.: Waist and hip circumferences have independent and opposite effects on cardiovascular disease risk factors: the Quebec Family Study. *Am. J. Clin. Nutr.*, 74:315, 2001.

Simkin-Silverman, L., et al.: Lifetime weight cycling and psychological health in normal-weight and overweight women. *Int. J. Eating Disord.*, 24:175, 1998.

Sims, E.A.H., and Horton, E.S.: Endocrine and metabolic adaptation to obesity and starvation. *Am. J. Clin. Nutr.*, 21:1455, 1968.

Siri, W.E.: Body volume measurement by gas dilution. In: *Techniques for Measuring Body Composition*. Brozek, J., and Henschel, A. (eds.). Washington, D.C.: National Academy of Sciences–National Research Council, 1961.

Smalls, L.K., et al.: Quantitative model of cellulite: three-dimensional skin surface topography, biophysical characterization, and relationship to human perception. *J. Cosmet. Sci.*, 56:105, 2005.

Solomons, N.W., and Kumanyika, S.: Implications of racial distinctions for body composition and its diagnostic assessment. *Am. J. Clin. Nutr.*, 71:1387, 2000.

Stern, L., et al.: The effects of low-carbohydrate versus conventional weight loss diets in severely obese adults: one-year follow-up of a randomized trial. *Ann. Intern. Med.*, 140:778, 2004.

Sternfeld, B., et al.: Menopause, physical activity, and body composition/fat distribution in midlife women. *Med. Sci. Sports Exerc.*, 37:1195, 2005.

Stewart, K.J., et al.: Exercise effects on bone mineral density relationships to changes in fitness and fatness. *Am. J. Prev. Med.*, 28(5):453, 2005.

Stollk, R.P., et al.: Ultrasound measurements of intraabdominal fat estimate the metabolic syndrome better than do measurements of waist circumference. *Am. J. Clin. Nutr.*, 77:857, 2003.

St-Onge, M.P., et al.: Changes in childhood food consumption patterns: a cause for concern in light of increasing body weights. *Am. J. Clin. Nutr.*, 78:1068, 2003.

Sun, G., et al.: Comparison of multifrequency bioelectrical impedance analysis with dual-energy X-ray absorptiometry for assessment of percentage body fat in a large, healthy population. *Am. J. Clin. Nutr.*, 81:74, 2005.

Torstveit, M.K., Sundgot-Borgen, J.: Participation in leanness sports but not training volume is associated with menstrual dysfunction: a national survey of 1276 elite athletes and controls. *Br. J. Sports Med.*, 39:14, 2005.

Tran, Z.V., and Weltman, A.: Generalized equation for predicting body density of women from girth measurements. *Med. Sci. Sports Exerc.*, 21:101, 1989.

Tran, Z.V., and Weltman, A.: Predicting body composition of men from girth measurements. *Hum. Biol.*, 60:167, 1988.

Treuth, M.S., et al.: Familial resemblance of body composition in prepubertal girls and their biological parents. *Am. J. Clin. Nutr.*, 74:529, 2001.

Treuth, M.S., et al.: Predictions of body fat gain in nonobese girls with a familial predisposition to obesity. *Am. J. Clin. Nutr.*, 78:1212, 2003.

Trichopoulou, A., et al.: Physical activity and energy intake selectively predict the waist-to-hip ratio in men but not in women. *Am. J. Clin. Nutr.*, 74:574, 2001.

Tuomilehto, J.: Cardiovascular risk: prevention and treatment of the metabolic syndrome. *Diabetes Res. Clin. Pract.*, 68:S28, 2005.

Utter, A.C., et al.: Evaluation of air displacement for assessing body composition of collegiate wrestlers. *Med. Sci. Sports Exerc.*, 35:500, 2003.

van Marken Lichtenbelt, et al. Body composition changes in bodybuilders: a method comparison. *Med. Sci. Sports Exerc.*, 36:490, 2004.

Wagner, D.R., and Heyward, V.H.: Measures of body composition in blacks and whites: A comparative review. *Am. J. Clin. Nutr.*, 71:1392, 2000.

Watts, K., et al.: Exercise training in obese children and adolescents: current concepts. *Sports Med.*, 35:375, 2005.

Weinsier, R.L., et al.: Free-living activity energy expenditure in women successful and unsuccessful at maintaining a normal body weight. *Am. J. Clin. Nutr.*, 75:499, 2002.

Weltman, A., et al.: Accurate assessment of body composition in obese females. *Am. J. Clin. Nutr.*, 48:1179, 1988.

Westerterp, K.R.: Alterations in energy balance with exercise. *Am. J. Clin. Nutr.*, 970S, 1998.

Weyers, A.M., et al.: Comparison of methods for assessing body composition changers during weight loss. *Med. Sci. Sports Exerc.*, 34:497, 2002.

Whitlock, E.P., et al.: Screening and interventions for childhood overweight: a summary of evidence for the US Preventive Services Task Force. *Pediatrics*, 116:e125, 2005.

Yancy, W.S. Jr, et al.: A low-carbohydrate, ketogenic diet versus a low-fat diet to treat obesity and hyperlipidemia: a randomized, controlled trial. *Ann. Intern. Med.*, 140:769, 2004.

Zoladz, J.A., et al.: Effect of moderate incremental exercise, performed in fed and fasted state on cardio-respiratory variables and leptin and ghrelin concentrations in young healthy men. *J. Physiol. Pharmacol.*, 56:63, 2005.

CHAPTER OBJECTIVES

* Describe what the term "healthspan" means.

* Explain the concept of successful aging compared to traditional views of the aging process.

* Distinguish between the terms exercise and physical activity.

* Explain the basis of the Physical Activity Pyramid.

* Answer the question: "How safe is exercise?"

* Describe the goals of Healthy People 2010.

* What is SeDS, and why is it important?

* List important age-related changes in: (1) muscular strength, (2) joint flexibility, (3) nervous system function, (4) cardiovascular function, (5) pulmonary function, (6) endocrine function, and (7) body composition.

* Describe five field tests to assess flexibility of major body areas.

* Describe research showing that regular physical activity protects against disease and may even extend life.

* List the three major causes of death in the United States.

* List and describe the four major coronary heart disease risk factors.

* List secondary and novel risk factors for coronary heart disease.

* List specific components of the blood lipid profile and give values considered desirable for each.

* Discuss factors that affect cholesterol lipoprotein levels.

* Explain how regular physical activity reduces coronary heart disease risk.

* Describe the occurrence of CHD risk factors in children.

* Explain interactions between CHD risk factors.

CHAPTER OUTLINE

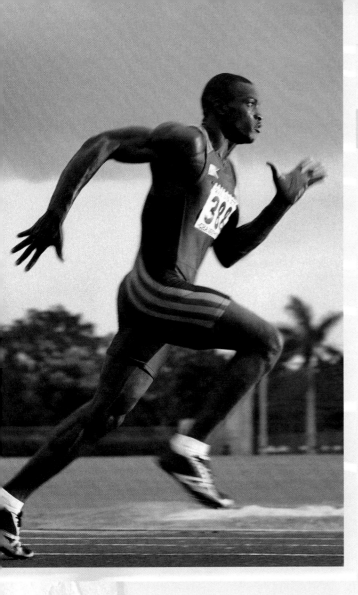

Exercise, Successful Aging, and Disease Prevention

THE GRAYING OF AMERICA

Elderly persons make up the fastest growing segment of American society. Thirty-five years ago, age 65 represented the onset of **old age**. Gerontologists now consider age 85 the demarcation of "**oldest-old**" and age 75, "**young-old**." Currently, nearly 12% or approximately 35 million Americans exceed age 65, and by the year 2030, 70 million Americans will exceed age 85. Some demographers project that one-half of the girls and one-third of the boys born in developed countries near the end of the 20th century will live in three centuries. In the short term, disease prevention, health care, and more effective treatment of age-related heart disease and osteoporosis help people live longer. Far fewer people now die from infectious childhood diseases, and those with the genetic potential actualize their proclivity for longevity. On a different but parallel front, anticipated breakthroughs in genetic therapies may slow the aging of individual cells. Cellular damage results from (1) accumulated mutations in mitochondrial DNA, perhaps produced by injury and deterioration from oxidative stress, and/or (2) gene alterations that depress telomerase synthesis, the enzyme that protects telomers at the ends of chromosomes, allow cells to divide properly. Gene therapies could boost human life spans to a much greater extent than improved medical treatment or even eradication of deadly diseases.

Figure 17.1A shows that proportionately, centenarians currently represent the fastest growing age group in the United States. Numbers range from 30,000 to 50,000, up from the estimated 15,000 in 1980 and almost none at the beginning of the 20th century. No longer viewed as a quirk of nature, 1 in 10,000 Americans now lives to the age of 100. Demographers project that by the middle of this cen-

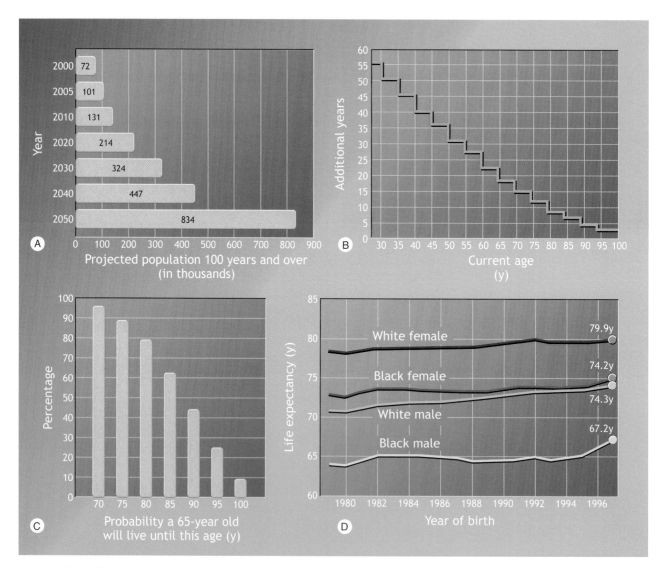

Figure 17.1.   The graying of America. (**A**) Growth in number of centenarians in the United States. (**B**) Additional life expectancy in years for individuals currently at a specific age. (**C**) Probability that a current 65-year old will live to a certain age. (**D**) Life expectancy trends by year of birth, race, and gender. (Data from U.S. Bureau of the Census, National Center for Health Statistics, Centers for Disease Control and Prevention: Washington, D.C., and acturial tables from insurance companies.)

tury, more than 800,000 Americans will exceed age 100, with many in relatively good health. Old-age mortality appears to be on the decline because death rate (number of people per 100 in a specific age group) levels off in the 90-year-old age category (approximately 11 per 100) and decreases to 8 per 100 after age 100. Figure 17.1, B and C, depicts longevity statistics that retirement-pension organizations use to calculate the payout of annuity dividends. For example, a typical 55-year-old person today can expect to live an additional 31.4 years for a life span of 86 years (Fig. 17.1B). But if this 55-year-old lives an additional 15 years to age 70, life expectancy extends to almost 89 years. Figure 17.1C indicates the proportion of individuals aged 65 years who survive to specified ages. Among current 65-year-olds, 95.5% will live to age 70, 63.3% will live to age 85, and nearly 10% will live to be 100 years old. A child born in 1996 should survive to age 95 or 100 years.

Cigarette smoking, elevated body mass index, excess body fatness, and reduced physical activity provide potent predictors of subsequent morbidity and mortality. Changing to a more physically active lifestyle significantly reduces mortality from common ailments and greatly improves cardiovascular and muscular functional capacities, quality of life, and capacity for independent living. At any age, behavioral changes, such as becoming more physically active, quitting cigarette smoking, and controlling body weight and blood pressure, act independently to delay all-cause mortality and extend life. Persons with more healthful lifestyles survive longer with a reduced risk of disability as life progresses.

THE NEW GERONTOLOGY: SUCCESSFUL AGING

Many gerontologists maintain that research on aging should not focus on increasing life span but rather on improving "**healthspan**," the total number of years a person remains in excellent health. The "**new gerontology**" addresses areas beyond age-related diseases and their prevention to recognize that successful aging requires maintenance of enhanced physiologic function and physical fitness. Much of the physiologic deterioration previously considered "normal aging" included deleterious changes in blood pressure, bone mass, body composition, and body fat distribution, insulin sensitivity, and homocysteine levels. These maladies convey increased health risk, dysfunction, or actual disease, and depend on lifestyle and environmental influences subject to considerable modification with proper diet and exercise. For those achieving older age, low muscular strength, diminished cardiovascular function, poor range of joint motion, and sleep disturbances relate directly to functional limitations regardless of disease status. Gerontologists consider that successful aging includes four components: (1) physical health, (2) spirituality, (3) emotional and educational health, and (4) social satisfaction.

Healthy Life Expectancy: A New Concept

Life expectancy estimates determine the overall length of life based on mortality data without considering the quality of life during aging. At some point during the life span, some level of disability detracts from longevity. For example, the Centers for Disease Control and Prevention (*http://www.cdc.gov/nchs/fastats/lifexpec.htm*) reports that nearly 1 in 10 Americans over age 70 requires help with daily activities, such as bathing, and 4 in 10 use assistive devices such as walkers or hearing aids. Approximately one-half of men and two-thirds of women over age 70 have arthritis; one-third of all Americans in this age group also have high blood pressure, and 11% have diabetes. Of all seniors, women over age 85 years are the most likely to need everyday help; 23% require assistance with at least one basic activity (such as dressing or going to the toilet).

To estimate healthful longevity, the World Health Organization (*http://www.who.int/whr/*) introduced the concept of **healthy life expectancy**, the expected number of years a person might live in the equivalent of full health. This involves computing the **disability-adjusted life expectancy** (**DALE**). DALE considers the years of ill health weighted according to severity and subtracted from expected

Questions & Notes

Give the age ranges for:

Old age –

Oldest-old –

Young-old –

What is the fastest growing age group in the United States?

What is the prognosis for how long you will live?

Explain the term "new gerontology."

FOR YOUR INFORMATION

Vigorous Exercisers

People who expend 200 to 300 kCal daily (walk, jog, or run at least 10 miles weekly or equivalent energy expenditure in swimming, cycling, racquet sports, or other "big muscle" activities) qualify as vigorous exercisers. This represents a reasonable exercise standard associated with beneficial health and health-related changes.

overall life expectancy to compute the equivalent years of healthy life. The WHO rankings by country show substantially more years lost to disability in poorer countries from the impact of injury, blindness, and paralysis and the debilitating effects of tropical diseases (such as malaria) that affect children and young adults more frequently. **Figure 17.2** shows the DALE for a sample of 14 countries. Of the 191 countries evaluated, DALE estimates reached 70 years in 24 countries and 60 years in more than half. Thirty-two countries were at the lower extreme, at which DALE estimates were less than 40 years. Many of these countries bear the burden of the major epidemics of HIV/AIDS and other causes of death and disability.

The Japanese experience the longest healthy life expectancy of 74.5 years. Surprisingly, the United States ranks only 24th worldwide with 70.0 years of healthy life for babies born in 1999 (72.6 years for females and 67.5 years for males). Native Americans, rural African-Americans, and the inner-city poor mimic the poor health characteristics of underdeveloped countries.

A comparison statistic to identify causes of reduced healthy life expectancy is termed attributable **years of life lost (YLL)**. The six most prominent factors (in order of importance) responsible for decreased life expectancy in non-Western countries include:

1. Low birth weight
2. Vitamin/mineral deficiency (particularly vitamin A and iron)
3. Unsafe water/sanitation procedures
4. Unsafe sex–HIV
5. Introduction of carcinogens
6. Work-related risk

In the Americas and Europe the six major factors contributing to YLL relate mostly to lifestyle patterns:

1. Tobacco use
2. High blood pressure
3. Increased cholesterol
4. Obesity
5. Low levels of physical activity
6. Low frequency of fruit and vegetable consumption

PHYSICAL ACTIVITY EPIDEMIOLOGY

Epidemiology involves quantifying factors that influence the occurrence of illness to better understand, modify, and/or control a disease pattern in the general population. The specific field of **physical activity epidemiology** applies the general research strategies of epidemiology to study physical activity as a health-related behavior linked to disease and other outcomes.

Terminology

Physical activity epidemiology applies specific definitions to characterize behavioral patterns and outcomes of the groups under investigation. Relevant terminology includes the following:

- **Physical activity:** Body movement produced by muscle action that increases energy expenditure
- **Exercise:** Planned, structured, repetitive, and purposeful physical activity
- **Physical fitness:** Attributes related to how well one performs physical activity

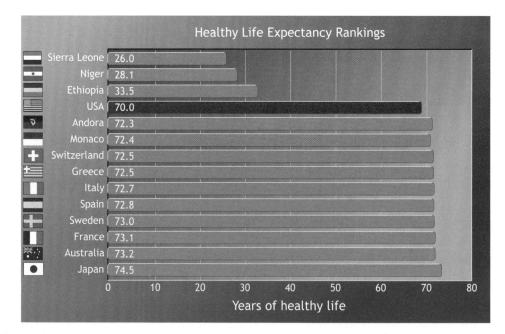

Healthy Life Expectancy Rankings

Country	Years of healthy life
Sierra Leone	26.0
Niger	28.1
Ethiopia	33.5
USA	70.0
Andora	72.3
Monaco	72.4
Switzerland	72.5
Greece	72.5
Italy	72.7
Spain	72.8
Sweden	73.0
France	73.1
Australia	73.2
Japan	74.5

Figure 17.2.   Disability-adjusted life expectancy (DALE, an estimate of healthy life expectancy) ranking of populations of selected countries as assessed by the World Health Organization. Of all countries surveyed, the U.S. ranked 24th, with Japan ranked highest.

- **Health:** Physical, mental, and social well-being, not simply absence of disease
- **Health-related physical fitness:** Components of physical fitness associated with some aspect of good health and/or disease prevention (**Fig. 17.3**)
- **Longevity:** Length of life

Within this framework, physical activity becomes a generic term with exercise its major component. Similarly, the definition of health focuses on the broad spectrum of well-being that ranges from complete absence of health (near death) to the highest levels of physiologic function. Such definitions often challenge our ability to measure and quantify health and physical activity objectively. They do provide a broad perspective to study the role of physical activity in health and disease.

The trend in physical fitness assessment during the past 30 years de-emphasizes tests stressing motor performance and athletic fitness (i.e., speed, power, balance, agility). Instead, current assessment focuses on functional capacities related to overall good health and disease prevention. The four most common components included in health-related physical fitness are aerobic and/or cardiovascular fitness, body composition, abdominal muscular strength and endurance, and lower back and hamstring flexibility (see Close Up, *How to Assess Joint Flexibility in Common Body Areas, page 634*).

Physical Activity Participation

More than 30 different methods can assess physical activity. They include direct and indirect calorimetry, self-reports and questionnaires, job classifications, physiologic markers, behavioral observations, mechanical or electronic monitors, and activity surveys. Each approach offers unique advantages, but also has disadvantages, depending on the situation and population studied. Obtaining valid estimates of physical activity of large groups remains difficult because such studies by necessity apply self-reports of daily activity and exercise participation rather than direct monitoring or objective measurement. Despite limitations in assessment, a discouraging picture of physical activity participation worldwide consistently emerges. In the United States, adult participation in any physical activity is quite low:

- Only about 15% engage in regular, vigorous physical activity during leisure time, 3 times a week for at least 30 minutes
- More than 60% do not engage in any regularly physical activity
- About 25% lead sedentary lives (i.e., do not exercise)
- Walking, gardening, and yard work are the most popular leisure-time activities

Questions & Notes

Explain the concept of healthy life expectancy.

List 3 factors responsible for decreased life expectancy in non-Western countries.

1.

2.

3.

List 3 factors responsible for decreased life expectancy in the Americas and European countries.

1.

2.

3.

Distinguish between the terms physical activity and exercise.

List the 4 components of health-related physical fitness.

1.

2.

3.

4.

List 4 methods to assess physical activity.

1.

2.

3.

4.

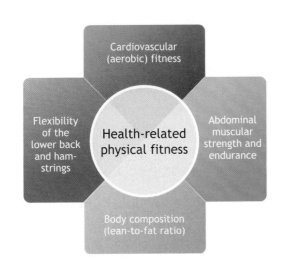

Figure 17.3. Health-related physical fitness components.

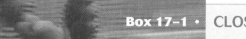

Box 17–1 • CLOSE UP

HOW TO ASSESS JOINT FLEXIBILITY IN COMMON BODY AREAS

Two types of flexibility include: (1) **static**—full range of motion (ROM) of a specific joint, and (2) **dynamic**—torque or resistance encountered as the joint moves through its ROM. Improper alignment of the vertebral column accounts for more than 80% of all lower back and pelvic girdle ailments; this often results from poor flexibility in regions of the lower back, trunk, hip, and posterior thigh (common in runners) and weak abdominal and erector spinae muscles.

SPECIFICITY AND FLEXIBILITY

Considerable specificity exists for joint ROM depending on joint structure. Triaxial joints (ball and socket) of the hip and shoulder afford a greater degree of movement than either uniaxial or biaxial joints (wrist, knee, elbow, and ankle). "Tightness" of the soft tissue structures of the joint capsule, muscle, and its fascia, tendons, ligaments, and skin constitute major factors that influence static and dynamic flexibility. Other influences include a well-developed musculature and excess fatty tissue of adjacent body segments. Flexibility progressively decreases with advancing age, due mainly to decreased soft-tissue extensibility. How decrements in flexibility reflect true aging or result from a "disuse" effect of an increasingly sedentary lifestyle remains unclear. On average, women remain more flexible than men at any age.

FIVE COMMON FIELD TESTS OF STATIC FLEXIBILITY

Field tests assess static flexibility indirectly through linear measurement of ROM. Administer a minimum of three trials after a warm-up.

Test 1: Hip and Trunk Flexibility (Modified Sit-and-Reach Test)

Starting Position   Sit on the floor with the back and head against a wall; legs are fully extended with the bottom of the feet against the sit-and-reach box. Place the hands on top of each other, stretching the arms forward while keeping the head and back against the wall (**A**). Measure the distance from the fingertips to the box edge with a yardstick. This becomes the zero or starting point.

Movement   Slowly bend and reach forward as far as possible (head and back move away from the wall), sliding the fingers along the yardstick; hold the final position for 2 seconds (**B**).

Score   The score is the total distance reached to the nearest one-tenth inch.

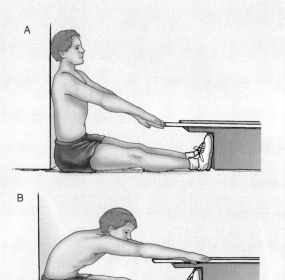

Test 2: Shoulder-Wrist Flexibility (Shoulder and Wrist Elevation Test)

Starting Position   Lay prone on the floor with the arms fully extended overhead; grasp a yardstick with the hands shoulder width apart.

Movement   Raise the stick at high as possible.

- Measure the vertical distance (nearest 1/2 in) the yardstick rises from the floor.
- Measure arm length from the acromial process to the tip of longest finger.
- Subtract the best vertical score from arm length.

Score
- Arm length − best vertical score (nearest 1/4 in).

Box 17–1 • CLOSE UP *(Continued)*

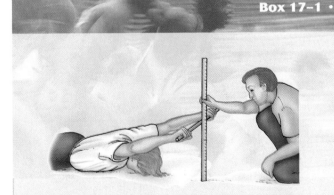

Test 3: Trunk and Neck Flexibility (Trunk and Neck Extension Test)

Starting Position Lay prone on the floor with the hands clasped together behind the head.

Movement Raise the trunk as high as possible while keeping the hips in contact with the floor. An assistant can hold the legs down.

Score
- Vertical distance (nearest 1/4 in) from the tip of the nose to the floor.

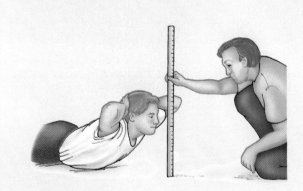

Test 4: Shoulder Flexibility (Shoulder Rotation Test)

Starting Position Grasp one end of a rope with the left hand; four inches away, grasp the rope with the right hand.

Movement Extend both arms in front of the chest, and rotate the arms overhead and behind the back; as resistance occurs, slide the right hand further from the left hand along the rope until the rope touches against the back.
- Measure the distance on the rope between the thumb of each hand after successfully rotating overhead with the rope against the back.

- Measure shoulder width from deltoid to deltoid. Subtract the rope distance from the shoulder width distance.

Score
- Shoulder width distance − rope distance (nearest 1/4 in).

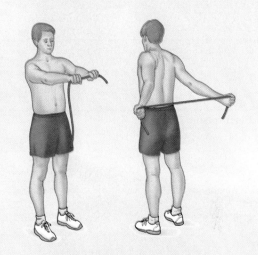

Test 5: Ankle Flexibility (Ankle Flexion Test)

Starting Position Stand facing a wall. With feet flat on the floor, lean into the wall.

Movement Slowly slide back from the wall as far as possible while keeping the feet flat on the floor, body and knees fully extended, and chest in contact with the wall.

Score
- Distance between the toe line and the wall (nearest 1/4 in).

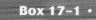

Box 17–1 • CLOSE UP *(Continued)*

Table 1 Static Flexibility Classifications

TEST ITEM	MEN		PERFORMANCE RATING	WOMEN	
Shoulder and wrist elevation	6.00 or less		Excellent	5.50 or less	
	8.25–6.25		Good	7.50–5.75	
	11.50–8.50		Average	10.75–7.75	
	12.50–11.75		Fair	11.75–11.0	
	12.75 or more		Poor	12.00 or more	
Trunk and neck extension	3.00 or less		Excellent	2.00 or less	
	6.00–3.25		Good	5.75–2.25	
	8.00–6.25		Average	7.75–6.00	
	10.00–8.25		Fair	9.75–8.00	
	10.25 or more		Poor	10.00 or more	
Shoulder rotation	7.00 or less		Excellent	5.00 or less	
	11.50–7.25		Good	9.75–5.25	
	14.50–11.75		Average	13.00–10.00	
	19.75–14.75		Fair	17.75–13.25	
	20.00 or more		Poor	18.00 or more	
Ankle flexion	26.50 or less		Excellent	24.25 or less	
	29.50–26.75		Good	26.50–24.50	
	32.50–29.75		Average	30.25–26.75	
	35.25–32.75		Fair	31.75–30.50	
	35.50 or more		Poor	32.00 or more	
Modified sit-and-reach, age range	<35 y	36–49 y		<35 y	36–49 y
	>17.9	>16.1	Excellent	>17.9	>17.4
	17.0–17.9	14.6–16.1	Good	16.7–17.9	16.2–17.4
	15.8–17.0	13.9–14.6	Average	16.2–16.7	15.2–16.2
	15.0–15.8	13.4–13.9	Fair	15.8–16.2	14.5–15.2
	<15.0	<13.4	Poor	<15.4	<14.5

Adapted from Johnson, B.L., Nelson, J.K.: *Practical Measurements for Evaluation in Physical Education.* 4th Ed. New York: Macmillan Publishing, 1986.

- About 22% engage in light-to-moderate physical activity regularly during leisure time (5 times/wk for at least 30 min)
- Physical inactivity occurs more frequently among: women than men, blacks and Hispanics than whites, older than younger adults, and less-affluent than wealthier persons
- Participation in fitness activities declines with age; older citizens typically have such poor functional capacity that they cannot rise from a chair or bed, walk to the bathroom, or climb a single stair without assistance

Equally discouraging data emerge for children and teenagers:

- Nearly one-half of those between ages 12 and 21 do not exercise vigorously on a regular basis regardless of gender
- About 14% report no recent physical activity; this is more prevalent among females, particularly black females
- About 25% engage in light-to-moderate physical activity (e.g., walk or bicycle) nearly every day
- Participation in all types of physical activity declines strikingly as age and school grade increase
- More males than females participate in vigorous physical activity, strengthening activities, and walking or bicycling

Getting America More Physically Active

On July 11, 1996, in a landmark announcement, the Surgeon General of the United States acknowledged the importance of physical activity to the nation with the release of the **First Surgeon General's Report on Physical Activity and Health.** This encompassing report summarized the benefits of regular physical activity in disease prevention. The Surgeon General proposed a national agenda that urged the nation to adopt and maintain a physically active lifestyle to combat ailments associated with the country's generally low level of energy expenditure. The report stated that men and women of all ages benefit from regular physical activity. It became a stated goal of the government to encourage all citizens to include moderate physical activity (e.g., 30 min of brisk walking or raking leaves, 15 min of running, or 45 min of playing volleyball) on most, if not all, days of the week.

The **Physical Activity Pyramid** (**Fig. 17.4**) summarizes major goals for increasing the level of regular physical activity in the general population; the pyramid emphasizes diverse forms of behavioral and lifestyle options.

Healthy People 2010

The **Healthy People 2010** initiative launched on January 25, 2000 and builds on the initiatives of the previous two decades as an instrument to improve national health for the first decade of the 21st century. Healthy People 2010 outlines a comprehensive, nationwide health promotion and disease prevention agenda as a roadmap to promote health and prevent illness, disability, and premature death among all people in the United States.

Healthy People 2010 (*http:www.healthypeople.gov/*) attempts to achieve two primary goals:

1. Increase quality and years of healthy life
2. Eliminate health disparities among the nation's citizens

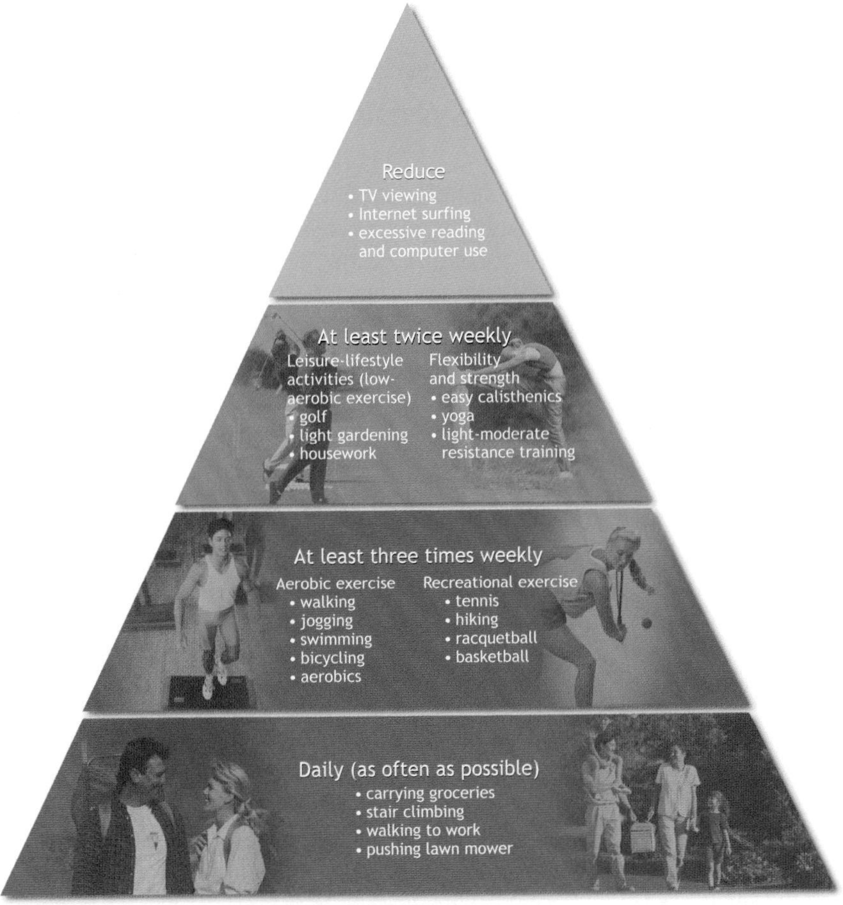

Questions & Notes

List 3 objectives of the Healthy People 2010 initiative.

    1.

    2.

    3.

List 2 major goals of the Healthy People 2010 initiative.

    1.

    2.

Briefly describe the physical activity pyramid.

What is the risk of dying suddenly during exercise?

Identify the most prevalent medical complication from exercising.

List 4 factors that increase the likelihood of an exercise-related catastrophe.

    1.

    2.

    3.

    4.

Figure 17.4. The Physical Activity Pyramid.

Progress will be monitored through achievements within 467 objectives in 28 focus areas. Many goals and objectives, several of which either directly or indirectly involve upgrading the national level of regular physical activity, converge on interventions designed to reduce or eliminate illness, disability, and premature death among individuals and communities. Other objectives focus on broader issues such as improving access to quality health care, strengthening public health services, and improving availability and dissemination of health-related information. Each objective has a target for specific improvements and explicit guidelines on how to achieve the stated goal by the year 2010.

Safety of Exercising

Several well-publicized reports of sudden death during exercise raises the question of exercise safety. It may surprise some that the death rate during exercise has declined over the past 25 years despite an overall increase in exercise participation. In one report of cardiovascular episodes over a 65-month period, 2935 exercisers recorded 374,798 hours of exercise that included 2,726,272 km of running and walking. No deaths occurred during this time, and only two nonfatal cardiovascular complications occurred. This amounts to two complications per 100,000 hours of exercise for women and three complications for men.

In other research, the relative risk of sudden death among athletes versus nonathletes was 1.95 for males and 2.00 for females. The higher risk of sudden death in athletes strongly related to underlying cardiovascular diseases (congenital coronary artery anomaly, arrhythmogenic right ventricular cardiomyopathy, premature coronary artery disease). Interestingly, athletic participation did not cause the enhanced mortality, but it triggered sudden death in athletes affected by cardiovascular conditions predisposing them to life-threatening ventricular arrhythmias during physical exercise.

Intense physical exertion poses a small risk of sudden death (e.g., one sudden death per 1.51 million episodes of exertion) during the activity, compared with resting an equivalent time, particularly for sedentary people with a genetic predisposition to sudden death. The longer-term reduction in overall death risk from regular exercise far outweighs the small potential for acute cardiovascular complications.

Prospective epidemiologic research evaluated clinically significant medical incidents and emergencies for 7725 low-risk, apparently healthy corporate fitness enrollees in a supervised facility at a major medical center. Over 2.5 years of surveillance, there were 15 medically significant events (0.048 per 1000 participant-hours) and two medical emergencies (both recovered; 0.0063 per 1000 participant-hours). This extremely low rate of medical incidents in a supervised health-fitness facility shows that the health-related fitness benefits far outweigh the small risk of participation.

The most recently published report (July 2000–June 2001) from the National Electronic Injury Surveillance System All Injury Program (*http://www.webapp.icpsr.umich.edu/cocoon/icpsr-series/00198.xml*) that characterizes sports- and recreation-related injuries among the U.S. population revealed that 4.3 million nonfatal injuries were treated in U.S. hospital emergency departments (comprising 6% of all unintentional injury-related emergency room visits). Injury rates varied by sex and age and were highest for persons aged 10 to 14 years (51.5% for boys and 38% for girls) and lowest for persons aged 45 years and older (6.4% for men and 3.1% for women). The overall rate of sports- and recreation-related injuries was 15.4 per 1000 population. For persons 20 to 24 years of age, basketball and bicycle-related injuries ranked among the three leading types of injury. Basketball-related injuries ranked highest for men aged 25 to 44 years. Exercise (e.g., weight lifting, aerobics, stretching, walking, jogging, and running) was the leading injury-related activity for women 20 years and older and ranked among the top four types of injuries for men 20 years and older. The most frequent injury diagnosis included strains/sprains (29.1%), fractures (20.5%), contusions/abrasions (20.1%), and lacerations (13.8%). The body parts injured most commonly were ankles (12.2%), fingers (9.5%), face (9.2%), head (8.2%), and knees (8.1%). Overall, hospitalizations included 2.3% of persons with sports- and recreation-related injuries.

SEDENTARY ENVIRONMENTAL DEATH SYNDROME (SeDS)

A review of the world literature over the last 55 years has led to the conclusion that physical inactivity produces a constellation of problems and conditions that eventually lead to premature death. The term **sedentary environmental death syndrome (SeDS)** (*http://hac.missouri.edu*) identifies this condition. In summary:

- SeDS will cause 2.5 million Americans to die prematurely in the next decade.
- SeDS will cost $2 to $3 trillion in healthcare expenses in the United States in the next decade.
- Chronic diseases have increased because of physical inactivity. In the United States, type 2 diabetes has increased ninefold since 1958, obesity has doubled since 1980, and heart disease remains a leading cause of death.
- Children are now getting SeDS related diseases. American children are increasingly overweight, showing fatty streaks in their arteries, and developing type 2 diabetes.
- SeDS relates to 23 medically related conditions, including high blood triglyceride, high blood cholesterol, high blood glucose, type 2 diabetes, hypertension, myocardial ischemia, arrhythmias, congestive heart failure, obesity, breast cancer, depression, chronic back pain, spinal cord injury, stroke, disease

cachexia, debilitating illnesses, falls resulting in a broken hip, and vertebral/femoral fractures.

Increased research efforts are trying to understand the biological link between physical inactivity and disease by exploring the molecular and genetic basis of this link. The biological research thrust has coupled with new research into the behavioral and epidemiological components of SeDS. More medical-based evidence must convince American citizens that *physical inactivity* promotes unhealthy gene expression. As such, regular physical activity should play an increasingly more important role in the lives of all individuals.

AGING AND BODILY FUNCTION

Figure 17.5 shows that bodily functions improve rapidly during childhood and reach a maximum at about age 30; thereafter, a decline in functional capacity occurs. A similar age trend exists for physically active persons; physiologic function averages about 25% higher compared with sedentary counterparts at each age category (e.g., an active 50-year-old man or woman often maintains the functional level of a 30-year-old). All physiologic measures eventually decline with age, but not all decrease at the same rate.

Nerve conduction velocity, for example, declines only 10% to 15% from age 30 to 80 years, whereas resting cardiac index (ratio of cardiac output to body surface area) and joint flexibility decline 20% to 30%; maximum breathing capacity at age 80 averages 40% of values for a 30-year-old. Brain cells die at a fairly constant rate until age 60, whereas the liver and kidneys lose 40% to 50% of their function between ages 30-and-70. By the seventh decade, the average female has lost 30% of her bone mass, whereas men lose only 15%. Unfortunately, some gerontologists consider these aging patterns the "normal" and "expected" decreases in structure and function.

Aging and Muscular Strength

Men and women achieve maximum strength between ages 20 to 30 years, when muscle cross-sectional area achieves maximum size. Thereafter, strength progressively declines for most muscle groups; by age 70, overall "general" strength decreases by 30%.

Questions & Notes

What do the initials SeDS stand for?

List 5 statistics related to SeDS.

1.

2.

3.

4.

5.

Give the approximate age when bodily functions reach their maximum.

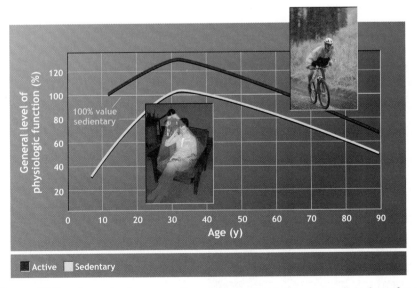

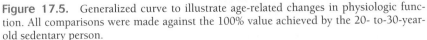

Figure 17.5. Generalized curve to illustrate age-related changes in physiologic function. All comparisons were made against the 100% value achieved by the 20- to-30-year-old sedentary person.

FOR YOUR INFORMATION

Heart Attack Versus Cardiac Arrest
- *Heart attack:* Caused by (1) blockage in one or more arteries supplying the heart, thus cutting off myocardial blood supply, or (2) sudden spasms (constrictions) of a coronary vessel, causing part of the heart muscle to die (necrosis) from lack of oxygen (anoxia).
- *Cardiac arrest:* Caused by irregular neural-electrical transmission within the myocardium. This produces chaotic, unregulated beating in the heart's upper chambers (atrial fibrillation) or lower chambers (ventricular fibrillation).

Decrease in Muscle Mass *Strength decreases with age because of reduced muscle mass, a condition termed sarcopenia.* The smaller muscle mass in older adults reflects a loss of total muscle protein induced by physical inactivity, aging, or the combined effects of both. Some loss in muscle fiber number also takes place with aging. For example, the biceps of a newborn contains about 500,000 individual fibers, whereas the same muscle for an 80-year-old man contains 300,000 fibers, or 40% less.

Muscle Trainability Among the Middle Aged and Elderly *Regular exercise training retains body protein and blunts the loss of muscle mass and strength with aging.* Healthy men between age 60 and 72 years participated in a 12-week standard resistance-training program. **Figure 17.6** shows that the men's muscle strength increased progressively throughout the program, averaging about 5% each exercise session (a training response similar to young adults). Many exercise specialists who work with the elderly believe that improving strength effectively maintains muscle mass, increases mobility, and reduces injury incidence.

Aging and Joint Flexibility

With advancing age, connective tissue (cartilage, ligaments, and tendons) becomes stiffer and more rigid, which reduces joint flexibility. It is unclear whether these changes result from biologic aging or reflect the impact of chronic disuse through sedentary living and/or degenerative tissue diseases of specific joints. Regardless of the cause, appropriate exercises that regularly move joints through their full range of motion increase flexibility 20% to 50% in men and women at all ages.

Endocrine Changes with Aging

Endocrine function changes with age, particularly the pituitary, pancreas, adrenal, and thyroid glands. About 40% of individuals between ages 65 and 75 years and 50% of individuals older than age 80 have impaired glucose tolerance that leads to type 2 diabetes, the most common form of diabetes. Impaired glucose metabolism leading to high blood glucose levels in type 2 diabetes results from three factors:

1. Decreased effect of insulin on peripheral tissue (**insulin resistance**)
2. Inadequate insulin production by the pancreas to control blood sugar (**relative insulin deficiency**)
3. Combined effect of insulin resistance and relative insulin deficiency

With the exception of a genetic predisposition, increased prevalence of type 2 diabetes largely relates to "controllable" factors like poor diet, inadequate physical activity, and increased body fat (particularly in the visceral-abdominal region).

Thyroid dysfunction from lowered pituitary gland release of the thyroid-stimulating hormone thyrotropin (and reduced output of thyroxine from the thyroid gland) commonly occurs among the elderly. This affects metabolic function, including decreased glucose metabolism and protein synthesis.

Figure 17.7 depicts changes in three additional hormonal systems associated with aging: (1) the hypothalamic-pituitary-gonadal axis, (2) adrenal cortex, and (3) growth hormone/insulin-like growth factor 1 axis.

Hypothalamic-Pituitary-Gonadal Axis Alteration in the interaction among stimulating hormones from the hypothalamus and anterior pituitary gland and gonads decreases estradiol output from the ovaries. This effect probably initiates permanent cessation of the menses (**menopause**) in the aging female. Changes in hypothalamic-pituitary-gonadal axis activity in males occur more slowly and subtly. For example, serum total and free testosterone decline with aging in males. Age-related de-

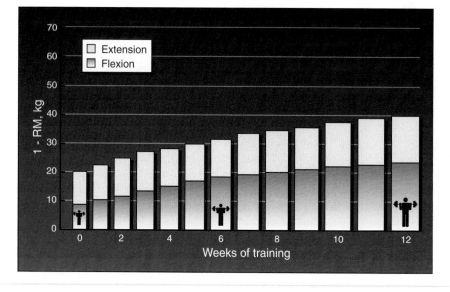

Figure 17.6. Weekly measurement of dynamic muscle strength (1-RM) in left knee extension (yellow) and flexion (red) during a 12-week period of resistance training in men aged 60–72 y. (Data from Frontera, W.R., et al.: Strength conditioning in older men: skeletal muscle hypertrophy and improved function. *J. Appl. Physiol.,* 64:1038, 1988.)

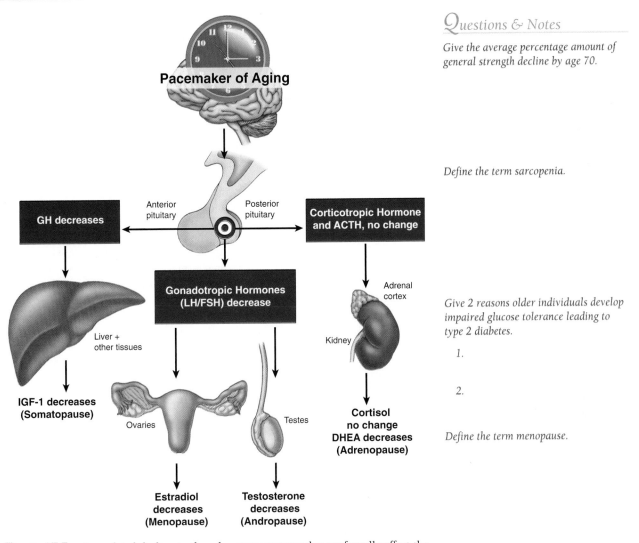

Figure 17.7.   Age-related decline in three hormone systems that profoundly affect the rate of biological aging. **Left,** Decreased growth hormone (GH) (released by the anterior pituitary) depresses production of IGF-1 to inhibit cellular growth (a condition of aging termed somatopause). **Middle,** Decreased output of LH and FSH by the anterior pituitary, coupled with reduced estradiol secretion from ovaries and testosterone from testes, causes menopause (females) and andropause (males). **Right,** Adrenocortical cells responsible for DHEA production decrease their activity (termed adrenopause) without clinically evident changes in this gland's corticotrophin (ACTH) and cortisol secretion. A central "pacemaker" in the hypothalamus and/or higher brain areas probably mediates these processes to produce aging-related changes in the ovaries, testicles, and adrenal cortex.

Questions & Notes

Give the average percentage amount of general strength decline by age 70.

Define the term sarcopenia.

Give 2 reasons older individuals develop impaired glucose tolerance leading to type 2 diabetes.

1.

2.

Define the term menopause.

Define the term andropause.

Define the term adrenopause.

creases in gonadotropic secretions from the anterior pituitary gland characterize male **andropause.**

Adrenal Cortex   **Adrenopause** refers to the significant decrease in output of dehydroepiandrosterone (DHEA) and its sulfated ester (DHEAS) from the adrenal cortex. In contrast to the glucocorticoid and mineralocorticoid adrenal steroids whose plasma levels remain relatively high with aging, a long, progressive, but slow decline in DHEA occurs after about age 30. This has led to speculation concerning DHEA's role in aging, prompting a dramatic increase in unregulated supplementation of this hormone.

Growth Hormone/Insulin-Like Growth Factor-1 Axis   Mean pulse amplitude, duration, and fraction of secreted growth hormone (GH) gradually decrease with aging, a condition termed **somatopause**. A parallel decrease in circulating levels of insulin-like growth factor (IGF-1) also takes place. IGF-1, produced by the liver and other cells, stimulates tissue growth and protein synthesis. The trigger for the age-related GH decrease probably lies in the interaction between the hypothalamus and anterior pituitary gland.

To what extent changes in gonadal function (menopause and andropause) contribute to adrenopause and somatopause in both sexes remains unknown. A growing body of evidence indicates that functional correlates, such as muscle size and strength, body composition, bone mass alterations, and progression of atherosclerosis, directly relate to hormonal changes with aging. Hormonal replacement therapy, nutritional supplementation, and regular exercise may suppress aspects of hormone-related aging dysfunction.

Aging and Nervous System Function

A 37% decline in the number of spinal cord axons and 10% decline in nerve conduction velocity reflect cumulative effects of aging on central nervous system function. Such changes partially explain age-related decrements in neuromuscular performance. Partitioning reaction time into central processing time and muscle contraction time indicates that aging exerts the greatest effect on stimulus detection and information processing to produce a response. For example, the knee-jerk reflex does not require central nervous system processing; it becomes less affected by aging than voluntary responses and movement patterns.

Despite the real effects of aging on reaction and movement time, physically active young or old groups move faster than a corresponding less active age group. These observations fuel speculation that regular participation in physical activity thwarts biologic aging of certain neuromuscular functions.

Aging and Pulmonary Function

Will regular exercise throughout one's life override pulmonary system "aging?" Cross-sectional studies indicate that dynamic pulmonary capacity of older endurance-trained athletes exceeds that of sedentary peers. Although longitudinal studies will provide a definitive answer, available data suggests that regular physical activity retards pulmonary function deterioration associated with aging. Much of this effect probably relates to the maintenance of power and endurance of the ventilatory musculature promoted by regular exercise.

Aging and Cardiovascular Function

Different indices of cardiovascular function and exercise endurance decline with age, yet regular physical activity can exert a profound influence on age-related decrements.

Maximal Oxygen Uptake Maximal oxygen uptake ($\dot{V}O_{2max}$) declines steadily after age 20, decreasing by 35%

to 40% at age 65 years (slightly less than 1% per year). A slower rate of decline occurs for individuals who maintain an active lifestyle that includes regular aerobic training, particularly with a decrease in fat-free body mass (FFM). *Physical activity, however, does not entirely offset aging's effect on $\dot{V}O_{2max}$, even when adjusting for a person's quantity of muscle mass.*

Figure 17.8 shows the relationship between $\dot{V}O_{2max}$ and active appendicular muscle mass for younger (average age, 25 years) and older (average age, 63 years) aerobically trained men and women. Younger subjects had trained for 9 consecutive years and older subjects had trained for 20 consecutive years. Older men and women exhibited about a 14% lower $\dot{V}O_{2max}$ than their younger counterparts throughout the broad range of variation in muscle mass among subjects. In other words, despite an equivalence in appendicular muscle mass between a young and older subject, the young subject exhibited a *higher* $\dot{V}O_{2max}$.

Age-associated loss of muscle mass, increase in body fat, and altered cardiovascular and pulmonary functions partially account for the deterioration in $\dot{V}O_{2max}$ with aging. The reductions in aerobic power per kg of active muscle mass with aging displayed in Figure 17.8 can reflect only age-associated reduced oxygen delivery and/or reduced oxygen extraction at the active muscle. Skeletal muscle oxidative capacity and capillarization (important components of oxygen extraction) remain similar in older and younger individuals with comparable physiologic characteristics and training histories. Consequently, the well-documented reduction in cardiac output (decreases in both maximum heart rate and stroke volume) represents the most likely explanation for the decrease in $\dot{V}O_{2max}$ per kg of active muscle that accompanies aging.

Aging Response to Exercise Training *For the healthy elderly, exercise training enhances the heart's capacity to pump blood and increases aerobic capacity to the same relative degree as in younger adults.* Nine to 12 months of endurance training in healthy older adults increased $\dot{V}O_{2max}$ 19% in men and 22% in women. These values represent the high end of the typical training response for young adults. Middle-age men who regularly engaged in aerobic training for more than 20 years significantly delayed the usual 10% to 15% decline in exercise capacity and aerobic fitness. At age 55, these active men maintained nearly the same values for blood pressure, body mass, and $\dot{V}O_{2max}$ as at age 35; by age 70, their $\dot{V}O_{2max}$ equaled values for individuals 25 years younger. These remarkable findings attest to the adaptability of the aerobic system to training at any age.

Other Age-Related Variables

Figure 17.9 shows longitudinal changes for maximum heart rate, minute pulmonary ventilation, and oxygen pulse (mL O_2 per heart beat; to estimate stroke volume) of 21 men tested at ages 50 (T1), 60 (T2), and 70 years (T3). The men trained continuously throughout the 20-year pe-

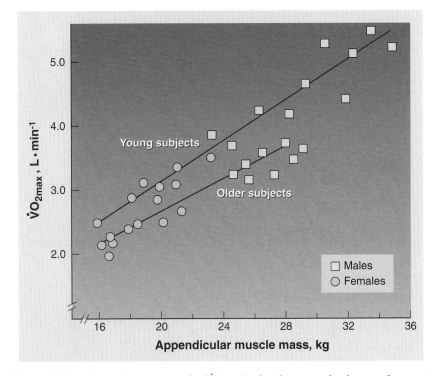

Figure 17.8. Maximal oxygen uptake ($\dot{V}O_{2max}$) related to appendicular muscle mass in young and older endurance-trained men and women. $\dot{V}O_{2max}$ per kg of active muscle mass decreases with age, independent of training status. (Modified from Proctor, D.N., Joyner, J.: Skeletal muscle mass and the reduction of $\dot{V}O_{2max}$ in trained older subjects. *J. Appl. Physiol.*, 82:1411, 1997.)

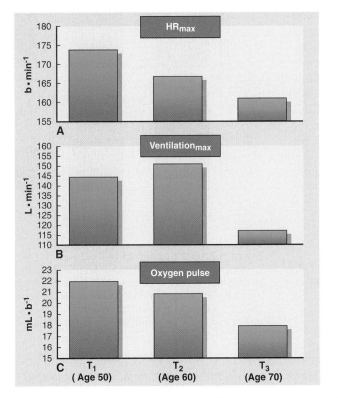

Figure 17.9. Changes in maximum **(A)** heart rate, **(B)** minute ventilation, and **(C)** oxygen pulse ($\dot{V}O_2$, mL·min^{-1} ÷ HR, b·min^{-1}) of 21 endurance athletes who continued to train over a 20-year period, beginning at age 50 years. (Modified from Pollock, M.L., et al.: Twenty-year follow-up of aerobic power and body composition of older track athletes. *J. Appl. Physiol.*, 82:1508, 1997.)

Questions & Notes

Define the term somatopause.

Give the percentage rate decline in $\dot{V}O_{2max}$ between age 20 and age 60.

Describe the general relationship between $\dot{V}O_{2max}$, L·min^{-1} and appendicular muscle mass, kg.

True or False:

The healthy elderly cannot enhance their cardiovascular capacity with exercise training to the same relative extent as younger counterparts.

Chapter 17 Exercise, Successful Aging, and Disease Prevention • 643

riod; each had placed either first, second, or third in regional, national, or international competition in running events during a 10-year measurement interval. With the exception of pulmonary ventilation (small increase at T2), each variable decreased over time. Maximum heart rate decreased by 5 to 7 beats per minute at each measurement over the 20 years (a smaller decrease than generally reported for nonathletes). Age-related decrements in maximum heart rate have been attributed to three factors:

1. Alterations in the innate activity of the sinoatrial (S-A) node
2. Reduced sympathetic activity output from the medulla
3. Reluctance of researchers to encourage older, nonathletic individuals to go "all-out" to achieve a maximal effort during testing

Reduction in the heart's stroke volume (indicated by the change in the oxygen pulse measurements) most likely reflects changes in myocardial contractility with aging. Other age-related cardiovascular changes include reduced blood flow capacity to peripheral tissues, narrowing of the coronary arteries (30% obstruction by middle age), and decreased elasticity of major blood vessels.

Aging and Body Composition

Excess body fat accumulation usually begins in childhood or develops slowly during adulthood. Middle-age men and women invariably weigh more than college-age counterparts of the same stature, with differences in body fat accounting for the weight difference. Researchers do not know whether gains in body fat during adulthood represent a normal biologic pattern. Observations of physically active older individuals suggest that the typical individual grows fatter with age, but those who remain physically active (1) counter the "normal" age-related loss in FFM, while (2) depressing the typical increase in body fat percentage.

Figure 17.10 shows body composition changes over a 20-year period for the same 21 elite master's runners depicted in Figure 17.9. Despite maintaining a relatively constant body mass during the prolonged period of exercise training (T1 = 70.1 kg; T2 = 69.4 kg; T3 = 70.8 kg), gains occurred in body fat while FFM declined. The roughly 3% body fat unit increase per decade paralleled similar increases in waist girth. These data support an argument that some alterations in body composition and body fat distribution represent a normal aging response.

In addition to preservation of FFM, a real concern about the lack of weight-bearing (mechanical loading) exercise deserves concern because it impacts on osteoporosis with aging. Longitudinal research of bone mineral content assessed every 6 months in children from age 6 to 12 years showed that 26% of adult total body bone mineral accrued during just 2 years of peak bone mineral deposition. Such direct evidence seems self-evident for its long range implications. Perhaps the eventual "cure" for osteo

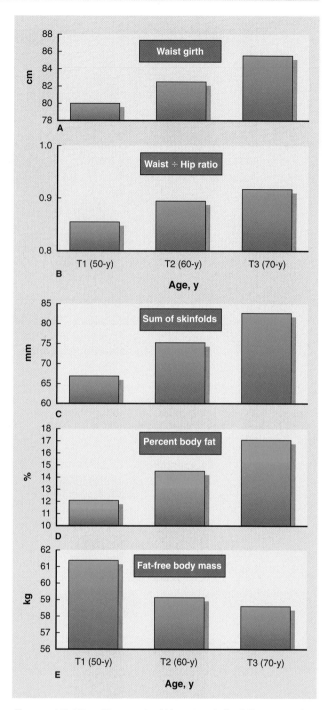

Figure 17.10. Changes in **(A)** waist girth, **(B)** waist-to-hip girth ratio, **(C)** sum of skinfolds, **(D)** percent body fat, and **(E)** fat-free body mass for 21 endurance athletes who continued to train over a 20-year period, starting at age 50 years. (Modified from Pollock, M.L., et al.: Twenty-year follow-up of aerobic power and body composition of older track athletes. *J. Appl. Physiol.*, 82:1508, 1997.)

porosis and its attendant medical and societal costs really should be viewed as a problem of young age (pediatric medicine) and not older age (geriatric medicine). From our perspective, we strongly endorse the position that increased physical activity should play an increasingly more important role as children grow into adolescence and adulthood. In this scenario, daily required classroom physical education begun in kindergarten seems worthwhile and entirely justified.

REGULAR EXERCISE: A FOUNTAIN OF YOUTH?

Exercise may not necessarily represent a "fountain of youth," yet the preponderance of evidence shows that regular physical activity retards the decline in functional capacity associated with aging and disuse. Exercise participation can reverse the loss of function regardless of when a person becomes active.

Actual Causes of Death in the United States

During the last two decades, substantial changes in lifestyle have led to variations in actual causes of death in the United States. Mortality rates from heart disease, stroke, and cancer have declined. Concurrently, behavioral changes have increased the prevalence of obesity and type 2 diabetes. The latest research detailing actual cause of death in the United States in the year 2000 is summarized in **Table 17.1**. Diseases of the heart (710,760), malignant neoplasma and cancers (555,091), and cerebrovascular disease (167,661) account for the majority of deaths.

Table 17.2 compares the **actual causes of deaths** in 1990 and 2000. The most striking finding is the substantial increase in the number of estimated deaths attributable to poor diet and physical inactivity. The gap between deaths due to poor diet and physical inactivity and those due to cigarette smoking has narrowed substantially. *Clearly, about one-half of all deaths that occurred in the United States in 2000 could be attributed to a limited number of largely preventable behaviors and exposures, most of which relate directly to physical inactivity and overfatness.* Unless curtailed, the increasing trend of overfatness, poor diet and physical inactivity will likely overtake tobacco as the leading preventable cause of mortality in the United States. Clearly, the need exists to establish a more preventive orientation in health care and public health systems in the United States.

Does Exercise Improve Health and Extend Life?

Medical experts have debated whether a lifetime of regular exercise contributes to good health and perhaps longevity compared with a sedentary "good life." Because older, fit individuals exhibit many functional characteristics of younger people, one could argue that improved physical fitness and a vigorous lifestyle in older age retard biologic aging and confer health benefits later in life.

Questions & Notes

Give 2 reasons for age-related decrements in maximum heart rate.

1.

2.

Describe what happens to waist girth, percentage body fat, and FFM with aging, independent of physical activity level.

List the 3 leading causes of death in the U.S. in the year 2000.

1.

2.

3.

Table 17•1	Leading Causes of Death in the United States in 2000		
CAUSE OF DEATH		**NUMBER OF DEATHS**	**DEATH RATE PER 100,000 POPULATION**
Heart disease		710,760	258.2
Malignant neoplasm		553,091	200.9
Cerebrovascular disease		167,661	60.9
Chronic lower respiratory tract disease		122,009	44.3
Unintentional injuries		97,900	35.6
Diabetes mellitus		69,301	25.2
Influenza and pneumonia		65,313	23.7
Alzheimer disease		49,558	18.0
Nephritis, nephritic syndrome, nephrosis		37,251	13.5
Septicemia (bacterial infections)		31,224	11.3
Other		449,283	181.4
Total		**2,403,351**	**873.1**

From Mokdad, A.H., et al.: Actual causes of death in the United States, 2000. *JAMA*, 291:1238, 2005.

FOR YOUR INFORMATION

Should Cholesterol Be Measured in Children?

Guidelines issued by the National Cholesterol Education Program (http://www. americanheart.org) conclude "yes" if a family history of high cholesterol or heart disease exists (particularly if a parent suffered a heart attack before age 50). Shockingly, this parental "cardiac proneness" includes up to one-fourth of the United States adult population! Research with children age 10 to 15 years indicates that lifestyle habits like regular exercise, improved cardiovascular fitness, and a prudent nutritional profile contribute to favorable lipid profiles similar to effects with adults.

Table 17•2	Actual Causes of Death in the United States in 1990 and 2000	
ACTUAL CAUSE	**NUMBER (%) 1990[a]**	**NUMBER (%) 2000[b]**
Tobacco	400,000 (19%)	435,000 (18.1%)
Poor diet and physical inactivity	**300,000 (14%)**	**400,000 (16.6%)**
Alcohol consumption	100,000 (5%)	85,000 (3.5%)
Microbial agents	90,000 (4%)	75,000 (3.1%)
Toxic agents	60,000 (3%)	55,000 (2.3%)
Motor vehicle	25,000 (1%)	43,000 (1.8%)
Firearms	35,000 (2%)	29,000 (1.2%)
Sexual behavior	30,000 (1%)	20,000 (0.8%)
Illicit drug use	20,000 (<1%)	17,000 (0.7%)

[a] Data from McGinnis, J.M., Foege, W.H.: Actual causes of death in the United States, 1990. *JAMA*, 270:2207, 1993.
[b] Date from Mokdad, A.H., et al.: Actual causes of death in the United States, 2000. *JAMA*, 291:1238, 2005.

Research concerning current lifestyles and exercise habits of 17,000 Harvard alumni who entered college between 1916 and 1950 *indicates that only moderate aerobic exercise, equivalent to jogging 3 miles a day, promotes good health and adds time to life.* Men who expended 2000 kCal in weekly exercise had up to one-third lower death rates than classmates who did little or no exercise. To achieve a 2000 kCal energy output weekly requires moderate additional physical activity such as a daily 30- to 45-minute brisk walk or a moderate run, cycle, swim, cross-country ski, or aerobic dance participation. The following summarizes the results of the long-term study of alumni:

1. Regular exercise counters the life-shortening effects of cigarette smoking and excess body weight
2. Even for people with high blood pressure (a primary heart disease risk), those who exercised regularly reduced their death rate by one-half
3. Regular exercise countered genetic tendencies toward an early death. Individuals with one or both parents who died before age 65 (another significant but non-modifiable risk), reduced death risk by 25% with a lifestyle that included regular exercise
4. A 50% reduction in mortality rate occurred for active men whose parents lived beyond 65 years

Figure 17.11 shows that, among physically active people, a person who exercises more reduces risk of death. For example, men who walked 9 or more miles a week had a 21% lower mortality rate than men who walked 3 miles or less. Exercising in light sports activities increased life expectancy 24% over men who remained sedentary. From a

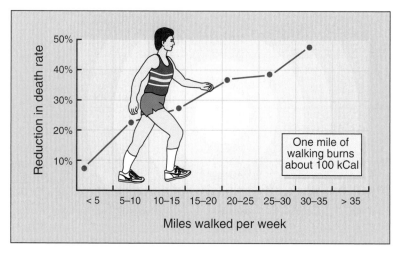

Figure 17.11. Reduced risk of death with regular exercise. (Data from Paffenbarger, R.S., Jr, et al.: Physical activity, all-cause mortality, and longevity of college alumni. *N. Engl. J. Med.*, 314:605, 1986.)

perspective of energy expenditure, the life expectancy of Harvard alumni increased steadily from a weekly exercise energy output of 500 kCal to 3500 kCal, the equivalent of 6 to 8 hours of strenuous weekly exercise. In addition, active men lived an average of 1 to 2 years longer than sedentary classmates. (Other research estimates a life expectancy increase of about 10 months with regular exercise.)

No additional health or longevity benefits accrued beyond weekly exercise of 3500 kCal. Men who performed extreme exercise had higher death rates than less active colleagues (another example of why *more* does not necessarily indicate *better* exercise benefits).

Improved Fitness: A Little Goes a Long Way

A study of more than 13,000 men and women over an 8-year interval indicates that even modest amounts of exercise substantially reduce the risk of death from heart disease, cancer, and other causes. The study evaluated fitness performance directly rather than by relying on verbal or written reports of physical activity habits. To isolate the effect of physical fitness per se, the researchers considered factors of smoking, cholesterol and blood sugar levels, blood pressure, and family history of coronary heart disease. **Figure 17.12**, based on age-adjusted death rates per 10,000 person-years, illustrates that the least fit group died at a 3 times greater rate than the most fit subjects.

The most striking finding was that the group rated just above the most sedentary category derived the greatest change in health benefits. The decrease in death rate for men from the least fit to the next category equaled 38 (64.0 vs. 25.5 deaths per 10,000 person-years), whereas the decline from the second group to the most fit category equaled only 7. Women obtained similar benefits as men. The amount of exercise required moving from the most sedentary category to the next more fit category (the jump showing the greatest increase in health benefits) was moderate-intensity exercise like walking briskly for 30 minutes several times weekly. *If life-extending benefits of exercise exist, they are associated more with preventing early mortality than improving overall life span.* Although the maximum life span may not extend greatly, only moderate exercise enables individuals to live a more productive and healthy life.

Changes in Physical Activity and Mortality Among Older Women
Studies of changes in physical activity and mortality have mostly examined middle-

Questions & Notes

Give 2 major findings of the Harvard Alumni Study of physical activity and health.

1.

2.

This amount of exercise (distance jogged per day) is necessary to promote good health and add time to life, according to the Harvard Health Study.

The life-extending benefits of exercise associate more with preventing early _____ than improving overall _____.

True or False:

Health benefits from regular exercise are about the same for men and women.

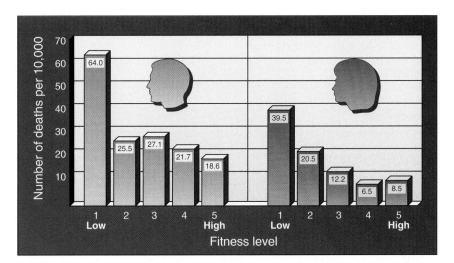

Figure 17.12. Physical fitness and risk of death. The greatest reduction in death rate risk occurs when going from the most sedentary category to a moderate fitness level. (Data from Blair, S.N., et al.: Physical fitness and all-cause mortality: A prospective study of healthy men and women. *JAMA*, 262:2395, 1989.)

aged male populations. It remains unclear whether adoption of a physically active lifestyle by previously sedentary older women, particularly those with chronic cardiovascular disease, diabetes, and physical frailty, produces similar benefits typically observed for men. **Figure 17.13** summarizes a unique study of 9704 mostly white women aged at least 65 years who were followed for 12.5 years. They were classified at baseline and 4.0 to 7.7 years later into one of four groups (quintiles, from highest to lowest) based on physical activity level (amount of walking per day and frequency and duration of other leisure time activities such as dancing, gardening, aerobics, swimming). The four groups were (1) active at baseline and stayed active during follow-up; (2) active at baseline but became sedentary during the follow-up; (3) sedentary at baseline and remained sedentary at follow-up; and (4) sedentary at baseline but became active at follow-up. All-cause mortality data were compared between groups up to 12.5 years after baseline (6.7 years after the follow-up visit).

Compared with continually sedentary women, women who were active or who become active had lower all-cause mortality. Notably, sedentary women who increased daily physical activity to the equivalent of 1 mile of walking between baseline and follow-up had 40% to 50% lower all-cause mortality rates than chronically sedentary women. These findings take on added importance because the population of older women in the U.S. will double in the next 30 years, and more than one-third is now sedentary. *Modest increases in physical activity would improve the risk factor profile.*

CORONARY HEART DISEASE

Table 17.1 illustrated that diseases of the heart and blood vessels cause the majority of total deaths in the United States. Deaths from coronary heart disease have declined more than 35% since 1970, yet heart disease still remains the leading cause of death in the Western world. For every American who dies of cancer, almost two die of heart-related diseases. Death rates for women lag about 10 years behind men, but the gap has rapidly closed for women who smoke; for them, heart disease is now the leading cause of death. Despite limited heart disease research on women, available evidence indicates that disease symptoms, progression, and outcome differ in women and men. Four gender-related heart disease differences include:

1. Women usually die sooner after a heart attack
1. Women who survive a heart attack frequently experience a second episode
2. Women become more incapacitated by heart disease-related pain and disability
3. Women are less likely to survive coronary artery bypass surgery

Changes on the Cellular Level

Coronary heart disease (CHD) involves degenerative changes in the intima or inner lining of the larger arteries that supply the myocardium. Damage to arterial walls begins as a low-grade chronic inflammatory response to injury, perhaps from hypertension, cigarette smoking, infection, homocysteine, elevated cholesterol, free radicals, reaction to obesity-related substances, or immunologically mediated factors. One response triggers the chemical modification of various compounds, including oxidation of low-density lipoprotein cholesterol (LDL-C). LDL-C oxidation represents a crucial step in a complex series of changes that produce lesions that sometimes bulge into the vessel lumen or protrude into the arterial wall. Lesions

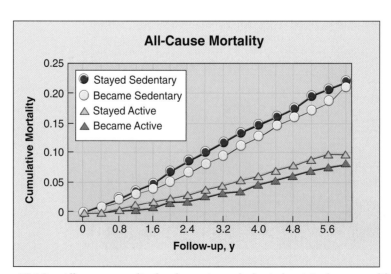

Figure 17.13. All-cause mortality by change in total physical activity by years of follow-up in older women. (Gregg, E.W., et al.: Relationship of changes in physical activity and mortality among older women. *JAMA*, 289:2379, 2003.)

initially take the form of fatty streaks, the first signs of atherosclerosis. With further inflammatory damage from continued lipid deposition and proliferation of smooth muscle and connective tissue, the vessels congest with lipid-filled plaques, fibrous scar tissue, or both. Progressive occlusion gradually reduces blood flow capacity, causing the myocardium to become ischemic or poorly supplied with oxygen.

Vulnerable Plaque: Difficult to Detect yet Lethal Vulnerable plaque, a soft type of metabolically active, unstable plaque, does not necessarily produce significant coronary artery narrowing but tends to fissure and burst. The rupture of unstable plaque—the sudden breakdown of fatty plaques in the lining of the coronary arteries—exposes the blood to thrombogenic compounds. This triggers a cascade of chemical events that culminates in clot formation (thrombus) and leads to myocardial infarction and possible death. The sudden, complete obstruction of a coronary artery frequently occurs in blood vessels with only mild-to-moderate obstructions (~70% blockage). Arterial blockage often occurs before the coronary vessel has narrowed enough to produce angina symptoms or electrocardiographic (ECG) abnormalities or to indicate the need for revascularization procedures (e.g., coronary bypass surgery or balloon angioplasty). Acute disruption and rupture of arterial plaque provides a plausible explanation for sudden death from acute physical and emotional exertion in middle-aged men with coronary artery disease compared with sudden death under resting conditions. The beneficial effects of cholesterol-lowering strategies on heart disease risk do not always improve coronary blood flow. A reduction in overall blood cholesterol may improve the stability of vulnerable plaque. This stabilizing effect would reduce the likelihood of future rupture of existing coronary artery plaque.

A Life-Long Process

Landmark studies of atherosclerosis in 22-year-old American soldiers killed in Korea showed they had advanced lesions. These findings surprised the medical community and focused attention on the possible childhood origins of atherosclerosis. Researchers now know that fatty streaks and clinically significant fibrous plaques develop rapidly during adolescence through the third decade of life.

Body mass index, systolic and diastolic blood pressure, and total serum cholesterol, triacylglycerols, and low-density lipoprotein cholesterol (LDL-C) strongly and positively related (high-density lipoprotein cholesterol [HDL-C] related negatively) to the extent of vascular lesions in the deceased young people. History of cigarette smoking magnified the vascular damage. As the number of risk factors increased, so did the severity of atherosclerosis. Analyses of microscopic qualities of coronary atherosclerosis in teenagers and young adults who died as a result of accidents, suicide, and murder indicated that many had arteries so clogged that they could suffer a myocardial infarction. Two percent of those aged 15 to 19 years and 20% of those aged 30 to 34 years had advanced plaque formation, the blockages considered most likely to tear away from the arterial walls and trigger a heart attack or stroke. Collectively, these and other data support the wisdom of primary prevention of atherosclerosis through risk factor identification and intervention early in childhood or adolescence.

Figure 17.14 shows the progressive occlusion of an artery from a buildup of calcified fatty substances in atherosclerosis. The first overt sign of atherosclerotic change occurs when lipid-laden macrophage cells cluster under the endothelial lining to form a bulge (fatty streak) in the artery. Over time, proliferating smooth muscle cells accumulate to narrow the artery's lumen (center). Typically, a clot (**thrombus**) forms and plugs the artery, depriving the myocardium of normal blood flow with its oxygen supply. When the thrombus blocks one of the smaller coronary vessels, a portion of the heart muscle dies (necrosis), and the person suffers a heart attack or **myocardial infarction** (**MI**). MIs are caused by (1) blockage in one or more arteries supplying the heart, thus cutting off myocardial blood supply, or (2) sud-

Questions & Notes

Name the leading cause of death in the western world.

Give 2 gender-specific differences related to heart disease.

  1.

  2.

What is vulnerable plaque and why is it important?

List 4 variables that positively relate to vascular lesions.

  1.

  2.

  3.

  4.

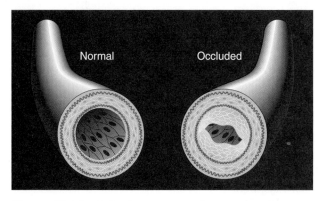

Figure 17.14. Left, Cross-section of a normal coronary artery. **Right,** Deterioration of a coronary artery in atherosclerosis; deposits of fatty substances roughen the vessel's center.

den spasms (constrictions) of a coronary vessel, which causes tissue necrosis from lack of oxygen. MI contrasts with **cardiac arrest** caused by irregular neural–electrical transmission within the myocardium. Cardiac arrest results from chaotic, unregulated beating of the heart's upper chambers (atrial fibrillation) or lower chambers (ventricular fibrillation).

If coronary artery narrowing leads to brief periods of inadequate myocardial perfusion, the person may experience temporary chest pains termed **angina pectoris** (see Chapter 18). These pains usually emerge during exertion because increased physical activity creates a great demand for myocardial blood flow. Anginal attacks provide painful, dramatic evidence of the importance of adequate myocardial oxygen supply.

Seven Heart Attack Warning Signs The American Heart Association (*http://www.aha.org*) and other medical experts say that one or more of these seven warning signs can help to identify an impending heart attack:

1. Uncomfortable pressure, fullness, squeezing, or pain in the center of the chest lasting more than a few minutes
2. Pain spreading to the shoulders, neck, or arms. The pain ranges from mild to intense. It may feel like pressure, tightness, burning, or heavy weight. It may be located in the chest, upper abdomen, neck, jaw, or inside the arms or shoulders.
3. Chest discomfort with lightheadedness, fainting, sweating, nausea, or shortness of breath
4. Anxiety, nervousness, and/or cold, sweaty skin
5. Paleness or pallor
6. Increased or irregular heart rate
7. Feeling of impending doom

Cardiovascular Disease Epidemic

Each year, cardiovascular diseases top the list of the country's most serious health problems. Coronary heart disease

remains the leading health problem and the primary cause of death. It represents the most expensive condition to treat as it exemplifies a resource-intensive chronic condition. Consider recent (2001–2002) statistics released by the American Heart Association (AHA) (**Fig. 17.15**):

- At least 64.4 million people (one person in four) in the United States suffer from some form of cardiovascular disease.
- Cardiovascular disease is the primary killer of women and men. Diseases of the cardiovascular system claim the lives of more than half a million females every year, about a death a minute.
- Cardiovascular disease accounts for almost 1 of every 2.4 deaths.
- Since 1900, cardiovascular disease was the leading cause of death in every year but 1918, and it caused more deaths than the next seven causes combined.
- Every 34 seconds, an American suffers a coronary event; each minute, someone dies from one.
- No previous symptoms of the disease existed in 57% of men and 64% of women who died suddenly from cardiovascular disease.
- In 2004, cardiovascular disease cost an estimated $368.4 billion.

CORONARY HEART DISEASE RISK FACTORS: DEBUNKING THE "ONLY 50%" MYTH

Research over the past 40 years has identified four major modifiable cardiovascular risk factors: **cigarette smoking, diabetes mellitus, hypertension,** and **hypercholesterol-**

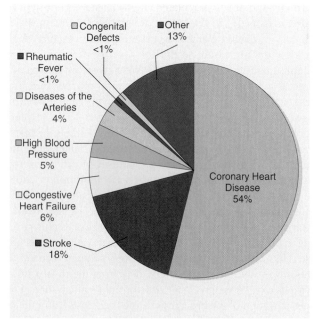

Figure 17.15. Deaths due to cardiovascular diseases.

emia. These factors supposedly account for only about 50% of those individuals who subsequently develop coronary heart disease. Thus, researchers have spent considerable time and energy investigating novel markers and other nontraditional risk factor candidates to increase cardiovascular risk predictability. **Table 17.3** presents different novel risk factors that independently associate with atherosclerotic vascular disease.

Several reports directly challenge this "only 50%" claim for the aforementioned four risk factors. Analysis of data from 14 randomized clinical trials (n = 122,458) and three observational studies (n = 386,915) showed that, in contrast to previous belief, 80% to 90% of patients who developed clinically significant CHD and more than 95% of patients who experienced a fatal CHD event in fact had at least one of the four traditional major risk factors, including overweight/obesity and a sedentary lifestyle. Remarkably, these findings may even underestimate the true extent of this relationship, given the self-report design of the observational studies because a number of patients were likely unaware or not diagnosed as having risk factors at the time of evaluation. These findings have enormous public health implications for targeting a large segment of the population at risk of developing CHD. Smoking is arguably the single most important modifiable and preventable cardiovascular disease risk factor and one of the strongest predictors of premature CHD. *Obesity and physical inactivity may turn out as equally important predictors of CHD.*

None of the factors listed in Table 17.3 conclusively adds prognostic information for accurate CHD prediction beyond determining suboptimal levels of cholesterol, blood pressure, cigarette smoking, diabetes, physical inactivity and overweight/obesity.

Cigarette Smoking

Cigarette smoking, either active or passive through environmental exposure, directly increases CHD risk. Smokers experience twice the risk of death from heart disease as nonsmokers. The risk increases further for smokers with diabetes and hypertension. The Centers for Disease Control and Prevention estimates that every cigarette smoked steals 7 minutes from a smoker's life. This adds up to 5

FOR YOUR INFORMATION

Diabetes Risk Significantly Lowered with Regular Exercise

Men who exercise five or more times a week show a 42% lower risk of type 2 diabetes than men who exercise less than once a week. The exercise benefits become most pronounced among obese participants. The risk of diabetes decreases approximately 6% for every 500 kCal of additional weekly exercise.

FOR YOUR INFORMATION

Exercise Is Good Medicine for the Colon

Research based on the health and exercise habits of Harvard alumni indicates that physically active men had about one-half the risk of colon cancer as inactive classmates. The protection disappeared if the men stopped exercising. One mechanism proposes that exercise protects against this major killer by speeding the passage of food residues through the digestive tract that reduces the colon's exposure to any potential food carcinogens.

Table 17·3	Novel Risk Factors for Atherosclerotic Vascular Disease			
INFLAMMATORY MARKERS	**HEMOSTASIS/ THROMBOSIS MARKERS**	**PLATELET-RELATED FACTORS**	**LIPID-RELATED FACTORS**	**OTHER FACTORS**
• C-reactive protein • Interleukins (e.g., IL-6) • Serum amyloid A • Vascular and cellular adhesion molecules • Soluble CD40 ligand • Leukocyte count	• Fibrinogen • Von Willebrand factor antigen • Plasminogen activator inhibitor 1 (PAI-1) • Tissue-plasminogen activator • Factors V, VII, VIII • D-dimer • Fibrinopeptide A • Prothrombin fragment	• Platelet aggregation • Platelet activity • Platelet size and volume	• Low-density lipoprotein (LDL) • Lipoprotein(a) • Remnant lipoproteins • Apolipoproteins A1 and B • High-density lipoprotein (HDL) • Oxidized LDL	• Homocysteine • Lipoprotein-associated phospholipase A(2) • Microalbuminuria • Insulin resistance • PAI-1 genotype • Angiotensin-converting enzyme genotype • ApoE genotype • Infectious agents (cytomegalovirus, chlamydia, pneumonia, helicobacter pylori, herpes simplex virus) • Psychosocial factors

million years of potential life Americans lose to cigarettes yearly. CHD risk increases the more one smokes (or receives passive exposure), the deeper one inhales, and the stronger the cigarette (for tars and noxious byproducts). The increasing death rate from heart disease among women in the United States almost parallels their increased cigarette use. British researchers estimate that smokers between age 30 and 40 years suffer five times as many heart attacks as nonsmokers in the same age range. When these relatively young smokers suffer a heart attack, an 80% chance exists that smoking caused it; this percentage averages nearly 70% for smokers in their 50s and 50% for smokers in their 60s and 70s. Also, smokers run a five times greater risk for stroke than nonsmokers, and those who smoke one pack or more each day are 11 times more likely to suffer a specific type of sudden, deadly stroke most common in younger men and women. Surprisingly, the CHD risk from smoking correlates with more deaths than the excess mortality of cigarette smokers from lung cancer.

Smoking risk usually remains independent of other risk factors. If additional risk factors exist, then smoking accentuates their influence. Cigarette smoking facilitates heart disease through its potentiating effect on serum lipoproteins; individuals who smoke have lower levels of HDL-C than nonsmokers. When smokers quit, the HDL-C and heart disease risk return to levels of nonsmokers. A frightening statistic predicts that by the year 2030, smoking will become the world's single leading cause of death and disability.

Blood Lipid Abnormalities

An abnormal blood lipid level or hyperlipidemia provides a crucial component in the genesis of atherosclerosis. Figure 17.16 shows the rate of increase in death risk from CHD related to total serum cholesterol. Current guidelines focus less on total cholesterol and more on its lipoprotein components (see How to Classify Cholesterol, Lipoproteins, and Triacylglycerol Values on page 655). Early treatment becomes crucial because of a strong association between high serum cholesterol as a young adult and cardiovascular disease in middle age. A cholesterol level of 200 mg·dL^{-1} or lower is usually desirable, although risk for a fatal heart attack begins to rise at 150 mg·dL^{-1}. A cholesterol level of 230 mg·dL^{-1} increases heart attack risk to about twice that of 180 mg·dL^{-1}, and 300 mg·dL^{-1} increases the risk fourfold. For triacylglycerols, the National Cholesterol Education Program considers 200 mg·dL^{-1} an upper limit of normal triacylglycerol level, with 200 to 400 mg·dL^{-1} considered borderline, requiring changes in exercise, diet, and possibly drug treatment if accompanied by other CHD risk factors. More than likely, triacylglycerol levels above 100 mg·dL^{-1} pose a cardiac risk. Individuals with triacylglycerol levels above 100 mg·dL^{-1} (after a 12-h fast) show a 50% greater CHD risk than those with triacylglycerols below 100 mg·dL^{-1}, even after controlling for HDL-C.

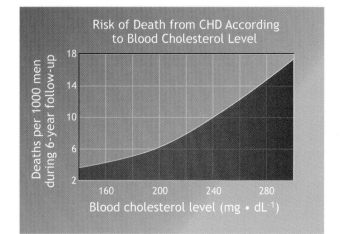

Figure 17.16. Generalized risk for death from coronary heart disease (CHD) in relation to total serum cholesterol level. (Adapted from Martin, M.J., et al.: Serum cholesterol, blood pressure and mortality: Implications from a cohort of 361,662 men. *Lancet*, 2:933, 1986.)

Major clinical drug trials show conclusively that reducing cholesterol lowers death rates and prevents heart attacks. Medications that affect blood lipids include (1) bile acid sequestrants (e.g., cholestyramine resin and colestipol hydrochloride), which bind bile acids and stimulate conversion of cholesterol to bile acids and facilitate removal of cholesterol from serum; (2) fibric acid derivatives (e.g., gemfibrozil, probucol, clofibrate), which lower triacylglycerols and LDL-C (5% to 20%) and elevate HDL-C (average 6% per year); and (3) the remarkably effective statins (e.g., lovastatin, pravastatin, simvastatin, atorvastatin), which inhibit an enzyme that controls cholesterol synthesis by the cell, increase LDL-C receptors in the liver, and facilitate LDL-C removal from serum (18% to 55% reduction). Raising HDL-C by 34 mg·dL^{-1} via a 5-year gemfibrozil therapy trial reduced heart attacks, strokes, and death by 24% in patients with initially low HDL-C levels.

In July, 2004, the National Cholesterol Education Program (*http://www.nhlbi.nih.gov/ chd/*), based on a review of five recent studies involving more than 50,000 patients, recommended more intensive drug treatment (statins) to help meet new guidelines established for LDL cholesterol. The update identifies a subset of patients as very high risk and suggests they reduce LDL cholesterol to below 70 mg·dL^{-1}. Only 5% of women and 2% of men in the United States have an LDL cholesterol level below 70; the average is 130. In 2001, the program lowered the LDL cholesterol goal for high-risk patients to below 100. A risk assessment calculator from the National Cholesterol Education Program uses information from the Framingham Heart Study to predict a person's chance of having a heart attack in the next 10 years. This internet-based tool is designed for adults aged 20 and older without heart disease or diabetes (*http://www.nhlb.nih.gov/about/ncep*).

Lipids do not circulate freely in blood plasma; they combine with a carrier protein to form lipoproteins composed of a hydrophobic cholesterol core and coat of free cholesterol, phospholipid, and a regulatory protein (apolipoprotein [Apo]). Table 17.4 lists the four different lipoproteins, their approximate gravitational densities, and their percentage of composition in the blood. Serum cholesterol is a composite of the total cholesterol contained in each of the different lipoproteins. Although discussions commonly refer to hyperlipidemia, the more meaningful focus addresses the different types of hyperlipoproteinemias.

Cholesterol distribution among the various lipoproteins provides a more powerful predictor of heart disease risk than total blood cholesterol. Specifically, elevated HDL-C levels relate causally with a *lower* heart disease risk, even among individuals with total cholesterol below 200 mg·dL^{-1}. Overwhelming evidence links high LDL-C and apolipoprotein (B) levels with *increased* CHD risk. A more effective evaluation of heart disease risk than either total cholesterol or LDL-C levels divides total cholesterol by HDL-C. A ratio greater than 4.5 indicates high heart disease risk; a ratio of 3.5 or lower represents a more desirable risk level.

LDL-C (synthesized in the liver) and very low–density lipoprotein cholesterol (VLDL-C) provide the transport medium for fats to cells, including the smooth muscle walls of arteries. Upon oxidation, LDL-C participates in artery-clogging, plaque-forming atherosclerosis by stimulating monocyte-macrophage infiltration, and lipoprotein deposition. LDL-C's surface coat contains the specific apolipoprotein (Apo B) that facilitates cholesterol removal from the LDL-C molecule by binding to LDL-C receptors of specific cells. Prevention of LDL-C oxidation slows the progression of CHD. In this regard, the potential benefit of the dietary antioxidants vitamins C and E and β-carotene on heart-disease risk reflect how well they blunt LDL-C oxidation.

LDL-C targets peripheral tissue and contributes to arterial damage, and HDL-C (also produced in the liver and whose levels relate to genetic factors) facilitates reverse cholesterol transport. HDL-C promotes surplus cholesterol removal from peripheral tissues (including arterial walls) for transport to the liver for bile synthesis and subsequent excretion via the digestive tract. The apolipoprotein A-1 (Apo A-1) in HDL-C activates the enzyme lecithin acetyl transferase (LCAT) that converts free cholesterol into cholesterol esters. This facilitates removal of cholesterol from lipoproteins and other tissues.

Factors that Affect Blood Lipids

Six diverse behaviors favorably impact the blood lipid profile:

1. Weight loss
2. Regular aerobic exercise (independent of weight loss)
3. Increased intake of water-soluble fibers (fibers in beans, legumes, and oat bran)
4. Increased dietary intake of polyunsaturated to saturated fatty acid ratio and monounsaturated fatty acids

FOR YOUR INFORMATION

Most Popular Exercises for Americans

Activity	Percentage	
	Male	Female
Walking	39	48
Resistance training	20	9
Cycling	16	15
Running	12	6
Stair climbing	10	12
Aerobics	3	10

FOR YOUR INFORMATION

Physical Activity and Women: How Much Is Good Enough?

Scientific data now shows conclusively that modest and achievable levels of physical activity (30 minutes per day on most days) decreases the risk of chronic diseases including breast cancer. Appropriate dietary restraint (and this is essential), coupled with increased physical activity, can help overweight women reduce weight. When prescribing physical activity, allied health professionals should set a goal of 30 minutes per day of moderate-intensity activity. This can be accumulated in bouts of at least 10 minutes most days of the week. For those willing to do more and for whom no contraindications exist, greater duration and increased intensity of activity confers additional benefits. (Jakicic, J.M. *JAMA*, 290:1323, 2003; Lee, I.-M. *JAMA*, 290:1377, 2003; and Manson, J.E. *N. Engl. J. Med.*, 347:716, 2002.)

Table 17·4   Approximate Composition of Lipoproteins in the Blood

	CHYLOMICRONS	VERY LOW-DENSITY LIPOPROTEINS (VLDL: PREBETA)	LOW-DENSITY LIPOPROTEINS (LDL: BETA)	HIGH-DENSITY LIPOPROTEINS (HDL: ALPHA)
Density, g·cm^{-3}	0.95	0.95–1.006	1.006–1.019	1.063–1.210
Protein, %	0.5–1.0	5–15	25	45–55
Lipid, %	99	95	75	50
Cholesterol, %	2–5	10–20	40–45	18
Triacylglycerol, %	85	50–70	5–10	2
Phospholipid, %	3–6	10–20	20–25	30

5. Increased dietary intake of unique polyunsaturated fatty acids in fish oils (omega-3 fatty acids)
6. Moderate alcohol consumption

Four variables adversely affect cholesterol and lipoprotein levels:

1. Cigarette smoking
2. Diet high in saturated fatty acids, *trans* fatty acids, and preformed cholesterol
3. Emotionally stressful situations
4. Oral contraceptives

Hypertension

More than 35 million Americans currently have systolic blood pressure that exceeds 140 mm Hg (systolic hypertension) or diastolic pressure that exceeds 90 mm Hg (diastolic hypertension). These values form the lower limit for the classification of *borderline* high blood pressure. One out of every four or five people experience chronic, abnormally high blood pressure sometime during their life. Uncorrected hypertension can precipitate heart failure, heart attack, stroke, and kidney failure.

Modification of lifestyle behaviors can lower blood pressure, often called the *"silent killer"*; important modifications include weight loss, cessation of smoking (nicotine constricts peripheral blood vessels that elevates blood pressure), and reducing salt intake (excess sodium retains fluid that elevates blood pressure in susceptible individuals). Unfortunately, the cause(s) of hypertension remains unknown in more than 90% of individuals. Men and women age 30 to 54 years with mild hypertension modestly lowered systolic (2.9 mm Hg) and diastolic (2.3 mm Hg) blood pressure when they reduced body weight and salt intake over an 18-month period. No blood pressure changes occurred for subjects who undertook only stress reduction and relaxation techniques or consumed calcium, magnesium, phosphorus, and fish oil dietary supplements. Prescription drugs that either reduce fluid volume or decrease peripheral resistance to blood flow effectively treat high blood pressure. Experts estimate that each 2 mm Hg reduction in blood pressure decreases CHD risk by 4% and stroke by 6%.

Diabetes

Diabetics are two to four times more likely to develop cardiovascular disease from multiple risk factors usually coincident with the diabetic condition. These factors include:

1. *Obesity* represents a major risk factor for cardiovascular disease that strongly associates with insulin resistance. Insulin resistance may be a mechanism by which obesity leads to cardiovascular disease. Weight loss improves cardiovascular risk, decreases insulin concentration, and increases insulin sensitivity.

2. *Physical inactivity* is a modifiable major risk factor for insulin resistance and cardiovascular disease. Exercising more while reducing excess body weight (and fat) prevents or delays the onset of type 2 diabetes, reduces blood pressure, and helps to reduce heart attack and stroke risk.

3. *Hypertension* positively correlates with insulin resistance in diabetes. When a person possesses hypertension and diabetes, a common combination, their risk for cardiovascular disease doubles.

4. *Atherogenic dyslipidemia*, often called diabetic dyslipidemia in diabetics, relates to insulin resistance characterized by high levels of triacylglycerols (hypertriglyceridemia) and high levels of small LDL particles and low levels of HDL. This lipid triad often occurs in patients with premature coronary heart disease. All of the components of the *lipid triad* contribute to atherosclerotic risk. Most diabetics do not have elevated LDL cholesterol, yet their LDL levels are high enough to support the development of atherosclerosis.

Other CHD Risk Factor Candidates

The following factors, (not causally linked) are potentially potent CHD risk predictors.

Age, Gender, and Heredity Age represents a CHD risk factor because it is associated with other risk factors—hypertension, elevated blood lipid levels, and glucose intolerance. After age 35 years in men and age 45 years in women, the chances of dying from CHD increase progressively and dramatically. Heredity also represents a risk factor, in that heart attacks that strike at an early age tend to run in families. Such familial predisposition probably relates to a genetic role in determining risk of heart disease.

Immunologic Factors An immune response may trigger plaque development within arterial walls. During this process, mononuclear immune cells produce proteins called cytokines, some of which stimulate plaque buildup while others inhibit plaque formation. Within this framework, regular exercise may stimulate the immune system to inhibit agents that facilitate arterial disease. For example, 2.5 hours of weekly exercise for 6 months decreased cytokine production that aids plaque development by 58%, while cytokines that inhibit plaque formation increased by nearly 36%. A fruitful line of research should pursue whether regular exercise stimulates the immune system in a way that inhibits infectious agents from initiating arterial disease.

Homocysteine Homocysteine, a highly reactive, sulfur-containing amino acid, forms as a byproduct of methionine metabolism. Researchers in the 1960s and 1970s described three different inborn errors of homocysteine

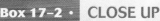

Box 17–2 • CLOSE UP

HOW TO CLASSIFY CHOLESTEROL, LIPOPROTEINS, AND TRIACYLGLYCEROL VALUES

Important risk factors for development of atherosclerosis include high levels of serum cholesterol, triacylglycerol, and low-density lipoprotein cholesterol (LDL-C) and a low level of high-density lipoprotein cholesterol (HDL-C). The primary sites for artery-narrowing plaque formation (i.e., incorporation of connective tissue, smooth muscle, cellular debris, minerals, and cholesterol) include the aorta and carotid, coronary, femoral, and iliac arteries. Specific cut-off values for total cholesterol, LDL-C, HDL-C, and triacylglycerol relate to varying levels of increased coronary heart disease risk. The following tables present current guidelines for the various blood lipids and lipoproteins.

Table 1	Classification of Serum Total Cholesterol, LDL-C, and HDL-C Levels
TOTAL CHOLESTEROL	**CLASSIFICATION**
<200 mg·dL^{-1}	Desirable cholesterol
200–239 mg·dL^{-1}	Borderline high cholesterol
>240 mg·dL^{-1}	High cholesterol
LDL CHOLESTEROL	**CLASSIFICATION**
<70 mg·dL^{-1}	Optimal (recommended for people with CHD or diabetes)
<130 mg·dL^{-1}	Desirable
130–159 mg·dL^{-1}	Borderline high
160–189 mg·dL^{-1}	High
>190 mg·dL^{-1}	Very High
HDL CHOLESTEROL	**CLASSIFICATION**
<35 mg·dL^{-1}	Low
>60 mg·dL^{-1}	High

Table 2	Classification of Triacylglycerol Levels	
SERUM TRIACYLGLYCEROLS	**CLASSIFICATION**	**COMMENTS**
<150 mg·dL^{-1}	Normal	
150–199 mg·dL^{-1}	Borderline high	Check for accompanying primary or secondary dyslipidemias
200–499 mg·dL^{-1}	High	Check for accompanying primary or secondary dyslipidemias
>500 mg·dL^{-1}	Very high	Increased risk for acute pancreatitis

From Diabetes Education Research Center and American Heart Association, 2004.

metabolism involving B-vitamin enzymes. High levels of homocysteine in the blood and urine were common to all three disorders of the inflicted individuals, and half of these individuals developed arterial or venous thrombosis by age 30. It was postulated that moderate elevation of homocysteine in the general population predisposes individuals to atherosclerosis similarly to elevated cholesterol concentration.

Numerous studies have shown a nearly lockstep association between plasma homocysteine levels and heart attack and mortality in men and women. This metabolic abnormality is present in nearly 30% of CHD patients and 40% of patients with cerebrovascular disease. Excessive homocysteine causes blood platelets to clump, fostering blood clots and deterioration of smooth muscle cells that line the arterial wall. Chronic homocysteine exposure eventually scars and thickens arteries and provides a fertile medium for circulating LDL-C to initiate damage. In the presence of other conventional CHD risks (e.g., smoking and hypertension), synergistic effects magnify the negative impact of homocysteine on cardiovascular health. Resting homocysteine levels exert a significant independent increased risk (on a continuum) for vascular disease similar to that of smoking and hyperlipidemia. A powerful multiplicative interaction effect also emerged in the presence of other risks, particularly cigarette smoking and hypertension. In general, people in the highest quartile for homocysteine levels have nearly twice the risk of heart attack or stroke compared with those in the lowest quartile. Why some people accumulate homocysteine is uncertain, but the evidence points to a deficiency of B vitamins (B_6, B_{12}, and particularly folic acid); cigarette smoking, drinking coffee, and high meat intake, associated with elevated homocysteine concentrations.

Excessive Body Fat

Excess body fat has received attention as a CHD risk factor, but its relationship is often codependent with hypertension, elevated cholesterol level, type 2 diabetes, and cigarette smoking. The number of annual deaths attributable to overfatness in the United States adult population ranges between about 263,000 and 383,000. Weight loss and accompanying body fat reduction, whether through diet or exercise, usually normalize cholesterol and triacylglycerol levels and exert beneficial effects on blood pressure and type 2 diabetes.

Physical Inactivity

Prospective research studies show clearly that regular physical activity offers protection against heart disease. Sedentary men and women are approximately twice as likely to suffer a fatal heart attack as more physically active counterparts. Maintenance of aerobic fitness (independent of actual activity level) throughout life also provides protection against CHD risk factors and disease occurrence. One could argue that genetic factors contribute more to fitness level than to daily exercise patterns. Fitness level relates closely to individual differences in physical activity level among most individuals, making regular exercise assume greater importance than genetics in determining physical fitness and related health benefits. **Table 17.5** summarizes possible biologic mechanisms for how regular aerobic exercise confers protection against CHD progression.

C-Reactive Protein

C-reactive protein (CRP) is a circulating acute-phase reactant that increases during the inflammatory response to tissue injury or infection. The liver primarily synthesizes CRP with its release stimulated by interleukin 6 (IL-6) and other proinflammatory cytokines. Small increases in CRP within the normal range predict future vascular events in apparently healthy, asymptomatic individuals. Such predictive accuracy of CRP extends to patients with pre-existing vascular disease. CRP correlates

Table 17·5	Possible Mechanisms for Beneficial Effects of Regular Aerobic Exercise on Risk of Coronary Heart Disease and Mortality

- Improves myocardial circulation and metabolism to protect the heart from hypoxic stress. Improvements include enhanced vascularization and increased coronary blood flow capacity via altered control of coronary vascular smooth muscle and increased reactivity of coronary resistance vessels. Modest increases in cardiac glycogen stores and glycolytic capacity also prove beneficial if the heart's oxygen supply suddenly becomes compromised.
- Enhances the mechanical properties of the myocardium to enable the exercise-trained heart to maintain or increase contractility during a specific challenge.
- Establishes more favorable blood-clotting characteristics and other hemostatic mechanisms, including increased fibrinolysis and production of endothelial prostacyclin.
- Normalizes the blood lipid profile to slow or reverse atherosclerosis.
- Favorably alters heart rate and blood pressure so myocardial work significantly decreases during rest and exercise.
- Suppresses age-related body weight gain and promotes a more desirable body composition and body fat distribution (particularly a reduced level of intra-abdominal adipose tissue).
- Establishes a more favorable neural–hormonal balance to conserve oxygen for the myocardium; improves the mixture of carbohydrate and fat metabolized by the body.
- Provides a favorable outlet for psychological stress and tension.

greater than chance with abdominal obesity, and raised levels predict the risk of developing type 2 diabetes.

The utility of CRP as a tool in CHD risk assessment has several severe limitations, including poor specificity in the setting of coexisting inflammatory states (e.g., rheumatoid arthritis, chronic pulmonary disease, and infections), and only minimal data are available for non-white populations. The independent predictive power of CRP has not been firmly established.

Lipoprotein(a)

Lipoprotein(a) [Lp(a)] is an LDL-like particle largely under genetic control; it varies substantially between individuals depending on the size of the apo(a) isoform present; Lp(a) levels vary little with diet or exercise, unlike the other lipoproteins LDL and HDL. The biological function of Lp(a) remains unclear, but strong evidence suggests its phylogenetic role to respond to tissue injury and vascular lesions, to prevent infectious pathogens from invading cells, and to promote wound healing. Lp(a) is an acute-phase reactant, more than doubling in concentration in response to the proinflammatory cytokine IL-6; it binds readily to endothelial cells, macrophages, fibroblasts, platelets, and subendothelial matrix. Lp(a)'s most important role in atherothrombosis may be to inhibit clot fibrinolysis at sites of tissue injury. These properties make Lp(a) a highly atherothrombotic lipoprotein.

Fibrinogen   Fibrinogen, a circulating glycoprotein, acts at the final step in the coagulation response to vascular tissue injury. Fibrinogen has other functions that make it biologically plausible as a possible participant in vascular disease: (1) regulation of cell adhesion, chemotaxis (movements of cells in response to substances exhibiting chemical properties), and cell proliferation; (2) vasoconstriction at sites of vessel wall injury; (3) stimulation of platelet aggregation; and (4) determinants of blood viscosity. Fibrinogen, like CRP, is an acute-phase reactant.

Epidemiological data support an independent association between elevated fibrinogen levels and cardiovascular morbidity and mortality. Elevated blood fibrinogen, independent of classic CHD risk factors, correlates with ischemic stroke and peripheral vascular disease. Several factors other than inflammation modulate fibrinogen levels. A dose-response relationship exists between number of cigarettes smoked and fibrinogen level. Fibrinogen tends to be higher in patients with diabetes, hypertension, obesity, and a sedentary lifestyle.

CHD RISK FACTOR INTERACTIONS

Smoking generally acts independently of other risk factors to increase CHD risk. The other risk factors interact with each other and CHD itself to accentuate disease risk. **Figure 17.17** quantifies the interaction of three primary CHD risk factors in the same person. With one risk factor, a 45-year-old man's chance for CHD symptoms during the year averages about twice that of a man without risks. The chance for chest pain, heart attack, or sudden death with three risk factors increases five times compared with no risk factors.

RISK FACTORS IN CHILDREN

The frequent occurrence of multiple CHD risk factors in young children emphasizes the need for early CHD initiatives to reduce atherosclerosis risk later in life. Obesity and family history of heart disease represent the two most common risk factors in physically active and apparently healthy boys and girls. A relatively large percentage of these children also show abnormally high blood lipid concentrations.

Questions & Notes

List 6 factors not causally linked that are nevertheless potent CHD risk factors.

1.

2.

3.

4.

5.

6.

List 3 possible exercise-induced mechanisms for reducing CHD risk.

1.

2.

3.

Briefly explain the role of C-reactive protein as a CHD risk factor.

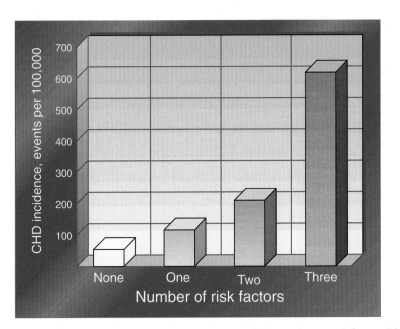

Figure 17.17.   Relationship between a combination of abnormal CHD risk factors (cholesterol >250 mg·dL^{-1}; systolic blood pressure >160 mm Hg; smoking >1 pack a day) and incidence of coronary heart disease.

> FOR YOUR INFORMATION
>
> **Fiber Intake and CHD in the Elderly**
> There is an inverse association between consumption of fiber from cereal sources (including whole grains and bran) and CHD risk in elderly men and women (average age 72+ years). Compared with medical or surgical interventions, increasing fiber intake by the equivalent of two slices of whole grain bread per day is easy to incorporate into the daily routine, is low cost, and is widely available.

> FOR YOUR INFORMATION
>
> **Apoprotein**
> **Apoproteins** represent a class of specific proteins embedded in the outer shell of a lipoprotein particle that (1) increase the solubility of the lipoprotein's cholesterol and triacylglycerol components, (2) act as ligands for specific lipoprotein receptors in cell membranes, and (3) serve as important cofactors to activate enzymes in lipoprotein metabolism. Researchers believe that specific apoproteins more reliably predict heart disease proneness than total cholesterol level.

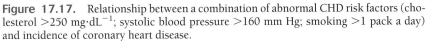

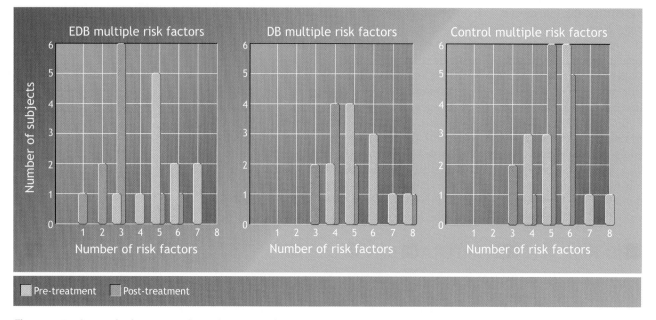

Figure 17.18.   Multiple coronary heart disease risk factors for obese adolescents before and after treatment. *DB*, diet + behavior change group; *EDB*, exercise + diet + behavior change group. (From Becque, M.D., et al.: Coronary risk incidence of obese adolescents: Reduction by exercise plus diet intervention. *Pediatrics*, 81:605, 1988.)

As with adults, the association between body fat and serum lipid levels becomes apparent in overfat children. The fattest children usually have the highest levels of serum cholesterol and triacylglycerols. For these children, general adiposity and visceral adipose tissue relate to unfavorable hemostatic factors that increase CHD morbidity and mortality in adulthood. Of 62 overfat children aged 10 to 15 years, only one child had just one CHD risk factor. Of the remaining children, 14% had two risk factors, 30% had three risk factors, 29% had four risk factors, 18% had five risk factors, and the remaining five children (8%) had six risk factors. A subsample of these children were then enrolled in a 20-week program to evaluate the effects on the risk profile of either (1) diet plus behavior therapy, or (2) regular exercise plus diet and behavior therapy. No changes resulted in multiple-risk reduction in the control group or in those receiving diet with behavior treatment. In contrast, children who exercised, dieted, plus underwent behavior therapy dramatically reduced multiple risks (**Fig. 17.18**). These encouraging findings demonstrate that supervised programs of moderate food restriction and exercise with behavior modification reduces CHD risk factors in obese adolescents. Adding regular exercise augmented the effectiveness of risk-factor intervention.

The most sedentary children (e.g., those who watch the most TV) typically have more body fat and higher BMI than physically active peers. School-based programs aimed at increasing the level of daily physical activity and/or reducing risk factors in children and adolescents increase students' knowledge about risk factors and benefits of physical activity without impairing academic performance. Such programs also may produce a long-term positive effect on exercise habits and overall health. If regular physical activity upgrades or at least stabilizes a poor risk factor profile, then school curricula at all grade levels, particularly at the kindergarten and elementary grades, should strongly encourage more physically active lifestyles. In this regard, not implementing required daily physical education seems counterproductive from a public health policy standpoint.

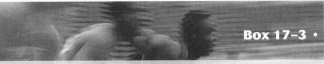

Box 17–3 • CLOSE UP

CALCULATING YOUR CHD RISK

Coronary heart disease risk inventories assess an individual's susceptibility to CHD. Such qualitative risk tools are valuable for assessing general lifestyle behaviors and current heart disease risk.

The table below presents the Framingham 10-year CHD risk estimate. This is the most widely used "traditional" risk analysis system.

To determine risk profile, review each risk factor and accompanying numerical "point" value. Insert the respective points into the applicable box at the top of the table. The total number of points represents the 10-year risk for developing CHD expressed as a percentage.

Framingham 10-Year CHD Risk Estimate Worksheet

☐	+	☐	+	☐	+	☐	+	☐	+	☐	=	☐
Age		**HDL-C**		**SBP**		**TC**		**Smoking**		**Total Points**		**10-y Risk (%)**

Age (y)				Systolic Blood Pressure (SBP), mmHg					
Women	Points	Men	Points	Women	Points		Men	Points	
				mmHg	Treated	Untreated	mmHg	Treated	Untreated
20–34	−7	20–34	−9	<120	0	0	<120	0	0
35–39	−3	35–39	−4	120–129	1	3	120–129	0	1
40–44	0	40–44	0	130–139	2	4	130–139	1	2
45–49	3	45–49	3	140–159	3	5	140–159	1	2
50–54	6	50–54	6	>160	4	6	>160	2	3
55–59	8	55–59	8						
60–64	10	60–64	10						
65–69	12	65–69	11						
70–74	14	70–74	12						
75–79	16	75–79	13						

Points for Total Cholesterol (TC) At Each Age Category (y)						Points for Total Cholesterol (TC) At Each Age Category (y)					
Women						Men					
$TC(mg \cdot dL^{-1})$	20–39	40–49	50–59	60–69	70–79	$TC(mg \cdot dL^{-1})$	20–39	40–49	50–59	60–69	70–79
<160	0	0	0	0	0	<160	0	0	0	0	0
160–199	4	3	2	1	1	160–199	4	3	2	1	0
200–239	8	6	4	2	1	200–239	7	5	3	1	0
240–279	11	8	5	3	2	240–279	9	6	4	2	1
>280	13	10	7	4	2	>280	11	8	5	3	1

Points for Smoking At Each Age Category (y)						Points for Smoking At Each Age Category (y)					
Women						Men					
	20–39	40–49	50–59	60–69	70–79		20–39	40–49	50–59	60–69	70–79
Nonsmoker	0	0	0	0	0	Nonsmoker	0	0	0	0	0
Smoker	9	7	4	2	1	Smoker	8	5	3	1	1

Predicted 10-Year CHD Risk From Point Total			
Women		Men	
Point Total	10-Year Risk (%)	Point Total	10-Year Risk (%)
<9	<1	0	<1
9–12	1	1–4	1
13–14	2	5–6	2
15	3	7	3
16	4	8	4
17	5	9	5
18	6	10	6
19	8	11	8
20	11	12	10
21	14	13	12
22	17	14	16
23	22	15	20
24	27	16	25
≥25	≥30	≥17	≥30

SUMMARY

1. Elderly persons make up the fastest growing segment of American society. Thirty years ago, age 65 represented the onset of old age. Gerontologists now consider 85 the demarcation of "oldest-old" and age 75 "young-old."

2. Nearly 12% or approximately 35 million Americans exceed age 65; by the year 2030, 70 million Americans will exceed age 85.

3. "Healthspan" refers to the total number of years a person remains in excellent health.

4. The "new gerontology" addresses areas beyond age-related diseases and their prevention to recognize that successful aging maintains enhanced physiologic function and physical fitness.

5. "Healthy life expectancy" refers to the expected number of years a person might live in the equivalent of full health. This involves computing disability-adjusted life expectancy (DALE).

6. DALE considers the years of ill health weighted according to severity, and subtracted from expected overall life expectancy to compute the equivalent years of healthy life.

7. The specific field of physical activity epidemiology applies the general research strategies of epidemiology to study physical activity as a health-related behavior linked to disease and other outcomes.

8. The Physical Activity Pyramid summarizes major goals for increasing the level of regular physical activity in the general population; it emphasizes many forms of behavioral and lifestyle options.

9. Healthy People 2010 describes a comprehensive, nationwide health promotion and disease prevention agenda as a roadmap for promoting health and preventing illness, disability, and premature death among all people in the United States.

10. Inactivity alone produces a constellation of problems and conditions eventually leading to premature death. The term "sedentary death syndrome" (SeDS) identifies this condition.

11. Physiologic and performance capabilities generally decline after age 30. The decline rates of various functions differ within and among individuals. Regular exercise enables older persons to retain higher levels of functional capacity, particularly cardiovascular and muscular functions.

12. Aging alters endocrine function, particularly for the pituitary, pancreas, adrenal, and thyroid glands.

13. A physically active lifestyle throughout life confers significant health-related benefits.

14. About half of all deaths that occurred in the United States in 2000 can be attributed to a limited number of largely preventable behaviors and exposures, most of which relate directly to physical inactivity and overweight and obesity.

15. Life-extending benefits of exercise correlate more with preventing early mortality than improving overall life span. While the maximum life span may not extend greatly, only moderate exercise enables many men and women to live a more productive and healthy life.

16. Sedentary white women who increase their physical activity to the equivalent of about 1 mile/day of walking exhibit approximately 40% to 50% lower all-cause mortality rates than chronically sedentary white women.

17. Coronary heart disease (CHD) represents the single largest cause of death in the Western world. The pathogenesis of CHD involves degenerative changes in the inner lining of the arterial wall that leads to progressive occlusion.

18. Four major modifiable cardiovascular risk factors (smoking, diabetes mellitus, hypertension, and hypercholesterolemia) account for 80% to 90% of coronary heart disease cases. Physical inactivity and excessive body weight also contribute to disease risk.

19. Cigarette smoking, either active or passive through environmental exposure, directly relates to CHD risk. Smokers experience twice the risk of death from heart disease as nonsmokers.

20. A cholesterol level of 200 mg·dL^{-1} or lower is usually desirable, although risk for a fatal heart attack begins to rise at 150 mg·dL^{-1}. A cholesterol level of 230 mg·dL^{-1} increases heart attack risk to about twice that of 180 mg·dL^{-1}, and 300 mg·dL^{-1} increases the risk fourfold.

21. For triacylglycerols, less than 150 mg·dL^{-1} is considered a nominal level, with 200 to 499 mg·dL^{-1} considered high.

22. Behaviors that favorably affect cholesterol and lipoprotein levels include weight loss, regular aerobic exercise (independent of weight loss), increased intake of water-soluble fibers (fibers in beans, legumes, and oat bran), increased intake of polyunsaturated to saturated fatty acid ratio and monounsaturated fatty acids, increased intake of unique polyunsaturated fatty

acids in fish oils (omega-3 fats), and moderate alcohol consumption.

23. Variables that adversely affect cholesterol and lipoprotein levels include cigarette smoking, diet high in saturated fatty acids and preformed cholesterol, emotionally stressful situations, and oral contraceptives.

24. A systolic blood pressure that exceeds 140 mm Hg or diastolic pressure that exceeds 90 mm Hg forms the lower limit for the classification of borderline high blood pressure (hypertension).

25. People with diabetes are two to four times more likely to develop cardiovascular disease from a variety of risk factors usually coincident with the diabetic condition, such as obesity, physical inactivity, hypertension, and atherogenic dyslipidemia.

26. The following variables are considered positive CHD predictors: age, gender, and heredity; immunologic factors; homocysteine; excessive body fat; physical inactivity; C-reactive protein; lipoprotein(a); and fibrinogen.

27. CHD risk factors interact with each other and CHD itself to accentuate disease risk.

28. The frequent occurrence of multiple CHD risk factors in young children emphasizes the need for early CHD initiatives to reduce atherosclerotic risk later in life

29. Implementing required daily physical education to reduce the risk of CHD in children seems imperative from a public health policy standpoint.

THOUGHT QUESTIONS

1. Does risk factor modification always change disease risk?

2. If regular physical activity contributes little to overall life span, what other reasons exist for maintaining a physically active lifestyle throughout middle and old age?

3. Respond to the question: "Overwhelming epidemiological evidence links physical activity on the job or in leisure time to reduced CHD risk, but does this prove that exercise benefits cardiovascular health?"

SELECTED REFERENCES

Abdollahi, M.R., et al.: Angiotensin II type I receptor gene polymorphism: anthropometric and metabolic syndrome traits. *J. Med. Genet.*, 42:396, 2005.

ACSM: ACSM Position Stand on Exercise and Physical Activity for Older Adults. *Med. Sci. Sports Exerc.*, 30:992, 1998.

ACSM: ACSM Position Stand on Exercise and Type 2 Diabetes. *Med. Sci. Sports Exerc.*, 32:1345, 2000.

ADA/ACSM: ADA/ACSM Diabetes Mellitus and Exercise Joint Position Paper. *Med. Sci. Sports Exerc.*, 29:I, 1997.

Albert, C.M., et al.: Triggering of sudden death from cardiac causes by vigorous exertion. *N. Engl. J. Med.*, 9:343, 2000.

Blair, S.N., and Connelly, J.C.: How much physical activity should we do? The case for moderate amounts and intensities of physical activity. *Res. Q. Exerc. Sport*, 67:193, 1996.

Blair, S.N., et al.: Changes in physical fitness and all cause mortality: A prospective study of healthy and unhealthy men. *JAMA*, 273:1093, 1995.

Blair, S.N., et al.: Influences of cardiorespiratory fitness and other precursors on cardiovascular disease and all-cause mortality in men and women. *JAMA*, 276:205, 1996.

Blair, S.N., et al.: Physical activity, nutrition, and chronic disease. *Med. Sci. Sports Exerc.*, 28:335, 1997.

Blair, S.N.: Physical activity, physical fitness, and health. *Res. Q. Exerc. Sport*, 64:365, 1993.

Bodegard, J., et al.: Reasons for terminating an exercise test provide independent prognostic information: 2014 apparently healthy men followed for 26 years. *Eur. Heart J.*, 26:1394, 2005.

Bolad, I., Delafontaine, P.: Endothelial dysfunction: its role in hypertensive coronary disease. *Curr. Opin. Cardiol.*, 20:270, 2005.

Booth, F.W., et al.: Waging war on modern chronic diseases: Primary prevention through exercise biology. *J. Appl. Physiol.*, 88:774, 2000.

Canto, J.G., and Iskandrian, A.E.: Major risk factors for cardiovascular disease: Debunking the "only 50%" myth. *JAMA*, 290:947, 2003.

Carnethon, M.R., et al.: A longitudinal study of physical activity and heart rate recovery: CARDIA, 1987–1993. *Med. Sci. Sports Exerc.*, 37:606, 2005.

Corrado, D., et al.: Does sport activity enhance the risk of sudden death in adolescent and young adults? *J. Am. Coll. Cardio.*, 42:1959, 2003.

Croom, K.F., Plosker, G.L.: Atorvastatin: a review of its use in the primary prevention of cardiovascular events in patients with type 2 diabetes mellitus. *Drugs*, 65:137, 2005.

DiBrezzo, R., et al.: Exercise intervention designed to improve strength and dynamic balance among community-dwelling older adults. *J. Aging Phys. Act.*, 13:199, 2005.

Djousse, L., et al.: Dietary linolenic acid is associated with a lower prevalence of hypertension in the NHLBI Family Heart Study. *Hypertension*, 45:368, 2005.

Frontera, W.R., et al.: Aging of skeletal muscle: A 12-yr longitudinal study. *J. Appl. Physiol.*, 88:1321, 2000.

Giovannucci, E.L., et al.: A prospective study of physical activity and incident and fatal prostate cancer. *Arch. Intern. Med.*, 165:1005, 2005.

Gotsch, K., et al.: Nonfatal sports- and recreation-related injuries treated in emergency departments—United States, July 2000-June 2001. *MMWR*, 51:736, 2002.

Greenland, P., et al.: Major risk factors as antecedents of fatal and nonfatal coronary heart disease events. *JAMA*, 290:891, 2003.

Greenland, P.: Improving risk of coronary heart disease: Can a picture make the difference. *JAMA*, 289:2270, 2003.

Hankam, D.G., and Anand, S.S.: Emerging risk factors for atherosclerotic vascular disease. *JAMA*, 290:932, 2003.

Hay, J.W., Sterling, K.L.: Cost effectiveness of treating low HDL-cholesterol in the primary prevention of coronary heart disease. *Pharmacoeconomics*, 23:133, 2005.

Health, United States 2002. Rockville, MD: Department of Health and Human Services, Centers for Disease Control and Prevention. DHHS Publication No. 1232, 2002.

Holmes, J.S., et al.: Heart disease and prevention: race and age differences in heart disease prevention, treatment, and mortality. *Med. Care*, 43:133, 2005.

Hu, F.B., et al.: Trends in the incidence of coronary heart disease and changes in diet and lifestyle in women. *N. Engl. J. Med.*, 343:530, 2000.

Ingram, D.K.: Age-related decline in physical activity: generalization to nonhumans. *Med. Sci. Sports Exerc.*, 32:1623, 2000.

Jouven, X., et al.: Heart-rate profile during exercise as a predictor of sudden death. *N. Engl. J. Med.*, 352:1951, 2005.

Karsten, S.L., Geschwind, D.H.: Exercise your amyloid. *Cell*, 120:572, 2005.

Kelley, G.A., et al.: Walking and Non-HDL-C in adults: a meta-analysis of randomized controlled trials. *Prev. Cardiol.*, 8:102, 2005.

Kemmler, W., et al.: Exercise effects on menopausal risk factors of early postmenopausal women: 3-yr erlangen fitness osteoporosis prevention study results. *Med. Sci. Sports Exerc.*, 37:194, 2005.

Khot, U.N., et al.: Prevalence of conventional risk factors in patents with coronary heart disease. *JAMA*, 290:898, 2003.

Kurl, S., et al.: Cardiac power during exercise and the risk of stroke in men. *Stroke*, 36:820, 2005.

Kurozawa, Y., et al.: JACC Study Group. Levels of physical activity among participants in the JACC study. *J. Epidemiol.*, 15:S43, 2005.

Lauer, M.S., and Fontanarosa, P.B.: Updated guidelines for cholesterol management. *JAMA*, 285:2508, 2001.

Lee, I.M.: Physical activity in women: How much is good enough? *JAMA*, 290:1377, 2003.

Lee, S., et al.: Cardiorespiratory fitness attenuates metabolic risk independent of abdominal subcutaneous and visceral fat in men. *Diabetes Care*, 28:895, 2005.

Li, D., et al.: Lean meat and heart health. *Asia Pac. J. Clin. Nutr.*, 14:113, 2005.

Lloyd-Jones, D.M., et al.: Parental cardiovascular disease as a risk factor for cardiovascular disease in middle-aged adults. *JAMA*, 291:2204, 2004.

Martinez, M.E.: Primary prevention of colorectal cancer: lifestyle, nutrition, exercise. *Recent Results Cancer Res.*, 166:177, 2005.

McGill, H.C., et al.: Starting earlier to prevent heart disease. *JAMA*, 290:2320, 2003.

Miller, M.G., et al.: Aspirin under fire: aspirin use in the primary prevention of coronary heart disease. *Pharmacotherapy*, 25:847, 2005.

Mokdad, A.H., et al.: Actual causes of death in the United States, 2000. *JAMA*, 291:1238, 2004.

Morris, J.N., et al.: Coronary heart disease and physical activity of work. *Lancet*, 265:1053, 1953.

Morris, J.N.: Exercise in the prevention of coronary heart disease: Today's best bet in public health. *Med. Sci. Sports Exerc.*, 26:807, 1994.

Mozaffarian, D., et al.: Cereal, fruit, and vegetable fiber intake and the risk of cardiovascular disease in elderly individuals. *JAMA*, 289:1659, 2003.

Nelson, R.: Exercise could prevent cerebral changes associated with AD. *Lancet. Neurol.*, 4:275, 2005.

Nestel, P.J., et al.: Relation of diet to cardiovascular disease risk factors in subjects with cardiovascular disease in Australia and New Zealand: analysis of the Long-Term Intervention with Pravastatin in Ischaemic Disease trial. *Am. J. Clin. Nutr.*, 81:1322, 2005.

Oguma, Y., Shinoda-Tagawa, T.: Physical activity decreases cardiovascular disease risk in women: review and meta-analysis. *Am. J. Prev. Med.*, 26:407, 2004.

Ornish, D., et al.: Intensive lifestyle changes for reversal of coronary heart disease. *JAMA*, 280:2001, 1998.

Panagiotakos, D.B., Polychronopoulos, E.: The role of Mediterranean diet in the epidemiology of metabolic syndrome; converting epidemiology to clinical practice. *Lipids Health Dis.*, 12; 4:7, 2005.

Pollock, M.L., et al.: Twenty-year follow-up of aerobic power and body composition of older track athletes. *J. Appl. Physiol.*, 82:1508, 1997.

Regan, C., et al.: Relationship of exercise and other risk factors to depression of Alzheimer's disease: the LASER-AD study. *Int. J. Geriatr. Psychiatry*, 20:261, 2005.

Reid, R.D., et al.: Impact of program duration and contact frequency on efficacy and cost of cardiac rehabilitation: results of a randomized trial. *Am. Heart J.*, 149:862, 2005.

Robinson, J.G., Maheshwari, N.: A "poly-portfolio" for secondary prevention: a strategy to reduce subsequent events by up to 97% over five years. *Am. J. Cardiol.*, 1; 95:373, 2005.

Simon, A., et al.: Differences between markers of atherogenic lipoproteins in predicting high cardiovascular risk and subclinical atherosclerosis in asymptomatic men. *Atherosclerosis*, 179:339, 2005.

Smith, D.A., et al.: Abdominal diameter index: a more powerful anthropometric measure for prevalent coronary heart disease risk in adult males. *Diabetes Obes. Metab.*, 7:370, 2005.

Smith, J.K.: Exercise and atherogenesis. *Exerc. Sport Sci. Rev.*, 29:49, 2001.

Smith, S.C., Jr, et al.: Principles for national and regional guidelines on cardiovascular disease prevention: A scientific statement from the World Heart and Stroke Forum. *Circulation*, 109:3112, 2004.

Spirduso, W.W., Clifford, P.: Replication of age and physical activity effects on reaction and movement time. *J. Gerontol.*, 33:26, 1978.

Stefan, M.A., et al.: Effect of activity restriction owing to heart disease on obesity. *Arch. Pediatr. Adolesc. Med.*, 159:477, 2005.

Tully, M.A., et al.: Brisk walking, fitness, and cardiovascular risk: A randomized controlled trial in primary care. *Prev. Med.*, 41:622, 2005.

Van den Hoogen, P.C., et al.: Blood pressure and long-term coronary heart disease mortality in the Seven Countries study: Implications for clinical practice and public health. *Eur. Heart J.*, 21:1639, 2000.

Visser, M., et al.: Muscle mass, muscle strength, and muscle fat infiltration as predictors of incident mobility limitations in well-functioning older persons. *J. Gerontol. A. Biol. Sci. Med. Sci.*, 60:324, 2005.

Williams, P.T.: Physical fitness and activity as separate heart disease risk factors: A meta-analysis. *Exerc. Sport Sci. Rev.*, 33:754, 2001.

Young, D.R., et al.: Physical activity, cardiorespiratory fitness, and their relationship to cardiovascular risk factors in African Americans and non-African Americans with above-optimal blood pressure. *J. Community Health*, 30:107, 2005.

CHAPTER OBJECTIVES

- List six clinical areas and corresponding diseases and disorders where physical activity (exercise) therapy exerts positive influence.

- List three different diseases of the heart muscle.

- Categorize two diseases that affect heart valves and the cardiac nervous system.

- Describe the major steps in cardiac disease assessment.

- List different laboratory-based coronary heart disease screening tools.

- List reasons for including stress testing to evaluate coronary heart disease.

- List several indicators of coronary heart disease during an exercise stress test.

- Give advantages and limitations of different modes of exercise for graded exercise stress testing.

- Define the following terms for stress test results: true-positive, false-negative, true-negative, and false-positive.

- List four reasons for stopping an exercise stress test.

- Outline the approach for individualizing an "exercise prescription."

- Give advantages and disadvantages of submaximal versus maximal exercise stress testing.

- Give the pros and cons of the different stress test protocols.

- Discuss of the role of physical activity and exercise prescription in pulmonary rehabilitation.

- Describe the role of exercise in the diagnosis and treatment for diseases and disorders of the cardiovascular system.

- Describe the role of exercise in the diagnosis and treatment for diseases and disorders of the neuromuscular system.

- Describe the role of exercise in the diagnosis and treatment for cancer.

- Describe the role of exercise in the diagnosis and treatment for depression.

CHAPTER OUTLINE

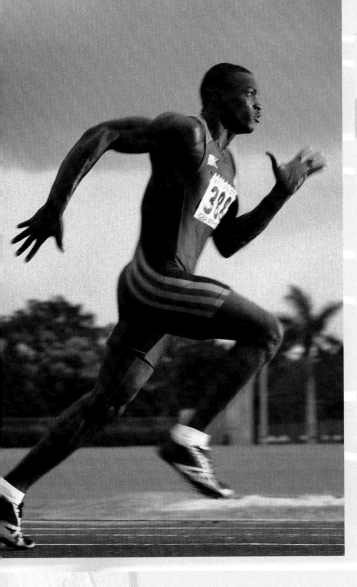

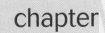

chapter

18

Clinical
Aspects of
Exercise
Physiology

The use of regular exercise in the global prevention of disease, in the rehabilitation from injury, and as adjunctive therapy for diverse medically related disorders is widespread and increasing. Attention now focuses on understanding the mechanisms by which exercise improves health, physical fitness, and rehabilitation potential of patients challenged by chronic disease and disability. This chapter highlights several clinical applications of exercise interventions for some of the medical/health conditions that exercise positively influences, which are listed in **Table 18.1**.

CARDIOVASCULAR DISEASES AND DISORDERS

As detailed in Chapter 17, diseases of the cardiovascular system account for the greatest number of deaths in industrialized nations. Because increased physical activity represents the prudent first line of defense to combat cardiovascular diseases, the exercise physiologist needs to become familiar with all aspects of this disease. **Table 18.2** lists three categories of heart disease that lead to functional disability—diseases affecting the heart muscle, diseases affecting heart valves, and diseases affecting the cardiac nervous system. Diseases of the myocardium become most prevalent with advancing age. The following terms frequently describe these diseases: degenerative heart disease (DHD), atherosclerotic cardiovascular disease, arteriosclerotic cardiovascular disease, coronary artery disease (CAD), and coronary heart disease (CHD).

Diseases of the Myocardium

Advances in molecular biology have isolated a possible genetic link to CHD. This gene (on chromosome 19 near the gene related to LDL cholesterol receptor functioning), called the **atherosclerosis susceptibility gene (ATHS)**, accounts for almost 50% of all CHD cases. The ATHS gene causes a set of characteristics (abdominal obesity, low HDL cholesterol levels, and high levels of LDL cholesterol) that triple a person's risk of myocardial infarction.

CHD pathogenesis progresses along the following sequence:

1. Injury to the coronary artery's endothelial cell wall
2. Fibroblastic proliferation of the artery's inner lining or intima
3. Accumulation of lipids at the junction of the arterial intima and middle lining, further obstructing blood flow
4. Deterioration and formation of hyaline (a clear, homogeneous substance formed in degeneration) in the vessel's intima
5. Calcium deposition at the edges of the hyalinated area

The major disorders from reduced myocardial blood supply include angina pectoris, myocardial infarction, and congestive heart failure.

Angina Pectoris Angina pectoris is characterized by acute chest pain from an imbalance between the oxygen demands of the heart and its' oxygen supply. The pain results from metabolite accumulation within an ischemic segment of heart muscle. The sensation of angina pectoris, often confused with simple heartburn, includes squeezing, burning, and pressing or "choking" in the chest region (**Table 18.3**). The pain usually lasts up to 3 minutes but can continue for longer intervals. One-third of all individuals who suffer from angina will die suddenly from myocardial infarction. Several types of angina exist, including **chronic stable angina** (often referred to as "walk-through" angina); it occurs at a predictable level of physical exertion (e.g., MET level). Vasodilators like nitroglycerin reduce cardiac work-load (and thus oxygen requirement) to effectively control this uncomfortable and potentially debilitating condition.

Table 18•1	Clinical Areas and Their Corresponding Diseases and Disorders Where Exercise Therapy Applies
Cardiovascular diseases and disorders	Ischemia; chronic heart failure; dyslipidemias; cardiomyopathies; cardiac valvular disease; heart transplantation; congenital
Pulmonary diseases and disorders	Chronic obstructive pulmonary disease; cystic fibrosis; asthma and exercise-induced asthma
Neuromuscular diseases and disorders	Stroke; multiple sclerosis; Parkinson's disease; Alzheimer's disease; polio; cerebral palsy
Metabolic diseases and disorders	Obesity (adult and pediatric); diabetes; renal disease; menstrual dysfunction
Immunological and hematological diseases and disorders	Cancer; breast cancer; immune deficiency; allergies; sickle cell disease; HIV and AIDS
Orthopedic diseases and disorders	Osteoporosis; osteoarthritis and rheumatoid arthritis; back pain; sports injuries
Aging	Sarcopenia
Cognitive and emotional disorders	Anxiety and stress disorders; mental retardation; depression

Table 18•2	Three Categories of Heart Disease that Lead to Functional Disability		
DISEASES AFFECTING THE HEART MUSCLE	**DISEASES AFFECTING THE HEART VALVES**	**DISEASES AFFECTING THE CARDIAC NERVOUS SYSTEM**	
CHD Angina Myocardial infarction Pericarditis Congestive heart failure Aneurysms	Rheumatic fever Endocarditis Mitral valve prolapse Congenital deformations	Arrhythmias Tachycardia Bradycardia	

Table 18•3	Similarity of Symptoms of Angina and Heartburn	
ANGINA	**HEARTBURN**	
• Gripping, viselike feelings of pain or pressure behind the breast bone • Pain that radiates to the neck, jaw, back, shoulders, or arms (usually left) • Toothache • Burning indigestion • Shortness of breath • Nausea • Frequent belching	• Frequent feeling of heartburn • Frequent use of antacids to relieve pain • Waking up at night • Acid or bitter taste in mouth • Burning sensation in chest • Discomfort after eating spicy food • Difficulty swallowing	

Figure 18.1 shows the usual pattern of pain associated with an episode of acute angina pectoris. Pain frequently occurs in the left shoulder or along the arm to the elbow. Occasionally, angina pain emanates in the back area of the left scapula along the spinal cord.

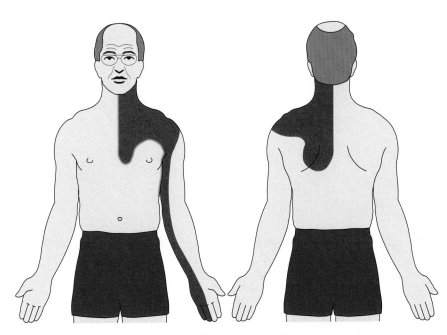

Figure 18.1   Location of pain generally associated with angina pectoris.

Myocardial Infarction Myocardial infarction (MI, heart attack, or coronary occlusion) results from a severely inadequate perfusion of blood in the coronary arteries and/or a dramatic imbalance in myocardial oxygen demand and supply from occlusion of a portion of the coronary vasculature. Sudden occlusion results from prior clot formation initiated by plaque accumulation in one or more coronary arteries. Severe fatigue for several days without specific pain usually precedes the onset of an MI.

Figure 18.2 displays the locations of early warning signs of the onset of an MI. Severe, unrelenting chest pain can last up to 1 hour during an MI.

Pericarditis Pericarditis, an inflammation of the heart's outer pericardial lining, is classified as either acute or chronic (recurring or constrictive). Acute pericarditis symptoms vary but usually include chest pain, shortness of breath (dyspnea), and elevated resting heart rate and body temperature. In chronic pericarditis, inflammation creates extreme chest pain due to fluid accumulation in the pericardial sac, which prevents the heart from fully expanding during diastole. The prognosis for acute viral pericarditis is excellent, whereas chronic pericarditis from bacterial origin presents a persistent serious pathology.

Congestive Heart Failure Congestive heart failure (CHF or chronic decompensation) occurs when cardiac output cannot keep pace with venous return. The heart fails from intrinsic myocardial disease, chronic hypertension, or structural defects that impair pump performance. Left ventricular output diminishes and blood accumulates in the pulmonary vasculature. This causes dyspnea and eventual flooding of the pulmonary alveoli with plasma filtrate, a condition termed **pulmonary congestion**. Common CHF symptoms include dyspnea, coughing with large amounts of frothy blood-tinged sputum, pulmonary edema, general fatigue, and overall muscle weakness. Heart failure can occur from the right or left side of the heart, each with different symptoms and prognosis depending on initiation of treatment.

Aneurysm Aneurysm represents an abnormal dilatation in the wall of an artery or vein or within the myocardium itself. Vascular aneurysms occur when a vessel's wall weakens from trauma, congenital vascular disease, infection, or atherosclerosis. Aneurysms are identified as either "arterial" or "venous" and classified according to the specific vasculature area affected (e.g., thoracic aneurysm). A routine chest x-ray uncovers most aneurysms. Common

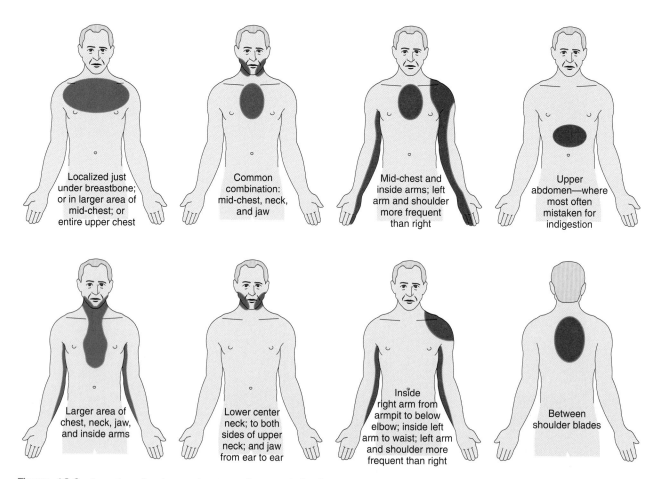

Figure 18.2 Location of early warning signs of myocardial infarction. Note diverse locations of pain.

symptoms include chest pain with a specific, palpable, pulsating mass in the chest, abdomen, or lower back.

Heart Valve Diseases

Diseases and abnormalities that affect heart valve structure and function include:

- **Stenosis**: Valve narrowing or constriction that prevents the valve from opening fully; caused by growths, scars, or abnormal mineral deposits.
- **Insufficiency** (also called regurgitation): Heart valves do not close properly, causing blood to flow back into the heart's chambers during diastole.
- **Prolapse** (only affects mitral valve): Enlarged valve leaflets bulge backward into the left atrium during the cardiac cycle.

Valvular abnormalities increase myocardial work-load, requiring the heart to generate greater force to pump blood through a constricted valve or to maintain cardiac output if blood seeps back into a chamber. **Rheumatic fever**, a potentially fatal infection by streptococcal bacteria that can lead to rheumatic heart disease (causing valvular scarring and heart valve deformity), usually causes heart valve stenosis. The two most common symptoms of this heart valve pathology include fever and joint pain.

Endocarditis
Endocarditis, an inflammation of the innermost layer of the heart (endocardium) usually of bacterial origin, damages the tricuspid, aortic, or mitral valves from direct invasion of bacteria into the tissue. Patients initially have musculoskeletal symptoms, including arthritis, low back pain, and general weakness in one or more joints. Antibiotic drugs effectively treat this disease.

Congenital Malformations
Congenital heart defects appear in one of every 100 births; they include defects of the heart valves, such as ventricular or atrial septal defects (hole between the ventricles and atria) and patent ductus arteriosus (shunt caused by an opening between the aorta and pulmonary artery). These defects require surgical repair.

Mitral Valve Prolapse
Mitral valve prolapse (MVP) occurs in about 10% of Americans and involves variations in either the mitral valve's shape or structure. This defect has been called "floppy valve syndrome," "Barlow's syndrome," and the "click-murmur syndrome." MVP usually remains benign, but frequency of diagnosis has increased over the past decade due to MVP's association with endocarditis, atherosclerosis, and muscular dystrophy. MVP probably results from connective tissue abnormalities in mitral valve leaflets. Sixty percent of patients with MVP have no symptoms; the remainder experience profound fatigue during exercise.

Cardiac Nervous System Diseases

Diseases that affect the heart's electrical conduction system include **dysrhythmias (arrhythmias)** that cause the heart to beat too quickly (tachycardia), beat too slowly (bradycardia), generate extra beats (ectopic, extrasystole, or premature ventricular contractions), or fibrillate (fine rapid contractions or twitching of cardiac muscle fibers).

Dysrhythmias usually change circulatory dynamics and can result in low blood pressure, heart failure, and shock. They often occur following a stroke induced by physical exertion or other stressor.

In adults, **sinus tachycardia** represents a resting heart rate greater than 100 $b \cdot min^{-1}$, whereas in **sinus bradycardia**, resting heart rate decreases below 60 $b \cdot min^{-1}$. Asymptomatic sinus bradycardia often occurs in endurance athletes.

Questions & Notes

List 3 common symptoms of angina pectoris.

1.

2.

3.

Name 3 locations generally associated with early warning signs of myocardial infarction.

1.

2.

3.

Name the major cause of a myocardial infarction.

Name a symptom of acute pericarditis.

Name a symptom of chronic pericarditis.

Give 2 reasons for congestive heart failure.

1.

2.

Give 2 common symptoms of congestive heart failure.

1.

2.

This benign dysrhythmia may reflect a beneficial training adaptation because it provides a longer diastole for ventricular filling during the cardiac cycle.

CARDIAC DISEASE ASSESSMENT

A thorough cardiac disease assessment includes the following:

- Patient medical history
- Physical examination
- Laboratory tests
- Physiological tests

Patient Medical History A proper patient history documents the most common complaints and establishes a basis for CHD risk profiling. Because CHD symptoms frequently include chest pain, this pain's differential diagnosis becomes a primary focus. **Table 18.4** lists a limited differential diagnosis of chest pain, including possible causes and pathogenesis.

Physical Examination A physician, nurse, or physician's assistant usually conducts the physical examination that includes the patient's vital signs (body temperature, heart rate, breathing rate, and blood pressure; see accompanying Close Up on page 672).

For purposes of prescribing exercise and identifying early warning signs of CHD, the clinical exercise physiologist must know a patient's customary heart rate and blood pressure response to incremental exercise. For example, an increase in systolic blood pressure of 20 mm Hg or more (**hypertensive response**) in low-level physical activity (2 to 4 METs) would indicate overall cardiovascular impairment and warn of an increased myocardial oxygen demand (suggestive of potential coronary ischemia). In contrast, failure for systolic blood pressure to increase (**hypotensive response**) during moderate physical activ-

ity would indicate left ventricular dysfunction; a hypotensive response in intense exercise signals serious mortality risk. Individuals unable to elevate systolic blood pressures above 140 mm Hg during maximal exercise often have serious but dormant cardiac disease.

Heart Auscultation Listening to heart sounds (**auscultation**) provides important information about cardiac function. The exercise physiologist should become familiar with abnormal heart sounds, including how to identify those related to heart murmurs. Auscultation can readily diagnose valvular diseases (e.g., MVP diagnosed by the classic click-murmur sounds) and congenital abnormalities (e.g., regurgitation sounds in ventricular septal defects).

Laboratory-Based Screening/Assessment

The following laboratory-based screenings provide considerable information for confirming and documenting the extent of CHD:

- **Chest x-ray:** Chest x-rays reveal the size and shape of the heart and lungs.
- **Electrocardiogram (ECG):** Resting and exercise ECG provide essential information to assess myocardial electrical conductivity and oxygenation. Correctly reading and interpreting an ECG requires specialized training and considerable practice. **Table 18.5** lists the six different categories of ECG interpretations. Later in this chapter, various ECG abnormalities and abnormal physiologic responses to exercise are described; how to count heart rate from ECG tracings is also detailed. Careful monitoring of ECG changes during exercise targets individuals with potential CHD for further evaluation. **Table 18.6** lists common ECG changes associated with CHD.
- **Blood lipid and lipoproteins:** Routine laboratory testing for CHD risk includes analysis of the blood

Table 18·4 Chest Pain Diagnosis

PAIN/COMPLAINT/FINDINGS	POSSIBLE CAUSES	STIMULI	POSSIBLE PATHOLOGY
Pressure, ache, tightness or burning in midsternum, left shoulder, arm; diaphoresis; nausea; vomiting; S-T segment changes	MI	Exertion; cold; smoking; heavy meal; fluid overload	CHD
Sharp pain worsens with inspiration, improves with sitting	Inflammation	Acute MI	Pericarditis
Chest tightness with breathlessness; low-grade fever	Infection	IV drug use; microbes	Myocarditis; endocarditis
Sharp, stabbing pain; breathlessness; cough; loss of consciousness	Pulmonary	Recent surgery	Pulmonary embolism
Burning pain in stomach; indigestion relieved by antacids	Referred pain	Heavy meal; spicy food	Esophageal reflux
Angina pain; breathlessness; wide pulse pressure; ventricular hypertrophy on ECG	Ventricular outflow tract obstruction	Exertion; CHD	Aortic stenosis; Mitral valve prolapse

Table 18·5	Six Categories for ECG Interpretation

1. **Measurements**
   - Heart rate (atrial and ventricular)
   - PR interval (0.12 to 0.20 s)
   - QRS duration (0.06 to 0.10 s)
   - QT interval (HR dependent)
   - Frontal plane QRS Axis (−30° to +90°)
2. **Rhythm diagnosis**
3. **Conduction diagnosis**
4. **Wave form description**
   - P wave (atrial enlargement)
   - QRS complex (ventricular hypertrophy, infarction)
   - S-T segment (elevated or depressed)
   - T wave (flattened or inverted)
   - U wave (prominent or inverted)
5. **ECG diagnosis**
   - Within normal limits
   - Borderline abnormal
   - Abnormal
6. **Comparison with previous ECG**

From Fardy, P., and Yanowitz, F.G.: *Cardiac Rehabilitation, Adult Fitness and Exercise Testing.* Baltimore, MD: Williams & Wilkins, 1996.

lipid and lipoprotein profiles. Individuals with heart disease often have elevated cholesterol and LDL cholesterol.

- **Serum enzymes:** Alterations in serum enzymes can diagnose or rule out an acute MI. When myocardial cell death (**necrosis**) or prolonged lack of blood flow (**ischemia**) occur, enzymes from the damaged muscle leak into the blood because of the plasma membrane's increased permeability. This leakage increases serum levels of three enzymes: (1) **creatine phosphokinase (CPK)**, which reflects either skeletal or cardiac muscle necrosis depending on one of three isoenzymes that form, (2) **lactate dehydrogenase (LDH)**, which also fractionates into different isoenzyme markers, one of which increases during an MI, and (3) **serum glutamic oxaloacetic transaminase (SGOT)**, which elevates during an MI.

Table 18·6	Normal and Abnormal ECG Changes Commonly Observed During Exercise

NORMAL ECG CHANGES IN HEALTHY INDIVIDUALS	ABNORMAL ECG CHANGES WITH CHD
1. Slight increase in P wave amplitude	1. Appearance of bundle branch block at a critical HR
2. Shortening of PR interval	2. Recurrent or multifocal PVCs during exercise and recovery
3. Shift to the right of QRS axis	3. Ventricular tachycardia
4. S-T segment depression <1.0 mm	4. Appearance of bradyarrhythmias, tachyarrhythmias
5. Decreased T wave amplitude	5. S-T segment depression/elevation of >1.0 mm 0.08 s after J point
6. Single or rare PVC during exercise and recovery	6. Exercise bradycardia
7. Single or rare PVC or PAC	7. Submaximal exercise tachycardia
	8. Increase in frequency or severity of any known arrhythmia

PVC, premature ventricular contraction; PAC, premature atrial contraction.

Questions & Notes

List the 3 diseases that affect heart valves.

1.

2.

3.

Floppy valve syndrome is another name for _____.

Name the 2 types of dysrhythmias.

1.

2.

Give a typical heart rate for sinus tachycardia.

Give a typical heart rate for sinus bradycardia.

List 3 common laboratory-based screening tests for CHD.

1.

2.

3.

Define the term ischemia.

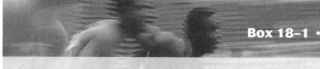

Box 18-1 • CLOSE UP

HOW TO RECOGNIZE VITAL SIGNS

Proper handling of potentially critical situations requires recognition of the following nine **vital signs**:

1. Heart (pulse) rate
2. Breathing rate
3. Blood pressure
4. Body temperature
5. Skin color
6. Pupils of the eye
7. State of consciousness
8. Movement
9. Pain and/or abnormal nerve response

HEART (PULSE) RATE

A normal pulse rate for adults ranges between 60 and 80 b·min^{-1}, and 80 to 100 b·min^{-1} in children. Any alteration from normal can indicate the presence of a pathological condition. For example, a rapid but weak pulse could indicate shock, bleeding, diabetic coma, or heat exhaustion. A rapid and strong pulse may indicate heatstroke or severe fright. A strong but abnormally slow pulse could indicate a skull fracture or stroke, whereas no pulse means cardiac arrest or death.

BREATHING RATE

The normal breathing rate in adults is approximately 12 breaths per minute, and 20 to 25 breaths per minute in children. Breathing can be shallow, irregular, or gasping. Frothy blood from the mouth indicates a chest injury involving the lung. *Look, listen, and feel;* look to ascertain whether the chest is rising or falling; listen for air passing in and out of the mouth or nose or both; and feel how the chest is moving.

BLOOD PRESSURE

Normal systolic blood pressure for 15- to 20-year-old males ranges from 115 to 120 mm Hg; the diastolic pressure ranges from 75 to 80 mm Hg. Blood pressure for females is usually 8 to 10 mm Hg lower for both systolic and diastolic pressures. Between the ages of 15 to 20 years, a systolic pressure of 135 mm Hg and above may be excessive; while a pressure of 110 mm Hg or lower may be considered too low. Diastolic pressure should not exceed 60 mm Hg for females and 85 mm Hg for males. A dramatically lowered blood pressure can indicate hemorrhage, shock, heart attack, or internal organ injury.

BODY TEMPERATURE

Normal body temperature at rest averages 98.6°F (37°C). Temperature can be measured under the tongue, in the armpit, or in the rectum. Changes in body temperature can also be palpated. Hot dry skin can indicate disease, infection, or overexposure to environmental heat. Cool, clammy skin can indicate trauma, shock, or heat exhaustion. Cool, dry skin can be the result of overexposure to cold. A rise or fall of the internal temperature can be caused by a variety of circumstances such as the onset of a communicable disease, cold exposure, pain, fear, or nervousness.

SKIN COLOR

For individuals who are lightly pigmented, the skin can be a good indicator of the state of health. Three skin colors are commonly identified in medical emergencies:

1. *Red:* may indicate heatstroke, high blood pressure, or carbon monoxide poisoning
2. *White:* a pale, ashen, or white skin can mean insufficient circulation, shock, fright, hemorrhage, heat exhaustion, or insulin shock
3. *Blue:* usually means that circulating blood is poorly oxygenated, indicating an airway obstruction or respiratory insufficiency

Assessing a dark skinned individual is complicated. They normally have pink coloration of the nail beds and inside the lips, mouth, and tongue. Changes in these areas can indicate a medical emergency.

PUPILS OF THE EYE

The pupils are extremely sensitive to situations affecting the nervous system. Most persons have pupils of regular outline and equal size. A constricted pupil can indicate a central nervous system response to a depressant drug. If one or both pupils are dilated, the individual may have sustained a head injury, may be experiencing shock, heat stroke, or hemorrhage, or may have ingested a stimulant drug. The pupil's response to light should also be noted. If one or both pupils fail to accommodate to light, there may be brain injury or alcohol or drug poisoning. Pupil response is more critical in evaluation than pupil size.

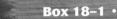

Box 18-1 • CLOSE UP (Continued)

STATE OF CONSCIOUSNESS

Normally, individuals are alert, aware of their environment, and respond quickly to vocal stimulation. Head injury, heatstroke, and diabetic coma can vary an individual's level of conscious awareness.

MOVEMENT

Inability to move a body part can indicate a serious central nervous system injury. Inability to move one side of the body can result from a head injury or cerebrovascular accident. Paralysis of the upper limb can indicate a spinal injury; inability to move the lower extremities

could mean an injury below the neck; and pressure on the spinal cord could lead to limited use of the limbs.

PAIN AND/OR ABNORMAL NERVE RESPONSE

Numbness or tingling in a limb with or without movement can indicate nerve or cold damage. Blocking of a main artery can produce severe pain, loss of sensation, or lack of a pulse in a limb. A complete lack of pain or of awareness of serious but obvious injury can be caused by shock, hysteria, drug usage, or spinal cord injury. Generalized or localized pain in an injured region probably means there is no spinal cord injury.

Noninvasive Physiologic Screening/Assessment

Noninvasive physiologic tests can identify specific cardiovascular/cardiac dysfunction with minimal patient discomfort and risk.

Echocardiography Echocardiography uses pulses of reflected ultrasound to evaluate heart function and morphology; it identifies the heart's structural components and measures distances within the myocardial chambers. This allows estimation of various chamber sizes (volumes), in addition to blood vessel dimensions and thickness of various myocardial components. The echocardiogram has surpassed the ECG in recognizing chamber enlargement, myocardial hypertrophy, and other structural abnormalities. Echocardiograms can diagnose heart murmurs, evaluate valvular lesions, and determine the extent of congenital heart diseases and cardiomyopathies.

Graded Exercise Stress Test A graded exercise stress test (GXT) describes the systematic use of exercise for two purposes:

1. Observe cardiac rhythm abnormalities during exercise
2. Assess physiologic adjustments to increased metabolic demands

The most common modes for exercise stress testing include multistage bicycle and treadmill tests. The test, "graded" for exercise intensity, includes submaximal exercise levels of 3 to 5 minutes in duration, each level progressing up to self-imposed fatigue or a specific target heart rate. The graded nature of testing allows detection of ischemic manifestations and rhythm disorders with small increments in exercise intensity. The stress test provides a reliable, quantitative index of the person's level of functional impairment. *For most screening purposes, the test does not need to be maximal; instead, the person exercises to at least 85% of age-predicted maximum heart rate.* Laboratory-based GXTs remain preferable to field tests (walking or running tests) because of control over test environment and exercise intensity.

A resting ECG precedes the GXT to establish whether the person can engage safely in subsequent graded exercise. The resting ECG also provides an important baseline measure for subsequent comparisons.

Questions & Notes

List 5 vital signs.

1.

2.

3.

4.

5.

Name 2 common noninvasive physiologic CHD screening tests.

1.

2.

Give the 2 purposes for administering a GXT.

1.

2.

Why Stress Test? Stress testing serves an important role in an overall CHD evaluation to:

- **Detect heart disease:** An exercise ECG can diagnose overt heart disease and screen for possible "silent" coronary disease in seemingly healthy individuals. Between 25% and 40% of people with confirmed coronary artery disease have normal resting electrocardiograms. ECG analysis during exercise uncovers about 80% of these abnormalities.
- **Reproduce and assess exercise-related chest symptoms:** Individuals older than age 40 often suffer angina symptoms with physical exertion. ECG analysis during graded exercise provides a more objective and valid diagnosis of exercise-induced chest discomfort.
- **Screen candidates for preventive and rehabilitative exercise programs:** Stress test results help design an exercise program within the person's functional capacity and health status. Repeated testing evaluates training progress and safely modifies the initial exercise prescription.
- **Detect abnormal blood pressure responses:** Exercise hypertension often signifies underlying cardiovascular complications.
- **Monitor responses to various therapeutic interventions designed to improve cardiovascular health and function:** Periodic stress testing often objectifies the degree of benefit derived from pharmacologic, surgical, or dietary treatment of heart disease.

- **Quantify functional aerobic capacity and evaluate its degree of deviation from established standards:** Metabolic measurements during the GXT allow determination of the $\dot{V}O_{2max}$ or $\dot{V}O_{2peak}$.

Who Should Be Stress Tested? **Table 18.7** shows a classification system by age and health status for screening and supervisory procedures for both stress testing and participation in a regular exercise program. These guidelines apply for healthy individuals and those at higher risk. Healthy young adults can begin moderate intensity exercise at 40% to 60% $\dot{V}O_{2max}$ without an exercise stress test or medical examination. Men above age 40 and women above age 50 should have a medical examination that includes a stress test before starting an exercise program. A GXT that precedes exercise training takes on added importance for higher risk individuals of any age. *This pertains to people with two or more major CHD risk factors and/or symptoms suggestive of cardiopulmonary or metabolic disease.*

Informed Consent All testing and exercise training must be performed by "informed volunteers." *Informed consent raises awareness about all potential risks of participation.* Informed consent must include a written statement that the person had an opportunity to ask questions about the procedures with sufficient information clearly provided so consent occurs from a knowledgeable (in-

Table 18·7	Recommendations for Medical Examination, Graded Exercise Stress Testing (GXT) and Physician Supervision of GXT Before Participation in an Exercise Program	
RISK CATEGORY	**MEDICAL EXAMINATION AND GXT**	**M.D. SUPERVISION**
Low risk Men <45 years Women <55 years; asymptomatic with ≤1 risk factor[a,b]	Moderate exercise; not necessary Vigorous exercise; not necessary	Moderate exercise; not necessary Vigorous exercise; not necessary
Moderate risk Men ≥45 Women ≥55, with ≥2 risk factors[a,b]	Moderate exercise; not necessary Vigorous exercise; recommended	Moderate exercise; not necessary Vigorous exercise; recommended
High risk Individuals with ≥1 sign/symptom of cardiovascular or pulmonary disease[c] or known cardiovascular (cardiac, peripheral vascular, or cerebrovascular), pulmonary (obstructive pulmonary disease, asthma, cystic fibrosis), or metabolic (diabetes, thyroid disorder, renal or liver) disease	Moderate exercise; recommended Vigorous exercise; recommended	Moderate exercise; recommended Vigorous exercise; recommended

[a] Risk factors: family history of heart disease, cigarette smoking, hypertension, hypercholesterolemia, impaired fasting glucose, obesity, and sedentary lifestyle.
[b] HDL>60 mg·dL^{-1} (subtract 1 risk factor from the sum of other risk factors because high HDL decreases CHD risk).
[c] Signs and symptoms of cardiovascular and pulmonary disease: pain, discomfort in chest, neck, jaw, left arm; shortness of breath at rest or with mild exertion; dizziness or syncope; orthopnea or paroxysmal nocturnal dyspnea; ankle edema; tachycardia; intermittent claudication; heart murmur; and unusual fatigue or shortness of breath with mild activity.

formed) perspective. A minor requires prior legal consent from a legal guardian or parent. Individuals need assurance that test results remain confidential. Minors must understand that they may terminate the exercise testing or training program at any time and for any reason. **Table 18.8** presents a sample informed consent statement.

Contraindications to Stress Testing   Certain conditions preclude administering a stress test (absolute contraindications), whereas other conditions require the GXT be administered under more closely monitored conditions (relative contraindications).

Absolute Contraindications to Stress Testing

Under no circumstances should a stress test be administered without direct medical supervision if any of the following conditions exist:

- Resting ECG suggestive of acute cardiac disease
- Recent complicated myocardial infarction
- Unstable angina pectoris
- Uncontrolled ventricular arrhythmia
- Uncontrolled atrial arrhythmia that compromises cardiac function
- Third-degree AV heart block without pacemaker
- Acute congestive heart failure
- Severe aortic stenosis
- Active or suspected myocarditis or pericarditis
- Recent systemic or pulmonary embolism
- Acute infections
- Acute emotional distress

Questions & Notes

Give 2 reasons for stress testing.

  1.

  2.

Give a reason for obtaining informed consent.

List 4 absolute contraindications to stress testing.

  1.

  2.

  3.

  4.

Table 18·8   Informed Consent Example for a Graded Exercise Stress Test

Name _____

1. **Explanation of the exercise test**
   You will perform an exercise test on a cycle ergometer or a motor-driven treadmill. The exercise intensity begins at a level you can easily accomplish and will advance in stages of difficulty depending on your fitness level. We may stop the test at any time because of signs of fatigue, or you may stop the test when you wish because of fatigue or discomfort that you feel, particularly at the higher exercise levels.

2. **Risks and Discomforts**
   The possibility exists that certain abnormal changes can occur during the test. These include abnormal blood pressure, fainting, disorder of heart beat, and in rare instances, heart attack, stroke, or death. Every effort will be made to minimize these risks by evaluating preliminary information related to your health and fitness, and by observations during testing. Emergency equipment and available trained personnel can deal with unusual situations that may arise.

3. **Responsibilities of the Participant**
   Information you possess about your health status or previous experiences of unusual feelings with physical effort may affect the safety and value of your exercise test and you should report this information now. Your prompt reporting of how you feel during the exercise test also is important. You are responsible for fully disclosing such information when requested to do so by the testing staff.

4. **Expected Benefits from the Test**
   The results obtained from the exercise test may assist in diagnosing your illness, or evaluating what type of physical activities you might do with low risk.

5. **Inquires**
   We encourage you to ask any questions about the procedures used in the exercise test or in the estimation of your functional capacity. If you have doubts or questions, please ask us for further explanations.

6. **Freedom of Consent**
   Your permission to perform this exercise test is voluntary. You are free to deny consent or stop the test at any point.
   I have read this form and understand the test procedures. I voluntarily consent to participate in this test.

Date: _____

Signature of Patient: _____

Signature of Witness: _____

Questions: _____

_____

Responses: _____

Signature of Physician or Delegate: _____

Relative Contraindications to Stress Testing

Administer a GXT with caution and with medical personnel in close proximity to the test area if any of the following conditions exist:

- Resting diastolic blood pressure >115 mm Hg or systolic blood pressure = 200 mm Hg
- Moderate valvular disease
- Electrolyte abnormalities
- Frequent or complex ventricular ectopic beats
- Ventricular aneurysm
- Uncontrolled metabolic disease (diabetes, thyrotoxicosis)
- Chronic infectious disease (hepatitis, mononucleosis, AIDS)
- Neuromuscular or musculoskeletal disorders
- Pregnancy (complicated or in the last trimester)
- Psychological distress/apprehension about taking the test

Maximal Versus Submaximal Stress Testing *A maximal GXT (GXT_{max}) represents the most common noninvasive method to screen for CHD and determine $\dot{V}O_{2max}$ or $\dot{V}O_{2peak}$.* Individuals exercise until they decide to stop or develop abnormal symptoms that signal test termination (**Table 18.9**). The term **symptom limited** describes such stress tests.

GXT_{max} normally progresses through several stages (multistage); the duration, starting point, and increments between stages vary with the person (e.g., young active, healthy sedentary, and questionable health status). Advantages of a GXT_{max} include direct determination of $\dot{V}O_{2max}$ and maximal cardiovascular responses, screening for ab-

normal ECG patterns not revealed during rest or low-intensity exercise, and establishing more precise training levels. Disadvantages include the considerable stress placed on the person; although GXT_{max} exhibits low risk, the discomfort of being pushed to maximum without prior physical conditioning may deter some persons from participating in a subsequent exercise fitness program. For most healthy people, about the same physiologic information can be obtained from a submaximal test as from an intense submaximal test (80–90% HR_{max}) requiring all-out effort.

The criteria for stopping a test distinguish one GXT protocol from another; otherwise, any of the protocols are effective. In all instances, an abnormal response should result in test termination.

Important factors that influence a person's physiologic response to submaximal or maximal exercise include:

- Ambient temperature and relative humidity
- Subject's sleep state (number of sleep hours prior to testing)
- Emotional state
- Medication
- Time of day
- Caffeine intake
- Time since last meal
- Time since last exercise
- Testing environment (type and appearance of testing room, physical appearance and behavior of test personnel)

Stress Test Protocols Test duration, initial exercise intensity level, and increments of intensity between stages for GXT protocols dictate the test to administer. In a national survey of 1400 exercise stress test centers, 71% used treadmills, 17% use bicycle ergometers, and only 12% use step tests. No statistics exist for arm-cranking or swimming stress tests.

Treadmill Tests

Treadmill tests accommodate individuals through a broad spectrum of fitness using the "natural" activities of walking and running. (See Chapter 7, page 246, for a discussion of the different treadmill protocols.) **Table 18.10** presents adaptations of the **Naughton** (best for deconditioned persons), **Balke** (best for normal, inactive persons), and **Bruce** (best for active, young persons) treadmill test protocols.

Each protocol has advantages and disadvantages. The Bruce test, for example, uses a more abrupt increase in exercise intensity between stages. This may benefit sensitivity to ischemic ECG responses, but it also necessitates that the person tolerate the increased exercise level. A stress test should begin at a relatively low level, with 2- to 3-minute increments in exercise intensity. A warm-up should be used either separately or incorporated into the test. Total test duration should last at least 8 minutes. A test longer than 20 minutes provides no additional useful ECG or physiologic data. However, a longer test establishes more precise end points.

Table 18•9	Criteria for Stopping a GXT in Apparently Healthy Adults

1. Onset of angina or angina-like symptoms
2. Ventricular tachycardia
3. Significant decrease in systolic blood pressure of 20 mm Hg or more
4. Failure of systolic blood pressure and/or heart rate to rise with an increase in exercise load
5. Light-headedness, confusion, ataxia, pallor, cyanosis, nausea, or signs of severe peripheral circulatory insufficiency
6. Early onset horizontal or downsloping S-T segment depression or elevation (>4 mm)
7. Increasing ventricular ectopy, multiform PVCs
8. Excessive increase in blood pressure: systolic > 260 mm Hg; diastolic > 115 mm Hg
9. Increase in heart rate < 25 b·min^{-1} of predicted normal value (in the absence of beta blockade medication)
10. Sustained supraventricular tachycardia
11. Subject requests to stop test for whatever reason
12. Equipment failure

From *ACSM's Guidelines for Exercise Testing and Prescription.* 7th Ed. Baltimore: Lippincott, Williams & Wilkins, 2006.

Table 18·10	Adaptations of the Naughton, Balke, and Bruce Treadmill Protocols for Different Populations				
STAGE	METs	SPEED[a] km·h⁻¹	GRADE %	TIME MIN
For very sedentary adults (modified Naughton test[b])				
1	2.5	3.2	0	3
2	3.5	3.2	3.5	3
3	4.5	3.2	7	3
4	5.4	3.2	10.5	3
5	6.4	3.2	14	3
6	7.3	3.2	17.5	3
7	8.5	4.8	12.5	3
8	9.5	4.8	15	3
9	10.5	4.8	17.5	3
For normal sedentary adults (modified Balke test[c])				
1	4.3	4.8	2.5	2
2	5.4	4.8	5	2
3	6.4	4.8	7.5	2
4	7.4	4.8	10	2
5	8.5	4.8	12.5	2
6	9.5	4.8	15	2
7	10.5	4.8	17.5	2
8	11.6	4.8	20	2
9	12.6	4.8	22.5	2
10	13.6	4.8	25	2
For young active adults (modified Bruce test[d])				
1	5	2.7	10	3
2	7	4	12	3
3	9.5	5.4	14	3
4	13	6.7	16	3
5	16	8	18	3

[a] 1 km = 0.625 miles.
[b] Naughton, J.P.: Methods of Exercise Testing. In: *Exercise Testing and Exercise Training in Coronary Heart Disease*. New York: Academic Press, 1973.
[c] Balke, B.: *Advanced Exercise Procedures for Evaluation of the Cardiovascular System*. Monograph. Milwaukee: The Burdick Corp., 1970.
[d] Bruce, R.A.: Multi-stage treadmill test of maximal and submaximal exercise. In: *AHA: Exercise Testing and Training of Apparently Healthy Individuals: A Handbook for Physicians*. New York: 1972.

Questions & Notes

List 4 relative contraindications to stress testing.

1.

2.

3.

4.

List 3 factors that influence a person's physiologic response to submaximal or maximal exercise.

1.

2.

3.

Describe the Bruce GXT protocol.

Describe the Balke GXT protocol.

Bicycle Ergometer Tests

Bicycle ergometers have distinct advantages over other exercise devices. In contrast to treadmills, power output (easily calculated and regulated) on the ergometer is independent of body mass. Most ergometers are portable, safe, and relatively inexpensive. Electrically braked and weight-loaded, friction-type devices represent the two most common cycle ergometers. For electrically braked ergometers, preselected power output remains fixed within a range of pedaling frequencies. Power output with weight-loaded ergometers relates directly to frictional resistance and pedaling rate.

The same general guidelines for treadmill testing apply to testing on a bicycle ergometer (and arm-crank ergometer). Power output on a bicycle ergometer is expressed in kg-m·min⁻¹ or watts (1 W = 6.12 kg-m·min⁻¹). Bicycle ergometer tests generally use 2- to 4-minute stages of graded exercise. Initial resistance ranges between 0 and 30 W; power output generally increases 15 to 30 W per stage. Pedaling at 50 or 60 revolutions per minute (rpm) represents the typical rpm for weight-loaded ergometers.

Arm-Crank Ergometer Tests

Stress testing can use arm cranking (**Fig. 18.3**) as the exercise stressor when formulating the exercise prescription for upper-body exercise. Arm-crank exercise

Box 18–2 • CLOSE UP

DETERMINING HEART RATE FROM AN ELECTROCARDIOGRAPHIC TRACING

The **electrocardiogram (ECG)** depicts the pattern of electrical activity across the myocardium recorded by an **electrocardiograph**. As the wave of depolarization travels throughout the heart, electrical currents spread through the highly conductive body fluids for monitoring by electrodes placed on the skin's surface. Standard markings on the ECG paper allow time interval and voltage measurements during ECG propagation.

STANDARD ECG TRACING

Figure 1 shows a standard ECG tracing with time recorded on the horizontal axis. The paper normally moves at 25 mm per second. A repeating grid marks the ECG paper; major grid lines occur 5 mm apart (at 25 mm·s^{-1} paper speed, 5 mm = 0.20 s), minor grid lines occur 1 mm apart (at 25 mm·s^{-1} paper speed,

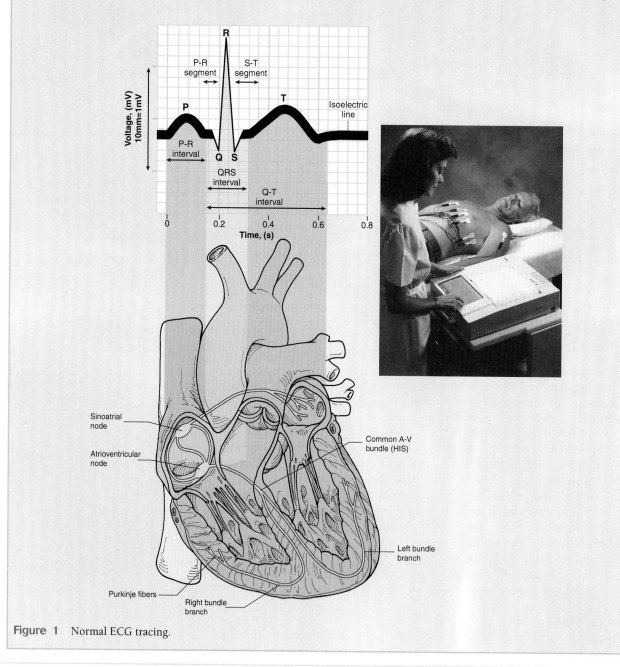

Figure 1   Normal ECG tracing.

Box 18–2 •   CLOSE UP *(Continued)*

1 mm = 0.04 s). The graph's vertical axis indicates electrical voltage. The standard calibration factor equals 0.1 mV (millivolt) per mm of vertical deflection.

DETERMINING HEART RATE

Three methods determine heart rate from the standard ECG tracing.

Method 1

Figure 2A shows the standard **R-R method**. The R-R interval indicates the time between successive R waves. An approximate heart rate in beats per minute ($b \cdot min^{-1}$) can be determined by dividing 1500 (60 s ÷ 25 $mm \cdot s^{-1}$) by the number of mm between adjacent R waves. In the example, heart rate equals 125 $b \cdot min^{-1}$ because 12 mm occurs between two successive R waves.

Method 2

This method begins with an R wave that falls on a thick blue line of the tracing (Fig. 2B). Moving to the right, the next six thick lines represent heart rates of 300, 150, 100, 75, 60, and 50 $mm \cdot s^{-1}$ (these numbers need to be memorized). If the next R wave (after the first one falling on the thick line) falls on either the first through sixth subsequent thick lines, the corresponding number (300 to 50) indicates heart rate in $mm \cdot s^{-1}$. Interpolation becomes necessary if the next R wave falls between two thick lines. In this instance, the first R wave falls between points 60 and 75 at 70 $mm \cdot s^{-1}$.

Method 3

This method (Fig. 2C) is often used with irregular heart rates, counts the number of complete R-R intervals in a 6-second ECG strip multiplied by 10. In this example, six complete R-to-R intervals occur in 6 seconds; this equals a heart rate of 60 $b \cdot min^{-1}$ (6 × 10 = 60).

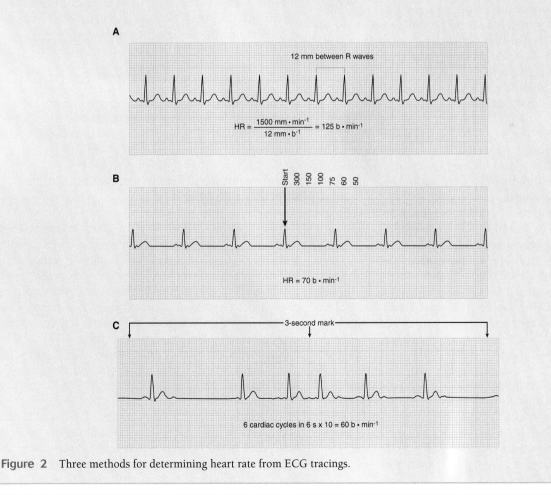

Figure 2   Three methods for determining heart rate from ECG tracings.

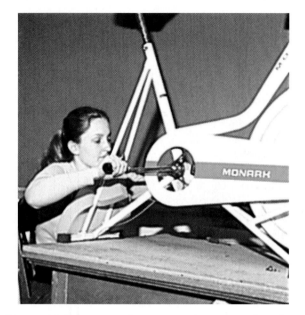

Figure 18.3   Arm-crank ergometer for testing physiologic and metabolic responses to upper-body exercise.

generally produces up to 30% lower $\dot{V}O_{2max}$ values and 10 to 15 b·min^{-1} lower maximum heart rates compared with treadmill or bicycle exercise. Unfortunately, arm-crank exercise interferes with conventional blood pressure measurement during exercise. Blood pressure, heart rate, and oxygen uptake values remain higher during submaximal arm-cranking compared to the same power output in leg exercise. Protocols developed for leg cycling tests can evaluate a patient's response to upper-body exercise. The starting frictional resistance will be less with incremental power output levels adjusted accordingly.

Safety of Stress Testing   The yearly death rate from stress testing ranges between 2% to 12% for men with clinical evidence of heart disease. Such broad variation in expected mortality directly relates to the number and severity of diseased coronary arteries.

In approximately 170,000 submaximal and maximal stress tests, only 16 high-risk but apparently healthy patients suffered coronary episodes. This represents about one person per 10,000, or approximately 0.01% of the total group. In more than 9000 stress tests, no cardiovascular episodes occurred for subjects with increased heart disease risk. In other reports, risk of coronary episodes for healthy, middle-aged adults during a maximum stress test equaled about 1 in 3000. In most middle-aged men and women, test risk generally increases about 6 to 12 times higher than for young adults. For patients with documented CHD (including previous myocardial infarction or episodes of angina), risk of cardiovascular incident in stress testing increases 30 to 60 times above normal. Based on total risk analyses, many experts believe that a *lower* "overall risk" exists for those who take a GXT and then initiate a regular exercise program than for those who take no GXT and remain sedentary.

Stress Test Outcomes   The clinical value of a stress test depends on how well it detects heart disease, or its degree of **sensitivity**. *Sensitivity of a stress test refers to the percentage of people with actual disease who have an abnormal test result.* Four possible outcomes from a graded exercise stress test include:

- **True-Positive**: Test results correctly diagnose heart disease (test successful).
- **False-Negative**: Normal test results, but heart disease is present (test unsuccessful; heart disease undiagnosed).
- **True-Negative**: Test results normal; no heart disease (test successful).
- **False-Positive**: Test results abnormal, but person does not have heart disease (test unsuccessful; healthy person diagnosed with heart disease).

False-negative results occur 25% of the time, and false-positives occur 15% of the time. False-negatives and false-positives have dramatic ramifications, particularly a false-negative result. Whenever a stress test indicates presence of heart disease, subsequent thallium imaging or angiocardiography confirms the diagnosis. Similarly, a normal stress test does not rule out heart disease. Despite these limitations, the predictive value of an abnormal stress test exceeds the predictive value of a normal test.

Exercise-Induced Indicators of CHD

The prognostic value of exercise testing in asymptomatic individuals is based on observations of electrocardiographic ischemia (and other abnormalities) and from fitness-related variables obtained during the GXT.

Exercise-Induced Electrocardiographic Indicators of CHD

Angina Pectoris   Approximately 30% of initial manifestations of CHD during exercise are revealed from chest-related pain (angina pectoris). This condition indicates insufficiency of coronary blood flow, where oxygen supply momentarily reaches critically low levels. Myocardial ischemia (insufficient oxygen supply caused by coronary atherosclerosis) stimulates sensory nerves in the walls of coronary arteries and myocardium. (Refer to Fig. 18.3 for locations of angina pain.) After resting a few minutes, the pain usually subsides without permanent damage to the heart muscle.

ECG Disorders   Alterations in the heart's normal pattern of electrical activity rarely show up until the heart's metabolic (and blood flow) requirements increase above the resting level. The most common ECG abnormalities observed during exercise indicate myocardial ischemia (coronary artery obstruction accounts for most myocardial ischemia). Significant arterial obstruction refers to more than 50% diameter reduction from occlusion. A 50% diameter reduction equals a 75% loss in the arterial lumen. A significantly obstructed coronary artery can still maintain adequate blood flow at rest but cannot deliver sufficient blood (and oxygen) to meet increased myocardial needs with exercise. Ischemia does not always produce angina pectoris; its diagnosis most readily occurs through depressions of the S-T segment of the ECG. **Figure 18.4** shows three types of **S-T segment depressions**: upsloping, horizontal, and downsloping.

Alterations in cardiac rhythm (**arrhythmia**) with exercise frequently appear as **premature ventricular contractions** (**PVCs; Fig. 18.5**). In this case, the ventricles demonstrate disorganized electrical activity. The ECG shows this as an "extra" ventricular beat (QRS complex), which occurs without a P wave normally preceding it.

Exercise PVCs generally herald the presence of severe ischemic atherosclerotic heart disease, often involving two or more major coronary vessels. Individuals who experience frequent PVCs have a high risk of sudden death from ventricular fibrillation, an electrical instability when ventricles fail to contract synchronously. This disrupts myocardial function, causing cardiac output to fall dramatically.

Exercise-Induced Non-Electrocardiographic Indicators of CHD

Two useful non-electrocardiographic indicators of possible CHD include blood pressure and heart rate response to exercise.

Hypertensive Response/Hypotensive Response

During a graded exercise test, a normal, progressive transition in systolic blood pressure occurs from about 120 mm Hg at rest to 160 to 190 mm Hg during peak exercise. Diastolic pressure generally changes less than 10 mm Hg. A hypertensive response in strenuous exercise can elevate systolic blood pressure to 250 mm

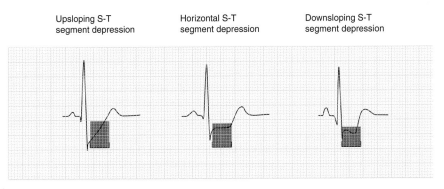

Upsloping S-T segment depression   Horizontal S-T segment depression   Downsloping S-T segment depression

Figure 18.4   Three types of S-T segment depression: upsloping, horizontal, and downsloping.

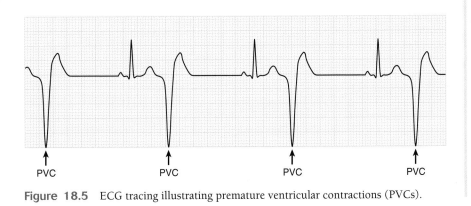

PVC   PVC   PVC   PVC

Figure 18.5   ECG tracing illustrating premature ventricular contractions (PVCs).

Questions & Notes

Give the units of measurement for power on a bicycle ergometer.

Name an exercise-induced electrocardiographic indicator of CHD.

FOR YOUR INFORMATION

Chronic Fatigue Syndrome and Exercise

Chronic fatigue syndrome (CFS) involves continual and severe fatigue. Its prevalence has been estimated at between 75 and 265 people per 100,000 population. The cause(s) of CFS remain unknown, but may represent a common end point from multiple causes that include infectious agents (similar to Epstein-Barr virus), immunological variables (perhaps inappropriate production of cytokines such as interleukin-1), hypothalamic-pituitary-adrenal (HPA) axis stimulation leading to increased release of cortisol and other hormones that influence the immune system and other body systems, neurally mediated hypotension, and possible nutritional deficiencies.

Treatment for CFS focuses on relief of symptoms with the goal of regaining some level of pre-existing function. Modest regular exercise to avoid deconditioning is important for all CFS patients. A key consideration involves modulating exercise intensity and duration and knowing when to stop activity at the first signs of fatigue. Regardless of activity level, the individual must avoid increasing the level of fatigue. A regular, manageable daily routine of light to moderate physical activity helps avoid the "push-crash" phenomenon characterized by overexertion during periods of better health, followed by a relapse of symptoms initiated by the excessive physical activity (*http://www.ncpad.org/*).

Box 18–3 • CLOSE UP

RECOGNIZING MAJOR SIGNS AND SYMPTOMS OF CARDIOPULMONARY DISEASE

Individuals with undiagnosed cardiopulmonary diseases exhibit specific signs and symptoms during rest and exercise. Signs and symptoms of cardiopulmonary disease in the clinical context help identify individuals in need of further evaluation.

MAJOR SIGNS AND SYMPTOMS

- Pain or discomfort (or other angina equivalent) in the chest, neck, or arms
- Shortness of breath at rest or with mild exertion
- Dizziness or syncope (feeling of light-headedness or faintness)

- Dyspnea (shortness of breath or labored breathing) on rising from supine position or at night during sleep
- Palpitations or tachycardia (unexplained increased heart rate) during rest or mild exercise
- Ankle edema (swelling)
- Intermittent claudication (ischemic pain described as an aching, weakness, tightness or cramping sensation during physical activity) in the calf of the leg
- Known heart murmur
- Unusual fatigue accompanied by moderate to extreme dyspnea during usual activities

---

Hg or higher, whereas diastolic pressure can approach 150 mm Hg. Abnormal blood pressure responses to exercise often provide an important clue to cardiovascular disease.

Failure of blood pressure to increase with graded exercise (hypotensive response) can indicate cardiovascular malfunction. For example, diminished cardiac reserve may exist if systolic blood pressure does not increase by at least 20 or 30 mm Hg during graded exercise.

Heart Rate Response

An abnormally rapid heart rate (tachycardia) early in submaximal exercise often foretells cardiac problems. Likewise, abnormally low exercise heart rate (bradycardia) can reflect sinus node malfunction (**sick sinus node syndrome**). Inability of heart rate to increase during exercise, especially when accompanied by extreme fatigue, indicates cardiac strain and underlying heart disease.

In asymptomatic adult women, heart rate recovery (peak HR minus HR 2 minutes after exercise; higher value [poorer recovery] = greater risk) provides the most sensitive predictor of cardiovascular and all-cause mortality than S-T segment depression, as occurs with men, even when considering other diagnostic variables. Because nearly two-thirds of women who die suddenly from cardiovascular disease have no previous symptoms, the important potential role of treadmill testing this population should be recognized.

Invasive Physiologic Tests

Invasive physiologic tests provide diagnostic information unavailable through noninvasive procedures. This infor-

mation includes the extent, severity, and location of coronary atherosclerosis, degree of ventricular dysfunction, and specific cardiac abnormalities. The three most common invasive physiologic tests include:

1. **Radionucleotide studies** include two types: (1) **thallium imaging**, which evaluates areas of myocardial blood flow and tissue perfusion to differentiate between a true- and a false-positive S-T segment depression (by ECG evaluation), and (2) **ventriculography**, an imaging procedure that provides information about left ventricular functional dynamics.
2. **Cardiac catheterization** involves threading a small-diameter, flexible tube (catheter), guided by x-ray, directly into an arm or leg vein and/or artery into the right or left side of the heart. Sensors on the catheter tip accurately measure pressure gradients at various locations within the heart's chambers or large vessels and also assess the heart's electrical patterns to determine coronary artery blockage. The oxygen content of arterial and mixed-venous blood comes from blood sampled from the ventricles or atria. Cardiac catheterization takes place under local anesthesia, depending on the point of catheter entry (arm or leg). The patient remains awake during the procedure, and test results usually become available on the day of testing.
3. **Coronary angiography** provides an intracardiac x-ray after a radiopaque contrast medium enters the coronary blood vessels, and its passage is viewed during a cardiac cycle. This technique accurately assesses the extent of atherosclerosis and serves as the criterion "gold standard" for viewing coronary blood flow.

It also creates a baseline for other test comparisons and validations. Angiography does not show how readily blood flows within local portions of the myocardium (does not measure capillary blood flow), and it cannot be used during exercise.

Functional Classification of Heart Disease

Table 18.11 shows a system for classifying the functional and therapeutic characteristics of various stages of heart disease. Substantial individual differences exist in symptoms, functional capacities, and appropriate rehabilitation requirements. Whenever patients undertake rehabilitation, their classification should include available medical screening information and recent GXT.

Exercise Prescription for Cardiac Patients

Heart rate and oxygen uptake data obtained during the GXT form the basis for an individualized exercise prescription. Many people who start exercising do not recognize their limitations and exercise above a prudent level. Even group exercise programs that require medical clearance may not be appropriate because all members often exercise at about the *same* work level (walk, jog, or swim at a similar pace) without much attention paid to individual differences in fitness status.

Figure 18.6 illustrates a practical approach for functional translation of treadmill or cycle ergometer exercise test responses to an exercise prescription. Heart rate (A) during the Bruce test is plotted as a function of time. Line B depicts a mathematical line of "best fit" drawn through the data points. A target zone for heart rate equals 60% to 75% of maximum heart rate (167 b·min^{-1}; shaded portion represented as C). The individualized prescription includes pace (14.0 to 15.4 min per mile and/or 3.9 to 5.9 METs) (E). The acceptable range of exercise

Table 18·11	Functional Capacity and Therapeutic Classifications of Heart Disease	
Functional Capacity Classification		
Class I		No limitation of physical activity. Ordinary physical activity does not cause undue fatigue, palpitation, dyspnea, or anginal pain
Class II		Slight limitation of physical activity. Comfortable at rest, but ordinary physical activity results in fatigue, palpitation, dyspnea, or anginal pain
Class III		Marked limitation of physical activity. Comfortable at rest, but less than ordinary activity causes fatigue, palpitation, dyspnea, or anginal pain
Class IV		Unable to carry on any physical activity without discomfort. Symptoms of cardiac insufficiency or angina may be present even at rest. If any physical activity is undertaken, discomfort increases
Therapeutic Classification		
Class A		Physical activity need not be restricted
Class B		Ordinary physical activity need not be restricted, but unusually severe or competitive efforts should be avoided
Class C		Ordinary physical activity should be moderately restricted, and more strenuous efforts should be discontinued
Class D		Ordinary physical activity should be markedly restricted
Class E		Patient should be at complete rest and confined to bed or a chair

Questions & Notes

Draw and label a typical ECG tracing.

FOR YOUR INFORMATION

Fibromyalgia and Exercise
Fibromyalgia (FM) represents a complex condition experienced by 3.4% of women and 0.5% of men in the United States. FM causes persistent pain in muscles, ligaments, tendons, and joints. FM may cause other symptoms including disturbed sleep, and headaches. Symptoms can worsen with anxiety, cold environments, depression, hormonal changes, physical overexertion, and increased stress. FM can exist by itself, but it usually accompanies rheumatoid arthritis, hypothyroidism, and chronic fatigue syndrome.

Individuals with FM benefit from tailored exercise programs that condition muscles and decrease symptoms by countering the effects of prolonged deconditioning. Primary exercises combine slow stretching, light resistance exercise for all major muscle groups, and low-intensity aerobic activity. Low-impact walking, stair climbing, or swimming is particularly well suited for FM patients. Avoid exercises that include high-impact or high-loading, jogging, aerobic dancing, weight training, racquet sports, basketball, or other activities that involve repetitive jumping (*http://www.ncpad.org/*).

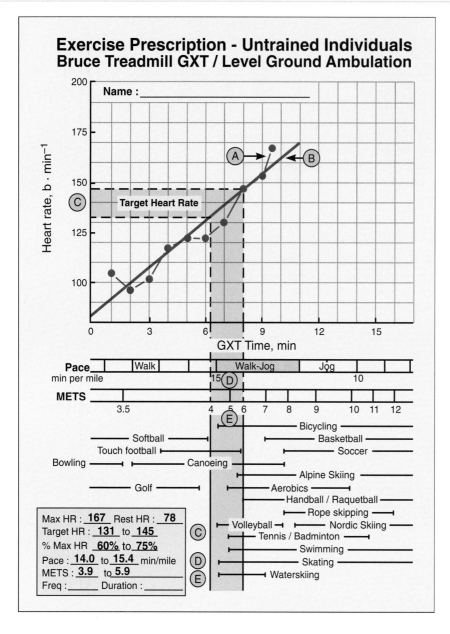

Figure 18.6 Exercise prescription based on functional translation algorithm for level ground ambulation. (Courtesy of Dr. C. Foster, Professor, Department of Exercise and Sport Science; Director, Department of Exercise and Sport Science, University of Wisconsin-La Crosse, La Crosse, WI.

intensity in area C, based on heart rate response during the graded exercise test, includes the following recreational activities: bicycling, canoeing, alpine skiing, aerobics, volleyball, tennis and badminton, swimming, skating, and waterskiing. This quantitative method of assigning exercise improves exercise prescription specificity and precision for previously sedentary, healthy individuals and patients with diagnosed cardiovascular diseases.

Guidelines Any exercise prescription should begin with 5 to 15 minutes of light stretching and range-of-motion activities followed by several minutes of light to moderate preliminary, rhythmic "warm-up" movements. The aerobic conditioning phase should progress in duration so individuals eventually perform 30 to 45 minutes of continuous activity at the prescribed intensity followed by

5 to 15 minutes of low-intensity walking or other rhythmic cool-down activities.

Most cardiac rehabilitation patients tolerate exercising 3 days per week with no more than a 2-day lapse between exercise sessions. For elderly patients or those with poor functional capacity (<5 METs), low-intensity exercise should be performed daily or twice daily. As a patient's functional capacity improves, exercise intensity and duration can increase progressively with little fear of complications. The most recent GXT serves as the basis for updating the exercise prescription.

Three other important components of cardiac rehabilitation include (1) patient education, (2) appropriate pharmacologic intervention, and (3) family support counseling. A trained social worker often coordinates these aspects of the rehabilitative process.

Box 18–4 • CLOSE UP

THE REVISED rPAR-Q TO ASSESS READINESS FOR PHYSICAL ACTIVITY

The original Par-Q (1978) was first recommended as *minimal* screening for entry into moderate-intensity exercise programs. It was designed to identify the small number of adults for whom physical activity might be inappropriate or those who should receive medical advice concerning the most suitable type of activity. The revised Par-Q (rPar-Q, 1994) presented here was developed to reduce the number of unnecessary exclusions (false-positives). The revision can determine the exercise readiness of apparently healthy middle-aged adults with no more than one major risk factor for coronary heart disease.

If You Answered *Yes* to One or More Questions

Talk with your doctor by phone or in person BEFORE you start becoming much more physically active or BEFORE you have a fitness appraisal. Tell your doctor about the rPar-Q and which questions you answered YES to.

- You may be able to do any activity you want—as long as you start slowly and build up gradually. Or, you may need to restrict your activities to those that are safe for you. Talk with your doctor about the kinds of activities you wish to participate in, and follow his or her advice.

- Find out which community programs are safe and helpful for you.

If You Answered *No* to All Questions

If you answered NO honestly to all rPar-Q questions, you can be reasonably sure that you can:

Start becoming much more physically active—begin slowly and build up gradually; this is the safest and easiest way to go.

Take part in a fitness appraisal—this is an excellent way to determine your basic fitness so that you can plan the best way for you to live actively.

DELAY BECOMING MUCH MORE ACTIVE

If you are not feeling well because of a temporary illness such as a cold or a fever, wait until you feel better, or if you are or may be pregnant, talk to your doctor before you start becoming more active.

Note, if your health changes so that you then answer YES to any of the questions on the rPar-Q, tell your fitness or health professional. Ask whether you should change your physical activity plan.

YES ___ NO ___ 1. Has your doctor ever said that you have a heart condition and recommended only medically supervised activity?

YES ___ NO ___ 2. Do you have chest pain brought on by physical activity?

YES ___ NO ___ 3. Have you developed chest pain in the past month?

YES ___ NO ___ 4. Do you lose your balance because of dizziness, or do you ever lose consciousness?

YES ___ NO ___ 5. Do you have a bone or joint problem that could be worsened by a change in your physical activity?

YES ___ NO ___ 6. Is your doctor currently prescribing drugs (for example, water pills) for high blood pressure or a heart condition?

YES ___NO ___ 7. Do you know of any other reason why you should not do physical activity?

NOTE: Postpone testing if you have a temporary illness such as a common cold or are not feeling well.

REFERENCE

Canadian Society for Exercise Physiology: *Par-Q and You.* Gloucester, Ontario, Canada: Canadian Society for Exercise Physiology, 1994.

Beneficial Effects of Resistance Exercise Resistance exercise helps restore and maintain muscular strength and preserve fat-free body mass as part of a comprehensive cardiac rehabilitation program. Because blood pressure increases substantially with straining-type exercises, resistance training for the cardiac patient should consist of relatively light resistance (30% to 60% estimated 1-RM) with at least 15 repetitions. Progression should be slow, starting with one set and advancing to three sets, depending on the patient's fitness level. For heart transplant patients, a carefully supervised total body (including back) resistance training program (3 days weekly for 6 months) increases functional strength and muscle mass to counter the generally debilitating effects of immunosuppressive medication.

The Rehabilitation Program The most effective preventive and rehabilitative programs emphasize individualized exercise. Some CHD patients have a reduced heart rate response to exercise with a corresponding decrease in maximum heart rate. Use of population-based target heart rates for these individuals overestimates a prudent training intensity. This argues for exercise testing to each patient's symptom-limited maximum and then formulating the exercise prescription based on the patient's *actual* heart rate data.

Patients should engage in endurance-type activities at least three times weekly for 20 to 40 minutes each exercise session at 50% to 75% of exercise capacity or at a similar oxygen uptake capacity measured on the GXT. This "target zone" puts individuals at or above a threshold level to achieve a training effect. Ideally, the personalized exercise prescription includes recommendations for weight loss and dietary modification (if necessary), warm-up and cool-down activities, and a developmental total-body or muscle-specific strength improvement program.

PULMONARY DISEASES AND DISORDERS

The exercise physiologist's involvement in treating patients with pulmonary disease focuses primarily on improving ventilation, decreasing the work of breathing, and increasing overall level of functional capacity. The exercise physiologist applies clinical information from the personal history, physical examination, pertinent laboratory data, and imaging studies. Disorders of the cardiovascular system usually impair pulmonary function. Conversely, cardiovascular complications often follow pulmonary disease onset.

Restrictive (reduced lung volume dimensions) and obstructive (impeded air flow) lung diseases represent two common classifications for pulmonary dysfunction. Although a convenient classification system, several pulmonary disorders combine both restrictive and obstructive impairments.

Restrictive Lung Dysfunction

Restrictive lung dysfunction (RLD), characterized by an abnormal reduction in pulmonary ventilation, includes diminished lung expansion and decreased tidal volume. The chest and lung tissues in RLD tend to stiffen and offer considerable resistance to expansion under normal pulmonary pressure differentials. This represents a reduction in **lung compliance**, that is, a change in lung volume per unit change in intra-alveolar pressure. Decreased pulmonary compliance increases the energy cost of ventilation, even at rest. Eventually, RLD progresses to a point where considerable decreases occur in all lung volumes and capacities.

Table 18.12 lists major RLDs, along with causes, signs and symptoms, and treatments. Other known causes of RLD include rheumatoid arthritis, immunologic impairment, massive obesity, diabetes mellitus, trauma from impact injuries, penetrating wounds, burns and other inhalation injuries, radiation trauma, poisoning, and complications from drug therapy (including negative reactions to antibiotics and anti-inflammatory drugs).

Chronic Obstructive Pulmonary Disease

Chronic obstructive pulmonary disease (COPD), also termed chronic airflow limitations (CAL), includes respiratory diseases that produce airflow obstruction. This ultimately affects the lung's mechanical function and compromises alveolar gas exchange. In the United States, COPD ranks as the fifth leading cause of death and the second leading cause of morbidity. The natural history of COPD spans 20 to 50 years and is closely linked with chronic cigarette smoking.

COPD is usually diagnosed from changes in pulmonary function, most notably a decrease in expiratory flow rates and an increase in residual lung volume. Classic symptoms include spontaneous spasms of bronchial smooth muscle that produce chronic coughing, inflammation and thickening of the mucosal lining of the bronchi and bronchioles, increased mucus production, wheezing, and dyspnea upon physical exertion. **Table 18.13** summarizes the differences among major COPD conditions.

In all forms of COPD, airways narrow to obstruct airflow. Airway narrowing hinders alveolar ventilation by trapping air in the bronchi and alveoli; in essence, COPD increases physiologic dead space. Obstruction principally increases resistance to airflow during expiration, impairs normal alveolar gas exchange, diminishes exercise capacity, and reduces ventilatory capacity.

The following brief discussion centers on three major COPD diseases: (1) chronic bronchitis, (2) emphysema, and (3) cystic fibrosis. Chapter 11 discussed the obstructive conditions of asthma and exercise-induced bronchospasm.

Chronic Bronchitis **Acute bronchitis** refers to self-limiting and short duration inflammation of the trachea

Table 18·12	Major Restrictive Lung Diseases and Their Causes, Signs and Symptoms, and Treatment		
CAUSES/TYPE	**ETIOLOGY**	**SIGNS AND SYMPTOMS**	**TREATMENT**
I. Maturational			
a. *Abnormal fetal lung development*	Premature birth (hypoplasia-reduced lung tissue)	Asymptomatic; pulmonary insufficiency	No specific treatment
b. *Respiratory distress syndrome* (hyaline membrane disease)	Insufficient maturation of lungs due to premature birth	↑ respiration rate; ↓ lung volumes; ↓ PaO_2; acidemia; rapid and labored respiration pressure	Treat mother prior to birth (corticosteroids); hyperalimentation; continuous positive airway
c. *Aging*	Aging and cumulative effects of pollution, noxious gas, inhaled drug use, and cigarette smoking	↑ residual volume; ↓ vital capacity; repetitive periodic apnea	No specific treatment; increase physical activity
II. Pulmonary			
a. *Idiopathic pulmonary fibrosis* (IPF)	Unknown origin (perhaps viral or genetic)	↓ lung volumes; pulmonary hypertension; dyspnea; cough; weight loss, fatigue	Corticosteriods; maintain adequate nutrition and ventilation
b. *Coal workers' pneumoconiosis*	Repeated inhalation of coal dust over 10–12 y	↓ TLC, VC, FRC; ↓ lung compliance; dyspnea; ↓ PaO_2; pulmonary hypertension; cough	Nonreversible, no known cure
c. *Asbestosis*	Chronic exposure to asbestos	↓ lung volumes; abnormal x-ray; ↓ PaO_2; dyspnea on exertion; shortness of breath	Nonreversible, no known cure
d. *Pneumonia*	Inflammatory process caused by various bacteria, microbes, viruses	↓ lung volumes; abnormal x-ray; tachypneic dyspnea; high fever, chills, cough; pleuritic pain	Drug therapy (antibiotic)
e. *Adult respiratory distress syndrome*	Acute lung injury (fat emboli, drowning, drug induced, shock, blood transfusion, pneumonia)	Abnormal lung function tests; PaO_2 < 60 mm Hg; extreme dyspnea; cyanotic; headache; anxiety	Intubation and mechanical ventilation
f. *Bronchogenic carcinoma*	Tobacco use	Variable depending on type and location of growth	Surgery; radiation; chemotherapy
g. *Pleural effusions*	Accumulation of fluid within pleural space; heart failure; cirrhosis	Shortness of breath; pleuritic chest pain; ↓ PaO_2	Specific drainage
III. Cardiovascular			
a. *Pulmonary edema*	↑ pulmonary capillary hydrostatic pressure secondary to left ventricular failure	↑ respiration rate; ↓ lung volumes; ↓ PaO_2; arrhythmias; feeling of suffocation, shortness of breath, cyanotic, cough	Drug therapy; diuretics; supplemental O_2
b. *Pulmonary emboli*	Complications of venous thrombosis	↓ lung volumes, ↓ PaO_2; tachycardia; acute dyspnea, shortness of breath; syncope	Heparin therapy; mechanical ventilation

and bronchi. In contrast, **chronic bronchitis** mostly occurs with long-term exposure to non-specific irritants. Increases in mucus secretion accompany prolonged respiratory tract inflammation. Over time, the swollen mucous membranes and thick sputum obstruct airways, causing wheezing and persistent coughing. Partial or complete airway blockage from mucus secretion causes insufficient arterial oxygen saturation and edema, which produces the characteristic look known as the "Blue Bloater" (**Fig. 18.7**). Chronic bronchitis develops slowly and worsens over time. Patients usually have been long-term smokers. Functional exercise capacity remains low, and fatigue occurs readily with only moderate effort. If left untreated, the disease can lead to death.

Emphysema   Abnormal, permanent enlargement of air spaces distal to the terminal bronchi characterizes **emphysema**. This disease often develops from chronic

Table 18•13	Differences Among Major COPD Diseases	
NAME	**AREA AFFECTED**	**RESULT**
Bronchitis	Membrane lining bronchial tubes	Inflammation of bronchial lining
Bronchiectasis	Bronchial tubes (bronchi or air passages)	Bronchial dilation with inflammation
Emphysema	Air spaces beyond terminal bronchioles (aleveoli)	Breakdown of alveolar walls; air spaces enlarged
Asthma	Bronchioles (small airways)	Bronchioles obstructed by muscle spasm; swelling of mucosa; thick secretions
Cystic fibrosis	Bronchioles	Bronchioles become obstructed and obliterated; plugs of mucus cling to airway walls leading to bronchitis, atelectasis, pneumonia, or pulmonary abscess

bronchitis and occurs frequently in long-term cigarette smokers. Symptoms include extreme dyspnea, abnormally increased arterial carbon dioxide tension (hypercapnia), persistent cough, cyanosis, and digital clubbing (evidence of chronic hypoxemia; **Fig. 18.8**). Patients frequently appear thin; they lean forward with arms braced on the knees to support their shoulders and chest for easier breathing. The effects of trapped air and alveolar distention change the size and shape of the chest, causing the characteristic emphysemic "barrel chest" appearance (**Fig. 18.9**).

Although exercise cannot "cure" emphysema, it does enhance cardiovascular fitness and strengthens respiratory musculature. Regular exercise also improves a patient's psychological state.

Cystic Fibrosis The term **cystic fibrosis (CF)** originated from observing cysts and scar tissue on the pancreas of autopsied patients. Although pancreatic cysts and scar tissue often exist, they are not primary characteristics of the disease (although the term cystic fibrosis remains in use). **Table 18.14** lists clinical signs and symptoms of CF. CF, characterized by thickened secretions of all exocrine glands (e.g., pancreatic, pulmonic, and gastrointestinal), eventually obstructs pulmonary airflow. The most common inherited genetic disease in Caucasians, CF afflicts approximately one in 2000 white newborn infants in the United States. The disease, inherited as a recessive trait (both parents are carriers), has no current cure and remains fatal.

Pulmonary system involvement represents the most common and severe manifestation of CF. Airway obstruction leads to a chronic state of hyperinflation. Over time, RLD superimposes on the obstructive disorder, leading to chronic hypoxia, hypercapnia, and acidosis. Pneumothorax and pulmonary hypertension eventually follow and cause death.

Treatment of CF includes antibiotics, enzyme supplements, nutritional intervention, and frequent secretion

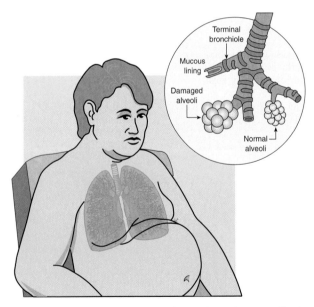

Figure 18.7 Individuals with chronic bronchitis usually develop cyanosis and pulmonary edema with the characteristic appearance known as "Blue Bloater." The effects of chronic bronchitis displayed in the insert illustrate misshapen or large alveolar sacs with reduced surface for oxygen and carbon dioxide exchange.

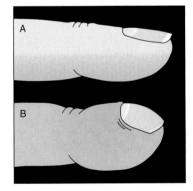

Figure 18.8 Normal digit configuration **(A)** and example of digital clubbing **(B)**, indicating chronic tissue hypoxia, a common physical symptom of emphysema.

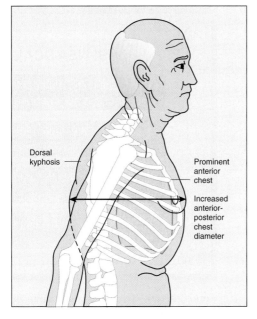

Dorsal
kyphosis

Prominent
anterior
chest

Increased
anterior-
posterior
chest
diameter

Figure 18.9 Emphysema traps air in the lungs, making exhalation difficult. With time, changes in the patient's physical features include a "barrel chest" appearance.

removal. Regular physical activity can provide beneficial outcomes: Twenty minutes of aerobic exercise replaces one session of secretion removal in some children. Increased minute ventilation with aerobic exercise helps clear excessive secretions from the airways. Improved physical fitness may play a role in delaying the crippling effects of CF.

Pulmonary Assessments

Chest and lung imaging provide the most common pulmonary assessment techniques. These include conventional x-ray and computed tomography (CT) scanning to (1) screen for abnormalities, (2) provide a baseline for subsequent assessments, and (3) monitor disease progression. Magnetic resonance imaging (MRI) plays a limited role because the density of large portions of the lungs cannot generate clear magnetic signals. Static and dynamic tests of lung function,

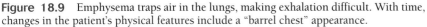

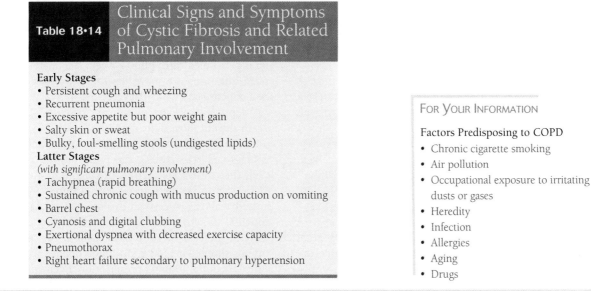

Table 18·14	Clinical Signs and Symptoms of Cystic Fibrosis and Related Pulmonary Involvement

Early Stages
- Persistent cough and wheezing
- Recurrent pneumonia
- Excessive appetite but poor weight gain
- Salty skin or sweat
- Bulky, foul-smelling stools (undigested lipids)

Latter Stages
(with significant pulmonary involvement)
- Tachypnea (rapid breathing)
- Sustained chronic cough with mucus production on vomiting
- Barrel chest
- Cyanosis and digital clubbing
- Exertional dyspnea with decreased exercise capacity
- Pneumothorax
- Right heart failure secondary to pulmonary hypertension

Questions & Notes

Briefly describe 3 COPD symptoms.

1.

2.

3.

List 3 different COPD diseases.

1.

2.

3.

List 3 symptoms of cystic fibrosis.

1.

2.

3.

List 2 factors that predispose a person to COPD.

1.

2.

FOR YOUR INFORMATION

Factors Predisposing to COPD
- Chronic cigarette smoking
- Air pollution
- Occupational exposure to irritating dusts or gases
- Heredity
- Infection
- Allergies
- Aging
- Drugs

pulmonary diffusing capacity, and flow-volume loops also provide diagnostic information.

Pulmonary Rehabilitation and Exercise Prescription

Pulmonary rehabilitation receives considerably less attention than programs for cardiovascular and musculoskeletal diseases. Perhaps de-emphasis has resulted from rehabilitation's failure to markedly improve pulmonary function or reverse the natural progression of these debilitating and often deadly diseases. Pulmonary rehabilitation can have marked, positive effects on exercise capacity, respiratory muscle function, psychological status, quality of life variables (e.g., self-esteem and self-efficacy), frequency of hospitalization, and disease progression. Major goals for pulmonary rehabilitation include the following:

- Improve health status
- Improve respiratory symptoms (shortness of breath and cough)
- Recognize early signs requiring medical intervention
- Decrease frequency and severity of respiratory problems
- Obtain maximal arterial oxygen saturation
- Improve daily functional capacity through enhanced muscular strength, joint flexibility, and cardiorespiratory endurance
- Improve strength and power of the ventilatory musculature
- Improve body composition
- Improve nutritional status

Pulmonary rehabilitation programs include the following five components:

1. General care
2. Pulmonary respiratory care
3. Exercise and functional training
4. Education
5. Psychosocial management

The exercise and functional training aspects of rehabilitation are particularly important to individuals with end-stage disease because the effects of weakness, fatigue, and severe dyspnea profoundly limit physical activity. Physiologic monitoring during exercise rehabilitation should asses heart rate, blood pressure, respiratory rate, arterial oxygen saturation by pulse oximetry (indicates arterial oxygen desaturation), and dyspnea.

Dyspnea monitoring involves a perceived dyspnea scale (**Fig. 18.10**), similar to scales for rating of perceived exertion. Extreme shortness of breath, fatigue, palpitations, chest discomfort, or a decrease of 3% to 5% on pulse oximetry indicates the need to terminate the exercise test.

The pretraining GXT and spirometric analyses govern the exercise prescription. Exercise stress test interpretation includes determining: (1) whether the test termi-

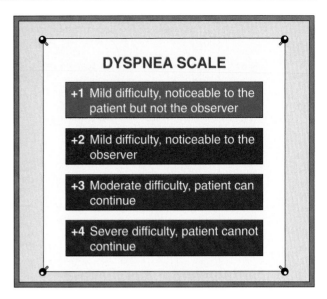

Figure 18.10 Dyspnea scale. Grading of subjective ratings of dyspnea intensity during exercise testing occurs on a scale of 1 to 4. Dyspnea usually accompanies poor exercise capacity and impaired ability to increase systolic blood pressure during graded exercise testing.

nated for cardiovascular or ventilatory end points, (2) the difference between pre- and postexercise pulmonary function (e.g., a decrease of 10% in $FEV_{1.0}$ indicates the need for bronchodilator therapy before exercise), and (3) the need for supplemental oxygen from arterial oxygen desaturation during exercise (e.g., a decrease in PaO_2 of more than 20 mm Hg or a PaO_2 of less than 55 mm Hg).

The exercise prescription for a patient with mild pulmonary disease (shortness of breath with heavy exercise) mirrors that for a healthy individual. For patients with moderate disease (shortness of breath with normal daily activities or clinical symptoms of RLD or COPD), exercise training can proceed: (1) at an intensity no greater than 75% of ventilatory reserve, (2) in the middle of the calculated training heart rate range (50% to 70% of age-predicted HR_{max}), or (3) at the point where the patient becomes noticeably dyspneic. For most individuals, dyspnea occurs between 40% to 85% of maximum MET level on a GXT. Under these circumstances, exercise duration usually lasts 20 minutes, and is performed three times a week. If 5- to 15-minute exercise durations are more desirable, exercise frequency should increase to 5 to 7 days weekly.

Patients with severe pulmonary disease (shortness of breath during most daily activities, and FVC and $FEV_{1.0}$ below 55% of predicted values) require a modified approach to exercise testing and prescription. Usually low-level, discontinuous testing can begin at two to three METs with increments every several minutes. Symptom-limited walking speeds and distances provide helpful guidelines for formulating an exercise prescription. Brief bouts of interval exercise often benefit this population. Patients should exercise a minimum of once daily because of the low initial training prescription. Even small gains in exercise tolerance improve an individual's functional capacity and quality of life indices.

For all pulmonary disease patients, regular exercise contributes to improved respiratory muscle function. Two approaches achieve this goal:

1. Resistance training improves strength and power of ventilatory muscles by use of a **continuous positive airway pressure (CPAP) device.** This overloads ventilatory muscles in a manner similar to progressive resistance exercise for other skeletal muscles.
2. Increases in endurance performance capacity of respiratory muscles through regular and progressive aerobic exercise training.

NEUROMUSCULAR DISEASES AND DISORDERS

Neuromuscular diseases represent conditions affecting the brain in one way or another. Progressive nerve degeneration or trauma to specific brain neurons result in specific impairment that ranges from simple to complex. *More Americans are hospitalized with neurological and mental disorders than any other major disease group, including heart disease and cancer.* The economic costs of brain dysfunction are enormous, but they pale in comparison with the staggering emotional toll on victims and their families.

The pace of neuroscience research is truly breathtaking and raises hopes that new treatments will be found for the wide range of nervous system disorders that debilitate and cripple millions of people. Exercise and physical activity play a unique role in this endeavor.

Stroke

Stroke refers to a potentially fatal reduction or cutoff of the blood supply to part of the brain from restricted blood supply (ischemia) or bleeding (hemorrhage). The resulting brain injury affects multiple systems depending on injury site and the amount of damage sustained. Effects include motor and sensory impairment and language, perception, and affective and cognitive dysfunction. Strokes can cause severe limitations in mobility and cognition or can be mild with only short-term, non-permanent consequences.

Clinical Features   Clinical features of stroke depend on location and severity of the injury. Signs of a hemorrhagic stroke include altered levels of consciousness, severe headache, and elevated blood pressure. Cerebellar hemorrhage usually occurs unilaterally and is associated with disequilibrium, nausea, and vomiting. **Table 18.15** presents the typical physical and psychological traits and comorbidities associated with stroke.

Cerebral blood flow (CBF) represents the primary marker for assessing ischemic strokes. When CBF drops below 10 mL·100 g·min^{-1} (normal CBF = 50–55 mL·100 g·min^{-1}), synaptic transmission failure occurs, and a CBF of $\leq$8 mL·100 g·min^{-1} results in cell death.

Strokes cause physical and cognitive damage. Left-hemisphere lesions typically are associated with expressive and receptive language deficits compared to right-hemisphere lesions. Motor impairment from a stroke usually results in hemiplegia (paralysis) or hemiparesis (weakness). Damage to descending neural pathways produces an abnormal regulation of spinal motor neurons, resulting in adverse changes in postural and stretch reflexes and difficulty with voluntary movement. Deficits in motor control may involve muscle weakness, abnormal synergistic organization of movement, impaired regulation of force, decreased reaction times, abnormal muscle tone, and loss of active range of joint motion.

Exercise Prescription   The emphasis for stroke survivors centers on rehabilitation of movement (flexibility, passive and active-assisted, strength) during

Questions & Notes

List 3 goals for pulmonary rehabilitation.

1.

2.

3.

List 3 components of a pulmonary rehabilitation program.

1.

2.

3.

List 2 variables that require monitoring during exercise rehabilitation.

1.

2.

Briefly describe the dyspnea grading scale.

Give the best marker for assessing ischemic stroke.

Table 18·15	Physical and Psychological Conditions and Comorbidities Associated with Stroke Patients		
PHYSICAL CONDITIONS	**PSYCHOLOGICAL CONDITIONS**	**COMORBIDITIES**	
Aphasia	Cognitive impairment	Coronary heart disease	
Balance problems	Emotional instability	Diabetes mellitus	
Falls	Depression	Hypertension	
Fatigue	Memory loss	Hyperlipidemia	
Muscle weakness	Low self-esteem	Obesity	
Obesity	Social isolation	Peripheral vascular disease	
Paralysis			
Paresis			
Spasticity			
Visual impairments			

the first 6 months of recovery. The few exercise-training studies with stroke patients support using exercise to improve mobility and functional independence and prevent or reduce further disease and functional impairment. Since stroke survivors vary widely in age, degree of disability, motivational level, and number and severity of comorbidities, secondary conditions, and associated circumstances, the specific exercise prescription focuses on reducing these conditions and improving functional capacity.

Multiple Sclerosis

Multiple sclerosis (MS) represents a chronic, often disabling disease characterized by destruction of the myelin sheath (demyelination) that surrounds nerve fibers of the central nervous system. Lesions of inflammatory demyelination can be present in any part of the brain and spinal cord.

Clinical Features Two or more areas of demyelination confirm the diagnosis of MS. MS usually develops between the ages of 20 and 40 years. Frequently, a history emerges of transient neurological deficits, such as numbness of an extremity, weakness, blurring of vision, and diplopia (double vision) in childhood or adolescence prior to the development of more persistent neurological deficits that lead to the definitive diagnosis. MS occurs worldwide at a higher frequency in latitudes further from the equator. Prevalence of MS in the U.S. below the 37th parallel occurs at a rate of 57 to 78 cases per 100,000, whereas the prevalence rate above the 37th parallel averages 140 cases per 100,000. Reasons for these differences remain unknown. Patients with a definite MS diagnosis more likely have a variety of other autoimmune illnesses, such as systemic lupus erythematosus, rheumatoid arthritis, polymyositis, and myasthenia gravis. A person with a first-degree relative with MS has a 12- to 20-fold increased chance of developing MS.

Fatigue is the most common symptom of MS. Other symptoms include one or all of the following: painful blurring or loss of vision in one eye; muscle weakness in the extremities; clumsiness; numbness and tingling; bowel and bladder dysfunction; sexual dysfunction; joint contractures; urinary tract infection; osteoporosis; and spasticity.

Exercise Prescription MS patients benefit from a comprehensive health prescription involving aerobic, strength, balance, and flexibility exercises. One important factor hindering endurance training is that about 80% of MS patients report adverse effects to heat, whether generated environmentally by outside climatic changes or internally via fever or exercise-induced thermogenesis. This makes continuous exercise training difficult and not well tolerated. Nevertheless, MS patients still can improve cardiovascular function. Stationary cycling, walking, and low-impact chair or water aerobics provide ideal training choices, depending on personal interest and level and nature of physical impairment. Ideal exercise consists of walking in a climate-controlled area that provides stable temperatures, a level surface, and the opportunity to rest frequently. Controlling body temperature represents a primary consideration in the exercise prescription. A realistic and achievable goal for structured exercise provides training three times per week for a minimum of 30 minutes each session, which can be divided into three 10-minute sessions.

Parkinson's Disease

Parkinson's disease (PD), a common neurodegenerative disease, has a prevalence of 60 to 187 per 100,000 people worldwide (no population is immune to the disease). The risk of developing PD increases with age; 10% of patients become symptomatic before age 40 years, 30% become symptomatic before age 50 years, and 40% become symptomatic between 50 and 60 years.

Clinical Features Clinical symptoms of PD include varying degrees of tremor, a decrease in spontaneity and movement (bradykinesia), rigidity, and impaired postural reflexes. These conditions produce extreme gait and postural instability, resulting in increased episodes of falling and/or freezing and great difficulty walking. Some patients exhibit a complete lack of movement (**akinesia**). Functional problems also include difficulty getting out of bed or a car and rising from a chair. Other problems include difficulties dressing, writing, talking, and swallowing. The person with PD generally experiences difficulty with more than one task at a time. As the disease progresses, these problems usually become more pronounced and the person eventually loses the ability to perform activities of daily living. In the last stage of the disease, the person becomes wheelchair and/or bed bound.

Exercise Prescription   Most exercise prescriptions for PD patients are individualized and directed toward interventions that impact associated motor control problems. They emphasize slow, controlled movements for specific tasks through various ranges of motion while lying, sitting, standing, and walking. Treatment protocols include range of motion exercises that use slow static stretches for all major muscle/joint areas, balance and gait training, mobility, and/or coordination exercises. Little research has assessed the effects of training on aerobic capacity, and there are no guidelines established. Anecdotal reports indicate that swimming provides a well-tolerated exercise mode.

RENAL DISEASE AND DISORDERS

Like cardiovascular diseases, treatment modalities for the major metabolic diseases of obesity, diabetes, and renal disease use regular exercise as adjunctive therapy. Obesity and diabetes have been discussed in different chapters of this text. In this section, we review aspects of renal (associated with kidney function) disease related to exercise physiology.

Renal Disease

Chronic kidney disease occurs when kidneys no longer adequately filter toxins and waste products from the blood. Acute renal failure occurs from a toxin (e.g., drug allergy or poison) or severe blood loss or trauma. Diabetes is the number one cause of kidney disease and is responsible for about 40% of all kidney failures; high blood pressure is the second greatest cause of kidney disease and is responsible for about 25% of all kidney failures. Genetic diseases, autoimmune diseases, birth defects, and other problems also cause kidney ailments.

Clinical Features   Common symptoms of chronic kidney disease, sometimes referred to as **uremia** (retention in the blood of waste products normally excreted in urine), include the following:

- *Changes in urination*: making more or less urine than usual, feeling pressure when urinating, changes in the color of urine, foamy or bubbly urine, or having to get up at night to urinate.
- *Swelling of the feet, ankles, hands, or face*: fluid that the kidneys are unable to remove may stay in the tissues.
- *Fatigue or weakness*: a build-up of wastes or a shortage of red blood cells (anemia) can cause these problems as the kidneys begin to fail.
- *Shortness of breath*: kidney failure is sometimes confused with asthma or heart failure because fluid can build up in the lungs.
- *Ammonia breath or an ammonia or metal taste in the mouth*: waste build-up can cause bad breath, changes in taste, or an aversion to protein foods like meat.
- *Back or flank pain*: the kidneys are located on either side of the spine in the back.
- *Itching*: waste accumulation can cause severe itching, especially of the legs.
- *Loss of appetite*

Questions & Notes

Give the age range when multiple sclerosis usually develops.

Give the most common symptom of multiple sclerosis.

Give 2 clinical symptoms of Parkinson's disease.

  1.

  2.

_____ is the number one cause of kidney disease.

Common symptoms of chronic kidney disease are usually referred to as

_____.

List 3 common symptoms of kidney disease.

  1.

  2.

  3.

- *Nausea and vomiting*
- *Increased hypoglycemic episodes, if diabetic*: patients with chronic uremia eventually progress to **end-stage renal disease (ESRD)** requiring life-long dialysis or a kidney transplant. The number of renal transplants has increased steadily in the last decade worldwide and generally offers a more normal lifestyle and full rehabilitation. Nearly 80% of transplant patients function at near normal levels compared with 40% to 60% of those treated with various forms of dialysis. Almost 75% of transplant patients are able to resume work compared to about 50% to 60% of dialysis patients.

Exercise Prescription   Exercise training does not accentuate progression of kidney disease. Decreases in cardiovascular function and exercise performance relate to associated anemia in ESRD; this can improve somewhat with the blood-building hormone erythropoietin (EPO) therapy (injections at the end of each three-time per week dialysis session). Regular exercise serves an important role in rehabilitating dialysis and transplant patients to better adapt to their illness. The rehabilitation program should begin prior to the start of dialysis to optimize beneficial effects. Normal low-level endurance training reduces muscle protein degradation in moderate renal insufficiency, reduces resting blood pressure in some hemodialysis patients, and modestly improves aerobic capacity in patients undergoing hemodialysis.

No longitudinal data exist on the effects of aerobic training or a more physically active lifestyle on the survival of patients with chronic uremia or kidney transplants. However, those uremic patients who maintain a lifetime of diverse physical activity do report an enhanced quality of life. Despite lack of quantitative, long-term quality of live and survival data, more than 23 years have passed since initiation of the first U.S. Transplant Games (*http://www.kidney.org/recips/athletics/tgames/index.cfm*). Participants in these games, which are open to recipients of a currently functioning solid organ or tissue transplant, train rigorously and perform at world record levels.

DISEASES AND DISORDERS OF UNCONTROLLED GROWTH OF ABNORMAL CELLS

Cancer represents a group of diseases collectively characterized by uncontrolled growth of abnormal cells. More than 100 different types of cancers exist, most occurring in adults. **Carcinomas** are cancers that develop from epithelial cells that line the surface of the body, glands, and internal organs. They account for 80% to 90% of all cancers including prostate, colon, lung, cervical, and breast cancer. Cancers also can arise from cells of the blood (**leukemias**), the immune system (**lymphomas**), and connective tissues such as bones, tendons, cartilage, fat, and muscle (**sarcomas**).

Cancer remains the second leading cause of death in the United States; approximately one-third of the population has some type of cancer. Minorities (with different cultural backgrounds and health-nutrition beliefs) consistently have higher cancer rates, although the reasons remain unknown. Cancer represents the leading cause of death in women between the ages of 25 and 44 years.

The current population of more than 8 million cancer survivors (many initially diagnosed in the 1970s and 1980s) illustrates the ongoing need for rehabilitative and maintenance options in this important area of medicine. The most serious outcomes for most cancer patients and survivors include loss of muscle mass and functional status. Depressed functional status encompasses difficulty walking (even a short distance) and serious fatigue that limits completion of simple household chores. Approximately 75% of cancer survivors report extreme fatigue during and following radiotherapy or chemotherapy, accompanied by weight loss and decreased muscular strength and cardiovascular endurance. Maintaining and restoring functional capacity challenges the cancer survivor, even those patients considered "cured." Sufficient rationale now justifies exercise intervention for cancer patients during and following different treatment modalities.

Epidemiological evidence shows that regular exercise can reduce risk for certain cancers by:

- Reducing levels of plasma glucose and insulin
- Increasing levels of corticosteroid hormones
- Increasing anti-inflammatory cytokines
- Augmenting insulin-receptor expression in cancer-fighting T cells
- Increasing interferon production
- Stimulating glycogen synthetase activity
- Augmenting leukocyte function
- Improving ascorbic acid metabolism
- Benefiting pro-virus or oncogene activation

Clinical Features   Clinical features of cancer relate to the effects of the three primary cancer treatment modalities: **surgery**, **radiation**, and **systemic** (**pharmacologic**) therapy. Surgery represents the oldest and most common modality in cancer therapy. Surgeries include operations to remove high-risk tissues to prevent cancer development, biopsies of abnormal tissue to diagnose cancer, excision of tumors with curative intent, insertion of central venous catheters to support chemotherapy infusions, reconstruction after definitive surgery, and palliative or symptom relief for incurable disease (i.e., partial bowel removal). Radiation treatment occurs in over 50% of all cancer survivors. It involves photon penetration into specific tissue, which produces an ionized (electrically charged) particle that damages DNA to inhibit cell replication and produce cell death. Radiation treatment typically is given daily for between 5 and 8 weeks. Pharmacologic therapy is prescribed for many advanced solid tumors if cancer cells are suspected of metastasizing beyond the primary site and regional lymph nodes. Chemotherapy, endocrine therapy, and biologic therapy represent the three major types of systemic therapy. Table 18.16 presents common clinical symptoms resulting from surgery, radiation therapy, and systemic therapy interventions.

Exercise Prescription Lance Armstrong's 7th consecutive Tour de France victory in July, 2005 serves as a testament to the remarkable adaptability of the human body. Armstrong survived cancer's potentially lethal effects, including the following years of demanding exercise training that transformed him into one of the greatest endurance athletes. Armstrong did not "beat" cancer—rather, he is successfully surviving it. A legitimate question arises: What constitutes the proper exercise prescription for cancer patients? Unfortunately, little research exists on the timing of exercise relative to various phases of carcinogenesis. This makes it difficult to determine when to initiate exercise intervention. With such little objective information on exercise prescription and cancer rehabilitation, health-fitness professionals generally recommend a symptom-limited, progressive, and individualized exercise prescription. Prudent ambulation of any kind proves beneficial for the most sedentary and deconditioned patient.

Exercise intervention during treatment produces meaningful benefits. Diverse types of research (randomized control, descriptive, and prospective) demonstrate beneficial effects of exercise during cancer treatment in multiple domains of functioning. Benefits include decreased fatigue symptoms, improved functional capacity, decreased neutropenia (abnormally small numbers of neutrophils in circulating blood), reduced severity of pain and diarrhea, and a shortened hospital

Table 18·16 Cancer Therapies and Their Complications	
TYPE OF TREATMENT	**DESCRIPTION AND EFFECTS/OUTCOME**
Surgery	**Lung** – reduced lung capacity, dyspnea, deconditioning **Neck** – reduced range of motion, muscle weakness, occasional cranial nerve palsy **Pelvic region** – urinary incontinence, erectile dysfunction, deconditioning **Abdomen** – deconditioning, diarrhea **Limb amputation** – chronic pain, deconditioning
Radiation Therapy	**Skin** – redness, pain, dryness, peeling, sloughing, reduced elasticity **Brain** – nausea, vomiting, fatigue, memory loss **Thorax** – some degree of irreversible lung fibrosis, heart may receive radiation causing pericardial inflammation or fibrosis, premature atherosclerosis, cardiomyopathy **Abdomen** – vomiting, diarrhea **Pelvis** – diarrhea, pelvic pain, bladder scarring, occasional incontinence, sexual dysfunction **Joints** – connective tissue and joint capsule fibrosis, possible decreased range of motion
Systemic Therapy	**Chemotherapies** [depending on type and amount] – extreme fatigue, anorexia, nausea, anemia, neutropenia, muscle pain, sensory and motor peripheral neuropathy, ataxia, anemia, vomiting, loss of muscle mass, deconditioning, infection **Endocrine Therapies** [depending on type and amount] – fat redistribution (truncal and facial obesity), proximal muscle weakness, osteoporosis, edema, infection, weight gain, extreme fatigue, hot flashes, loss of muscle mass **Biologic Therapies** [depending on type and amount] – fevers or allergic reactions, chills, fever, headache, extreme fatigue, low blood pressure, skin rash, anemia

Reference: Courneya, K.S., et al.: *ACSM's Resource Manual for Clinical Exercise Physiology for Special Populations*. In: Myers, J. (ed.). Baltimore: Lippincott Williams & Wilkins, 2002.

Questions & Notes

Give 3 ways exercise can reduce certain cancer risks.

1.

2.

3.

FOR YOUR INFORMATION

Decreased Cancer Prevalence Associated with Increased Physical Activity
Evidence from more than 25 research studies on humans (from different continents with different diets, ways of life, environmental circumstances, race, ethnicity, and socio-economic backgrounds) and laboratory animals (undergoing voluntary or forced exercise) show that a reduced risk of cancer development is associated with higher levels of regular physical activity.

FOR YOUR INFORMATION

Possible Mechanisms for Breast Cancer Protection with Exercise
1. Alteration in cumulative exposure to estrogen (a primary risk factor for the disease)
   - Changes in menstrual/ovulatory patterns
   - Delayed onset of menarche
   - Increased number of menstrual cycles without ovulation
   - Increased menstrual irregularity results in fewer cycles
   - Decreased levels of body fat
2. Immune system enhancement
3. Healthy lifestyle that accompanies regular exercise
   - Prevention of excess body fat
   - Consumption of low-fat diets
   - Consumption of fruits and vegetables
   - Abstinence from cigarette smoking
   - Attention to preventive health practices
   - Less depression and anxiety
   - Greater self-esteem

stay. Exercise intervention also decreases psychological distress (improves mood state) and enhances immune function.

Current research focuses on psychosocial outcomes such as general fatigue, satisfaction with life, level of depression, self-concept, and quality of life. Such studies report positive associations between regular exercise and improvement in psychosocial outcomes.

Cancer patients can participate in an exercise stress test, which also serves as a basis for the exercise prescription. Similar testing procedures apply as with healthy individuals, except feelings of fatigue require greater attention. **Table 18.17** presents special precautions to consider when testing the functional capacity of cancer patients.

The exercise prescription should encourage ambulation if the patient has no specific exercise contraindications. Also encouraged are range of motion and flexibility exercises and exercises to improve muscular strength and overall mobility (e.g., submaximal static exercises for antigravity muscles, deep breathing exercises, and dynamic trunk rotation movements). In most cases, preference goes to low-level exercise for short periods, performed several times daily. Exercise progression and intensity are individualized, with initial work to rest ratios of 1:1 progressing to 2:1. Eventually, continuous exercise can be prescribed, as tolerated, starting with 3 to 5 minutes, then 10 minutes, and moving up to 30 to 45 minutes per session whenever possible. **Table 18.18** presents general aerobic exercise guidelines for otherwise healthy cancer survivors.

Breast Cancer

Carcinoma of the breast, one of the most common forms of cancer in white females age 40 years and older, represents the leading cause of death in women between ages 40 to 60 years. In 2004, nearly 217,440 new cases of breast cancer were reported (1450 men and 215,990 women) with 40,590 deaths (470 men and 40,110 women); this means that one of every nine females develops breast cancer at some time during her life, with a high rate of reoccurrence. Only heart disease and lung cancer kill more women yearly. Primary breast cancer risk factors include a positive family history of breast cancer, a personal history of cancer, first menstrual period at an early age, menopause at a late age, first childbirth after age 30 or no childbirth, and a high-fat diet.

Numerous studies indicate that daily low- to moderate-intensity aerobic exercise reduces fatigue in women with breast cancer undergoing chemotherapy and improves a wide range of quality of life outcomes from breast cancer treatment. Regular exercise produces positive improvements in functional capacity, body composition, side effects of treatment, mood, and self-image.

A study from one of our laboratories illustrates the benefits of regular exercise in breast cancer survivors. The program, conducted 4 days per week, consisted of self-paced hydraulic resistance exercises performed in a 14-station aerobic exercise circuit by 28 patients recovering from breast cancer surgery.

Figure 18.11 illustrates that exercisers exhibited a 38% decrease in depression compared with a 13% increase for

Table 18·17	Special Precautions for Testing the Functional Capacity of Cancer Patients	
COMPLICATION	**PRECAUTION**	
Ataxia/dizziness/peripheral sensory neuropathy	Avoid tests that require balance and coordination (treadmill, weights)	
Bone pain	Avoid high-impact tests that increase risk of fracture (treadmill, weights)	
Low blood count (hemoglobin ≤ 8.0 g·dL^{-1}; neutrophil count $\leq 0.5 \times 10^9$·L^{-1})	Avoid tests that require high oxygen uptake or high impact (risk of bleeding); ensure proper sterilization of equipment	
Dyspnea	Avoid maximal tests	
Fever ≥ 38°C (100.4°F)	May indicate systemic infection; avoid exercise testing	
Mouth sores/ulcerations	Avoid mouthpieces; use face masks	
Low functional status	Avoid exercise testing	
Surgical wounds/tenderness	Avoid pressure/trauma to surgical site	
Severe nausea/vomiting	Avoid/postpone exercise testing	

Modified from Courneya, K.S., et al.: Coping with cancer: Can exercise help? *Phys. Sports Med.*, 28:49, 2000.

Table 18•18	General Aerobic Exercise Guidelines for Otherwise Healthy Cancer Survivors	
PRESCRIPTION VARIABLE	**GUIDELINES**	
Frequency	At least 3 to 5 times per week; daily activity may be optimal for deconditioned patients	
Intensity	Depends on fitness status and GXT results; usually 50% to 70% $\dot{V}O_{2peak}$; or 60% to 80% HR_{max}; or RPE = 11–14	
Type (mode)	Large muscle group activity, particularly walking and cycling in some cases	
Time (duration)	20 to 30 continuous minutes per session; this goal can be achieved through multiple intermittent shorter sessions with adequate rest intervals	
Progression	May not always be linear; rather it may be cyclical with periods of regression, depending on treatments, etc.	

Modified from Courneya, K.S., et al.: Coping with cancer: Can exercise help? *Phys. Sports Med.*, 28:49, 2000.

Questions & Notes

List 3 primary breast cancer risk factors.

1.

2.

3.

List the 5 major classifications of cognitive and emotional diseases.

1.

2.

3.

4.

5.

List 2 variables common in cancer prevalence.

1.

2.

Name the neurochemical substance usually associated with the "runners high."

List 3 cognitive and emotional diseases.

1.

2.

3.

non-exercising controls who were also recovering from breast cancer surgery. Exercisers decreased trait anxiety by 16% and state anxiety by 20% compared with increases in both variables for controls. These results demonstrate that a planned, moderate aerobic resistance exercise program exerts positive effects on psychosocial variables during breast cancer rehabilitation.

COGNITIVE AND EMOTIONAL DISEASES AND DISORDERS

The National Institutes of Mental Health report that nearly 18.8 million Americans over the age of 18 suffer from major depression. Suicide, closely linked to depression, represents the third leading cause of death among 10- to 24-year olds. Also, 6% to 8% of all outpatients in primary care settings suffer from major depression. According to the National Ambulatory Medical Care Survey, more than 7 million primary care visits were made annually in the early 1990s for the treatment of depression, which is double the number from 10 years earlier. Depression remains underdiagnosed, and only about one-third of those diagnosed with it receive treatment.

The major classifications of cognitive and emotional diseases include:

- **Major depressive disorder**: commonly referred to as "depression."
- **Dysthymia**: mildly depressed on most days over a period of at least 2 years; symptoms resemble major depression but are less severe.
- **Seasonal affective disorder**: recurrence of the depressive symptoms during certain seasons (e.g., winter).
- **Postpartum depression**: in women who have recently given birth; typically occurs in the first few months after delivery, but can happen within the first year after giving birth.
- **Bipolar disorder** (previously known as manic-depressive illness): characterized by extremes in mood and behavior, lasting for at least 2 weeks. Disorder includes manic episodes (mania) of an abnormally and constantly elevated, expansive, or irritable mood and, at the opposite extreme, a major depressive episode

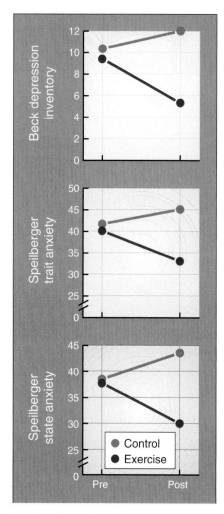

Figure 18.11   Effects of 10 weeks of moderate aerobic circuit resistance exercise on depression (top) and trait (middle) and state (lower) anxiety in women recovering from breast cancer surgery. (Data courtesy of M. Segar, Applied Physiology Laboratory, University of Michigan, Ann Arbor, MI, 1996.)

(depression) of either depressed mood or the loss of interest or pleasure in nearly all activities.z

Clinical Features   Depression has no single cause; often it results from a combination of factors and events. Whatever its cause, depression is not just a state of mind. It is related to physical changes in the brain and is connected to a chemical imbalance of neurotransmitters.

Women are almost twice as likely to become depressed as men, due partly to hormonal changes brought on by puberty, menstruation, menopause, and pregnancy. Men are more likely go undiagnosed and are less likely to seek help. Men may show the typical symptoms of depression, but they tend to be angry and hostile or to mask their condition with alcohol or drug abuse. Suicide becomes an especially serious risk for depressed men, who are four times more likely than women to kill themselves. Depression among the elderly poses a unique situation. Older people often lose loved ones and have to adjust to living alone.

Physical illness decreases normal levels of physical activity. These changes can all contribute to depression. Loved ones may attribute the signs of depression to the normal results of aging, and many older people are reluctant to talk about their symptoms. As a result, older people may not receive proper treatment for their depression.

Common factors in depression include:

- **Family situation**: trauma and stress from financial problems, breakup of a relationship, death of a loved one, or other major life changes
- **Pessimistic personality**: higher risk for individuals who have low self-esteem and a negative outlook
- **Health status**: medical conditions like heart disease, cancer, and HIV contribute to depression
- **Other psychological disorders**: anxiety disorders, eating disorders, schizophrenia, and (especially) substance abuse often appear with depression

Table 18.19 presents common signs and symptoms of depression.

Exercise Prescription   Studies in clinically depressed populations include hospitalized and ambulatory patients. Overall, the data support the positive effects of exercise on depressive symptoms. In most, but not all studies, depression scores significantly decreased in exercising patients.

No one kind of exercise has a greater impact on depression than other types of exercise, although most studies have used running or other aerobic-type activities. Interestingly, positive psychological outcomes do not depend on achieving physical fitness, although fitness-related indicators, like lower blood pressure and increased aerobic capacity, frequently do improve.

How exercise alleviates depression remains unclear. Different psychological and physiologic mechanisms have been suggested. Psychologically, exercise enhances one's sense of mastery and self-esteem, which is important for the depressed individual who feels a loss of control over his or her life. Exercise also provides a therapeutic distraction that diverts a patient's attention from areas of worry, concern, and guilt. Improving one's health,

Table 18•19	Common Signs and Symptoms of Depression

- Loss of enjoyment from things that were once pleasurable
- Loss of energy
- Feelings of hopelessness or worthlessness
- Difficulty concentrating
- Difficulty making decisions
- Insomnia or excessive sleep
- Stomach ache and digestive problems
- Sexual problems (e.g., decreased sex drive)
- Aches and pains (e.g., recurrent headaches)
- A change in appetite causing weight loss or gain
- Thoughts of death or suicide
- Attempting suicide

Box 18–5 • CLOSE UP

PHYSICAL AND HEALTH BENEFITS OF REGULAR PHYSICAL ACTIVITY[a]

PHYSICAL ACTIVITY BENEFIT	SURETY RATING	PHYSICAL ACTIVITY BENEFIT	SURETY RATING
Fitness of body		**Cigarette smoking**	
Improves heart and lung function	****	Improves success in quitting	**
Improves muscular strength/size	****	**Diabetes**	
Cardiovascular disease		Prevention of type 2	****
Coronary heart disease prevention	****	Treatment of type 2	***
Regression of atherosclerosis	**	Treatment of type 1	*
Treatment of heart disease	***	Improvement in life quality	***
Prevention of stroke	**	**Infection and immunity**	
Cancer		Prevention of the common cold	**
Prevention of colon cancer	****	Improves overall immunity	**
Prevention of breast cancer	**	Slows progression of HIV to AIDS	*
Prevention of uterine cancer	**	Improves life quality of infected	****
Prevention of prostate cancer	**	**Arthritis**	
Prevention of other cancers	*	Prevention of arthritis	*
Treatment of cancer	*	Treatment/cure of arthritis	*
Osteoporosis		Improvement life quality/fitness	****
Helps increase bone mass and density	****	**High blood pressure**	
Prevention of osteoporosis	***	Prevention of high blood pressure	****
Treatment of osteoporosis	**	Treatment of high blood pressure	****
Blood cholesterol/lipoproteins		**Asthma**	
Lowers blood total cholesterol	*	Prevention/treatment of asthma	*
Lowers LDL cholesterol	*	Improvement in life quality	***
Lowers triacylglycerols	***	**Sleep**	
Raises HDL cholesterol	***	Improvement in sleep quality	***
Low back pain		**Psychological well-being**	
Prevention of low back pain	**	Elevation in mood	****
Treatment of low back pain	**	Buffers effects of mental stress	***
Nutrition and diet quality		Alleviates/prevents depression	****
Improvement in diet quality	**	Anxiety reduction	****
Increase in total energy intake	***	Improves self-esteem	****
Weight management		**Special issues for women**	
Prevention of weight gain	****	Improves total body fitness	****
Treatment of obesity	**	Improves fitness while pregnant	****
Helps maintain weight loss	***	Improves birthing experience	**
Children and youth		Improves health of fetus	**
Prevention of obesity	***	Improves health during menopause	***
Controls disease risk factors	***		
Reduction of unhealthy habits	**		
Improves odds of adult activity	**		
Elderly and the aging process			
Improvement in physical fitness	****		
Counters loss in heart/lung fitness	**		
Counters loss of muscle	***		
Counters gain in fat	***		
Improvement in life expectancy	****		
Improvement in life quality	****		

Surety Rating Scale
**** Strong consensus, with little or no conflicting data
*** Most data supportive, but more research needed for clarification
** Some supportive data, but much more research needed
* Little or no data to support

[a] Based on a total physical fitness program that includes physical activity designed to improve both aerobic and musculoskeletal fitness.
From Newman, C.C.: The human body. *ACSM's Health Fitness J.*, 2:30, 1998.

physique, flexibility, and body weight can also enhance mood. Large-muscle activity in exercise may help to discharge feelings of pent-up frustration, anger, and hostility.

Researchers continue to study exercise effects on the neurochemistry of mood regulation, specifically turnover of monoamines and other central neurotransmitters at presynaptic and postsynaptic sites. Antidepressant medications, including the selective serotonin reuptake inhibitors (SSRIs), are believed to exert their effect by increasing the availability of neurotransmitters at receptor sites. Exercise may exert its beneficial effect on mood by influencing the metabolism and availability of these central neurotransmitters.

The role of beta-endorphins in mood regulation has received considerable attention. These endogenous chemicals that reduce pain and can induce euphoria have been linked to the "runner's high" experienced by intensive exercisers. The ability of exercise to produce enough beta-endorphins to affect depression remains questionable, but the possibility still exists for depressed patients.

Because disturbed sleep represents both a symptom of depression and an aggravating factor, the beneficial effects of exercise on sleep take on added importance. Recent controlled clinical trials in individuals with depression demonstrate improved subjective sleep quality and a corresponding improvement in depression measures.

The exercise prescription for patients with depression considers the following:

- **Anticipate barriers**. Common symptoms of depression, such as fatigue, lack of energy, and psychomotor retardation, pose formidable barriers to physical activity. Feelings of hopelessness and worthlessness also interfere with motivation to exercise.
- **Keep expectations realistic**. Make exercise recommendations with caution. Depressed patients often self-blame and may view exercise as another occasion for failure. Do not raise false expectations that can arouse anxiety and guilt. Explain that exercise provides an adjunct to, not a substitute for, primary treatment.
- **Design a feasible plan**. Make the exercise prescription realistic and practical, not an additional burden to compound the patient's sense of futility. Consider the individual's background and history. For severely

depressed patients, exercise may need to be postponed until medication and psychotherapy can alleviate symptoms. Previously sedentary patients should start with a light exercise schedule (for example, just a few minutes of walking each day).

- **Accentuate pleasurable aspects**. Guide the choice of exercise by the patient's preferences and circumstances. Use pleasurable activities that are easily added to the patient's schedule.
- **Include group activities**. Depressed patients who are isolated and withdrawn are most likely to benefit from increased social involvement. The stimulation of being outdoors in a pleasant setting can enhance mood; exposure to light exerts therapeutic effects for seasonal depression.
- **State specifics**. Walking is almost universally acceptable, carries minimal risk of injury, and benefits mood enhancement. In keeping with recent ACSM recommendations for healthy adults, a goal of 20 to 60 minutes of walking or other aerobic exercise, three to five times a week, remains reasonable. The ACSM also recommends resistance training 2 to 3 days per week and flexibility training 2 to 3 days per week.
- **Encourage compliance**. Improved fitness may be a valuable consequence of exercise participation but not necessary for an antidepressant effect. Compliance increases with less physically demanding exercise programs.
- **Integrate exercise with other treatments**. The primary treatments for depression should not present exercise obstacles. Antidepressant medication is frequently prescribed when depression impairs a patient's ability to function. It is important to ensure the compatibility of a particular medication with exercise.

Combatting depression relies on a spectrum of brief and longer term psychotherapies, either alone or with antidepressant medication. An exercise prescription complements psychotherapy when the goal increases the patient's overall activity level and adds pleasurable, satisfying experiences. The patient's difficulties with exercise, (motivational problems, fear of interpersonal situations, and/or a tendency to transform exercise into a burdensome chore), may shed light on dysfunctional attitudes that psychotherapy can explore.

SUMMARY

1. In clinical settings, an exercise physiologist health-fitness professional becomes part of a team approach to comprehensive patient health care. The exercise physiologist focuses on restoring the patient's mobility and functional capacity.

2. The major cardiovascular diseases affect the heart muscle directly, the heart valves, or the neural regulation of cardiac function. Each disease category has its specific pathogenesis and intervention strategies.

3. Advances in molecular biology have isolated a possible genetic link to CHD. This gene (on chromosome 19 near the gene related to LDL-cholesterol receptor functioning), called the atherosclerosis susceptibility gene (ATHS), accounts for almost 50% of all CHD cases.

4. An imbalance between the oxygen demands of the heart and its oxygen supply causes acute chest pain (angina pectoris).

5. Myocardial infarction (MI, heart attack, or coronary occlusion) results from inadequate perfusion of blood in the coronary arteries and/or imbalance in myocardial oxygen demand and supply during physical activity. MI generally relates to occlusion of coronary vasculature.

6. Pericarditis, an inflammation of the heart's outer pericardial lining, is classified as either acute or chronic (recurring or constrictive).

7. Congestive heart failure occurs when cardiac output cannot keep pace with venous return. The heart fails from intrinsic myocardial disease, chronic hypertension, or structural defects that impair pump performance.

8. Aneurysm represents an abnormal dilatation in the wall of an artery or vein or the myocardium itself. Vascular aneurysms occur when a vessel's wall weakens from trauma, congenital vascular disease, infection, or atherosclerosis.

9. Aerobic exercise programs implemented for cardiac patients should consider specific disease pathophysiology, mechanisms that can limit exercise capacity, and individual differences in functional capacity.

10. Heart valve diseases include stenosis, insufficiency (regurgitation), and prolapse.

11. Dysrhythmias (bradycardia, tachycardia, and premature ventricular contractions) represent diseases of the heart's nervous system.

12. A thorough cardiac disease assessment includes medical history, physical examination, laboratory assessments (chest x-ray, ECG, blood lipid analyses, and serum enzyme testing), and physiologic tests.

13. The term "stress test" describes systematic exercise for two purposes: (1) ECG observations, and (2) evaluation of physiologic adjustments to metabolic demands that exceed resting requirements.

14. Multistage bicycle and treadmill tests represent the most common modes for exercise stress testing. These tests, graded for exercise intensity, include several levels of 3 to 5 minutes of exercise that bring the person to self-imposed, symptom-limited fatigue.

15. Reasons for including a stress test (and ECG observations) in an overall CHD evaluation include: (1) diagnose overt heart disease, (2) screen for possible "silent" coronary disease in seemingly healthy individuals, (3) reproduce and assess exercise-related chest symptoms, (4) screen candidates for preventive and cardiac rehabilitative exercise programs, (5) detect an abnormal blood pressure response, (6) monitor responses to various therapeutic interventions for improving cardiovascular function, and (7) evaluate functional aerobic capacity in relation to normative standards.

16. Graded exercise stress testing provides a low-risk screening for CHD preventive and rehabilitative exercise programs. Stress test results provide the objective framework to design an exercise program within a person's current functional capacity and health status.

17. A single stress test cannot diagnose heart disease perfectly. Four possible outcomes from a stress test are true-positive (test a success), false-negative (heart disease not diagnosed when present), true-negative (test a success), and false-positive (healthy person diagnosed with heart disease).

18. Exercise-induced indicators of CHD include angina pectoris, ECG disorders, cardiac rhythm abnormalities, and abnormal blood pressure and heart rate responses.

19. Invasive physiologic tests that include radionucleotide studies, cardiac catheterization, and coronary angiography provide diagnostic information unavailable through noninvasive procedures.

20. Cardiac patients can improve functional capacity similar to healthy people of the same age.

21. Based on diagnosis, patients enter different cardiac rehabilitation phases depending on disease severity and degree of risk.

22. Restrictive lung disease (RLD) and chronic obstructive pulmonary disease (COPD) represent two major pulmonary disease categories. RLD increases chest-lung resistance to lung inflation. COPD (including bronchitis, emphysema, asthma, exercise-induced bronchospasm, and cystic fibrosis) affects expiratory flow capacity and ultimately impedes aeration of alveolar blood.

23. Pulmonary disease assessment requires different diagnostic tools, including chest x-ray, CT scanning, MRI, and standard spirometric lung volume testing.

24. Exercise contributes to pulmonary disease management if close attention focuses on exercise intensity, patient monitoring, and exercise progression.

25. The most prominent neuromuscular diseases affecting the brain are stroke, multiple sclerosis (MS), and Parkinson's disease.

26. Patients who suffer chronic kidney disease can benefit from an individualized and structured exercise program.

27. More than 100 different types of cancers affect adults: (1) carcinomas (develop from epithelial cells that line

the body surface), (2) leukemias (arise from cells of the blood), (3) lymphomas (immune system), and (4) sarcomas (bones, tendons, cartilage, fat, and muscle).

28. The exercise prescription for cancer patients is symptom limited, progressive, and individualized, with improved ambulation as the primary goal.

29. For women recovering from breast cancer surgery, a carefully planned, aerobic circuit resistance exercise program decreases depression and state and trait anxieties.

30. Whatever its cause, depression is not just a state of mind. It is related to physical changes in the brain produced by neurotransmitter imbalance.

31. No evidence indicates that any one kind of exercise has a greater impact on depression than others.

32. Exercise-related positive psychological outcomes do not depend on achieving physical fitness, although fitness-related indicators, like lower blood pressure and increased aerobic capacity, improve with regular exercise in depressed individuals.

THOUGHT QUESTIONS

1. Give two recommendations to a middle-aged man who wants to begin an aerobic training program because he feels breathless and experiences chest discomfort while walking the golf course.

2. What type of aerobic training exercise prescription would prove most beneficial for a CHD patient who

experiences angina during upper-body work as a plasterer and paper hanger.

3. List two possible mechanisms that might account for the experience of a mildly depressed person who states: "Whenever I begin to feel 'down,' I take a brisk walk and my mental attitude perks right back up."

SELECTED REFERENCES

Ahluwalia, I.B., et al.: Report from the CDC. Changes in Selected Chronic Disease-Related Risks and Health Conditions for Nonpregnant Women 18-44 Years Old BRFSS. *J. Womens Health* (Larchmt); 14:382, 2005.

Akabas, S.R., Dolins, K.R.: Micronutrient requirements of physically active women: what can we learn from iron? *Am. J. Clin. Nutr.*, 81:1246S, 2005.

Aldana, S.G., et al.: The effects of a worksite chronic disease prevention program. *J. Occup. Environ. Med.*, 47:558, 2005.

Alexander, K.P., et al.: Value of exercise treadmill testing in women. *J. Am. Col. Cardiol.*, 32:1657, 1998.

American Association of Cardiovascular and Pulmonary Rehabilitation: *Guidelines For Cardiac Rehabilitation Programs*. Champaign, IL: Human Kinetics, 1995.

American Psychiatric Association: Diagnostic and Statistical Manual of Mental Disorders: *DSM-IV*. 4th Ed. Washington, D.C.: American Psychiatric Association, 1994.

ASCM's Guidelines to Exercise Testing and Prescription. 7th Ed. Baltimore, MD: Lippincott Williams & Wilkins, 2006.

Askew, C.D., et al.: Skeletal muscle phenotype is associated with exercise tolerance in patients with peripheral arterial disease. *J. Vasc. Surg.*, 41:802, 2005.

Bauman, A.E.: Updating the evidence that physical activity is good for health: an epidemiological review 2000–2003. *J. Sci. Med. Sport*, 7(1 Suppl):6, 2004.

Blain, G., et al.: Assessment of ventilatory thresholds during graded and maximal exercise test using time varying analysis of respiratory sinus arrhythmia. *Br. J. Sports Med.*, 39:448, 2005.

Blair, S.N., et al: Physical activity, nutrition, and chronic disease. *Med. Sci. Sports Exerc.*, 28:335, 1996.

Bobkowski, W., et al.: The importance of magnesium status in the pathophysiology of mitral valve prolapse. *Magnes. Res.*, 18:35, 2005.

Bodegard, J., et al.: Reasons for terminating an exercise test provide independent prognostic information: 2014 apparently healthy men followed for 26 years. *Eur. Heart J.*, 26:1394, 2005.

Braith, R.W., et al.: Exercise training in patients with CHF and heart transplant recipients. *Med. Sci. Sports Exerc.*, 30(Suppl):S367, 1998.

Brown, T.R., Kraft, G.H.: Exercise and rehabilitation for individuals with multiple sclerosis. *Phys. Med. Rehabil. Clin. N. Am.*, 16:513, 2005.

Camacho, T.C., et al.: Physical activity and depression: Evidence from the Alameda County Study. *Am. J. Epidemiol.*, 13:220, 1991.

Carnethon, M.R., et al.: A longitudinal study of physical activity and heart rate recovery: CARDIA, 1987–1993. *Med. Sci. Sports Exerc.*, 37:606, 2005.

Cerin, E., et al.: Levels of physical activity for colon cancer prevention compared with generic public health recommendations: population prevalence and sociodemographic correlates. *Cancer Epidemiol. Biomarkers Prev.*, 14:1000, 2005.

Clark, C.J., et al.: Low intensity peripheral muscle conditioning improves exercise tolerance and breathlessness in COPD. *Eur. J. Respir. J.*, 9:2590, 1996.

Cooper, C.B.: Determining the role of exercise in patients with chronic pulmonary disease. *Med. Sci. Sports Exerc.*, 27:147, 1995.

D'Andrea, A., et al.: Prognostic value of supine bicycle exercise stress echocardiography in patients with known or suspected coronary artery disease. *Eur. J. Echocardiogr.*, 6:271, 2005.

Dimeo, F., et al.: Aerobic exercise as therapy for cancer fatigue. *Med. Sci. Sports Exerc.*, 30:475, 1998.

Doyne, E.J., et al.: Running versus weight lifting in the treatment of depression. *J. Consult Clin. Psychol.*, 55:748, 1987.

Franco, M.J., et al.: Comparison of dyspnea ratings during submaximal constant work exercise with incremental testing. *Med. Sci. Sports Exerc.*, 30:479, 1998.

Frazer, C.J., et al.: Effectiveness of treatments for depression in older people. *Med. J. Aust.*, 182:627, 2005.

Friedenreich, C.M.: Physical activity and breast cancer risk: The effect of menopausal status. *Exerc. Sport Sci. Rev.*, 2004;32:180, 2004.

Gallagher, M.J., et al.: Comparative impact of morbid obesity vs heart failure on cardiorespiratory fitness. *Chest*, 127:2197, 2005.

Galvao, D.A., Newton, R.U.: Review of exercise intervention studies in cancer patients. *J. Clin. Oncol.*, 1;23:899, 2005.

Giovannucci, E.L., et al.: A prospective study of physical activity and incident and fatal prostate cancer. *Arch. Intern. Med.*, 165:1005, 2005.

Hebestreit, H., et al.: Oxygen uptake kinetics are slowed in cystic fibrosis. *Med. Sci. Sports Exerc.*, 37:10, 2005.

Holmes, M.D., et al.: Physical activity and survival after breast cancer diagnosis. *JAMA*, 293:2479, 2005.

Hu, F.B., et al.: Adiposity as compared with physical activity in predicting mortality among women. *Obstet. Gynecol. Surv.*, 60:311, 2005.

Jarrell, L.A., et al.: Gender differences in functional capacity following myocardial infarction: an exploratory study. *Can. J. Cardiovasc. Nurs.*, 15:28, 2005.

King, W.C., et al.: Objective measures of neighborhood environment and physical activity in older women. *Am. J. Prev. Med.*, 28:461, 2005.

Kohl, H.W., et al.: Maximal exercise hemodynamics and risk of mortality in apparently healthy men and women. *Med. Sci. Sports Exerc.*, 28:601, 1998.

Kumar, N.B., et al.: A case-control study evaluating the association of purposeful physical activity, body fat distribution, and steroid hormones on premenopausal breast cancer risk. *Breast J.*, 11:266, 2005.

Leroux, A.: Exercise training to improve motor performance in chronic stroke: effects of a community-based exercise program. *Int. J. Rehabil. Res.*, 28:17, 2005.

Lobstein, D.D., et al.: Beta-endorphin and components of depression as powerful discriminators between joggers and sedentary and middle-aged men. *J. Psychosom. Res.*, 33:293, 1989.

Malin, A., et al.: Energy balance and breast cancer risk. *Cancer Epidemiol. Biomarkers Prev.*, 14:1496, 2005.

McCartney, N.: Role of resistance training in heart disease. *Med. Sci. Sports Exerc.*, 30(Suppl):S396, 1998.

Mirza, M.A.: Anginalike pain and normal coronary arteries. Uncovering cardiac syndromes that mimic CAD. *Postgrad. Med.*, 117:41, 2005.

Mock, V., et al.: Exercise manages fatigue during breast cancer treatment: a randomized controlled trial. *Psychooncology*, 14:464, 2005.

Morris, J.N.: Exercise in the prevention of coronary heart disease: Today's best bet in public health. *Med. Sci. Sports Exerc.*, 26:807, 1994.

Paffenbarger, R.S., Jr, et al.: Physical activity and personal characteristics associated with depression and suicide in American college men. *Acta. Psychiatr. Scand.*, 377(Suppl):16, 1994.

Pelletier, A.R., et al.: Revisions to chronic disease surveillance indicators, United States, 2004. *Prev. Chronic Dis.*, 2:A15, 2005.

Resnick, B.: Research review: exercise interventions for treatment of depression. *Geriatr. Nurs.*, 26:196, 2005.

Saitoh, M., et al.: Comparison of cardiovascular responses between upright and recumbent cycle ergometers in healthy young volunteers performing low-intensity exercise: assessment of reliability of the oxygen uptake calculated by using the ACSM metabolic equation. *Arch. Phys. Med. Rehabil.*, 86:1024, 2005.

Samad, A.K., et al.: A meta-analysis of the association of physical activity with reduced risk of colorectal cancer. *Colorectal Dis.*, 7:204, 2005.

Schwartz, A.L., et al.: Exercise reduces daily fatigue in women with breast cancer receiving chemotherapy. *Med. Sci. Sports Exerc.*, 33:718, 2001.

Sesso, H.D., et al.: Physical activity and breast cancer risk in the College Alumni Health Study (United States). *Cancer Causes Control*, 9:433, 1998.

Shephard, R.J., and Baldy, G.J.: Exercise as cardiovascular therapy. *Circulation*, 99:963, 1999.

Singh, N.A., et al.: A randomized controlled trial of the effect of exercise on sleep. *Sleep,* 20:95, 1997.

Spence, J.C., et al.: The effect of physical-activity participation on self-concept: A meta-analysis. *J. Sport Exerc. Psychol.,* 19:S109, 1997.

Theisen, V., et al.: Blood pressure Sunday: introducing genomics to the community through family history. *Prev. Chronic Dis.,* 2:A23, 2005.

Vallebona, A., et al.: Heart rate response to graded exercise correlates with aerobic and ventilatory capacity in patients with heart failure. *Clin. Cardiol.*, 28:25, 2005.

Verrill, D.E., and Ribisl, P.M.: Resistive exercise training in cardiac rehabilitation (an update). *Sports Med.*, 21:371, 1996.

Visovsky, C., Dvorak, C.: Exercise and cancer recovery. *Online J. Issues Nurs.*, 10:7, 2005.

White, L.J., Dressendorfer, R.H.: Exercise and multiple sclerosis. *Sports Med.*, 34:1077, 2004.

Wilson, D.B., et al.: Anthropometric changes using a walking intervention in African American breast cancer survivors: a pilot study. *Prev. Chronic Dis.*, 2:A16, 2005.

Yach, D., et al.: Improving diet and physical activity: 12 lessons from controlling tobacco smoking. *BMJ*, 330:898, 2005.

Yamazaki, T., et al.: Circadian dynamics of heart rate and physical activity in patients with heart failure. *Clin. Exp. Hypertens.*, 27:241, 2005.

Yang, P.S., Chen, C.H.: Exercise stage and processes of change in patients with chronic obstructive pulmonary disease. *J. Nurs. Res.*, 13:97, 2005.

Youngstedt, S.D.: Effects of exercise on sleep. *Clin. Sports Med.*, 24:355, 2005.

Appendix A

Reliable Information Resources and Exercise Physiology

Appendix B

The Internet and Exercise Physiology
Part 1. Search Engines
Part 2. Government-Related Sites
Part 3. Exercise Physiology-Related Sites
Part 4. General Science Sites
Part 5. Science and Technology News
Part 6. Useful Resources

Appendix C

The Metric System and Conversion Constants in Exercise Physiology

Appendix D

Metabolic Computations in Open-Circuit Spirometry

Appendix E

Frequently Cited Journals in Exercise Physiology

Appendix F

Evaluation of Body Composition—Girth Method

Appendix G

Evaluation of Body Composition—Skinfold Method

RELIABLE INFORMATION RESOURCES AND EXERCISE PHYSIOLOGY

American Alliance for Health, Physical Education, Recreation & Dance (AAHPERD)
1900 Association Drive
Reston, VA 20191
Phone: (800) 213-7139
E-mail: info@aahperd.org
http://www.aahperd.org

American College of Sports Medicine (ACSM)
401 West Michigan Street
Indianapolis, IN 46202-3233
(Mailing address: PO Box 1440; Indianapolis, IN 46202-1440)
Phone: (317) 637-9200
Fax: (317) 634-7817
http://www.acsm.org

American Heart Association
Inquiries Coordinator
7272 Greenville Avenue
Dallas, TX 75231-4596
Phone: (800) 242-8721
Fax: (214) 706-1341
E-mail: dstokes@amhrt.org
http://www.americanheart.org

American Institute for Cancer Research
1759 R Street NW
Washington, DC 20009
Phone: (800) 843-8114; (202) 328-7744
Fax: (202) 328-7226
E-mail: aircrweb@aicr.org
http://www.aicr.org

Anorexia Nervosa and Related Eating Disorders
PO Box 5102
Eugene, OR 97405
Phone: (541) 344-1144
http://www.anred.com

American Obesity Association
1250 24th Street NW, Suite 300
Washington, DC 20037
Phone: (202) 776-7711
Fax: (202) 776-7712
http://www.obesity.org

American Public Health Association
1015 18th Street NW
Washington, DC 20036
Phone: (202) 789-5600
Fax (202) 789-5661
E-mail: comments@apha.com
http://www.apha.org

American Running and Fitness Association
4405 East West Highway, Suite 405
Bethesda, MD 20814
Phone: (800) 776-2732

American Society for Nutritional Sciences and American Society for Clinical Nutrition
9650 Rockville Pike
Bethesda, MD 20814
Phone: (301) 530-7050
Fax: (301) 571-1892
http://www.faseb.org/asns/

Canadian Association for Health, Physical Education, Recreation, and Dance (CAHPERD)
1600 James Naismith Drive
Gloucester, Ontario KIB 5N4, Canada
Phone: (613) 748-5622; (800) 663-8708
Fax: (613) 748-5737
E-mail: cahperd@activeliving.ca
http://www.activeliving.ca/cahperd

Canadian Society for Exercise Physiology
185 Somerset Street West, Suite 202
Ottawa, Ontario K2P OJ2, Canada
Phone: (613) 234-3755
Fax: (613) 234-3565
E-mail: info@csep.ca
http://www.csep.ca

Canadian Society for Nutritional Sciences
Department of Foods and Nutrition
University of Manitoba
Winnipeg, Manitoba R3T 2N2, Canada

Cancer Research Foundation
1600 Duke Street
Alexandria, VA 22314
Phone: (703) 836-4412
http://www.preventcancer.org/

Centers for Disease Control and Prevention
Natural Institutes of Health
1600 Clifton Road, NE
Atlanta, GA 30333
Phone: (404) 639-3311
http://www.cdc.gov/

Food and Drug Administration (FDA)
Center for Food Safety and Applied Nutrition
Room 4405B, Federal Building, 200 C Street SW
Washington, DC 20204
Phone: (202) 205-4168
Fax: (202) 205-5295
http://www/fda/gov/

Food Insight
International Food Information Council
E-mail: foodinfo@ific.health.org
http://www.ificinfo.health.org/

Food and Nutrition Information Center
National Agriculture Library
Agriculture Research Service, USDA
10301 Baltimore Avenue
Beltsville, MD 20705-2351
Phone: (301) 504-5719
Fax: (301) 504-6409
E-mail: fnic@nal.usda.gov/fnic/
http://www.nal.usda.gov/fnic/

Food Research and Action Center (FRAC)
1875 Connecticut Avenue NW #540
Washington, DC 20009
Phone: (202) 986-2200
Fax: (202) 986-2525
http://www.frac.org

Food Safety and Inspection Service
FSIS Food Safety Education and Communications Staff
U.S. Department of Agriculture
Room 1175, South Building
1400 Independence Avenue, SW
Washington, DC 20250
Phone: (202) 720-7943
Fax: (202) 720-1843
E-mail: fsis.webmaster@usda.gov
http://www.fsis.usda.gov

Health and Welfare Canada
Canadian Government Publishing Center
Minister of Supply and Services
Ottawa, Ontario KIA 0S9, Canada

International Association of Eating Disorders Professionals
123 NW 13th Street #206
Boca Raton, FL 33432-1618
Phone: (800) 800-8126

IDEA Health and Fitness Association
10455 Pacific Center Court
San Diego, CA 92121-4339
Phone: (800) 999-4332
Fax: (619) 535-8234
http://www.iaedp.com

International Society of Sports Nutrition
Executive Director
600 Pembrook Drive
Woodland Park, CO 80863
Phone: (866) 472-4650
Fax: (719) 395-5615
E-mail: issn@sportsnutritionsociety.org
http://www.theissn.org

Jean Mayer U.S. Department of Agriculture Human Nutrition Research Center on Aging
Tufts University
711 Washington Street
Boston, MA 02111-1524
Phone: (617) 556-3000
Fax: (617) 556-3344
http://hnrc.tufts.edu/

Massachusetts Eating Disorders Association, Inc.
1162 Beacon Street
Brookline, MA 02146
Phone: (617) 738-6332

National Academy of Sciences/Institute of Medicine Food and Nutrition Board
2101 Constitution Avenue NW
Washington, DC 20418
Phone: (202) 334-2000
Fax: (202) 334-2316
E-mail: Fnb@nas.edu
http://www.nas.edu/fnb/

National Association of Anorexia Nervosa and Associated Disorders
PO Box 7
Highland Park, IL 60035
Phone: (847) 831-3438
Fax: (847) 433-4632
http://www.anad.org/site/anadweb/

National Cancer Institute
Office of Cancer Communications
Building 31, Room 10A-24
Bethesda, MD 20892
Phone: (800) 422-6237
E-mail: cis@icicc.nci.nih.gov
http://www.nci.nih.gov

National Center for Nutrition and Dietetics
The American Dietetic Association
216 West Jackson Boulevard
Chicago, IL 60606-6995
Phone: (312) 899-0040, ext. 4653
Fax: (312) 899-1739
http://www.eatright.org

National Center for Health Statistics (NCHS)
National Institutes of Health
6525 Belcrest Road
Hyattsville, MD 20782
Phone: (301) 436-8500
http://www.cdc.gov/nchswww/default.htm

National Dairy Council
10255 W. Higgins Rd
Rosemont, IL 60018-4233

National Diabetes Information Clearinghouse
1 Information Way
Bethesda, MD 20892-3560
Phone: (301) 654-3327
Fax: (301) 907-8906
E-mail: ndic@info.niddk.nih.gov
http://www.niddk.nih.gov/health/diabetes/diabetes/
diabetes.htm

National Eating Disorders Organization (NEDO)
6655 South Yale Avenue
Tulsa, OK 74136
Phone: (918) 481-4044
Fax: (918) 481-4076
http://www.laureate.com

National Eating Disorders Screening Program
One Washington Street, Suite 304
Wellesley, MA 02181-1706
http://www.nmisp.org

National Heart, Lung, and Blood Institute Information Center
PO Box 30105
Bethesda, MD 20842-0105
Phone: (301) 251-1222
Fax: (301) 251-1223
E-mail: nhlbiic@dgsys.com
http://www.nhlbi.nih.gov/nhlbi/nhlbi.htm

National Institute on Aging
Information Office
Building 31, Room 5C35
Bethesda, MD 20205
http://www.nia.nih.gov/

National Institute of Diabetes and Digestive and Kidney Diseases
31 Center Drive, MSC-2560
Building 31, Room 9A-04
Bethesda, MD 20892-2560
Phone: (301) 496-3583
Fax: (301) 496-7422
http://www.niddk.nih.gov

National Institutes of Health (NIH)
9000 Rockville Pike
Bethesda, MD 20892
Phone: (301) 496-4461
Fax: (301) 496-0017
http://www.nih.gov/

National Institute of Nutrition
1335 Carling Avenue, Suite 210
Ottawa, Ontario K1Z OL2, Canada

National Library of Medicine
8600 Rockville Pike
Bethesda, MD 20894
Phone: (888) 346-3656
Fax: (301) 594-5983
http://www.nlm.nih.gov

National Kidney and Urologic Diseases Information Clearinghouse (NKUDIC)
3 Information Way
Bethesda, MD 20892-3580
(301) 654-4415; Fax: (301) 907-8906
http://kidney.niddk.nih.gov/

National Mental Health Association
1201 Prince Street
Alexandria, VA 22314-2971
Phone: (703) 684-7722
Fax: (703) 684-5968
http://www.nmha.org

National Osteoporosis Foundation
1150 17th Street, NW, Suite 500
Washington, DC 20036-4603
Phone: (202) 223-2226
Fax: (202) 223-2237
http://www.nof.org

National Strength and Conditioning Association (NSCA)
PO Box 38909
Colorado Springs, CO 80937-8909
Phone: (719) 632-6722
Fax: (719) 632-6367
E-mail: nsca@usa.net
http://www.nsca-lift.org

North American Association of the Study of Obesity (NAASO)
Executive Office
8630 Fenton Street, Suite 918
Silver Spring, MD 20910
Phone: (301) 563-6526
Fax: (301) 563-6595
http://www.naaso.org

Nutrition Programs
446 Jeanne Mance Building
Tunney's Pasture
Ottawa, Ontario K1A 1B4, Canada

Office of Disease Prevention and Health Promotion (ODPHP)
National Institutes of Health
2131 Switzer Building, 330 C Street SW
Washington, DC 20201
Phone: (202) 205-9007
Fax: (202) 205-9478

Overeaters Anonymous
World Service Office
6075 Zenith Court, NE
Rio Rancho, NM 87124
Phone: (505) 891-4320
Fax: (505) 891-4320
E-mail: Overeattn@technet.run.org
http://www.overeatersanonymous.org

Public Health Resource Service
15 Overlea Boulevard, 5th Floor
Toronto, Ontario M4H IA9, Canada

Sports Information Resource Centre (SIRC)
107-1600 James Naismith Drive
Gloucester, Ontario K1B 5N4, Canada
Phone: (800) 664-6413; (613) 748-5658
Fax: (613) 748-5701
E-mail: moreinfo@sirc.ca
http://www.sirc.ca/

Sports, Cardiovascular, and Wellness Nutritionists (SCAN)
90 S Cascade #1190
Colorado Springs, CO 80903
Phone: (719) 475-7751
Fax: (719) 475-8748
http://www.scandpg.org/

The Weight-Control Information Network
National Institute of Diabetes and Digestive
and Kidney Diseases
1 Win Way
Bethesda, MD 20892-3665
Phone: (301) 570-2177; (800) 946-8098
Fax: (301) 570-2186
http://win.niddk.nih.gov/

U.S. Department of Health and Human Services (DHHS)
200 Independence Avenue SW
Washington, DC 20201
Phone: (202) 619-0257
Fax: (202) 619-3363
http://www.os.dhhs.gov

U.S. Department of Agriculture (USDA)
12th and Independence Avenue SW
Washington, DC 20250
Phone: (202) 720-3631
Fax: (202) 720-5437
http://www.usda.gov

Vitamin Nutrition Information Service (VNIS)
Hoffmann-LaRoche
340 Kingsland Avenue
Nutley, NJ 07110

World Health Organization (WHO)
Headquarter Offices
Avenue Appia 20
1211 Geneva 27, Switzerland
Phone: (141 22) 791 21 11
Fax: (141 22) 791 0746
E-mail: info@who.cho
http://www.who.int/

THE INTERNET AND EXERCISE PHYSIOLOGY

The Internet provides a phenomenal information resource about millions of topics covering every facet of our society. In the basic and applied sciences, the information explosion has spawned an inordinately large number of websites in a relatively short time period. No one person can ever hope to keep current with the most up-to-the minute information about a particular topic. Just six years ago, when we began our own web searches about the relatively new topic of exercise and molecular biology, we had difficulty locating websites because so few sites dealt with the topic, particularly related to exercise. What a difference six years makes!

On September 7, 2005 when we turned to the AltaVista search engine (www.altavista.com) to locate available sites for the term molecular biology, over 30,300,000 sites emerged about this topic. Then (October 6, 1999) "only" two million sites were listed for molecular biology and exercise. Quite frankly, that second number seemed shocking to contend with-and even more so now. During that early search, we discovered that many of the established disciplines had considerably more websites associated with their fields. Now, in performing the same search, we discovered the following number of sites for these key terms: biology—112,000,000; chemistry—104,000,000; physics—121,000,000; statistics—447,000,000; computers—723,000,000. A search on *exercise physiology* showed 4,500,000 websites, while general areas typically associated with exercise physiology produced a huge list of sites (health—1,620,000,000—yes, that's billion; *fitness*—421,000,000; *exercise*—4,520,000; *human biology*—41,200,000; *wellness*—126,000,000). A search on *exercise science* yielded 37,000,000 websites, while 3,940,000 matches were available for *kinesiology*. Obviously, the growth of the Internet has been nothing short of phenomenal. Just think of it—six years ago a search on the term *health* yielded an "astounding" 27,536,356 sites—a number that today exceeds one billion! Even the newly minted term *kinesiology* had roughly 104,000 sites in 1999—a number that now has increased about 40-fold to almost four million.

Obviously, this textbook appendix can only provide an eclectic collection of relatively few sites germane to exercise physiology, no matter how selectively we identify the categories. Many of us who relied on the Internet less than a decade ago to gather information for our various projects felt pretty comfortable with the few search engines we routinely tapped for information. Now, that comfort level has

all but vanished-for those so inclined, 160,000,000 listings now exist on AltaVista to search worldwide for search engines! Daunting yes, but impossible no. We have added a few of the newer search engines (i.e., Google, not available six years ago, and several others). We also reviewed each of the listed sites and updated many of the URLs, deleted several dozen of the sites that changed focus, and added new ones we hope you will find useful in your own searches.

The websites we highlight in this section have been placed into one of six parts: (1) Search Engines; (2) Government-Related Sites; (3) Exercise Physiology-Related Sites; (4) General Science Sites; (5) Science and Technology News; and (6) Useful Resources.

Part 1. Search Engines

A2Z Online
   www.a2z.com

All-In-One Search Page
   www.albany.net/allinone/

AltaVista
   www.altavista.com/

AOL Search
   www.aol.com/

Ask Jeeves
   askjeeves.com/

Beaucoup!
   www.beaucoup.com/

ComFind
   www.comfind.com/

Dejanews
   www.dejanews.com/

Directory Guide
   www.directoryguide.com/

Dogpile
   www.dogpile.com

eBLAST
   www.eblast.com/

Excite
   www.excite.com/

Galaxy
   galaxy.einet.net/

Google
   www.google.com/

GoTo
   www.goto.com/

Hardin Meta Directory of Internet Health Sources
www.lib.uiowa.edu/hardin/md/index.html

HealthFinder
www.healthfinder.gov/

Hotbot
www.hotbot.com

Inference Find
www.infind.com/

Infoseek
www.infoseek.com/

Internet Grateful Med
igm.nlm.nih.gov/

Internet Sleuth
www.isleuth.com/

Linkstar
www.linkstar.com/

Lycos
www.lycos.com/

Magellan
www.mckinley.com/

Mayo Clinic Health Oasis
www.mayohealth.org/

MedExplorer
www.medexplorer.com/

MedHunt
www.hon.ch/cgi-bin/find?1

Medical Matrix
www.medmatrix.org/index.asp

MedSurf
www.medsurf.com/

MedWeb Plus
www.medwebplus.com/

MedWeb
www.MedWeb.Emory.Edu/MedWeb/

MedWorld
www-med.stanford.edu/medworld/home/

MetaCrawler
www.metacrawler.com/

MSN
www.msn.com/

Multimedia Medical Reference Library
www.med-library.com/medlibrary/

Netscape
www.netscape.com/

Northern Light
www.northernlight.com/

Pathfinder
www.pathfinder.com/welcome/

Savvy Search
www.cs.colostate.edu/~dreiling/smartform.html

Search Tools for the Internet
www.nal.usda.gov/other_internet_sites/
srchtool.html

Searching the Internet
jan.ucc.nau.edu/~bwp2/isearch.html

The New PubMed
www.ncbi.nlm.nih.gov/entrez/query.fcgi

Unified Computer Science TR Index
www.cs.indiana.edu:800/cstr/

Various Search Engines
ic.net/~baustin/search/search.html

Webcrawler
webcrawler.com/

Welcome to PubMed
www.ncbi.nlm.nih.gov/PubMed/

Yahoo!
search.yahoo.com/bin/search/options

Part 2. Government-Related Sites

Administration for Children and Families
www.acf.dhhs.gov/

Agency for Health Care Policy and Research
www.ahcpr.gov/

Agency for Toxic Substances and Disease Registry
atsdr1.atsdr.cdc.gov:8080

Agricultural Network Information Center
www.agnic.org/

Berkeley Lab Research Review Magazine
www.lbl.gov/Science-Articles/Research-
Review/newsstand.html

Biology Information Center
www.er.doe.gov/production/ober/ober_top.html

Cancer Genome Anatomy Project
www.ncbi.nlm.nih.gov/ncicgap/

Center for Food Safety and Applied Nutrition
vm.cfsan.fda.gov/list.html

Center for Nutrition Policy and Promotion
www2.hqnet.usda.gov/cnpp/

Centers for Disease Control and Prevention
www.cdc.gov/

Centers for Disease Control Genomics and Disease
Prevention
www.cdc.gov/genomics/

Clinical Guidelines for Treatment of Overweight
and Obesity in Adults
www.nhlbi.nih.gov/nhlbi/cardio/obes/prof/
guidelns/ob_home.htm

Code of Federal Regulations
www.access.gpo.gov/nara/cfr/cfr-table-search.html

Consumer Information Center
www.pueblo.gsa.gov/

Department of Health and Human Services
www.os.dhhs.gov/

Dietary Guidelines for Americans
www.nalusda.gov/fnic/dga/dguide95.html

Dietary Supplements
www.cfsan.fda.gov/~dms/supplmnt.html

DNA From the Beginning
vector.cshl.org/dnaftb/

Environmental Protection Agency
www.epa.gov/

Exercise Physiology Laboratory at NASA-
Johnson Space Center
www.jsc.nasa.gov/sa/sd/sd3/exl/index.htm

FDA Consumer
www.fda.gov/fdac/698_toc.html

Federal Directory: Government Information Xchange
www.info.gov/

Federal Trade Commission
www.ftc.gov/

FedStats
www.fedstats.gov/search.html

FedWorld Network
www.fedworld.gov/

Food and Agriculture Organization of the
United Nations (FAO)
www.fao.org/

Food and Drug Administration
www.fda.gov/default.htm

Food and Nutrition Information Center
www.nalusda.gov/fnic/

Food and Nutrition Service
www2.hqnet.usda.gov/fcs/

Food Guide Pyramid Information
www.nalusda.gov/fnic/Fpyr/pyramid.html

Food Labeling and Nutrition
vm.cfsan.fda.gov/label.html

Food Labeling Education
www.nal.usda.gov/fnic/Label/label.html

Food Surveys Research Group
www.barc.usda.gov/bhnrc/foodsurvey/home.htm

Gene Map of the Human Genome
www.ncbi.nlm.nih.gov/SCIENCE96/

Genes and Disease
www.ncbi.nlm.nih.gov/disease/

Grants.Gov
www.grants.gov/

Health Care Financing Administration
www.hcfa.gov

Health Finder
www.healthfinder.gov/

Health Resources and Services Administration
www.hrsa.dhhs.gov

Human Genome Project Information
www.ornl.gov/TechResources/Human_Genome/home.
html

Indian Health Service
www.ihs.gov

International Space Station
station.nasa.gov/

Internet Health Resources
www.health-library.com/index.html

Internet Sites Related to Food and Nutrition
www.barc.usda.gov/bhnrc/foodsurvey/Sites.html

Lawrence Berkeley National Laboratory Human
Genome Sequencing
www-hgc.lbl.gov/

Library of Congress Catalogs
lcweb.loc.gov/catalog/

Library of Congress
www.loc.gov/

Medline Plus
medlineplus.gov/

Medline (PubMed)
www.ncbi.nlm.nih.gov/PubMed/

Mental Health
www.mentalhealth.org/cornerstone/index.cfm

Molecular Biology Desk Reference
molbio.info.nih.gov/molbio/desk.html

Morbidity and Mortality Weekly Report
www2.cdc.gov/mmwr/

NASA Scientific and Technical Information (STI)
www.sti.nasa.gov/STI-public-homepage.html

National Academy of Sciences
www.nas.edu/

National Aeronautics and Space Administration
www.nasa.gov/

National Agricultural Library
www.nal.usda.gov/

National Air and Space Museum
www.nasm.edu/

National Center for Biotechnology Information
www.ncbi.nlm.nih.gov/

National Center for Health Statistics Web Search
www.cdc.gov/nchswww/search/search.htm

National Highway Traffic Safety Administration
www.nhtsa.dot.gov

National Institute for Occupational Safety and Health
www.cdc.gov/niosh/homepage.html

National Institute on Aging
www.nih.gov/nia/

National Institutes of Health
www.nih.gov/index.html

National Institutes of Health Food and Nutrition Board
www2.nas.edu/fnb/

National Institutes of Health Sleep, Sleep Disorders, and
Biological Rhythms
science.education.nih.gov/supplements/nih3/sleep/
default.htm

National Institutes of Health Stem Cell Information
stemcells.nih.gov/index.asp

National Library of Medicine
www4.ncbi.nlm.nih.gov/

National Science Foundation (NSF)
www.nsf.gov/

National Women's Health Information Center
www.4woman.gov/

NCBI Entrez Genomes List
www.ncbi.nlm.nih.gov/Entrez/Genome/org.html

NIH Library Online
libwww.ncrr.nih.gov/

NSF Science and Technology Centers
www.cs.brown.edu/stc/allstc.html

Nutrient Data laboratory: Agricultural Research Service
www.nal.usda.gov/fnic/foodcomp/

Nutrition and Physical Activity Topic Index
www.cdc.gov/nccdphp/dnpa/site_index.htm

Occupational Safety and Health Administration
www.osha.gov

Office of Biological and Environmental Research
www.er.doe.gov/production/ober/ober_top.html

Office of Disease Prevention and Health Promotion
odphp.osophs.dhhs.gov/

Office of Health Affairs: U.S. Food and Drug Administration
www.fda.gov/oc/oha/

Office of Naval Research
web.fie.com/fedix/onr.html

Office of Science and Technology Policy
www.whitehouse.gov/OSTP.html

Physical Activity and Health: Surgeon General Report
www.cdc.gov/nccdphp/sgr/sgr.htm

Profiles in Science
www.profiles.nlm.nih.gov/

Science and Technology Web Sites
www.harvardhealthpubs.org/frindex.html

State Departments of Public Health
www.fsis.usda.gov/OPHS/stategov.htm

Statistical Abstract of the United States
www.census.gov/prod/www/abs/cc97stab.html

Superintendent of Documents (GPOAccess)
www.access.gpo.gov/su_docs/

Team Nutrition
www2.hqnet.usda.gov/cnpp/team.htm

The Genome Database
www.gdb.org/

U.S. Copyright Office
lcweb.loc.gov/copyright/

U.S. Census Bureau
www.census.gov/

U.S. Consumer Gateway
www.consumer.gov/

U.S. Department of Agriculture
www.usda.gov/

U.S. Department of Agriculture Center for Nutrition Policy and Promotion
www.usda.gov/fcs/cnpp.htm

U.S. Department of Agriculture Cooperative State Research, Education, and Extension Service
www.reeusda.gov/

U.S. Department of Agriculture Food and Nutrition Service
www.usda.gov/fcs/

U.S. Department of Agriculture Healthy Eating Index
www2.hqnet.usda.gov/cnpp/usda_healthy_eating_index.htm

U.S. Department of Agriculture MyPyramid.gov
www.mypyramid.gov/

U.S. Department of Agriculture Nutrient Data Laboratory
www.nal.usda.gov/fnic/foodcomp/

U.S. Department of Education
www.ed.gov/

U.S. Department of Health and Human Services Agency for Healthcare Research and Quality
www.ahrq.gov/

U.S. Department of Health and Human Services Office of Research Integrity
www.cdc.gov/nccdphp/dnpa/site_index.htm

U.S. Department of Health and Human Services President's Council on Physical Fitness and Sports
www.fitness.gov/pcpfs_research_digs.htm

U.S. Government Printing Office
www.access.gpo.gov/su_docs/

U.S. Indian Health Service
www.ihs.gov/

U.S. Military Network
www.military-network.com/MainSite.htm

U.S. Patent and Trademark Office
www.uspto.gov/

U.S. Pharmacopeia
www.usp.org/

U.S. State and Local Gateway: Federal Funding
www.statelocal.gov/funding.html

Visible Human Project
www.nlm.nih.gov/research/visible/visible_human.html

Walk Through Time
physics.nist.gov/GenInt/Time/time.html

Zip Code Lookup
www.usps.gov/ncsc/lookups/lookup_zip14.html

Part 3. Exercise Physiology-Related Sites

ADIPOS: Publication in Obesity
www.adipos.com/index.html

Aging Research Centre (ARC)
www.arclab.org/

Alberta Centre for Active Living
www.centre4activeliving.ca/

American Alliance for Health, Physical Education, Recreation and Dance
www.aahperd.org/

American College of Sports Medicine
www.acsm.org/

American Dietetic Association
www.eatright.org/

American Heart Association
www.americanheart.org/

American Journal of Clinical Nutrition
www.faseb.org/ajcn/

American Medical Association
www.ama-assn.org/

American Red Cross: CPR Training
www.redcross.org/hss/cpraed.html

American Society for Nutritional Sciences
www.nutrition.org/

Ancient Medicine/Medicina Antiqua
www.medicinaantiqua.org.uk/medant/

Ancient Olympic Games Virtual Museum
minbar.cs.dartmouth.edu/greecom/olympics/

Applied Exercise Science Websites
www.edb.utexas.edu/abraham/Links.html

Artificial Muscle Project
www.ai.mit.edu/projects/muscle/overview.html

Artigen Health News
www.artigen.com/newswire/health.html

Ask an Expert
www.askanexpert.com/askanexpert/catscitec.shtml

Ask the Dietician
www.dietitian.com/

Audiovisuals about Basic Nutrition
www.nal.usda.gov/fnic/pubs/bibs/av/basic-av.htm

Beginners Guide to Molecular Biology
www.tiac.net/users/pmgannon/

Biomechanics Worldwide
www.per.ualberta.ca/biomechanics/bwwframe.htm

Blonz Guide: Nutrition, Food and Health Resources
www.blonz.com/blonz/nfindex2.htm

Body Composition Tutorial
nuts.uvm.edu/nusc/uww/

Canadian Academy of Sport Medicine
www.casm-acms.org/

Canadian Diabetes Association
www.diabetes.ca/Section_Main/welcome.asp

Canadian Journal of Applied Physiology
www.humankinetics.com/infok/journals/cjap/intro.htm

Cell and Molecular Biology Online
www.cellbio.com/

Cells Alive!
www.cellsalive.com/

Center for Cancer Biology and Nutrition
www.tamu.edu/ccbn/ccbnweb/ccbn.htm

CHID Online (Combined Health Information Database)
chid.nih.gov/

Clinical Guidelines About Overweight and
Obesity in Adults
www.nhlbi.nih.gov/nhlbi/cardio/obes/prof/guidelns/
ob_home.htm

Coaching Science Abstracts
www-rohan.sdsu.edu/dept/coachsci/intro.html

Community of Science (COS)
www.cos.com/

Complete Home Medical Guide
cpmcnet.columbia.edu/texts/guide/

Comprehensive Medical Indexes
www.ama-assn.org/med_link/links.htm

Cycling Performance Tips
www.halcyon.com/gasman/

Dieticians of Canada
www.dietitians.ca/index.html

DOCINFO
www.docinfo.com/

Donald B. Brown Research Chair on Obesity
obesity.chair.ulaval.ca/welcome.html

Electric Library: Encyclopedia
www.encyclopedia.com/

Exercise Physiology Digital Image Archive
www.abacon.com/dia/exphys/home.html

Exercise Physiology: The Methods and Mechanisms
Underlying Performance
home.hia.no/~stephens/exphys.htm

Fatfree: The Low Fat Vegetarian Archive
www.fatfree.com/index.shtml

Federation of American Societies for Experimental Biology
www.faseb.org/

Fitness Links Page
www.general.uwa.edu.au/u/rjwood/links.htm

Food Composition Resource List for Professionals
www.nal.usda.gov/fnic/pubs/bibs/gen/97fdcomp.htm

Food Finder
www.olen.com/food/

Food Guide Pyramid
www2.hqnet.usda.gov/cnpp/pyramid2.htm

Free Medical Journals
www.freemedicaljournals.com/

From Quackery to Bacteriology
www.cl.utoledo.edu/canaday/quackery/quack1.html

GastroSource
www.gastrosource.com/

Gatorade Sports Science Institute
www.gssiweb.com/

GeroWeb
www.iog.wayne.edu/govlinks.html

Guide to Eating Disorders
eatingdisorders.miningco.com/

Guide to Medical Information and Support
on the Internet
www.geocities.com/HotSprings/1505/guide.html

Health A to Z
www.healthatoz.com/

Health Activity Center: Researchers Against Inactivity-
related Disorders (RID)
hac.missouri.edu/RID/index.htm

Health Directory Worldwide
www.healthdirectory.com/

Health on the Net Foundation
www.hon.ch/

Healthgate
www.healthgate.com/

Herbal Medicine Resource List
http://library.uchc.edu/departm/hnet/altmedres.html/

HMS Beagle: The BioMedNet Magazine
biomednet.com/hmsbeagle/index.htm

Home of the Glycemic Index
www.glycemicindex.com/

Horus' Web Links to History Resources
www.ucr.edu/h-gig/horuslinks.html

Hosford Muscle Tables: Skeletal Muscles of the
Human Body
www.ptcentral.com/muscles/

Human Muscle Gene Map
www.bio.unipd.it/~telethon/Hmgm/HMGM.html

Hypermuscle: Muscles in Action
www.med.umich.edu/lrc/Hypermuscle/Hyper.html

In Vivo Sarcomere Length Measurement
www-neuromus.ucsd.edu/surgery/surgery.html

Institute of Medicine
www.iom.edu/

Intelihealth
www.intelihealth.com/IH/ihtIH

International Food Composition Tables Directory
www.fao.org/infoods/directory_en.stm

International Food Information Council
ificinfo.health.org/

International Journal of Sport Nutrition
www.humankinetics.com/infok/journals/ijsn/intro.htm

Internet Drug Index
www.rxlist.com/

Introduction to Muscle Physiology and Design
muscle.ucsd.edu/MusIntro/

John B. Pierce Laboratory, Inc.
www.jbpierce.org/jbp/default.htm

Journal of Applied Physiology
jap.physiology.org/

Journal of Food Composition and Analysis
www.academicpress.com/jfca

Journal of Sports Science & Medicine
www.jssm.org/

KEGG Metabolic
www.genome.ad.jp/kegg/metabolism.html

KidsHealth
KidsHealth.org/index2.html

Kinesiology and Health Science Links
www.tahperd.sfasu.edu/links3.html

Link to Electronic Journals
www.eurekalert.org/links/Journals_public.html

Lipids Online
www.glycemicindex.com/

Marathoning Start to Finish
www.teamoregon.com/publications/marathon/

Masters Athlete Physiology and Performance
www.krs.hia.no/~stephens/index.html

MayoClinic
www.mayohealth.org/

Medfacts
www.medfacts.com/

MedFinder
www.netmedicine.com/medfinder.htm

Medical History on the Internet
www.anes.uab.edu/medhist.htm

Medical World Search
www.mwsearch.com/

Medicine and Science in Sports and Exercise
www.wwilkins.com/MSSE/

Medicine- and Sports-Related Links
www.mspweb.com/

MedicineNet
www.medicinenet.com/

Medscape
www.medscape.com/

Medsite
www.medsite.com/

MedWeb Biomedical Internet Resources
www.cc.emory.edu/WHSCL/medweb.html

MedWeb Physiology
www.gen.emory.edu/MEDWEB/keyword/
physiology.html

MedWeb Sports Medicine
www.gen.emory.edu/medweb/medweb.sportsmed.html

Merck Frosst/CIHR Research Chair in Obesity
obesity.chair.ulaval.ca/

Metabolic Pathways of Biochemistry
www.gwu.edu/~mpb/

Multilingual Glossary of Technical and Popular
Medical Terms
allserv.rug.ac.be/~rvdstich/eugloss/welcome.html

Muscle Physiology and Design
www-neuromus.ucsd.edu/MusIntro/Jump.html

Museum of Health and Medical Science
www.mhms.org/

NASA
www.nasa.gov/

National Fraud Information Center
www.fraud.org/

National Research Council
www.nas.edu/nrc/

National Sports Medicine Institute of the
United Kingdom
www.nsmi.org.uk/publ.html

Net Doctor
www.net-doctor.com/

NetBiochem
www-medlib.med.utah.edu/NetBiochem/
NetWelco.htm

Neuromuscular Research Lab
nmrc.bu.edu/

New England Journal of Medicine
www.nejm.org/

Nutrition and Fitness Links
www.lifelines.com/ntnlnk.html

Nutrition Analysis Tool
www.ag.uiuc.edu/~food-lab/nat/

Nutrition Navigator: Rating Guide to Nutrition Websites
navigator.tufts.edu/

Obesity
www.obesity.com/

Obesity, Health, and Metabolic Fitness
www.mesomorphosis.com/exclusive/gaesser/
obesity01.htm

Olympic Centennial: Athletic, Sport, Recreation
Bibliography Project
www-nutrition.ucdavis.edu/Olympics/

Pedro's Biomolecular Research Tools
www.biophys.uni-duesseldorf.de/bionet/
research_tools.html

Pennington Biomedical Research Center
www.pbrc.edu/default.htm

Perseus Project: The Ancient Olympic
www.perseus.tufts.edu/Olympics

Physical Activity and Health Network
www1.pitt.edu/pahnet/

Physician and Sports Medicine Online
www.physsportsmed.com/

Physiology and Biophysics (Biosciences)
physiology.med.cornell.edu/WWWVL/PhysioWeb.html

Primer on Molecular Genetics
www.bis.med.jhmi.edu/Dan/DOE/intro.html

Professional Resources about Eating Disorders
www.nal.usda.gov/fnic/pubs/bibs/gen/anorhpbr.htm

Quackwatch: Guide to Health Fraud, Quackery, and
Intelligent Decisions
www.quackwatch.com/

Quick'Ndex: Your Own Medical Librarian on the Internet
www.healthy.net/welcome/quick.htm

Reedy's Muscle Database
note.cellbio.duke.edu/Faculty/~Reedy/Muscle/
MuscleDB.html

Resources for Medical History Papers
www.usuhs.mil/meh/histres.html

Runner's World Online
www.runnersworld.com/

Science of Foods
osu.orst.edu/instruct/nfm236/head/glossary/index.html

Science of Obesity and Weight Control
www.loop.com/~bkrentzman/index.html

Scientific American
www.sciam.com/

Shape Up America
www.shapeup.org/

SIRC Sport Research
www.sirc.ca/

Something Fishy Website on Eating Disorders
www.something-fishy.com/ed.htm

Sportscience
www.sportsci.org/

Swiss Food Composition Database
food.ethz.ch/swifd/

The Fédération Internationale de Médecine
du Sport (FIMS)
www.fims.org/

The Heart: An Online Exploration
sln.fi.edu/biosci/heart.html

The Journal of the American Medical Association
www.ama-assn.org/public/journals/jama/

The Lancet Interactive
www.thelancet.com/

The Online Medical Dictionary
www.graylab.ac.uk/omd/index.html

The Physiologist
www.faseb.org/aps/tphys.htm

The Sleep Well
www.stanford.edu/dement/

The Spine Institute
www.espineinstitute.com/

Today's Dietitian
www.todaysdietitian.com/

United States Sports Academy
www.sport.ussa.edu/

University of Wisconsin Medical School Anatomy
Dissections
www.anatomy.wisc.edu/courses/gross/

U.S. Department of Agriculture Food Safety
and Inspection Service
www.fsis.usda.gov/

Useful Links for Endurance Athletes
www.krs.hia.no/~stephens/coolinks.htm

Vegetarian Resource Group
www.vrg.org/

Virtual Anatomy
hyperion.advanced.org/16421/

Virtual Body
www.medtropolis.com/vbody/

WebMedLit
www.webmedlit.com/

WebSearch: Health and Medicine
websearch.miningco.com/

Wellness Web: Nutrition and Fitness
www.wellweb.com/nutrition_fitness_homepage.htm

Women in Health and Medicine
www.netsrq.com/~dbois/health.html

Women's Health Matters
www.womenshealthmatters.ca/

World Health Organization
www.who.int/

Part 4. General Science Sites

American Association for the Advancement of Science
www.aaas.org/

American Institute of Physics
www.aip.org/history/

Bioinformatics Links
www.ii.uib.no/~inge/list.html

BioMedNews
www.biomednet.com/biomednews

Biosciences
vlib.org/Biosciences

BioSites
www.library.ucsf.edu/biosites/

BioTech Life Sciences Resources and Reference Tools
biotech.icmb.utexas.edu/

Boston Museum of Science
www.british-museum.ac.uk/

BrainPop
www.brainpop.com/indexgen.asp

Cell and Molecular Biology Online
www.cellbio.com/

Center for Human Simulation
www.uchsc.edu/sm/chs/

Center of Science and Industry
cosi.org/

Charles Darwin Origin of Species and Voyage of the Beagle
www.literature.org/Works/Charles-Darwin/

Chicago Academy of Sciences
www.chias.org/

Discover Magazine
www.discover.com/

Discovery Channel Online
www.discovery.com/

Exploratorium
www.exploratorium.org/

Franklin Institute Science Museum
sln.fi.edu/

History of the Health Sciences World Wide Web Links
www.mia_hhss.org/histlink.htm

HMS Beagle
www.biomednet.com/hmsbeagle/current/about/index

How Things Work
howthingswork.virginia.edu/

Human Anatomy Online
www.innerbody.com/indexbody.html

International Museum of Surgical Science
www.imss.org/

International Space Station
station.nasa.gov/

Journals, Conferences, and Current Awareness Services
mcb.harvard.edu/BioLinks.html

Life Science Dictionary
biotech.chem.indiana.edu/pages/dictionary.html

Marching Through the Visible Man
www.crd.ge.com/esl/cgsp/projects/vm/

Mayo Clinic Health Oasis
www.mayohealth.org/

Medical Breakthroughs
www.ivanhoe.com/

MedWeb: History
www.gen.emory.edu/MEDWEB/alphakey/history.html

Monterey Bay Aquarium Online
www.mbayaq.org

NASA
www.nasa.gov

National Academy of Sciences
www.nas.edu/

National Academy Press
www.nap.edu/

National Geographic
www.nationalgeographic.com/

National Science Teachers Association
www.nsta.org/

Natural History on the WWW
www.nhm.ac.uk/info/links/general.htm

Nature.com
www.nature.com/

New Scientist
www.newscientist.com/

Nobel Foundation
www.nobel.se/

Nobel Laureates in the Sciences
www.lib.lsu.edu/sci/chem/guides/srs118.html

NOVA Online
www.pbs.org/wgbh/nova/

Paleontology Without Walls
www.ucmp.berkeley.edu/exhibit/exhibits.html

People and Discoveries
www.pbs.org/wgbh/aso/databank/

Periodic Table on the WWW
www.shef.ac.uk/~chem/web-elements/

Popular Science
www.popsci.com/

Science and Technology
www.artigen.com/newswire/scitech.html

Science Direct
www.sciencedirect.com/

Science in the Headlines
www.nas.edu/headlines/

Science Magazine
www.sciencemag.org/

Science Now
sciencenow.sciencemag.org/

Science Online
www.scienceonline.org/

Science Resources
biotech.chem.indiana.edu/pages/scitools.html

Scientific American
www.scientificamerican.com/

Sirs Web Guide
www.sirs.com/tree/science.htm

Smithsonian Institution
www.si.edu/start.htm

Tech Museum of Innovation
www.thetech.org/

The Genome Database
gdbwww.gdb.org/

The John Hopkins University BioInformatics Web Server
www.bis.med.jhmi.edu/

The Why Files
whyfiles.news.wisc.edu/index.html

Visible Human Viewer
www.npac.syr.edu/projects/vishuman/VisibleHuman.html

Welcome to Nye Labs OnLine
nyelabs.kcts.org/flash_go.html

Wellcome Institute for the History of Medicine
www.wellcome.ac.uk/wellcomegraphic/a2/index.html

WorldOrtho
worldortho.com/

Part 5. Science and Technology News

ABC News: Science
www.abcnews.com/sections/science/

American Medical News
www.ama-assn.org/public/journals/amnews/amnews.htm

CBS News SciTech
www.cbsnews.com/sections/tech/main205.shtml

CNN Interactive Sci-Tech
www.cnn.com/TECH/

EurekAlert
www.eurekalert.org/

FDA News and Publications
www.fda.gov/opacom/hpnews.html

Fox News: Sci-Tech
www.foxnews.com:80/nav/stage_scitech.sml

Institute for Scientific Information
www.isinet.com/

Los Angeles Times: Health
www.latimes.com/

MSNBC Health
www.msnbc.com/news/HEALTH_Front.asp?a

News File Top News Stories
www.newsfile.com/topcwh.htm

News Scientist
www.newscientist.com/

NY Times on the Web: National Science
www.nytimes.com/yr/mo/day/national/
index-science.html
Reuters Health
www.reutershealth.com/
Science Daily
www.sciencedaily.com/
Science News Update
www.ama-assn.org/sci-pubs/sci-
news/1997/pres_rel.htm
Science Technology News
www.topix.net/tech
SciSeek
www.sciseek.com/
The Chronicle of Higher Education Information
Technology
chronicle.com/infotech/index.htm
The National Academies
www.nationalacademies.org/
The Philadelphia Inquirer Health and Science
sln.fi.edu/inquirer/inquirer.html
UniSci
www.comfind.com/
Up to the Minute News
www.size-acceptance.org/news/
USAToday Science
www.usatoday.com/life/science/lsd1.htm
World Tech News
www.worldtechnews.com/

Part 6. Useful Resources

4000 Years of Women in Science
www.astr.ua.edu/4000WS/4000WS.html
Active Living Leadership
www.leadershipforactiveliving.org/
African Americans in the Sciences
www.lib.lsu.edu/lib/chem/display/faces.html
Albert Einstein Online
www.westegg.com/einstein/
All About the Internet
home.rmi.net/~kgr/internet/
AltaVista Translation
babelfish.altavista.digital.com/cgi-bin/translate?
American Cancer Society
www.cancer.org/
American Diabetes Association
www.diabetes.org/
American Lung Association
www.lungusa.org/
Arthritis Foundation
www.arthritis.org/
Australian Sports Commission
www.ausport.gov.au/
Aviation, Space, and Environmental Medicine
www.asma.org/html/journal.htm
Best Medical Resources on the Web
www.priory.com/other.htm

Beyond Discovery
www.beyonddiscovery.org/
Bio Online
www.bio.com/os/start/home.html
Biochemist On-line
www.biochemist.com/home.htm
BioLinks
www.biolinks.com/
Biology Labs Virtual Courseware
vcourseware2.calstatela.edu/
Biomechanics World Wide
www.per.ualberta.ca/biomechanics/
BioMedNet
www.biomednet.com/
BioResearch Online
www2.bioresearchonline.com/content/homepage/
Brain.com
www.brain.com/home.cfm
British Journal of Sports Medicine
bjsm.bmjjournals.com/
Bugs in the News!
falcon.cc.ukans.edu/~jbrown/bugs.html
Build it Yourself
northshore.shore.net/biy/
Canadian Health Network
www.canadian-health-network.ca/
Chem4Kids
chem4kids.com/
Classics in the History of Psychology
www.yorku.ca/dept/psych/classics/
Coaching Science Abstracts
www-rohan.sdsu.edu/dept/coachsci/index.htm
Contributions of 20th Century Women to Physics
www.physics.ucla.edu/~cwp/index.html
Diabetes.com
www.diabetes.com/
Educational Package in Molecular Biology
www.bis.med.jhmi.edu/Dan/DOE/intro.html
Email List Server
www.tile.net/listserv/
English Weights and Measures
home.clara.net/brianp/index.html
Enter Evolution: Theory and History
www.ucmp.berkeley.edu/history/evolution.html
Ergoworld
www.interface-analysis.com/ergoworld/
EurekAlert!
www.eurekalert.org/
GeneBrowser
www.natx.com/
Global Medic
www.globalmedic.com/
Harvard Molecular and Cell Biology Links
mcb.harvard.edu/BioLinks.html
Health and Fitness Links: Professional Societies
www.tc.columbia.edu/academic/movement/links/
societies.html
Healthgate.com
www.healthgate.com/

Heart and Stroke Foundation
ww2.heartandstroke.ca/

HighWire Press
highwire.stanford.edu/

HospitalWeb
neuro-www.mgh.harvard.edu/hospitalweb.shtml

HyperHistory Online
www.hyperhistory.com/

International Association for Sports Information
www.iasi.org/

International Council of Sport Science and Physical
Education
www.icsspe.org/

International Institute for Sport and Human Performance
Darkwing.uoregon.edu/~iishp/

International Museum of Surgical Science
www.imss.org/

International Olympic Committee
www.olympic.org/map/index.html

International Society for Aging and Physical Activity
www.isapa.org/

Internet Pathology Laboratory for Medical Education
www-medlib.med.utah.edu/WebPath/webpath.html

Internet@address.finder
iaf.net/

Journal of Medical Genetics
jmg.bmjjournals.com/

Medical/Health Science Libraries on the Web
www.lib.uiowa.edu/hardin-www/hslibs.html

Medical Breakthroughs
www.ivanhoe.com/

Medicine Through Time
www.bbc.co.uk/education/medicine/

MendelWeb
www.netspace.org/MendelWeb/

MolecularVision
www.molvis.org/molvis/

Museums Around the World
www.comlab.ox.ac.uk/archive/other/museums/world.html

NASA Astrobiology
astrobiology.arc.nasa.gov/index.cfm

National Academy Press
www.nap.edu/

National Academy for State Health Policy
www.nashp.org/

National Center on Physical Activity and Disability
www.ncpad.org/

National Institute of Diabetes and Digestive and Kidney
Diseases
www.niddk.nih.gov/

National Inventors Hall of Fame
www.invent.org/book/

Neurosciences on the Internet
www.neuroguide.com/

Newspapers Online!
www.newspapers.com/

Newton's Apple
www.pbs.org/ktca/newtons/

Nobel Prize Internet Archive
www.almaz.com/

Oxford English Dictionary
www.oed.com/

People Finder: Netscape
database.rsnz.govt.nz/sportsci/indexnew.html

Publicly Accessible Mailing Lists
www.neosoft.com/internet/paml/

Quicktime VR for Macintosh and Windows
www.apple.com/quicktime/qtvr/index.html

Referencing Online Documents in Scientific Publications
www.beadsland.com/weapas/

Roget's Thesaurus
humanities.uchicago.edu/forms_unrest/ROGET.html

Society for Human Performance in Extreme Environments
www.hpee.org/

Sport and the European Union
europa.eu.int/comm/sport/

The Aging Research Center
www.graylab.ac.uk/omd/index.html

The Biology Place
www.biology.com/

The Chemistry Place
www.chemplace.com/

The Cooper Institute
www.cooperinst.org/

The Educational Resources Information Center
www.accesseric.org:81/

The Galileo Project
es.rice.edu/ES/humsoc/Galileo/

The Medieval Science Page
members.aol.com/mcnelis/medsci_index.html

The Nephron Information Center
www.nephron.com/

The Tech Museum of Innovation
www.thetech.org/

The Virtual Resource Centre for Sport Information
www.sportquest.com/

Three Dimensional Medical Reconstruction
www.crd.ge.com/esl/cgsp/projects/medical/

University of Michigan Documents Center
www.lib.umich.edu/libhome/Documents.center/
index.html#doctop

WhoWhere? People Finder
www.whowhere.lycos.com/

Yahoo! People Search
people.yahoo.com/

Yellow.com (includes white pages)
www.yellow.com

THE METRIC SYSTEM AND CONVERSION CONSTANTS IN EXERCISE PHYSIOLOGY

Appendix C has two parts. Part 1 deals with the metric system, and Part 2 discusses the Système International d'Unités (SI units).

The Metric System

Most measurements in science are expressed in terms of the metric system. This system uses units that are related to one another by some power of 10. The prefix centi means one-hundredth, milli means one-thousandth, and kilo is derived from a word that means one thousand. In the following sections, we show the relationship between metric units and English units of measurement that are relevant to the material presented in this book.

UNITS OF LENGTH

Metric Unit	Equivalent Metric Units	Equivalent English Units
meter (m)	100 cm; 1000 mm	39.37 in; 3.28 ft; 1.09 yd
centimeter (cm)	0.01 m; 10 mm	0.3937 in
millimeter (mm)	0.001 m; 0.1 cm	0.03937 in

Units of Weight

Use the following conversions for common units of mass (weight) and volume. For example, 1 ounce = 0.06 pound. Therefore, two ounces would equal 2 × 0.06 = 0.12 pound, and 16 ounces = 0.96 pound (16 × 0.06).

Metric Unit	Equivalent Metric Units	Equivalent English Units
kilogram (kg)	1000 g; 1,000,000 mg	35.3 oz; 2.2046 lb
gram (g)	0.001 kg; 1000 mg	0.353 oz
milligram (mg)	0.000001 kg; 0.001 g	0.0000353 oz

UNITS OF VOLUME

Metric Unit	Equivalent Metric Units	Equivalent English Units
liter (L)	1000 mL	1.057 qt
milliliter (mL) or cubic centimeter (cc)	0.001 L	0.001057 qt

TEMPERATURE

To convert Fahrenheit to Celsius: $°C = (°F − 32) ÷ 1.8$
To convert Celsius to Fahrenheit: $°F = (1.8 ÷ °C) + 32$

On the Fahrenheit scale, water freezes at 32°F and boils at 212°F. On the Celsius scale, water freezes at 0°C and boils at 100°C.

UNITS OF SPEED

mph	$km·h^{-1}$	$m·s^{-1}$
1	1.6	0.47
2	3.2	0.94
3	4.8	1.41
4	6.4	1.88
5	8.0	2.35
6	9.6	2.82
7	11.2	3.29
8	12.8	3.76
9	14.4	4.23
10	16.0	4.70
11	17.7	5.17
12	19.3	5.64
13	20.9	6.11
14	22.5	6.58
15	24.1	7.05
16	25.8	7.52
17	27.4	7.99
18	29.0	8.46
19	30.6	8.93
20	32.2	9.40

COMMON EXPRESSIONS OF WORK, ENERGY, AND POWER

Watts	Kilocalories (kCal)	Foot-Pounds (ft·lb)
1 watt = 0.73756 ft-lb·s^{-1}	1 kCal = 3086 ft-lb	1 ft·lb = 3.2389 $\times$ 10^{-3} kCal
1 watt = 0.01433 kCal·min^{-1}	1 kCal = 426.8 kg-m	1 ft·lb = 0.13825 kg-m
1 watt = 1.341 $\times$ 10^{-3} hp or 0.0013 hp	1 kCal = 3087.4 ft-lb	1 ft·lb = 5.050 $\times$ 10^{-3} hp·h^{-1}
1 watt = 6.12 kg-m·min^{-1}	1 kCal = 1.5593 $\times$ 10^{-3} hp·h^{-1}	

Terminology and Units of Measurement

The American College of Sports Medicine suggests that the following terminology and units of measurement be used in scientific endeavors to promote consistency and clarity of communication and to avoid ambiguity. The following terms are defined using the units of measurement of the Système International d'Unités (SI units).

Exercise: Any and all activity involving generation of force by the activated muscle(s) that results in disruption of a homeostatic state. In dynamic exercise, the muscle may perform shortening (concentric) contractions or be overcome by external resistance and perform lengthening (eccentric) contractions. When muscle force results in no movement, the contraction should be termed static or isometric.

Exercise intensity: A specific level of maintenance of muscular activity that can be quantified in terms of power (energy expenditure or work performed per unit of time), isometric force sustained, or velocity of progression.

Endurance: The time limit of a person's ability to maintain either a specific isometric force or a specific power level involving combinations of concentric or eccentric muscular contractions.

Mass: A quantity of matter of an object; a direct measure of the object's inertia (note: mass = weight ÷ acceleration due to gravity; unit: gram or kilogram).

Weight: The force with which a quantity of matter is attracted toward Earth by normal acceleration of gravity (traditional unit: kilogram of weight).

Energy: The capability of producing force, performing work, or generating heat (unit: joule or kilojoule).

Force: That which changes or tends to change the state of rest or motion in matter (unit: Newton).

Speed: Total distance traveled per unit of time (unit: meters per second).

Velocity: Displacement per unit of time. A vector quantity requiring that direction be stated or strongly implied (unit: meters per second or kilometers per hour).

Work: Force expressed through a distance but with no limitation on time (unit: joule or kilojoule). Quantities of energy and heat expressed independently of time should also be presented in joules. The term "work" should *not* be employed synonymously with muscular exercise.

Power: The rate of performing work; the derivative of work with respect to time; the product of force and velocity (unit: watt). Other related processes, such as energy release and heat transfer, should, when expressed per unit of time, be quantified and presented in watts.

Torque: Effectiveness of a force to produce axial rotation (unit: Newton meter).

Volume: A space occupied, for example, by a quantity of fluid or gas (unit: liter or milliliter). Gas volumes should be indicated as ATPS, BTPS, or STPD.

Amount of a substance: The amount of a substance is frequently expressed in moles. A mole is the quantity of a chemical substance that has a weight in mass units (e.g., grams) numerically equal to the molecular weight or that, in the case of a gas, has a volume occupied by such a weight under specified conditions. One mole of a respiratory gas is equal to 22.4 liters at STPD.

SI Units

The uniform numerical value system is known as the Système International d'Unités (SI units). SI was developed through international cooperation to create a universally acceptable system of measurement. SI ensures that units of measurement are uniform in concept and style. The SI system permits quantities in common use to be more easily compared. Many scientific organizations endorse the concept of the SI, and leading journals in nutrition, health, and exercise science now require that laboratory data be presented in SI units. The information in this appendix has been summarized from a detailed description about the SI published in the following article: Young DS: Implementation of SI units for clinical laboratory data. Style specifications and conversion tables. *Ann. Intern. Med.*, 106:114, 1987.

DEFINITIONS OF COMMON SI UNITS

Degree Celsius (°C)	The degree Celsius (centigrade) is equivalent to K − 273.15.
Radian (rad)	The radian is the plane angle between two radii of a circle that subtend on the circumference of an arc equal in length to the radius.
Joule (J)	The joule is the work done when the point of application of a force of 1 Newton is displaced through a distance of 1 meter in the direction of the force. 1 J = 1 Nm.
Kelvin (K)	The kelvin is the fraction 1/273.16 of the thermodynamic temperature of the triple point of water.
Kilogram (kg)	The kilogram is a unit of mass equal to the mass of the international prototype of the kilogram.
Meter (m)	The meter is the length equal to 1,650,763.73 wavelengths in vacuum of the radiation that corresponds to the transition between the levels $2p_{10}$ and $5d_5$ of the krypton 86 atom.
Newton (N)	The Newton is the force that, when applied to a mass of 1 kilogram, gives it an acceleration of 1 meter per second squared. $1\ N = 1\ kg \cdot m^{-1} \cdot s^{-2}$.
Pascal (Pa)	The Pascal is the pressure produced by a force of one Newton applied, with uniform distribution, over an area of 1 square meter. $1\ Pa = 1\ N \cdot m^{-2}$.
Second (s)	The second is the duration of 9,192,631,770 periods of the radiation that corresponds to the transition between the two hyperfine levels of the ground state of the cesium 133 atom.
Watt (W)	The watt is the power that, in 1 second, gives rise to the energy of 1 joule. $1\ W = 1\ J \cdot s^{-1}$.

BASE UNITS OF SI NOMENCLATURE

Physical Quantity	Base Unit	SI Symbol
Length	meter	m
Mass	kilogram	kg
Time	second	s
Amount of substance	mole	mol
Thermodynamic temperature	kelvin	K
Electric current	ampere	A
Luminous intensity	candela	cd

BASE UNITS OF SI STYLE GUIDLINES

Guidelines	Example	Incorrect Style	Correct Style
Lowercase letters are used for symbols or abbreviations	kilogram	Kg	kg
Exceptions:	kelvin	k	K
	ampere	a	A
	liter	l	L
Symbols are not followed by a period	meter	m.	m
Exception: end of sentence	mole	mol.	mol
Symbols are not to be pluralized	kilograms	kgs	kg
	meters	ms	m
Names and symbols are not to be combined	force	kilogram·meter·s^{-2}	kg−m·s^{-2}
			kg−m/s^2
When numbers are printed, symbols are preferred		100 meters	100 m
		2 moles	2 mol
A space should be placed between number and symbol		50ml	50 mL
The product of units is indicated by a dot above the line		kg × m/s^2	kg−m·s^{-2}
			kg−m/s^2
Only one solidus (/) should be used per expression		mmol/L/s	mmol/(L·s)
A zero should be placed before the decimal		.01	0.01
Decimal numbers are preferable to fractions		$^3/_4$	0.75
		75%	0.75
Spaces are used to separate long numbers		1,500,000	1 500 000
Exception: optional with four-digit number		1,000	1000 or 1 000

For SI units in exercise physiology, the term body weight is properly referred to as mass (kg), height should be referred to as stature (m), second is s, minute is min, hour is h, week is wk, month is mo, year is y, day is d, gram is g, liter is L, hertz is Hz, joule is J, kilocalorie is kCal, ohm is V, pascal is Pa, revolutions per minute is rpm, volt is V, and watt is W. These abbreviations or symbols are used for the singular or plural form.

METABOLIC COMPUTATIONS IN OPEN-CIRCUIT SPIROMETRY

Standardizing Gas Volumes: Environmental Factors

Gas volumes obtained during physiologic measurements are usually expressed in one of three ways: *ATPS*, *STPD*, or *BTPS*.

ATPS refers to the volume of gas at the specific conditions of measurement, which are, therefore, at Ambient Temperature (273°K + ambient temperature°C), ambient Pressure, and Saturated with water vapor. Gas volumes collected during open-circuit spirometry and pulmonary function tests are measured initially at ATPS.

The volume of a gas varies depending on its temperature, pressure, and content of water vapor, even though the absolute number of gas molecules remains constant. These environmental influences are summarized as follows:

Temperature: The volume of a gas varies *directly* with temperature. Increasing the temperature causes the molecules to move more rapidly; the gas mixture expands, and the volume increases proportionately (*Charles' law*).
Pressure: The volume of a gas varies *inversely* with pressure. Increasing the pressure on a gas forces the molecules closer together, causing the volume to decrease in proportion to the increase in pressure (*Boyle's law*).
Water vapor: The volume of a gas varies depending on its water vapor content. The volume of a gas is greater when the gas is saturated with water vapor than it is when the same gas is dry (i.e., contains no moisture).

These three factors—temperature, pressure, and the relative degree of saturation of the gas with water vapor—must be considered, especially when gas volumes are to be compared under different environmental conditions and used subsequently in metabolic and physiologic calculations. The standards that provide the frame of reference for expressing a volume of gas are either STPD or BTPS.

STPD refers to the volume of a gas expressed under Standard conditions of Temperature (273°K or 0°C), Pressure (760 mm Hg), and Dry (no water vapor). Expressing a gas volume STPD, for example, makes it possible to evaluate and compare the volumes of expired air measured while running in the rain at high altitude, along a beach in the cold of winter, or in a hot desert environment below

sea level. *In all metabolic calculations, gas volumes are always expressed at STPD.*

1. To reduce a gas volume to standard temperature (ST), the following formula is applied:

$$\text{Gas volume ST} = V_{\text{ATPS}} \times \frac{273°K}{273°K + T°C} \quad (1)$$

where T°C = temperature of the gas in the measuring device and 273°K = absolute temperature kelvin, which is equivalent to 0°C.

2. The following equation is used to express a gas volume at standard pressure (SP):

$$\text{Gas volume SP} = V_{\text{ATPS}} \times \frac{P_B}{760 \text{ mm Hg}} \quad (2)$$

where P_B = ambient barometric pressure in mm Hg and 760 = standard barometric pressure at sea level, mm Hg.

3. To reduce a gas to standard dry (SD) conditions, the effects of water vapor pressure at the particular environmental temperature must be subtracted from the volume of gas. Because expired air is 100% saturated with water vapor, it is not necessary to determine its percent saturation from measures of relative humidity. The vapor pressure in moist or completely humidified air at a particular ambient temperature can be obtained in Table D.1 and is expressed in mm Hg. This vapor pressure (P_{H_2O}) is then subtracted from the ambient barometric pressure (P_B) to reduce the gas to standard pressure dry (SPD) as follows:

$$\text{Gas volume SPD} = V_{\text{ATPS}} \times \frac{P_B - P_{H_2O}}{760} \quad (3)$$

By combining equations (1) and (3), any volume of moist air can be converted to STPD as follows:

Gas volume STPD

$$= V_{\text{ATPS}}\left(\frac{273}{273 + T°C}\right)\left(\frac{P_B - P_{H_2O}}{760}\right) \quad (4)$$

TABLE D.1
VAPOR PRESSURE (P_{H_2O}) OF WET GAS AT TEMPERATURES NORMALLY ENCOUNTERED IN THE LABORATORY

T (°C)	P_{H_2O} (mm Hg)	T (°C)	P_{H_2O} (mm Hg)
20	17.5	31	33.7
21	18.7	32	35.7
22	19.8	33	37.7
23	21.1	34	39.9
24	22.4	35	42.2
25	23.8	36	44.6
26	25.2	37	47.1
27	26.7	38	49.7
28	28.4	39	52.4
29	30.0	40	55.3
30	31.8		

TABLE D.2
FACTORS TO REDUCE MOIST GAS TO A DRY GAS VOLUME AT 0°C AND 760 MM HG

Barometric Pressure	Temperature (°C)																	
	15	16	17	18	19	20	21	22	23	24	25	26	27	28	29	30	31	32
700	0.855	851	847	842	838	834	829	825	821	816	812	807	802	797	793	788	783	778
702	857	853	849	845	840	836	832	827	823	818	814	809	805	800	795	790	785	780
704	860	856	852	847	843	839	834	830	825	821	816	812	807	802	797	792	787	783
706	862	858	854	850	845	841	837	832	828	823	819	814	810	804	800	795	790	785
708	865	861	856	852	848	843	839	834	830	825	821	816	812	807	802	797	792	787
710	867	863	859	855	850	846	842	837	833	828	824	819	814	809	804	799	795	790
712	870	866	861	857	853	848	844	839	836	830	826	821	817	812	807	802	797	792
714	872	868	864	859	855	851	846	842	837	833	828	824	819	814	809	804	799	794
716	875	871	866	862	858	853	849	844	840	835	831	826	822	816	812	807	802	797
718	877	873	869	864	860	856	851	847	842	838	833	828	824	819	814	809	804	799
720	880	876	871	867	863	858	854	849	845	840	836	831	826	821	816	812	807	802
722	882	878	874	869	865	861	856	852	847	843	838	833	829	824	819	814	809	804
724	885	880	876	872	867	863	858	854	849	845	840	835	831	826	821	816	811	806
726	887	883	879	874	870	866	861	856	852	847	843	838	833	829	824	818	813	808
728	890	886	881	877	872	868	863	859	854	850	845	840	836	831	826	821	816	811
730	892	888	884	879	875	871	866	861	857	852	847	843	838	833	828	823	818	813
732	895	890	886	882	877	873	868	864	859	854	850	845	840	836	831	825	820	815
734	897	893	889	884	880	875	871	866	862	857	852	847	843	838	833	828	823	818
736	900	895	891	887	882	878	873	869	864	859	855	850	845	840	835	830	825	820
738	902	898	894	889	885	880	876	871	866	862	857	852	848	843	838	833	828	822
740	905	900	896	892	887	883	878	874	869	864	860	855	850	845	840	835	830	825
742	907	903	898	894	890	885	881	876	871	867	862	857	852	847	842	837	832	827
744	910	906	901	897	892	888	883	878	874	869	864	859	855	850	845	840	834	829
746	912	908	903	899	895	890	886	881	876	872	867	862	857	852	847	842	837	832
748	915	910	906	901	897	892	888	883	879	874	869	864	860	854	850	845	839	834
750	917	913	908	904	900	895	890	886	881	876	872	867	862	857	852	847	842	837
752	920	915	911	906	902	897	893	888	883	879	874	869	864	859	854	849	844	839
754	922	918	913	909	904	900	895	891	886	881	876	872	867	862	857	852	846	841
756	925	920	916	911	907	902	898	893	888	883	879	874	869	864	859	854	849	844
758	927	923	918	914	909	905	900	896	891	886	881	876	872	866	861	856	851	846
760	930	925	921	916	912	907	902	898	893	888	883	879	874	869	864	859	854	848
762	932	928	923	919	914	910	905	900	896	891	886	881	876	871	866	861	856	851
764	936	930	926	921	916	912	907	903	898	893	888	884	879	874	869	864	858	853
766	937	933	928	924	919	915	910	905	900	896	891	886	881	876	871	866	861	855
768	940	935	931	926	922	917	912	908	903	898	893	888	883	878	873	868	863	858
770	942	938	933	928	924	919	915	910	905	901	896	891	886	881	876	871	865	860

As was the case with the correction to STPD, appropriate BTPS *correction factors* are available for converting a moist gas volume at ambient conditions to a volume BTPS. These BTPS factors for a broad range of ambient temperatures are presented in Table D.3. These factors have been computed assuming a barometric pressure of 760 mm Hg, and small deviations ($\pm$10 mm Hg) from this pressure introduce only a minimal error.

TABLE D.3
BTPS FACTORS

T (°C)	BTPS[a]	T (°C)	BTPS
20	1.102	29	1.051
21	1.096	30	1.045
22	1.091	31	1.039
23	1.085	32	1.032
24	1.080	33	1.026
25	1.075	34	1.020
26	1.068	35	1.014
27	1.063	36	1.007
28	1.057	37	1.000

[a]Body temperature, ambient pressure, and saturated with water vapor.

Calculation of Oxygen Uptake

In determining oxygen uptake by open-circuit spirometry, we are interested in knowing how much oxygen has been removed from the *inspired air*. Because the composition of inspired air remains relatively constant ($CO_2 = 0.03\%$, $O_2 = 20.93\%$, $N_2 = 79.04\%$), it is possible to determine how much oxygen has been removed from the inspired air by measuring the amount and composition of the expired air. When this is done, the expired air contains more carbon dioxide (usually 2.5 to 5.0%), less oxygen (usually 15.0 to 18.5%), and more nitrogen (usually 79.04 to 79.60%). It should be noted, however, that nitrogen is inert in terms of metabolism; any change in its concentration in expired air reflects the fact that the number of oxygen molecules removed from the inspired air is not replaced by the same number of carbon dioxide molecules produced in metabolism. This results in the volume of expired air (V_E, STPD) being unequal to the inspired volume (V_I, STPD). For example, if the respiratory quotient is less than 1.00 (i.e., less CO_2 produced in relation to O_2 consumed), and 3 liters of air are inspired, *less than* 3 liters of air will be expired. In this case, the nitrogen concentration is higher in the expired air than in the inspired air. This is not to say that nitrogen has been produced, only that nitrogen molecules now represent a larger percentage of V_E compared to V_I. In fact, V_E differs from V_I in direct proportion to the change in nitrogen concentration between the inspired and expired volumes. Thus, V_I can be determined from V_E using the relative change in nitrogen in an equation known as the *Haldane transformation*.

$$V_I, STPD = V_E, STPD \times \frac{\%N_{2_E}}{\%N_{2_I}} \quad (5)$$

where $\%N_{2_I} = 79.04$ and $\%N_{2_E}$ = percent nitrogen in expired air computed from gas analysis as:

$$[(100 - (\%O_{2_E} + \%CO_2)].$$

The volume of O_2 in the inspired air (VO_{2_I}) can then be determined as follows:

$$VO_{2_I} = V_I \times \%O_{2_I} \quad (6)$$

Substituting equation (5) for V_I,

$$VO_{2_I} = V_E \times \frac{\%N_{2_E}}{79.04\% \times \%O_{2_I}} \quad (7)$$

where $\%O_{2_I} = 20.93\%$

The amount or volume of oxygen in the expired air (VO_{2_E}) is computed as:

$$VO_{2_E} = V_E \times \%O_{2_E} \quad (8)$$

where $\%O_{2_E}$ is the fractional concentration of oxygen in expired air determined by gas analysis (chemical or electronic methods).

The amount of O_2 removed from the inspired air each minute ($\dot{V}O_2$) can then be computed as follows:

$$\dot{V}O_{2_E} = (\dot{V}_I \times \%O_{2_I}) - (\dot{V}_E \times \%O_{2_E}) \quad (9)$$

By substitution

$$\dot{V}O_2 = \left[\left(\dot{V}_E \times \frac{\%N_{2_E}}{79.04\%} \right) \times 20.93\% \right] - (\dot{V}_E \times \%O_{2_E}) \quad (10)$$

where $\dot{V}O_2$ = volume of oxygen consumed per minute, expressed in milliliters or liters, and $\dot{V}_E$ = expired air volume per minute expressed in milliliters or liters.
Equation 10 can be simplified to:

$$\dot{V}O_2 = \dot{V}_E \left[\left(\frac{\%N_{2_E}}{79.04\%} \times 20.93\% \right) - \%O_{2_E} \right] \quad (11)$$

The final form of the equation is:

$$\dot{V}O_2 = \dot{V}_E [(\%N_{2_E} \times 0.265) - \%O_{2_E}] \quad (12)$$

The value obtained within the brackets in equations 11 and 12 is referred to as the *true O_2*; this represents the "oxygen extraction" or, more precisely, the percentage of oxygen consumed for any volume of air *expired*.

Although equation 12 is the equation used most widely to compute oxygen uptake from measures of expired air, it is also possible to calculate $\dot{V}O_2$ from direct measurements of both $\dot{V}_I$ and $\dot{V}_E$. In this case, the Haldane transformation is not used, and oxygen uptake is calculated directly as:

$$\dot{V}O_2 = (\dot{V}_I \times 20.93) - (\dot{V}_E \times \%O_{2_E}) \quad (13)$$

In situations in which only $\dot{V}_I$ is measured, the $\dot{V}_E$ can be calculated from the Haldane transformation as:

$$\dot{V}_E = \dot{V}_I \frac{\%N_{2_E}}{\%N_{2_I}}$$

By substitution in equation 13, the computational equation is:

$$\dot{V}O_2 = \dot{V}_I\left[\%O_{2_I} - \left(\frac{\%N_{2_I}}{\%N_{2_E}} \times \%O_{2_E}\right)\right] \quad (14)$$

Calculation of Carbon Dioxide Production

The carbon dioxide production per minute ($\dot{V}CO_2$) is calculated as follows:

$$\dot{V}CO_2 = \dot{V}_E(\%CO_{2_E} - \%CO_{2_I}) \quad (15)$$

where $\%CO_{2_E}$ = percent carbon dioxide in expired air determined by gas analysis, and $\%CO_{2_I}$ = percent carbon dioxide in inspired air, which is essentially constant at 0.03%.

The final form of the equation is:

$$\dot{V}CO_2 = \dot{V}_E(\%CO_{2_E} - 0.03\%) \quad (16)$$

Calculation of Respiratory Quotient

The respiratory quotient (RQ) is calculated in one of two ways:
1. $RQ = \dot{V}CO_2/\dot{V}O_2$ $\qquad\qquad$ (17)
or
2. $RQ = \dfrac{(\%CO_{2_E} - 0.03\%)}{\text{"True" } O_2}$ $\qquad$ (18)

Sample Metabolic Calculations

The following data were obtained during the last minute of a steady-rate, 10-minute treadmill run performed at 6 miles per hour at a 5% grade.

$\dot{V}_E$: 62.1 liters, ATPS
Barometric pressure: 750 mm Hg
Temperature: 26°C
$\%O_2$ expired: 16.86 (O_2 analyzer)
$\%CO_2$ expired: 3.60 (CO_2 analyzer)
$\%N_2$ expired: $[100 - (16.86 + 3.60)] = 79.54$

Determine the following:

1. $\dot{V}_E$, STPD
2. $\dot{V}O_2$, STPD
3. $\dot{V}CO_2$ STPD
4. RQ
5. kCal·min^{-1}

1. $\dot{V}_E$, STPD (use equation 4 or STPD correction factor in Table D.2).

$$\dot{V}_E, \text{STPD} = \dot{V}_E, \text{ATPS}\left(\frac{273}{273 + T°C}\right)\left(\frac{P_B - P_{H_2O}}{760}\right)$$

$$= 62.1\left(\frac{273}{299}\right)\left(\frac{750 - 25.2}{760}\right)$$

$$= 54.07 \text{ L} \cdot \text{min}^{-1}$$

2. $\dot{V}O_2$, STPD (use equation 12)

$$\dot{V}O_2, \text{STPD} = \dot{V}_E, \text{STPD}[(\%N_{2_E} \times 0.265) - \%O_{2_E}]$$

$$= 54.07[(0.7954 \times 0.265) - 0.1686]$$

$$= 54.07(0.0422)$$

$$= 2.281 \text{ L} \cdot \text{min}^{-1}$$

3. $\dot{V}CO_2$, STPD (use equation 16)

$$\dot{V}CO_2, \text{STPD} = \dot{V}_E, \text{STPD}(CO_{2_E} - 0.03\%)$$

$$= 54.07(0.0360 - 0.0003)$$

$$= 54.07(0.0357)$$

$$= 1.930 \text{ L} \cdot \text{min}^{-1}$$

4. RQ (use equation 17 or 19)

$$RQ = \dot{V}CO_2/\dot{V}O_2$$

$$= \frac{1.930}{2.281}$$

$$= 0.846$$

or

$$RQ = \frac{(\%CO_{2_E} - 0.03\%)}{\text{"true" O}}$$

$$= \frac{3.60 - 0.03}{4.22}$$

$$= 0.846$$

Because the exercise was performed in a steady-rate of aerobic metabolism, the obtained RQ of 0.846 can be applied in Table 7.2 to obtain the appropriate caloric transformation. In this way, the exercise oxygen uptake can be transposed to kCal of energy expended per minute as follows:

5. Energy expenditure (kCal·min^{-1}) = $\dot{V}O_2$ (L·min^{-1}) × caloric equivalent per liter O_2 at the given steady-rate RQ:

Energy expenditure $= 2.281 \times 4.862$

$$= 11.09 \text{ kCal} \cdot \text{min}^{-1}$$

Assuming that the RQ value reflects the nonprotein RQ, a reasonable estimate of both the percentage and quantity of lipid and carbohydrate metabolized during each minute of the run can be obtained from Table 7.2.

Percentage kCal derived from lipid = 50.7%

Percentage kCal derived from carbohydrate = 49.3%

Grams of lipid utilized = 0.267 g per liter of oxygen, or approximately 0.61 g per minute (0.267×2.281 L O_2)

Grams of carbohydrate utilized = 0.580 g per liter of oxygen, or approximately 1.36 g per minute (0.580×2.281 L O_2)

FREQUENTLY CITED JOURNALS IN EXERCISE PHYSIOLOGY

In our own writing to produce this text and others, we rely on many sources of information that fall into two main categories: (1) research journals, and (2) Internet resources (six categories of resources are presented in Appendix B). The more than 100 journals listed in this appendix range in scope from molecular biology (an ever increasing presence in exercise physiology) to biological chemistry (focus on the chemistry of pharmacologic agents and drug-related mechanisms) to radiology (dose-response curves for medical and space biology applications) to experimental brain research (motor memory and learning). The entire gamut of what constitutes "exercise physiology" can be searched from this list of journals to provide a wealth of timely information about numerous topics of interest. To discover the intimate details about an article (if the full article is not available via the Internet), access to a library can provide that information if the library subscribes to the journal. Unfortunately, the escalating cost of journal subscriptions often makes this route unavailable as libraries frequently rely on "electronic" journal subscriptions. The two types of electronic subscriptions include "free" access (available to anyone via the Internet) and paid subscriptions (individuals, library, or organization pays the required fees). Here is a salient example for *Medicine and Science in Sports and Exercise* (*Med Sci Sports Exerc*) published by the American College of Sports Medicine (www.acsm.org). Navigate to "newsroom and publica-tions" and select the journal MSSE; you will obtain the following information:

> ACSM members and *MSSE®* subscribers have access to full-text articles from *MSSE®* issues from 2000 to the latest issue. To view the full-text, you must first activate your online subscription at the *MSSE®* Web Site (www.acsm-msse.org).

> For the *MSSE®* Web site, which contains contents (non-members and non-subscribers may view abstracts only), a search feature, position stands, journal information, author guide (containing information for authors), and a feedback feature, click here.

If you want to access the *Journal of Applied Physiology* (*J Appl Physiol*) published by the American Physiological Society (www.the-aps.org/), you must subscribe to gain access to the electronic versions of publications. Check with your reference librarian about electronic subscriptions and access privileges. As a "shot gun" approach, use Google (www.google.com) to find the URL for the journal. Many journals allow free access to all issues (i.e., National Library of Medicine free medical journals: www.lib.uiowa.edu/hardin/md/ej.html; Free Access to Science: www.dcprinciples.org/), while some journals permit viewing of the abstract only or the full text and abstract for a particular year from the journal's electronic archives (i.e., *American Journal of Clincial Nutrition*; www.ajcn.org/contents-by-date.0.shtml).

Journal	Abbreviation	Journal	Abbreviation
Acta Medica Scandinavica	Acta Med Scand	British Heart Journal	Br Heart J
Acta Physiologica Scandinavica	Acta Physiol Scand	British Journal of Nutrition	Br J Nutr
American Journal of Clinical Nutrition	Am J Clin Nutr	British Journal of Sports Medicine	Br J Sports Med
American Heart Journal	Am Heart J	British Medical Journal	Br Med J
American Journal of Anatomy	Am J Anat	Canadian Journal of Applied Physiology	Can J Appl Physiol
American Journal of Cardiology	Am J Cardiol		
American Journal of Epidemiology	Am J Epidemiol	Canadian Journal of Applied Sports Sciences	Can J Appl Sport Sci
American Journal of Human Biology	Am J Hum Biol		
American Journal of Physical Anthropology	Am J Phys Anthropol	Cellular Physiology and Biochemistry	Cell Physiol Biochem
		Circulation Research	Circ Res
American Journal of Physiology	Am J Physiol	Circulation: Journal of the American Heart Association	Circulation
American Journal of Public Health	Am J Public Health		
American Journal of Sports Medicine	Am J Sports Med	Clinical Biomechanics	Clin Biomech
Annals of Human Biology	Ann Hum Biol	Clinical Chemistry	Clin Chem
Annals of Internal Medicine	Ann Intern Med	Clinical Nutrition	Clin Nutr
Annals of Nutrition and Metabolism	Ann Nut Met	Clinical Science	Clin Sci
Appetite	Appetite	Clinical Sports Medicine	Clin Sports Med
Archives of Environmental Health	Arch Environ Health	Diabetes	Diabetes
Atherosclerosis	Atherosclerosis	Diabetologia	Diabetologia
Aviation and Space Environmental Medicine	Aviat Space Environ Med	Endocrinology	Endocrinology
		Ergonomics	Ergonomics
Brain: Journal of Neurology	Brain	European Journal of Applied Physiology	Eur J Appl Physiol

Journal	Abbreviation	Journal	Abbreviation
Exercise Immunology Review	Exerc Immun Rev	Journal of Strength and Conditioning Research	JSCR
Experientia	Experientia	Journal of the American Dietetic Association	J Am Diet Assoc
Experimental Brain Research	Exp Brain Res		
FASEB Journal	FASEB J	Journal of the American Medical Association	JAMA
Fertility and Sterility	Fertil Steril		
Geriatrics	Geriatrics	Journal of Sports Medicine	J Sports Med
Growth	Growth	Journal of Sports Science and Medicine	JSSM
Human Biology	Hum Biol	Lancet	Lancet
Human Heredity	Hum Her	Medicine and Science in Sports and Exercise	Med Sci Sports Exerc
Human Movement Science	Hum Mov Sci		
International Journal of Fitness	I J Fitness	Medicine and Sport Science	Med Sport Sci
International Journal of Obesity	Int J Obes	Molecular Genetics and Metabolism	Mol Gen Metabol
International Journal of Sports Medicine	Int J Sports Med		
		Muscle and Nerve	Muscle Nerve
International Journal of Sport Nutrition	IJSN	Molecular Medicine Today	Mol Med Today
		Nature	Nature
International Journal for Vitamin and Nutrition Research	Int J Vitam Nutr Res	Neuroscience Letters	Neurosci Lett
		New England Journal of Medicine	N Engl J Med
Journal of Aging and Physical Activity	J Aging Phys Act	Nutrition Abstracts and Reviews	Nutr Abstr Rev
Journal of Applied Physiology	J Appl Physiol	Nutrition and Metabolism	Nutr Metab
Journal of Biological Chemistry	J Biol Chem	Nutrition Reviews	Nutr Rev
Journal of Biomechanics	J Biomech	Pediatric Exercise Science	Pediatr Exerc Sci
Journal of Bone and Joint Surgery	J Bone Joint Surg	Pediatrics	Pediatrics
Journal of Clinical Endocrinology and Metabolism	J Clin Endocrinol Metab	Physical Therapy Reviews	Phys Ther Rev
		Physician and Sports Medicine	Physician Sports Med
Journal of Clinical Investigation	J Clin Invest	Physiological Reviews	Physiol Rev
Journal of Gerontology	J Gerontol	Preventive Medicine	Prev Med
Journal of Human Movement Studies	J Hum Mov Stud	Proceedings of the Nutrition Society	Proc Nutr Soc
Journal of Laboratory and Clinical Medicine	J Lab Clin Med		
		Psychosomatic Medicine	Psychosom Med
Journal of Lipid Research	J Lipid Res	Public Health Reports	Public Health Rep
Journal of Molecular Biology	J Mol Biol	Radiology	Radiology
Journal of Neurophysiology	J Neurophysiol	Research Quarterly for Exercise and Sports	Res Q Exerc Sport
Journal of Nutrition	J Nutr		
Journal of Parenteral and Enteral Nutrition	JPEN	Scandinavian Journal of Sports Science	Scand J Sports Sci
		Science	Science
Journal of Pediatrics	J Pediatr	Science in Sport	Sci Sport
Journal of Physical and Medical Rehabilitation	J Phys Med Rehabil	Scientific American	Sci Am
		Sports Medicine	Sports Med
Journal of Physiology	J Physiol	Sports Medicine, Training and Rehabilitation	Sports Med Train Rehabil
Journal of Sport and Exercise Psychology	J Sport Exerc Psychol		
		Sport Science Review	Sport Sci Rev
Journal of Sport Psychology	J Sport Psychol	World Review of Nutrition and Dietetics	World Rev Nutr Diet
Journal of Sports Medicine and Physical Fitness	J Sports Med Phys Fitness		
Journal of Sports Sciences	J Sports Sci		

EVALUATION OF BODY COMPOSITION–GIRTH METHOD

This appendix contains the age- and sex-specific equations to predict body fat percentage based on three girth measurements. There are four charts, one each for younger and older men and women. In our experience, it is important to calibrate the tape measure prior to its use. Use a meter stick as the standard and check the markings on the cloth tape at 10-cm increments. A cloth tape is preferred over a metal one because there is little skin compression when applying a cloth tape to the skin's surface at a relatively constant tension.

To use the charts, measure the three girths for your age and gender as follows:

Age (years)	Sex	Site A	Site B	Site C
18–26	M	Right upper arm	Abdomen	Right forearm
	F	Abdomen	Right thigh	Right forearm
27–50	M	Buttocks	Abdomen	Right forearm
	F	Abdomen	Right thigh	Right calf

A step-by-step explanation of how to compute the relative and absolute values for body fat, lean body mass, and desirable body mass from the Appendix F charts is presented in Chapter 16. The specific equation to predict percentage body fat with its corresponding constant is presented at the bottom of each of the Appendix F charts.

CHART F.1
CONVERSION CONSTANTS TO PREDICT PERCENTAGE BODY FAT FOR YOUNG MEN[a]

Upper Arm			Abdomen			Forearm		
in	cm	Constant A	in	cm	Constant B	in	cm	Constant C
7.00	17.78	25.91	21.00	53.34	27.56	7.00	17.78	38.01
7.25	18.41	26.83	21.25	53.97	27.88	7.25	18.41	39.37
7.50	19.05	27.76	21.50	54.61	28.21	7.50	19.05	40.72
7.75	19.68	28.68	21.75	55.24	28.54	7.75	19.68	42.08
8.00	20.32	29.61	22.00	55.88	28.87	8.00	20.32	43.44
8.25	20.95	30.53	22.25	56.51	29.20	8.25	20.95	44.80
8.50	21.59	31.46	22.50	57.15	29.52	8.50	21.59	46.15
8.75	22.22	32.38	22.75	57.78	29.85	8.75	22.22	47.51
9.00	22.86	33.31	23.00	58.42	30.18	9.00	22.86	48.87
9.25	23.49	34.24	23.25	59.05	30.51	9.25	23.49	50.23
9.50	24.13	35.16	23.50	59.69	30.84	9.50	24.13	51.58
9.75	24.76	36.09	23.75	60.32	31.16	9.75	24.76	52.94
10.00	25.40	37.01	24.00	60.96	31.49	10.00	25.40	54.30
10.25	26.03	37.94	24.25	61.59	31.82	10.25	26.03	55.65
10.50	26.67	38.86	24.50	62.23	32.15	10.50	26.67	57.01
10.75	27.30	39.79	24.75	62.86	32.48	10.75	27.30	58.37
11.00	27.94	40.71	25.00	63.50	32.80	11.00	27.94	59.73
11.25	28.57	41.64	25.25	64.13	33.13	11.25	28.57	61.08
11.50	29.21	42.56	25.50	64.77	33.46	11.50	29.21	62.44
11.75	29.84	43.49	25.75	65.40	33.79	11.75	29.84	63.80
12.00	30.48	44.41	26.00	66.04	34.12	12.00	30.48	65.16
12.25	31.11	45.34	26.25	66.67	34.44	12.25	31.11	66.51
12.50	31.75	46.26	26.50	67.31	34.77	12.50	31.75	67.87
12.75	32.38	47.19	26.75	67.94	35.10	12.75	32.38	69.23
13.00	33.02	48.11	27.00	68.58	35.43	13.00	33.02	70.59
13.25	33.65	49.04	27.25	69.21	35.76	13.25	33.65	71.94
13.50	34.29	49.96	27.50	69.85	36.09	13.50	34.29	73.30

(continued)

CHART F.1 *(Continued)*

Upper Arm			Abdomen			Forearm		
in	cm	Constant A	in	cm	Constant B	in	cm	Constant C
13.75	34.92	50.89	27.75	70.48	36.41	13.75	34.92	74.66
14.00	35.56	51.82	28.00	71.12	36.74	14.00	35.56	76.02
14.25	36.19	52.74	28.25	71.75	37.07	14.25	36.19	77.37
14.50	36.83	53.67	28.50	72.39	37.40	14.50	36.83	78.73
14.75	37.46	54.59	28.75	73.02	37.73	14.75	37.46	80.09
15.00	38.10	55.52	29.00	73.66	38.05	15.00	38.10	81.45
15.25	38.73	56.44	29.25	74.29	38.38	15.25	38.73	82.80
15.50	39.37	57.37	29.50	74.93	38.71	15.50	39.37	84.16
15.75	40.00	58.29	29.75	75.56	39.04	15.75	40.00	85.52
16.00	40.64	59.22	30.00	76.20	39.37	16.00	40.64	86.88
16.25	41.27	60.14	30.25	76.83	39.69	16.25	41.27	88.23
16.50	41.91	61.07	30.50	77.47	40.02	16.50	41.91	89.59
16.75	42.54	61.99	30.75	78.10	40.35	16.75	42.54	90.95
17.00	43.18	62.92	31.00	78.74	40.68	17.00	43.18	92.31
17.25	43.81	63.84	31.25	79.37	41.01	17.25	43.81	93.66
17.50	44.45	64.77	31.50	80.01	41.33	17.50	44.45	95.02
17.75	45.08	65.69	31.75	80.64	41.66	17.75	45.08	96.38
18.00	45.72	66.62	32.00	81.28	41.99	18.00	45.72	97.74
18.25	46.35	67.54	32.25	81.91	42.32	18.25	46.35	99.09
18.50	46.99	68.47	32.50	82.55	42.65	18.50	46.99	100.45
18.75	47.62	69.40	32.75	83.18	42.97	18.75	47.62	101.81
19.00	48.26	70.32	33.00	83.82	43.30	19.00	48.26	103.17
19.25	48.89	71.25	33.25	84.45	43.63	19.25	48.89	104.52
19.50	49.53	72.17	33.50	85.09	43.96	19.50	49.53	105.88
19.75	50.16	73.10	33.75	85.72	44.29	19.75	50.16	107.24
20.00	50.80	74.02	34.00	86.36	44.61	20.00	50.80	108.60
20.25	51.43	74.95	34.25	86.99	44.94	20.25	51.43	109.95
20.50	52.07	75.87	34.50	87.63	45.27	20.50	52.07	111.31
20.75	52.70	76.80	34.75	88.26	45.60	20.75	52.70	112.67
21.00	53.34	77.72	35.00	88.90	45.93	21.00	53.34	114.02
21.25	53.97	78.65	35.25	89.53	46.25	21.25	53.97	115.38
21.50	54.61	79.57	35.50	90.17	46.58	21.50	54.61	116.74
21.75	55.24	80.50	35.75	90.80	46.91	21.75	55.24	118.10
22.00	55.88	81.42	36.00	91.44	47.24	22.00	55.88	119.45
			36.25	92.07	47.57			
			36.50	92.71	47.89			
			36.75	93.34	48.22			
			37.00	93.98	48.55			
			37.25	94.61	48.88			
			37.50	95.25	49.21			
			37.75	95.88	49.54			
			38.00	96.52	49.86			
			38.25	97.15	50.19			
			38.50	97.79	50.52			
			38.75	98.42	50.85			
			39.00	99.06	51.18			
			39.25	99.69	51.50			
			39.50	100.33	51.83			
			39.75	100.96	52.16			
			40.00	101.60	52.49			
			40.25	102.23	52.82			
			40.50	102.87	53.14			
			40.75	103.50	53.47			
			41.00	104.14	53.80			
			41.25	104.77	54.13			
			41.50	105.41	54.46			
			41.75	106.04	54.78			
			42.00	106.68	55.11			

Note: Percentage Fat = Constant A + Constant B − Constant C − 10.2.

CHART F.2
CONVERSION CONSTANTS TO PREDICT PERCENTAGE BODY FAT FOR OLDER MEN[a]

Buttocks			Abdomen			Forearm		
in	cm	Constant A	in	cm	Constant B	in	cm	Constant C
28.00	71.12	29.34	25.50	64.77	22.84	7.00	17.78	21.01
28.25	71.75	29.60	25.75	65.40	23.06	7.25	18.41	21.76
28.50	72.39	29.87	26.00	66.04	23.29	7.50	19.05	22.52
28.75	73.02	30.13	26.25	66.67	23.51	7.75	19.68	23.26
29.00	73.66	30.39	26.50	67.31	23.73	8.00	20.32	24.02
29.25	74.29	30.65	26.75	67.94	23.96	8.25	20.95	24.76
29.50	74.93	30.92	27.00	68.58	24.18	8.50	21.59	25.52
29.75	75.56	31.18	27.25	69.21	24.40	8.75	22.22	26.26
30.00	76.20	31.44	27.50	69.85	24.63	9.00	22.86	27.02
30.25	76.83	31.70	27.75	70.48	24.85	9.25	23.49	27.76
30.50	77.47	31.96	28.00	71.12	25.08	9.50	24.13	28.52
30.75	78.10	32.22	28.25	71.75	25.29	9.75	24.76	29.26
31.00	78.74	32.49	28.50	72.39	25.52	10.00	25.40	30.02
31.25	79.37	32.75	28.75	73.02	25.75	10.25	26.03	30.76
31.50	80.01	33.01	29.00	73.66	25.97	10.50	26.67	31.52
31.75	80.64	33.27	29.25	74.29	26.19	10.75	27.30	32.27
32.00	81.28	33.54	29.50	74.93	26.42	11.00	27.94	33.02
32.25	81.91	33.80	29.75	75.56	26.64	11.25	28.57	33.77
32.50	82.55	34.06	30.00	76.20	26.87	11.50	29.21	34.52
32.75	83.18	34.32	30.25	76.83	27.09	11.75	29.84	35.27
33.00	83.82	34.58	30.50	77.47	27.32	12.00	30.48	36.02
33.25	84.45	34.84	30.75	78.10	27.54	12.25	31.11	36.77
33.50	85.09	35.11	31.00	78.74	27.76	12.50	31.75	37.53
33.75	85.72	35.37	31.25	79.37	27.98	12.75	32.38	38.27
34.00	86.36	35.63	31.50	80.01	28.21	13.00	33.02	39.03
34.25	86.99	35.89	31.75	80.64	28.43	13.25	33.65	39.77
34.50	87.63	36.16	32.00	81.28	28.66	13.50	34.29	40.53
34.75	88.26	36.42	32.25	81.91	28.88	13.75	34.92	41.27
35.00	88.90	36.68	32.50	82.55	29.11	14.00	35.56	42.03
35.25	89.53	36.94	32.75	83.18	29.33	14.25	36.19	42.77
35.50	90.17	37.20	33.00	83.82	29.55	14.50	36.83	43.53
35.75	90.80	37.46	33.25	84.45	29.78	14.75	37.46	44.27
36.00	91.44	37.73	33.50	85.09	30.00	15.00	38.10	45.03
36.25	92.07	37.99	33.75	85.72	30.22	15.25	38.73	45.77
36.50	92.71	38.25	34.00	86.36	30.45	15.50	39.37	46.53
36.75	93.34	38.51	34.25	86.99	30.67	15.75	40.00	47.28
37.00	93.98	38.78	34.50	87.63	30.89	16.00	40.64	48.03
37.25	94.61	39.04	34.75	88.26	31.12	16.25	41.27	48.78
37.50	95.25	39.30	35.00	88.90	31.35	16.50	41.91	49.53
37.75	95.88	39.56	35.25	89.53	31.57	16.75	42.54	50.28
38.00	96.52	39.82	35.50	90.17	31.79	17.00	43.18	51.03
38.25	97.15	40.08	35.75	90.80	32.02	17.25	43.81	51.78
38.50	97.79	40.35	36.00	91.44	32.24	17.50	44.45	52.54
38.75	98.42	40.61	36.25	92.07	32.46	17.75	45.08	53.28
39.00	99.06	40.87	36.50	92.71	32.69	18.00	45.72	54.04
39.25	99.69	41.13	36.75	93.34	32.91	18.25	46.35	54.78
39.50	100.33	41.39	37.00	93.98	33.14			
39.75	100.96	41.66	37.25	94.61	33.36			
40.00	101.60	41.92	37.50	95.25	33.58			
40.25	102.23	42.18	37.75	95.88	33.81			
40.50	102.87	42.44	38.00	96.52	34.03			
40.75	103.50	42.70	38.25	97.15	34.26			
41.00	104.14	42.97	38.50	97.79	34.48			
41.25	104.77	43.23	38.75	98.42	34.70			
41.50	105.41	43.49	39.00	99.06	34.93			
41.75	106.04	43.75	39.25	99.69	35.15			
42.00	106.68	44.02	39.50	100.33	35.38			
42.25	107.31	44.28	39.75	100.96	35.59			
42.50	107.95	44.54	40.00	101.60	35.82			
42.75	108.58	44.80	40.25	102.23	36.05			
43.00	109.22	45.06	40.50	102.87	36.27			

(continued)

CHART F.2 (Continued)

Buttocks			Abdomen			Forearm		
in	cm	Constant A	in	cm	Constant B	in	cm	Constant C
43.25	109.85	45.32	40.75	103.50	36.49			
43.50	110.49	45.59	41.00	104.14	36.72			
43.75	111.12	45.85	41.25	104.77	36.94			
44.00	111.76	46.12	41.50	105.41	37.17			
44.25	112.39	46.37	41.75	106.04	37.39			
44.50	113.03	46.64	42.00	106.68	37.62			
44.75	113.66	46.89	42.25	107.31	37.87			
45.00	114.30	47.16	42.50	107.95	38.06			
45.25	114.93	47.42	42.75	108.58	38.28			
45.50	115.57	47.68	43.00	109.22	38.51			
45.75	116.20	47.94	43.25	109.85	38.73			
46.00	116.84	48.21	43.50	110.49	38.96			
46.25	117.47	48.47	43.75	111.12	39.18			
46.50	118.11	48.73	44.00	111.76	39.41			
46.75	118.74	48.99	44.25	112.39	39.63			
47.00	119.38	49.26	44.50	113.03	39.85			
47.25	120.01	49.52	44.75	113.66	40.08			
47.50	120.65	49.78	45.00	114.30	40.30			
47.75	121.28	50.04						
48.00	121.92	50.30						
48.25	122.55	50.56						
48.50	123.19	50.83						
48.75	123.82	51.09						
49.00	124.46	51.35						

Note: Percentage Fat = Constant A + Constant B − Constant C − 15.0.

[a]Copyright © 1986, 1991, 1996, 2000, 2006 by Frank I. Katch, Victor L. Katch, and William D. McArdle, and Fitness Technologies, Inc., 5043 Via Lara Ln. Santa Barbara, CA 93111. No part of this appendix may be reproduced in any manner without written permission from the copyright holders.

CHART F.3
CONVERSION CONSTANTS TO PREDICT PERCENTAGE BODY FAT FOR YOUNG WOMEN[a]

Abdomen			Thigh			Forearm		
in	cm	Constant A	in	cm	Constant B	in	cm	Constant C
20.00	50.80	26.74	14.00	35.56	29.13	6.00	15.24	25.86
20.25	51.43	27.07	14.25	36.19	29.65	6.25	15.87	26.94
20.50	52.07	27.41	14.50	36.83	30.17	6.50	16.51	28.02
20.75	52.70	27.74	14.75	37.46	30.69	6.75	17.14	29.10
21.00	53.34	28.07	15.00	38.10	31.21	7.00	17.78	30.17
21.25	53.97	28.41	15.25	38.73	31.73	7.25	18.41	31.25
21.50	54.61	28.74	15.50	39.37	32.25	7.50	19.05	32.33
21.75	55.24	29.08	15.75	40.00	32.77	7.75	19.68	33.41
22.00	55.88	29.41	16.00	40.64	33.29	8.00	20.32	34.48
22.25	56.51	29.74	16.25	41.27	33.81	8.25	20.95	35.56
22.50	57.15	30.08	16.50	41.91	34.33	8.50	21.59	36.64
22.75	57.78	30.41	16.75	42.54	34.85	8.75	22.22	37.72
23.00	58.42	30.75	17.00	43.18	35.37	9.00	22.86	38.79
23.25	59.05	31.08	17.25	43.81	35.89	9.25	23.49	39.87
23.50	59.69	31.42	17.50	44.45	36.41	9.50	24.13	40.95
23.75	60.32	31.75	17.75	45.08	36.93	9.75	24.76	42.03
24.00	60.96	32.08	18.00	45.72	37.45	10.00	25.40	43.10
24.25	61.59	32.42	18.25	46.35	37.97	10.25	26.03	44.18
24.50	62.23	32.75	18.50	46.99	38.49	10.50	26.67	45.26
24.75	62.86	33.09	18.75	47.62	39.01	10.75	27.30	46.34
25.00	63.50	33.42	19.00	48.26	39.53	11.00	27.94	47.41
25.25	64.13	33.76	19.25	48.89	40.05	11.25	28.57	48.49
25.50	64.77	34.09	19.50	49.53	40.57	11.50	29.21	49.57

(continued)

CHART F.3 (*Continued*)

Abdomen			Thigh			Forearm		
in	cm	Constant A	in	cm	Constant B	in	cm	Constant C
25.75	65.40	34.42	19.75	50.16	41.09	11.75	29.84	50.65
26.00	66.04	34.76	20.00	50.80	41.61	12.00	30.48	51.73
26.25	66.67	35.09	20.25	51.43	42.13	12.25	31.11	52.80
26.50	67.31	35.43	20.50	52.07	42.65	12.50	31.75	53.88
26.75	67.94	35.76	20.75	52.70	43.17	12.75	32.38	54.96
27.00	68.58	36.10	21.00	53.34	43.69	13.00	33.02	56.04
27.25	69.21	36.43	21.25	53.97	44.21	13.25	33.65	57.11
27.50	69.85	36.76	21.50	54.61	44.73	13.50	34.29	58.19
27.75	70.48	37.10	21.75	55.24	45.25	13.75	34.92	59.27
28.00	71.12	37.43	22.00	55.88	45.77	14.00	35.56	60.35
28.25	71.75	37.77	22.25	56.51	46.29	14.25	36.19	61.42
28.50	72.39	38.10	22.50	57.15	46.81	14.50	36.83	62.50
28.75	73.02	38.43	22.75	57.78	47.33	14.75	37.46	63.58
29.00	73.66	38.77	23.00	58.42	47.85	15.00	38.10	64.66
29.25	74.29	39.10	23.25	59.05	48.37	15.25	38.73	65.73
29.50	74.93	39.44	23.50	59.69	48.89	15.50	39.37	66.81
29.75	75.56	39.77	23.75	60.32	49.41	15.75	40.00	67.89
30.00	76.20	40.11	24.00	60.96	49.93	16.00	40.64	68.97
30.25	76.83	40.44	24.25	61.59	50.45	16.25	41.27	70.04
30.50	77.47	40.77	24.50	62.23	50.97	16.50	41.91	71.12
30.75	78.10	41.11	24.75	62.86	51.49	16.75	42.54	72.20
31.00	78.74	41.44	25.00	63.50	52.01	17.00	43.18	73.28
31.25	79.37	41.78	25.25	64.13	52.53	17.25	43.81	74.36
31.50	80.01	42.11	25.50	64.77	53.05	17.50	44.45	75.43
31.75	80.64	42.45	25.75	65.40	53.57	17.75	45.08	76.51
32.00	81.28	42.78	26.00	66.04	54.09	18.00	45.72	77.59
32.25	81.91	43.11	26.25	66.67	54.61	18.25	46.35	78.67
32.50	82.55	43.45	26.50	67.31	55.13	18.50	46.99	79.74
32.75	83.18	43.78	26.75	67.94	55.65	18.75	47.62	80.82
33.00	83.82	44.12	27.00	68.58	56.17	19.00	48.26	81.90
33.25	84.45	44.45	27.25	69.21	56.69	19.25	48.89	82.98
33.50	85.09	44.78	27.50	69.85	57.21	19.50	49.53	84.05
33.75	85.72	45.12	27.75	70.48	57.73	19.75	50.16	85.13
34.00	86.36	45.45	28.00	71.12	58.26	20.00	50.80	86.21
34.25	86.99	45.79	28.25	71.75	58.78			
34.50	87.63	46.12	28.50	72.39	59.30			
34.75	88.26	46.46	38.75	73.02	59.82			
35.00	88.90	46.79	29.00	73.66	60.34			
35.25	89.53	47.12	29.25	74.29	60.86			
35.50	90.17	47.46	29.50	74.93	61.38			
35.75	90.80	47.79	29.75	75.56	61.90			
36.00	91.44	48.13	30.00	76.20	62.42			
36.25	92.07	48.46	30.25	76.83	62.94			
36.50	92.71	48.80	30.50	77.47	63.46			
36.75	93.34	49.13	30.75	78.10	63.98			
37.00	93.98	49.46	31.00	78.74	64.50			
37.25	94.61	49.80	31.25	79.37	65.02			
37.50	95.25	50.13	31.50	80.01	65.54			
37.75	95.88	50.47	31.75	80.64	66.06			
38.00	96.52	50.80	32.00	81.28	66.58			
38.25	97.15	51.13	32.25	81.91	67.10			
38.50	97.79	51.47	32.50	82.55	67.62			
38.75	98.42	51.80	32.75	83.18	68.14			
39.00	99.06	52.14	33.00	83.82	68.66			
39.25	99.69	52.47	33.25	84.45	69.18			
39.50	100.33	52.81	33.50	85.09	69.70			
39.75	100.96	53.14	33.75	85.72	70.22			
40.00	101.60	53.47	34.00	86.36	70.74			

Note: Percentage Fat = Constant A + Constant B − Constant C − 19.6.

CHART F.4
CONVERSION CONSTANTS TO PREDICT PERCENTAGE BODY FAT FOR OLDER WOMEN[A]

Abdomen			Thigh			Forearm		
in	cm	Constant A	in	cm	Constant B	in	cm	Constant C
25.00	63.50	29.69	14.00	35.56	17.31	10.00	25.40	14.46
25.25	64.13	29.98	14.25	36.19	17.62	10.25	26.03	14.82
25.50	64.77	30.28	14.50	36.83	17.93	10.50	26.67	15.18
25.75	65.40	30.58	14.75	37.46	18.24	10.75	27.30	15.54
26.00	66.04	30.87	15.00	38.10	18.55	11.00	27.94	15.91
26.25	66.67	31.17	15.25	38.73	18.86	11.25	28.57	16.27
26.50	67.31	31.47	15.50	39.37	19.17	11.50	29.21	16.63
26.75	67.94	31.76	15.75	40.00	19.47	11.75	29.84	16.99
27.00	68.58	32.06	16.00	40.64	19.78	12.00	30.48	17.35
27.25	69.21	32.36	16.25	41.27	20.09	12.25	31.11	17.71
27.50	69.85	32.65	16.50	41.91	20.40	12.50	31.75	18.08
27.75	70.48	32.95	16.75	42.54	20.71	12.75	32.38	18.44
28.00	71.12	33.25	17.00	43.18	21.02	13.00	33.02	18.80
28.25	71.75	33.55	17.25	43.81	21.33	13.25	33.65	19.16
28.50	72.39	33.84	17.50	44.45	21.64	13.50	34.29	19.52
28.75	73.02	34.14	17.75	45.08	21.95	13.75	34.92	19.88
29.00	73.66	34.44	18.00	45.72	22.26	14.00	35.56	20.24
29.25	74.29	34.73	18.25	46.35	22.57	14.25	36.19	20.61
29.50	74.93	35.03	18.50	46.99	22.87	14.50	36.83	20.97
29.75	75.56	35.33	18.75	47.62	23.18	14.75	37.46	21.33
30.00	76.20	35.62	19.00	38.26	23.49	15.00	38.10	21.69
30.25	76.83	35.92	19.25	48.89	23.80	15.25	38.73	22.05
30.50	77.47	36.22	19.50	49.53	24.11	15.50	39.37	22.41
30.75	78.10	36.51	19.75	50.16	24.42	15.75	40.00	22.77
31.00	78.74	36.81	20.00	50.80	24.73	16.00	40.64	23.14
31.25	79.37	37.11	20.25	51.43	25.04	16.25	41.27	23.50
31.50	80.01	37.40	20.50	52.07	25.35	16.50	41.91	23.86
31.75	80.64	37.70	20.75	52.70	25.66	16.75	42.54	24.22
32.00	81.28	38.00	21.00	53.34	25.97	17.00	43.18	24.58
32.25	81.91	38.30	21.25	53.97	26.28	17.25	43.81	24.94
32.50	82.55	38.59	21.50	54.61	26.58	17.50	44.45	25.31
32.75	83.18	38.89	21.75	55.24	26.89	17.75	45.08	25.67
33.00	83.82	39.19	22.00	55.88	27.20	18.00	45.72	26.03
33.25	84.45	39.48	22.25	56.51	27.51	18.25	46.35	26.39
33.50	85.09	39.78	22.50	57.15	27.82	18.50	46.99	26.75
33.75	85.72	40.08	22.75	57.78	28.13	18.75	47.62	27.11
34.00	86.36	40.37	23.00	58.42	28.44	19.00	48.26	27.47
34.25	86.99	40.67	23.25	59.05	28.75	19.25	48.89	27.84
34.50	87.63	40.97	23.50	59.69	29.06	19.50	49.53	28.20
34.75	88.26	41.26	23.75	60.32	29.37	19.75	50.16	28.56
35.00	88.90	41.56	24.00	60.96	29.68	20.00	50.80	28.92
35.25	89.53	41.86	24.25	61.59	29.98	20.25	51.43	29.28
35.50	90.17	42.15	24.50	62.23	30.29	20.50	52.07	29.64
35.75	90.80	42.45	24.75	62.86	30.60	20.75	52.70	30.00
36.00	91.44	42.75	25.00	63.50	30.91	21.00	53.34	30.37
36.25	92.07	43.05	25.25	64.13	31.22	21.25	53.97	30.73
36.50	92.71	43.34	25.50	64.77	31.53	21.50	54.61	31.09
36.75	93.35	43.64	25.75	65.40	31.84	21.75	55.24	31.45
37.00	93.98	43.94	26.00	66.04	32.15	22.00	55.88	31.81
37.25	94.62	44.23	26.25	66.67	32.46	22.25	56.51	32.17
37.50	95.25	44.53	26.50	67.31	32.77	22.50	57.15	32.54
37.75	95.89	44.83	26.75	67.94	33.08	22.75	57.78	32.90
38.00	96.52	45.12	27.00	68.58	33.38	23.00	58.42	33.26
38.25	97.16	45.42	27.25	69.21	33.69	23.25	59.05	33.62
38.50	97.79	45.72	27.50	69.85	34.00	23.50	59.69	33.98
38.75	98.43	46.01	27.75	70.48	34.31	23.75	60.32	34.34
39.00	99.06	46.31	28.00	71.12	34.62	24.00	60.96	34.70
39.25	99.70	46.61	28.25	71.75	34.93	24.25	61.59	35.07
39.50	100.33	46.90	28.50	72.39	35.24	24.50	62.23	35.43
39.75	100.97	47.20	28.75	73.02	35.55	24.75	62.86	35.79
40.00	101.60	47.50	29.00	73.66	35.86	25.00	63.50	36.15

(continued)

CHART F.4

Abdomen			Thigh			Forearm		
in	cm	Constant A	in	cm	Constant B	in	cm	Constant C
40.25	101.24	47.79	29.25	74.29	36.17			
40.50	102.87	48.09	29.50	74.93	36.48			
40.75	103.51	48.39	29.75	75.56	36.79			
41.00	104.14	48.69	30.00	76.20	37.09			
41.25	104.78	48.98	30.25	76.83	37.40			
41.50	105.41	49.28	30.50	77.47	37.71			
41.75	106.05	49.58	30.75	78.10	38.02			
42.00	106.68	49.87	31.00	78.74	38.33			
42.25	107.32	50.17	31.25	79.37	38.64			
42.50	107.95	50.47	31.50	80.01	38.95			
42.75	108.59	50.76	31.75	80.64	39.26			
43.00	109.22	51.06	32.00	81.28	39.57			
43.25	109.86	51.36	32.25	81.91	39.88			
43.50	110.49	51.65	32.50	82.55	40.19			
43.75	111.13	51.95	32.75	83.18	40.49			
44.00	111.76	52.25	33.00	83.82	40.80			
44.25	112.40	52.54	33.25	84.45	41.11			
44.50	113.03	52.84	33.50	85.09	41.42			
44.75	113.67	53.14	33.75	85.72	41.73			
45.00	114.30	53.44	34.00	86.36	42.04			

Note: Percentage Fat = Constant A + Constant B − Constant C − 19.6.

EVALUATION OF BODY COMPOSITION–SKINFOLD METHOD

Skinfold equations to predict body density (Db) and/or percentage body fat (%BF) use regression analyses in which scores obtained on several variables are multiplied by constants to arrive at a predicted Db or %BF. Solving these equations requires extensive computations that are ill suited for field work and are subject to error, particularly when done by hand or with calculators.

A nomogram is a pictorial method that simplifies computations by providing a simple "look-up" method to solve the equation.

The Nomogram

Figure G-1 presents the nomogram to estimate percentage body fat for college-aged men and women from the sum of three skinfolds plus age using the generalized equations (see next page) of Jackson and colleagues.

Variables

- For men, obtain the following variables: skinfolds in mm (chest, abdomen, thigh); age in years.
- For women, obtain the following variables: skinfolds in mm (triceps, thigh, suprailiac); age in years.

Using the Nomogram

1. Sum the three skinfolds.
2. Locate on the right scale (sum of the three skinfolds, mm).
3. Locate on the left scale (age in y).
4. With a ruler, connect the two points (right scale and left scale); read the resulting percentage body fat from the center scale (male or female).

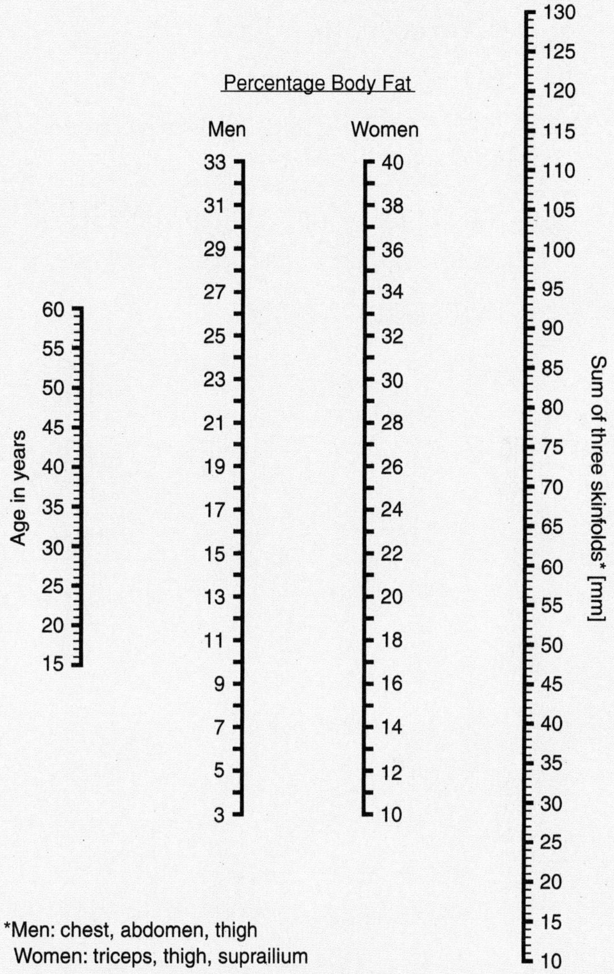

Example

Data for a women, age 30 y; triceps skinfold = 15 mm; thigh skinfold = 15 mm; suprailiac skinfold = 25 mm.

1. Sum skinfolds = 55 mm.
2. Place rule on right scale over 55 mm; connect to left scale at age 30 y.
3. Read percentage body fat: 23%.

Caution

Although nomograms can save time, they are subject to error, particularly interpolation error where precision and accuracy can be compromised. At best, interpolation of the %BF value for males and females in the present nomogram becomes limited to no more than one-half of a whole percentage. Also, because the nomogram uses the Siri equation to convert body density to percentage body fat, it should not be used with populations where other density-to-percentage fat conversions are more appropriate.

*Men: chest, abdomen, thigh
 Women: triceps, thigh, suprailium

Figure G-1. Nomogram to estimate percentage body fat of college-aged men and women using the Jackson et al. generalized equations. *Note:* From Baun, W.B., and Baun, M.R.: A Nomogram for the Estimate of Percent Body Fat From Generalized Equations. *Res. Q. Exerc. Sport,* 52:382, 1981. Copyright 1981 by AAHPERD. Reprinted by permission.

Equations

Check the accuracy of using the nomogram by solving the following equations to predict percentage body density. Convert body density to percentage body fat using the Siri equations (%BF = 495 ÷ Db − 450).

1. Equation for males: $\sum$3SKF equals sum of chest, abdomen, and thigh skinfolds:

$$Db = 1.10938 - (0.0008267 \times \textstyle\sum 3SKF)$$
$$+ ([0.0000016 \times \textstyle\sum 3SKF]^2)$$
$$- (0.0002574 \times age)$$

2. Equation for females: $\sum$3SKF equals sum of triceps, thigh, and suprailiac skinfolds:

$$Db = 1.0994921 - (0.0009929 \times \textstyle\sum 3SKF)$$
$$+ ([0.0000023 \times \textstyle\sum 3SKF]^2)$$
$$- (0.0001392 \times age)$$

REFERENCES

Baun, W.B., Baun M.R.: A nomogram for the estimate of percent body fat from generalized equations. *Res. Quart. Exerc. Sport*, 52:382, 1981.

Jackson, A.S., et al.: Generalized equations for predicting body density of women. *Med. Sci. Sports Exerc.*, 12:175, 1980

Jackson, A.S., Pollock, M.L.: Generalized equations for predicting body density of men. *Br. J. Nutr.*, 40:497, 1978.

Note: Page numbers in *italics* denote figures; those followed by a t denote tables.